Outcomes Assessment in Cancer
Measures, Methods, and Applications

Cancer touches the lives of millions worldwide each year. This is reflected not only in well-publicized mortality statistics but also in the profound – though much more difficult to measure – effects of cancer on the health-related quality of life, economic status, and overall well-being of patients and their families. In 2001, the US National Cancer Institute established the Cancer Outcomes Measurement Working Group to evaluate the state of the science in measuring the important and diverse impacts of this disease on individuals and populations. The findings and recommendations of the working group's 35 internationally recognized members are reported in *Outcomes Assessment in Cancer*, lucidly written and accessible to both researchers and policy makers in academia, government, and industry. This volume provides the most penetrating yet practical discussion to date of alternative approaches for comprehensively measuring the burden of cancer and the effectiveness of preventive and therapeutic interventions.

Joseph Lipscomb is Professor of Public Health at Emory University (Atlanta, GA, USA) and formerly Chief of the Outcomes Research Branch within the Applied Research Program of the Division of Cancer Control and Population Sciences at the National Cancer Institute (Bethesda, MD, USA).

Carolyn C. Gotay is a professor within the Cancer Research Center of Hawai'i at the University of Hawai'i (Honolulu, HI, USA).

Claire Snyder is an expert in outcomes research in the Outcomes Research Branch within the Applied Research Program of the Division of Cancer Control and Population Sciences at the National Cancer Institute (Bethesda, MD, USA).

Outcomes Assessment in Cancer

Measures, Methods, and Applications

EDITED BY

Joseph Lipscomb

Emory University, Atlanta, GA, USA and formerly
National Cancer Institute, Bethesda, MD, USA

Carolyn C. Gotay

Cancer Research Center of Hawai'i, University of Hawaii,
Honolulu, HI, USA

Claire Snyder

National Cancer Institute, Bethesda, MD, USA

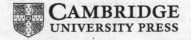

CAMBRIDGE
UNIVERSITY PRESS

CAMBRIDGE UNIVERSITY PRESS
Cambridge, New York, Melbourne, Madrid, Cape Town,
Singapore, São Paulo, Delhi, Tokyo, Mexico City

Cambridge University Press
The Edinburgh Building, Cambridge CB2 8RU, UK

Published in the United States of America by Cambridge University Press, New York

www.cambridge.org
Information on this title: www.cambridge.org/9781107403161

First published 2005
Reprinted 2006
First paperback edition 2011

A catalogue record for this publication is available from the British Library

Library of Congress Cataloguing in Publication data
Outcomes assessment in cancer / edited by Joseph Lipscomb, Carolyn C. Gotay, Claire Snyder.
    p. ; cm.
Includes bibliographical references and index.
ISBN (invalid) 052183890 (hardback: alk. paper)
1. Cancer – Treatment – Evaluation.   2. Outcome assessment (Medical care)   I. Lipscomb, Joseph, 1948–
II. Gotay, Carolyn C., 1951–   III. Snyder, Claire, 1973–
[DNLM: 1. Neoplasms – therapy.   2. Health Status Indicators.   3. Quality of Life.   4. Treatment Outcome.
QZ 266 O94 2005]
RC270.8.O93   2005
616.99'406 – dc22   2004054539

ISBN 978-0-521-83890-0 Hardback
ISBN 978-1-107-40316-1 Paperback

Contents

List of contributors   *page* ix
Acknowledgments   xiii

1   Introduction to *Outcomes Assessment in
    Cancer*   1
    *Joseph Lipscomb, Ph.D., Carolyn C. Gotay,
    Ph.D., and Claire Snyder, M.H.S. (The Editors)*

**Health-related quality of life in
cancer: general concepts and
generic measures**

2   Definitions and conceptual models of
    quality of life   14
    Carol Estwing Ferrans, Ph.D., R.N., F.A.A.N.

3   Assessing health status and quality of life
    of cancer patients: the use of general
    instruments   31
    Pennifer Erickson, Ph.D.

4   The roles for preference-based measures
    in support of cancer research and policy   69
    David H. Feeny, Ph.D.

**Assessing health-related quality of life
during treatment**

5   Quality of life in breast cancer: what have
    we learned and where do we go from here?   93
    *Patricia A. Ganz, M.D., and Pamela J.
    Goodwin, M.D., M.Sc.*

6   Measuring quality of life in prostate
    cancer: progress and challenges   126
    Mark S. Litwin, M.D., M.P.H., and James A.
    Talcott, M.D., S.M.

7   The science of quality-of-life
    measurement in lung cancer   160
    Craig C. Earle, M.D., M.Sc., and Jane C.
    Weeks, M.D.

8   Treatment for colorectal cancer: impact
    on health-related quality of life   178
    Carol M. Moinpour, Ph.D., and Dawn
    Provenzale, M.D., M.S.

9   Instruments to measure the specific
    health impact of surgery, radiation, and
    chemotherapy on cancer
    patients   201
    Michael J. Barry, M.D., and Janet E. Dancey,
    M.D.

Assessing health-related quality of life across the cancer continuum

10 Short-term outcomes of
    chemoprevention, genetic susceptibility
    testing, and screening interventions:
    What are they? How are they measured?
    When should they be
    measured?   216
    Jeanne S. Mandelblatt, M.D., M.P.H., and Joe
    V. Selby, M.D., M.P.H.

11 Evaluating quality of life in cancer
    survivors   241
    Brad Zebrack, Ph.D., M.S.W., and David
    Cella, Ph.D.

12 Assessing health-related quality of life at
    end of life   264
    Betty R. Ferrell, Ph.D., F.A.A.N.

Measuring the experience and needs of cancer patients and caregivers

13 Patient advocate perspective on
    health-related quality of life issues with
    prostate cancer survivors   286
    (Col. Ret.) James E. Williams, Jr.

14 Measuring the patient's perspective on
    the interpersonal aspects of cancer care 290
    Charles Darby

15 Needs assessment in cancer   305
    David H. Gustafson, Ph.D.

16 Assessing the subjective impact of
    caregiving on informal caregivers of
    cancer patients   329
    Claire Snyder, M.H.S.

Methodological considerations in applications to cancer outcomes research

17 Practical considerations in outcomes
    assessment for clinical trials   346
    Diane L. Fairclough, Dr.P.H.

18 Statistical issues in the application of
    cancer outcome measures   362
    Jeff A. Sloan, Ph.D.

19 The clinical value and meaning of
    health-related quality-of-life outcomes
    in oncology   386
    David Osoba, B.Sc., M.D., F.R.C.P.C.

20 Cross-cultural use of health-related
    quality of life assessments in clinical
    oncology   406
    Neil K. Aaronson, Ph.D.

Modern psychometric theory in cancer outcomes research

21 Item response theory and its applications
    for cancer outcomes measurement   425
    Steven P. Reise, Ph.D.

22 Applications of item response theory to
    improve health outcomes assessment:
    developing item banks, linking
    instruments, and computer-adaptive
    testing   445
    Ronald K. Hambleton, Ph.D.

23 Subscales and summary scales: issues in
    health-related outcomes   465
    Mark Wilson, Ph.D.

Assessing the economic impact of cancer

24 On the definition and measurement of
    the economic burden of cancer   480
    Mark C. Hornbrook, Ph.D.

25 Cost-effectiveness analysis in cancer:
    toward an iterative framework for
    integration of evidence from trials and
    models   503
    Bernie J. O'Brien, Ph.D.

Research and policy implications

26 Data for cancer outcomes research:
    identifying and strengthening the
    empirical base   522
    *Carolyn C. Gotay, Ph.D., and Joseph
    Lipscomb, Ph.D.*

27 Use of health-related quality of life
    measures by industry and regulatory
    agencies in evaluating oncology
    therapies   550
    Dennis A. Revicki, Ph.D.

28 Reflections on COMWG findings and
    moving to the next phase   568
    *Carolyn C. Gotay, Ph.D., Joseph Lipscomb,
    Ph.D., and Claire Snyder, M.H.S.*

Invited papers

Invited Paper A The world of outcomes
research: yesterday, today, and tomorrow   584
Bert Spilker, Ph.D., M.D.

Invited Paper B The ten Ds of health
outcomes measurement for the
twenty-first century   590
*Colleen A. McHorney, Ph.D., and Karon F.
Cook, Ph.D.*

Invited Paper C The use of cognitive
interviewing techniques in quality of life
and patient-reported outcomes
assessment   610
*Gordon B. Willis, Ph.D., Bryce B. Reeve,
Ph.D., and Ivan Barofsky, Ph.D.*

Invited Paper D Industry perspective
regarding outcomes research in oncology   623
*Kati Copley-Merriman, M.S., M.B.A., Joseph
Jackson, Ph.D., J. Gregory Boyer, Ph.D.,
Joseph C. Cappelleri, Ph.D., M.P.H., Robert
DeMarinis, Ph.D., Joseph DiCesare, M.P.H.,
R.Ph., M. Haim Erder, Ph.D., Jean Paul
Gagnon, Ph.D., Lou Garrison, Ph.D.,
Kathleen Gondek, Ph.D., Kim A. Heithoff,
Sc.D., Tom Hughes, Ph.D., David Miller,
Ph.D., Margaret Rothman, Ph.D., Nancy
Santanello, M.D., M.S., Richard Willke,
Ph.D., and Bruce Wong, M.D.*

Index   639

Contributors

Members of the Cancer Outcomes Measurement Working Group (2001–2004)

Co-Chairs

Joseph Lipscomb, Ph.D.
Chief, Outcomes Research Branch
Applied Research Program
Division of Cancer Control and Population Sciences
National Cancer Institute

Carolyn C. Gotay, Ph.D.
Professor, Cancer Research Center of Hawai'i
University of Hawaii

Working Group Initiator

Claire Snyder, M.H.S
Expert, Outcomes Research Branch
Applied Research Program
Division of Cancer Control and Population Sciences
National Cancer Institute

Working Group Participants

Neil K. Aaronson, Ph.D.
Head, Division of Psychosocial Research &
Epidemiology
The Netherlands Cancer Institute
Professor, Faculty of Medicine
Vrije Universiteit

Michael J. Barry, M.D.
Chief, General Medicine Unit
Massachusetts General Hospital

David Cella, Ph.D.
Professor of Psychiatry and Behavioral Science
Northwestern University Feinberg School
of Medicine
Director, Center on Outcomes Research
and Education
Evanston Northwestern Healthcare

Janet E. Dancey, M.D.
Senior Clinical Investigator, Investigational Drug
Branch, Cancer Therapy Evaluation Program
Division of Cancer Treatment and Diagnosis
National Cancer Institute

Charles Darby
Social Science Administrator
Agency for Healthcare Research and Quality

Craig C. Earle, M.D., M.Sc.
Assistant Professor of Medicine, Harvard
Medical School
Dana-Farber Cancer Institute

Pennifer Erickson, Ph.D.
Associate Professor, Departments of Biobehavioral
Health and Health Evaluation Sciences
Pennsylvania State University

Diane L. Fairclough, Dr.P.H.
Professor, Colorado Health Outcomes Center and
Department of Preventive Medicine and Biometry
University of Colorado Health Sciences Center

David H. Feeny, Ph.D.
Professor of Pharmacy and Pharmaceutical
Sciences
Institute for Health Care Economics
and Departments of Economics
and Public Health Sciences
University of Alberta

Carol Estwing Ferrans, Ph.D., R.N., F.A.A.N.
Professor, College of Nursing
University of Illinois at Chicago

Betty R. Ferrell, Ph.D., F.A.A.N.
Research Scientist
City of Hope Medical Center

Patricia A. Ganz, M.D.
Professor, Schools of Medicine and Public Health
Director, Division of Cancer Prevention
and Control Research
Jonsson Comprehensive Cancer Center
University of California, Los Angeles

Pamela J. Goodwin, M.D., M.Sc., F.R.C.P. (C)
Senior Scientist, Samuel Lunenfeld Research
Institute, Mount Sinai Hospital
Professor of Medicine, University of Toronto

David H. Gustafson, Ph.D.
Robert Ratner Professor of Industrial Engineering
Director, Center of Excellence in Cancer
Communications Research
University of Wisconsin, Madison

Ronald K. Hambleton, Ph.D.
Distinguished University Professor, School
of Education
University of Massachusetts

Mark C. Hornbrook, Ph.D.
Chief Scientist, Center for Health Research,
Northwest and Hawaii
Kaiser Permanente, Northwest Region

Mark S. Litwin, M.D., M.P.H.
Professor of Urology and Health Services
Schools of Medicine and Public Health
University of California, Los Angeles

Jeanne S. Mandelblatt, M.D., M.P.H.
Director, Cancer & Aging Research
Lombardi Comprehensive Cancer Center
and Departments of Oncology and Medicine
Georgetown University Medical Center

Mary S. McCabe, R.N., M.A.
Director, Office of Education and Special
Initiatives
National Cancer Institute

Carol M. Moinpour, Ph.D.
Behavioral Scientist
Southwest Oncology Group Statistical Center
Associate Member, Division of Public
Health Sciences
Fred Hutchinson Cancer Research Center

Bernie J. O'Brien, Ph.D.
Professor, Department of Clinical Epidemiology
and Biostatistics
McMaster University
Associate Director, Centre for Evaluation of
Medicines
St. Joseph's Healthcare

David Osoba, B.Sc., M.D., F.R.C.P.C.
Quality of Life Consultant
QOL Consulting, West Vancouver, BC

Dawn Provenzale, M.D., M.S.
Associate Professor of Medicine and
Director GI Outcomes Research
Duke University Medical Center

Steven P. Reise, Ph.D.
Professor, Department of Psychology
University of California, Los Angeles

Dennis A. Revicki, Ph.D.
Vice President and Director, Center for
Health Outcomes Research
MEDTAP International

Joe V. Selby, M.D., M.P.H.
Director, Division of Research
Kaiser Permanente Northern California

Jeff A. Sloan, Ph.D.
Lead Statistician, Cancer Center Statistics
Mayo Clinic, Rochester (MN)

James A. Talcott, M.D., S.M.
Assistant Professor and Director, Center
for Medical Outcomes
Massachusetts General Hospital

Jane C. Weeks, M.D., M.Sc.
Associate Professor of Medicine
Chief, Division of Population Science
Dana-Farber Cancer Institute

James E. Williams, Jr. (Col. Ret.) USA
Co-Chairman, Pennsylvania Prostate
Cancer Coalition
Vice President, Intercultural Cancer
Council Caucus

Mark Wilson, Ph.D.
Professor, Graduate School of Education
University of California, Berkeley

Brad Zebrack, Ph.D., M.S.W.
Cancer Survivor/Advocate
NCI Director's Consumer Liaison Group
Assistant Professor, School of Social Work
University of Southern California

Authors of invited papers

Ivan Barofsky, Ph.D.
The Quality of Life Institute, East Sandwich, MA

J. Gregory Boyer, Ph.D.
Assistant Executive Director, Accreditation
Evaluation and Research
The Accreditation Council for Pharmacy Education

Joseph C. Cappelleri, Ph.D., M.P.H.
Director, Biostatistics
Pfizer, Inc.

Karon F. Cook, Ph.D.
Associate Director for Research, Parkinson's Disease,
Research & Education Center
Houston Veterans Affairs Medical Center
Assistant Professor, Department of Neurology
Baylor College of Medicine

Kati Copley-Merriman, M.S., M.B.A.
Senior Director/Site Leader, Global Outcomes
Research
Pfizer, Inc.

Robert M. DeMarinis, Ph.D.
Assistant Vice President, Global Health Outcomes
Assessment
Wyeth Research

Joseph DiCesare, M.P.H., R.Ph.
Executive Director, Health Economics &
Outcomes Research
Novartis Pharmaceuticals Corporation

M. Haim Erder, Ph.D.
Director, Health Economics & Epidemiology
Amgen Inc.

Jean Paul Gagnon, Ph.D.
Director, Public Policy
Aventis Pharmaceuticals Inc.

Lou Garrison, Ph.D.
Vice President and Head, Health Economics
& Strategic Pricing
F. Hoffmann-La Roche AG.

Kathleen Gondek, Ph.D.
Director, Health Economics and Outcomes
Research
Bayer Corporation

Kim Allen Heithoff, Sc.D.
Director, Health Economics
Schering-Plough Pharmaceuticals

Tom Hughes, Ph.D.
Director, Health Outcomes
Global Economic Affairs
Eli Lilly and Company

Joseph D. Jackson, Ph.D.
Group Director, Outcomes Research
Bristol-Myers Squibb

Colleen A. McHorney, Ph.D.
Professor of Medicine
Indiana University School of Medicine
and Regenstrief Institute for Health Care;
Research Career Scientist and Senior Scientist
Roudebush Veterans Affairs Medical Center

David W. Miller, Ph.D.
Vice President, Global Health Outcomes
GlaxoSmithKline

Bryce B. Reeve, Ph.D.
Psychometrician, Outcomes Research Branch
Applied Research Program
Division of Cancer Control and Population Sciences
National Cancer Institute

Margaret L. Rothman, Ph.D.
Executive Director, HE&P, PGSM
Johnson & Johnson Pharmaceutical Services, LLC

Nancy Santanello, M.D., M.S.
Executive Director, Epidemiology
Merck Research Laboratories

Bert Spilker, Ph.D., M.D.
President
Bert Spilker & Associates, LLC

Richard Willke, Ph.D.
Senior Director/Group Leader, OR Product
Development Group B
Worldwide Outcomes Research
Pfizer, Inc.

Gordon B. Willis, Ph.D.
Cognitive Psychologist, Applied Research Program
Division of Cancer Control and Population Sciences
National Cancer Institute

Bruce Wong, M.D.
Vice President, Global Outcomes Research
Bristol-Myers Squibb

Acknowledgments

This volume reflects the contributions of a host of individuals who devoted time, intellectual energy, and substantive expertise towards the common goal of better understanding how to assess the outcomes of cancer and cancer care. While we mention only a few names below, we are extremely grateful to everyone who provided support and scientific guidance to the Cancer Outcomes Measurement Working Group (COMWG), established in early 2001 by the US National Cancer Institute (NCI) and whose work continued well into 2004.

First and foremost, we salute the members of the COMWG. *Outcomes Assessment in Cancer* is the product of their hard work, always under tight deadlines and sometimes under difficult circumstances. We also heartily thank the authors of the invited chapters, whose contributions fill important gaps in the working group's coverage of topics to create a stronger overall product.

We note that the work of each COMWG member who was not a US government employee was supported under an NCI contract; participation by Federal members was regarded as an "official duty" activity. The National Cancer Institute also provided limited financial support for research assistance for any COMWG member requesting it. Non-Federal authors of the invited chapters were likewise supported under NCI contract, except the members of the PhRMA Health Outcomes Committee, whose efforts were contributed. Consistent with the operating principles of an NCI-approved working group (see Chapter 1), the views expressed in each chapter are solely those of the author(s) and are not intended to reflect working group opinions or consensus positions. Chapters authored by one or more Federal employees were subject to internal clearance review by each author's agency to evaluate factual accuracy and editorial quality. These internal review policies applied to both working group and invited chapters.

Staff scientists in NCI's Outcomes Research Branch supported the working group's operations in a number of important ways. Most especially, we acknowledge the invaluable contributions of Bryce Reeve, Ph.D., a psychometrician who provided expert review and commentary on chapters dealing with application of modern measurement concepts like item response theory to improve cancer outcomes assessment. Similarly, Neeraj Arora, Ph.D., offered important perspectives on chapters examining individuals' perceptions about cancer care and approaches to assessing patient needs.

Created as one component of the NCI-wide initiative to improve the quality of cancer care, the COMWG's administrative home was NCI's Division of Cancer Control and Population Sciences (DCCPS). The project began under the leadership of DCCPS Director Barbara Rimer, Dr.P.H., and Deputy Director Robert Hiatt, M.D., Ph.D., and continued to receive unfailing support and sound guidance from Robert Croyle, Ph.D., when he became DCCPS Director in 2003. Throughout, valuable substantive direction and editorial advice was provided by Rachel Ballard-Barbash, M.D., Associate Director Applied Research, DCCPS.

In the course of the COMWG's three on-site meetings, there were stimulating presentations by Robert Wittes, M.D., NCI Deputy Director; Laurie B. Burke, R.Ph., M.P.H., Director, Endpoints and Labeling Development at the US Food and Drug Administration; Julia Rowland, Ph.D., Director of the NCI Office of Cancer Survivorship; and also members of the working group and invited chapter authors.

Two contractors provided critically important assistance. The late Ellen Tobin, President of Cancer Care Strategies, conducted a number of focus groups to deepen the COMWG's understanding of how cancer patients and survivors perceive and cope with this disease and its aftermath. Jane Kolimaga worked rapidly, tirelessly, and with unerring accuracy in copy-editing the book's chapters.

We note with great sadness the untimely passing in early 2004 of COMWG member Bernie O'Brien, Ph.D., an internationally recognized health economist whose contributions to the profession are well exemplified by, but extend far beyond, the superb chapter he produced for this volume.

Over the months since the COMWG began, cancer touched our lives through family, friends, and colleagues. We have seen first-hand the impact on patients and their loved ones. It is our sincere hope that the work presented here will stimulate additional research and application to improve the lives of all those affected by cancer.

Introduction to *Outcomes Assessment in Cancer*

Joseph Lipscomb, Ph.D.,[1] Carolyn C. Gotay, Ph.D.,[2] and Claire Snyder, M.H.S.[3]

[1] National Cancer Institute, Bethesda, MD
[2] Cancer Research Center of Hawai'i, Honolulu, HI
[3] National Cancer Institute, Bethesda, MD

Understanding how a disease and its associated health care interventions affect the lives of individuals is important whatever the medical condition, but especially so for diseases that are chronic or incurable and for which treatments often have toxic and long-lasting consequences. For this reason, cancer provides an exceptionally compelling model for examining the impact of disease on individual well-being. It is the second leading cause of death in the US, with one out of every four deaths in 2004 (over 560 000 in total) projected to be attributable to cancer. Many more individuals (an estimated 9.6 million in 2000) will be undergoing cancer treatment, coping with progressive disease, or living cancer-free in the aftermath of diagnosis and treatment.[1]

The principal means of treating cancer – surgery, chemotherapy, and radiation – are powerful and toxic. All of these treatments, and additional ones like hormonal therapy, have side effects, which may be short-term or time-limited, or chronic and persistent, or else generate late effects emerging only after treatment is completed and sometimes not evident until many years later. Efforts to prevent, screen for, and treat cancer are all aimed at maximizing the chances for a healthy life while, at the same time, minimizing the associated side effects. In addition to its mortality and morbidity impact, cancer inflicts an enormous economic burden on society. Total direct medical care costs attributable to cancer in the US in 2003 were projected to be $64.2 billion (or 4.5% of all direct medical costs), while the total economic burden (measured as direct costs plus the indirect costs associated with cancer-attributable

morbidity and premature mortality) for 2003 was projected at nearly $190 billion (or 8.4% of all disease-generated costs).[1] Consequently, documenting how cancer and cancer-related interventions affect the individual becomes crucial for determining whether these interventions are tolerable and acceptable, provide significant clinical benefits, and are economically viable.

"Outcomes research" may be defined generally as the scientific field devoted to measuring and interpreting the impact of medical conditions and health care on individuals and populations. According to the Agency for Healthcare Research and Quality, "outcomes research seeks to understand the end results of particular health care practices and interventions. . . . End results include effects that people experience and care about, such as change in the ability to function . . . and include quality of life as well as mortality."[2] The Outcomes Research Branch of the US National Cancer Institute (NCI) (within the National Institutes of Health) states that "outcomes research describes, interprets, and predicts the impact of various influences, especially (but not exclusively) interventions on 'final' endpoints that matter to decision makers: patients, providers, private payers, government agencies, accrediting organizations, and society at large."[3] Such final endpoints, according to NCI, may include survival or disease-free survival (with or without an adjustment for variations in quality of life); health-related quality of life (HRQOL), as captured through either generic (non-disease specific), general cancer, or cancer site-specific measures; perceptions about and satisfaction with health care; and economic burden, as felt by patients, caregivers, payers (public and private), or society at large.

Consequently, the central task of outcomes assessment in cancer is to enhance our understanding about the impact of interventions (and possibly other factors) on these final endpoints from a variety of potential decision perspectives. Elsewhere, NCI has proposed a three-part categorization of these decision perspectives that, together, comprise the arenas of application for cancer outcomes research. These arenas have been defined as macro (population surveillance of progress against the cancer burden); meso (descriptive and analytical studies to understand the impact of cancer, patterns of service use, and the effects of interventions on outcomes); and micro (use of outcomes measurement and clinical decision modeling to facilitate patient-provider choice making).[4]

However, before outcomes research can be used in these arenas, it is essential to know that cancer outcomes can be measured in a scientifically sound manner. Some outcomes, such as survival and disease-free survival, are relatively straightforward to assess. Other measures commonly used in health care may involve more interpretation and calibration but be no less useful – for example, measurement of blood pressure. This assessment has a long and successful history in health care. There are standard, well-calibrated instruments yielding numerical values that have, over time, taken on comparatively clear meaning for purposes of diagnosing hypertension and identifying (through clinical research) effective interventions that reduce, delay, or eliminate serious target organ damage. Although there is much intra-individual variation in blood pressure readings (posing a threat to reliability), there is enough accumulated research and observational experience to conclude confidently that (for example) a sustained change in diastolic from 105 mmHg to 85 mmHg for a given individual is both a "clinically meaningful" and "clinically important" difference. Moreover, knowledge of the 105 mmHG reading undoubtedly would bring "added value" to the clinical deliberations leading the provider to prescribe and the patient to accept the medication and behavioral health changes generating such an improvement.

It is worth remembering that the first measurement of blood pressure occurred in 1733 (measured intra-arterially in a horse), and it took until 1905 for a technique to be developed that is similar to what is used today.[5] Further, it was only in the 1960s that hypertension was recognized as a cardiac risk factor and medical interventions developed accordingly. The pathway to scientific consensus can be lengthy and serpentine, even for a comparatively "hard" endpoint like blood pressure. It should not be surprising, therefore, that we do not yet have definitively established, widely accepted, and extensively used measures for health-related quality of life, perceptions of and satisfaction with health care, and many aspects of economic burden. To be sure, there has been significant progress over the past two decades, as many chapters in this volume attest, with the result that certain HRQOL and satisfaction instruments are being used with increasing frequency and sophistication in clinical trials and observational studies. Still, there remains much that is not understood, and is currently under debate, about the scientific foundations, clinical utility, and overall decisional relevance of such patient-reported outcome measures. In blood pressure assessment, the relevant data are transmitted straight from the patient's arm, as it were, into the sphygmomanometer. In HRQOL assessment, it is the patient who must perceive, interpret, and evaluate his or her own health-related circumstances at the moment and then map this assessment to a candidate survey item or some other form of evaluation (e.g., preference score). Thus, the measurement challenges here include not only obtaining an adequate physiological "pulse" about the health condition of interest, but also a cognitively meaningful sorting and evaluation of the data, so that a coherent assessment of something called "quality of life" emerges. Doing this successfully is arguably required for achieving the type of patient-centered health care long advocated by many public and private decision makers.[6] Indeed, much of this volume is devoted to the review and evaluation of where the field stands in developing and applying such patient-reported (and patient-centered) outcome measures.

As a review of publication trends in the peer-review literature indicates, there has been increasing attention to cancer-related outcomes in recent years. A MEDLINE search crossing the terms "cancer" with "quality of life" identified 2416 articles for the five-year period 1990–1994, 4683 articles over the 1995–99 period, and 5676 articles between 2000 and 2003. A similar trend was seen when "cancer" was crossed with "patient satisfaction," with the number of citations across these three periods being 214, 666, and 970, respectively.

Despite this substantial and apparent growing interest in cancer outcomes measurement, there have been only limited efforts to review and synthesize the literature from a methodological perspective to understand what has been well-established, what remains unknown or equivocal, and what research is needed to accelerate progress. In fact, determining how best to address these issues became a first order of business for NCI's Outcomes Research Branch after it was created in 1999. In the same year, NCI established a new research initiative (which continues today on a number of fronts) to improve the quality of cancer care. This has served to accentuate the potential policy import of cancer outcomes measurement. Specifically, this initiative has defined quality cancer care "as the provision of evidence-based, patient-centered services throughout the continuum of care in a timely and technically competent manner, with good communication, shared decision making, and cultural sensitivity. The ultimate aim is to improve a range of outcomes important to patients, families, and other decision makers, including patient survival and quality of life."[7] Consequently, it is centrally important to have scientifically sound, patient-centered outcome measures for assessing whether specific cancer interventions lead to the end results desired by decision makers.

For these measurement tools to be as useful as possible to NCI and other organizations that attempt to evaluate cancer care from a broad perspective, they would ideally possess several characteristics. One is parsimony: for any given outcomes research application, there would be a small "core" set of measures available that meet rigorous scientific standards. Among other things, such a core would improve the comparability of outcome findings across studies, thus enhancing the quality and usefulness of meta-analyses by strengthening the statistical robustness and representativeness of conclusions about the impact of interventions. Another important characteristic is sensitivity: that is, that the outcome measure(s) in any given application are known to reflect what is important to patients. By the same token, it is also essential to know when such measures are detecting changes that are not in fact meaningful to the patient. Questions regarding what constitutes a "truly meaningful" change in a patient-reported outcome like HRQOL, and how to recognize and utilize such data, point to some thorny issues. There may be an unavoidable tradeoff between selecting measures that promote comparability across studies versus those that are sensitive to change within studies. On the other hand, might there be analytical approaches, either available now or in development, that would allow us to sidestep this tradeoff? More broadly, what are the methodological tools and research strategies for effectively tackling the broad range of challenges arising in outcomes measurement?

To address these and many other related issues, the NCI established in 2001 the Cancer Outcomes Measurement Working Group (COMWG). Comprising 35 experts drawn from academia, government, industry, and the cancer patient and survivorship communities, the COMWG was charged with evaluating the state of the science in outcomes measurement and recommending approaches to improve the scientific quality and usefulness of measures. This volume reports the findings and recommendations of the COMWG members. In the remaining sections of this chapter, we describe the development and operation of the COMWG, suggest an organizational framework for analyzing cancer outcomes measurement, provide operational definitions for key terms used throughout the book, and finally present an overview of the book's organization and its individual chapters.

Development of the working group

With the state of the science in cancer outcomes measurement still evolving and diverse in its approaches and perspectives, NCI determined that the appropriate way forward was to establish a "working group" rather than a Federal advisory committee or some other mechanism geared to produce consensus recommendations to guide policy. As defined and formally chartered by NCI, a working group is not a decisional body. Rather, it is a group convened for the purpose of exchanging facts or information and reviewing data, with group members being expected to provide their "individual opinions on the information being reviewed."[8] Consequently (and as the reader will readily discern), individual chapters addressing broadly similar topics may concur on some points, disagree on others, or even take varying perspectives on what the important issues are. An important question, further discussed in the book's concluding chapter, is whether there emerges from the COMWG analyses certain "natural pockets" of consensus that point the way to future consensus development.

The membership of the COMWG was carefully constituted to reflect a variety of perspectives on cancer outcomes measurement and to provide a broad range of clinical and methodological expertise. The working group members, with their affiliations, are listed at the beginning of this volume. They were selected on the basis of their contributions to the literature and to the conduct of clinical and outcomes research through major cancer-related organizations. The aim was to create a group whose skills, insights, and experiences would be complementary and sufficient, taken together, to address the many topics within the working group's purview. The majority of members were cancer researchers, many of whom were also clinicians representing medicine (with 9 of the 12 clinicians being oncologists),

nursing, psychology, and social work. There was expertise in economics, biostatistics, psychometrics, and health services research generally. The perspectives of the cancer patient and survivor were given particular focus through the appointment of two members nominated by the NCI Director's Consumer Liaison Group.

To chair the COMWG, NCI named Joseph Lipscomb, Ph.D., Chief of the Outcomes Research Branch (ORB), and Carolyn C. Gotay, Ph.D., a psychosocial oncology researcher at the University of Hawai'i. Claire Snyder, M.H.S., an ORB staff member with a background in health services research, served as the COMWG "initiator" (NCI's term for working group convenor) and provided both technical and scientific input throughout the process.

To obtain additional, complementary insight on particular topics in cancer outcome measures development and application, NCI commissioned the four invited chapters published in this volume.

Framework for COMWG cancer outcomes assessment

Evaluating the state of the science in cancer outcomes measurement is both a daunting task and potentially an ill-defined one, unless some additional structure is imposed. To focus the COMWG's work while striving to maintain adequate breadth of coverage, four key issues about content and scope were addressed early on, and their resolution effectively defined the framework for the working group's research.

1. Outcome measures of prime interest. Among outcome measures important for decision making in cancer, we believed those that pose the largest methodological challenges fall under the broad headings of health-related quality of life, patient perceptions of and satisfaction with care, and economic burden. Survival and disease-free survival are centrally important, but the challenge today lies with how to improve these outcomes, not how to measure them. Intermediate outcomes such as

time to tumor progression or time to recurrence were not a COMWG focus since they do not incorporate the patient's point of view or evaluation.

2. Disease focus. Cancer is not one disease but well over a hundred now, and our rapidly expanding understanding of the biological mechanisms of cancer will likely lead to ever more refined categorizations in years to come. As a practical matter, we elected to focus on a manageable number of cancer types that collectively account for a substantial portion of the total US cancer burden: breast (female), colorectal, lung, and prostate. In 2003, about 55% of all new cancer cases and just over 50% of all cancer deaths were attributable to these four diseases (with those proportions virtually the same, respectively, in men and women).[1] Moreover, the majority of cancer outcomes research studies published to date have examined one or more of these disease sites.

3. Continuum of care. The COMWG was charged with examining outcomes measurement across the entire cancer trajectory: prevention and screening, diagnosis and treatment, survivorship, and end of life. We believed that, especially for HRQOL, the appropriate choice of measure may vary along this continuum of cancer care. One could not assume, for example, that HRQOL measures designed to detect symptom relief and toxicity burdens during initial treatment would necessarily be appropriate for outcomes assessment in survivorship, or for evaluating the short-term impacts of preventive interventions.

4. Arenas of application. Cancer outcomes assessment can contribute to decision making at multiple levels in multiple ways. Consequently, the COMWG collectively was charged with examining progress across the three arenas of application (as defined above) – but with the implied proviso that the search was to be largely confined to the peer-review literature. As it turned out, that literature is dominated by meso-level papers with a clinical or health services research orientation: randomized trials, observational studies of interventions, investigations of cancer burden in particular populations, and economic evaluations including cost-effectiveness analyses. With respect to macro-level studies on the cancer burden using the outcome measures of interest here, there are many government reports, but comparatively few papers in the peer-review literature. While there is increasing discussion of the role cancer outcome measures can, or should, play in patient-provider decision making and clinical care, the scientific literature on these micro-level applications is small (though growing), as the recent analysis by Donaldson confirms.[9]

In sum, the COMWG was asked to examine current practices, and identify best practices, for assessing the three outcomes of interest in the four selected cancers across the continuum of care, with attention also to likely decision-making applications. As will be seen, some chapters in this volume evaluated the published literature at various points of intersection implied by these four factors (e.g., assessment of HRQOL in initial treatment of breast cancer, with implications for clinical decision making). Other chapters focused on the methodological underpinnings of outcomes assessment (e.g., defining and modeling HRQOL, patient satisfaction, or economic burden; psychometric advances to improve HRQOL measurement generally; or statistical considerations in evaluating the impact of interventions on outcomes).

However, the work of the COMWG, and the book that flows from it, was never intended to address all of the questions and needs of the cancer outcomes researcher. Additional cancer disease sites await evaluation. We do not provide here a detailed guide or tutorial for how to develop, test, or actually use outcome measures; nor how to carry out psychometric analyses step-by-step; nor how to conduct statistical evaluations of outcomes data. For lucid discussions on such matters, the reader is referred to such texts as Fayers and Machin[10] and Spilker.[11] We note also that the chapters in this volume reviewing and evaluating the outcomes measurement instruments employed to date for a particular purpose generally do not "pick a winner." Rather, they attempt to provide an objective, side-by-side comparison of the strengths and limitations of competing instruments to provide a basis for choosing among instruments for a particular application. It will be clear in many cases that certain measures and instruments are the strongest and most promising, but these conclusions emerge from the analysis and discussion, rather than from directives to make recommendations for particular approaches to measurement.

Operations of the working group

COMWG members were asked to review and evaluate specific aspects of cancer outcomes measurement, to meet periodically as a group to discuss their findings, and to prepare written reports for submission to the NCI. These reports, collectively, constitute the basis for Chapters 2–27 of this book.

Given the outcomes assessment framework noted above, we developed "question sets" that were assigned to COMWG members, either individually or in pairs. The question sets were intended to encompass the major issues arising from consideration of the four dimensions defining the framework, as well as cross-cutting methodological topics. For example, members addressing the performance of a particular type of outcome measure (e.g., HRQOL) at a specific point along the cancer continuum (e.g., treatment) for a specified cancer type (e.g., lung) were asked to assess the psychometric properties of the commonly used instruments, their overall strengths and weaknesses, their value-added compared with biomedical outcome measures, and the additional research now needed. To the extent appropriate, we attempted to standardize the question sets so that inquiries about the same broad topic (e.g., HRQOL) were as comparably phrased as possible. As the working group proceeded, we also developed common definitions for key terms and standardized approaches to data abstraction, and table construction, as discussed below.

The process of report generation and chapter preparation was an iterative one: research, initial manuscript drafts, group discussions, electronic communication between editors and authors, revision and re-revision, and final editing. The three working group meetings (February 2001, December 2001, and December 2002) provided important opportunities for presentations, panel discussions, and small-group sessions. In addition, each COMWG member was assigned to an "affinity group" consisting of COMWG members with allied methods or application interests, in order to promote interdisciplinary peer review and discussion.

Throughout the period from early 2001 until the final assigned chapter was completed in 2004, the editors had both the responsibility and the remarkable opportunity to work closely with the other 32 members of the COMWG in a number of respects. Beyond the initial designation of topic areas, this involved tailoring question sets in response to author suggestions, reviewing chapter drafts, and working interactively through the multi-step review and editing process that led to the chapters found here.

Sources of data

The primary source of data for the majority of findings reported in this book is the peer-review literature. Some authors performed re-analysis of existing data bases (see the chapters by Hambleton,[12] Reise,[13] and Wilson[14]), and one relied heavily on websites and government reports (Gotay and Lipscomb[15]).

Early on, some COMWG members noted the paucity of data on certain topics. In response, we organized a series of focus groups under NCI sponsorship during the summer of 2001. A professional focus group facilitator (Ellen Tobin) led the effort, working with COMWG members to define the eligibility criteria for group participation, develop discussion guides, and analyze and report the results.

A total of 92 cancer patients and survivors each participated in one of 12 focus groups conducted at a facility designed for such research in suburban Washington, DC. These groups included diverse participation with respect to gender, site of disease, and time since diagnosis.

In addition, a focus group comprising 11 national experts in outcomes data development, linkage, and analysis was convened, by electronic video-conference, in the summer of 2001 in support of the COMWG chapter on data for cancer outcomes research.[15]

Establishing a common approach

Standardized definitions of key terms and procedures for data abstraction and reporting were developed in the course of the working group, are used throughout this book, and are briefly described below.

Defining health-related quality of life

We were aware that an entire chapter of this volume (Ferrans[16]) would be devoted to identifying and evaluating alternative definitions and conceptual models of HRQOL, so we imposed no fixed definition of HRQOL on the COMWG at the start. However, it became evident over time that varying definitions were being used in the literature and by different working group members, and that some consistency was needed. In this book, a key defining feature of a HRQOL measure is that it must be patient-reported and thus involve the patient's (or, more generally, the individual respondent's) subjective assessment or evaluation. The potential usefulness of the patient-reported outcome concept for cancer outcomes assessment has been noted by both the US Food and Drug Administration (FDA)[17] and the pharmaceutical industry.[18]

In the guidelines we developed with the COMWG members analyzing HRQOL, we defined patient-reported measures of HRQOL to include symptoms, functional status, and/or global well-being. Symptom measures include patient reports on the frequency, severity, bother, or impact of symptoms (both disease-related and treatment-related). Toxicities are distinct from patient-reported symptoms, in that they involve the clinician's evaluation and recording; the clinician's evaluation may result from discussion with the patient or in other ways (e.g., laboratory test values). Functional status measures include patient reports on the impact of cancer and its treatment on everyday life and overall well-being. Functional status measures may be multidimensional and thus include more than one domain of HRQOL and/or symptoms (e.g., the FACT-G or the EORTC QLQ-C30), or unidimensional and focus on a single domain of HRQOL (e.g., a measure of pain or fatigue). Global rating measures capture the individual's overall assessment of personal well-being. These can be preference-based (involving utility scores) or non-preference based (involving an overall rating or summary score on a unidimensional psychometric scale).

Identifying the desirable properties of outcome measurement instruments

The comprehensive instrument review criteria assembled by the Medical Outcomes Trust (MOT)[19] were adopted as the basis for evaluating the psychometric properties of the patient-reported outcome measures analyzed by the COMWG. As constructed, the MOT criteria are to be applied in assessing the adequacy of an instrument on the following eight attributes: conceptual and measurement model, reliability, validity, responsiveness, interpretability, burden of administration, alternative forms (modes of administration), and cultural and language adaptations. The MOT attributes and criteria were distributed to all COMWG members in the early months of the project.

Categorizing HRQOL measures by breadth of application

For the purposes of this book, *generic* measures of HRQOL are not specific to cancer but can be applied to healthy and ill individuals, or populations, regardless of health state. Examples include the SF-36, the Sickness Impact Profile, and the Brief Pain Inventory. *General cancer* measures are designed to assess HRQOL in cancer regardless of disease site.

Examples include the FACT-G and the EORTC QLQ-C30. *Cancer site-specific* measures assess HRQOL in a particular type (disease site) of cancer. For example, the general FACT and the core of the EORTC can be supplemented with questionnaires developed for patients with particular cancers; for example, the FACT-B and EORTC-LC13 are cancer site-specific measures for breast and lung cancer, respectively.

Approach to tables

For reporting on the development of commonly used HRQOL instruments and their psychometric properties, a standardized table shell, modeled after similar reports in other studies,[20] was constructed and distributed to COMWG members early in the project. In addition, we worked closely with the authors of the disease-specific chapters (breast, colorectal, lung, and prostate) to develop table shells for abstracting data from the literature to identify the most commonly used measures of HRQOL and biomedical outcomes, and to facilitate an assessment of the added value of HRQOL outcomes compared with biomedical outcomes. For purposes of the COMWG's deliberations, and this book, we defined HRQOL ratings as providing "added value" when they were instrumental in interpreting the study's conclusions and therefore would be expected to influence recommendations about appropriate intervention(s). Consequently, a given study needed to include both HRQOL and biomedical outcomes (e.g., survival, disease-free survival, toxicities) to facilitate a direct determination of whether HRQOL data did provide added value. That said, we acknowledge that HRQOL data may provide added value in other ways and encourage the reader to keep in mind the specific way the term is being used here.

Organization of the book

This book evaluates the state of the science in cancer outcomes assessment and offers perspectives on what is required to advance the field. The chapters collectively cover a diverse set of topics, which are examined in a sequence suggested by the broad section headings below. Developed as stand-alone documents, the chapters can be read in any order. Cross-citations to other relevant chapters are provided throughout. Each chapter presents a number of findings and recommendations, and the previews below provide only a flavor of the full range of results.

HRQOL in cancer: general concepts and generic measures

Carol Ferrans[16] discusses alternative definitions and conceptual models for HRQOL, emphasizing the distinction between measuring the patient's perceived health state descriptively and obtaining also the patient's evaluation of the state. She urges further work on causal models to understand better the determinants of HRQOL and also the possibility that patient perceptions and evaluations of health may shift over time. The chapter's recommendations are directed towards developing a common understanding of the meaning of HRQOL.

Pennifer Erickson[21] analyzes the use of the most common generic and general cancer HRQOL measures in cancer outcomes research. The chapter reviews the development and psychometric properties of these measures, and assesses their relative strengths and weaknesses and their application to specific cancers and across the continuum of care. It discusses the merits of new measurement systems that would combine generic or general cancer measures with modules of additional items tailored to specific applications.

David Feeny[22] reviews the foundations of health state preference measurement, its importance in cancer outcomes assessment, and the major available preference measurement systems currently available to researchers. Preference-based measures are already employed in most economic evaluations and many clinical decision analysis studies of cancer care. He discusses how, and why, such measures should also be used routinely in cancer clinical trials and observational studies of the effectiveness of interventions.

Assessing HRQOL during treatment

By far, the most extensive application of HRQOL in cancer to date has occurred in randomized clinical trials of biomedical or psychosocial therapies. Across tumor types, the greatest number of applications are found in breast cancer.

Patricia Ganz and Pamela Goodwin[23] examine the relative performance of HRQOL and biomedical outcome measures across a wide range of breast cancer trials. They recommend that the decision about whether to measure HRQOL in any given study, as well as the choice of specific measure(s), should be driven by the study's specific aims and hypotheses. They conclude that, based on the studies reviewed, HRQOL has contributed greater value added to psychosocial trials than to biomedical trials in breast cancer, and that routine use of HRQOL measures in breast cancer biomedical trials is not supported by the existing evidence. But they also note that future studies using breast cancer-specific measures of HRQOL will provide additional empirical insight about value added.

In their analysis of HRQOL applications in prostate cancer, Mark Litwin and James Talcott[24] discuss the importance of and challenges in measuring the impact of alternative therapies on disease symptoms (sexual, urinary, and bowel dysfunction). They conclude that the role of quality-of-life considerations in treatment choice is highly personal and find that prostate cancer-specific measures of HRQOL are often more useful than global measures in detecting important changes for prostate cancer patients.

Craig Earle and Jane Weeks[25] compare the most commonly used lung cancer-specific HRQOL measures, and note that the choice among them in a given application will depend on the purpose of the trial (biomedical versus psychosocial therapy) and the saliency of respondent burden; rapid patient deterioration is a major problem in lung cancer studies. They discuss the potential value added of HRQOL measurement in describing the balance between symptomatic improvement with treatment and its toxicity.

In their assessment of HRQOL applications to colorectal cancer treatment trials, Carol Moinpour and Dawn Provenzale[26] find that many studies to date have suffered from small sample sizes or missing data, hampering one's ability to draw clear conclusions about the value added of HRQOL. They make important recommendations about improving the content validity of HRQOL measures for colorectal cancer application.

Michael Barry and Janet Dancey[27] examine treatment-specific measures of HRQOL that cut across cancer types. They find only a very limited number of measures available that assess the morbidity and side effects attributable to specific treatments (e.g., radiation, chemotherapy). While they conclude it is premature to recommend a definitive measurement strategy, they suggest exploration of treatment-specific modules that could be linked to general cancer or cancer site-specific instruments.

Assessing HRQOL across the cancer continuum

Jeanne Mandelblatt and Joe Selby[28] propose a framework for assessing the short-term HRQOL outcomes associated with cancer prevention and screening, review the small literature to date on how measures have been applied in particular areas (e.g., chemoprevention), and consider specific recommendations for improvement. For example, they suggest that many generic HRQOL measures may not be sufficiently sensitive, and recommend further research to examine whether preference-based measures might perform well in capturing the net impact of such effects as relief, anxiety, reassurance, and discomfort.

Brad Zebrack and David Cella[29] evaluate the HRQOL measures commonly used in survivorship studies, comparing generic and general cancer measures with those developed specifically for survivorship populations. They find that while the generic and general cancer measures have generally performed adequately, they tend not to encompass such survivor-specific issues as fear of disease recurrence, chronic physical compromise, and post-traumatic growth.

Betty Ferrell[30] discusses how HRQOL assessment can play a vital role in end-of-life care, helping to evaluate and improve the quality of care. Measuring HRQOL at end of life, and appropriately interpreting the findings, poses challenges because one should take into account not only the patient's disease status, but a variety of personal, family, and environmental circumstances. At present, there are several viable HRQOL instruments appropriate to this point on the cancer continuum.

Measuring the experience and needs of cancer patients and caregivers

James Williams[31] discusses how HRQOL information can be helpful to patients and families, as well as some of the barriers that presently prevent wider use of such data. His remarks have particular credence since he himself is a prostate cancer survivor.

Charles Darby[32] examines the emerging literature on measuring the patient's perspectives on cancer care, including both descriptive reports and ratings of the care received (or not received). He proposes the development of new instrumentation that would include a core set of items for application across all cancer disease sites and the continuum of care, supplemented by additional items tailored to the application at hand.

David Gustafson[33] reviews current methods for assessing patient needs and proposes innovative new approaches (such as conjoint analysis) that would apply modern statistical techniques to survey data to create tighter links between perceived needs and constructive strategies for meeting them. He also probes the complex interconnections among patient needs, satisfaction with care, and HRQOL.

Claire Snyder[34] examines caregiver impact. She seeks to identify the positive and negative impacts that caring for a loved one with cancer can have on the informal caregiver, evaluates the most commonly used measures, and proposes additional research on instruments designed to assess these effects.

Methodological considerations in applications to cancer outcomes research

Diane Fairclough[35] looks at a host of practical considerations in planning and executing a cancer outcomes research study. These include identifying the appropriate role of HRQOL assessment (and noting this may vary in drug evaluations depending on the phase of development), the mode and medium of questionnaire administration, and approaches to the problem of missing data. While there are sophisticated statistical techniques for coping with a variety of missing data dilemmas, she emphasizes that the best policy is prevention – through careful study design and conscientious execution.

Jeff Sloan[36] provides a brief yet relatively comprehensive overview of statistical modeling and analysis techniques relevant to cancer outcomes research. To promote thoughtful and transparent analysis, he recommends simple, robust analytical models; careful attention to subtle patterns of variations in the underlying data; and methods of presentation (such as graphical approaches) that provide a more descriptive picture of findings than summary statistics alone.

David Osoba[37] assays the various potential ways that HRQOL information can be useful to clinical decision making in oncology. He urges that HRQOL data be analyzed for both statistical and clinical significance (using both distribution-based and anchor-based approaches), and points to recent convergent evidence on what *may* constitute a perceptible and clinically meaningful difference in HRQOL scores.

Neil Aaronson[38] reviews the need for and challenges in adapting HRQOL instruments for use across different populations and cultures. He concludes there are several available instruments meeting minimum psychometric requirements, with the choice among these depending on the study at hand. There should be greater attention to standardization and quality monitoring in the instrument translation process, and he also recommends greater application of modern psychometric techniques to detect and correct for problems that arise when a given survey item is interpreted differently across populations or cultures (differential item functioning).

Modern psychometric theory in cancer outcomes research

The chapters in this section examine innovative approaches to measuring unobservable (latent) constructs such as HRQOL, focusing on techniques that have become well-established in the field of educational assessment and are just beginning to be applied in the health arena. The findings and recommendations emerging from these chapters may be particularly important in shaping the research agenda in cancer outcomes measurement, and we explore these issues in some detail in the book's concluding chapter.

Steven Reise[13] introduces the basic concepts and techniques of item response theory (IRT) modeling, including the frequently used Rasch model variant, and compares these approaches to the more traditional classical test theory model for measuring HRQOL. He points to the potential advantages of modern over classical approaches, including enhanced reliability and the capability of cross-walking scores between alternative instruments, and urges additional empirical studies to investigate these issues.

HRQOL is generally regarded as a multidimensional concept, and Mark Wilson[14] takes up two important, related issues: how best to estimate HRQOL scores for each (single dimensional) subscale, and how best to derive a summary score across dimensions. He proposes a multidimensional IRT model for doing this, and illustrates with survey data.

Ronald Hambleton[12] reviews and then illustrates with a data analysis how IRT provides both a theoretical framework and practical way forward for developing survey item banks, setting the stage for computer-adaptive assessment of HRQOL to enhance both reliability and feasibility.

Assessing the economic impact of cancer

The economic implications of cancer and cancer interventions at the individual level have received considerably less attention to date than the impacts on HRQOL and other patient-reported outcomes.

Mark Hornbrook[39] analyzes the key components of the economic burden of cancer and illustrates from the literature how to measure them. He develops a comprehensive typology of economic burden and uses it to discuss how to select the relevant measures for the particular research application at hand.

Bernie O'Brien[40] discusses the role of cost-effectiveness analysis in economic evaluations of cancer care. He emphasizes the potential (and under-exploited) interplay between randomized clinical trials and decision analytic models in the assessment of interventions. Trials can provide valuable data for these decision models, while they, in turn, permit the time frame of the analysis to extend across the patient's life cycle (and thus well beyond the boundaries of most trials). Such interactive analyses are best conducted through Bayesian statistical modeling.

Research and policy implications

The focus of this section is on outcomes data development and its application to policy decisions. Carolyn Gotay and Joseph Lipscomb[15] review the currently available sources of data for conducting cancer outcomes research, including registries, medical records, administrative files, and surveys of patients, providers, and individuals at risk of cancer. They illustrate by example how these sources can be linked to strengthen the empirical foundation of analyses, and discuss possible mechanisms for strengthening the national data infrastructure for cancer outcomes assessment.

Dennis Revicki[17] examines the actual and potential use of HRQOL data by the pharmaceutical industry and regulatory agencies, particularly the US FDA. He concludes that for drug labeling and marketing, HRQOL data can add meaningfully to biomedical outcome measures. He emphasizes both the importance of transparency and scientific rigor in industry-sponsored studies, and the need for explicit guidance from governments about the conduct of these studies.

A final chapter by Carolyn Gotay, Joseph Lipscomb, and Claire Snyder[41] assays the key findings and recommendations across the chapters of the book, as well as from other relevant literature, and identifies important considerations in moving to the "next phase" of cancer outcomes assessment.

The book is supplemented with four invited chapters that augment the perspectives and findings provided by COMWG members. Bert Spilker[42] provides an overview of the history, current state, and future of health outcomes research. This chapter provides a broad perspective of where the field has been in the past, progress to date, and areas requiring further development.

Gordon Willis, Bryce Reeve, and Ivan Barofsky[43] discuss the use of cognitive interviewing techniques in HRQOL and other research using patient-reported outcomes. They emphasize that these techniques can improve the ways that questions are developed and asked, and thus reduce respondent bias and burden.

Colleen McHorney and Karon Cook[44] provide an analysis of the role of modern psychometric methods that complements the chapters by Reise, Hambleton and Wilson. The chapter examines the many potential benefits offered by item banks and computer-adaptive assessments in outcomes research, and discusses the challenges that will have to be addressed before this potential is realized.

A chapter by members of the Health Outcomes Committee of the Pharmaceutical Research and Manufacturers of America[18] offers an industry perspective on the uses of and value added provided by patient-reported outcomes such as HRQOL, as well as the analytical challenges in collecting and using such data effectively and appropriately.

Conclusions

Cancer touches the lives of millions worldwide each year. This is reflected not only in well-publicized mortality statistics but also in the profound – though much more difficult to measure – effects of cancer on the health-related quality of life, economic status, and overall well-being of patients and families. Meanwhile, the field of cancer outcomes research is at an exciting point in its development. Much research has been reported already, as witnessed by the voluminous reference lists that accompany every chapter. At the same time, the science of patient self-report and its application in cancer is still relatively new. This book is intended to provide a comprehensive review and evaluation of the state of this science, with an eye to new developments on the horizon that will strengthen our capacity to measure, evaluate, and improve the outcomes of cancer care. Our hope is that readers will have a sense of where the field is now and will be encouraged to participate in its future growth.

REFERENCES

1 American Cancer Society (2004). *Cancer Facts & Figures 2004.* Atlanta, GA: ACS.

2 Agency for Healthcare Research and Quality. "Outcomes research fact sheet: What is outcomes research." Available at http://www.ahrq.gov/clinic/outfact.htm. Last accessed on September 9, 2004.

3 National Cancer Institute. "Defining the emerging field of outcomes research." Available at http://outcomes.cancer.gov/aboutresearch/defining.html/. Last accessed on September 9, 2004.

4 Lipscomb, J., Donaldson, M. S., Hiatt, R. A. (2004). Cancer outcomes research and the arenas of application. *Journal of the National Cancer Institute Monograph* 33:1–7.

5 Braun (GmbH) Health Care Information Center. "History of Blood Pressure Measurement." Available at http://www.braun.com/medical/bloodpressure/infocenter/background/history.html. Last accessed on January 30, 2004.

6 Clancy, C. M., Eisenberg, J. M. (1998). Outcomes research: measuring the end results of health care. *Science* **282**(5387):245–6

7 National Cancer Institute. "The Nation's Investment in Cancer Research: a Plan and Budget Proposal for Fiscal Year 2005." Available at http://plan.cancer.gov. Last accessed on September 13, 2004.

8 National Cancer Institute. "Guidelines for the Conduct of Working Groups that Are Not Subject to the Federal Advisory Committee Act." Available at http://deaintranet.nci.nih.gov/ncipolicy/non-faca-final.htm. Last accessed on September 12, 2004.

9 Donaldson, M. S. (2004). Taking stock of health-related quality of life measurement in oncology practice in the United States. *Journal of the National Cancer Institute Monograph (Cancer Outcomes Research: the Arenas of Application).* In press.

10 Fayers, P. M., Machin, D. (2002). *Quality of Life: Assessment, Analysis and Interpretation.* Chichester: John Wiley & Sons Ltd.

11 Spilker, B. (Ed.) (1996). *Quality of Life and Pharmacoeconomics in Clinical Trials* (2nd Edition). Philadelphia: Lippincott-Raven.

12 Hambleton, this volume, Chapter 22.

13 Reise, this volume, Chapter 21.

14 Wilson, this volume, Chapter 23.

15 Gotay, Lipscomb, this volume, Chapter 26.

16 Ferrans, this volume, Chapter 2.

17 Revicki, this volume, Chapter 27.

18 Copley-Merriman *et al.*, this volume, Invited Paper D.

19 Lohr, K. N. (2002). Assessing health status and quality-of-life instruments: attributes and review criteria. *Quality of Life Research* **11**:193–205.

20 Damiano A. M., Snyder, C. F., Strausser, B. *et al.* (1999). A review of health-related quality-of-life concepts and measures for Parkinson's disease. *Quality of Life Research* **8**: 236–43.

21 Erickson, this volume, Chapter 3.

22 Feeny, this volume, Chapter 4.

23 Ganz, Goodwin, this volume, Chapter 5.

24 Litwin, Talcott, this volume, Chapter 6.

25 Earle, Weeks, this volume, Chapter 7.

26 Moinpour, Provenzale, this volume, Chapter 8.

27 Barry, Dancey, this volume, Chapter 9.

28 Mandelblatt, Selby, this volume, Chapter 10.

29 Zebrack, Cella, this volume, Chapter 11.

30 Ferrell, this volume, Chapter 12.

31 Williams, this volume, Chapter 13.

32 Darby, this volume, Chapter 14.

33 Gustafson, this volume, Chapter 15.

34 Snyder, this volume, Chapter 16.

35 Fairclough, this volume, Chapter 17.

36 Sloan, this volume, Chapter 18.

37 Osoba, this volume, Chapter 19.

38 Aaronson, this volume, Chapter 20.

39 Hornbrook, this volume, Chapter 24.

40 O'Brien, this volume, Chapter 25.

41 Gotay, Lipscomb, Snyder, this volume, Chapter 28.

42 Spilker, this volume, Invited Paper A.

43 Willis, Reeve, Barofsky, this volume, Invited Paper C.

44 McHorney, Cook, this volume, Invited Paper B.

2

Definitions and conceptual models of quality of life

Carol Estwing Ferrans, Ph.D., R.N., F.A.A.N.

University of Illinois at Chicago, Chicago, IL

Over the past 30 years, quality of life has evolved into a respected construct for evaluating the effectiveness of treatment in health care. The field has grown in methodological rigor and in the sophistication of instrument development. Researchers in oncology have been at the forefront in the evaluation of quality of life, recognizing the need to assess outcomes more broadly than tumor response and length of survival. In 1985, quality of life was identified as a key parameter of efficacy to be used for approval of new anticancer drugs for advanced metastatic disease in the USA.[1] In 1988, the Division of Cancer Treatment (CTEP) of the National Cancer Institute (USA) identified improving quality of life as one of its highest priorities.[2] Quality-of-life endpoints are integral components of cancer clinical trials throughout the world, and are required for all phase III clinical trials by the National Cancer Institute of Canada Clinical Trials Group.[3]

But what is quality of life? The literature contains a bewildering array of characterizations. The term "quality of life" is commonly used to mean health status, physical functioning, symptoms, psychosocial adjustment, well-being, life satisfaction, or happiness. Introducing the term "health-related quality of life" has not solved the problem. Because the terms have meaning in everyday language, they are frequently used without explicit definition. At the heart of the problem is the very nature of the idea of quality of life, which is uniquely personal in its essence. The difficulty lies in the need to define quality of life for groups of people, in order to provide some sort of approximation of quality of life for evaluation of health care outcomes.

In this effort, clarity in the meaning of the term quality of life is critically important, because confusion hinders progress in research and application to clinical practice. Differences in meaning make it difficult to compare findings across studies and interpret the literature. The purpose of this chapter is to examine the ways in which quality of life has been conceptualized, in order to provide a framework for categorizing various approaches to the use of the construct. The definitions and conceptual models presented are limited to those that are related to health care, and specifically cancer care. The conceptualizations used by major quality-of-life instruments also are examined in this chapter, because the instruments used to measure the construct ultimately define it for any particular study.

Quality of life versus health-related quality of life

When defining quality of life as it applies to health care, the term *health-related quality of life* (HRQOL) commonly is used to focus on the effects of illness and treatment. It is used to distinguish these aspects of life from those that are beyond the realm of health care, such as education, standard of living, quality of the environment, public safety, transportation, political freedom, and cultural amenities. Thus, the term HRQOL draws a line between those facets of life that are primarily health related and those that are not.

Quality of life as it relates to political, societal, or cultural issues generally qualifies as non-health-related quality of life and falls within the domain of fields such as sociology, economics, anthropology, criminology, and demography. Spilker and Revicki[4] developed a taxonomy for non-HRQOL, composed of four domains: (a) personal-internal (facets within the individual that influence perceptions and interactions with the environment); (b) personal-social (the individual's social network and immediate social environment); (c) external-natural environment (geographical and natural environment); and (d) external-societal environment (organizations and institutions created by society). They note that the distinction between HRQOL and non-HRQOL is fluid, in that each component can become health related. For example, at the level of the external-natural environment, long dark winters contribute to seasonal affective disorder and air pollution contributes to chronic respiratory disease. In addition, when an individual becomes ill, almost all areas of life can become health related.[5]

Domains of health-related quality of life

There is general agreement that HRQOL is a multi-dimensional construct, which at a minimum consists of physical, mental, and social domains. These three domains appear in the definition of health of the World Health Organization (WHO),[6] which has been used to enlarge the notion of HRQOL beyond the absence of illness to that of complete physical, mental, and social well-being. In addition to these domains, economic and spiritual domains are commonly included. For example, these five broad domains are included in Spilker's[7] representation of quality of life, which summarizes the prevailing views of the dimensions of HRQOL found in the literature (Figure 2.1). It is a pyramid divided into three levels: the middle level consists of the five domains, the bottom level shows the components of each domain, and the top is one's overall sense of well-being.

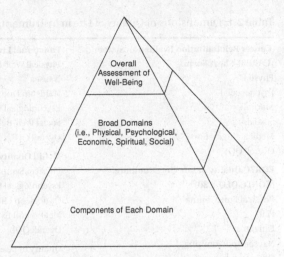

Figure 2.1. Three levels of quality of life.
Used with permission: Spilker, B. (1996). Introduction. In *Quality of Life and Pharmacoeconomics in Clinical Trials* (2nd Edition), ed. B. Spilker, Philadelphia, PA: Lippincott-Raven Publishers, pp. 1–10.

Overall well-being represents the integration of the levels below it, and thus is also multidimensional in nature.

Instruments used to measure HRQOL vary in the number and characterization of the dimensions they assess. Many of these differences stem from the fact that the instruments were developed to target different populations and purposes, and so are appropriately tailoring the concept. For example, a cluster of dimensions that reflects important concerns for patients receiving chemotherapy may be less pertinent for patients in a hospice. These sorts of differences can be seen in the domains measured by instruments used to measure quality of life in cancer patients (Table 2.1). For example, the EORTC QLQ-C30 was initially developed for use in clinical trials of therapeutic agents, and the majority of dimensions focus on functioning and symptom assessment.[8] The intent of the CARES was to focus on day-to-day problems and rehabilitation needs of cancer patients, and so includes content on disruption of daily activity caused by disease and treatment, including relationship, marital, and sexual problems.[9] The McGill Quality of Life Questionnaire

Table 2.1. Dimensions of Quality of Life in Instruments for Cancer Care

Cancer Rehabilitation Evaluation System (CARES)-Short Form[9]	**Functional Living Index – Cancer (FLIC)**[68-70]
Physical	Physical Well-Being and Ability
Psychosocial	Nausea
Marital	Hardship Due to Cancer
Sexual	Psychological Well-Being
Medical Interaction	Social Well-Being
Overall QOL	Overall QOL
EORTC Quality of Life Questionnaire (EORTC QLQ-C30)[8,30]	**McGill Quality of Life Questionnaire (MQOL)**[10]
Physical Functioning	Physical Symptoms
Pain	Psychological Symptoms
Fatigue	Outlook on Life
Nausea and Vomiting	Meaningful Existence
Other Symptoms	Overall QOL
Role Functioning	**Quality of Life Scale for Cancer (QOL-CA)**[12,13]
Cognitive Functioning	Physical Well-Being
Psychological Functioning	Psychological Well-Being
Social Functioning	Spiritual Well-Being
Financial Impact	Social Well-Being
Overall QOL	Overall QOL
Ferrans and Powers Quality of Life Index-Cancer Version (QLI)[14-16]	**SF-36 Health Survey**[71,72]
Health and Functioning	Physical Function
Psychological/Spiritual	Physical Role Function
Social and Economic	Vitality
Family	Bodily Pain
Overall QOL	Mental Health
	Emotional Role Function
Functional Assessment of Cancer Therapy (FACT)[31,32]	Social Function
	General Health Perceptions
Physical Well-Being	**Spitzer Quality of Life Index (QL-Index)**[73]
Social/Family Well-Being	Health
Emotional Well-Being	Activity
Functional Well-Being	Daily Living
Overall QOL	Support (social)
	Outlook (psychological)
	Overall QOL

Note: All the instruments listed were developed for use with cancer populations, except for the SF-36, which was designed for the general population. Dimensions of core instruments only are listed: additional dimensions can be added to the EORTC QLQ-C30 and FACT through modules developed for specific cancers.

(MQOL) was developed for patients with advanced disease and so emphasizes meaning in life and existential concerns.[10]

Leplege and Hunt[11] stressed the importance of addressing the concerns of patients in measure-ment of HRQOL, and efforts have been made to capture these in various instruments. For example, both the Quality of Life Scale for Cancer (QOL-CA)[12,13] and the Ferrans and Powers Quality of Life Index (QLI)[14-16] were developed based on patient-oriented conceptual models. (The components of these models are listed in Table 2.1.) Both models were based on qualitative analysis of patients' perspectives of quality of life, and the models were validated with additional patient data. The City of Hope model[17] was based initially on information from cancer patients with pain,[12,18] and it was validated with data from patients with breast cancer, bone marrow transplantation, and cancer survivors.[13,19-21] The Ferrans model[15,22] was based initially on descriptions of the components of life that were important to dialysis patients.[14,22] It was then modified to include the concerns of cancer patients and validated using information from patients with breast cancer, sarcoma, bone marrow transplantation, and other chronic illnesses.[16,22-29] Other instruments also have been developed based directly on information provided by patients (e.g., CARES,[9] EORTC QLQ-C30,[8,30] FACT,[31,32] MQOL[10]).

In some situations a subset of domains may be used to assess outcomes. However, measurement of only one or two domains does not provide a comprehensive evaluation of HRQOL, and this distinction should be made clear in research reports to reduce confusion.[33] There are valid reasons for investigators to choose to measure a single dimension of HRQOL, particularly if it is expected to be differentially affected by an intervention. As shown by the review of Ganz and Goodwin[34] in this volume, in clinical trials of breast cancer, measures of symptom control (e.g., pain, fatigue, treatment toxicities, performance status, nausea) were the most useful in determining the effectiveness of pharmacologic agents, while psychosocial assessments were most valuable in trials of psychosocial interventions. Gotay[35] has pointed out that a number of the domains commonly included in HRQOL instruments are unlikely to be differentially affected by therapies in clinical trials, such as spiritual concerns or family functioning. On the other hand, aspects of life that are expected to be affected, such as sleep patterns or fatigue, may be measured inadequately by a single question or not measured at all. Because of this, Gotay[35] cautioned that some HRQOL instruments may not be sensitive enough to show

differences between treatments, which was seen in the review by Ganz and Goodwin.

It is critically important to choose instruments that are sufficiently sensitive to change, so that they can be used to show differences among treatments or to conclude with confidence that there are no differences. For this reason, the selection of instruments needs to be driven primarily by the purpose of the study. This means that no one instrument will be appropriate for all studies. Having said this, it also must be acknowledged that the use of different instruments makes it difficult to compare findings across studies. However, newer analytic techniques may provide a solution to this problem. Chang and Cella[36] demonstrated that Rasch analysis could be used to convert raw scores from different instruments to a common metric. They produced equivalent scores for five HRQOL measures (CARES, EORTC QLQ-C30, FACT, Spitzer QL-Index, and SF-36). In addition, the analysis showed variation in the strengths and weaknesses of the instruments, providing further support for the notion that it is unrealistic to expect one instrument to be appropriate for all studies.

Comprehensive assessment of HRQOL also has produced important unanticipated findings. For example, measurement of HRQOL has identified patients who may be at greater risk, over and above what would be expected based on their disease status alone. In a study of treatment for primary brain tumors, Weitzner et al.[37] found expected relationships, such as a poorer HRQOL for patients who had bilateral tumor involvement, poorer functional status, or more aggressive treatment. However, they also found that patients who were female, divorced, or unable to work were at greatest risk for poorer HRQOL while receiving treatment. HRQOL studies of survivors of Hodgkin's disease also produced unexpected findings. Although treatment for Hodgkin's disease does not commonly cause changes in appearance, 26% of long-term survivors felt they were less physically attractive because of their cancer, and this belief was associated with depression and decreased sexual activity.[38] Another Hodgkin's study[39] found that 22% of survivors

Table 2.2. Scope of HRQOL: Categories of Definitions

Quality of Life within the Purview of Health Care

Schipper *et al.*, 1996[40]

Quality of life in clinical medicine represents *the functional effect of an illness and its consequent therapy* upon a patient, as perceived by the patient.

Impact of Illness on Quality of Life

Cella, 1995[74]

HRQOL refers to the extent to which one's usual or expected physical, emotional, and social well-being *are affected by a medical condition or its treatment*.

Ebrahim, 1995[75]

HRQOL may be thought of as those aspects of self-perceived well-being that are *related to or affected by the presence of disease or treatment*.

Revicki *et al.*, 2000[76]

HRQOL is defined as the subjective assessment of *the impact of disease and its treatment* across the physical, psychological, social, and somatic domains of functioning and well-being.

Quality of Life during Illness

Osoba, 1994[33]

HRQOL is a multidimensional construct encompassing *perceptions of both positive and negative aspects of dimensions*, such as physical, emotional, social, and cognitive functions, as well as the negative aspects of somatic discomfort and other symptoms produced by a disease or its treatment.

Padilla *et al.*, 1996[77]

HRQOL is defined as a personal, evaluative statement summarizing *the positivity or negativity of attributes* that characterize one's psychological, physical, social, and spiritual well-being at a point in time when health, illness, and treatment conditions are relevant.

Note: Italics were added for this table. "Health related quality of life" has been abbreviated "HRQOL" for all definitions.

experienced psychological distress severe enough to meet the criterion suggested for psychiatric diagnosis. In addition, 39% still experienced conditioned nausea triggered by smells and sights associated with chemotherapy. They reported problems with sex life, employment, income, education, and denial of health and life insurance. Moreover, the problems identified in these two Hodgkin's disease studies had persisted for a substantial number of years after treatment (a median of 9 years and a mean of 6.3 years, respectively).

Definitions of HRQOL

Definitions of HRQOL can be classified into three groups based on their scope, ranging from the most narrow to the most broad. Examples of these are listed in Table 2.2. The question of scope in this case is not one of domains, but instead refers to the perspective taken in the definition. The first category

provides the most restricted view and limits HRQOL to things that are within the purview of physicians and the health care system, such as physical dysfunction, symptoms, mental health problems, and work-related disability. The health care system is concerned primarily with the correction of problems, and so this category is essentially negative in nature, focusing on dysfunction and its resolution. This delineation for HRQOL is found commonly in the literature, and the definition provided by Schipper *et al.*[40] is an excellent example for its focus on the functional effects of illness and treatment.

The second category focuses on the impact of illness and treatment on quality of life. This includes the typical concerns of health care providers, but also allows for consideration of the effects of disease on other aspects of life. For example, the financial impact of illness for the individual is of interest, rather than just the ability to work. Instead of focusing only on sexual functioning, the broader impact of illness on a marital relationship is of concern.

The effects of mastectomy include consideration of degradation of body image and self-concept, in addition to arm function and prevention of lymphedema. Worries about cancer recurrence also fall within this category. It should be noted that the definitions used as examples refer explicitly to well-being, which is a broader notion than functioning. The term "well-being" has a positive connotation; however, the focus is the impact of illness on well-being, which is primarily negative.

The third category is the most comprehensive in scope, in that it focuses on quality of life for the individual who has an illness. This broad perspective is consistent with the notion that illness can affect all aspects of life. However, in addition to the concerns of the two previous categories, it also explicitly extends the scope to positive aspects of life. For example, it may include improved relationships, changes in values and priorities, or increased faith in God, all of which have been reported to result from an experience with cancer and treatment.[23] It also includes existential concerns such as finding meaning in life and peace of mind, which are of particular importance at the end of life.

Definitions, like instruments, should be selected based on the fit with a study's purpose and population. For example, a definition for use in a clinical trial of two chemotherapeutic agents may be more narrow in scope, focusing on toxicity and interference with functioning. For a study whose focus is rehabilitation, a definition focusing on the impact of illness and treatment may be appropriate. For a study of hospice care, the broadest type of definition would provide a balance between physical comfort and existential concerns.

Objective conditions, perceived status, and evaluations

In the assessment of HRQOL there is yet a more fundamental issue to consider, one that concerns the nature of the information desired within the domains. The distinction is commonly made between objective and subjective indicators of quality of life. Subjective indicators rely on patient self-report, whereas objective indicators are directly measurable, such as blood pressure, hemoglobin levels, tumor size, income, or years of education. Occasionally, there is a mistaken notion that all patient-reported data are subjective, and all data reported by an outside observer are objective. However, it is the nature of the information, rather than who reports it, that is the distinguishing characteristic. Information concerning objective indicators can be reported by patients and still remain objective. Similarly, an outside observer can make subjective judgments about another individual. Items in HRQOL instruments occasionally may assess things that are directly observable, but more often they are neither directly observable nor measurable. For example, to assess nausea and vomiting, the number of emeses can be counted objectively, but the severity of nausea cannot. Moreover, experts[41] point out that even for vomiting, counting the number of emeses does not sufficiently characterize the experience, and used alone is inadequate for determining the effectiveness of antiemetics. Thus, most of the items in HRQOL instruments of necessity depend on subjective assessment.

Within the realm of subjective assessment, there are two types of information, both of which are provided by the patient: one concerns the perceived state (or status) of the components within the domains, and the other concerns the patient's personal evaluation of those components. An evaluation provides different information than perceived status and requires additional steps in cognitive processing. To provide an evaluation, a person first must think of the state of a particular aspect of life and then make a judgment about it, good or bad, satisfied or dissatisfied. This is different from the commonly made distinction between objective and subjective indicators of quality of life, in that both perceived status and evaluations are within the subjective arena of patient-reported outcomes.

Definitions of quality of life vary in their focus on objective conditions, perceived status, and evaluation. For example, in Table 2.2, the definition of Schipper et al. is concerned with perceived status,

Table 2.3. Perceived Status and Evaluation in Definitions of Quality of Life

Evaluation Definitions	
Calman, 1987[78]	Quality of life therefore measures the *difference, at a particular period of time, between the hopes and expectations* of the individual and the individual's present experience. It is concerned with the *difference between perceived goals and actual goals.*
Campbell *et al.*, 1976[44]	Quality of life is defined in terms of satisfaction of needs, and "level of satisfaction can be precisely defined as the *perceived discrepancy between aspiration and achievement*, ranging from the perception of fulfillment to that of deprivation."
Ferrans, 1990[15]	QOL is defined as a person's sense of well-being that stems from *satisfaction or dissatisfaction* with the areas of life that are important to him/her.
Felce and Perry, 1996[79]	Quality of life is defined as an overall general well-being that is comprised of *objective and subjective evaluations* of physical, material, social, and emotional well-being together with the extent of personal development and purposeful activity, all weighted by a personal set of values.
Frisch, 1993[52]	Life satisfaction is equated with quality of life and refers to a person's subjective *evaluation of the degree to which his or her most important needs, goals, and wishes have been fulfilled.*
Patrick and Erickson, 1993[80]	Health related quality of life is the *value assigned to duration of life* as modified by the impairments, functional states, perceptions and social opportunities that are influenced by disease, injury, treatment, or policy.
Perceived Status and Evaluation Definitions	
Gotay *et al.*, 1992[81]	Quality of life is a state of well-being which is a composite of two components: 1) the *ability to perform* everyday activities which reflect physical, psychological, and social well-being and 2) *patient satisfaction* with levels of functioning and the control of disease and/or treatment-related symptoms.
Roy, 1992[82]	The expression "quality of life" refers both to the *experiences that make life meaningful* and to the *conditions* that allow people to have such experiences.
World Health Organization, 1995[83]	Quality of life was defined, therefore, as *individuals' perception of their position in life* in the context of the culture and value systems in which they live and *in relation to their goals, expectations, standards, and concerns.*

Note: Italics were added for this table.

in that it focuses on the functional effect of illness and therapy as perceived by the patient. Examples of definitions that focus primarily on evaluation are found in Table 2.3. The definitions of Calman, Campbell *et al.* and Frisch are concerned with the degree to which expectations, goals, or aspirations have been fulfilled, and therefore explicitly refer to internal standards used for evaluation. Internal standards are implied in Ferrans' definition with its focus on satisfaction with aspects of life important to the individual. Patrick and Erickson's definition adds a dimension that focuses on the value assigned to the length of life, which clearly concerns a type of evaluation.

In addition, Table 2.3 presents definitions that can be characterized both in terms of perceived status and evaluation. Gotay *et al.* provide a balanced definition that focuses on subjective well-being in terms of the ability to perform everyday activities (perceived status) and patient satisfaction (evaluation).

Another example is provided in the World Health Organization's definition of quality of life, which differs from its definition of health cited earlier in this chapter. The definition focuses on both individuals' perceptions of their position in life (perceived status) and the correspondence with their standards, goals, and expectations (evaluation). Roy's definition is unique in its focus on experiences that make life meaningful, but also represents both categories. The determination of meaning in life is evaluative in nature. The conditions that allow people to have such experiences could be considered in terms of objective conditions or perceived status. However, the examples provided by Roy were freedom from pain and tormenting symptoms, which are subjective and thus would be characterized in terms of perceived status.

In HRQOL instruments, the wording of questions determines which type of information is obtained. For example, the question, "how much pain did you have," would elicit perceived pain status, whereas the question, "how satisfied are you with the amount of pain you have," (or stated another way, "how satisfied are you with the amount of pain relief you have") would elicit an evaluation. Both provide subjective information that requires a judgment regarding quantity (severity of pain); however, the second question also asks for a personal evaluation. Evaluations can be elicited in a variety of ways, such as asking how distressing something is, how bothered you are by it, whether it is sufficient, how much of a problem it is, or how happy you are with it.

Table 2.4 presents examples of HRQOL instruments that provide patient self-reported information. The table shows that there are differences among instruments in the type of information they elicit, even when they assess the same domains. Some instruments produce perceived status information only, such as the SF-36 and the EORTC QLQ-C30. Others produce evaluations only, such as the Ferrans and Powers Quality of Life Index (QLI) and the Quality-of-Life Scale for Cancer (QOL-CA). Some contain items that elicit both perceived status and evaluation information, such as the Functional Assessment of Cancer Therapy (FACT).

There are two major reasons why we need to be concerned about the nature of HRQOL and the type of information provided by instruments that measure it. First, as would be expected, scores differ depending on whether perceived status or evaluations are measured, which has been shown in studies that have used two HRQOL instruments with the same sample. For example, in patients with angina[42] or HIV,[43] scores were only moderately correlated between the SF-36 and QLI, even though they measured many of the same domains. Similarly, in patients with brain cancer,[37] only moderate correlations were found between scores for the FACT and the QLI.

The second reason is that the two types of subjective information are influenced by different factors, and these need to be considered when interpreting results. Campbell, Converse, and Rodgers published one of the earliest and most influential conceptual models that describes the relationships among objective conditions, perceived status, and evaluation in assessment of quality of life.[44] Their model begins with the objective characteristics of an attribute. The person's perception of the attribute does not necessarily represent the objective attribute as it actually is, but is distinct. This is because the individual's perception is influenced by personal characteristics, such as demographic characteristics, general optimism or pessimism, as well as other attributes of personality. Thus, the *perceived status* (our term) of an attribute provides a reflection of the objective attribute, albeit not a pure one. On the other hand, a person's *evaluation* of an attribute is dependent both on the perceived status of the attribute and on internal standards by which that perception is judged. Internal standards include personal values, expectation levels, aspiration levels, personal needs, and comparisons with others.

More recently, other conceptual models[35,45–48] have been published that highlight the complex nature of evaluation in quality-of-life assessment. On the whole, they are similar in nature to the model of Campbell *et al.*,[44] although some differences in terminology exist. The important point is that evaluations are influenced by many more factors than

Table 2.4. Measurement of Perceived Status and Evaluation in Quality of Life Instruments

Instrument	Physical Status	Physical Evaluation	Psychological Status	Psychological Evaluation	Social Status	Social Evaluation	Spiritual Status	Spiritual Evaluation
Cancer Rehabilitation Evaluation System (CARES) – Short Form[9]	X	X	X	X		X		
Quality-of-Life Scale for Cancer (QOL-CA)[12,13]		X		X		X		X
EORTC Quality of Life Questionnaire (EORTC QLQ-C30)[8,30]	X		X		X			
Quality-Adjusted Time Without Symptoms and Toxicity (Q-TWIST)[85]	X							
Functional Assessment of Cancer Therapy (FACT)[31,32]	X	X	X	X		X		
Functional Living Index-Cancer (FLIC)[68–70]	X	X	X	X	X	X		
Karnofsky Performance Status (KPS)[84]	X							
SF-36 Health Survey[71,72]	X		X		X			
Spitzer Quality of Life Index (QL-Index)[73]	X				X			
World Health Organization Quality of Life Assessment (WHOQOL)[83]	X	X	X	X	X	X	X	X
Quality of Life Inventory (QOLI)[52]		X		X		X		
Ferrans and Powers Quality of Life Index – Cancer Version (QLI)[14–16]		X		X		X		X
McGill Quality of Life Questionnaire (MQOL)[10]	X	X	X	X		X		X

• X's indicate that at least one item in a category is included in an instrument, and so do NOT indicate whether or not a domain is addressed adequately. X's do not indicate that a score is obtained for that domain.

• Generic or core instruments were examined. Different modules or versions may measure additional or different domains.

perceived status. Gotay[35] pointed out these factors are not typically the variables under study in therapeutic trials, which may make it difficult to detect differences in treatment arms on the basis of evaluation data. This could result in erroneous conclusions of no differences between groups. The problem of inadequate sensitivity in terms of selecting the domains to measure has already been noted above; however, the nature of the questions asked within the domains may compound the problem. These issues require focused study to clarify the differences in sensitivity between evaluation and perceived status information and the appropriate use for each.

A better understanding also is needed of the factors that influence evaluations. The majority of information about these variables is found in the literature focusing on subjective well-being (specifically life satisfaction and happiness) and its determinants, and substantial progress has been made in this area. Based on a review of research over the past 30 years, Diener *et al.*[49] concluded that the current challenge is to develop theories to explain the causal relationships among the factors that affect subjective well-being and to understand the processes underlying adaptation to events.

As a result of adaptation, the factors influencing evaluations potentially may change over time. Evaluations are based on internal standards and values, which are dynamic and can change in response to significant life events. These changes are referred to as "response shift" and can occur as a result of behavioral, cognitive, and affective processes necessary for accommodating to illness.[50] The implication for clinical trials and other longitudinal studies is the possibility that changes in patient evaluations, such as ratings of satisfaction or distress, may partially reflect changes in internal standards. Because of this potential for change (which may be confounding), evaluations should not be used alone to assess the effectiveness of treatment, but should be supplemented by other types of information.[35]

One way to deal with potential changes in internal standards is to measure them. This would make it possible to determine whether changes actually occurred and to account for them in the statistical analysis. Either preference-based measures or psychometric instruments could be used to measure values. Some preference-based measures directly ask patients to think of a particular state of health and then to value it in reference to perfect health. Examples are the standard gamble and the time-tradeoff techniques. (For a more complete discussion of utility/preference-based measures, see Chapter 4 by Feeny in this volume.[51]) Psychometric instruments provide an assessment of patient values in terms of individual aspects of life or domains. For example, the Quality of Life Inventory[52] and the Quality of Life Index[15] ask patients to rate the importance of individual aspects of life. Entire domains are rated in the FACT (original version)[31] and the Prostate Cancer Index[53] in terms of how much they affect patients' quality of life or bother them, respectively.

Nevertheless, there are several reasons to continue to pursue patients' evaluations of their quality of life. First, it is the incorporation of patients' values that sets quality of life assessment apart from measures of health status.[54] Quality of life in its essence is uniquely personal. It conveys the idea of a value judgment about a person's life. People use their own internal standards for what they consider a desirable or undesirable quality of life. In the final analysis, when determining the quality of life of an individual, that person's own judgment is the only one that is ethically justifiable. If one's values are not to be imposed on another, there is no substitute for personal appraisals of well-being.[55]

Second, personal evaluations provide an understanding of the impact of illness from the viewpoint of the patient, which are different from health status and physical functioning. These evaluations provide an important tool for understanding individual differences in response to illness. This includes individual changes that occur in the process of adapting to cancer and its treatment, including the re-evaluation of one's life in the context of a life-threatening disease.[56] Individuals can consider their quality of life to be good, even when faced with physical disabilities, as found in the studies by Covinsky *et al.*[57] and Patrick *et al.*[58]

Third, the ultimate objective for assessment of HRQOL is enhanced well-being, as pointed out recently by Barofsky.[59] (Also see Chapter 19 by David Osoba in this volume.[60]) Focusing on health problems, loss of abilities, or deficits in comparison to a normative ideal do not promote the positive objective of enhanced well-being.[59] This has been recognized in end-of-life and palliative care, when current health status measures tend to exhibit floor effects. Interventions instead are aimed at providing comfort and emotional support, to maximize quality of life at the end of life.

Causal models

The majority of conceptual models of HRQOL focus on the identification of domains and their components. However, relationships among domains

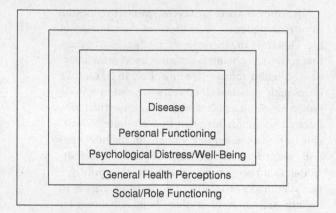

Figure 2.2. Framework for discussing disease and its impact. Used with permission: Ware, J. E., Jr. (1984). Conceptualizing disease impact and treatment outcomes. *Cancer* **53 Suppl**:2316–23.

in these models are usually not specified, other than to say there are mutual simultaneous interactions among them. In addition, the identification of domains does not necessarily make clear what exactly is of interest. For example, the term "physical domain" can refer to a wide range of variables, such as pathophysiological changes, symptoms, functional deficits, or perceived health status. The current challenge is to develop causal models that identify relationships among critical elements of HRQOL and the variables that are determinants of them. This is important because it will allow for the distinction between process and outcome variables.[61] Three models are presented below to examine the nature of the variables and the relationships among them, as well as studies that examine the proposed relationships.

A figure that has been widely cited as a characterization of HRQOL was published by Ware in 1984.[62] The figure is based on his four dimensions of health status: physiological status, personal (physical) functioning, mental health, and social well-being. The figure represents five categories of measures of these, which are presented as a series of nested boxes (Figure 2.2). Each box influences all the boxes outside of it. The center box refers to measurable physiologic parameters of disease. The second box, personal

functioning, refers to the performance of daily tasks related to self-care, mobility, and physical activity. The third box consists of psychological concepts that are affected by disease and treatment. Psychological distress refers to negative effects, such as depression or anxiety, and well-being refers to positive affect. The fourth box is the individual's evaluation of personal health, which requires consideration of the three preceding boxes. The final box is social/role functioning, which is the performance of usual activities related to employment, school, or homemaking.

The figure is referred to as a picture of health status and quality of life, but it is actually only meant to represent health status. Quality of life is described in the text as encompassing the dimensions of health status shown in the figure, as well as a broader set of concepts, such as housing, finances, and employment. The term "HRQOL" is not used by Ware in this article, but since the figure is called a framework for discussing disease and its impact, others have used the term subsequently in reference to the figure. In an evaluation of Ware's model, Bloom[56] considered it to be an acceptable characterization of health status, but thought it failed to provide a model for understanding the impact of illness. The reason was that it lacked the personal interpretation from the viewpoint of the patient.

Wilson and Cleary[63] developed a conceptual model of HRQOL that integrated patient perceptions more fully by including symptoms and overall quality of life, as well as values (Figure 2.3). Its purpose was to provide a taxonomy for measures of health outcomes. The arrows indicate the dominant causal associations. Reciprocal relationships are recognized to exist, but are not characterized in the figure. The model focuses on five levels of measures of patient outcomes. The first level, biological and physiological variables, includes traditional clinical variables, such as medical diagnoses, laboratory tests, and physical examinations. The second level is symptom status, which refers to physical, emotional, and cognitive symptoms perceived by the patient. The third level, functional status, includes four domains of functioning: physical,

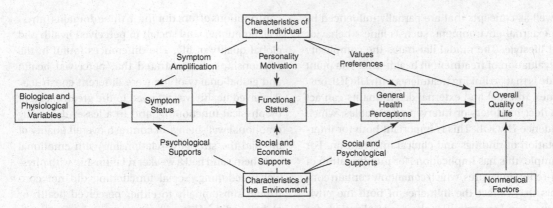

Figure 2.3. Relationships among measures of patient outcomes in a health-related quality of life conceptual model.
Used with permission: Wilson, I. B., Cleary, P. D. (1995). Linking clinical variables with health-related quality of life: a conceptual model of patient outcomes. *Journal of the American Medical Association* 273:59–65.

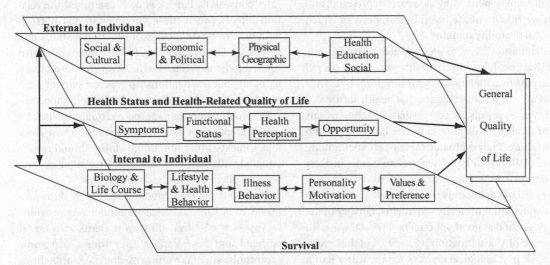

Figure 2.4. Relations among quality of life and health concepts.
Used with permission: Patrick, D. L., Chiang, Y. P. (2000). Measurement of health outcomes in treatment effectiveness evaluations: conceptual and methodological challenges. *Medical Care* 38 (Suppl. II):14–25.

social, role, and psychological function. General health perceptions, the fourth level, refers to a subjective rating that integrates all of the health concepts preceding it. The fifth level is overall quality of life, described as general measures of subjective well-being assessed by how happy or satisfied someone is with life as a whole. The values and preferences of patients are recognized as contributing to general health perceptions and overall quality of life.

Patrick and Chiang[64] recently published a model that incorporates these health concepts into quality of life in general (Figure 2.4). The model shows the complexity of linking clinical variables with health-related quality of life and then integrating them with the internal and external environments. External to the individual are aspects of the social and cultural environment. Internal to the individual are fixed traits such as genetic endowment and age, as well as concepts that are partially influenced by the external environment, such as illness behavior and lifestyle. The model illustrates the complexity of evaluation of treatment in health care. The point made is that, in linking treatments with HRQOL outcomes, internal and external determinants can act as effect modifiers or intervening variables, which influence HRQOL. This is important both for interpretation of findings and clinical intervention. For example, this has implications for interpretation of self-report measures, which commonly contain concepts that reflect the influence of both the environment and treatment. It also has implications for interventions, in that environmental modification, such as increased community participation or meaningful employment, may decrease depression and improve quality of life, even in situations in which physical disability remains.

Wilson and Cleary, as well as Patrick and Chiang, specifically address both health status and overall quality of life in their models. A recent study by Covinsky et al.[57] provides evidence that health status and quality of life are distinct constructs, and conclusions about quality of life should not be based on health status alone. They evaluated the concordance among global quality-of-life and health status scales in older patients (n = 493). They found that health status indicators did not accurately reflect overall quality of life for a substantial minority of patients. Quality of life was described as good or better by 43% of those with the worst physical functioning and 47% of those with the most psychological distress. On the other hand, quality of life was described as fair or poor for 15% of those who had the best physical functioning and 21% of those who had the least psychological distress. It should be noted that the findings also suggest that conclusions regarding the effectiveness of treatment may differ depending on whether outcomes are measured in terms of overall quality of life or health status.

A meta-analysis of 12 studies in chronic disease also provided evidence that patients considered perceived health and global quality of life to be two distinct constructs. Based on the meta-analysis, Smith et al.[65] developed path models to show the contributions of functioning in three domains (physical, emotional, and social) to perceived health and global quality of life. The differences found in the relationships demonstrated that perceived health and global quality of life were different constructs. Perceived health was affected to the greatest extent by physical functioning, and to a lesser degree by emotional well-being. In contrast, overall quality of life had the strongest relationship with emotional well-being and had a weaker relationship with physical functioning. Social functioning did not contribute substantially to either perceived health or global quality of life.

Another recent study provided evidence that functional status and perceived quality of life also are distinct constructs. Patrick et al.[58] examined the relationships between these variables in 454 persons with widely varying levels of functional status and disability. They found that lower functional status tended to be associated with lower perceived quality of life, but the relationship was not perfect. Self-rated health and depressive symptoms made substantial contributions to perceived quality of life that were independent of functional status. These findings indicated that functional status should not be equated with quality of life, and that other characteristics play a contributory role as well.

A test of the overall direction of relationships proposed in Wilson and Cleary's model was provided by Fayers et al.[66] In a study of patients with breast or head and neck cancer, they found that some symptoms, such as vomiting, diarrhea, and shortness of breath, were causal variables of overall quality of life, which was consistent with the Wilson and Cleary model. However, they found that other symptoms, such as weakness, tiredness, and feeling depressed, were not causal variables, but rather were indicators of overall quality of life. This meant that they were behaving as a reflection of quality of life, which conflicted with the dominant causal relationships proposed by Wilson and Cleary's model. Fayers and Hand[67] point out that symptoms in general tend to be causal variables, but they may sometimes shift to become indicator variables, as seen in this example. The findings of Fayers et al. indicate that, for this sample, the model should be revised to show some types of symptoms to be indicators of quality of life rather than as causal variables. These findings also have implications for HRQOL instruments, in that causal variables and indicator variables should not be aggregated together to produce a single score. This example illustrates (1) the complexity of relationships and the difficulty in characterizing clusters of variables under one rubric, such as symptoms; and (2) the need for testing proposed relationships with various groups of patients. It is likely that other samples, different types of cancer, or other illnesses would reveal other variations in relationships.

Conclusions and recommendations

The field of HRQOL has proceeded generally in an atheoretical manner, with little awareness of related progress in other fields. This chapter has presented some of the important work accomplished in the development of the construct. However, more research is needed to provide a better understanding of the causal relationships among critical elements of HRQOL (indicator variables) and the variables that are determinants of them (causal variables). The differences between health status and overall quality of life need to be made clear, along with the influence of other variables such as values and expectations and the role of adaptation. This complex task is essentially in its infancy. The majority of HRQOL models go no further than identifying domains, and thus provide insufficient guidance for research and clinical practice.

There are a number of well-established instruments available for assessment of HRQOL in cancer care. However, no single instrument is able to measure HRQOL adequately across the continuum of cancer care, nor is this a reasonable expectation. The characteristics of each instrument make it more or less appropriate for any particular study's purpose and population. A better understanding is needed of what HRQOL instruments measure and how this differentially affects outcomes. The domains of various instruments have been well characterized in the literature, but less attention has been paid to their conceptual approach. Both have implications for sensitivity, specificity, and interpretability of the instruments, and hence affect the outcomes they produce. Head-to-head comparisons of instruments within the same studies are needed to provide better empirical justification for the selection of instruments.

Studies comparing two HRQOL instruments have provided preliminary evidence to support the idea that scores differ depending on whether perceived status or evaluations are measured. The concern for clinical trials and other longitudinal studies is the possibility that changes in patient evaluations, such as ratings of distress, may partially reflect changes in internal standards, rather than the effect of the intervention. More research is needed to determine whether the distinction between perceived status and evaluation is important in clinical outcomes and, if so, what factors contribute to differences between them. In addition, the notion of response shift needs to be explored further to understand its effect, particularly in studies without random assignment to treatment groups.

Conceptual issues in HRQOL have pragmatic implications. There is a close interplay between theoretical work (development of conceptual models) and measurement of HRQOL: the two endeavors are part of the same process. Conceptual models provide the starting point for generation of instruments, as well as the template by which the final outcome is judged.

Acknowledgments

The author is grateful to Drs. Neil Aaronson, Ivan Barofsky, David Cella, David Feeny, David Osoba, and Donald Patrick for their thoughtful critique of the original draft of this chapter. The author also thanks Deborah Bruley, doctoral candidate, for her valuable help in preparing this manuscript, assisting in the literature review, and evaluation of the instruments.

REFERENCES

1 Johnson, J. R., Temple, R. (1985). Food and Drug Administration requirements for approval of new anticancer drugs. *Cancer Treatment Reports* **69**:1155–7.

2 National Cancer Institute (1988). *Clinical Trials Cooperative Group Program, Cancer Therapy Evaluation Program: Guidelines*. Bethesda, MD, Division of Cancer Treatment, National Cancer Institute, February 29, 1988. Cited in: Varricchio, C. (1990). Relevance of quality of life to clinical nursing practice. *Seminars in Oncology Nursing* **6**:255–9.

3 Osoba, D. (1992). The quality of life committee of the clinical trials group of the National Cancer Institute of Canada: Organization and functions. *Quality of Life Research* **1**: 211–8.

4 Spilker, B., Revicki, D. (1996). Taxonomy of quality of life. In *Quality of Life and Pharmacoeconomics in Clinical Trials* (2nd Edition), ed. B. Spilker, pp. 25–31. Philadelphia, PA: Lippincott-Raven Publishers.

5 Guyatt, G. H., Feeny, D. H., Patrick, D. L. (1993). Measuring health-related quality of life. *Annals of Internal Medicine* **118**:622–8.

6 World Health Organization (1958). *The First Ten Years of the World Health Organization*. Geneva: World Health Organization.

7 Spilker, B. (1996). Introduction. In *Quality of Life and Pharmacoeconomics in Clinical Trials* (2nd Edition), ed. B. Spilker, pp. 1–10. Philadelphia, PA: Lippincott-Raven Publishers.

8 Aaronson, N., Ahmedzai, S., Bergman, B. *et al.* (1993). The European Organization for Research and Treatment of Cancer QLQ-C30: A quality of life instrument for use in international clinical trials in oncology. *Journal of the National Cancer Institute* **85**:365–76.

9 Shag, C., Ganz, P. A., Heinrich, R. (1991). Cancer Rehabilitation Evaluation System – Short Form (CARES-SF). *Cancer* **68**:1406–13.

10 Cohen, S., Mount, B., Strobel, M. *et al.* (1995). The McGill Quality of Life Questionnaire: A measure of quality of life appropriate for people with advanced disease. *Palliative Medicine* **9**:207–19.

11 Leplege, A., Hunt, S. (1997). The problem of quality of life in medicine. *Journal of the American Medical Association* **278**:47–50.

12 Padilla, G., Ferrell, B., Grant, M. *et al.* (1990). Defining the content domain of quality of life for cancer patients with pain. *Cancer Nursing* **13**:108–15.

13 Grant, M., Ferrell, B., Schmidt, G. *et al.* (1992). Measurement of quality of life in bone marrow transplantation survivors. *Quality of Life Research* **1**:375–84.

14 Ferrans, C., Powers, M. (1985). Quality of Life Index: development and psychometric properties. *Advances in Nursing Science* **8**:15–24.

15 Ferrans, C. E. (1990). Development of a quality of life index for patients with cancer. *Oncology Nursing Forum* **17**:15–19.

16 Ferrans, C., Powers, M. (1992). Psychometric assessment of the Quality of Life Index. *Research in Nursing and Health* **15**:29–38.

17 Ferrell, B. R. (1996). The quality of lives: 1,525 voices of cancer. *Oncology Nursing Forum* **26**:907–16.

18 Ferrell, B., Wisdom, C., Wenzl, C. (1989). QOL as an outcome variable in the management of cancer pain. *Cancer* **63**:2321–7.

19 Ferrell, B., Grant, M., Padilla, G. (1991). Experience of pain and perceptions of quality of life: Validation of a conceptual model. *Hospice Journal* **7**:9–24.

20 Ferrell, B., Grant, M., Schmidt, G. *et al.* (1992). The meaning of quality of life for bone marrow transplant survivors. Part 1: The impact of bone marrow transplant on QOL. *Cancer Nursing* **15**:153–60.

21 Ferrell, B., Dow, K., Leigh, S. *et al.* (1995). Quality of life in long term cancer survivors. *Oncology Nursing Forum* **22**:915–22.

22 Ferrans, C. (1996). Development of a conceptual model of quality of life. *Scholarly Inquiry for Nursing Practice: An International Journal* **10**:293–304.

23 Ferrans, C. (1994). Quality of life through the eyes of survivors of breast cancer. *Oncology Nursing Forum* **21**: 1645–51.

24 Ferrans, C., Powers, M. (1993). Quality of life of hemodialysis patients. *American Nephrology Nurses Association Journal* **20**:575–81.

25 Ferrans, C., Cohen, F., Smith, K. (1992). Quality of life of persons with narcolepsy. *Grief, Loss, and Care* **5**:23–32.

26 Warnecke, R., Ferrans, C., Johnson, T. *et al.* (1996). Measuring quality of life in culturally diverse populations. *Journal of the National Cancer Institute Monographs* **20**:29–38.

27 Anderson, J., Ferrans, C. (1997). The quality of life of persons with chronic fatigue syndrome. *Journal of Nervous and Mental Disease* **106**:359–67.

28 Arzouman, J., Dudas, S., Ferrans, C. *et al.* (1991). Quality of life of patients with sarcoma post-chemotherapy. *Oncology Nursing Forum* **18**:889–94.

29 Belec, R. (1992). Quality of life: Perceptions of long-term survivors of bone marrow transplantation. *Oncology Nursing Forum* **19**:31–7.

30 Aaronson, N. K., Cull, A. M., Kaasa, S. *et al.* (1996). The European Organization for Research and Treatment of Cancer (EORTC) modular approach for quality of life assessment

in oncology: An update. In *Quality of Life and Pharmacoeconomics in Clinical Trials* (2nd Edition), ed. B. Spilker, pp. 179–89. Philadelphia: Lippincott-Raven.

31 Cella, D., Tulsky, D., Gray, G. *et al.* (1993). The Functional Assessment of Cancer Therapy (FACT) Scale: Development and validation of the general version. *Journal of Clinical Oncology* **11**:570–9.

32 Cella, D., Bonomi, A., Lloyd, S. *et al.* (1995). Reliability and validity of the Functional Assessment of Cancer Therapy-Lung (FACT-L) quality of life instrument. *Lung Cancer* **12**:199–220.

33 Osoba, D. (1994). Lessons learned from measuring health-related quality of life in oncology. *Journal of Clinical Oncology* **12**:608–16.

34 Ganz, Goodwin, this volume, Chapter 5.

35 Gotay, C. C. (1996). Trial-related quality of life: using quality-of-life assessment to distinguish among cancer therapies. *Journal of the National Cancer Institute Monographs* **20**: 1–6.

36 Chang, C., Cella, D. (1997). Equating health-related quality of life instruments in applied oncology settings. *Physical Medicine and Rehabilitation* **11**:397–406.

37 Weitzner, M., Meyers, C., Byrne, K. (1996). Psychosocial functioning and quality of life in patients with primary brain tumors. *Journal of Neurosurgery* **84**:29–34.

38 Fobair, P., Hoppe, R. T., Bloom, J. *et al.* (1986). Psychosocial problems among survivors of Hodgkin's disease. *Journal of Clinical Oncology* **4**:805–14.

39 Kornblith, A. B., Anderson, J., Cella, D. F. *et al.* (1992). Hodgkin's disease survivors at increased risk for problems in psychosocial adaptation. *Cancer* **70**:2214–24.

40 Schipper, H., Clinch, J., Olweny, C. (1996). Quality of life studies: Definitions and conceptual issues. In *Quality of Life and Pharmacoeconomics in Clinical Trials* (2nd Edition), ed. B. Spilker, pp. 11–23. Philadelphia, PA: Lippincott-Raven Publishers.

41 Rhodes, V. A., McDaniel, R. W. (1997). Measuring nausea, vomiting, and retching. In *Instruments for Clinical Health-Care Research*, ed. M. Frank-Stromborg and S. J. Olsen, pp. 509–18. Sudbury, MA: Jones and Bartlett.

42 Dougherty, C., Dewhurst, T., Nichol, P. *et al.* (1998). Comparison of three quality of life instruments in stable angina pectoris: Seattle Angina Questionnaire, Short Form Health Survey (SF-36), and Quality of Life Index – Cardiac Version III. *Journal of Clinical Epidemiology* **51**:569–75.

43 Schlenk, E., Erlen, J., Dunbar-Jacob, J. *et al.* (1998). Health-related quality of life in chronic disorders: a comparison across studies using the MOS SF-36. *Quality of Life Research* **7**:57–65.

44 Campbell, A., Converse, P. E., Rodgers, W. L. (1976). *The Quality of American Life: Perceptions, Evaluations, and Satisfactions.* New York: Russell Sage.

45 Day, H. and Jankey, S. G. (1996). Lessons from the literature: toward a holistic model of quality of life. In *Quality of Life in Health Promotion and Rehabilitation: Conceptual Approaches, Issues, and Applications*, pp. 39–50. Thousand Oaks, CA: Sage.

46 Frisch, M. B. (1998). Quality of life therapy and assessment in health care. *Clinical Psychology Science and Practice* **5**: 19–40.

47 Selby, P. (1993). Measurement of quality of life in cancer patients. *Journal of Pharmacy & Pharmacology* **45** (Suppl. 1):384–6.

48 Zissi, A., Barry, M. M., Cochrane, R. A. (1998). A mediational model of quality of life for individuals with severe mental health problems. *Psychological Medicine* **28**:1221–30.

49 Diener, E., Suh, E. M., Lucas, R. E. *et al.* (1999). Subjective well-being: three decades of progress. *Psychological Bulletin* **125**:276–302.

50 Sprangers, M. A. G., Schwartz, C. E. (1999). Integrating response shift into health-related quality of life research: a theoretical model. *Social Science and Medicine* **48**: 1507–15.

51 Feeny, this volume, Chapter 4.

52 Frisch, M. B. (1993). The Quality of Life Inventory: a cognitive-behavioral tool for complete problem assessment, treatment planning, and outcome evaluation. *Behavior Therapy* **16**:42–4.

53 Litwin, M. (1994). Measuring health related quality of life in men with prostate cancer. *Journal of Urology* **152**:1882–7.

54 Gill, T., Feinstein, A. (1994). A critical appraisal of the quality of quality-of-life measurements. *Journal of the American Medical Association* **272**:619–26.

55 Felce, D., Perry, J. (1995). Quality of life: its definition and measurement. *Research in Developmental Disabilities* **16**:51–74.

56 Bloom, J. R. (1984). Response to J. E. Ware, Jr., Conceptualizing disease impact and treatment outcomes. *Cancer* **53** (Suppl.):2323–6.

57 Covinsky, K. E., Wu, A. W., Landefeld, S. *et al.* (1999). Health status versus quality of life in older patients: does the distinction matter? *American Journal of Medicine* **106**:435–40.

58 Patrick, D. L., Kinne, S., Engleberg, R. A. *et al.* (2000). Functional status and perceived quality of life in adults with and without chronic conditions. *Journal of Clinical Epidemiology* **53**:779–85.

59 Barofsky, I. (2003). Patient's rights, quality of life, and health care system performance. *Quality of Life Research* **12**:473–84.

60 Osoba, this volume, Chapter 19.

61 Barofsky, I. (1996). Cancer: psychosocial aspects. In *Quality of Life and Pharmacoeconomics in Clinical Trials* (2nd Edition), ed. B. Spilker, pp. 993–1002. Philadelphia, PA: Lippincott-Raven.

62 Ware, J. E., Jr. (1984). Conceptualizing disease impact and treatment outcomes. *Cancer* 53 (Suppl.):2316–23.

63 Wilson, I. B., Cleary, P. D. (1995). Linking clinical variables with health-related quality of life: a conceptual model of patient outcomes. *Journal of the American Medical Association* 273:59–65.

64 Patrick, D. L., Chiang, Y. P. (2000). Measurement of health outcomes in treatment effectiveness evaluations: conceptual and methodological challenges. *Medical Care* 38 (Suppl. II):14–25.

65 Smith, K. W., Avid, N. E., Assmann, S. F. (1999). Distinguishing between quality of life and health status in quality of life research: a meta-analysis. *Quality of Life Research* 8:447–59.

66 Fayers, P. M., Hand, D. J., Bjordal, K. *et al.* (1997). Causal indicators in quality of life research. *Quality of Life Research* 6:393–406.

67 Fayers, P. M., Hand, D. J. (2002). Causal variables, indicator variables, and measurement scales: an example from quality of life. *Journal of the Royal Statistical Society* 165 (Part 2):1–21.

68 Schipper, H., Clinch, J., McMurray, A. *et al.* (1984). Measuring the quality of life of cancer patients: the Functional Living Index – Cancer: Development and validation. *Journal of Clinical Oncology* 2:472–83.

69 Morrow, G., Lindke, J., Black, P. *et al.* (1992). Measurement of quality of life in patients: psychometric analysis of the Functional Living Index-Cancer (FLIC). *Quality of Life Research* 1:287–96.

70 Clinch, J. (1996). The Functional Living Index-Cancer: ten years later. In *Quality of Life and Pharmacoeconomics in Clinical Trials* (2nd Edition), ed. B. Spilker, pp. 215–25. Philadelphia, PA: Lippincott-Raven Publishers.

71 Ware, J. E., Jr., Sherbourne, C. D. (1992). The MOS 36-item short-form health survey (SF-36). *Medical Care* 30:473–83.

72 Stewart, A. L., Hays, R. D., Ware, J. E. (1988). The MOS short-form general health survey. *Medical Care* 26:724–35.

73 Spitzer, W., Dobson, A., Hall, J. *et al.* (1981). Measuring the quality of life of cancer patients: a concise QL-Index for use by physicians. *Journal of Chronic Disease* 34:585–97.

74 Cella, D. (1995). Measuring quality of life in palliative care. *Seminars in Oncology* 22:73–81.

75 Ebrahim, S. (1995). Clinical and public health perspectives and applications of health-related quality of life measurement. *Social Science and Medicine* 41:1383–94.

76 Revicki, D., Osoba, D., Fairclough, D. *et al.* (2000). Recommendations on health-related quality of life research to support labeling and promotional claims in the United States. *Quality of Life Research* 9:887–900.

77 Padilla, G. V., Grant, M. M., Ferrell, B. R. *et al.* (1996). Quality of Life – Cancer. In *Quality of Life and Pharmacoeconomics in Clinical Trials* (2nd Edition), ed. B. Spilker, pp. 301–8. Philadelphia, PA: Lippincott-Raven.

78 Calman, K. C. (1987). Definitions and dimensions of quality of life. In *The Quality of Life of Cancer Patients*, ed. N. K. Aaronson and J. H. Beckmann, pp. 1–9. New York: Raven Press.

79 Felce, D., Perry, J. (1996). *Quality of Life in Health Promotion and Rehabilitation: Conceptual Approaches, Issues, and Applications*. Thousand Oaks, CA: Sage.

80 Patrick, D. L., Erickson, P. (1993). *Health Status and Health Policy: Allocating Resources to Health Care*. Oxford: Oxford University Press.

81 Gotay, C., Korn, E., McCabe, M. *et al.* (1992). Quality-of-life assessment in cancer treatment protocols: Research issues in protocol development. *Journal of the National Cancer Institute* 84:575–9.

82 Roy, D. J. (1992). Measurement in the service of compassion. *Journal of Palliative Care* 8:3–4.

83 World Health Organization (1995). The World Health Organization Quality of Life Assessment (WHOQOL): Position paper from the World Health Organization. *Social Science and Medicine* 41:1403–9.

84 Karnofsky, D., Abelman, W., Craver, L. F. *et al.* (1948). The use of nitrogen mustards in the palliative treatment of carcinoma with particular reference to bronchogenic carcinoma. *Cancer* 1:634–56.

85 Gelber, R., Goldhirsch, A., Cavelli, F. (1991). Quality-of-life-adjusted evaluation of adjuvant therapies for operable breast cancer. *Annals of Internal Medicine* 114:621–8.

3

Assessing health status and quality of life of cancer patients: the use of general instruments

Pennifer Erickson, Ph.D.

Pennsylvania State University, State College, PA

Introduction

In response to the increasing demand for high quality, affordable health care, policy makers are beginning to consider the burden of disease on patients and their families, as well as on society, more generally.[1-4] Within the continuum of cancer care, these concerns are often expressed in terms of health promotion and disease prevention initiatives, evaluations of alternative treatments or other interventions, and provision of compassionate care for survivors of cancer or those living with terminal illness.[5] Traditionally, morbidity and mortality measures have been used for assessing disease and policy impacts, but as more people are living longer, many with chronic disease such as cancer, decision makers are recognizing the need for indicators that inform them not only about quantity of life but also about multiple aspects of quality of life such as physical, social, and mental well-being.[6]

Over the past 30 years, instruments have been developed that provide decision makers with profiles of scores that indicate people's capacity or performance on important domains and subdomains of health status and quality of life. Profiles, rather than a battery of single indicators, have the advantage of using a single scoring system so that domain scores can be easily compared, thereby giving clinicians and policy makers systematic information about well-being and function across the key domains. Generic profiles, such as the Sickness Impact Profile[7-8] and the short forms from the Medical Outcomes Study,[9-11] are used in demographically and diagnostically diverse populations, whereas general cancer measures, e.g., the European Organization for Research and Treatment of Cancer Core Quality of Life Questionnaire (EORTC QLQ-C30)[12] and the Functional Assessment of Cancer Therapy (FACT-G),[13] have been developed for use across the spectrum of cancer diagnoses. In addition to allowing comparisons across groups defined by socioeconomic or disease status, the general content of both generic and general cancer profiles facilitates comparison across a range of applications that comprise the continuum of cancer care. For example, instruments that are applicable to patients with various types of cancer have been used to evaluate treatments (e.g., palliative care) or to describe the relative burden of cancer across patients with different diagnoses.[14-17]

This chapter reviews generic and general cancer measures that have been used to assess health-related quality of life of persons with cancer, regardless of site or stage of disease. Results from the conceptual and methodological stages of each instrument's development, and its subsequent applications, give important evidence on the instrument's performance in diverse study settings. This chapter summarizes the published evidence for evaluating the state of the art of instrument usage and for guiding the development of agendas for research, policy, and applications development.

Methods

Generic profiles and general cancer instruments, as well as the literature that documents their development and use within the cancer care continuum, were identified using OLGA, The On-Line Guide to Quality-of-Life Assessment.[18] We have selected instruments that contain multiple domains and use a psychometrically rather than a utility-based scoring system; utility measures are discussed in Chapter 4 by Feeny in this volume.[19] By "instrument," we mean a questionnaire or rating scale that has a well-defined format, set of administration procedures and scoring algorithms, and documentation that supports the instrument development and guides the interpretation of results.[20]

The discussion of each instrument is organized by the developmental and post-developmental stages in its life cycle.[21] The former encompasses the conceptual and measurement properties that are essential for developing an instrument for a given application. These properties specify theoretical foundations and assumptions, as well as reliability, validity, and responsiveness, that are essential for interpreting results obtained from an instrument's use. In the post-development stage, investigators other than the developers may conduct studies specifically to assess measurement properties of an instrument. More commonly, however, instruments are used in diverse studies, whether defined by research design, target population, or both. These applications provide additional information on an instrument's performance, especially its construct validity. Articles that address cultural adaptation are discussed in Chapter 20 by Aaronson in this volume.[22]

In the review of post-development studies involving cancer patients, articles were included when an instrument was used without modification, thereby making comparisons between post-developmental studies meaningful and also allowing findings from developmental and post-developmental studies to be compared. OLGA allows for a comprehensive survey of the use of these instruments; however, references cited in this chapter were selected based on recency of publication and relevance of topic and do not include the full range of each instrument's applications.

Generic measures

By definition, generic instruments are developed for use in various populations to assess important core domains and subdomains of function and well-being. Of the multidimensional, generic profile-type measures developed for use with persons 18 years of age and older, five that have been commonly used with cancer patients are reviewed below: Hospital and Anxiety Depression Scale (HAD Scale); Medical Outcomes Study Short Form 36 (SF-36); Profile of Mood States (POMS); Quality of Life Index (QL Index); and Sickness Impact Profile (SIP). Table 3.1 includes more detailed information on each measurement instrument. Table 3.1 also includes descriptions of the Nottingham Health Profile (NHP) and Quality of Life Index (QLI), which are not reviewed comprehensively due to lack of extensive use with cancer patients.

Hospital Anxiety and Depression Scale

Conceptual, practical, and measurement features

The HAD Scale (the abbreviation recommended by its developers) was developed as a brief, patient self-report instrument to assess the two most common aspects of neurosis seen in non-psychiatric hospital departments.[23-24] The depression items were based on states that were known to respond to treatment with antidepressant medication, whereas items in the anxiety subscale were based on a review of selected instruments and the investigators' research experiences. The HAD Scale consists of brief statements that describe feelings such as the following: "I feel cheerful," "I feel as if I am slowed down," and "I get sudden feelings of panic." The HAD Scale's structure and measurement properties are more fully described in Table 3.1.

The scale, originally developed in the United Kingdom, was translated into several European and non-European languages to facilitate its widespread use in hospital and clinic populations. Its availability in several languages and the brief time it takes to administer has made this a popular instrument, leading to its recommended use in cancer clinical trials sponsored by the British Medical Research Council.[25]

Performance across the cancer continuum

Of the empirical studies documenting use of the HAD Scale, approximately one-third involve patients with cancer, with several studies from the post-development stage which were explicitly designed to validate this scale in cancer patients; these findings are summarized in Table 3.1.

The HAD Scale has been used across all stages of the cancer continuum. Most uses, however, report on randomized clinical trials that assess the effectiveness of alternative chemotherapies for a range of cancer diagnoses.[26–33] As examples of its ability to detect change, depression scores were found to improve after treatment in patients with colorectal and ovarian cancer,[30,33] and anxiety scores improved for the colorectal cancer patients.[33] In addition, change from baseline differed according to degree of toxicity.[34] In studies using radiotherapy for head and neck and lung cancer,[35–37] the scale showed no change over the course of treatment. Improvement in levels of both anxiety and depression was observed in a study of the effective dose of radiotherapy for painful bone metastases,[38] and levels of both anxiety and depression also improved in patients with lymphoma who participated in a trial to examine the effectiveness of stem cell transplantation.[39]

In about 5% of the reports, the HAD Scale was used to examine relationships between anxiety and depression and issues important to cancer survivors. For example, Loge et al.[40] studied fatigue in Hodgkin's disease survivors, finding that approximately 50% of the survivors had levels of distress that might benefit from treatment. Others have examined the psychological impact of cancer survivorship

and its treatment.[41–43] Similar types of studies have looked at anxiety and depression in breast, lung, and ovarian cancer patients at the end of life.[29,44–46] The HAD Scale has also been used to assess reactions to screening programs targeted at identifying and preventing disease in persons at high risk for developing breast and prostate cancer and melanoma.[47–49] The widespread use of the HAD Scale is attributed to its ease of use, general acceptance by patients, and ability to detect change in affective well-being that may occur due to a disease or its treatment.[23]

Medical Outcomes Study Short Form 36

Conceptual, practical, and measurement features

The SF-36 was derived primarily from longer questionnaires that were included in a general population study of the health impact of alternative health insurance plans.[50] Data from the original battery of measures fielded in the follow-on study, the Medical Outcomes Study (MOS),[51] were reanalyzed to form shortened versions consisting of 18, 20, and 36 items.[9,52] Subsequently, a 12-item version has been developed.[11] This chapter reviews the 36-item version since it is viewed by the developers as representing a suitable trade-off between breadth and depth of coverage.[53] Sample items from the SF-36 Mental Health subscale are: "Have you been a very nervous person?" and "Have you felt downhearted and blue?" More detailed information on the format and measurement properties of the SF-36 is given in Table 3.1.

The SF-36 is the most widely used of the five generic measures reviewed here, with over 50% of health outcomes applications, regardless of diagnosis, using the SF-36. However, of the empirical studies documenting use of the SF-36, less than 10% involve cancer patients.

Performance across the cancer continuum

Within the cancer literature, the SF-36 is used in about 25% of the reports in which at least one of the five generic measures is used, making it second

Table 3.1. Generic measures: supporting data on psychometrics and validation

Instrument name:	Hospital Anxiety and Depression Scale (HAD Scale)	Profile of Mood States (POMS)	Medical Outcomes Study Short Form-36 (SF-36)	Quality of Life Index (QL Index)	Sickness Impact Profile (SIP)	Nottingham Health Profile (NHP)	Quality of Life Index (Ferrans)
Purpose for which developed	To detect depression and anxiety in the hospital outpatient clinic setting	To assess mood states and mood changes associated with psychotherapeutic interventions in research and clinical evaluation	To express health outcomes from a wide range of interventions on a common scale, for purposes of managing patient care, evaluating health services, and monitoring population health	To assess health outcomes in persons with chronic disease	To assess health outcomes from a wide range of interventions on a common scale	To assess health problems in an adult general population	To assess quality of life in healthy persons, as well as those with illness
Length	14 items. Time frame: past week	65 items. Time frame: one week	36 items. Time frame: one week for acute version; one month for chronic version	5 items. Time frame: past week	136 items. Time frame: "today"	45 items in 2 parts that may be administered separately. Part 1, 38 items; Part 2, 7 items. Time frame: present time	64 items. Time frame: "present time"
Administration time	2–3 minutes	Cited variously as 3–5, 5–7 minutes in healthy people; up to 20 minutes for physically ill	5–10 minutes	1 minute on average	20–30 minutes	5–15 minutes	8–10 minutes

	Depression	Tension-Anxiety	Physical Functioning	Activities of Daily Living	Alertness Behavior	Part I. Emotional	General
Domains included	Depression (7 items); Anxiety (7 items). Response options represent frequency	Tension-Anxiety (9 items); Depression-Dejection (15 items); Anger-Hostility (12 items); Vigor-Activity (8 items); Fatigue-Inertia (7 items); Confusion-Bewilderment (7 items). Response options: not at all, a little, moderately, quite a bit, and extremely	Physical Functioning (10 items); Role-Physical (4 items); Bodily Pain (2 items); General Health (5 items); Vitality (4 items); Social Functioning (2 items); Role-Emotional (3 items); Mental Health (5 items); Health Change (1 item). Response options vary according to domain	Activities of Daily Living (1 item); Health Perceptions (1 item); Outlook on Life (1 item); Physical Activity (1 item); Social Support (1 item). Response options vary depending on the domain	Alertness Behavior (10 items); Ambulation (12 items); Body Care and Movement (23 items); Communication (9 items); Eating (9 items); Emotional Behavior (9 items); Home Management (10 items); Mobility (10 items); Recreation and Pastimes (8 items); Sleep and Rest (7 items); Social Interaction (20 items); Work (9 items). Response option: item is checked off if applicable	Part I. Emotional Reactions (9 items); Energy Level (3 items), Physical Mobility (8 items), Pain (8 items), Sleep (5 items), and Social Isolation (5 items). Part II. Problems in Daily Life (7 items)	General Satisfaction, Family Relations, Health and Functioning, Psychological and Spiritual Well-Being, Social Well-Being, and Economic Well-Being
Scoring	0–3 scale. Item scores are summed to form subscale scores that range from 0–21. Higher scores indicate more dysfunction	Item scores range from 0–4. Scores are summed to form subscale scores that range from 0–60, depending on number of items. Total Mood Disturbance score = sum of subscale scores. Higher scores more mood disturbance	Item scores are summed to form subscale scores that range from 0–100, with higher scores indicating less dysfunction. Subscales are used to form Physical and Mental Component scores. No overall score. Scoring algorithms are available from RAND (www.rand.org) and QualityMetric, Inc. (www.sf-36.com). Ware scoring forces physical and mental summary scales to be uncorrelated; RAND scoring allows them to correlate	3-point categorical scaling, with item scores ranging from 0–2. Item scores are summed to form an overall score that ranges from 0–10. Higher scores indicate less dysfunction	Item weights are summed and divided by the sum of weights and transformed to 0–100% scale to form subscale, Physical and Psychosocial dimension and overall scores. Lower scores indicate less dysfunction	Item weights are summed and divided by the sum of weights and transformed to 0–100% scale to form subscale scores	Item scores are adjusted to center the score around 0, and then summed. To avoid negative scores, all scores are increased by 15. Overall scores range from 0 to 30. Higher scores indicate less dysfunction. Computer scoring is available

(cont.)

Table 3.1. (*cont.*)

Developmental Evidence:

Instrument name:	Hospital Anxiety and Depression Scale (HAD Scale)	Profile of Mood States (POMS)	Medical Outcomes Study Short Form-36 (SF-36)	Quality of Life Index (QL Index)	Sickness Impact Profile (SIP)	Nottingham Health Profile (NHP)	Quality of Life Index (Ferrans)
Validated modes of administration	Self-administered	Self-administered	Self-administered, in person or telephone interview, computer administration	Rating by health professional and self-administered	Self- and interviewer-administered	Self- and interviewer-administered	Self- and interviewer-administered
Validated translations/ cultural adaptations	English (UK), Arabic, Chinese, Danish, Dutch, Finnish, French, German, Hebrew, Icelandic, Italian, Japanese, Norwegian, Portuguese, Spanish, Swedish, Thai, Turkish, Urdu	English (US), Africanni, Bulgarian, Chinese, Croatian, Dutch, Finnish, French, German, Greek, Haitian Creole, Italian, Japanese, Korean, Polish, Russian, Spanish, Swedish	English (US), Afrikaans, Bengali, Bulgarian, Chinese (China, Hong Kong, Singapore, Taiwan, United States), Croatian, Czech, Danish, Dutch (Belgium & The Netherlands), Estonian, Finnish, French (Belgium, Canada, France), Greek, German, English (Australia/New Zealand, Canada, United Kingdom) Hebrew, Hungarian, Icelandic, Indonesian, Italian, Japanese, Kiswahili, Korean, Norwegian, Polish, Portuguese (Brazil & Portugal), Romanian, Russian, Slovack, Spanish (Argentina, Columbia, Mexico, Spain, United States), Swedish, Turkish, US Japanese, US Vietnamese, Welsh, Yugoslavian	English, Dutch, French, French-Canadian, German, Hebrew, Italian, Spanish, Thai	English (US), Arabic, Chinese, Danish, Dutch, English (UK), Finnish, Flemish, French, German, Italian, Norwegian, Portuguese, Russian, Spanish, Swedish, Tamil, Thai, Turkish	English (UK), Arabic, Danish, Dutch, English (US), Finnish, French, German, Italian, Japanese, Norwegian, Portuguese, Spanish, Swedish	English (US), Chinese, French, Hungarian, Japanese, Korean, Norwegian, Polish, Portuguese, Romanian, Russian, Spanish, Swedish, Thai

Evidence of reliability (internal consistency, test-retest, other)							
Internal consistency was assessed in a sample of 50 general medical outpatients who were 16–65 years of age. Intra-class correlation for anxiety items = 0.41–0.76; for depression = 0.30–0.60. These findings were replicated in a second sample of 50 patients.[24]	Internal consistency: (1) ranged from 0.87–0.95 for the six subscales in a group of 350 male psychiatric outpatients; (2) ranged from 0.84–0.95 in a group of 650 female psychiatric outpatients. For both groups the lowest coefficients were obtained on the Confusion-Bewilderment concept and the highest on the Depression-Dejection concept. Test-retest: ranged from 0.65–0.74 between evaluation and first therapy session (median 20 days) in 100 patients undergoing psychiatric treatment; finding treatment probably associated with change in emotional states. In another study of 150 outpatients, test-retest coefficients ranged from 0.61–0.69.	Internal consistency: assessed in a general population (n=1692) Cronbach's alpha ranged from 0.63–0.94. Also assessed in a sample of 3445 persons with at least 1 chronic disease; Cronbach's alpha ranged from 0.78–0.93. Test-retest reliability exceeds 0.80. An extensive bibliography is available at www.sf-36.com.	Internal consistency: assessed in a sample of 91 patients; Cronbach's alpha was 0.78.[92] Interrater: assessed in a sample of 64 patients by two physicians who rated patients independently within 7 days; correlation between the 2 ratings was 0.81. Correlation of agreement for the English version was 0.84; for the French version, the coefficient was 0.74.[92]	Internal consistency: assessed in a sample of 307 outpatients; using self-administered version, Cronbach's alpha for the overall SIP score was 0.94. For the interviewer-administered version, alpha = 0.94 in samples of 53 and 299 outpatients.[8] Test-retest: assessed in same samples: self-administered version (n = 307), r = 0.87; interviewer-administered (n = 299), r = 0.97.[8]	Test-retest: assessed in sample of 58 patients with osteoarthritis: retest interval, 4 weeks; correlation coefficients for the 6 concepts in Part I ranged from 0.77 to 0.85. For Part II, coefficients ranged from 0.44 to 0.86.[212]	Internal consistency: for graduate students (n = 69), the coefficient was 0.93; for dialysis patients (n = 349), internal consistency was 0.90.[220] Test-retest: for graduate students (n = 69) tested two weeks apart, the correlation was 0.87. In a group of 20 dialysis patients, the correlation was 0.81.[220]

(cont.)

Table 3.1. (*cont.*)

Instrument name:	Hospital Anxiety and Depression Scale (HAD Scale)	Profile of Mood States (POMS)	Medical Outcomes Study Short Form-36 (SF-36)	Quality of Life Index (QL Index)	Sickness Impact Profile (SIP)	Nottingham Health Profile (NHP)	Quality of Life Index (Ferrans)
Evidence of validity (content, construct, criterion-related)	Validated in 50 patients attending general medical clinics, age 16–65.[24] Content: Anxiety items based on a review of related instruments and the investigator's research experience and need to achieve separation between anxiety and depression concepts. Construct: Compared with patients evaluated to have distinctly different levels of anxiety vs depression, insignificant correlation between depression, anxiety scores. Physically ill patients without mood disorders had scores similar to normal sample. Criterion: Compared with psychiatric evaluation, depression scale yielded 99% sensitivity, 99% specificity; anxiety scale had 99% sensitivity, 95% specificity.	Construct validity: Factor analysis congruent in 6 patient and normal samples. Highly correlated with Hopkins Symptom Distress Scales, especially Anxiety and Depression ($r >= 0.60$ for most POMS factors). Tension-Anxiety factor correlated with Taylor Manifest Anxiety Scale, $r = 0.80$.	Content: comparisons with other generic health surveys indicates SF-36 includes 8 of most frequently used health concepts with exception of sexual functioning. Construct validity demonstrated through factor analysis. Known groups validation demonstrated for patients with depression, heart disease, other conditions, as well as by gender and age group for a general population sample.	Content: assessed by one panel of 34 healthy patients and persons with chronic disease, and relatives and another of health professionals and researchers. A majority of panel members approved of the content and format of the instrument. Construct: assessed in 5 study groups encompassing healthy people (n = 84, 101), patients with chronic illness other than cancer (n = 108), cancer patients (n = 105), and critically ill and terminal patients (n = 78). Correlations between QL Index and the UNISCALE ranged from 0.28 to 0.63. Also, the mean scores were directly related to the health of the 5 groups, that is, ranging from highest for the healthiest to lowest for the critically and terminally ill group.	Construct validity was assessed by correlating the SIP with self-reported dysfunction and sickness. The validity coefficients were 0.69 for dysfunction and 0.63 for sickness, based on a sample consisting largely of prepaid group plan enrollees. In a sample of inpatients and outpatients, coefficients were 0.52 for dysfunction and 0.54 for sickness.[8]	Construct validity for Part I was assessed by observing discrimination of scores between 4 groups of elderly persons; NHP scores were related to health status, the identifying criterion. Validity has also been assessed in other groups, including pregnant women, persons with rheumatoid arthritis, and mine rescue workers.[213]	Criterion-related validity was assessed by correlating overall QLI scores with responses to a global rating of satisfaction with life. The coefficients were 0.75 for graduate students and 0.65 for dialysis patients.[220]

Evidence of responsiveness/sensitivity to change	Correlation with clinical assessment of severity: depression = 0.70, anxiety = 0.74, p < .0001 for both.	Multiple studies showing sensitivity to change reported in Manual[75] including psychotherapy interventions, drug trials, emotion-inducing conditions.	MHI (mental health scale), MCS shown to be useful in screening for psychiatric disorders (sensitivity = 74%, specificity = 81%). Sensitivity to change shown for overall change in health status, and in knee replacement, hip replacement, heart valve surgery, depression treatment.	Sensitivity to change over time was demonstrated in a sample of patients with total hip replacement and a sample of hyperthyroid patients.[8]	In a sample of 141 adults recovering from fracture, mean subscale scores on Part I declined indicating less dysfunction after 9-weeks; for spouses of the patients, there was no change in scores.[214]
Interpretability (availability of normative data, clinically meaningful difference)	Suggests cut-off scores to be used for presence of mood disorders, based on study purpose. Cutpoints: <7 indicate non-cases; 8–10 indicate doubtful cases; and >10 indicate definite cases.[24]	Normative data in Manual[75] dated (1960s) and limited: 350 male and 650 female English-speaking psychiatric outpatients, including demographics; also 340 male, 516 female volunteer undergraduate college students.	Norms published in QualityMetric manual and online at www.sf-36.com include US general population by age, gender; chronic conditions from MOS; one-year change scores for hypertension, CHF, MI, diabetes, depression from MOS. International norms also available. Minimally clinically meaningful difference approximately 3 to 5 points (0–100 scale), 0.09–0.28 effect size.	Correlations of SIP scores with clinical measures, e.g., the Harris Analysis of Hip Function, were generally high. For example, the correlation between the overall SIP score and the Harris scale was −0.81.[8]	

(cont.)

Table 3.1. (*cont.*)

Post-Development Evidence in Cancer Patients:

Instrument name:	Hospital Anxiety and Depression Scale (HAD Scale)	Profile of Mood States (POMS)	Medical Outcomes Study Short Form-36 (SF-36)	Quality of Life Index (QL Index)	Sickness Impact Profile (SIP)	Nottingham Health Profile (NHP)	Quality of Life Index (Ferrans)
Reliability	Internal consistency: Cronbach's alphas were above 0.75 for breast clinic attendees (n = 258), persons with MI (n = 108), and acute stroke patients (n = 68).[196] Cronbach's alphas for Anxiety and Depression subscales were 0.87 and 0.83, respectively, in a sample of 568 cancer patients.[197]	Internal consistency for 11-item short form assessed in 619 cancer patients; Cronbach's alpha was 0.91. In a second sample of 295 patients with small cell lung cancer; alpha was 0.92.[76] Cronbach's alphas for the 37-item short form (Shacham) were over 0.85 in cancer patient samples.[200]	Internal consistency assessed in a sample of 156 persons with laryngeal cancer. Cronbach's alpha ranged from 0.69 (General Health) to 0.91 (Social Functioning).[201]				
Validity	Exploratory and confirmatory factor analysis supported the basic structure of the scale.[196] Comparison of HAD Scale and RSCL scores were considered to have good predictive value for identifying those with affective disorder in a sample of women with advanced breast cancer (n = 81).[198] HAD Scale scores were positively associated with subscale scores of the EORTC QLQ-C30 in a sample of 568 cancer patients.[199]	Validity of the 11-item short form was demonstrated in a sample of 119 patients with pancreatic cancer and 128 with gastric cancer.[76] Correlations between original and 37-item short form were at least 0.95 for all subscale scores and the total mood disturbance.[200]	Convergent and discriminant validity assessed in a sample of 156 persons with laryngeal cancer; the percent of correlations at least 0.40 was over 90 for the 8 subscales.[201] Mean scores for all but the Mental Health subscale were higher for oral and oro-pharyngeal squamous cell carcinoma patients who had less dysfunction as measured by the University of Washington head and neck cancer questionnaire (UW-QOL) and who were awaiting surgery.[60]	Correlations between QLI and UNISCALE scores ranged from 0.57 to 0.81, with observations taken at baseline and monthly through 4 months of treatment for patients with advanced cancer.[208]	In a sample of 15 patients treated surgically for oral and pharyngeal cancer, the overall as well as domain scores showed change from pre-surgery to 2–4 and 12 months post-surgery. Outcomes were poorer for patients with more extensive surgery.[114] In a sample of 25 patients who had a Whipple procedure; 25 who had undergone cholecystectomy served as a control group. The overall SIP score indicated less dysfunction for those with the Whipple procedure.[117] In a sample of 16 patients with neoplasia; 16 who had pelvic pouch surgery due to medical failure served as a matched control group. The overall SIP score indicated less dysfunction for the control group as did the Physical and Psychological Function subscale scores.[62]	Subscale scores for Part I indicated that patients with non-Hodgkin's lymphoma who were treated with ABMT had less dysfunction 2 years after initial treatment, except for the Social Isolation subscale which indicated more dysfunction. Part I scores also detected change in function among a sample treated with standard chemotherapy. Items in Part II were more likely to detect change among the patients treated with chemotherapy than with ABMT.[215]	

Responsiveness	Improvement at 3, 6, and 12 months following surgery for oral cancer.[202] Significant improvement in Role-Emotional function following conformal radiation therapy for 41 patients with prostate carcinoma. No significant improvement for the other 7 subscales in the same group.[65]	Subscale scores for Part I indicated that patients with non-Hodgkin's lymphoma who were treated with ABMT had less dysfunction 2 years after initial treatment, except for the Social Isolation subscale which indicated more dysfunction. Part I scores also detected change in function among a sample treated with standard chemotherapy.[215] Change in Part I scores in response to treatment was also found in 33 patients with carcinoid syndrome.[216]	
Interpretability	Mean scores for a sample of 35 patients with esophageal cancer or those with esophagogastric junction did not differ from reference values obtained from a national sample of adults for the Bodily Pain and Mental Health subscales; for the other 6 subscales, the patients had higher scores.[61] Subscale scores for patients with neoplasia (n = 16) and matched controls (n = 16) did not differ, except for the Role-Physical subscale, with the controls having a higher mean score.[62]	For the Swedish version, group means have been published in graphical form for a general population reference group as well as for 7 patient groups, including one sample of colorectal cancer patients post-surgery and another of oropharyngeal cancer post-surgery.[114]	

(cont.)

Table 3.1. (*cont.*)

Instrument name:	Hospital Anxiety and Depression Scale (HAD Scale)	Profile of Mood States (POMS)	Medical Outcomes Study Short Form-36 (SF-36)	Quality of Life Index (QL Index)	Sickness Impact Profile (SIP)	Nottingham Health Profile (NHP)	Quality of Life Index (Ferrans)
Key reference(s)	Snaith, 1987[23] Zigmund, Snaith, 1983[24] Skarstein, Aass, Fossa et al., 2000[199] Hopwood, Howell, Maguire, 1991[198] Johnston, Pollard, Hennessey, 2000[196]	McNair, Lorr, Droppleman, 1981[75] Cella, Jacobsen, Orav et al., 1987[76] Shacham, 1983[78] Curran, Andrykowski, Studts, 1995[200]	Ware, Sherbourne, 1992[10] Ware, Snow, Kosinski et al., 1993[53] McHorney, Ware, Raczek, 1993[203] McHorney, Ware, Lu et al., 1994[204] Ware, Kosinski, Bayliss et al., 1995[205] Stewart, Greenfield, Hays et al., 1989[206] Rogers, Lowe, Brown et al., 1998[202] Quality Metric, Inc., 2002[207]	Spitzer, Dobson, Hall et al., 1981[92] Sloan, Loprinzi, Kuross et al., 1998[208]	Gilson, Gilson, Bergner et al., 1975[7] Bergner, Bobbitt, Carter et al., 1981[8] Thompson-Fawcett, Richard, O'Connor et al., 2000[62] Langius, Bjorvell, Lind et al.,1994[114] McLeod, Taylor, O'Connor et al., 1995[117] Bergner, Bobbitt, Pollard et al., 1976[209] Carter, Bobbitt, Bergner. et al., 1976[210] Pollard, Bobbitt, Bergner et al., 1976[211]	Hunt, McEwen, 1980[217] Hunt, McEwen, McKenna et al., 1984[218] Hunt, McEwen, McKenna et al., 1982[219] Hunt, McKenna, McEwen et al., 1980[213] Hunt, McKenna, McEwen et al., 1981[212] McKenna, McEwen, Hunt et al., 1984[214] Uyl-de Groot, Hagenbeek, Verdonck et al., 1995[215] O'Toole, Ducreux, Bommelaer et al., 2000[216]	Ferrans, Powers, 1985[220] Ferrans, Powers, 1992[221] Ferrans, 1990[222]

in usage to the HAD Scale. Several studies have been explicitly designed to validate the SF-36 in cancer patients in the post-development stage; these findings are summarized in Table 3.1.

The SF-36, like the HAD Scale, has been used across all stages of the cancer continuum. It is widely used in the evaluation of treatment effectiveness, and is more likely to be used to evaluate surgical and radiation treatments than in clinical trials of alternative chemotherapies.[54-67] The SF-36 is more likely to be used in studies of cancer survivors than are other generic measures.[54,61,68-72] Regardless of use, there is no apparent clustering of diagnoses. It has been used, albeit rarely, in screening and prevention studies as well as those designed to assess health status and quality of life among terminally ill cancer patients. Its infrequent use among patients at the end of life is consistent with its purpose for development, that is, to assess health outcomes in a general population. The widespread use of this scale in general, and with cancer patients specifically, can be attributed at least in part to the developers' continued support of its use and promotional activities.[73-74]

Profile of Mood States

Conceptual, practical, and measurement features

The POMS was developed over 30 years ago as a self-report instrument to assess transient affective states in psychiatric outpatients.[75] Each subscale contains a list of adjectives that describe various feelings, e.g., friendly, listless, peeved, muddled, anxious, desperate, and weary. Respondents select the response option that best describes the frequency of feeling during the past week. Information on the format and measurement properties of the POMS is presented in Table 3.1.

The POMS has been modified for use with cancer patients.[76-78] For example, Shacham has developed a 37-item version after terminally ill cancer patients found the original 65-item version difficult to complete, taking 3 to 5 times longer than the time reported for healthy people.[78] Although less burden-some, these modified versions do not seem to have been widely adopted for use.

Performance across the cancer continuum

Of the generic instruments, the POMS has been used in less than 20% of published empirical references that purport to measure health-related quality of life in cancer patients. In about 30% of these, a modified version of the full instrument has been used. Articles addressing post-development validation relating to short forms are summarized in Table 3.1.

Of the articles that report on the use of the POMS with cancer patients, about 40% cite its use in assessing treatment effectiveness, most frequently in chemotherapy[79-81] and transplantation.[82,83] The POMS has been used to a lesser extent in studies that evaluate the psychological impact of surgery[84,85] and radiation.[67,86] While the POMS has been used to assess mood states in cancer survivors,[84,87-90] it has been rarely if ever used in programs designed for screening and prevention of cancer and in patients receiving terminal care;[91] this lack of use may be due to its length, difficulty, and inclusion of subscales that are thought to be irrelevant to these groups.[78]

Quality-of-Life Index

Conceptual, practical, and measurement features

The QL Index, which is modeled after the Apgar Scale for newborns, was developed as a simple, easy to use and understand way of assessing health outcomes in persons with chronic disease. Although originally published as a clinician-reported rating scale, the QL Index is also available as a patient self-report instrument. Each item has three descriptive statements; for example, the three options in the Health domain are: "the patient has been appearing to feel well or reporting feeling 'great' most of the time," "has been lacking energy or not feeling entirely 'up to par' more than just occasionally," and "has been feeling very ill or 'lousy,' seeming weak and washed out most of the time or was unconscious."[92]

Spitzer et al.[92] suggest that the QL Index is suitable for assessing treatment options, including for seriously ill persons such as those receiving palliative care or hospice service, but not for assessing health status and quality of life of healthy individuals. In two outpatient, basically healthy population samples, over 50% of those who completed the QL Index had the highest possible score,[92] thus demonstrating that this instrument would be unresponsive to interventions designed to improve outcome in relatively healthy individuals.

Performance across the cancer continuum

The QL Index has been used in studies involving cancer patients with a diversity of diagnoses.[93–97] It has been widely used with breast, colorectal, and lung cancer patients; however, it is used infrequently with prostate cancer patients. Of all reports, regardless of cancer diagnosis, approximately 30% provide information on either the QL Index's reliability and validity or its use to demonstrate these properties in other instruments. Table 3.1 presents information about the QL Index's measurement properties in its post-development stage.

As with the other generic measures, the QL Index has been most frequently used in studies of treatment effectiveness. These include clinical trials of persons with prevalent forms of cancer such as breast, colorectal, and lung, as well as with less prevalent diagnoses such as adenocarcinoma and bile duct and bone neoplasms.[93,94] While there is no apparent clustering of use of the QL Index by diagnosis, there is an observed tendency for the QL Index to be primarily used in trials to assess chemotherapeutic[93,98–100] and surgical interventions.[101–104] This scale has rarely been used in studies evaluating treatment with radiation or transplantation.

Less frequently, the QL Index has been used to assess outcomes of treatment designed to improve palliative care and extend survival,[93,94,105] and to examine relationships between quality of life and physical and psychological symptoms as well as caregiver reaction in home care settings for terminally ill patients.[106,107] The QL Index has rarely if ever been used in studies of cancer survivorship or prevention which, in part, can be attributed to the developers' recognition of its lack of sensitivity in relatively healthy people.[92]

Sickness Impact Profile

Conceptual, practical, and measurement features

Development of the SIP began in 1972 with the aim of creating a measure of self-reported health status capable of detecting changes that occur either between groups or over time, especially for use in clinical practice.[7,8] Items for the SIP were derived from measures of physical, social, and mental dysfunction that were available in the early 1970s. The Emotional Behavior subscale includes the following items: "I laugh or cry suddenly," "I often moan and groan in pain or discomfort," and "I talk about the future in a hopeless way." Additional information about the format and measurement properties of the SIP is provided in Table 3.1.

To overcome respondent burden, a 68-item version of the SIP, the Short Form-Sickness Impact Profile (SF-SIP), has been derived from a factor analysis of a Dutch translation of the original 136-item questionnaire.[108] Although developed almost 10 years ago, the SF-SIP has been rarely used in clinical research or epidemiologic investigations. Other than the SF-SIP, few if any attempts have been made to reduce the length of the SIP, which is considered to be a barrier to its use.

Performance across the cancer continuum

Of all articles reporting on the use of the SIP in empirical studies, less than 10% provide evidence of its relevance for use with cancer patients. The SIP has been used in a range of cancer diagnoses, but fewer than for the other generic instruments. The SIP has been used in patients with lung, liver, colorectal, and head and neck cancer,[63,109–115] but these studies contribute evidence supporting the construct validity of the SIP, rather than explicitly reporting on measurement properties in the post-development stage.

Within the context of the cancer care continuum, the SIP has been used almost exclusively in studies of treatment effectiveness.[63,111,116,117] As an example of SIP performance, in a sample of surgically treated stomach cancer patients, the overall and physical subscale scores increased between baseline and three months post-surgery, with the decline in physical function contributing to the change in the overall score.[118] The SIP's lack of use in palliative care settings is probably due to its length and inclusion of items that might be unacceptable to terminally ill persons.

Even though recommended as a standard,[119] the SIP has not been adopted as such in the cancer arena. In evaluating the SIP for possible use in a trial treating premenopausal women with breast cancer, Nystedt *et al.* found the items in the SIP too general.[26] The SIP can also be considered as less than ideal for use in cancer screening initiatives involving relatively healthy populations due to its initial purpose of assessing outcomes in people with dysfunction and its observed ceiling effect.[7,120]

Summary: use of generic instruments within the cancer arena

These generic instruments were used with many different cancer diagnoses, with no apparent instrument-by-diagnosis clustering. There was a definite pattern of use, however, by stage of the continuum of cancer care. Namely, most applications are treatment related, whether for assessing chemotherapeutic or surgical interventions. There was a tendency for the HAD Scale to be used more in evaluations of chemotherapy, while the SF-36 tends to be used with either surgery or radiation treatments; no apparent patterns emerged for the other instruments.

While the instruments were most widely used in studies to assess cancer treatments, there was relatively little use for cancer screening, understanding the impacts of these prevention programs on healthy people, and examining health status and quality of life among cancer survivors and patients at the end of life. Of the five generic instruments, the HAD Scale and SF-36 were the most likely to be used across all stages of the cancer continuum.

General cancer measures

General cancer instruments have been designed to consider that cancer patients have been diagnosed with malignant disease; thus, they focus on distinguishing functional status and well-being specific to cancer patients regardless of site or stage of disease. Five multidimensional measures that have been developed for persons 18 years of age and older have been identified: Cancer Rehabilitation Evaluation System (CARES); European Organization for Research and Treatment of Cancer Core Quality of Life Questionnaire (EORTC QLQ-C30); Functional Assessment of Cancer Therapy-General (FACT-G); Functional Living Index-Cancer (FLIC); and Rotterdam Symptom Checklist (RSCL). Each instrument is reviewed below according to developmental and post-developmental evidence, with additional detail on each provided in Table 3.2.

Cancer Rehabilitation Evaluation System

Conceptual, practical, and measurement features

The CARES, which was developed to assess cancer patients' ability to cope with their disease and its treatment, consists of a list of problems typically encountered by patients on a day-to-day basis as they live with cancer and its treatment.[121-125] Representative items from the Psychosocial Function subscale are: "I become nervous when I am waiting to see the doctor," and "I do not know what to say to friends or relatives." For ease of completion, all items in the CARES have the same response options which range from "not at all" to "very much." Other information about the structure and format of the CARES is given in Table 3.2.

Table 3.2. General cancer measures: supporting data on psychometrics and validation

Instrument name:	Cancer Rehabilitation Evaluation System (CARES; formerly Cancer Inventory of Problem Situations, CIPS)	Functional Assessment of Cancer Therapy-General (FACT-G)	Functional Living Index – Cancer (FLIC)	European Organization for Research and Treatment of Cancer Quality of Life Questionnaire (EORTC QLQ-C30)	Rotterdam Symptom Check List (RSCL)
Purpose for which developed	To document psychosocial and physical problems of cancer patients; for both clinical and research use	To measure functional status and well-being in cancer patients	To compare groups of patients with respect to overall functional response to their cancer and to different treatment approaches	To assess health outcomes in cancer-specific clinical trials	To measure symptoms reported by cancer patients participating in clinical research; subsequently, to evaluate impact of psychosocial interventions and detect psychiatric illness
Length	Long form: 93 to 132 items out of 142, rating problems during past month. Short Form: 38 to 57 items out of 59 items	27 items (Version 4). Time frame: past 7 days	22 items. Time frames range from "today" to "past month"	30 items. Revised from 36 items in initial validation study. Time frame: past week	38 items. 30 symptoms, 8 activity items. Time frame: past week
Administration time	Long form: Mean 18 minutes	5 minutes or less	Less than 10 minutes	15 minutes or less	Less than 10 minutes
Domains included	Physical (26 items, 7 subscales); Psychosocial (44, 9 subscales); Medical Interaction (11, 3 subscales); Marital (18, 5 subscales); Sexual (8, 2 subscales); Miscellaneous (32, 5 subscales)	Version 4: Emotional Well-Being (6 items); Functional Well-Being (7 items); Physical Well-Being (7 items); Social/Family Well-Being (7 items). Response options range from "not at all" to "very much"	Physical Well-Being and Ability (9 items); Psychological Well-Being (7 items); Social Well-Being (2); Nausea (2); Hardship due to Cancer (3). Response options represent disease impact	Functioning domains: physical (5 items); role (2); emotional (4); cognitive (2) social (2); global QOL(2). Symptom domains/items: 3 fatigue, 2 nausea/vomiting, 2 pain, 1 each dyspnea, sleep disturbance, appetite loss, constipation, diarrhea, financial impact	Activity (8 items); response options range from "unable" to "with difficulty without help." Symptoms: psychological distress (8 items); physical distress (19); disease-specific symptoms (3). Response options represent bother and range from "not at all" to "very much"

Scoring	0–4 scale. Summary scores: total number of endorsed problems, total severity rating, average severity score, global score, 5 higher-order scale scores. Higher scores indicate more dysfunction	0 to 4 scale. Item scores are summed to form overall and subscale scores. Global score, FACT-G score, subscale scores. Higher scores indicate less dysfunction	Mixed 7-point Likert/VAS. Item scores range from 1–7 with items scored to the "nearest even whole integer." Item scores are summed to form an overall score that ranges from 22–154	Physical and role function, dichotomous; 4-point ("not at all, a little, quite a bit, very much") scale for other items; global questions on 7-point scale. Scale scores = mean of item scores, rescaled to 0-to-100 with higher function subscale scores indicating less dysfunction and higher symptom subscale scores indicating more dysfunction	Symptoms rated on 4-point scale. Item scores are summed to form overall and subscale scores. Domain scores rescaled to 0–100 scale in some studies. Higher scores indicate more dysfunction
Validated modes of administration	Face-to face interview, telephone interview, self-administered, mail, computer-assisted	Self-administered	Self-administered	Self-administered, interviewer-administered; touch sensitive video monitor[234]	Self-administered. Can be mailed
Validated translations/ cultural adaptations	English, Dutch, Spanish	English, Afrikaans, Arabic, Bulgarian, Chinese (Mainland), Chinese (Hong Kong, Taiwan), Czech, Danish, Dutch, Estonian, Finnish, French, Georgian, German, Greek, Hebrew, Hungarian, Italian, Japanese, Malay, Norwegian, Pedi, Polish, Portuguese, Romanian, Russian, Slovakian, Spanish, Swedish, Thai, Tswana, Turkish, Zulu	English (Canada), Afrikaans, Austrian German, Chinese (Mandarin), Danish, Dutch, Finnish, Flemish, French, French Canadian, German, Greek, Italian, Japanese, Luganda, Malay, Ndebele, Portuguese, Shona, Spanish, Swedish	Bulgarian, Chinese, Czech, Danish, Dutch, English (US, UK), Finnish, French, German, Greek, Hebrew, Hindi, Hungarian, Italian, Japanese, Korean, Malay, Norwegian, Persian, Polish, Portuguese, Russian, Slovak, Slovenian, Sotho, Spanish, Swedish, Turkish	Dutch, Czech, English (Australia, Ireland and UK), Finnish, French (France, Belgium), German, Hungarian, Italian, Portuguese, Slovak, Spanish (Argentina, Spain)

(cont.)

Table 3.2. (cont.)

Instrument name:	Cancer Rehabilitation Evaluation System (CARES; formerly Cancer Inventory of Problem Situations, CIPS)	Functional Assessment of Cancer Therapy-General (FACT-G)	Functional Living Index – Cancer (FLIC)	European Organization for Research and Treatment of Cancer Quality of Life Questionnaire (EORTC QLQ-C30)	Rotterdam Symptom Check List (RSCL)
Developmental Evidence:					
Evidence of reliability (internal consistency, test-retest, other)	Internal consistency: assessed in a sample of 479 cancer patients, over 60% of whom had a diagnosis of either breast, colorectal, lung, or prostate cancer. Cronbach's alpha for Physical = 0.92, Psychosocial = 0.94, Medical interaction = 0.87, Marital = 0.92, Sexual = 0.88.[223] Test-retest was assessed in a subsample of 120 patients. r > 0.80; agreement with problem present/ absent = 0.84–0.88.[223]	Internal consistency: assessed in 4 groups of in- and outpatients who were being treated for cancer; 466 persons were in the combined sample. FACT-G (Version 3) subscales ranged from 0.65 (Relationship with Doctor) to 0.82 (Physical Well-Being); for Overall score, alpha = 0.89. Test-retest: in a subsample of 60 patients, correlations for subscale scores ranged from 0.82 to 0.88; for Overall score, the correlation was 0.92.		Internal consistency: assessed in 305 lung cancer patients in 12 countries. Cronbach's alpha at baseline: physical = 0.68, role = 0.54, emotional = 0.73, cognitive = 0.56, social = 0.68, fatigue 0.80, pain = 0.82, nausea = 0.65, global = 0.86. Alpha during treatment: physical = 0.71, role = 0.52, emotional = 0.80, cognitive = 0.73, social = 0.77, fatigue = 0.85, pain = 0.76, nausea = 0.73, global = 0.89. Reliability generally improved with repeated measurement.[12] Also, assessed in Canadian sample of breast, ovarian, and lung cancer patients. Alpha > 0.70 except for role, cognitive function.[235] Test-retest: assessed in a sample of 180–189 cancer patients:[236] r = 0.82–0.91 for functional scales and global scores; r = 0.63–0.86 for symptom scales; and r = 0.72–0.84 for single items. Interval of re-administration was at least 4 days.	Internal consistency: 34-item symptom version assessed in a sample of 95 breast cancer patients and 56 advanced ovarian cancer patients. Cronbach's alphas ranged from 0.72–0.94. In cross-cultural study, Cronbach's alpha for psychologic = 0.83–0.89 at baseline, 0.85–0.90 at 3 months; physical = 0.68–0.85 at baseline, 0.77–0.85 at 3 months; activity scale 0.57 – 0.80 at baseline, 0.41–0.89 at 3 months. Significant differences in scores between cultures.

Evidence of validity (content, construct, criterion-related)				
Content validity: Items based on literature search, open-ended interviews with patients, significant others, professionals. Factor analysis used to develop scales.[224] Construct validity was assessed in the same sample of 479 cancer patients as was reliability. Correlation between the CARES global score and the SCL-90 = 0.76; with KPS = −0.46.[223] In a sample of 109 newly diagnosed breast cancer patients, Pschosocial, Physical summary scales strongly correlated with FLIC score; number of CARES problems reported were inversely associated with low, middle, high FLIC scores.[124]	Content validity: FACT-G: Generated candidate questions based on open-ended interviews with 45 stage II or IV patients (breast, lung, colorectal) and 15 oncology professionals. Item reduction used relevance rating by 90 different patients. Construct validity: Factor analysis used to establish FACT-G subscales. Correlation with FLIC: FACT-G global, r = 0.86. Significant correlations between Emotional Well-Being and POMS Depression (−0.53), Tension (−0.57), Anger (−0.45); Physical (0.46), Functional Well-Being (0.57) with POMS Vigor; Physical Well-Being with POMS Fatigue (−0.54); POMS-SF total correlated with Emotional (−0.60). Divergent validity: Lack of correlation with Marlowe-Crown Social Desirability Scale. Known groups: All scales except Relationship with Doctor differentiated groups by self-rated PSR category. All scales in expected direction relative to extent of disease, only Physical Well-Being was significant.	Content validity: Panel of patients, spouses, providers, clergy developed initial question list. Construct validity: Assessed in a sample of 175 hospital and outpatients. Overall FLIC score correlated with KPS (0.62), GHQ (−0.77), and BDI (−0.77). Physical well-being and ability subscale correlated with KPS (0.55), GHQ (−0.57) and BDI (−0.64). Psychological well-being correlated with KPS (0.55), GHQ (−0.57), and BDI (−0.64). The other domains were not correlated with these measures.[173] Average scores decreased with extent of disease.	Content validity: Position papers prepared for each domain, circulated among multicultural study group members, discussed at plenary sessions. Known groups: few differences in pre-treatment scores by disease stage, contrary to expectation. Explained based on finding stage not related to ECOG PSR and weight loss in this lung cancer sample. High discriminant validity based on clinical status (measured by ECOG performance status, weight loss, treatment toxicity) for physical, role, fatigue, global scales; moderate validity for pain, emotional, social. Cognitive, nausea did not discriminate well. Construct validity: With GHQ, r = 0.70,[237] r = 0.61,[238] Emotional function score with HADS, r = 0.71.[239]	Content validity: Based on secondary analysis of data from studies using Dutch version of the Hopkins Symptom Checklist,[187] McCorkle and Young Symptom Distress Scale,[189] Linssen[188] study of BC patients, plus opinions of oncologists, answer distribution. Construct, criterion validity not reported in 1990 paper. Factor analysis in cross-cultural sample consistent with original validation studies.

(cont.)

Table 3.2. (cont.)

Instrument name:	Cancer Rehabilitation Evaluation System (CARES; formerly Cancer Inventory of Problem Situations, CIPS)	Functional Assessment of Cancer Therapy-General (FACT-G)	Functional Living Index – Cancer (FLIC)	European Organization for Research and Treatment of Cancer Quality of Life Questionnaire (EORTC QLQ-C30)	Rotterdam Symptom Check List (RSCL)
Evidence of responsiveness/ sensitivity to change	CARES showed significant HRQOL improvement between one month and one year after breast cancer diagnosis.[121,224]	Sensitivity to 2-month changes in PSR found for FACT-B global, FACT-G global, Physical Well-Being, Functional Well-Being, BCS, TOI-PFB, as expected. Social, Emotional Well-Being, Relationship with Doctor not responsive to PSR change, also as expected.		With CARES, physical = 0.71, emotional = 0.56, social = 0.46, pain = 0.69.[238] In Canadian sample, physical, role, social, fatigue, pain, global changed significantly with change in ECOG PSR.[235] Construct validity was also assessed in three ways: item discriminant validity; inter-scale correlations; and responsiveness to patient clinical status. Validity has also been assessed by determining the extent to which patients and health raters agreed in their responses to items in the EORTC QLQ-C30. Did not find significant changes for total sample from pretreatment to on-treatment (mean 28 days); explained by heterogeneity of health status of sample over time. Did find significant differences in physical, role, fatigue, nausea, and global scores when sample grouped according to increase, decline, no change in PSR. Core questionnaire anticipates development of disease-specific modules.	

Interpretability (availability of normative data, clinically meaningful difference)	Scores for validation sample of 479 heterogeneous cancer patients.[223]	Kemmler et al. 1999[226] compared FACT-G, EORTC QLQ-C30; concluded they measure significantly different aspects of HRQOL and results should not be compared.	Niezgoda and Pater provide correlations of QLQ-C30 domains with SIP, CARES, GHQ, McGill Pain in 96 English-speaking cancer patients in Canada.[238] King compared FLIC, QLQ-C30; found convergent validity for global, role, emotional, pain, nausea scales but not social.[233] Kemmler compared FACT-G, EORTC QLQ-C30; concluded they measure significantly different aspects of HRQOL and results should not be compared.[226] Skarstein examined relation between QLQ-C30 and HAD Scale; recommends use of additional instrument to screen for depression.[199]	Normative data for 216 patients under treatment, 192 survivors (>= 3 years), 201 random Dutch population sample.[186]

Post-Developmental Evidence in Cancer Patients:

Reliability	Test-retest: assessed in 46 brain tumor patients using version 2; two administrations were 1 week apart. Correlation coefficients ranged from 0.60 to 0.83 for the subscales. For the overall score, the correlation was 0.80.[227] Internal consistency: assessed in 36 men with metastatic prostate cancer. Cronbach's alphas for the subscales ranged from 0.75–0.83.[97] Assessed in 231 rural cancer patients; Cronbach's alpha for overall score = 0.92.[228]	In Morrow et al. (489 American cancer patients, 44% with breast cancer): Cronbach's alpha = 0.64 to 0.87.[231]	Internal consistency: assessed in breast, lung, ovarian cancer patients (n=535); subscale coefficients at least 0.70 except for Cognitive and Role Function.[235] Assessed in long-term cancer survivors; Cronbach's alpha ranged from 0.58–0.90 for the subscales.[240]	Internal consistency: assessed in a multinational trial of women with early breast cancer. For activity subscale scores across subsamples, Cronbach's alphas range from 0.57–0.80 for assessment at baseline (n = 689) and from 0.42 – 0.83 after 3 months (n = 519). For symptoms, the coefficients ranged from 0.71–0.89 at baseline and from 0.77–0.90 after 3 months.[194]

(cont.)

Table 3.2. (*cont.*)

Instrument name:	Cancer Rehabilitation Evaluation System (CARES; formerly Cancer Inventory of Problem Situations, CIPS)	Functional Assessment of Cancer Therapy-General (FACT-G)	Functional Living Index – Cancer (FLIC)	European Organization for Research and Treatment of Cancer Quality of Life Questionnaire (EORTC QLQ-C30)	Rotterdam Symptom Check List (RSCL)
Validity		Assessed in 101 brain tumor patients using version 2. The correlation between the FACT-G and Quality of Life Index (Ferrans and Powers) was 0.41. Correlations between FACT-G and depression and anxiety scores were −0.71 and −0.70, respectively. Correlation between the FACT-G and KPS was 0.21. Correlations with non-health status measures were low, indicating divergent construct validity.[228] Assessed in 36 men with metastatic prostate cancer using version 3. Correlation between FACT-G and KPS was 0.67 and between FACT-G and Quality of Life Index (Spitzer), 0.77. Correlations between subscale scores and KPS ranged from 0.18–0.74; between subscale scores and QLI (Spitzer), the range was 0.16–0.77.[97] Overall, Physical and Emotional subscale scores differentiated patients with stable from progressive metastatic prostate cancer.[97] Convergent construct validity and factor structure supported in a sample of 231 rural cancer patients.[228]	Morrow *et al.*, using somewhat different factor structure, concluded psychometric properties were better if 4 cancer-specific questions were excluded. Recommends using FLIC without these items as a core generic measure with development of disease-specific modules.[231] Butow *et al.* (1991) found that 8 VAS items, the GLQ-8, explained 57% of the variance in FLIC scores. Of the 8 items, only hair loss was a non-significant predictor.[232] Correlations between FLIC and UNISCALE scores ranged from 0.49 to 0.83, with observations taken at baseline and monthly through 4 months of treatment for patients with advanced cancer.[208]	Validity assessed in cancer patients by comparing with medical records.[197] Subscale scores were systematically lower for less functional categories based on the ECOG-PS, demonstrating construct validity.[234] Within and between scale correlation coefficients were, generally, of the predicted levels, indicating convergent and discriminant validity.[240]	Factor analysis data from early breast cancer patients resulted in a two factor solution.[194] Comparison of RSCL and HAD Scale scores were considered to have good predictive value for identifying those with affective disorder in a sample of women with advanced breast cancer (n = 81).[198]

Responsiveness		Physical, Emotional and Functional subscales showed change from 1 week prior to thyroid scan to 4 weeks after scan in 34 thyroid cancer patients.[229]	FLIC showed significant HRQOL improvement over one year.[126] All FLIC subscores except emotional discriminated across health gradient of patients with metastatic breast, colon, and ovarian cancer.[233]	On an individual level, function scores observed to change over time.[197] Scores declined after the first 8 days patients received intravenous chemotherapy.[235]	
Interpretability			King (1996) compared FLIC, QLQ-C30; found convergent validity for global, role, emotional, pain, nausea scales but not social.[233]	Low to moderate effect sizes observed in a sample of long-term cancer survivors.[240]	
Key reference(s)	Ganz, Schag, Lee et al., 1992[121] Ganz, Schag, Cheng, 1990[124] Schag, Heinrich, 1989[225] Schag, Heinrich, Aadland et al., 1990[223]	Cella, Tulsky, Gray et al., 1993[13] Kemmler, Holzner, Kopp et al., 1999[226] Dow, Ferrell, Anello, 1997[229] Knight, Chmiel, Sharp et al., 2001[230] Weitzner, Meyers, Gelke et al., 1995[227]	Schipper, Clinch, McMurray et al., 1984[173] Clinch, 1996[174] Morrow, Lindke, Black, 1992[231] King, Dobson, Harnett, 1996[233] Sloan, Loprinzi, Kuross et al., 1998[208] Butow, Coats, Dunn et al., 1991[232] Winstead-Fry, Schultz, 1997[228]	Aaronson, Ahmedzai, Bergman et al., 1993[12] Osoba, Zee, Pater et al., 1994[235] Hjermstad, Fossa, Bjordal et al., 1995[236] Groenvold, Klee, Sprangers et al., 1997[241] Buxton, White, Osoba, 1998[234] Skarstein, Aass, Fossa et al., 2000[199]	de Haes, Pruyn, van Knippenberg, 1983[185] de Haes, van Knippenberg, Neift et al., 1990[186] de Haes, Olschewski, 1998[194] Hopwood, Howell, Maguire, 1991[198] Ravaioli, Buda, Fava et al., 1996[242] Skarstein, Aass, Fossa et al., 2000[199] Velikova, Wright, Smith et al., 2001[197] Apolone, Filberti, Cifani et al., 1998[240]

To overcome respondent burden, a 59-item CARES-Short Form, CARES-SF, has been derived from a reanalysis of data collected using the 142-item long form; the abbreviated version has the same subscales and scoring format.[126] Reliability, validity, and responsiveness, which were calculated using the original data, resulted in similar coefficients for the short and long forms. Although shorter than the original version, the CARES-SF is still longer than many short forms that have been recently developed and are commonly used.[9,10,127,128]

Performance across the cancer continuum

Since development, the original and short form versions of the CARES have been used to assess outcomes in persons with various types of cancer and in various stages of the care continuum. These studies contribute evidence to support the construct validity of the CARES, rather than explicitly reporting on measurement properties done by other investigators in the post-development stage. Frost and colleagues[129] used the CARES, along with the SF-36 and Brief Symptom Inventory, to study the impact of breast cancer across several stages of the continuum, from newly diagnosed to recurrent disease. Levels of physical and affective well-being were found to differ according to phase of disease.

Although rarely if ever used to assess the effectiveness of alternative forms of chemotherapy, the CARES has been used to study the effect of alternative behavioral,[130,131] surgical,[132,133] and nutritional interventions.[134] Differences were found between baseline and end-of-treatment scores, supporting developmental evidence that the CARES is responsive to change over time. A cross-sectional study in patients treated with interleukin for advanced renal cancer demonstrated the ability of CARES to differentiate between diagnoses.[135]

Survivorship was studied among persons with breast, colon, lung, and prostate cancer and acute myelogenous leukemia,[136–138] as well as with persons with head and neck cancer.[69,139] The infrequent use of the CARES in end-of-life studies suggests that its focus on problems of day-to-day living represents concerns that are secondary to terminally ill patients.

European Organization for Research and Treatment of Cancer Core Quality of Life Questionnaire

Conceptual, practical, and measurement features

The EORTC QLQ-C30 was developed for use in multinational clinical trials of cancer patients as part of the activities of the EORTC Study Group on Quality of Life.[12,140] The goal was to develop a multidimensional, cancer-specific assessment that was practical to administer across national and cultural boundaries. The core questionnaire is based on items included in other functional status assessments that were available in the early 1980s. Sample items in the Emotional Function section of the core questionnaire are: "Could you sit at ease and feel relaxed?" and "Did you get sudden feelings of panic?" Information about the format of the EORTC QLQ-C30 and its reliability, validity, and responsiveness is presented in Table 3.2.

In addition, disease-specific modules have been developed to supplement the general information collected in the core questionnaire, including modules for breast cancer, colorectal cancer, head and neck cancer, leukemia, and prostate cancer.[141–143]

Although originally developed for use in clinical trials, EORTC investigators are exploring the feasibility of using the core questionnaire in clinical practice settings to improve doctor-patient communication and enhance treatment.[144]

Performance across the cancer continuum

The EORTC QLQ-C30 has been used in over half of the empirical articles in which the five general cancer instruments have been used; this literature includes a range of diagnoses, notably esophageal, gastrointestinal and stomach, head and neck, and ovarian cancer, in addition to breast, colorectal, lung, and prostate cancer. Of these, several studies have been designed to explicitly validate the EORTC QLQ-C30 in the post-development stage; these findings are summarized in Table 3.2.

The EORTC QLQ-C30 has been used across all stages of the continuum of cancer care. Most articles, however, report on studies of the effectiveness of chemotherapy in multi-center randomized trials. In addition to trials to treat the four most prevalent forms of cancer, this instrument has been used in trials of less prevalent forms, e.g., adenocarcinoma and glioma, and bladder, biliary tract, bone, brain, liver, and ovarian cancer.[82,145-152] The QLQ-C30 was able to detect change in health status and quality of life over time[145,153,154] and to differentiate between patients with different diagnoses.[150]

The QLQ-C30 has been used less frequently to assess health status and quality of life in cancer survivors.[57,70,155-158] Of the five general cancer instruments, the EORTC QLQ-C30 is the one most likely to have been used in end-of-life studies to examine effectiveness and patient expectations of palliative treatments.[44,146,159-163] Few if any studies, however, have used the QLQ-C30 for assessing the health status and quality-of-life impacts of cancer screening and prevention initiatives.

Functional Assessment of Cancer Therapy-General Questionnaire

Conceptual, practical, and measurement features

The FACT-G is the general questionnaire of a measurement system designed to assess outcomes in clinical trials and practice settings. This core questionnaire is supplemented with tumor-specific modules for various types of cancer, including breast, brain, colorectal, lung, and prostate, as well as for problems associated with cancer treatment such as anemia and toxicity.[13,164,165] Items for the FACT-G and its modules were obtained from persons undergoing cancer treatment and from health professionals who were asked to identify significant quality-of-life concerns of cancer patients. Sample items from the Emotional Well-Being subscale are: "I feel sad," "I worry about dying," and "I am satisfied with how I am coping with my illness." For ease of completion, all items in the FACT-G have the same response options. Other information about the structure and format of the FACT-G is given in Table 3.2.

The naming convention used in the literature leads to a certain confusion regarding the use of the FACT-G and/or its modules. For example, the FACT for breast cancer notation, the FACT-B, may be used to represent the nine items specific to breast cancer or to represent the FACT-G plus the nine specific items. Thus, the decision to report on the FACT-G only when explicitly stated underrepresents the use of this instrument, but it is considered to be unbiased in terms of either diagnoses or usage across the continuum of cancer care.

Performance across the cancer continuum

In addition to being frequently used in persons with breast, colorectal, lung, and prostate cancer, the FACT-G has been used in persons with other diagnoses, including cervical, ovarian, and head and neck cancer.[166-168] Most reports document its use in methodologic studies to validate other instruments or linguistic or cultural adaptations. Information on post-development measurement properties of the FACT-G is given in Table 3.2.

As with the other general cancer instruments, most of the applications that relate to the continuum of cancer care have dealt with measuring treatment effectiveness. Recent longitudinal studies of men with prostate cancer[169,170] and persons with hepatocellular cancer[171] support findings from the development stage that the FACT-G is responsive to change in functional status and well-being over time. The FACT-G has rarely if ever been used in studies of screening, survivorship, or end of life, although some reports describe the use of different modules, possibly with or without the FACT-G, in either survivorship or end-of-life situations.[156,160,172]

Functional Living Index-Cancer

Conceptual, practical, and measurement features

The FLIC, like the CARES, was one of the first general cancer measures. It was developed to overcome major conceptual shortcomings of existing measures for assessing patient outcome in oncology, specifically, by addressing the need for psychometric validation and incorporating the patient's perspective.[173,174] Items in the FLIC have been selected as those most likely to be meaningful to cancer patients. For example, the psychological well-being subscale includes: "How much time do you spend thinking about your illness?" and "Rate how often you feel discouraged about your life." Information about the FLIC's format and measurement properties is given in Table 3.2.

Performance across the cancer continuum

Use of the FLIC is reported in about 15% of the articles in which general cancer instruments are used with cancer patients, with almost all of these reporting on the use of the original 22-item version of the FLIC without modifications. Of these, several studies have been designed to explicitly validate the FLIC in the post-development stage; findings are summarized in Table 3.2.

In addition to being frequently used with persons with breast, colorectal, lung, and prostate cancer, the FLIC has been used in patients with diverse diagnoses, including AIDS-related lymphoma and astrocytoma and bone and mouth cancer.[86,175–177] Of the clinical research reports, almost one-half were based on data collected to assess performance of alternative forms of chemotherapy.[175,178–182] For example, in a study of postmenopausal women with advanced breast cancer, the FLIC showed change from baseline in the vorozole treatment arm but not in the megestrol acetate arm, and worsening in scores as the disease progressed;[178] similar findings were reported in a trial of women with metastatic breast cancer.[179] In a study of persons with AIDS-related non-Hodgkin's lymphoma, FLIC scores declined in a subset of patients who developed febrile neutropenia.[175] These studies illustrate that, although not assessed in its developmental stage, the FLIC is responsive to change in response to treatment and disease state. FLIC scores have also been shown to be responsive in studies of surgical and radiologic interventions.[177,183,184] Like other general

cancer instruments, the FLIC has been used less frequently in the other three stages of the cancer care continuum. As illustrated above by the question examples, the content of the FLIC seems less suitable for use with relatively healthy individuals and patients with advanced disease than for persons receiving cancer treatment.

Rotterdam Symptom Checklist

Conceptual, practical, and measurement features

The RSCL was developed to assess symptoms experienced by cancer patients who were participating in clinical research studies.[185,186] Symptoms included in the RSCL were derived from the Dutch version of the Symptom Check List[187] developed for use with breast cancer patients,[188] the Symptom Distress Scale,[189] and the advice of psychologists and oncologists. The RSCL psychological distress symptom subscale includes depressed mood, irritability, nervousness, tension, and worrying. Information about the format of the RSCL and its measurement properties is given in Table 3.2.

The RSCL was one of the first general cancer instruments developed in Europe. Familiarity plus ease of use helped to make this scale widely used in European studies, especially prior to the development of the EORTC QLQ-C30. This usage was boosted by the recommendation that the RSCL be adopted for use in cancer clinical trials sponsored by the British Medical Research Council.[25]

Performance across the cancer continuum

The RSCL has been used in slightly less than 15% of all empirical reports that discuss the measurement of health status and quality of life in cancer patients. There is a tendency, however, to use a modified instrument, this being the case in approximately one-third of articles that report on the use of the RSCL. Several articles assess measurement properties of the full RSCL in the post-development stage, as shown in Table 3.2.

In addition to being widely used in persons with breast, colorectal, and lung cancer, the RSCL has been used in a wide range of diagnoses which include esophageal, liver, and renal neoplasms;[32,190,191] it has rarely been used, however, in men with prostate cancer. The most common use of the RSCL within the context of the cancer continuum is in the study of alternative chemotherapeutic agents.[27,191–194] Clinical research study in persons with advanced or metastatic breast cancer showed differences in psychologic subscale scores according to degree of toxicity recorded.[27] The RSCL has infrequently been used to study outcomes of other types of treatments, including surgery and transplantation, as well as outcomes of cancer survivors and patients at the end of life.

Summary: use of general cancer instruments within the cancer arena

The five general cancer instruments discussed above have been used in people with different diagnoses with no apparent instrument-by-diagnosis clustering. As was observed for the generic measures, the general cancer measures are more likely to be used in the treatment stage than other stages of the cancer continuum. The tendency for some instruments to be more often used in studies involving chemotherapy is to some extent attributable to organizational units that have supported the use and interpretation of findings from the EORTC QLQ-C30, FACT-G, and the RSCL. In addition to lacking this support, the CARES and FLIC have had less extensive evaluation of their measurement properties in both the development and post-development stages of their development. More detailed information is provided in Table 3.2.

Methodological and practical issues for future research

This review indicates that researchers are using, and cancer patients are willing to complete, questionnaire-based instruments that use a common scoring system to provide information on two or more key domains of health-related quality of life to assess outcomes and status. Further, usage is observed across a wide range of cancer diagnoses and stages of disease for all of the instruments reviewed, demonstrating construct validity for both the generic and general cancer instruments beyond the population groups for which these instruments were initially developed.

While considerable empirical evidence in the post-development stage exists for validation across a variety of patient groups, the tendency for these instruments to be used almost exclusively in clinical research studies provides little validation evidence to support their use with cancer survivors or patients at the end of life or in cancer screening programs designed to prevent disease. This selectivity of use can be attributed to item content for some instruments; for example, the general statements of functioning and well-being in the SIP have been judged inappropriate for premenopausal women with breast cancer.[26] Preference for selected instruments might also stem from a content validation process that, for example, would reveal that instruments developed for use in clinical trials of cancer therapies might be less than ideal for screening programs of essentially healthy individuals.

Other possible factors responsible for the preponderance of use in the treatment stage of the cancer continuum are: (1) a relative paucity of policy initiatives directed at the other stages of the cancer continuum; (2) an emphasis on research reports rather than clinical practice applications by purveyors of routinely searched databases; and (3) inadequate attention to transferring the technology of outcomes assessment methods beyond the research community. While solutions to issues (1) and (2) are possible, it is the last that can most easily be changed by the oncology community, broadly defined. For example, use of outcomes measures in prevention and clinical applications might be encouraged through publication in non-research-oriented medical and health journals and presentations aimed at clinical practitioners.

This transfer of health-related quality-of-life assessment technology to wider use will also be enhanced as interpretability of findings becomes clearer. An important aspect for interpretation is the availability of normative data. Comparing findings from research studies with data from reference populations allows investigators, health care managers, and policy makers to better understand the implications of their decisions. Further, normative data that are routinely available across time can help with differentiating changes in health that may be due to treatment and policy from those that might be due to factors external to the health care system.[195] Without compromising patient confidentiality, data on health status and quality of life that have been privately collected might provide normative information if made publicly available. Research on these data, as well as on data from large-scale general population surveys, is important if we are to more fully understand impacts of health policies as well as of factors external to the health care system, such as periods of economic growth and recession, on health outcomes.

This review suggests that no currently available, single generic or general cancer instrument has been widely accepted for use across the cancer continuum. Findings from this evaluation indicate that measures are more likely to be used if they are relatively short and have content that is relevant to the target population. Existing instruments, especially those that combine general measures with specific modules, suggest a framework by which a measurement system for evaluating outcomes across the range of cancer concerns, i.e., from screening and prevention to end of life, can be developed. The development of such a measurement system deserves serious consideration if clinical, community, and national decision makers are to have information to implement treatment and intervention policies that are reflective of the quality-of-life concerns of cancer patients and their families.

REFERENCES

1 Brown, M. L., Lipscomb, J., Snyder, C. (2001). The burden of illness of cancer: economic cost and quality of life. *Annual Review of Public Health* **22**:91–113.

2 Janknegt, R. (2001). Using health outcomes data to inform decision-making: formulary committee perspective. *Pharmacoeconomics* **19**(Suppl. 2):49–52.

3 Lancry, P.-J., O'Connor, R., Stempel, D. *et al.* (2001). Using health outcomes data to inform decision-making: healthcare payer perspective. *Pharmacoeconomics* **19**(Suppl. 2):39–47.

4 Taylor, R. (2001). Using health outcomes data to inform decision-making: government agency perspective. *Pharmacoeconomics* **19**(Suppl. 2):33–8.

5 Lipscomb, J., Snyder, C. F. (2002). The outcomes of cancer outcomes research: focusing on the National Cancer Institute's Quality-of-Care Initiative. *Medical Care* **40**(Suppl. 6):III3–III10.

6 National Center for Health Statistics (2002). *Health, United States, 2002 With Chartbook on Trends in the Health of Americans.* Hyattsville, MD: National Center for Health Statistics.

7 Gilson, B. S., Gilson, J. S., Bergner, M. *et al.* (1975). The Sickness Impact Profile: development of an outcome measure of health care. *American Journal of Public Health* **65**(12):1304–10.

8 Bergner, M., Bobbitt, R. A., Carter, W. B. *et al.* (1981). The Sickness Impact Profile: development and final revision of a health status measure. *Medical Care* **19**(8):787–805.

9 Stewart, A. L., Hays, R. D., Ware, J. E., Jr. (1988). The MOS Short-Form General Health Survey: reliability and validity in a patient population. *Medical Care* **26**(7):724–32.

10 Ware, J. E., Jr., Sherbourne, C. D. (1992). The MOS 36-Item Short-Form Health Survey (SF-36): I. Conceptual framework and item selection. *Medical Care* **30**(6):473–83.

11 Ware, J. E., Kosinski, M., Keller, S. D. (1996). A 12-Item Short-Form Health Survey (SF-12): Scale Construction and preliminary tests of reliability and validity. Boston, MA: Medical Outcomes Trust.

12 Aaronson, N. K., Ahmedzai, S., Bergman, B. *et al.* (1993). The European Organization for Research and Treatment of Cancer QLQ-C30: a quality of life instrument for use in international clinical trials in oncology. *Journal of the National Cancer Institute* **85**(5):365–76.

13 Cella, D. F., Tulsky, D. S., Gray, G. *et al.* (1993). The Functional Assessment of Cancer Therapy Scale: development and validation of the general measure. *Journal of Clinical Oncology* **11**(3):570–9.

14 Grassi, L., Indelli, M., Marzola, M. *et al.* (1996). Depressive symptoms and quality of life in home-care-assisted cancer patients. *Journal of Pain and Symptom Management* **12**(5):300–7.

15 Klee, M. C., King, M. T., Machin, D. *et al.* (2000). A clinical model for quality of life assessment in cancer patients receiving chemotherapy. *Annals of Oncology* **11**(1):23–30.

16 McWhinney, I. R., Bass, M. J., Donner, A. (1994). Evaluation of a palliative care service: problems and pitfalls. *British Medical Journal* **309**(6965):1340–2.

17 Witteveen, P. O., Jacobs, H. M., van Groenestijn, M. A. C. *et al.* (1999). Assessment of the quality of life of patients with advanced and end-stage cancer or serious infections with a symptom-based or an impact-based instrument. *Supportive Care in Cancer* **7**(2):64–70.

18 Erickson, P., Scott, J. (1993). The On-Line Guide to Quality-of-Life Assessment (OLGA): Resource for Selecting Quality-of-Life Assessments. In *Quality of Life Assessment: Key Issues in the 1990s*, ed. S. R. Walker, R. M. Rosser, pp. 221–32. Dordrecht, The Netherlands: Kluwer Academic Publishers.

19 Feeny, this volume, Chapter 4.

20 Patrick, D. L., Erickson, P. (1993). *Health Status and Health Policy: Quality of Life in Health Care Evaluation and Resource Allocation.* New York: Oxford University Press.

21 Erickson, P. (2000). Assessment of the evaluative properties of health status instruments. *Medical Care* **38**(Suppl. 9): S95–9.

22 Aaronson, this volume, Chapter 20.

23 Snaith, R. P. (1987). The concepts and assessment of depression in oncology. *Journal of Psychosocial Oncology* **5**(3): 133–9.

24 Zigmond, A. S., Snaith, R. P. (1983). The Hospital Anxiety and Depression Scale. *Acta Psychiatrica Scandinavica* **67**(6): 361–70.

25 Maguire, P., Selby, P. (1989). Assessing the quality of life in cancer patients. *British Journal of Cancer* **60**:437–40.

26 Nystedt, M., Berglund, G., Bolund, C. *et al.* (2000). Randomized trial of adjuvant tamoxifen and/or goserelin in premenopausal breast cancer: self-rated physiological effects and symptoms. *Acta Oncologica* **39**(8):959–68.

27 Howell, S. J., Radford, J. A., Adams, J. E. *et al.* (2001). Randomized placebo-controlled trial of testosterone replacement in men with mild Leydig Cell Insufficiency following cytotoxic chemotherapy. *Clinical Endocrinology* **55**(3): 315–34.

28 Razavi, D., Kormoss, N., Collard, A. *et al.* (1999). Comparative study of the efficacy and safety of trazodone versus clorazepate in the treatment of adjustment disorders in cancer patients: a pilot study. *Journal of International Medical Research* **27**(6):264–72.

29 Ranson, M. R., Jayson, G., Perkins, S. *et al.* (1997). Single-agent paclitaxel in advanced non-small cell lung cancer: single-center phase II study using a 3-hour administration schedule. *Seminars in Oncology* **24**(4 Suppl. 12): 6–9.

30 Smyth, J. F., Bowman, A., Perren, T. *et al.* (1997). Glutathione reduces the toxicity and improves quality of life of women diagnosed with ovarian cancer treated with cisplatin: results of a double-blind, randomised trial. *Annals of Oncology* **8**(6):569–73.

31 Bleehen, N. M., Girling, D. J., Hopwood, P. *et al.* (1996). Randomised trial of four-drug vs less intensive two-drug chemotherapy in the palliative treatment of patients with small-cell lung cancer (SCLC) and poor prognosis. *British Journal of Cancer* **73**(3):406–13.

32 Joffe, J. K., Banks, R. E., Forbes, M. A. *et al.* (1996). A Phase II study of interferon-alpha, interleukin-2 and 5-fluorouracil in advanced renal carcinoma: clinical data and laboratory evidence of protease activation. *British Journal of Urology* **77**(5):638–49.

33 Seymour, M. T., Slevin, M. L., Kerr, D. J. *et al.* (1996). Randomized trial assessing the addition of interferon alpha-2a to fluorouracil and leucovorin in advanced colorectal cancer. *Journal of Clinical Oncology* **14**(8):2280–8.

34 Harper-Wynne, C., English, J., Meyer, L. *et al.* (1999). Randomized trial to compare the efficacy and toxicity of cyclophosphamide, methotrexate and 5-fluorouracil (CMF) with methotrexate mitoxantrone (MM) in advanced carcinoma of the breast. *British Journal of Cancer* **81**(2):316–22.

35 Hammerlid, E., Mercke, C., Sullivan, M. *et al.* (1997). A prospective quality of life study of patients with oral or pharyngeal carcinoma treated with external beam irradiation with or without brachytherapy. *Oral Oncology* **33**(3):189–96.

36 Gregor, A., Cull, A., Stephens, R. J. *et al.* (1997). Prophylactic cranial irradiation is indicated following complete response to induction therapy in small cell lung cancer: results of a multicentre randomised trial. *European Journal of Cancer* **33**(11):1752–8.

37 Griffiths, G. O., Parmar, M. K. B., Bailey, A. J. (1999). Physical and psychological symptoms of quality of life in the CHART randomized trial in head and neck cancer: short-term and long-term patient reported symptoms. *British Journal of Cancer* **81**(7):1196–205.

38 Gaze, M. N., Kelly, C. G., Kerr, G. R. *et al.* (1997). Pain relief and quality of life following radiotherapy for bone metastases: a randomised trial of two fractionation schedules. *Radiotherapy and Oncology* **45**(2):109–16.

39 Hjermstad, M. J., Loge, J. H., Evensen, S. A. *et al.* (1999). The course of anxiety and depression during the first year after allogeneic or autologous stem cell transplantation. *Bone Marrow Transplantation* **24**(11):1219–28.

40 Loge, J. H., Abrahamsen, A. F., Ekeberg, O. *et al.* (2000). Fatigue and psychiatric morbidity among Hodgkin's disease survivors. *Journal of Pain and Symptom Management* **19**(2):91–9.

41 Olweny, C. L. M., Juttner, C. A., Rofe, P. *et al.* (1993). Long-term effects of cancer treatment and consequences of cure: cancer survivors enjoy quality of life similar to their neighbours. *European Journal of Cancer* **29A**(6):826–30.

42 Cull, A., Gregor, A., Hopwood, P. *et al.* (1994). Neurological and cognitive impairment in long-term survivors of small cell lung cancer. *European Journal of Cancer* **30A**(8): 1067–74.

43 Molassiotis, A., Boughton, B. J., Burgoyne, T. *et al.* (1995). Comparison of the overall quality of life in 50 long-term survivors of autologous and allogeneic bone marrow transplantation. *Journal of Advanced Nursing* **22**:509–16.

44 Stromgren, A. S., Groenvold, M., Pedersen, L. *et al.* (2001). Does the medical record cover the symptoms experienced by cancer patients receiving palliative care? A comparison of the record and patient self-rating. *Journal of Pain and Symptom Management* **21**(3):189–96.

45 Payne, S. A. (1992). A study of quality of life in cancer patients receiving palliative chemotherapy. *Social Science and Medicine* **35**(12):1505–9.

46 Macbeth, F. R., Bolger, J. J., Hopwood, P. *et al.* (1996). Randomized trial of palliative two-fraction versus more intensive 13-fraction radiotherapy for patients with inoperable non-small cell lung cancer and good performance status. *Clinical Oncology* **8**(3):167–75.

47 Bratt, O., Damber, J.-E., Emanuelsson, M. *et al.* (2000). Risk perception, screening practice and interest in genetic testing among unaffected men in families with hereditary prostate cancer. *European Journal of Cancer* **36**(2): 235–41.

48 Brandberg, Y., Bolund, C., Michelson, H. *et al.* (1993). Psychological reactions in public melanoma screening. *European Journal of Cancer* **29A**(6):860–3.

49 Scaf-Klomp, W., Sanderman, R., van de Wiel, H. B. M. *et al.* (1997). Distressed or relieved? Psychological side effects of breast cancer screening in the Netherlands. *Journal of Epidemiology and Community Health* **51**(6):705–10.

50 Brook, R. H., Ware, J. E., Jr., Rodgers, W. H. *et al.* (1983). Does free care improve adults' health? Results from a randomized controlled trial. *New England Journal of Medicine* **309**(23):1426–34.

51 Tarlov, A. R., Ware, J. E., Jr., Greenfield, S. *et al.* (1989). The Medical Outcomes Study: an application of methods for monitoring the results of medical care. *Journal of the American Medical Association* **262**(7):925–30.

52 Ware, J. E., Sherbourne, C. D., Davies, A. R. (1992). Developing and Testing the MOS 20-Item Short Form Health Survey: A General Population Application. In *Measuring Functioning and Well-Being: The Medical Outcomes Study Approach*, ed. A. L. Stewart, J. E. Ware, pp. 277–290. Durham, NC: Duke University Press.

53 Ware, J. E., Jr., Snow, K. K., Kosinski, M. *et al.* (1993). *SF-36 Health Survey: Manual and Interpretation Guide*. Boston, MA: Health Institute.

54 Brandberg, Y., Malm, M., Blomqvist, L. A. (2000). Prospective and randomized study, "SVEA," comparing effects of three methods for delayed breast reconstruction on quality of life, patient-defined problem areas of life, and the cosmetic result. *Plastic and Reconstructive Surgery* **105**(1): 66–74.

55 McGuire, M. S., Grimaldi, G., Grotas, J. *et al.* (2000). The type of urinary diversion after radical cystectomy significantly impacts on the patient's quality of life. *Annals of Surgical Oncology* **7**(1):4–8.

56 Veenstra, K. M., Sprangers, M. A. G., van der Eyken, J.-W. (2000). Quality of life in survivors with a Van Ness-Borggreve rotationplasty after bone tumour resection. *Journal of Surgical Oncology* **73**(4):192–7.

57 Fujisawa, M., Isotani, S., Gotoh, A. *et al.* (2000). Health-related quality of life with orthotopic neobladder versus ileal conduit according to the SF-36 survey. *Urology* **55**(6):862–5.

58 Neil-Dwyer, G., Lang, D. A., Davis, A. (2000). Outcome from complex neurosurgery: an evidence-based approach. *Acta Neurochirurgica* **142**(4):367–71.

59 Naughton, C. K., Miller, D. C., Yan, Y. (2001). Impact of transrectal ultrasound guided prostate biopsy on quality of life: a prospective randomized trial comparing 6 versus 12 cores. *Journal of Urology* **165**(1):100–3.

60 Rogers, S. N., Lowe, D., Humphris, G. (2000). Distinct patient groups in oral cancer: a prospective study of perceived health status following primary surgery. *Oral Oncology* **36**(6):529–38.

61 de Boer, A. G. E. M., Onorbe Genovesi, P. I., Sprangers, M. A. G. *et al.* (2000). Quality of life in long-term survivors after curative transhiatal oesophagectomy for oesophageal carcinoma. *British Journal of Surgery* **87**(12): 1716–21.

62 Thompson-Fawcett, M. W., Richard, C. S., O'Connor, B. I. *et al.* (2000). Quality of life is excellent after a pelvic pouch for colitis-associated neoplasia. *Diseases of the Colon and Rectum* **43**(11):1497–502.

63 Clark, P. E., Schover, L. R., Uzzo, R. G. *et al.* (2001). Quality of life and psychological adaptation after surgical treatment

for localized renal cell carcinoma: impact of the amount of remaining renal tissue. *Urology* **57**(2):252–6.

64 Davis, A. M., Devlin, M., Griffin, A. M. *et al.* (1999). Functional outcome in amputation versus limb sparing patients with lower extremity sarcoma: a matched case-control study. *Archives of Physical Medicine and Rehabilitation* **80**(6):615–18.

65 Janda, M., Gerstner, N., Obermair, A. *et al.* (2000). Quality of life changes during conformal radiation therapy for prostate carcinoma. *Cancer* **89**(6):1322–8.

66 Sanchez-Ortiz, R. F., Broderick, G. A., Rovner, E. S. *et al.* (2000). Erectile function and quality of life after interstitial radiation therapy for prostate cancer. *International Journal of Impotence Research* **12**(Suppl. 3): S18–24.

67 Beard, C. J., Propert, K. J., Rieker, P. P. *et al.* (1997). Complications after treatment with external-beam irradiation in early-stage prostate cancer patients: a prospective multi-institutional outcomes study. *Journal of Clinical Oncology* **15**(1):223–9.

68 Ganz, P. A., Greendale, G. A., Petersen, L. *et al.* (2000). Managing menopausal symptoms in breast cancer survivors: results of a randomized controlled trial. *Journal of the National Cancer Institute* **92**(13):1054–64.

69 Hammerlid, E., Taft, C. (2001). Health-related quality of life in long-term head and neck cancer survivors: a comparison with general population norms. *British Journal of Cancer* **84**(2):149–56.

70 Vickberg, S. M. J., Duhamel, K. N., Smith, M. Y. *et al.* (2001). Global meaning and psychological adjustment among survivors of bone marrow transplant. *Psycho-Oncology* **10**(1):29–39.

71 Loge, J. H., Abrahamsen, A. F., Ekeberg, O. *et al.* (1999). Reduced health-related quality of life among Hodgkin's disease survivors: a comparative study with general population norms. *Annals of Oncology* **10**(1):71–7.

72 Litwin, M. S., Shpall, A. I., Dorey, F. *et al.* (1998). Quality-of-life outcomes in long-term survivors of advanced prostate cancer. *American Journal of Clinical Oncology* **21**(4): 327–32.

73 QualityMetrics, Inc. Medical Outcomes Study instruments and measurement tools. Available at: www.qualitymetric.com. Last accessed October 17, 2002.

74 Hyland, M. E. (2002). Recommendations from quality of life scales are not simple (letter). *British Medical Journal* **325**:599.

75 McNair, D. M., Lorr, M., Droppleman, L. F. (1971/1981). *EITS Manual for the Profile of Mood States*. San Diego, CA: Educational and Industrial Testing Service.

76 Cella, D. F., Jacobsen, P. B., Orav, E. J. *et al.* (1987). A brief POMS measure of distress for cancer patients. *Journal of Chronic Diseases* **40**(10):939–42.

77 Guadagnoli, E., Mor, V. (1989). Measuring cancer patients' affect: revision and psychometric properties of the Profile of Mood States (POMS). *Journal of Consulting and Clinical Psychology* **84**:907–15.

78 Shacham, S. (1983). A shortened version of the Profile of Mood States. *Journal of Personality Assessment* **47**(3): 305–6.

79 Bunevicius, R., Kazanavicius, G., Zalinkevicius, R. *et al.* (1999). Effects of thyroxine as compared with thyroxine plus triiodothyronine in patients with hypothyroidism. *New England Journal of Medicine* **340**(6):424–9.

80 Postma, T. J., Heimans, J. J., Luykx, S. A. *et al.* (2000). A phase II study of paclitaxel in chemonaive patients with recurrent high-grade glioma. *Annals of Oncology* **11**(4):409–43.

81 Ahles, T. A., Silberfarb, P. M., Herndon II, J. *et al.* (1998). Psychologic and neuropsychologic functioning of patients with limited small-cell lung cancer treated with chemotherapy and radiation therapy with or without warfarin: a study by the Cancer and Leukemia Group B. *Journal of Clinical Oncology* **16**(5):1954–60.

82 Heinonen, H., Volin, L., Uutela, A. *et al.* (2001). Quality of life and factors related to perceived satisfaction with quality of life after allogeneic bone marrow transplantation. *Annals of Hematology* **80**(3):137–43.

83 Fife, B. L., Huster, G. A., Cornetta, K. G. *et al.* (2000). Longitudinal study of adaptation to the stress of bone marrow transplantation. *Journal of Clinical Oncology* **18**(7):1539–49.

84 Nissen, M. J., Swenson, K. K., Ritz, L. J. *et al.* (2001). Quality of life after breast carcinoma surgery: a comparison of three surgical procedures. *Cancer* **91**(7):1238–46.

85 Braslis, K. G., Santa-Cruz, C., Brickman, A. L. *et al.* (1995). Quality of life 12 months after radical prostatectomy. *British Journal of Urology* **75**(1):48–53.

86 Jason, G. W., Pajurkova, E. M., Taenzer, P. A. *et al.* (1997). Acute effects on neuropsychological function and quality of life by high-dose multiple daily fractionated radiotherapy for malignant astrocytomas: assessing the tolerability of a new radiotherapy regimen. *Psycho-Oncology* **6**(2): 151–7.

87 Greenberg, D. B., Kornblith, A. B., Herndon, J. E. *et al.* (1997). Quality of life for adult leukemia survivors treated on clinical trials of cancer and leukemia Group B during the period 1971–1988: predictors for later psychologic distress. *Cancer* **80**(10):1936–44.

88 Gotay, C. C., Muraoka, M. Y. (1998). Quality of life in long-term survivors of adult-onset cancers. *Journal of the National Cancer Institute* **90**(9):656–67.

89 Haidet, P., Hamel, M. B., Davis, R. B. *et al.* (1998). Outcomes, preferences for resuscitation, and physician-patient communication among patients with metastatic colorectal cancer. *American Journal of Medicine* **105**(3):222–9.

90 Paterson, D. L., Gayowski, T., Wannstedt, C. F. *et al.* (2000). Quality of life in long-term survivors after liver transplantation: impact of recurrent viral hepatitis C virus. *Hepatitis. Clinical Transplantation* **4**(1):48–54.

91 Holland, J. C., Silberfarb, P., Tross, S. *et al.* (1986). Psychosocial research in cancer: the Cancer and Leukemia Group B (CALGB) experience. In *Assessment of Quality of Life and Cancer Treatment*, ed. V. Ventafridda, F. S. A. M. van Dam, R. Yancik *et al.*, pp. 89–101. New York, NY: Elsevier Science Publishers.

92 Spitzer, W. O., Dobson, A. J., Hall, J. *et al.* (1981). Measuring the quality of life of cancer patients: a concise QL-Index for use by physicians. *Journal of Chronic Diseases* **34**(12): 585–97.

93 Lipton, A., Theriault, R. L., Hortobagyi, G. N. *et al.* (2000). Pamidronate prevents skeletal complications and is effective palliative treatment in women with breast carcinoma and osteolytic bone metastases: long term follow-up of two randomized, placebo-controlled trials. *Cancer* **88**(5): 1082–90.

94 Berr, F., Wiedmann, M., Tannapfel, A. *et al.* (2000). Photodynamic therapy for advanced bile duct cancer: evidence for improved palliation and extended survival. *Hepatology* **31**(2):291–8.

95 Mor, V., Stalker, M. Z., Gralla, R. *et al.* (1988). Day hospital as an alternative to inpatient care for cancer patients: a random assignment trial. *Journal of Clinical Epidemiology* **41**(8):771–85.

96 Leo, E., Audisio, R. A., Belli, F. (1994). Total rectal resection and colo-anal anastomosis for low rectal tumours: comparative results in a group of young and old patients. *European Journal of Cancer* **30A**(8):1092–5.

97 Knight, S. J., Chmiel, J. S., Kuzel, T. *et al.* (1998). Quality of life in metastatic prostate cancer among men of lower socioeconomic status: feasibility and criterion related validity of 3 measures. *Journal of Urology* **160**(5):1765–9.

98 Hortobagyi, G. N., Theriault, R. L., Lipton, A. *et al.* (1998). Long-term prevention of skeletal complications of metastatic breast cancer with pamidronate. *Journal of Clinical Oncology* **16**(6):2038–44.

99 Riccardi, A., Tinelli, C., Brugnatelli, S. *et al.* (2000). Doubling of the epirubicin dosage within the 5-fluorouracil, epirubicin and cyclophosphamide regimen: a prospective, randomized, multicentric study on antitumor effect and quality of life in advanced breast cancer. *International Journal of Oncology* **16**(4):769–76.

100 Theriault, R. L., Lipton, A., Hortobagyi, G. N. (1999). Pamidronate reduces skeletal morbidity in women with advanced breast cancer and lytic bone lesions: a randomized, placebo-controlled trial. *Journal of Clinical Oncology* **17**(3):846–54.

101 Roseveare, C. D., Patel, P., Simmonds, N. *et al.* (1998). Nutrition and survival in malignant oesophageal stenosis: a randomized controlled trial comparing modified Gianturco Z-Stents with plastic Atkinson tubes. *European Journal of Gastroenterology and Hepatology* **10**(8):653–7.

102 Wu, C.-W., Hsieh, M.-C., Lo, Su-S. *et al.* (1997). Quality of life of patients with gastric adenocarcinoma after curative gastrectomy. *World Journal of Surgery* **21**(7): 777–82.

103 Wu, C.-W., Lo, S.-S., Shen, K.-H. *et al.* (2000). Surgical mortality, survival, and quality of life after resection for gastric cancer in the elderly. *World Journal of Surgery* **24**(4): 465–72.

104 Barr, H., Krasner, N., Raouf, A. *et al.* (1990). Prospective randomized trial of laser therapy only and laser therapy followed by endoscopic intubation for the palliation of malignant dysphagia. *Gut* **31**(1):252–8.

105 Donnelly, S., Rybicki, L., Walsh, D. (2001). Quality of life measurement in the palliative management of advanced cancer. *Supportive Care in Cancer* **9**(5):361–5.

106 Hinton, J. (1994). Can home care maintain an acceptable quality of life for patients with terminal cancer and their relatives? *Palliative Medicine* **8**(3):183–96.

107 Hinton, J. (1994). Which patients with terminal cancer are admitted from home care? *Palliative Medicine* **8**(3): 197–210.

108 de Bruin, A. F., Buys, M., de Witte, L. P. *et al.* (1994). The Sickness Impact Profile: SIP68, a short generic version. First evaluation of the reliability and reproducibility. *Journal of Clinical Epidemiology* **47**(8):863–71.

109 Dales, R. E., Belanger, R., Shamji, F. M. *et al.* (1994). Quality-of-life following thoracotomy for lung cancer. *Journal of Clinical Epidemiology* **47**(12):1443–9.

110 Wu, A. W., Damiano, A. M., Lynn, J. *et al.* (1995). Predicting future functional status for seriously ill hospitalized adults: the SUPPORT prognostic model. *Annals of Internal Medicine* **122**(5):342–50.

111 Tsevat, J., Cook, E. F., Green, M. L. *et al.* (1994). Health values of the seriously ill. *Annals of Internal Medicine* **122**(7): 514–20.

112 Durand-Zaleski, I., Earlam, S., Fordy, C. *et al.* (1998). Cost-effectiveness of systemic and regional chemotherapy for the treatment of patients with unresectable colorectal liver metastases. *Cancer* **83**(5):882–8.

113 Earlam, S., Glover, C., Davies, M. *et al.* (1997). Effect of regional and systemic fluorinated pyrimidine chemotherapy on quality of life in colorectal liver metastasis patients. *Journal of Clinical Oncology* **15**(5):2022–9.

114 Langius, A., Bjorvell, H., Lind, M. G. (1994). Functional status and coping in patients with oral and pharyngeal cancer before and after surgery. *Head and Neck* **16**(6): 559–68.

115 Hassan, S. J., Weymuller, Jr., E. A. (1993). Assessment of quality of life in head and neck cancer patients. *Head and Neck* **15**(6):485–96.

116 Tenover, J. L., Pagano, G. A., Morton, A. S. *et al.* (1997). Efficacy and tolerability of finasteride in symptomatic benign prostatic hyperplasia: a primary care study. *Clinical Therapeutics* **19**(2):243–58.

117 McLeod, R. S., Taylor, B. R., O'Connor, B. I. *et al.* (1995). Quality of life, nutritional status, and gastrointestinal hormone profile following the Whipple procedure. *American Journal of Surgery* **169**(1):179–85.

118 Svedlund, J., Sullivan, M., Liedman, B. *et al.* (1997). Quality of life after gastrectomy for gastric carcinoma: controlled study of reconstructive procedures. *World Journal of Surgery* **21**(4):422–33.

119 McDowell, I., Newell, C. (1987). *Measuring Health: A Guide to Rating Scales and Questionnaires*. New York: Oxford University Press.

120 Patrick, D. L., Deyo, R. (1989). Generic and disease-specific measures in assessing health status and quality of life. *Medical Care* **27**:S217–23.

121 Ganz, P. A., Schag, C. A. C., Lee, J. J. *et al.* (1992). The CARES: A generic measure of health-related quality of life for patients with cancer. *Quality of Life Research* **1**(1):19–29.

122 Heinrich, R. L., Schag, C. A. C., Ganz, P. A. (1984). Living with cancer: the cancer inventory of problem situations. *Journal of Clinical Psychology* **40**:972–80.

123 Schag, C. A. C., Heinrich, R. L., Ganz, P. A. (1983). Cancer inventory of problem situations: an instrument for assessing cancer patients' rehabilitation needs. *Journal of Psychosocial Oncology* **1**:11–24.

124 Ganz, P. A., Schag, C. A. C., Cheng, H.-L. (1990). Assessing the quality of life – a study in newly-diagnosed breast cancer patients. *Journal of Clinical Epidemiology* **43**(1):75–86.

125 Schag, C. A., Heinrich, R. L. (1990). Development of a comprehensive quality of life measurement tool: CARES. *Oncology* **4**:135–8.

126 Schag, C. A. C., Ganz, P. A., Heinrich, R. L. (1991). Cancer Rehabilitation Evaluation System – Short Form (CARES-SF): a cancer specific rehabilitation and quality of life instrument. *Cancer* **68**(6):1406–13.

127 Cramer, J. A., Arrigo, C., Van Hammee, G. *et al.* (2000). Comparison between the QOLIE-31 and Derived QOLIE-10 in a clinical trial of levetiracetam. *Epilepsy Research* **41**(1): 29–38.

128 Devinsky, O., Vickrey, B. G., Cramer, J. *et al.* (1995). Development of the quality of life in Epilepsy Inventory. *Epilepsia* **36**(11):1089–104.

129 Frost, M. H., Suman, V. J., Rummans, T. A. *et al.* (2000). Physical, psychological and social well-being of women with breast cancer: the influence of disease phase. *Psycho-Oncology* **9**(3):221–31.

130 Herth, K. (2000). Enhancing hope in people with a first recurrence of cancer. *Journal of Advanced Nursing* **32**(6):1431–41.

131 Rustoen, T., Wiklund, I., Hanestad, B. R. *et al.* (1998). Nursing intervention to increase hope and quality of life in newly diagnosed cancer patients. *Cancer Nursing* **21**(4): 235–45.

132 Hawighorst-Knapstein, S., Schonefuss, G., Hoffmann, S. O. *et al.* (1997). Pelvic exenteration: effects of surgery on quality of life and body image – a prospective longitudinal study. *Gynecologic Oncology* **66**(3):495–500.

133 Ganz, P. A., Schag, C. A. C., Lee, J. J. *et al.* (1992). Breast conservation versus mastectomy: is there a difference in psychological adjustment or quality of life in the year after surgery? *Cancer* **69**(7):1729–38.

134 Glimelius, B., Birgegard, G., Hoffman, K. *et al.* (1992). Improved care of patients with small cell lung cancer: nutritional and quality of life aspects. *Acta Oncologica* **31**(8): 823–31.

135 Litwin, M. S., Fine, J. T., Dorey, F. *et al.* (1997). Health related quality of life outcomes in patients treated for metastatic kidney cancer: a pilot study. *Journal of Urology* **157**(5): 1608–12.

136 Schag, C. A. C., Ganz, P. A., Wing, D. S. *et al.* (1994). Quality of life in adult survivors of lung, colon and prostate cancer. *Quality of Life Research* **3**:127–41.

137 Wellisch, D. K., Centeno, J., Guzman, J. *et al.* (1996). Bone marrow transplantation vs. high-dose cytorabine-based consolidation chemotherapy for acute myelogenous leukemia: a long-term follow-up study of quality-of-life measures of survivors. *Psychosomatics* **37**(2):144–54.

138 Ashing-Giwa, K., Ganz, P. A., Petersen, L. (1999). Quality of life of African-American and white long term breast carcinoma survivors. *Cancer* **85**(2):418–26.

139 Gritz, E. R., Carmack, C. L., de Moor, C. *et al.* (1999). First year after head and neck cancer: quality of life. *Journal of Clinical Oncology* **17**(1):352–60.

140 Sprangers, M. A. G., Cull, A., Groenvold, M. *et al.* (1998). The European Organization for Research and Treatment of Cancer approach to developing questionnaire modules: an update and overview. *Quality of Life Research* **7**:291–300.

141 Aaronson, N. K., Cull, A. M., Kaasa, S. *et al.* (1996). The European Organization for Research and Treatment of Cancer (EORTC) modular approach to quality of life assessment in oncology: an update. In *Quality of Life and Pharmacoeconomics in Clinical Trials* (2nd Edition), ed. B. Spilker, pp. 179–89. Philadelphia, PA: Lippincott-Raven Publishers.

142 Bjordal, K., Ahlmer-Elmqvist, M., Tollesson, E. *et al.* (1994). Development of a European Organization for Research and Treatment of Cancer (EORTC) questionnaire module to be used in quality of life assessments in head and neck cancer patients. *Acta Oncologica* **33**(8):879–85.

143 Borghede, G., Sullivan, M. (1996). Measurement of quality of life in localized prostatic cancer patients treated with radiotherapy. Development of a prostate cancer-specific module supplementing the EORTC QLQ-C30. *Quality of Life Research* **5**(2):212–22.

144 Detmar, S. B., Aaronson, N. K. (1998). Quality of life assessment in daily clinical oncology practice: a feasibility study. *European Journal of Cancer* **34**(8):1181–6.

145 Macquart-Moulin, G., Viens, P., Palangie, T. *et al.* (2000). High-dose sequential chemotherapy with recombinant granulocyte colony-stimulating factor and repeated stem-cell support for inflammatory breast cancer patients: does impact on quality of life jeopardize feasibility and acceptability of treatment? *Journal of Clinical Oncology* **18**(4):754–64.

146 Morant, R., Bernhard, J., Maibach, R. *et al.* (2000). Response and palliation in a phase II trial of gemcitabine in hormone-refractory metastatic prostatic carcinoma. *Annals of Oncology* **11**(2):183–8.

147 Rauch, D. P., Maurer, C. A., Aebi, S. *et al.* (2001). Activity of gemcitabine and continuous infusion fluorouracil in advanced pancreatic cancer. *Oncology* **60**(1):43–8.

148 Simons, J. P., Aaronson, N. K., Vansteenkiste, J. F. *et al.* (1996). Effects of medroxyprogesterone acetate on appetite, weight, and quality of life in advanced-stage non-hormone-sensitive cancer: a placebo-controlled multicenter study. *Journal of Clinical Oncology* **14**(4):1077–84.

149 Hoffman, K., Glimelius, B. (1998). Evaluation of clinical benefit of chemotherapy in patients with upper gastrointestinal cancer. *Acta Oncologica* **37**(7–8):651–9.

150 Osoba, D., Brada, M., Prados, M. D. *et al.* (2000). Effect of disease burden on health-related quality of life in patients with malignant gliomas. *Neuro-Oncology* **2**(4):221–8.

151 Huan, S. D., Natale, R. B., Stewart, D. J. *et al.* (2000). Multicenter phase II trial of losoxantrone (DuP-941) in hormone-refractory metastatic prostate cancer. *Clinical Cancer Research* **6**(4):1333–6.

152 Latreille, J., Pater, J., Johnston, D. *et al.* (1998). Use of dexamethasone and granisetron in the control of delayed emesis for patients who receive highly emetogenic chemotherapy. *Journal of Clinical Oncology* **16**(3):1174–8.

153 Genre, D., Protiere, C., Macquart-Moulin, G. *et al.* (2002). Quality of life of breast cancer patients receiving high-dose-intensity chemotherapy: impact of length of cycles. *Supportive Care in Cancer* **10**(3):222–30.

154 Greimel, E., Thiel, I., Peintinger, F. *et al.* (2002). Prospective assessment of quality of life of female cancer patients. *Gynecologic Oncology* **85**(1):140–7.

155 Bjordal, K., Mastekaasa, A., Kaasa, S. (1995). Self-reported satisfaction with life and physical health in long-term cancer survivors and a matched control group. *European Journal of Cancer: Oral Oncology* **31B**(5):340–5.

156 Joly, F., Henry-Amar, M., Arveux, P. *et al.* (1996). Psychosocial sequelae in Hodgkin's disease survivors: a French population-based case-control study. *Journal of Clinical Oncology* **14**(9):2444–53.

157 Holzner, B., Kemmler, G., Kopp, M. *et al.* (2001). Quality of life in breast cancer patients – not enough attention for long-term survivors? *Psychosomatics* **42**(2):117–23.

158 Norum, J., Wist, E. A. (1996). Quality of life in survivors of Hodgkin's disease. *Quality of Life Research* **5**(3):367–74.

159 Kallen, K.-J., Hofmann, M. A. K., Timm, A. *et al.* (2000). Weekly oxaliplatin, high-dose infusional 5-fluorouracil and folinic acid as palliative third-line therapy of advanced colorectal carcinoma. *Zeitschrift für Gastroenterologie* **38**(2):153–7.

160 Langendijk, J. A., ten Velde, G. P. M., Aaronson, N. K. *et al.* (2000). Quality of life after palliative radiotherapy in non-small cell lung cancer: a prospective sudy. *International Journal of Radiation Oncology Biology and Physics* **47**(1):149–55.

161 Radbruch, L., Sabatowski, R., Loick, G. *et al.* (2000). Constipation and the use of laxatives: a comparison between transdermal fentanyl and oral morphine. *Palliative Medicine* **14**(2):111–19.

162 Doyle, C., Crump, M., Pintilie, M. *et al.* (2001). Does palliative chemotherapy palliate? Evaluation of expectations, outcomes, and costs in women receiving chemotherapy

for advanced ovarian cancer. *Journal of Clinical Oncology* **19**(5):1266–74.

163 Geels, P., Eisenhauer, E., Bezjak, A. *et al.* (2000). Palliative effect of chemotherapy: objective tumor response is associated with symptom improvement in patients with metastatic breast cancer. *Journal of Clinical Oncology* **18**(12):2395–405.

164 Cella, D. F. (1997). *FACIT MANUAL: Manual of the Functional Assessment of Chronic Illness Therapy (FACIT) Measurement System, Version 4,* Evanston, IL: Evanston Northwestern Healthcare and Northwestern University.

165 Esper, P., Pienta, K., Cella, D. (1995). FACT-P: a new instrument for quality of life evaluation in prostate cancer (Abstract). *Journal of Urology* **153**(Suppl. 4):239A.

166 Carter, J. R., Chen, M. D., Fowler, J. M. *et al.* (1997). The effect of prolonged cycles of chemotherapy on quality of life in gynaecologic cancer patients. *Journal of Obstetrics and Gynaecological Research* **23**(2):197–203.

167 Lutgendorf, S. K., Anderson, B., Rothrock, N. *et al.* (2000). Quality of life and mood in women receiving extensive chemotherapy for gynecologic cancer. *Cancer* **89**(6): 1402–11.

168 Sehlen, S., Hollenhorst, H., Lenk, M. *et al.* (2002). Only sociodemographic variables predict quality of life after radiotherapy in patients with head and neck cancer. *International Journal of Radiation Oncology Biology and Physics* **52**(3):779–83.

169 Krupski, T., Petroni, G. R., Bissonette, E. A. *et al.* (2000). Quality-of-life comparison of radical prostatectomy and interstitial brachytherapy in the treatment of clinically localized prostate cancer. *Urology* **55**(5):736–42.

170 Small, E. J., Meyer, M., Marshall, M. E. *et al.* (2000). Suramin therapy for patients with symptomatic hormone-refractory prostate cancer: results of a randomized phase III trial comparing suramin plus hydrocortisone to placebo plus hydrocortisone. *Journal of Clinical Oncology* **18**(7): 1440–50.

171 Poon, R. T.-P., Fan, S. T., Yu, W. C. *et al.* (2001). A prospective longitudinal study of quality of life after resection of hepatocellular carcinoma. *Archives of Surgery* **136**(6):693–9.

172 Courneya, K. S., Friedenreich, C. M. (1997). Relationship between exercise pattern across the cancer experience and current quality of life in colorectal cancer survivors. *Journal of Alternative and Complementary Medicine* **3**(3): 215–26.

173 Schipper, H., Clinch, J., McMurray, A. *et al.* (1984). Measuring the quality of life of cancer patients: the Functional Living Index – Cancer: development and validation. *Journal of Clinical Oncology* **2**(5):472–83.

174 Clinch, J. J. (1996). The Functional Living Index – Cancer: Ten years later. In *Quality of Life and Pharmacoeconomics in Clinical Trials* (2nd Edition), ed. B. Spilker, pp. 215–25. Philadelphia, PA: Lippincott-Raven Publishers.

175 Remick, S. C., Sedransk, N., Haase, R. F. *et al.* (2001). Oral combination chemotherapy in conjunction with filgrastim (G-CSF) in the treatment of AIDS-related non-Hodgkin's lymphoma: evaluation of the role of G-CSF; quality-of-life analysis and long-term follow-up. *American Journal of Hematology* **66**(3):178–88.

176 Osoba, D. (2000). Health-related quality-of-life assessment in clinical trials of supportive care in oncology. *Supportive Care in Cancer* **8**(2):84–8.

177 Schliephake, H., Schmelzeisen, R., Schonweiler, R. *et al.* (1998). Speech, deglutition and life quality after intraoral tumour resection: a prospective study. *International Journal of Oral and Maxillofacial Surgery* **27**(2):99–105.

178 Goss, P. E., Winer, E. P., Tannock, I. F. *et al.* (1999). Randomized phase III trial comparing the new potent and selective third-generation aromatase inhibitor vorozole with megestrol acetate in postmenopausal advanced breast cancer patients. *Journal of Clinical Oncology* **17**(1): 52–63.

179 Goss, P. E., Strasser, K., Marques, R. *et al.* (2000). Liarozole fumarate (R85246): in the treatment of ER negative, tamoxifen refractory or chemotherapy resistant postmenopausal metastatic breast cancer. *Breast Cancer Research and Treatment* **64**(2):177–88.

180 Harvey, J., Cantrell, J., Jr., Campbell, M. *et al.* (2001). Mitoxantrone and paclitaxel combination chemotherapy in metastatic breast cancer. *Cancer Investigation* **19**(3): 225–33.

181 Goss, P. E., Oza, A., Goel, R. *et al.* (2000). Liarozole fumarate (R85246): a novel imidazole in the treatment of receptor positive postmenopausal metastatic breast cancer. *Breast Cancer Research and Treatment* **59**(1):55–68.

182 Laufman, L. R., Bukowski, R. M., Collier, M. A. *et al.* (1993). A randomized, double-blind trial of fluorouracil plus placebo versus fluorouracil plus oral leucovorin in patients with metastatic colorectal cancer. *Journal of Clinical Oncology* **11**(10):1888–93.

183 Clohisy, D. R., Le, C. T., Cheng, E. Y. *et al.* (2000). Evaluation of the feasibility of and results of measuring health-status changes in patients undergoing surgical treatment for skeletal metastases. *Journal of Orthopaedic Research* **18**(1):1.

184 Ruckdeschel, J. C., Piantadosi, S. (1994). Quality of life in lung cancer surgical adjuvant trials. *Chest* **106**(Suppl. 6):324S–8S.

185 de Haes, J. C. J. M., Pruyn, J. F. A., van Knippenberg, F. C. E. (1983). Complaint list for cancer patients: first experiences. *Nederlands Tijdschrift voor de Psychologie* **38**:403–22.

186 de Haes, J. C. J. M., van Knippenberg, F. C. E., Neijt, J. P. (1990). Measuring psychological and physical distress in cancer patients: structure and application of the Rotterdam Symptom Checklist. *British Journal of Cancer* **62**(6): 1034–8.

187 Luteijn, F., Kok, A. R., Hamel, L. F. *et al.* (1979). Enige Ervaringe met en Klachtenlijst. *Nederlands Tidjschrift voor Psychologie* **34**:167.

188 Linssen, A. C. G., van Dam, F. S. A. M., Engelsman, E. *et al.* (1979). Leven met cytostatica. *Pharmaceutisch Weekblad* **114**:501.

189 McCorkle, R., Young, K. (1978). Development of a symptom distress scale. *Cancer Nursing* **1**(5):373–8.

190 O'Hanlon, D. M., Harkin, M., Karat, D. *et al.* (1995). Quality-of-life assessment in patients undergoing treatment for oesophageal carcinoma. *British Journal of Surgery* **82**(12):1682–5.

191 Allen-Mersh, T. G., Earlam, S., Fordy, C. *et al.* (1994). Quality of life and survival with continuous hepatic-artery floxuridine infusion for colorectal liver metastases. *Lancet* **344**(8932):1255–60.

191 Kramer, J. A., Curran, D., Piccart, M. *et al.* (2000). Randomised trial of paclitaxel versus doxorubicin as first-line chemotherapy for advanced breast cancer: quality of life evaluation using the EORTC QLQ-C30 and the Rotterdam Symptom Checklist. *European Journal of Cancer* **36**(12):1488–97.

192 Kramer, J. A., Curran, D., Piccart, M. *et al.* (2000). Identification and interpretation of clinical and quality of life prognostic factors for survival and response to treatment in first-line chemotherapy in advanced breast cancer. *European Journal of Cancer* **36**(12):1498–506.

193 Ranson, M., Davidson, N., Nicolson, M. *et al.* (2000). Randomized trial of paclitaxel plus supportive care versus supportive care for patients with advanced non-small-cell lung cancer. *Journal of the National Cancer Institute* **92**(13):1074–80.

194 de Haes, J. C. J. M., Olschewski, M. (1998). Quality of life assessment in a cross-cultural context: use of the Rotterdam Symptom Checklist in a multinational randomised trial comparing CMF and Zoladex (Goserlin) treatment in early breast cancer. *Annals of Oncology* **9**(7): 745–50.

195 Erickson, P. (2001). Trends in population-based health-related quality of life: implications for interpretation of change. *Value in Health* **4**(6):418.

196 Johnston, M., Pollard, B., Hennessey, P. (2000). Construct validation of the Hospital Anxiety and Depression Scale with clinical populations. *Journal of Psychosomatic Research* **48**(6):579–84.

197 Velikova, G., Wright, P., Smith, A. B. *et al.* (2001). Self-reported quality of life of individual cancer patients: concordance of results with disease course and medical records. *Journal of Clinical Oncology* **19**(7):2064–73.

198 Hopwood, P., Howell, A., Maguire, P. (1991). Screening for psychiatric morbidity in patients with advanced breast cancer: validation of two self-report questionnaires. *British Journal of Cancer* **64**:353–6.

199 Skarstein, J., Aass, N., Fossa, S. D. *et al.* (2000). Anxiety and depression in cancer patients: relation between the Hospital Anxiety and Depression Scale and the European Organization for Research and Treatment of Cancer Core Quality of Life Questionnaire. *Journal of Psychosomatic Research* **49**(1):27–34.

200 Curran, S. L., Andrykowski, M. A., Studts, J. L. (1995). Short Form of the Profile of Mood States (POMS-SF): psychometric information. *Psychological Assessment* **7**(1):80–3.

201 Mosconi, P., Cifani, S., Crispino, S. *et al.* (2000). The performance of the SF-36 Health Survey in patients with laryngeal cancer. *Head and Neck* **22**(2):175–82.

202 Rogers, S. N., Lowe, D., Brown, J. S. *et al.* (1998). Comparison between the University of Washington Head and Neck Disease-Specific Measure and the Medical Short Form 36, EORTC-QLQ-C33, and EORTC Head and Neck 35. *Oral Oncology* **34**(5):361–72.

203 McHorney, C. A., Ware, J. E., Raczek, A. E. (1993). The MOS 36-Item Short-Form Health Status Survey (SF-36): II. Psychometric and clinical tests of validity in measuring physical and mental health constructs. *Medical Care* **31**(3):247–63.

204 McHorney, C. A., Ware, J. E., Lu, J. F. R. *et al.* (1994). The MOS 36-item Short-Form Health Survey (SF-36): III. Tests of data quality, scaling assumptions and reliability across diverse patient groups. *Medical Care* **32**(4):40–66.

205 Ware, J. E., Kosinski, M., Bayliss, M. S. *et al.* (1995). Comparison of methods for the scoring and statistical analysis of the SF-36 health profile and summary measures: results from the Medical Outcomes Study. *Medical Care* **33**:A5264–A5279.

206 Stewart, A. L., Greenfield, S., Hays, R. D. *et al.* (1989) Functional status and well-being of patients with chronic conditions: results from the Medical Outcomes Study. *Journal of the American Medical Association* **262**(7):907–13.

207 Quality Metric, Inc. includes an online version of the instrument, annotated bibliography, on-line article

searches, norms table downloads, open discussion groups, FAQs, and weekly SF e-mail newsletters. Available at http://www.sf36.com. Last accessed September 9, 2004.

208 Sloan, J. A., Loprinzi, C. L., Kuross, S. A. *et al.* (1998). Randomized comparison of four tools measuring overall quality of life in patients with advanced cancer. *Journal of Clinical Oncology* **16**(11):3662–73.

209 Bergner, M., Bobbitt, R. A., Pollard, W. E. *et al.* (1976). The Sickness Impact Profile: validation of a Health Status Measure. *Medical Care* **14**(1):57–67.

210 Carter, W. B., Bobbitt, R. A., Bergner, M. *et al.* (1976). Validation of an interval scaling: the Sickness Impact Profile. *Health Services Research* **11**(4):516–28.

211 Pollard, W. E. M., Bobbitt, R. A., Bergner, M. *et al.* (1976). The Sickness Impact Profile: reliability of a health status measure. *Medical Care* **14**(2):146–55.

212 Hunt, S. M., McKenna, S. P., McEwen, J. (1981). Reliability of a population survey tool for measuring perceived health problems: a study of patients with osteoarthrosis. *Journal of Epidemiology and Community Health* **35**: 297–300.

213 Hunt, S. M., McKenna, S. P., McEwen, J. *et al.* (1980). A quantitative approach to perceived health status: a validation study. *Journal of Epidemiology and Community Health* **34**(4):281–6.

214 McKenna, S. P., McEwen, J., Hunt, S. M. *et al.* (1984). Changes in the perceived health of patients recovering from fractures. *Public Health (London)* **98**:97–102.

215 Uyl-de Groot, C. A., Hagenbeek, A., Verdonck, L. F. *et al.* (1995). Cost-effectiveness of ABMT in comparison with CHOP chemotherapy in patients with intermediate- and high-grade malignant non-Hodgkin's lymphoma (NHL). *Bone Marrow Transplantation* **16**(3):463–70.

216 O'Toole, D., Ducreux, M., Bommelaer, G. I. *et al.* (2000). Treatment of carcinoid syndrome: a prospective crossover evaluation of lanreotide versus octreotide in terms of efficacy, patient acceptability, and tolerance. *Cancer* **88**(4): 770–6.

217 Hunt, S. M., McEwen, J. (1980). The development of a subjective health indicator. *Sociology of Health and Illness* **2**:231–46.

218 Hunt, S. M., McEwen, J., McKenna, S. P. *et al.* (1984). Subjective health assessments and the perceived outcome of minor surgery. *Journal of Psychosomatic Research* **28**(2):105–14.

219 Hunt, S. M., McEwen, J., McKenna, S. P. *et al.* (1982). Subjective health status of patients with peripheral vascular disease. *Practitioner* **226**(1363):133–6.

220 Ferrans, C. E., Powers, M. J. (1985). Quality of Life Index: development and psychometric properties. *Advances in Nursing Science* **8**(1):15–24.

221 Ferrans, C. E., Powers, M. J. (1992). Psychometric assessment of the Quality of Life Index. *Research in Nursing and Health* **15**(1):29–38.

222 Ferrans, C. E. (1990). Development of a quality of life index for patients with cancer. *Oncology Nursing Forum* **17**(3 Suppl.):15–21.

223 Schag, C. A. C., Heinrich, R. L., Aadland, R. L. *et al.* (1990). Assessing problems of cancer patients: psychometric properties of the Cancer Inventory of Problem Situations. *Health Psychology* **9**(1):83–102.

224 Schag, C. A. C., Ganz, P. A., Polinsky, M. L. *et al.* (1993). Characteristics of women at risk for psychosocial distress in the year after breast cancer. *Journal of Clinical Oncology* **11**(4):783–93.

225 Schag, C. A. C., Heinrich, R. L. (1989). *The CAncer Rehabilitation Evaluation System (CARES) Manual*. Los Angeles: CARES Consultants.

226 Kemmler, G., Holzner, B., Kopp, M. *et al.* (1999). Comparison of two quality-of-life instruments for cancer patients: the Functional Assessment of Cancer Therapy-General and the European Organization for Research and Treatment of Cancer Quality of Life Questionnaire-C30. *Journal of Clinical Oncology* **17**(9):2932–40.

227 Weitzner, M. A., Meyers, C. A., Gelke, C. K. *et al.* (1995). The Functional Assessment of Cancer Therapy (FACT) Scale: development of a brain subscale and revalidation of the General version (FACT-G) in patients with primary brain tumors. *Cancer* **75**(5):1151–61.

228 Winstead-Fry, P., Schultz, A. (1997). Psychometric analysis of the Functional Assessment of Cancer Therapy-General (FACT-G) Scale in a rural sample. *Cancer* **79**(12): 2446–52.

229 Dow, K. H., Ferrell, B. R., Anello, C. (1997). Quality-of-life changes in patients with thyroid cancer after withdrawal of thyroid hormone therapy. *Thyroid* **7**(4):613–19.

230 Knight, S. J., Chmiel, J. S., Sharp, L. K. *et al.* (2001). Spouse ratings of quality of life in patients with metastatic prostate cancer of lower socioeconomic status: an assessment of feasibility, reliability, and validity. *Urology* **57**(2):275–80.

231 Morrow, G. R., Lindke, J., Black, P. (1992). Measurement of quality of life in patients: psychometric analyses of the Functional Living Index-Cancer (FLIC). *Quality of Life Research* **1**:287–96.

232 Butow, P., Coates, A., Dunn, S. *et al.* (1991). On the receiving end. IV: Validation of quality of life indicators. *Annals of Oncology* **2**(8):597–603.

233 King, M. T., Dobson, A. J., Harnett, P. R. (1996). A comparison of two quality-of-life questionnaires for cancer clinical trials: the Functional Living Index-Cancer (FLIC) and the Quality of Life Questionnaire Core Module (QLQ-C30). *Journal of Clinical Epidemiology* **49**(1):21–9.

234 Buxton, J., White, M., Osoba, D. (1998). Patients' experiences using a computerized program with a touch-sensitive video monitor for the assessment of health-related quality of life. *Quality of Life Research* **7**(6):513–19.

235 Osoba, D., Zee, B., Pater, J. *et al.* (1994). Psychometric properties and responsiveness of the EORTC Quality of Life Questionnaire (QLQ-C30) in patients with breast, ovarian and lung cancer. *Quality of Life Research* **3**(5): 353–64.

236 Hjermstad, M. J., Fossa, S. D., Bjordal, K. *et al.* (1995). Test/retest study of the European Organization for Research and Treatment of Cancer Core Quality-of-Life Questionnaire. *Journal of Clinical Oncology* **13**(5):1249–54.

237 Bjordal, K., Kaasa, S. (1992). Psychometric validation of the EORTC Core Quality of Life Questionnaire, 30-Item Version, and a diagnosis-specific module for head and neck cancer patients. *Acta Oncologica* **31**(3):311–21.

238 Niezgoda, H. E., Pater, J. L. (1993). A validation study of the domains of the Core EORTC Quality of Life Questionnaire. *Quality of Life Research* **2**(5):319–25.

239 Ringdal, G. I., Ringdal, K. (1993). Testing the EORTC Quality of Life Questionnaire on cancer patients with heterogeneous diagnoses. *Quality of Life Research* **2**:129–40.

240 Apolone, G., Filberti, A., Cifani, S. *et al.* (1998). Evaluation of the EORTC QLQ-C30 Questionnaire: a comparison with SF-36 Health Survey in a cohort of Italian long-survival cancer patients. *Annals of Oncology* **9**(5):549–57.

241 Groenvold, M., Klee, M. C., Sprangers, M. A. G. *et al.* (1997). Validation of the EORTC QLQ-C30 Quality of Life Questionnaire through combined qualitative and quantitative assessment of patient-observer agreement. *Journal of Clinical Epidemiology* **50**(4):441–50.

242 Ravaioli, A., Buda, P., Fava, C. *et al.* (1996). Assessment of the RSCL quality of life instrument during chemotherapy in an Italian setting. *Quality of Life Research* **5**(5):491–5.

4

The roles for preference-based measures in support of cancer research and policy

David H. Feeny, Ph.D.

University of Alberta, Edmonton, AB, Canada

Introduction

Although not widely used yet in studies of breast, prostate, colorectal, or lung cancer, *preference-based* outcome measures are starting to play an important role in the assessment of health-related quality of life (HRQOL) in decision analyses about optimal treatment choice and in the economic evaluation of interventions for these cancers.

There is increasing emphasis now on "patient-reported" or "patient-centered" outcome measures, as noted throughout this volume, and a wide range of generic, general cancer, and cancer-site-specific HRQOL instruments are being applied. But virtually all of these are, from the perspective of this chapter, *non-preference-based*. Whether the instrument in question is single-dimensional (e.g., the Brief Pain Index), multi-dimensional yielding an aggregate score (e.g., FACT-G), or multi-dimensional yielding a profile of scores (e.g., SF-36; see Erickson),[1] the patient's summary score is derived through some form of psychometric scaling process that does not assume, and thus cannot convey, information about the patient's own relative valuation of the health states in question. By contrast, preference-based measures are derived from either direct statements about, or statistical inferences concerning, the relative value the patient places on her current state of health. In this chapter, patient-centered means patient preference-based.

There are two major families of preference-based measures: direct (the patient is queried straightforwardly about how she values the health states at issue) and indirect (the patient received an imputed preference score through a several step attribution process).[2] For reasons that will become clear, the indirect approach is generally referred to now as the "multi-attribute" approach. Prototypically under this approach, the patient completes a questionnaire whose items are designed to describe, but not value, the current state of health along several posited dimensions or attributes, e.g., physical, social, emotional. The responses are then fed into a (pre-existing) utility function that assigns a preference value score to the multi-attribute health state implied by the respondent's particular pattern of item responses. Typically, such a utility function has been estimated on the basis of preference scores obtained directly from population-based samples.

Many applications of this multi-attribute approach to cancer, as well as other diseases, use scoring systems in which preferences are attached to generic states of health. The latter, in turn, are mapped, i.e., linked as a matter of expert judgment, to cancer-specific states or outcomes, which then assume the preference weights associated with the generic states. For example, suppose we wish to assign a preference score to the overall state of health for a patient recovering from colorectal cancer surgery. We would choose a multi-attribute HRQOL measure (three measurement systems for this purpose will be discussed later), and then select the particular multi-attribute health state – defined, for example, in terms of physical, social, and emotional functioning – that best characterizes the condition of the surgery patient. The (previously estimated) preference weight associated with that multi-attribute state then becomes the preference value for the cancer patient's state of health. In real world applications of this indirect approach, the patient completes a questionnaire constructed for the multi-attribute preference measurement system of choice, and the score for the patient's implied health state is then computed using the system's multi-attribute utility function. Recently, work has begun on cancer-specific multi-attribute preference-based measures, and these will be discussed later in this chapter.

As a prelude to what follows, it may be useful to describe briefly how preference-based measures can be employed in the assessment of cancer interventions. Under either the direct or multi-attribute approach, the conventional scale for preference measurement ranges from 1.00 for perfect health for the individual to 0.00 for dead (or states of health regarded as bad as being dead). The efficacy or effectiveness of an intervention is gauged by its impact on moving the individual, or groups of individuals, from lower rated to higher rated states of health. For example, assume the cancer patient's state of health over the next year in the absence of palliative care has a preference score of 0.35; the state of health with palliative care has a preference score of 0.75. Thus, the effectiveness of this intervention is $0.75 - 0.35 = 0.40$ utility units per year. As discussed by O'Brien,[3] such a result is commonly reported in the literature as 0.40 "quality-adjusted life-years," or QALYs. The maximum QALY value for a year is 1.00 (excellent health throughout) and the minimum is 0.00 (dead throughout); one QALY is equivalent in value to a full year in excellent health.

While such preference-based measures can clearly be used in trials or observational studies as a type of patient-reported outcome, a common arena of application is cost-utility analysis, a variant of cost-effectiveness analysis wherein the effectiveness measure is preference based.[3] Continuing the example above and adopting O'Brien's notation, if total cost per patient per year with and without the palliative care option is $50 000 and $40 000, respectively, the incremental cost-utility ratio for this option is

$CEA = \Delta C/\Delta E = \$10\,000/0.40 = \$25\,000$ per QALY gained. The implication is that palliative care would be regarded as a "good buy" if the relevant decision maker is willing to pay at least $25 000 per QALY gained.

The effectiveness measure in cost-effectiveness analyses need not be preference based, of course. In fact, the most commonly employed effectiveness measure is life-years gained or some other measure of survival benefit. Very rarely, however, is ΔE expressed in terms of non-preference-based patient–reported outcomes, such as improvement in a general or site-specific cancer measure. This is partly because most of these measures have been developed for and used in clinical trials and observational studies whose primary focus is not cost-effectiveness analysis. But it likely also reflects the perception, which is for the most part correct, that for cost-effectiveness analysis to realize its full potential to inform resource allocation decisions, the states of health to which preferences are attached must be generic in order to facilitate both intra-disease and inter-disease comparisons of interventions. For an example of the former, see the application to non-small-cell lung cancer in the chapter by O'Brien in this volume;[3] for an example of the latter, see Neumann et al.'s cost-effectiveness analysis of treatments for Alzheimer's disease.[4]

In a cost-effectiveness analysis conducted alongside a clinical trial, the time horizon for analysis need not be one year, of course, but may be selected to coincide with the time horizon of the trial. Or, the cost-effectiveness analysis may be structured so that the horizon corresponds to the remaining life expectancy of the patients under study, in order to place the intervention's trial-observed effectiveness and cost into a more complete, life-cycle context.[3] What this means for the incremental cost-effectiveness ratio above is that ΔE and ΔC must now reflect the net changes in the time streams of QALYs and cost over the horizon of interest to the decision maker. (Note that once the CEA moves to a multi-year context, there are certain other analytical issues that must be dealt with, including the need to recognize the time cost of money and the decision maker's possible time preference for a QALY gained today over a QALY gained years hence. Such issues are discussed at length in Drummond *et al.*[2] and Gold *et al.*[5] and are beyond the purview of this chapter.)

All that said, the focus in this chapter is on how such preference-based measures are operationally defined and derived, and how they have been used to evaluate the effectiveness of cancer interventions; the natural extensions to cost-effectiveness analysis are explored by O'Brien.[3]

Direct preference-based measures

In the direct approach, the respondent is asked to place a value on a health state using one or more of a variety of elicitation techniques. The three most common techniques are the visual analogue scale, standard gamble, and time trade-off.

Visual analogue scale

One of the most commonly used elicitation techniques is a vertical visual analogue scale (VAS) known as the Feeling Thermometer (FT). (Descriptions of techniques for preference-elicitation surveys are found in Furlong *et al.*[6]). Some investigators rely on the VAS alone, while others regard the VAS as a step in the process of formulating and reporting preference scores for health states.[7]

Typically, the VAS is a vertical line divided into 101 equally spaced points, labeled from 0 to 100. Usually, the top anchor of the FT is labeled "Most Desirable" and the bottom anchor is labeled "Least Desirable" (Figure 4.1). The respondent is given a set of health states to value and asked to place the health states on the VAS, both to reflect the rank order of the states and to ensure that the relative position of the states on the VAS reflects the strength of preference for the states.

In much of the decision science literature, a distinction is made between value and utility scores. Both types reflect preferences. Value scores are obtained under conditions of certainty. The VAS and the time trade-off (discussed below) are, therefore,

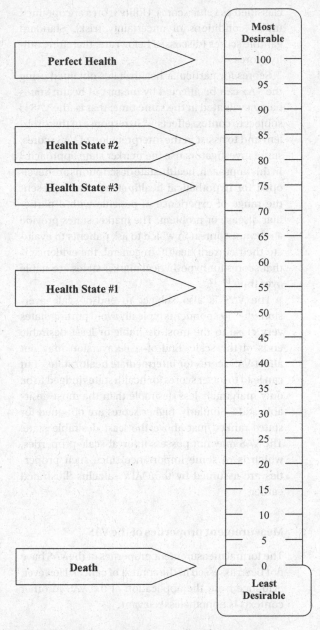

Figure 4.1. Visual Analogue Scale, or Feeling Thermometer, For Ordinal Ranking of Health States. Used with permission: Feeny, D. H., Torrance, G. W., Labelle, R. (1996). Integrating economic evaluations and quality of life assessments. In *Quality of Life and Pharmacoeconomics in Clinical Trials*, ed. B. Spilker, (2nd edition). Philadelphia, PA: Lippincott-Raven Publishers, pp. 85–95.

classified as value scores. Utility scores are obtained under conditions of uncertainty (risk). Standard gamble scores (discussed below) are, therefore, utility scores.

Scores for particular health states obtained using the VAS can be affected by the mix of health states being evaluated at the same time; that is, the VAS is subject to context effects.[7,8] In response to this problem and to assist in the interpretation of VAS scores, some investigators use the marker state approach.[9] In this approach, health-state descriptions are developed for hypothetical health states that represent the range of experience of patients with a particular disease or problem. The marker states provide a relevant context in which to ask patients to evaluate their current health. In general, the evidence is that scores for hypothetical marker states are stable over time.[10–12]

The VAS is also subject to end-of-scale aversion.[7,8,13] Respondents typically avoid putting states very close to the most desirable or least desirable ends of the scale. End-of-scale aversion may not affect VAS scores for intermediate health states, but can lead to lower scores for health states judged to be only marginally less desirable than the most desirable state. Similarly, higher scores are obtained for states ranked just above the least desirable state. The VAS may not possess interval-scale properties, which is of some importance since such properties are assumed by the QALY calculus illustrated earlier.

Measurement properties of the VAS

The formal measurement properties of the VAS have not been assessed in the context of cancer. However, evidence from the application of the VAS in other contexts is nonetheless relevant.

Content validity

Marker state descriptions are often constructed on the basis of an extensive search for evidence on the relevant domains of health status in a particular measurement context. For instance, descrip-
tions for health states associated with various stages of treatment for pediatric high-risk acute lymphoblastic leukemia were based on a review of the clinical literature and input from nurses, parents, child-life workers, and physicians.[14] Similarly, when respondents are asked to rate their current health, they are often prompted to think about pre-identified domains of interest.

Construct validity

Typically, the rank ordering of health states agrees across preference elicitation techniques such as the VAS, time trade-off, and standard gamble, which supports the construct validation of all three approaches. However, not all studies support this conclusion.[15]

VAS scores correlate moderately with time trade-off and standard gamble scores.[16,17] Time trade-off scores embody time preference; VAS scores do not. Standard gamble scores embody time and risk preferences; VAS scores do not. These underlying differences in the construct being measured account, in part, for the moderate correlation among scores observed. Similarly, standard gamble scores for the same health state are typically greater than time trade-off scores, which in turn are greater than VAS scores. Because of context effects and end-of-scale aversion, some investigators use the VAS as a warm-up exercise in the preference elicitation process but rely on choice-based techniques (standard gamble or time trade-off) as a more valid source of preference information.

Reliability

The test-retest reliability of VAS scores over time intervals of one week to 10 weeks has been assessed in a variety of contexts.[16–22] Correlations of 0.62 to 0.95 have been observed, with most ≥ 0.70, a level of test-retest reliability usually viewed as acceptable for group level comparisons.[23–25] The test-retest reliability of the VAS appears to be acceptable in a wide variety of contexts.

Internal consistency for the VAS has not been evaluated. Given that each "item" on the VAS is a health state that is often meant to be different from the other health states being evaluated at the same time, the degree of correlation among "items" (VAS scores) is not very meaningful.

Responsiveness

There is not a great deal of evidence on the responsiveness of VAS scores. Analysts who have collected VAS scores in longitudinal studies, and who have also collected time trade-off or standard gamble scores, often have not evaluated the responsiveness of the VAS scores. Nonetheless, in a number of contexts, VAS scores appear to have been moderately to highly responsive.[26-28]

Practical aspects

The VAS is seemingly easy to use. In practice, however, preference elicitation often requires interviewer administration using well-trained and well-supervised interviewers.[6] Although many regard the VAS to be more user friendly than the time trade-off and standard gamble, respondents in some studies have rated it as more difficult.[29] As the number of states on the VAS goes up, the number of pair-wise combinations increases rapidly, generating substantial cognitive demands. Ironically, the choice-based techniques (time trade-off, standard gamble) may be less demanding. In interview settings, a rule of thumb for the time of administration for the VAS is that each health state will take an average of five minutes, including the time for instructions, introductions, etc. Formats used for self-administration of the VAS often introduce additional measurement problems. For instance, because investigators cannot be sure which states the respondent will view as the most preferred and the least preferred, and because there is no interviewer present to assist, different respondents often use different top and bottom anchors for their idiosyncratic VAS. This can inhibit the aggregation of scores across respondents. Recently, computer-assisted preference elicitation

tools have become available. There do not seem to be any direct comparisons of scores obtained by traditional in-person interviewer administration with scores obtained with computer administration. For carefully trained respondents, computer-assisted administration may be quite useful.

Standard gamble

The standard gamble (SG) is a choice-based technique for preference elicitation.[2,18] The respondent is given the hypothetical choice between a specified period of time in the health state of interest and playing a specially constructed lottery. The lottery offers a probability p of spending that same specified period of time in perfect health and a probability (1-p) of immediate death (or, alternatively, some other health state not preferred to the health state of interest); see Figure 4.2. The probability p is varied until the respondent is indifferent (that is, unable to decide) between the lottery and the sure thing. The more desirable the state of interest, the higher the probability the respondent will require to be indifferent. The utility score for the health state of interest is derived from the indifference probability; in particular, when the undesirable outcome of the gamble is death, it can be shown that this utility value equals p.

The SG is directly tied to von Neumann-Morgenstern expected utility theory,[13,18,30-33] which assumes that people have stable well-formulated utility (preference) functions. Among the key axioms of expected utility theory are the requirements that utilities are transitive and continuous. Continuity implies that if A is preferred to B and B is preferred to C (and thus, by transitivity, A is preferred to C), there exists a lottery with outcomes of A or C such that the subject is indifferent to the lottery versus B. The SG is based directly on this continuity axiom. Conceptually, the SG is the gold standard for assessing preferences (and utilities) for health states because it is grounded in a coherent normative theory – the expected utility model – for how choices ought to be made under conditions of uncertainty.

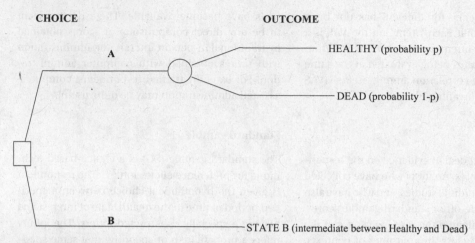

Figure 4.2.   Standard gamble approach for eliciting utility values. Used with permission: Feeny, D. H., Torrance, G. W., Labelle, R. (1996). Integrating economic evaluations and quality of life assessments. In *Quality of Life and Pharmacoeconomics in Clinical Trials*, ed. B. Spilker (2nd edition). Philadelphia, PA: Lippincott-Raven Publishers, pp. 85–95.

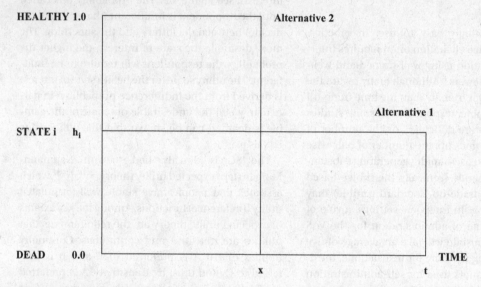

Figure 4.3.   Time trade-off approach for eliciting preference values. Used with permission: Feeny, D. H., Torrance, G. W., Labelle, R. (1996). Integrating economic evaluations and quality of life assessments. In *Quality of Life and Pharmacoeconomics in Clinical Trials*, ed. B. Spilker (2nd edition). Philadelphia, PA: Lippincott-Raven Publishers, pp. 85–95.

Time trade-off

The time trade-off (TTO) is a choice-based technique for preference elicitation.[2,16,18,34] Respondents are given a choice between a specified period of time in perfect health or a specified period of time in a health state (a hypothetical state or their current health state) (Figure 4.3). The period of time in perfect health is then varied until a point of indifference is found between a longer period (t) in the health state being evaluated and a shorter period of time in perfect health (x). The value score for the health state is then x/t, implying that life in the state for t years is "equivalent" to x years in perfect health. Like the SG, the TTO can be linked conceptually to expected utility theory by retaining all of the original axioms (assumptions) and adding the further requirement that utility in additional healthy time is linear with respect to time.

Measurement properties of SG and TTO

There have been relatively few evaluations of the measurement properties of the SG and TTO in the context of breast, prostate, colorectal, or lung cancer. However, evidence from other contexts is relevant. Because, for the most part, evidence on the measurement properties for the SG and TTO are similar, both sets of evidence will be described together.

Content validity

The marker state approach can provide a useful context within which respondents may assess the value that they attach to health states. Similarly, structured prompts may help respondents reflect on their current health and then value it.

Construct validity

In a wide variety of non-cancer studies, the SG and TTO have performed as one would expect them to perform, providing evidence of construct validity. There have also been several studies in breast, prostate, colorectal, and lung cancer, providing

evidence about the construct validity of these two approaches.

Ness et al.[35] constructed seven path states that described both treatment process and outcomes associated with colorectal cancer. Ratings were obtained using VAS and SG. Each health state description included information on tiredness and weakness, bowel habits, sexual problems, pain, thinking problems, social problems, and emotional problems. The ordering of mean SG scores agreed with a priori hypotheses.

Hayman et al.[36] used the SG to examine the health-related quality-of-life effects of risk reductions for local recurrence of breast cancer associated with radiation therapy versus the burden of that therapy. Results highlighted the importance of the reductions in risk and fear of recurrence. Albertsen et al.[37] report TTO estimates for health states associated with prostate cancer that conform to expectations about rank order. In a small study, Chapman et al.[38] used the TTO to obtain scores for three hypothetical health states and each patient's current health state. The rank ordering of the scores and the valuations of current health conformed to expectations. In another study, Chapman et al.[39] reported similar rankings to TTO questions concerning hypothetical health states associated with prostate cancer when states were described in personal versus impersonal terms, but the study also found greater willingness to trade survival for improved HRQOL when states were described impersonally. Bennett et al.[40] report that patients provided higher TTO scores than did physicians for three hypothetical health states associated with metastatic prostate cancer. (See also Sommers and Ramsey.[41]) Dominitz and Provenzale[42] report TTO scores for hypothetical health states associated with screening for colorectal cancer. Consistent with many other studies, they find considerable variability among patients in the values attached to particular health states.

TTO has been applied in several studies of breast cancer. One year or more after treatment for breast cancer, Ashby et al.[43] asked women to provide TTO scores for five scenarios as well as their current health state. They found considerable agreement in the ranking and valuation exercises. Jansen et al.[44] investigated the stability of TTO and SG scores for hypothetical health states among women undergoing treatment for breast cancer, and found, in most cases, the scores for hypothetical states were stable over time (see also[45–48]). Jansen et al.[44] also conclude that, in spite of conscientious efforts to produce realistic and accurate health-state descriptions, the descriptions may not reflect the experiences of patients adequately. Jansen et al. provide evidence that the health-state descriptions do not accurately reflect patients' perception of those same health states at the time during which patients are actually experiencing the states.

Patients undergoing therapy are often unwilling to trade-off any time or risk of survival.[49] This may attenuate the responsiveness of the TTO and SG when preference scores are obtained directly from patients undergoing therapy (for an example using TTO in colorectal cancer see Stiggelbout et al.;[50] for evidence using TTO in prostate cancer see Chapman et al.;[39] for evidence on TTO in genetic testing for risk of breast cancer see Grann et al.;[51,52] for evidence on TTO in advanced breast cancer see Hurny et al.[53]).

TTO has also been used to evaluate states associated with screening for breast cancer.[54] Because screening involves both temporary (process) and chronic (outcome) states, more complicated preference elicitation procedures have often been used. Hall et al.[55] asked subjects to evaluate "path states." In the path-state approach (see also[56]), subjects are asked to evaluate a health state that describes the process and outcome, in this case various health states associated with the screening and its consequences, lasting until death.

Reliability

In general, the test-retest reliability of the SG has been acceptable. O'Brien and Viramontes[20] report an intra-class correlation coefficient (ICC) of 0.82 for patients who assessed the same health states 4 weeks later. Green et al.[17] in their review paper report a range of results from various studies with correlations of 0.53 to 0.82. Shiell et al.[57] report ICCs between assessments (time 1 to time 2; time 2 to time 3) of 0.78 and 0.72 for one selected health state (F) and 0.60 and 0.81 for another (M).

Similarly, in general, test-retest reliability for the TTO has been acceptable. Correlations of 0.63 to 0.81 have been observed for intervals of four to six weeks.[18] Green et al.[17] found correlations of 0.63 to 0.87 for intervals of 1 to 16 weeks. In the context of caregivers' burden, Mohide et al. report an ICC of 0.79.[58] In the context of stroke, Gage et al.[59] report ICCs of 0.67 to 0.92. Tosteson et al.[60] report an ICC of 0.75 with automated TTO valuations in women's health.

In breast cancer patients, Ashby et al.[43] report correlations for test-retest reliability of 0.50 to 0.75 for the TTO for time intervals of 3 to 6 weeks. In prostate cancer patients, Albertsen et al.[37] report correlations of 0.22, 0.83, 0.91, 0.96, and 0.99 for five health states assessed one week later. Also in prostate cancer patients, Saigal et al.[61] report ICCs of 1.00 for all but one of the states (21 patients, 3 weeks later) for which the ICC was 0.56; see also Grann et al.[52] Test-retest reliability for the TTO appears acceptable.

Internal consistency for the SG and TTO have not been evaluated. As with the VAS, given that each "item" is a health state that is meant to be different from the other health states being evaluated at the same time, the degree of correlation among "items" (SG or TTO scores) is not very meaningful.

Responsiveness

Evidence of the responsiveness of SG and TTO scores is not abundant. A number of analysts who have collected SG scores in longitudinal studies have often found them to be moderately to highly responsive. For instance, in a double-blind placebo-controlled randomized clinical trial in arthritis of an oral gold compound, Bombardier et al.[26] found that a direct preference measure (using SG, time trade-off, and VAS) was among the most responsive of the wide variety of measures employed in the study. The evidence for the TTO is similar.

Practical aspects

The SG and TTO are choice-based techniques. Both involve complex cognitive processes and are more demanding than the completion of standardized health status assessment questionnaires.

The traditional technology for obtaining SG and TTO scores, and practical gold standard, is the in-person interview.[6] Interviews are supported by scripts and the use of props. Interviewers are well trained and carefully supervised; typically interviews are audio-taped for quality assurance. A rule of thumb is that one should budget 5 minutes of interview time per health state to be evaluated using the SG or TTO.

More recently, computer-assisted interview techniques have been developed. Results to date are promising,[62] although there appears to be a lack of evidence on agreement between scores from computer-assisted and in-person interviews. A crossover study involving expert interviewers and well-developed and properly supported computer-assisted interviews would help in determining the appropriate roles for the computer-assisted technology.

Standard gamble and TTO scores are not assessed with great precision. Differences in scores of 0.10 or larger are clearly important.[6] Many would regard differences in scores of 0.05 or larger as important.

Other variations on the theme of assigning preferences directly

While the standard approach to direct assessment is to obtain the individual's own preferences for the states of health relevant to the interventions being evaluated, some alternative strategies have been employed.

Hypothetical health states and surrogate informants

In a number of studies, a finite set of health states is identified and meaningful descriptions are developed for each. Preference scores for these hypothetical health states are then obtained, and sometimes the informants are health care professionals. For instance, a series of studies[63–65] obtained standard gamble scores for health states associated with chemotherapy for recurrent metastatic breast cancer from oncology nurses. An advantage of using nurses is that they are familiar with the health states experienced by patients. Further, one can obtain scores from nurses, or other health professionals, when patients are unable to respond on their own behalf.

In some studies, patients are asked to evaluate the hypothetical health states. For example, Goodwin et al.[66] obtained VAS and SG scores for six hypothetical health states associated with treatment for small cell lung cancer from a small group of patients and health care professionals. Similarly, Leung et al.[67] obtained TTO scores from patients, and health care professionals, for states associated with various chemotherapeutic regimes for anthracycline-resistant breast cancer. Results highlight the importance of quality-adjusted survival. Palliative chemotherapy offers a lower response rate but less toxicity. When feasible, obtaining preference scores from patients is desirable, but it may not always be feasible.

Direct assessment of treatment alternatives (not health states)

Because individuals may have different preferences about the trade-offs between quantity and quality of life, several investigators have used preference elicitation techniques to obtain information on treatment choices directly (rather than the values attached to particular health states, from which treatment preferences would be inferred).[49,68,69] For instance, Goel et al.[70] report results from a randomized controlled clinical trial in which patients were randomized to be offered, or not, a decision aid to assist with their choice of surgical technique for breast cancer. They found a formal decision aid had only modest effects on decisional conflict. Decision aids have also been developed for adjuvant chemotherapy for breast cancer.[71] Jansen et al.[47] investigate treatment preferences for adjuvant chemotherapy for early-stage breast cancer. Young *et al.*[72] examine patient treatment preferences in advanced colorectal cancer. Stigglebout *et al.*[73] assess patient preferences for follow up to detect recurrence after treatment for colorectal cancer. Cappelli *et al.*[74] assess preferences for health states associated with genetic testing for risk of breast cancer using the standard gamble.

Quality-Adjusted Time Without Symptoms or Toxicity (Q-TWiST)

The Quality-Adjusted Time Without Symptoms or Toxicity (Q-TWiST) offers a simple approach to adjusting the quantity of life for decrements in quality, namely, by subtracting the number of days with specified disease symptoms or treatment-induced toxicities from the total number of days of survival. In some studies, including early applications of Q-TWiST, no preference or utility scores are assigned directly to competing alternatives; instead, the analyst solves for the threshold value of utility scores for health states, i.e., that value such that quality-adjusted survival would be equal between the alternatives. Utility scores above or below that threshold would favor one treatment relative to another. One example is Gelber *et al.*[75] who examined adjuvant chemotherapy plus tamoxifen versus tamoxifen alone for postmenopausal breast cancer; the findings highlighted the burden of cytotoxic chemotherapy.

Multi-attribute preference-based measures

In the direct approach to the assessment of HRQOL, patients are asked to assess and value their current health state. As described earlier, an alternative strategy is to use an indirect, multi-attribute approach that assigns a preference score in two steps. First, the respondent completes a questionnaire that identifies (descriptively) her position along each relevant health status dimension or attribute. Then a utility function, generally estimated from a population-based sample of preferences for health states, is used to map this set of item endorsements into an imputed preference score. Multi-attribute measures that have been used in breast, prostate, colorectal, and lung cancer include the EuroQol EQ-5D,[76–79] the Health Utilities Index,[80–82] and the Quality of Well-Being scale.[83] Table 4.1 summarizes the characteristics of each of these systems (which will also be discussed below in alphabetical order).

EuroQol EQ-5D

The EQ-5D includes several components. First, there is a health status classification system. Health status in the EQ-5D consists of five dimensions (or attributes): mobility, self-care, usual activity, pain/discomfort, and anxiety/depression. There are three levels defined for each dimension of health status: no problem, some problem, or extreme problem. A standardized questionnaire based on the system is available. The health status of an individual at a point in time can be represented as a five-element vector, one level for each dimension.[84]

A score for that categorical information on health status can be obtained by using a scoring formula (the one described by Dolan[78] is probably the most commonly used one). That scoring system is based on preference scores using the TTO obtained from a representative sample of adults in the United Kingdom. Because some states, for instance, the state (3,3,3,3,3) with extreme problems in all five dimensions, were considered by respondents to be worse than dead, the scale runs from negative 0.59 to positive 1.00. Many refer to the scores derived from the scoring system as EQ-5D index scores. A modified linear additive functional form is used for the EQ-5D scoring function. A linear additive functional form implies that there are no important interactions in preferences among dimensions of health status. Thus, the disutility of a moderate problem with mobility ("I have some problems in walking about") does not depend on the degree of problem, if any, with respect to anxiety/depression.

Table 4.1. Description of EuroQol EQ-5D, Health Utilities Index Mark 2 (HUI2) and Mark 3 (HUI3), and Quality of Well-Being (QWB) multi-attribute preference-based measures

Measure	Dimension of health status (number of levels)	Number of unique health states	Scoring function
EQ-5D	mobility (3); self-care (3); usual activities (3); pain/discomfort (3); anxiety/depression (3)	243 plus unconscious and dead	*ad hoc* modified linear additive based on TTO scores from random sample of British population
HUI2	sensation (4); mobility (5); emotion (5); cognition (4); self-care (4); pain and discomfort (5); fertility (3)	24 000 plus dead	multiplicative multi-attribute based on SG scores from random sample of parents in general population in Canada
HUI3	vision (6); hearing (6); speech (5); ambulation (6); dexterity (6); emotion (5); cognition (5); pain and discomfort (5)	972 000 plus dead	multiplicative multi-attribute based on SG scores from random sample of general population in Canada
QWB	mobility (3); physical activity (3); social activity (5); symptom/problem complex (27)	1215 plus dead	linear additive based on VAS scores from random sample of general population in US

Another component of the EQ-5D system is a visual analogue scale on which respondents provide a direct rating of their own current health state. The general measurement properties of the visual analogue scale described earlier apply to EQ-5D VAS as well.

Measurement properties of the EQ-5D

There have been few assessments of the measurement properties of the EQ-5D in the context of breast, prostate, colorectal, and lung cancer, but evidence from applications in other areas is relevant.

Content validity

The five dimensions of health status included in the EQ-5D are of general relevance and importance in the context of breast, prostate, colorectal, and lung cancer. The omission of cognition has been identified as a problem with the EQ-5D.[85]

Construct validity

In general, there is evidence of the construct validity of the EQ-5D system in a variety of clinical applications.[86–88] In migraine patients, Essink-Bot

et al.[89] found that the Short Form 36 (SF-36) discriminated better between groups than a variety of other measures including the EQ-5D and Nottingham Health Profile. In general population surveys, the EQ-5D has substantially greater ceiling effects than the SF-36.[90] Ceiling effect problems are likely to be less prevalent in clinical studies, especially during acute phases of treatment. Ceiling effect problems may, however, be important in long-term follow-up studies of survivors or in studies on screening.

Trippoli et al.[91] used the EQ-5D and SF-36 in a cross-sectional study of patients with non-small-cell lung cancer, including recently and previously diagnosed patients. Both SF-36 summary scores (physical and mental) and EQ-5D index scores were able to distinguish among known groups.

Reliability

There is little evidence on the test-retest reliability of the EQ-5D system. There is also little evidence on internal consistency, but given that the standardized questionnaire for the system has one question per dimension of health status, the relevance of internal consistency is not clear. With respect to test-retest reliability, Dorman et al.[88] report kappa coefficients of 0.63 to 0.80 for the five dimensions of the EQ-5D in a group of stroke patients and an ICC of 0.86 for the index scores. Similar correlations were observed for the SF-36. In a review article, Coons et al.[90] report a two-week test-retest ICC of 0.78 for index scores in patients with rheumatoid arthritis.

Responsiveness

There is evidence that, in a variety of types of applications, the EQ-5D is responsive to large changes in health status. A number of investigators have commented that the coarseness of the system with only three levels per dimension may limit responsiveness.[86,87,92–93] For health status to improve, the person must change by at least one level on at least one dimension of health, for instance, move from an extreme problem to a moderate one. Brazier et al.[87] found that the EQ-5D was responsive to changes in health status associated with total knee replacement for osteoarthritis but was not responsive in detecting change in patients with osteoarthritis being treated in rheumatology clinics. The EQ-5D is subject to ceiling effect problems. In studies of patients undergoing therapy, ceiling effect problems may not be serious; however, in studies of population screening[94] or long-term follow up of survivors, ceiling effect issues may be more problematic.

Practical aspects

The EQ-5D is among the briefest of instruments. Missing values are more common with the EQ-5D VAS component of the system than with the health status classification system.[89,90] In a pre-test for the 1998 National Population Health Survey in Canada, Statistics Canada[95] found that, on average, the EQ-5D took 1.5 minutes to complete (computer-assisted telephone interviewer administration) with a 2.2% non-response rate.

Health Utilities Index (HUI)

There are three major versions of the Health Utilities Index: HUI Mark 1[19], HUI Mark 2,[96] and HUI Mark 3.[81,97] In all three versions, there is a health status classification system, a questionnaire to obtain information to classify subjects according to that system, and a multi-attribute utility function to provide utility scores of health-related quality of life. Because HUI2 and HUI3 have superceded HUI1 in most applications, discussion will focus on HUI2 and HUI3.

HUI2 consists of seven attributes (dimensions) of health status: sensation (vision, hearing, and speech), mobility, emotion, cognition, self-care, pain, and fertility. The original application of HUI2 was in childhood cancer. Because some survivors experience subfertility or infertility, fertility was included. In most applications, fertility is omitted from the standard questionnaire, but it has been included in a number of studies of breast and ovarian cancer prophylaxis.

The scoring function for the HUI2 system is based on preference measurements using the standard gamble obtained from a random sample of parents in the general population in Hamilton, Ontario, Canada.[98,99] Because the original application of HUI2 was cancer in childhood, parents were selected as respondents. A multiplicative functional form is used for the HUI2 multi-attribute utility function; the data rejected the simpler linear additive form. A multiplicative form implies that there are important interactions in preferences among attributes. More specifically, the parameter values for the HUI2 system imply that the attributes in the HUI2 system are preference complements. This interaction means that the disutility associated with a loss of function in two attributes is less than the sum of the "individual" disutilities associated with the independent loss of the function of each attribute.

The HUI3 system was originally designed for the 1990 Ontario Health Survey and includes eight attributes: vision, hearing, speech, ambulation, dexterity, emotion, cognition, and pain. There are five or six levels per attribute. The HUI3 has been widely used in population health surveys in Canada, including the 1994 and ongoing National Population Health Survey and the Canadian Community Health

Survey, and there is an abundance of data on population norms.

The HUI3 scoring system is based on preference scores obtained from a random sample of the general population in Hamilton, Ontario. As with the HUI2 function, the functional form is multiplicative, indicating that interactions in preferences among attributes are quantitatively important.[81,100]

Measurement properties of the HUI

There have been few assessments of the measurement properties of the HUI in the context of breast, prostate, colorectal, and lung cancer. However, evidence from applications in other areas is relevant.

Content validity

To facilitate applications in assessing health status and to ensure the feasibility of estimating a multi-attribute utility function (scoring function), it is necessary to limit the number of attributes or dimensions of health status included in a multi-attribute system. For instance, the Quality of Well-Being Scale (QWB) has four dimensions; the EQ-5D includes five. HUI2 includes seven dimensions; HUI3 includes eight. The attributes in HUI2 were chosen on the basis of their importance, as judged by members of the general population.[80,82] HUI3 was, in turn, based on HUI2, but with modifications to enhance descriptive power and to obtain structural independence. Structural independence means that logically a person can be in any level for one attribute and any other level for another attribute. A consequence of the structural independence of the HUI3 system is that there is relatively little overlap (much less than in EQ-5D) among attributes.[95] Thus, each item on the questionnaire provides new information.

Construct validity

HUI2 and HUI3 have demonstrated construct validity in a number of studies in pediatric oncology. HUI has distinguished the burden of morbidity in survivors of standard risk acute lymphoblastic leukemia (ALL) from that in survivors of high-risk ALL.[101] HUI has also been able to distinguish the burden of morbidity as a function of the dose of radiation in survivors of brain tumors in both adult and pediatric patients.[102,103] The importance of including cognition in the health status classification was evident in the applications in ALL and brain tumors. There is a substantial body of evidence on the construct validity of HUI2 and HUI3 in childhood cancer.[104]

Ramsey et al.[105] used the Functional Assessment of Cancer Therapy scale for Colorectal Cancer (FACT-C) and HUI3 in a cohort of survivors (n = 173) of colon cancer. HUI3 was able to detect trends in HRQOL over time. Stage 1–3 patients got better over time, while declines were observed for Stage 4 patients, as expected. FACT-C did not capture these same trends. Initial HUI3 and FACT-C scores were predictive of survival. HUI3 identified problems with vision and hearing (probably age related); FACT-C did not. FACT-C identified problems with social well-being that were not directly captured by HUI3. HUI3 identified problems with pain that did not diminish over time.

In a study of multiple sclerosis patients, Grima et al.[106] found that HUI2 was able to distinguish the stage of disease, as assessed by the expanded disability status scale. Similarly, Neumann et al.[107,108] found that HUI2 and HUI3 were able to distinguish the stage of disease, as assessed by the clinical dementia rating, in Alzheimer's disease patients. Bayoumi and Redelmeier[109] provide evidence of the construct validity of HUI2 in distinguishing among levels of severity in HIV infection and AIDS. Younossi et al.[110] report evidence of the construct validity of HUI2 in distinguishing among patients with chronic liver disease by degree of severity. Grootendorst et al.[111] provide evidence of construct validity for HUI3 in the context of a population health survey; HUI3 was able to distinguish respondents who had suffered a stroke from those who reported arthritis. Both groups were readily distinguishable from subjects without either condition.

Table 4.2. Illustration: mean scores and example patient, HUI3 in maintenance chemotherapy protocol

	Week 1	Week 2
Percent of patients with no problems	56	17
Mean HUI3 score (standard deviation)	0.94 (0.07)	0.74 (0.24)
HUI3 vector for patient "x" at week 1	(V1, H1, S1, A1, D1, E1, C1, P1)	
HUI3 score for patient "x" at week 1	1.00	
HUI3 vector for patient "x" at week 2		(V1, H1, S1, A2, D1, E3, C1, P4)
HUI3 score for patient "x" at week 2		0.46

Note: Patients assessed at week 1 had been off all therapy for one week; patients assessed at week 2 following the administration of high-dose corticosteroids and three other chemotherapeutic agents. V = vision, H = hearing, S = speech, A = ambulation, D = dexterity, E = emotion, C = cognition, P = pain; the number refers to the level. Level 1 is normal (no problem). Level 2 ambulation indicates the ability to walk but with difficulty (but without reliance on mechanical devices or the help of another person); level 3 emotion indicates some unhappiness; level 4 pain indicates moderate to severe pain that prevents some activities.[82] The HUI3 score for week 2 is calculated using the formula $u^* = 1.371 \ (b_1 \times b_2 \times b_3 \times b_4 \times b_5 \times b_6 \times b_7 \times b_8) - 0.371$ where b_i is the score for that level in the ith dimension of health status. The score for b_i for level 1 is 1.00; the score for A2 (level 2 ambulation) is 0.93; the score for E3 is 0.85; and the score for P4 is 0.77. HUI3 score for dead = 0.00, perfect health = 1.00; for more detail see Feeny et al.[81]

Reliability

Test-retest reliability for HUI3 has been examined in a population health survey.[112] Kappa values for attributes varied from 0.14 to 0.73, with most indicating substantial agreement. The ICC for overall scores (using the provisional scoring system) was 0.73.

In a small clinical study of stable systemic lupus erythematosus (SLE) patients (n = 23), kappa values between HUI2 attribute levels (two- to four-week intervals) were fair to excellent (0.46 to 0.88) with the exception of pain (kappa = 0.32).[113]

The standardized HUI2 and HUI3 questionnaires include the minimum number of questions to obtain information sufficient to classify subjects in the HUI2 and HUI3 systems. For some attributes there is only one question. For these dimensions of health status, it is not possible to assess internal consistency. In general, internal consistency has not been assessed for HUI. However, Le Gales et al.,[114] in a study of children with brain tumors, have examined the Spearman correlation coefficients among responses to the two questions that deal with the same attribute. Results varied from 0.47 (cognition, child self-report) to 1.00 (vision, physician assessment).

Responsiveness

HUI has been shown to be responsive in detecting changes in health status experienced by children on "maintenance" therapy for ALL.[82,115] Children experienced problems in pain, emotion, and ambulation and had lower overall scores in week 2 after taking high-dose corticosteroids. While 56% of patients experienced no problems (score of 1.00) in week 1 (off therapy), only 17% experienced no problems in week 2. Results from this study can be used to provide a brief illustration of how multi-attribute systems are employed in studies. The experiences of the cohort and a patient are summarized in Table 4.2.

Palmer et al.[116] found HUI2 to be highly responsive in a prospective study of hearing-impaired patients receiving cochlear implants (see also Krabbe et al.[117]). Grossman et al.[118] and Torrance et al.[119] found HUI2 and the St. George's Respiratory Questionnaire to be similarly responsive in detecting changes in chronic bronchitis patients treated with antibiotics. Suarez-Almazor et al.[120] found HUI2 and EQ-5D to be responsive in a cohort of patients being treated for lower back pain. Comerota et al.[121] found

HUI2 to be responsive in a study of treatment alternatives for deep venous thrombosis.

Like other multi-attribute preference-based measures, HUI is subject to ceiling effect problems. Given that HUI2 has 6 attributes (and 7 if fertility is also included) and HUI3 has 8, ceiling effect problems are less frequent than with the EQ-5D. In population screening and long-term follow-up studies, ceiling effect issues may be problematic.

Practical aspects

Standard questionnaires that include HUI2 and HUI3 usually require five to ten minutes for self completion. Typically, there are fewer problems and missing values than with the SF-36 questionnaire. In a pre-test of the National Population Health Survey, using computer-assisted telephone interviews, Statistics Canada found that completion of the HUI3 questionnaire took an average of 2.0 minutes with a 0.3% non-response rate.[95] Both self-completion and interviewer administration impose little burden, but these two modes of administration should not be regarded as interchangeable.

Quality of Well-Being Scale

The Quality of Well-Being (QWB) scale is the oldest of the multi-attribute systems.[122] The original system included 3 dimensions of health status and a problem/symptom complex: mobility (5 levels), physical activity (4 levels), social activity (5 levels), and problem/symptom (35 items). The original system described 3500 health states. The newer version has 3 levels for mobility, 3 for physical activity, 5 for social activity, and 27 problem/symptom items.

The scoring function is linear additive, based on visual analogue scale scores obtained from a random sample of the general population in San Diego, California. For an individual with multiple symptoms or problems, only the worst (among the 27 items) is scored.

Measurement properties of the QWB

There have been relatively few evaluations of the measurement properties of the QWB in breast, prostate, colorectal, and lung cancer; however, evidence from other settings is relevant.

Content validity

The mobility, physical activity, and social activity domains are of clear relevance for cancer. Symptoms include a number of items of potential relevance in cancer, for instance, trouble learning and remembering, pain, fatigue, difficulty sleeping, problems with sexual interest or performance, and excessive worry or anxiety.

Construct validity

Kaplan and Anderson[122] summarize evidence on the ability of the QWB to distinguish among known groups in population health and clinical studies. QWB scores varied by the degree of severity of patients with Alzheimer's disease.[122] QWB has been used extensively in studies of HIV and AIDS and has been able to discriminate among patients according to level of severity.[122] The QWB has been used in many clinical trials in a wide variety of areas, including chronic obstructive pulmonary disease, AIDS, cystic fibrosis, diabetes mellitus, lung transplantation, arthritis, and atrial fibrillation.[122] Frosch et al.[123] provide evidence on the performance of the German version of the QWB (newer self-administered questionnaire) in prostrate and colorectal cancer. Prostate cancer patients identified problems with sexual interest, loss of bladder control, difficulty urinating, and pain – evidence of the construct validity of the QWB. Problems with sleep and sexual interest were identified by both prostate and colorectal patients.

Reliability

Frosch et al.[123] report reliability of 0.90 or more in most populations. Given that each of the items in the problem/symptom complex is "unique," internal consistency is difficult to assess.

Responsiveness

Bombardier et al.[26] provide evidence on the responsiveness of the QWB in an evaluation of an oral gold compound for the treatment of arthritis. QWB has been responsive in a number of AIDS trials and in a trial evaluating sinus surgery.[122]

Practical aspects

The original version of the QWB required interviewer administration. The newer version provides both self- and interviewer-administered versions. Completion times for the newer version vary with the population being studied, but generally fall into the 10–15 minute range.

Choosing among the prominent multi-attribute systems

A number of criteria are relevant in selecting a multi-attribute system for application in a study. With respect to the time for completion, in general, EQ-5D probably takes the least amount of time, HUI is probably intermediate, and QWB takes the longest. All three, however, are not burdensome and are readily accommodated in study protocols.

It is important to examine the content validity of the system for application in the specific clinical area. Does the system cover most of the dimensions of health status relevant in that clinical context? For instance, the omission of cognition from the EQ-5D might make it less suitable for studies of brain tumor patients. If relevant symptoms are covered in the problem/symptom complex of the QWB, that instrument might be attractive. (Investigators may still wish to employ detailed specific HRQOL instruments and focused symptom checklists. It should also be noted that only the most severe problem is scored with the QWB.)

Have any of the multi-attribute systems been previously used in the relevant clinical context or a closely related one? Previous studies may provide evidence on cross-sectional and longitudinal construct validity. Evidence on responsiveness is of particular relevance in clinical trials. That the EQ-5D has only 3 levels per attribute may attenuate its responsiveness.

Investigators may also wish to consider the characteristics of the multi-attribute utility function for each measure. Many authors[2,5] have greater faith in the validity of choice-based (TTO and SG) preference scores than in VAS scores. The scoring function for the QWB is based on VAS scores. The scoring functions for the EQ-5D (based on TTO) and for HUI (based on SG) rely on choice-based preference scores.

Disease-specific multi-attribute preference systems

The EQ-5D, HUI, and QWB are generic preference-based multi-attribute systems. Generic measures cover a range of dimensions of health status and are applicable to virtually all adult populations. This facilitates broad comparisons and makes these measures especially well suited for cost-effectiveness and cost-utility analyses, including those that go across diseases to provide societal level rankings of competing interventions. The generic nature of these instruments may, however, reduce their specificity or responsiveness to particular diseases or health problems.

Recently, a number of teams of investigators have created disease-specific multi-attribute systems. These health status classification systems are designed to cover the most relevant dimensions of health status in a particular context. Two such systems have been devised for prostate cancer.

Chapman et al.[38] have produced a system for prostate cancer that includes five attributes: pain, mood, sexual function, bladder and bowel function, and fatigue and energy. Each attribute has three levels: high, moderate, and low. In a pilot study, using preference assessments obtained with the TTO, a linear additive multi-attribute utility function for the system was estimated.

Similarly, Krahn *et al.*[124] devised the patient-oriented prostate utility scale (PORPUS). PORPUS consists of 10 attributes: pain and disturbing body sensations, energy, support from family and friends, communication with doctor, emotional well-being, urinary frequency, leaking urine/poor bladder control, sexual function, sexual drive and interest, and bowel problems. Each attribute has either four or five levels. The attributes were selected after extensive investigation of the dimensions of health status that patients found troublesome. Work to estimate a multi-attribute utility function for the system is underway.

Both of these systems are promising. As yet, there is insufficient evidence to come to an informed judgment on their reliability, validity, and responsiveness.

Strengths and limitations of preference-based measures in cancer: direct approaches and multi-attribute systems

Direct measures have the advantage that patients can define their own health state and provide a valuation of it. That subjects define their own subjective state may overcome limitations associated with generic and even disease-specific multi-attribute systems. This advantage of the direct approach would be particularly important in a context in which patients have concerns about dimensions of health status that are entirely omitted or given little coverage in multi-attribute systems. The advantages come, however, at a cost. Direct assessments of preferences for health states are more burdensome, both for respondents and investigators. In addition, in acute situations, patients may not be willing to trade survival for improved health-related quality of life. Further, given standard preference-elicitation protocols, patients do not reveal the description of their current health state to the investigator. It would be interesting to investigate augmenting the standard elicitation approach to explore the feasibility of asking patients to reveal their subjective health-state descriptions. Doing so might, of course, increase the burden.

A key advantage of the preference-based multi-attribute measures is that they impose relatively small burdens on respondents and investigators. They can readily be used serially in prospective studies. Generic multi-attribute systems permit broad comparisons among cancers and other health problems. HUI3 and EQ-5D have been or are being included in major US, Canadian, and United Kingdom population health surveys, providing abundant data on population norms. Multi-attribute systems can also be useful in identifying unanticipated problems or the side effects of treatment that may not be covered adequately by disease-specific measures. For instance, using HUI2 and HUI3, Whitton *et al.*[103] identified an under-recognized burden of pain in survivors of brain tumors.

The preference-based generic systems such as the HUI, EQ-5D, and QWB may not, however, capture all of the important dimensions of health status. For instance, while emotional health is covered in each of the major multi-attribute systems, sexual function, which is clearly often relevant in prostate, colorectal, and breast cancer, is not directly captured.

Disease-specific multi-attribute systems may ameliorate some of these potential limitations in coverage. Typically, however, disease-specific multi-attribute measures do not produce scores on the conventional dead = 0.00 perfect health = 1.00 scale. Thus, disease-specific measures may not permit broad comparisons among cancers and with other diseases. These measures also have limited usefulness in cost-effectiveness and cost-utility analyses.

The generic multi-attribute systems are subject to ceiling effect problems. This may limit their usefulness in studies of alternative screening programs. These ceiling effect issues may also limit usefulness in long-term follow up of HRQOL in healthy survivors.

Implications for the research agenda

In spite of the potential promise of preference-based measures in breast, prostate, colorectal, and lung cancer, these measures have not been extensively used. In the absence of prospectively collected preference-based HRQOL scores, analysts have resorted to the use of threshold analyses or scores for hypothetical health states, often with scores provided by health care professionals.

To enhance the rigor of attempts to assess the quality of survival, treatment process, and screening programs, it is imperative that preference-based measures be included in clinical trials and related studies. The onus should be on investigators to justify why they have not chosen to use preference-based measures.

Direct or multi-attribute preference-based measures?

Multi-attribute measures such as the HUI impose relatively small burdens on patients (and investigators). Including this type of measure in studies would not, in general, be onerous. These measures provide valuable information on HRQOL. Scores from these measures can also be used to support economic evaluations, decision analyses, and adjustments of survival for its quality. However, because these measures are generic, they may not capture fully the burdens associated with treatment and outcome.

Direct preference measures are typically more burdensome for respondents (and investigators). The traditional technology requires highly trained and supervised interviewers. For reasons of practicality, direct measures such as the SG are unlikely to be incorporated routinely in studies. It is, however, important that such measures be used (along with generic preference-based multi-attribute measures) in selected studies. This application will be especially important in contexts (for instance, prostate cancer) where the content of the generic measures seems to be incomplete. The creation of a corpus of studies in which the SG (or TTO) and multi-attribute measures (such as the HUI or QWB) have been used simultaneously will enhance the ability to interpret results from the multi-attribute measures and make generalizations.

Importance of choice-based preference elicitation techniques

The VAS is useful as a key step in the process of preference elicitation. However, because of a number of well-documented problems with the VAS, it is preferable to rely upon choice-based techniques, the SG and the TTO. Further, because the SG is based directly on the underlying theory of expected utility maximization, it is the method of choice.

Preference-based measures complement other approaches

A number of guidelines for the assessment of health care technologies[5,125] recommend the use of preference-based measures alongside generic-profile and disease-specific measures. This advice is sound. Information from each type of measure can help in the interpretation of results from other measures. Given the coarseness of the generic multi-attribute systems, there is good reason to suspect that important aspects of HRQOL may not be captured by these measures. Concurrent use of site-specific cancer measures, with more targeted coverage of HRQOL aspects that are important in that context, will permit an assessment of the quantitative importance of this potential problem. For instance, if a decline in sexual function is captured by a disease-specific measure, in what attributes, if any, are declines in the attributes covered in a multi-attribute measure recorded? Further, do multi-attribute systems capture changes that are not captured by disease-specific measures (with their focused and limited coverage)?

A role for computer-assisted elicitation of preference scores?

Computer-assisted preference elicitation technologies have the potential to reduce the burden of obtaining direct preference scores, perhaps especially the burden borne by investigators. The computer algorithm does not, however, free the respondent from making difficult preference judgments. It is possible that patients could engage in face-to-face preference interviews at study baseline, be trained in the use of the computer-assisted technology, and then periodically report on their HRQOL throughout the study using computer or web-based technologies. As mentioned above, carefully conducted studies comparing scores from face-to-face interviews conducted by experienced experts, with scores from well-supported computer-assisted interviews using trained subjects, would provide valuable evidence on the extent to which computer-assisted technologies might replace the traditional in-person interview approach.

The field of preference-based measurement will continue to evolve

A prime case in point is the emergence of a new multi-attribute scoring system – the Short-Form (SF)-6D – based on the SF-36, one of the most widely used health status measures.[126–128] The SF-36 includes 36 items and generates a score for each of eight domains of health status: physical functioning, role-physical, bodily pain, general health, vitality, social functioning, role-emotional, mental health.[127] The SF-6D encompasses 7 of the 8 domains from the SF-36: physical functioning (with 6 levels), role limitations (4 levels), social functioning (5 levels), pain (6 levels), mental health (5 levels), and vitality (5 levels). Consequently, the SF-6D can describe up to 18 000 health states.

Summary utility scores for SF-6D are based on an *ad hoc* linear additive multi-attribute utility function estimated on the basis of standard gamble scores obtained from a random sample of the adult population in the United Kingdom; see Brazier *et al.*[129] Scores range from 0.00 (dead) to 0.29 (for the worst state derivable from items within the SF-6D system) to 1.00 (for perfect health as defined from items within the system). The lottery employed in the SG preference survey had as the best and worst outcomes the all-best SF-6D state and the all-worst SF-6D state; additional assumptions were required

to establish the utility positioning between the latter state and dead (0.00).

Preliminary evidence indicates that like the SF-36, the SF-6D is subject to floor and ceiling effects. In clinical studies in oncology the floor effect problems may be important. As with other generic preference-based measures, the ceiling effect problems of the SF-6D may be important in screening and prevention studies. Additional evidence on the measurement properties of the SF-6D and applications in the context of oncology is likely to be forthcoming.

Conclusions

Preference-based measures, both direct and multi-attribute, have a number of characteristics that make their use highly relevant and important in studies of breast, prostate, colorectal, and lung cancer (and more generally). Preference-based measures are designed to reflect what is important to patients, in particular, to capture the value that patients place on health states and survival and to explore the trade-offs between survival and morbidity. Moreover, preference-based measures can explore the trade-offs among different types of morbidity (chemotherapy versus radiation). To date, these measures have been underutilized in breast, prostate, colorectal, and lung cancer. It is important that preference-based measures be used prospectively in a wide variety of studies in these four types of cancers as part of the comprehensive assessment of HRQOL.

Acknowledgments

The author acknowledges the helpful comments and suggestions made by Heather-Jane Au, William Furlong, and George Torrance on earlier drafts. The author acknowledges the assistance of Janice Varney and Tania Stafinski in searching and retrieving the relevant literature.

REFERENCES

1 Erickson, this volume, Chapter 3.

2 Drummond, M. F., O'Brien, B., Stoddart, G. *et al.* (1997). *Methods for the Economic Evaluation of Health Care Programmes* (2nd Edition). Oxford: Oxford University Press.

3 O'Brien, this volume, Chapter 25.

4 Neumann, P. J., Hermann, R. C., Kuntz, M. *et al.* (1999). Cost-effectiveness of donepezil in treatment of mild or moderate Alzheimer's disease. *Neurology* **52**:1138–45.

5 Gold, M. R., Siegel, J. E., Russell, L. B. *et al.* (eds.) (1996). *Cost-Effectiveness in Health and Medicine.* New York: Oxford University Press.

6 Furlong, W., Feeny, D., Torrance, G. W. *et al.* (1990). *Guide to Design and Development of Health-State Utility Instrumentation.* McMaster University Centre for Health Economics and Policy Analysis Working Paper No. 90–9.

7 Torrance, G. W., Feeny, D., Furlong, W. (2001). Visual analogue scales: do they have a role in the measurement of preferences for health states? *Medical Decision Making* **21**:329–34.

8 Streiner, D. L., Norman, G. R. (1995). *Health Measurement Scales. A Practical Guide to their Development and Use* (2nd Edition). Oxford: Oxford University Press.

9 Bennett, K. J., Torrance, G. W. (1996). Measuring health state preferences and utilities: rating scale, time trade-off, and standard gamble techniques. In *Quality of Life and Pharmacoeconomics in Clinical Trials* (2nd Edition), ed. B. Spilker, pp. 253–65. Philadelphia, PA: Lippincott-Raven Press.

10 Llewellyn-Thomas, H. A., Sutherland, H. J., Thiel, E. C. (1993). Do patients' evaluations of a future health state change when they actually enter that state? *Medical Care* **31**:1002–12.

11 Feeny, D., Blanchard, C., Mahon, J. L. *et al.* (2001). Test-retest reliability and the interpretation of utility scores: evidence from elective total hip arthroplasty (abstract). *Quality of Life Research* **10**:264.

12 Laupacis, A., Bourne, R., Rorabeck, C. *et al.* (1993). The effect of elective total hip replacement upon health-related quality of life. *Journal of Bone and Joint Surgery* **75-A**:1619–26.

13 Torrance, G., Feeny, D., Furlong, W. (2002). Health utility estimation. *Expert Review in Pharmacoeconomics Outcomes Research* **2**:99–108.

14 Feeny, D., Barr, R. D., Furlong, W. *et al.* (1991). Quality of life of the treatment process in pediatric oncology: an approach to measurement. In *The Effect of Cancer on Quality of Life*, ed. D. Osoba, pp. 73–88. Boca Raton: CRC Press, Inc.

15 Giesler, R. B., Ashton, C. M., Brody, B. *et al.* (1999). Assessing the performance of utility techniques in the absence of a gold standard. *Medical Care* **37**:580–98.

16 Torrance, G. W. (1976). Social preferences for health states: an empirical evaluation of three measurement techniques. *Socio-Economic Planning Sciences* **10**:129–36.

17 Green, C., Brazier, J., Deverill, M. (2000). Valuing health-related quality of life: a review of health state valuation techniques. *Pharmacoeconomics* **17**:151–65.

18 Torrance, G. W. (1986). Measurement of health state utilities for economic appraisal – a review. *Journal of Health Economics* **5**:1–30.

19 Torrance, G. W., Boyle, M. H., Horwood, S. P. (1982). Application of multi-attribute utility theory to measure social preferences for health states. *Operations Research* **30**:1042–69.

20 O'Brien, B. J., Viramontes, J. L. (1994). Willingness to pay: a valid and reliable measure of health state preference? *Medical Decision Making* **14**:289–97.

21 van Agt, H. M. E., Essink-Bot, M.-L., Krabbe, P. F. *et al.* (1994). Test-retest reliability of health state valuations collected with the EuroQol Questionnaire. *Social Science and Medicine* **39**:1537–44.

22 Gudex, C., Dolan, P., Kind, P. *et al.* (1996). Health state valuations from the general public using the visual analogue scale. *Quality of Life Research* **5**:521–31.

23 Hays, R. D., Anderson, R., Revicki, D. (1993). Psychometric considerations in evaluating health-related quality of life measures. *Quality of Life Research* **2**:441–9.

24 Revicki, D. A., Osoba, D., Fairclough, D. *et al.* (2000). Recommendations on health-related quality of life research to support labeling and promotional claims in the United States. *Quality of Life Research* **9**:887–900.

25 McDowell, I., Newell, C. (1996). *Measuring Health: A Guide to Rating Scales and Questionnaires* (2nd Edition). New York: Oxford University Press.

26 Bombardier, C., Ware, J., Russell, I. J. *et al.* (1986). Auranofin therapy and quality of life in patients with rheumatoid arthritis: results of a multicenter trial. *American Journal of Medicine* **81**:565–78.

27 Feeny, D., Juniper, E. F., Ferrie, P. J. *et al.* (1998). Why not just ask the kids? Health-related quality of life in children with asthma. In *Measuring Health-Related Quality of Life in Children and Adolescents: Implications for Research, Practice, and Policy*, ed. D. Droter, pp. 171–85. Mahwah, NJ: Lawrence Erlbaum Associates.

28 Juniper, E. F., Guyatt, G. H., Feeny, D. H. *et al.* (1997). Minimum skills required by children to complete health-related quality of life instruments for asthma: comparison

of measurement properties. *European Respiratory Journal* **10**:2285–94.

29 Patrick, D. L., Starks, H. E., Cain, K. C. *et al.* (1994). Measuring preferences for health states worse than death. *Medical Decision Making* **14**:9–18.

30 von Neumann, J., Morgenstern, O. (1944). *Theory of Games and Economic Behavior.* Princeton: Princeton University Press.

31 Torrance, G. W., Feeny, D. (1980). Utilities and quality-adjusted life years. *International Journal of Technology Assessment in Health Care* **5**:559–75.

32 Feeny, D. H. (2000). A utility approach to assessing health-related quality of life. *Medical Care* **38**:II151–II154.

33 Feeny, D. H., Torrance, G. W. (1989). Incorporating utility-based quality-of-life assessments in clinical trials: two examples. *Medical Care* **27**:S190–204.

34 Torrance, G. W., Thomas, W. H., Sackett, D. L. (1972). A utility maximization model for evaluation of health care programs. *Health Services Research* **7**:118–33.

35 Ness, R. M., Holmes, A. M., Klein, R. *et al.* (1999). Utility valuations for outcome states of colorectal cancer. *American Journal of Gastroenterology* **94**:1650–7.

36 Hayman, J. A., Fairclough, D. L., Harris, J. R. *et al.* (1997). Patient preferences concerning the trade-off between the risks and benefits of routine radiation therapy after conservative surgery for early-stage breast cancer. *Journal of Clinical Oncology* **15**:1252–60.

37 Albertsen, P. C., Nease, R. F., Potosky, A. L. (1998). Assessment of patient preferences among men with prostate cancer. *Journal of Urology* **159**:158–63.

38 Chapman, G. B., Elstein, A. S., Kuzel, T. M. *et al.* (1999). A multi-attribute model of prostate cancer patients' preferences for health states. *Quality of Life Research* **8**:171–80.

39 Chapman, G. B., Elstein, A. S., Kuzel, T. M. *et al.* (1998). Prostate cancer patients' utilities for health states: how it looks depends on where you stand. *Medical Decision Making* **18**:278–86.

40 Bennett, C. L., Chapman, G., Elstein, A. S. *et al.* (1997). A comparison of perspectives on prostate cancer: analysis of the utility assessments of patients and physicians. *European Urology* **32**:86–8.

41 Sommers, S. D., Ramsey, S. D. (1999). A review of quality-of-life evaluations in prostate cancer. *Pharmacoeconomics* **16**:127–40.

42 Dominitz, J. A., Provenzale, D. (1997). Patient preferences and quality of life associated with colorectal cancer screening. *American Journal of Gastroenterology* **92**:2171–8.

43 Ashby, J., O'Hanlon, M., Buxton, M. J. (1994). The time tradeoff technique: how do the valuations of breast cancer

patients compare to those of other groups? *Quality of Life Research* **3**:257–65.

44 Jansen, S. T., Stiggelbout, A. M., Wakker, P. P. *et al.* (2000). Unstable preferences: a shift in valuation or an effect of the elicitation procedure? *Medical Decision Making* **20**:62–71.

45 Jansen, S. J. T., Stiggelbout, A. M., Nooij, M. A. *et al.* (2000). The effect of individually assessed preference weights on the relationship between holistic utilities and nonpreference-based assessment. *Quality of Life Research* **9**:541–57.

46 Jansen, S. J. T., Kievit, J., Nooij, M. A. *et al.* (2001). Stability of patients' preferences for chemotherapy: the impact of experience. *Medical Decision Making* **21**:295–306.

47 Jansen, S. J. T., Nooij, M. A., Overpelt, I. M. E. *et al.* (2001). Patients' preferences for adjuvant chemotherapy in early-stage breast cancer: is treatment worthwhile? *British Journal of Cancer* **84**:1577–85.

48 Perez, D. J., Williams, S. M., Christensen, E. A. *et al.* (2001). A longitudinal study of health related quality of life and utility measures in patients with advanced breast cancer. *Quality of Life Research* **10**:587–93.

49 O'Connor, A., Boyd, N. F., Warde, P. *et al.* (1987). Eliciting preferences for alternative drug therapies in oncology: influence of treatment outcome description, elicitation technique and treatment experience on preferences. *Journal of Chronic Disease* **40**:811–8.

50 Stiggelbout, A. M., Kiebert, G. M., Kievit, J. *et al.* (1995). The 'utility' of the time trade-off method in cancer patients: feasibility and proportional trade-off. *Journal of Clinical Epidemiology* **48**:1207–14.

51 Grann, V. R., Panageas, K. S., Whang, W. *et al.* (1998). Decision analysis of prophylactic mastectomy and oophorectomy in BRCA1-positive or BRCA2-positive patients. *Journal of Clinical Oncology* **16**:979–85.

52 Grann, V. R., Jacobson, J. S., Sundarajan, V. *et al.* (1999). The quality of life associated with prophylatic treatments for women with BRCA1/2 mutations. *Cancer Journal from Scientific American* **5**:283–92.

53 Hurny, C., van Wegberg, B., Bacchi, M. *et al.* (1998). Subjective health estimations (SHE) in patients with advanced breast cancer: an adapted utility concept for clinical trials. *British Journal of Cancer* **77**:985–91.

54 Johnston, K., Brown, J., Gerard, K. *et al.* (1998). Valuing temporary and chronic health states associated with breast screening. *Social Science and Medicine* **47**:213–22.

55 Hall, J., Gerard, K., Salkeld, G., Richardson, J. (1992). A cost utility analysis of mammography screening in Australia. *Social Science and Medicine* **34**:993–1004.

56 Kuppermann, M., Shiboski, S., Feeny, D. *et al.* (1997). Can preference scores for discrete states be used to derive preference scores for an entire path of events? An application to prenatal diagnosis. *Medical Decision Making* **17**:42–55.

57 Shiell, A., Seymour, J., Hawe, P. *et al.* (2000). Are preferences over health states complete? *Health Economics* **9**:47–55.

58 Mohide, E. A., Torrance, G. W., Streiner, D. L. *et al.* (1988). Measuring the wellbeing of family caregivers using the time trade-off technique. *Journal of Clinical Epidemiology* **41**:475–82.

59 Gage, B. F., Cardinalli, A. B., Owens, D. K. (1996). The effects of stroke and stroke prophylaxis with aspirin or warfarin on quality of life. *Archives of Internal Medicine* **156**:1829–36.

60 Tosteson, A. N. A., Kneeland, T. S., Nease, R. F. *et al.* (2002). Automated current health time trade-off assessments in women's health. *Value in Health* **5**:98–105.

61 Saigal, C. S., Gornbein, J., Nease, R., Litwin, M. S. (2001). Predictors of utilities for health states in early stage prostate cancer. *Journal of Urology* **166**:942–6.

62 Lenert, L., Kaplan, R. M. (2000). Validity and interpretation of preference-based measures of health-related quality of life. *Medical Care* **38**:II138–II150.

63 Hutton, J., Brown, R., Borowitz, M. *et al.* (1996). A new decision model for cost-utility comparisons of chemotherapy in recurrent metastatic breast cancer. *Pharmacoeconomics* **9**:8–22.

64 Launois, R., Reboul-Marty, J., Henry, B. *et al.* (1996). A cost-utility analysis of second-line chemotherapy in metastatic breast cancer: docetaxel versus paclitaxel versus vinorelbine. *Pharmacoeconomics* **10**:504–21.

65 Brown, R. E., Hutton, J., Burrell, A. (2001). Cost-effectiveness of treatment options in advanced breast cancer in the UK. *Pharmacoeconomics* **19**:1091–102.

66 Goodwin, P. J., Feld, R., Evans, W. K. *et al.* (1988). Cost-effectiveness of cancer chemotherapy: an economic evaluation of a randomized trial in small-cell lung cancer. *Journal of Clinical Oncology* **6**:1537–47.

67 Leung, P. P., Tannock, I. F., Oza, A. M. *et al.* (1999). Cost-utility analysis of chemotherapy using paclitaxel, docetaxel, or vinorelbine for patients with anthracycline-resistant breast cancer. *Journal of Clinical Oncology* **17**:3082–90.

68 Eckman, M. H. (2001). Patient-centered decision making: a view of the past and a look toward the future. *Medical Decision Making* **21**:441–7.

69 Lee, S. J., Earle, C. C., Weeks, J. C. (2000). Outcomes research in oncology: history, conceptual framework, and trends in the literature. *Journal of the National Cancer Institute* **92**:195–204.

70 Goel, V., Sawka, C. A., Thiel, E. C. *et al.* (2001). Randomized trial of a patient decision aid for choice of surgical treatment for breast cancer. *Medical Decision Making* **21**:1–6.

71 Levine, M. N., Gafni, A., Markham, B. *et al.* (1992). A bedside decision instrument to elicit patient's preference concerning adjuvant chemotherapy for breast cancer. *Annals of Internal Medicine* **117**:53–8.

72 Young, A., Topham, C., Turner, J., Wardle, J. *et al.* (1999). A patient preference study comparing raltitrexed ('Tomudex') and bolus or infusional 5-fluorouracil regimens in advanced colorectal cancer: influence of side-effects and administration attributes. *European Journal of Cancer* **8**:154–61.

73 Stiggelbout, A. M., de Haes, J. C. J. M., Vree, R. *et al.* (1997). Follow-up of colorectal patients: quality of life and attitudes towards follow-up. *British Journal of Cancer* **75**:914–20.

74 Cappelli, M., Surh, L., Humphreys, L. *et al.* (2001). Measuring women's preferences for breast cancer treatments and BRCA1/BRCA2 testing. *Quality of Life Research* **10**:595–607.

75 Gelber, R. D., Cole, B. F., Goldhirsh, A. *et al.* (1996). Adjuvant chemotherapy plus tamoxifen compared with tamoxifen alone for postmenopausal breast cancer: meta-analysis of quality-adjusted survival. *Lancet* **347**:1066–71.

76 Essink-Bot, M.-L., Stouthard, M. E. A., Bonsel, G. J. (1993). Generalizability of valuations on health states collected with the EuroQol questionnaire. *Health Economics* **2**:237–46.

77 EuroQol Group (1990). EuroQol: a new facility for the measurement of health-related quality of life. *Health Policy* **16**:199–208.

78 Dolan, P. (1997). Modeling valuations for EuroQol health states. *Medical Care* **35**:1095–108.

79 Rabin, R., de Charro, F. (2001). EQ-5D: a measure of health status from the EuroQol Group. *Annals of Medicine* **33**:337–43.

80 Feeny, D. H., Torrance, G. W., Furlong, W. J. (1996). Health Utilities Index. In *Quality of Life and Pharmacoeconomics in Clinical Trials* (2nd Edition), ed. B. Spilker, pp. 239–52. Philadelphia, PA: Lippincott-Raven Press.

81 Feeny, D., Furlong, W., Torrance, G. W. *et al.* (2002). Multiattribute and single-attribute utility functions for the Health Utilities Index Mark 3 System. *Medical Care* **40**:113–28.

82 Furlong, W. J., Feeny, D. H., Torrance, G. W. *et al.* (2001). The Health Utilities Index (HUI) System for assessing health-related quality of life in clinical studies. *Annals of Medicine* **33**:375–84.

83 Patrick, D. L., Bush, J. W., Chen, M. M. (1973). Methods for measuring levels of well-being for a health status index. *Health Services Research* **8**:228–45.

84 Kind, P. (1996). The EuroQol Instrument: an index of health-related quality of life. In *Quality of Life and Pharmacoeconomics in Clinical Trials* (2nd Edition), ed. B. Spilker, pp. 191–201. Philadelphia, PA: Lippincott-Raven Press.

85 Krabbe, P. F., Stouthard, M. E., Essink-Bot, M.-L. *et al.* (1999). The effect of adding a cognitive dimension to the EuroQol Multiattribute Health-Status Classification System. *Journal of Clinical Epidemiology* **52**:293–301.

86 Brazier, J. E., Walters, S. J., Nicholl, J. P. *et al.* (1996). Using the SF-36 and EuroQol on an elderly population. *Quality of Life Research* **5**:195–204.

87 Brazier, J. E., Harper, R., Munro, J. *et al.* (1999). Generic and condition-specific outcome measures for people with osteoarthritis of the knee. *Rheumatology* **38**:870–7.

88 Dorman, P., Slattery, J., Farrell, B. (1998). Qualitative comparison of the reliability of health status assessments with the EuroQol and the SF-36 questionnaires after stroke. *Stroke* **29**:63–8.

89 Essink-Bot, M.-L., Krabbe, P. F. M., Bonsel, G. J. *et al.* (1997). An empirical comparison of four generic health status measures: the Nottingham Health Profile, the Medical Outcomes Study 36-Item Short-Form Health Survey, the COOP/WONCA Charts, and the EuroQol Instrument. *Medical Care* **35**:522–37.

90 Coons, S. J., Rao, S., Keininger, D. L. *et al.* (2000). A comparative review of generic quality-of-life instruments. *Pharmacoeconomics* **17**:13–35.

91 Trippoli, S., Vaiani, M., Lucioni, C. *et al.* (2001). Quality of life and utility in patients with non-small cell lung cancer. *Pharmacoeconomics* **19**:855–63.

92 Brazier, J., Jones, N., Kind, P. (1993). Testing the validity of the EuroQol and comparing it with the SF-36 health survey questionnaire. *Quality of Life Research* **2**:167–8.

93 Lydick, E. (2000). Approaches to the interpretation of quality-of-life scales. *Medical Care* **38**:III 80–3.

94 Essink-Bot, M-L., De Koning, H. J., Nijs, H. G. T. *et al.* (1998). Short-term effects of population-based screening for prostate cancer on health-related quality of life. *Journal of the National Cancer Institute* **90**:925–31.

95 Houle, C., Berthelot, J.-M. (2000). A head-to-head comparison of the health utilities Mark 3 and the EQ-5D for the population living in private households in Canada. *Quality of Life Newsletter* **24**:5–6.

96 Feeny, D., Furlong, W., Barr, R. D. *et al.* (1992). A comprehensive multiattribute system for classifying the health status of survivors of childhood cancer. *Journal of Clinical Oncology* **10**:923–8.

97 Feeny, D., Furlong, W., Boyle, M. *et al.* (1995). Multi-attribute health status classification systems: Health Utilities Index. *Pharmacoeconomics* **7**:490–502.

98 Torrance, G. W., Furlong, W., Feeny, D. *et al.* (1995). Multi-attribute preference functions: Health Utilities Index. *Pharmacoeconomics* **7**:503–20.

99 Torrance, G. W., Feeny, D. H., Furlong, W. J. *et al.* (1996). Multi-attribute preference functions for a comprehensive health status classification system: Health Utilities Index Mark 2. *Medical Care* **34**:702–22.

100 Furlong, W., Feeny, D., Torrance, G. W. *et al.* (1998). *Multiplicative Multi-attribute Utility Function for the Health Utilities Index Mark 3 (HUI3) System: A Technical Report.* McMaster University Centre for Health Economics and Policy Analysis Working Paper No. 98-11.

101 Barr, R. D., Furlong, W., Dawson, S. *et al.* (1993). An assessment of global health status in survivors of acute lymphoblastic leukemia in childhood. *American Journal of Pediatric Hematology/Oncology* **15**:284–90.

102 Barr, R. D., Simpson, T., Whitton, A. *et al.* (1999). Health-related quality of life in survivors of tumours of the central nervous system in childhood – a preference-based approach to measurement in a cross-sectional study. *European Journal of Cancer* **35**:248–55.

103 Whitton, A. C., Rhydderch, H., Furlong, W. *et al.* (1997). Self-reported comprehensive health status of adult brain tumor patients using the Health Utilities Index. *Cancer* **80**: 258–65.

104 Pickard, A. S., Topfer, L.-A., Feeny, D. H. (2004). A structured review of studies on health-related quality of life and economic evaluation in pediatric acute lymphoblastic leukemia. *Journal of the National Cancer Institute Monographs*, in press.

105 Ramsey, S. D., Andersen, M. R., Etzioni, R. *et al.* (2000). Quality of life in survivors of colorectal carcinoma. *Cancer* **88**:1294–1303.

106 Grima, D. T., Torrance, G. W., Francis, G. *et al.* (2000). Cost and health related quality of life consequences of multiple sclerosis. *Multiple Sclerosis* **6**:91–8.

107 Neumann, P. J., Kuntz, K. M., Leon, J. *et al.* (1999). Health utilities and health status in Alzheimer's disease: a cross-sectional study of subjects and caregivers. *Medical Care* **37**:27–32.

108 Neumann, P. J., Sandberg, E. A., Araki, S. S. *et al.* (2000). A comparison of HUI2 and HUI3 utility scores in Alzheimer's disease. *Medical Decision Making* **20**:413–22.

109 Bayoumi, A. M., Redelmeier, D. A. (1999). Economic methods for measuring the quality of life associated with HIV infection. *Quality of Life Research* **8**:471–80.

110 Younossi, Z., Boparai, N., McCormick, M. *et al.* (2001). Assessment of utilities and health-related quality of life in patients with chronic liver disease. *American Journal of Gastroenterology* **96**:579–83.

111 Grootendorst, P., Feeny, D., Furlong, W. (2000). Health Utilities Index Mark 3: evidence of construct validity for stroke and arthritis in a population health survey. *Medical Care* **38**:290–9.

112 Boyle, M. H., Furlong, W., Feeny, D. *et al.* (1995). Reliability of the Health Utilities Index Mark III used in the 1991 Cycle 6 General Social Survey Health Questionnaire. *Quality of Life Research* **4**:249–57.

113 Moore, A. D., Clarke, A. E., Danoff, D. S. *et al.* (1999). Can health utility measures be used in lupus research? A comparative validation and reliability study of 4 utility indices. *Journal of Rheumatology* **26**:1285–90.

114 Le Gales, C., Costet, N., Gentet, J.-C. *et al.* (1999). Cross-cultural adaptation of a health status classification system in children with cancer. First results of the French adaptation of the Health Utilities Index Marks 2 and 3. *International Journal of Cancer* (Suppl.) **12**:112–8.

115 Barr, R. D., Petrie, C., Furlong, W. *et al.* (1997). Health-related quality of life during post-induction chemotherapy in children with acute lymphoblastic leukemia in remission: an influence of corticosteroid therapy. *International Journal of Oncology* **11**:333–9.

116 Palmer, C. S., Niparko, J. K., Wyatt, R. *et al.* (1999). A prospective study of the cost-utility of the multichannel cochlear implant. *Archives of Otolaryngology – Head and Neck Surgery* **125**:1221–8.

117 Krabbe, P. F. M., Hinderink, J. B., van den Broek, P. (2000). The effect of cochlear implant use in postlingually deaf adults. *International Journal of Technology Assessment in Health Care* **16**:864–73.

118 Grossman, R., Mukherjee, J., Vaughan, D. *et al.* (1998). A one-year community-based health economic study of ciprofloxacin versus usual antibiotic treatment in acute exacerbations of chronic bronchitis. *Chest* **113**:131–41.

119 Torrance, G. W., Walker, V., Grossman, R. *et al.* (1999). Economic evaluation of ciprofloxacin compared with usual antibacterial care for the treatment of acute exacerbations of chronic bronchitis in patients followed for 1 year. *Pharmacoeconomics* **16**:499–520.

120 Suarez-Almazor, M. E., Kendall, C., Johnson, J. A. *et al.* (2000). Use of health status measures in patients with low back pain in clinical settings. Comparison of specific, generic, and preference-based instruments. *Rheumatology* **39**:783–90.

121 Comerota, A. J., Throm, R. C., Mathias, S. D. *et al.* (2000). Catheter-directed thrombolysis for iliofemoral deep vein thrombosis improves health-related quality of life. *Journal of Vascular Surgery* **32**:130–7.

122 Kaplan, R. M., Anderson, J. P. (1996). The General Health Policy Model: an integrated approach. In *Quality of Life and Pharmacoeconomics in Clinical Trials* (2nd Edition), ed. B. Spilker, pp. 309–22. Philadelphia, PA: Lippincott-Raven Publishers.

123 Frosch, D., Porzsolt, F., Heicappell, R. *et al.* (2001). Comparison of German language versions of the QWB-SA and SF-36 evaluating outcomes for patients with prostate disease. *Quality of Life Research* **10**:165–73.

124 Krahn, M., Ritvo, P., Irvine, J. *et al.* (2000). Construction of the Patient-Oriented Prostate Utility Scale (PORPUS): a multi-attribute health status classification system for prostate cancer. *Journal of Clinical Epidemiology* **53**:920–30.

125 Canadian Coordinating Office for Health Technology Assessment. (1997). *Guidelines for Economic Evaluation of Pharmaceuticals: Canada, 2nd Edition.* Ottawa: Canadian Coordinating Office for Health Technology Assessment.

126 Ware, J. E., Sherbourne, C. D. (1992). The MOS 36-Item Short Form Health Survey (SF-36). *Medical Care* **30**:473–83.

127 Ware, J. E., Snow, K. K., Kosinski, M., Gandek, B. (1993). *SF-36 Health Survey Manual and Interpretation Guide.* Boston: New England Medical Center, The Health Institute.

128 Ware, J. E., Jr. (1996). The SF-36 Health Survey. In *Quality of Life and Pharmacoeconomics in Clinical Trials* (2nd Edition), ed. B. Spilker, pp. 337–45. Philadelphia, PA: Lippincott-Raven Press.

129 Brazier, J., Roberts, J., Deverill, M. (2002). The estimation of a preference-based measure of health status from the SF-36. *Journal of Health Economics* **21**:271–92.

5

Quality of life in breast cancer – what have we learned and where do we go from here?

Patricia A. Ganz, M.D.[1] and Pamela J. Goodwin, M.D., M.Sc.[2]

[1]University of California at Los Angeles, Los Angeles, CA
[2]University of Toronto, ON, Canada

Introduction

Breast cancer is the most common cancer in North American women, accounting for about a third of all incident cancers.[1] In 2004 in the USA, there are projected to be 215 900 newly diagnosed cases of female breast cancer and 40 110 deaths.[1] During the past 5 years, the mortality rate for breast cancer has declined significantly, most likely due to a combination of wider use of mammographic screening and the diffusion of adjuvant therapy for stage I and II disease.[2] In spite of this improvement in mortality, the number of incident cases of breast cancer is projected to rise with the continued aging of the population, as breast cancer peaks in women in the 8th decade of life.[2–4] Unless major advances in the prevention of breast cancer occur, using chemoprevention and other risk reduction strategies,[5] the absolute number of breast cancer patients and survivors will continue to increase as we move further into the 21st century.

The majority of women with breast cancer are diagnosed with early-stage localized disease.[1] In fact, tumor size at diagnosis has continued to decrease, with very small invasive and non-invasive cancers being detected through mammographic screening. Some series estimate that about 20% of incident cases are now non-invasive (stage 0) ductal carcinoma in situ. However, in spite of these decreases in tumor size and invasiveness, almost all patients diagnosed with breast cancer receive localized breast surgery (breast-conserving surgery and radiation to the breast or a modified radical mastectomy, with or without reconstruction). The choice of primary local therapy is usually determined by patient preference, clinical logistics, and other technical/medical factors. Mastectomy and/or breast-conserving surgery with radiation therapy are medically equivalent in most cases.[6] However, there are many decisions that must be made regarding adjuvant treatments for breast cancer,[7] and these are determined by tumor size, nodal status, metastatic spread, and tumor characteristics (histologic grade, receptor status). In addition to chemotherapy, hormone therapy, and radiation therapy, newer targeted therapies with monoclonal antibodies such as trastuzumab must now be considered. Fortunately, clinicians can draw on a quarter century of phase III randomized trials in the adjuvant therapy of breast cancer, as well as the overviews performed at Oxford for the Early Breast Cancer Collaborating Trialists, to help determine optimum therapy for early-stage breast cancer patients.[8,9] A recent NIH Consensus Conference updates these treatment recommendations.[7]

The vast majority of women with stage I breast cancer will have a life expectancy that is nearly equivalent to age-matched women without a breast cancer diagnosis.[10] Adjuvant therapy for both stage I and II breast cancer reduces the risk of recurrent cancer by about 30–40%, with absolute improvements in overall survival of about 7–11% depending on the stage of disease.[9] Thus, many women receive therapies with potential acute toxicities and late effects, but not all women benefit.[10] Understanding the impact of treatment on quality of life has been an important clinical and research question. Addressing the psychosocial and emotional concerns of women with breast cancer has been a focus of intervention research for the past quarter century. The natural history of breast cancer – large numbers of patients, with long disease-free and overall survival times, and effective treatments – has made this disease a central focus in the study of quality of life in cancer patients. Further, even women with metastatic disease may live productive lives for extended periods of time, in contrast to the experiences of patients with metastatic lung and colorectal cancer. Thus, there is an extensive literature on health-related quality-of-life (HRQOL) outcomes in breast cancer patients. A critical review of this literature is the focus of this chapter.

Quality-of-life outcomes should be considered across the breast cancer continuum, including women at high risk for the disease; women with non-invasive breast cancer; women newly diagnosed with early-stage breast cancer (stage I and II); women newly diagnosed with advanced local breast cancer (stage III or inflammatory); women with metastatic disease at diagnosis; women surviving disease-free beyond the first course of primary treatment; long-term disease-free breast cancer survivors (> 5 years since diagnosis); women with a first recurrence of breast cancer after a disease-free interval; and women living and dying with advanced metastatic disease. HRQOL studies have been conducted with women in all of these phases of the disease continuum. For the purposes of this chapter, the focus is only on women with a diagnosis of breast cancer.

The goal of this chapter is to give the reader an appreciation for the depth and breadth of research that measures HRQOL in breast cancer patients. Since this cancer was one of the first to attract investigators to measure HRQOL during cancer treatment,[11] an extensive literature was available to review and synthesize. Many of the cancer-specific quality-of-life instruments that were created in the past two decades were applied very early in their development to breast cancer patients, either in clinical trials or descriptive studies.[12–15] In parallel, a wide range of measures coming from the traditions of psychology and psychiatry were also used in breast cancer samples,[16] primarily because of a paucity of cancer-specific measures, but also because of the salience of using established measures of mood and depression in the evaluation of psychosocial intervention programs. Finally, in recent years, with the growing number of breast cancer survivors, more general measures of HRQOL have been applied to breast cancer patients to examine the impact of this disease compared to other chronic conditions and to see how much these survivors differ from healthy women.[17] A brief history of the measurement of HRQOL in breast cancer patients, a description of the methods, and information on the most commonly used HRQOL instruments in breast cancer studies are provided below. Then, studies that have used more than one HRQOL instrument are discussed, with emphasis on the strengths and weakness of various approaches, the role of HRQOL assessment in randomized controlled trials, and the value these measures add beyond biomedical outcome measures. Finally, comments on further research that is needed to develop a state of the art measurement model are provided.

History of measurement of HRQOL in breast cancer patients

Two streams of HRQOL research in breast cancer evolved during the last quarter of the twentieth century. The first stream emerges from the historic interest of psychiatrists and psychologists in the trauma associated with loss of the breast. In her classic 1980 review article, Meyerowitz examines the psychosocial correlates of breast cancer,[18] including psychosocial adjustment, quality of life, partner relationships, and the impact of treatments such as mastectomy and adjuvant chemotherapy. At about the same time, Spiegel et al. began to study the psychosocial support needs of women with advanced metastatic breast cancer, and they conducted a randomized psychosocial intervention trial to examine the effect of the intervention on pain and depression.[16] They found that psychological distress, as measured by a standardized psychological measure of mood (Profile of Mood States – POMS),[19] contributed substantially to the amount of pain experienced by these patients. This study was one of the first in breast cancer patients to use existing psychological measures to evaluate mood. Many subsequent studies with breast cancer patients drew extensively on a variety of standard psychological measures to describe and evaluate outcomes for women with breast cancer.[19,20]

The second stream of research comes from the realm of clinical trials, where, particularly in the case of metastatic breast cancer, there was an early interest in obtaining information on the subjective experience of chemotherapy treatment from the woman herself.[11,12,21] These initial scales were developed on an ad hoc basis for particular trials, and drew on the linear analogue self-assessment (LASA) approach that had been widely used to obtain subjective ratings in psychological assessments.[11] Subsequently, more rigorous development and evaluation of cancer-specific HRQOL instruments occurred, specifically for use in clinical trials, and these were then applied to clinical treatment trials in breast cancer. Examples of these cancer-specific measures include the Functional Living Index-Cancer (FLIC),[14] the European Organization for Research and Treatment of Cancer Quality of Life Questionnaire-30 item (EORTC QLQ-C30),[22] and the Functional Assessment of Cancer Therapy (FACT).[23] The Cancer Rehabilitation Evaluations System (CARES) was originally developed from a rehabilitation and needs assessment framework[13,15,24,25] and, later, a shortened version (CARES-SF) was adapted for potential use in clinical trials.[26] In 1988, Levine and colleagues reported on one of the first breast cancer-specific instruments for use in clinical trials, the Breast Cancer Chemotherapy Questionnaire (BCQ).[27] Subsequently, breast cancer-specific modules were developed for both the EORTC QLQ-C30[28] and the FACT.[29] These efforts paralleled the expanding clinical research on the use of adjuvant therapy in breast cancer, especially following the NIH Consensus Conference in 1985 which stressed the importance of considering HRQOL issues when selecting adjuvant therapy.[30]

During the past two decades, there has been increasing interest in describing the rehabilitation and recovery of breast cancer patients receiving complex therapies and facing stressful decisions regarding primary therapy (e.g., mastectomy versus breast conservation). There is an extensive literature on this topic, and a broad array of outcomes measurement strategies have been used in these studies, including standardized psychological measures and the cancer-specific HRQOL instruments. There have also been randomized trials of psychosocial interventions focusing on improvement in psychological well-being, symptoms, and even survival. These studies also were a focus for the literature reviewed in this paper.

Methods

In undertaking this review, a broad definition of HRQOL was used. Studies using instruments developed in the fields of psychiatry and psychology (which are unidimensional, in general) were included, as well as instruments developed for general or cancer-specific measurements of HRQOL (which are multidimensional, in general). All of the instruments considered for review use patient self-report for collection of data.

Studies that reported only symptoms were not included, unless those symptoms were measured as part of a broader measurement of HRQOL or if the impact of symptoms on function was also assessed. This decision was made to reduce the volume of literature being reviewed for this chapter; it does not reflect a lack of importance of patient-reported symptoms. Studies that included utilities as their only HRQOL outcomes were excluded, as they are covered in Chapter 4 by Feeny[31] in this volume. The literature search strategy was as comprehensive as possible in identifying all publications addressing HRQOL in breast cancer. Its main emphasis was on a series of MEDLINE searches of the National Library of Medicine conducted in May and June of 2000. The searches combined the term "breast cancer" with "quality of life" and with each of the known HRQOL instruments, as well as with the additional terms "clinical trials" and "randomized clinical trials". These strategies were supplemented by more focused MEDLINE searches, as well as review of articles in the authors' files and discussion with experts in the field.

Potentially relevant articles were identified and reviewed. Articles that did not provide new data were excluded (e.g., editorials, letters, some reviews, treatment trials that did not measure HRQOL). The articles thus identified were abstracted into detailed tables and formed the basis of this review.

A total of 256 references were systematically reviewed and categorized. Thirty papers that did not identify breast cancer patients as a distinct group, were methodological in nature, or did not include primary HRQOL data were excluded. The remaining 226 papers are included in this review.

Results

Literature review

The eight most frequently used HRQOL instruments in breast cancer identified in this process were the Profile of Mood States (POMS), the Hospital Anxiety and Depression Scale (HADS), the Rotterdam Symptom Checklist (RSCL), the European Organization for Research and Treatment of Cancer Quality of Life Questionnaire Core 30-item instrument (EORTC QLQ-C30), the Functional Living Index-Cancer (FLIC), the Functional Assessment of Cancer Therapy (FACT), the Cancer Rehabilitation Evaluation System (CARES), and the Medical Outcomes Study Short Form 36 survey (MOS SF-36). While the development, psychometric properties, and validation of these instruments were reviewed as part of this research, the details are presented in Chapter 3 by Erickson in this volume.[32] The current chapter will focus on the strengths and weaknesses of these instruments as used in breast cancer patients, and the added value of HRQOL assessment in breast cancer clinical trials.

Table 5.1 lists the key instruments selected for this review and describes the domains of HRQOL measured across instruments, including the total number of items in each instrument. This summary provides an overview of the range of constructs considered across instruments, from physical and emotional well-being to body image, sexuality, breast and arm symptoms, and treatment toxicities. These instruments were used in a wide range of studies and phases of the disease. The POMS[19] was one of the most widely used instruments (42 references identified). In contrast, the breast cancer-specific HRQOL tools – the EORTC QLQ-BR-23[28] or the FACT-B[29] – had many fewer citations (4–6 references identified). Because many clinical trials are in process using the FACT-B and the EORTC QLQ-BR-23, their psychometric properties are reviewed here.

Key HRQOL instruments used in studies of breast cancer

The eight HRQOL instruments most commonly used in breast cancer patients are generic and general cancer measures, and their psychometric properties are reviewed in Chapter 3 by Erickson in this volume. In this section, we discuss their use in breast cancer patient samples, and the breast cancer-specific modules of the EORTC QLQ-C30 and the FACT are described in detail.

The FLIC is the oldest of the cancer-specific HRQOL tools that have been used with breast cancer patients.[14] The FLIC has been found to be responsive to change,[33] and its total score correlates strongly with the number of problems endorsed by newly diagnosed breast cancer patients completing the CARES/CIPS.[34] Twenty-one studies in breast cancer were identified that used the FLIC, and several key references are noted here.[26,33,35–45] The FLIC has been supplanted by more recently developed measures.

The RSCL[46] has been found to be responsive to change[47] and has been widely used with breast cancer patients. There were 19 key breast cancer references, which are noted here.[48–66]

In the early 1980s, Schag and colleagues[13] developed a new cancer-specific instrument to capture the rehabilitation needs of cancer patients, initially

Table 5.1. Key instruments used in HRQOL research in breast cancer

Construct	SF-36	FLIC	RSCL	EORTC QLQ-C30	EORTC BR-23	FACT-G	FACT-B	CARES	POMS	HADS
Number of items included for each construct										
Physical functioning	10		4	5		2		4		
Role – physical	5	4	4	2		3		7		
Mental health										
Psychological distress/adjustment	3	4	8	4	1	7	2	5		
– Anxiety									9	7
– Depression									15	7
– Anger-hostility									12	
– Anxiety re cancer, treatment		2			1			4		
– Anxiety in medical situations								8		
Psychological well-being	2									
Role – emotional	3					2		2		
Social	2	2		2		6		14		
Energy/fatigue	4		2	3		1		3	15	
Cognitive				2				3	7	
Sleep			2	1		1		1		
Pain	2	3	1	2		1		4		
General health/global QOL	4	2		2	1	6	1			
Health change	1									
Body image					2		1	3		
Sexual interest/function/attractiveness			1		5	1	2	8		
Clothing								3		
Nausea/vomiting		2	2	2		2		6		
Hair loss					1		2	1		
Weight loss			1					2		
Appetite/taste/dry mouth/swallowing			1	1		2		3		
Other GI symptoms			3	2				1		
Shortness of breath			1	1			1			
Arm symptoms					3		1			
Breast symptoms					4					
Hot flashes					1					
Ostomy/prosthesis problems								2		
Other physical symptoms			8		1			4		
Medical interaction						2		11		
Patient compliance								4		
Relationship with partner								18		
Interaction with children								3		
Dating problems								5		
Employment concerns								7		
Hardship due to cancer (self)		1		1				3		
Hardship (family)		2								
Not scored									7	
Total items	36	22	38	30	23	34	10	139	65	14

called the Cancer Inventory of Problem Situations (CIPS). As the CIPS was further refined and developed, it became known as the Cancer Rehabilitation Evaluation System (CARES). Ganz and colleagues have used the CARES in a psychosocial intervention study with newly diagnosed breast cancer patients.[34,35,67] It has excellent reliability and validity,[24] as well as responsiveness to change in breast cancer patients and survivors.[17,33] Individual summary scales and subscales from the CARES have been used in studies of breast cancer patients.[68–70] There were 17 key references using the CARES or CARES-SF.[17, 33–35, 68–69, 71–81]

The EORTC QLQ-C30 is a general cancer HRQOL measure that is widely used in clinical trials in Europe and Canada.[22,82,83] It has been shown to be responsive to change[84,85] and to converge in a predictable fashion with other HRQOL and psychological questionnaires.[86] A recent exploratory factor analysis of psychosocial items identified and validated two factors, emotional distress and functional ability, in a sample of patients with metastatic breast cancer.[87] A disease-specific module (BR-23) (Table 5.2) has been developed for breast cancer. The BR-23 contains 23 items addressing body image, sexual functioning, arm symptoms, breast symptoms, systemic therapy side effects, sexual enjoyment, future perspective, and upset by hair loss.[28] It has good internal consistency and discriminates between patients receiving chemotherapy or not and between differing levels of performance status. It is sensitive to change in some, but not all, circumstances. Thirty key references were found that used the EORTC QLQ-C30, and six were found that used the EORTC QLQ-C30 and BR-23 module.[63,85,87–120]

The FACT, like the EORTC QLQ-C30, has a general core instrument and disease-specific modules. The FACT-G has evolved through several versions since its original description[23] and has been used in a number of studies with breast cancer patients. The FACT-B[29] (Table 5.2) includes a breast cancer-specific module with 9 items that relate to symptoms from treatment (short of breath, hair loss), body image and sexuality ("self-conscious about the way I dress," arms swollen or tender, sexual

attractiveness), and other miscellaneous concerns. These items are less extensive than the EORTC QLQ-breast cancer-specific module,[28] and the time interval is brief (7 days). When the breast module is used, it is added to the total score for the instrument. The FACT-B is currently being used in many multi-center trials, but there are few results available in the literature as yet. Four references used the FACT-G and 5 used the FACT-B.[43,44,118,121–126]

The MOS SF-36 is a widely used generic measure of HRQOL.[127–129] It has 8 scales (physical, emotional, role functioning-physical and emotional, bodily pain, vitality, social functioning, general health) and can be scored in two component domains of physical and mental health, with population reference norms. It does not have the precision for pain and symptoms that might be experienced by breast cancer patients, although it has great value for comparison of cancer patients to normative populations or other patients with chronic illness. For that reason, it has been adopted in studies of breast cancer survivors.[68,70,130–132] More targeted assessment tools for symptoms or specific problems associated with the breast cancer experience often supplement its use in these settings.[68] This review identified 39 references that used the MOS SF-36, subscales of the instrument, or variants of the instrument or the parent RAND instruments (e.g., MHI, MOS-20, SF-12).[17,36–38,42–44,50,68–70,74,78–81,88,97,103,105,109,116,131–147]

The HADS is a 14-item self-administered questionnaire developed for use in medically ill patients[148] to measure anxiety and depression. Its two subscales can be summed into a total score. In the UK it is commonly used in cancer trials in conjunction with the EORTC QLQ-C30 or the RSCL. Seventeen key references in breast cancer patients were found.[49,52,56,57,59,102,103,111,117,149–156]

The POMS, a 65-item self-administered adjectival checklist, has six domains (tension-anxiety, anger-hostility, depression-dejection, confusion-bewilderment, fatigue-inertia, vigor-activity) which can be summed into a Total Mood Disturbance (TMD) score.[19] It has been widely used in a large number of trials in breast cancer, especially in

Table 5.2. Description and psychometric properties of two breast cancer-specific questionnaires

Instrument name	EORTC Breast Module (BR-23)[28]	Functional Assessment of Cancer Therapy-General (FACT-G); Functional Assessment of Cancer Therapy – Breast (FACT-B) (version 3)[29]
Purpose for which developed	A breast cancer-specific questionnaire to be used in conjunction with the EORTC QLQ-C30.	To measure multidimensional HRQOL in patients with breast cancer. Includes FACT-General plus breast cancer-specific module.
Length	23 items. Time frame: past week for body image, symptom scales; past 4 weeks for sexual function.	44 items: 28 FACT-G, 9 BCS, 7 "additional concerns." Time frame past 7 days.
Administration time	On average, 9 minutes to complete both QLQ-C30 and BR-23.	10 minutes.
Domains included	Body image (4 items); sexual functioning (2); arm symptoms (3); breast symptoms (4); systemic therapy side effects (7); sexual enjoyment (1); future perspective (1); upset by hair loss (1).	Physical Well-Being (7 items), Emotional Well-Being (5), Social Well-Being (7), Functional Well-Being (7), Relationship with Doctor (2), Breast Cancer (9).
Scoring	4-point scale ("not at all, a little, quite a bit, very much"). Scale scores = mean of item scores, rescaled to 0-to-100.	0 to 4 scale ("not at all, a little bit, somewhat, quite a bit, very much"). Global score, FACT-G score, subscale scores. Trial Outcome Index-Physical/Functional/Breast (TOI-PFB) is a 28-item summary of FACT-B, not intended to be administered alone.
Validated modes of administration	Self-administered in clinic; self-administered mail; interviewer-administered.	Self-administered.
Validated translations/cultural adaptations	Dutch (initial development), Bulgarian, Danish, English, French, German, Greek, Hungarian, Italian, Norwegian, Persian, Polish, Portuguese, Spanish, Swedish, Turkish.	English (initial development), Spanish, Flemish, French (Canada, France, Belgium), German (Germany, Austria, Switzerland), Italian, Norwegian, Swedish, Japanese.
Evidence of reliability (internal consistency, test-retest, other)	Reliability and validity tested in 170 Dutch, 168 Spanish, 158 American patients. In American sample, Cronbach's alpha = 0.70 to 0.91; Dutch = 0.57 to 0.89 (arm, side effects < 0.70); Spanish 0.46 to 0.94 (arm, breast, side effects < 0.70). Spanish results attributed to homogeneity, good health status of sample. Missing data 1%–9% on sexuality items, especially among older women.	Internal: Cronbach's alpha for Breast Cancer Scale (BCS) = 0.63 (not intended to be a homogeneous scale); TOI-PFB = 0.88; FACT-G subscales = 0.60–0.86. FACT-G, FACT-B global scores, r = 0.90. Test-retest: BCS r = 0.88, FACT-G subscales 0.82–0.88, FACT-G global 0.92, FACT-B global 0.85 over 3 to 7 days.
Evidence of validity (content, construct, criterion-related)	Content developed by EORTC QOL Study Group, including lit review, interviews with patients and specialists. Multi-trait scaling analysis supported scales, except systemic therapy side effects.	Content (FACT-G, FACT-B, in turn): FACT-G: Generated candidate questions based on open-ended interviews with 45 stage II or IV patients (breast, lung, colorectal) and 15 oncology professionals. Item reduction used relevance rating by 90 different patients.

(cont.)

Table 5.2. (*cont.*)

Instrument name	EORTC Breast Module (BR-23)[28]	Functional Assessment of Cancer Therapy-General (FACT-G); Functional Assessment of Cancer Therapy – Breast (FACT-B) (version 3)[29]
	Known groups: In Dutch sample, discriminated between metastatic and other patients on sexual function, future perspective, therapy side effects (p < .001); same pattern in Spanish, American, but not significant. Discriminated based on KPS in Dutch patients; Spanish only significant for side effects.	FACT-B: Open-ended interview with 10 patients, 5 experts resulted in 137 candidate questions; relevance rated by 30 different patients.
		Construct: Factor analysis used to establish FACT-G subscales.
		Concurrent: Correlations with FLIC: FACT-B global, r = 0.87; FACT-G global, r = 0.86; BCS, r = 0.53. Also significant correlations between Emotional Well-Being and POMS Depression (−0.53), Tension (−0.57), Anger (−0.45); Physical (0.46), Functional Well-Being (0.57) with POMS Vigor; Physical Well-Being with POMS Fatigue (−0.54); POMS-SF total correlated with Emotional (−0.60).
		Divergent validity: Lack of correlation with Marlowe-Crown Social Desirability Scale.
		Known groups: All scales except Relationship with Doctor differentiated groups by self-rated ECOG Performance Status Rating (PSR) category. All scales in expected direction relative to extent of disease, only Physical Well-Being was significant.
Evidence of responsiveness/ sensitivity to change	Using improved, unchanged, worse KPS, significant difference over time found only in side effects in Dutch sample (p < .01) and body image in Spanish (p < .001). Responsiveness over time could not be demonstrated in American sample. Testing breast symptoms based on therapy (radiation vs chemo), Dutch and Spanish samples had significant differences; American was in expected direction.	Sensitivity to 2-month changes in PSR found for FACT-B global, FACT-G global, Physical Well-Being, Functional Well-Being, BCS, TOI-PFB, as expected. Social, Emotional Well-Being, Relationship with Doctor not responsive to PSR change, also as expected.
Interpretability (availability of normative data, clinically meaningful difference)	Effect sizes were moderate to large.	Norms from validation study published in Brady, 1997.[29]
		Kemmler compared FACT-G, EORTC QLQ-C30; concluded they measure significantly different aspects of HRQOL and results should not be compared.

psychosocial intervention trials. Norms and T scores (a T-score is a standardized score with a distribution whose mean is 50 and standard deviation is 10) are available for several populations, including non-psychiatrically ill patients and normal college students. There were 40 key references in breast cancer found.[16,17,33,35,40,71,72,76,121,124–126,131,138,145,153,154, 157–179]

In addition to these most commonly used HRQOL instruments, we identified two other instruments that were developed for individual studies and some instruments that have been used only by a few research groups. For example, the International Breast Cancer Study Group (IBCSG) has used a series of LASA scales, derived from the historical work of Priestman and Baum[11] and other groups.[21] These scales (described in a series of publications by the IBCSG)[180–182] are single-item measures of various symptoms (e.g., nausea, pain, appetite) and are reported as single item scores. Thus, they differ substantially from other symptom checklists (e.g., RSCL) or HRQOL instruments that are used in this research.

Another instrument that was developed specifically for monitoring the HRQOL of breast cancer patients is the Breast Cancer Chemotherapy Questionnaire (BCQ).[27] This brief instrument (N = 30 items) underwent rigorous psychometric evaluation, and was uniquely designed to capture the acute toxicity of breast cancer adjuvant therapy. In spite of the high specificity and responsiveness of this instrument, it has been used in very few clinical trials.[183–185] One limitation to the adoption of this instrument is that once patients are off treatment, the questions are no longer relevant (e.g., questions regarding alopecia, inconvenience coming for treatment, nausea, upset stomach). Thus, while this instrument meets important criteria for reliability, validity, and responsiveness, it has not been widely adopted and is not covered in detail in this chapter.

Studies that have used more than one HRQOL instrument simultaneously

We identified 44 papers that simultaneously used more than one HRQOL instrument. These papers included self-report mental health scales but excluded clinician-reported measures. These articles included validation studies,[27,29,64,87,93,180, 186] cross-sectional studies of breast cancer patients/survivors at various times along the disease trajectory,[34,36,45,68,81,116,132] and randomized clinical trials, e.g.,[40,42,52,103,173,187] as well as methodological studies that directly compared the measurement and content characteristics of two instruments in the same sample of patients.[49,92,98] Overall, in the validation studies, scales and instruments that were hypothesized to converge or diverge did so.[27,29,57,87,93,180,186] In these studies, classical test theory principles and factor analyses were used to examine aspects of reliability and validity. Similarly, in various cross-sectional studies at different phases of the disease, all of the mental health scales from various instruments (CES-D, POMS, HADS, RSCL, CARES, SF-36, EORTC QLQ-C30, FACT) demonstrated similar patterns of behavior in a wide variety of samples.[33,68,81,97,138] Specifically, younger patients uniformly showed greater psychological distress than older patients, and patients with more advanced disease showed more distress than disease-free survivors.[68,70,71,81] In several studies, HRQOL of breast cancer survivors was found to be good, using norms from generic HRQOL measures[17,68,70] and in direct comparison with control samples.[138] In several prospective longitudinal studies, various HRQOL scales demonstrated improving HRQOL in the year after breast cancer diagnosis and treatment,[33,132] and worsening of HRQOL at the time of recurrence.[70,188] Presentation of actual psychometric performance of scales within these papers was infrequent.

Table 5.3 shows representative ranges of scores for several of the major HRQOL instruments to provide normative reference information for those who may choose to use these instruments in new studies with breast cancer samples. Not all studies presented actual scores for each instrument within the published report. As can be seen, scores for most instruments are quite comparable across studies within phase of disease. For the EORTC QLQ-C30, patients with advanced metastatic breast cancer have poorer

Table 5.3. Representative scores for four commonly used HRQOL instruments in breast cancer

EORTC QLQ-C30

Author	Osoba, 1994[85] Canada		Fayers, 1998[*in 107]	Kramer, 2000[107]	Cohen, 2000[**105] Canada	Apolone, 1998[***97] Italy
	Primary and Metastatic		Metastatic	Metastatic RCT pre-treatment	Survivors 6–60 months	Survivors > 5 years; from RCT's
Disease Phase	Pre-treatment	During Chemo RCT				
Domain						
Physical	85.3	76.5	64.1	65.5	83.4	78.4
Role	79.2	68.9	63.4	63.6	85.5	84.0
Emotional	69.6	70.7	64.8	63.2	76.1	78.1
Social	78.1	67.4	70.1	76.0	90.9	90.7
Cognitive	82.5	80.3	81.1	82.4	83.7	81.6
Nausea/Vomiting	4.4	24.7	12.4	8.6	3.8	2.6
Fatigue	27.7	47.6	40.1	37.2	22.4	19.8
Pain	21.9	19.9	39.0	33.7	13.4	17.2
Global QOL	66.7	54.3	54.1	60.1	74.8	70.2

Mean scores, scale = 0–100; nr = not reported

*EORTC reference values for patients with advanced breast cancer (cited in Kramer 2000)

**Weighted average for radical, partial mastectomy groups

***Italian translation of the EORTC

FACT-B

Author	Brady, 1997[29] US	Wenzel, 1999[*123] US		Holzner, 2001[118] Austria		
	All phases; ages 28–86; 46% white, 51% black	Stage I, II, IIIA immediately after treatment; 90% white		Stage I, II; no recurrence; ages 30–70 Years since initial treatment:		
Disease Phase		Age ≤ 50	Age > 50	1–2	2–5	>5
Domain						
Physical well-being (28)	22.1	21.4	22.1	25	26.4	24.3
Emotional well-being (20)	16.3	17.9	19.9	18.7	20.5	18
Social well-being (28)	22.7	22.8	23.5	17.5	20.4	17.4
Functional well-being (28)	20.6	20.2	20.9	21.1	23.4	20.9
Relationship with doctor (8)	7.0	nr	nr	nr	nr	nr
FACT-G total (112)	88.8	89.2	93.3	82.3	91.1	80.3
Breast Cancer Subscale (36)	24.1	22.5	24.4	24.4	27.8	24.4
FACT-B total (148)	112.8	111.7	117.6	106.7	118.9	104.7

*Reported on 0–100 scale; retransformed for comparison

nr = not reported

SF-36

Author	MOS Norms*	Ganz, 1996[17] US (LA)		Ganz, 1998**[68] US (LA, DC)		Grunfeld, 1996***[103] England	Lindley, 1998[36] US (NC)				Broeckel, 2000[137] US (FL)	
		Stage I, II survivors		Stage 0, I, II survivors		Stage I, II, III survivors	Stage I, II survivors 2–5 years post-chemo				Stage I, II survivors < 3 years post-chemo	
							Age 45–54		Age 55–64			
Disease Phase	NA	2 years	3 years	Age < 50	Age ≥ 50	survivors	Study	US norms	Study	US norms	Patients	Controls
Domain												
Physical functioning	70.6	83.6	77.9	87.7	76.5	73.4	80.6	82.9	75.2	73.1	70.3	85.9
Role – physical	53.0	79.3	76.4	82.2	72.5	70.0	78.9	79.9	70.8	71.6	54.5	86.4
Role – emotional	65.8	84.5	83.6	73.9	80.8	74.0	82.3	81.9	84.7	79.5	70.5	80.2
Energy/fatigue	52.2	63.9	61.7	59.3	61.1	56.8	59.1	60.6	65.8	58.1	52.3	63.2
Emotional well-being	70.4	76.9	76.1	72.0	77.3	78.4	78.9	74.4	75.5	73.4	75.3	79.2
Social functioning	78.8	92.8	87.7	86.1	86.9	77.8	91.0	82.7	86.5	79.4	80.1	90.7
Pain	70.8	87.2	80.9	81.3	77.1	79.5	73.9	72.1	79.3	66.6	70.8	80.9
General heath	57.0	70.9	69.2	74.1	72.8	69.8	79.2	70.5	66.2	62.9	68.7	78.8
Health change	59.1	67.4	55.4	nr	nr							

* Based on outpatients in a physicians office

** ≥ 50 is weighted average of 50–59, ≥ 60

*** Weighted average of RCT baseline arms

Note: LA = Los Angeles; DC = Washington, DC; NC = North Carolina; FL = Florida; US = United States

FLIC

Author	Population	Disease Phase	Mean Score
FLIC norms*		Hospitalized	111.2–112.7
		Active Treatment	114.6
		Adjuvant Treatment	116.1
		Follow-up care	121.4
Edmonds, 1999[40] Canada	Metastatic patients in group therapy RCT		128.3
Ganz, 1996[17] US	Stage I, II survivors	1 month post-diagnosis	117.0
		Follow-up care	127.0
Winer, 1999[45] US	ABMT survivors	13–64 months	127.4
			128.6
			128.3
Lindley, 1998[36] US	Stage I, II, received adjuvant therapy	Survivors, 2–5 years	130.8
			138.3

* cited by Kornblith, 1993[42]

physical and emotional functioning than survivors. Scores on the SF-36 domains also show consistency across studies investigating the same stage of disease. These observations suggest that these measures are robust and perform well in various research settings across a broad range of breast cancer samples, countries, and differing data collection procedures.

What are the relative strengths and weaknesses of the most frequently used instruments? Fortunately, there are many reliable and valid instruments available for use in the evaluation of HRQOL outcomes with breast cancer patients. However, the multiplicity of instruments means there is no consensus on a single best instrument. To some extent, the choice of instrument depends on the clinical or research question, concerns about respondent burden, the phase of illness, and the type of intervention being assessed. For example, Table 5.1 shows that only one instrument assesses breast symptoms, but five address physical functioning. Evaluation of psychosocial interventions may require more detailed assessments of emotional well-being than currently provided by general cancer and generic instruments such as the EORTC QLQ-C30, FACT, FLIC, or SF-36 (see Table 5.1 for the number of items in each instrument addressing mental health). The POMS and HADS have been widely used for these purposes, but other validated measures from the psychological literature are often required to detect more specific changes in outcome.

Review of the existing literature allowed extraction of breast cancer norms by phase of illness to use as a reference point when studying a new patient sample, or for power calculations and sample size determinations (Table 5.3). The strength of the general cancer instruments (EORTC QLQ-C30, RSCL, FLIC, FACT, CARES) is that they are generally comprehensive in their inclusion of cancer-specific concerns related to physical and emotional functioning, and they capture some toxicities/symptoms of cancer and its treatment. These general cancer instruments also permit comparison of disease burden and outcomes across different cancers.[25] This type of instrument contrasts with the generic HRQOL measures (e.g., SF-36), which can be very insensitive to cancer-specific concerns,[189] although such measures may be very relevant for long-term survivors who are far removed from their cancer treatment and, thus, should be compared to healthy persons or those with other chronic health conditions.[17,68,70] The breast cancer-specific HRQOL instruments (FACT-B, EORTC QLQ-BR-23) and the BCQ[27] (not reviewed in detail because of its limited use) were designed primarily for use in clinical treatment trials, where they might be more sensitive to the unique toxicities associated with breast cancer treatments. These instruments often capture substantial differences in treatment toxicities expected by different treatment regimens and are responsive to treatment effects in longitudinal settings.[185] Because of their brevity, they may not capture some domains in as much depth as other cancer-specific instruments, e.g., the CARES, which includes body image, partner relationships, and sexuality concerns. There are many clinical trials underway using the FACT-B and the EORTC QLQ-BR-23; the future use of these questionnaires should be re-evaluated when results are available.

There have been few direct comparisons of most HRQOL instruments[98] from either a qualitative or quantitative perspective. Therefore, since the described instruments meet commonly accepted standards of reliability, validity, and responsiveness (in most cases),[190] the choice of instrument often depends on the specific item content a study requires because of study hypotheses. For example, if sexuality and body image are important considerations in a given study, a questionnaire that assesses these areas is warranted. Other considerations include the setting for administration of the questionnaire (e.g., in-person, mailed, telephone, clinical trial), language translations, and existing databases from other studies with breast cancer patients on which to build and compare. To some extent, international variations in use of these instruments primarily stem from habit and familiarity: the RSCL and HADS were combined in most British studies because this was selected as a standard approach across clinical trials; the EORTC QLQ-C30 is used in continental

Table 5.4. Use of HRQOL instruments in randomized clinical trials in breast cancer

	N	EORTC QLQ C-30	FLIC	FACT-B	POMS	HADS	RSCL	CARES	BCQ	SF-36	OTHER*
					Primary Instruments Used (NOTE: Some studies used >1 instrument)						
Biomedical Intervention											
Local Treatment	8	0	0	0	1	1	1	0	1	0	5
Adjuvant	7	2	0	0	0	1	0	0	2	1	2
Metastatic	20	8	2	0	0	1	5	0	0	0	6
Symptom Control	8	1	1	0	0	2	2	0	0	0	3
Follow-up	3	1	1	0	1	1	0	0	0	1	1
Subtotal	46	12	4	0	2	6	8	0	3	2	17
Psychosocial Intervention											
Adjuvant	12	0	1	2	5	1	1	2	0	2	3
Metastatic	7	1	1	0	7	1	0	0	0	0	0
Symptom Control	1	0	0	0	0	0	0	1	0	1	0
Subtotal	20	1	2	2	12	2	1	3	0	3	3
Grand Total	66	13	6	2	14	8	9	3	3	5	20

* None of the key instruments was used in these studies.

European and Canadian multi-center trials because of the extensive translation and validation efforts during its early development; the FLIC was used early on in US clinical studies, but then abandoned in favor of the FACT, which also became available in translated versions. Eventually, efforts at equating and item-banking across these questionnaires may succeed, and a common instrument may evolve from all of these measures. However, these options are not currently available, and the choice of measurement strategy is largely dependent on investigator preference.

HRQOL measurement in randomized trials in breast cancer

The literature review identified 66 randomized clinical trials that included HRQOL outcomes. Table 5.4 shows the HRQOL instruments most commonly used in these trials. There is considerable overlap with the instruments shown in Table 5.1, however, the use of specific HRQOL instruments varied according to the type of intervention and stage of disease. In biomedical intervention studies, the

EORTC QLQ-C30 and the RSCL were the most commonly used instruments. In psychosocial intervention studies, the POMS was used in the majority of studies; no other instrument was used in more than three studies. The use of novel (i.e., study-specific) HRQOL instruments was most common in biomedical intervention trials; however, the use of novel instruments hinders cross-study comparisons and, at times, makes interpretation of results difficult, especially when information regarding validation is limited.

To be useful in a clinical trial, a HRQOL instrument must have all of the methodological attributes discussed earlier in this chapter (e.g., validity, reliability) and must also be sensitive (responsive) to change over time.[190] Questionnaires that do not reflect changes in underlying HRQOL in a meaningful way are of little benefit in the clinical trial setting. Questionnaires measuring state rather than trait characteristics, and questionnaires that have scaling options that are sufficiently detailed to allow for identification of clinically important improvement or deterioration, are most likely to be useful in the clinical trials setting. All of the commonly used questionnaires in breast cancer trials have been shown to be sensitive to change in HRQOL; however, not all domains and/or items are equally responsive.

The focus of this review is on HRQOL that incorporates some aspect of function; symptoms are additional patient-reported outcomes often considered part of HRQOL measurement, even though they do not always include an assessment of function. In the randomized trials reviewed, the approach to symptom measurement was often poorly described, and it was not always clear whether symptom data were derived from patient reports only, provider observations, or both. When symptoms could be clearly identified as patient-reported using a standardized (preferably validated) instrument (e.g., diary, checklist), they were included as HRQOL outcomes; if not, they were included as medical outcomes.

Below, the results of randomized clinical trials in breast cancer are summarized, focusing on concordance of medical and HRQOL outcomes and on the contribution of the latter to selection of optimal treatments (Table 5.5). In the next section, the potential contributions of HRQOL measurements beyond selection of optimal treatments in clinical trials are discussed. A more detailed review of the contributions of HRQOL in selecting optimal treatments in clinical trials in breast cancer has been published elsewhere.[191]

Treatment of the primary breast tumor

Eight studies examined HRQOL in the primary management of breast cancer.[152,172,183,192–196] The majority (N = 5) compared mastectomy to breast-conserving surgery (BCS) with radiation treatment, although only two reported medical outcomes.[192,193] Neither study identified differences in recurrence or survival rates, in keeping with other published studies.[6] Four studies[192–195] reported enhancement of at least one aspect of body image (including emotional reaction to or satisfaction with body image), one[192] an improvement in sexual activity amongst older women, and one[193] reported enhanced satisfaction with treatment in women undergoing BCS.

One[195] also identified improvement in a broad variety of psychological reactions (feelings and concerns) using a novel HRQOL questionnaire when BCS was performed. There was frequent within-study discordance of HRQOL measures, with some scales and items identifying significant treatment effects and some showing no differences. Overall, these HRQOL outcomes help guide treatment recommendations by providing evidence that lumpectomy is preferable to mastectomy, even though medical outcomes are similar. However, the observation that not all aspects of HRQOL are improved in women undergoing BCS suggests that, for individual women, mastectomy may be a reasonable alternative.

The remaining three studies include a report of BCS, with or without radiation, which demonstrated a transient worsening of HRQOL during radiation therapy.[183] This was associated with reduced local recurrence but not reductions in mortality. Different radiation dose and fractionation schedules were examined in a second study;[152] the higher dose regimen was associated with transient adverse HRQOL effects, but medical outcomes were not reported. A final study[196] examined the role of surgery in elderly women receiving tamoxifen for primary breast cancer. Although local control was better when surgery was used, no differences in HRQOL were seen. In these three studies, enhanced local control or easier logistics of treatment were the primary factors influencing selection of optimal treatment; transient effects on HRQOL did not alter these therapeutic choices.

Systemic adjuvant therapy

A surprisingly small number of studies of adjuvant drug therapy have reported HRQOL outcomes.[104,109,184,197–199] Of note, none has provided information beyond 18 months after initiation of treatment. There are additional ongoing studies that have measured HRQOL whose data are not mature and have not yet been reported. There may be other studies that did not report HRQOL outcomes when treatment decisions were based on survival differences. All of these published studies

Table 5.5. Value-added of patient reported outcomes compared with clinical measures in breast cancer treatment trials

Phase of Study	Number of Studies	Most Commonly Used Patient Reported Outcomes Measures (#)	Most Commonly Used Clinical Measures (#)	Key Observations: Comments on the Value Provided by Patient-Reported Outcomes
Primary treatment	8	• STAI (2)	• Local Control (4) • Survival (4)	• Enhanced HRQOL (body image satisfaction, psychological or sexual function) identified in women receiving BCS (with radiation) in 4 of 5[192–195] studies, using novel body image questionnaires or items • HRQOL measured using multidimensional and unidimensional instruments was worse during XRT in 2 studies[152,183] (no concurrent clinical outcome measures available) • Differences in local recurrence rates were not reflected by HRQOL measures in 2 studies[183,196] • Frequent within-study discordance of HRQOL measures (some scales or items significant, others not)[52,183,192,194,195] • Overall, HRQOL results provide empiric support for use of BCS when clinical outcomes were equivalent
Adjuvant therapy	7	• EORTC QLQ-C30 (2) • BCQ (2) • LASA Scales (2) • PACIS (2)	• DFS (7) • OS (3) • Toxicity (4)	• All studies used at least one multidimensional HRQOL instrument • Significant heterogeneity of HRQOL outcomes was seen over time[109,184,197–199] (worse during treatment), between items/subscales[104,198] and with different methods of analysis[109,199] • HRQOL was found to be worse when treatment was more toxic[104,109,184,197,199] • HRQOL outcomes were not congruent with recurrence/survival outcomes in 3 studies,[104,184,198] congruent in 2 studies[197] and mixed in 2 studies (depending on analytic approach used)[109,199] • HRQOL and toxicity were congruent in 3 of 3 chemotherapy trials[104,184,199] • In all studies, selection of optimal treatment was driven by recurrence and survival outcomes, not by HRQOL differences • No HRQOL data beyond 18 months were reported in any study
Advanced disease	20	• EORTC QLQ-C30 (8) • RSCL (5) • LASA Scales (3) • FLIC (2)	• TTP/TTF (19) • Survival (19) • Response Rate (15) • Response Duration (5) • Toxicity (18) • Performance Status (3)	• Significant HRQOL effects seen for at least one subscale or item in 12[21,42,60–63,113,114,119,179,200,204] of 20 studies that used multidimensional instruments (in 9 of these studies, effects differed across subscale items) • Of the 12 studies identifying significant HRQOL effects, 9[21,42,63,112,114,119,179,200,204] also identified significant differences in TTP/TTF, OS, and/or response • Of the 19 studies that reported toxicity, HRQOL and toxicity results were congruent in 5[21,42,60,115,179] and mixed in 6[62,63,113,114,200,204]; in 8 studies toxicity was not reflected in HRQOL measurements[59,61,115,201–203,205,206]

(cont.)

Table 5.5. (*cont.*)

Phase of Study	Number of Studies	Most Commonly Used Patient Reported Outcomes Measures (#)	Most Commonly Used Clinical Measures (#)	Key Observations: Comments on the Value Provided by Patient-Reported Outcomes
				• Selection of optimal treatment was based on clinical outcomes in all but one study[61]; in the other 19 studies, HRQOL outcomes supported these selections in 5 studies[21,42,60,62,204] and provided mixed support in 4 additional studies[63,113,114,200]
Symptom control	8	• RSCL (2) • HADS (2)	• Emesis (4) • Nausea (1) • Fracture (3) • Radiation Use (3) • Pain (3) • Hypercalcemia (2)	• Multidimensional HRQOL instruments identified improvements in psychologic functioning in 3[51,53] of 4 anti-emetic trials; unidimensional instruments identified improvement in 1 additional trial[51] – all 4 trials identified reduced emesis using targeted questionnaires/diaries • Multidimensional HRQOL instruments identified beneficial effects in 1[207] of 3 bisphosphonate trials; all 3 trials identified beneficial effects on pain, fracture, need for palliative radiation, and/or hypercalcemia[110,207,208] • Overall QOL was enhanced when hot flashes were reduced by clonidine (10-point QOL Scale)[209] • Selection of optimal treatment was based on clinical outcomes in all 8 studies; HRQOL measurement provided support for these selections in 5 studies[51,53,207,209]
Follow-Up	3	• SIP (2)	• Survival (2)	• None of the studies (CT vs. MRI investigation of axillary symptoms; intensive vs. non-intensive radiologic and laboratory surveillance; specialist vs. general practice follow-up) identified any significant differences in clinical or HRQOL outcomes
Psychosocial	20	• POMS (12) • MAC (3) • IES (3) • HADS (2) • FLIC (2) • Coopersmith Self-Esteem Inventory (2) • Duke – UNC – FSSS (2)	• OS (4)	• Beneficial effects of psychosocial intervention were identified using unidimensional questionnaires in 15 of 20 studies (9[124,126,154,166,211,212,216,218,219] of 13 in the adjuvant setting, 5[16,177,178,214,220] of 6 in advanced disease, 1[69] of 1 symptom control); beneficial effects of intervention were identified in 3[69,212,219] of 9 studies using multidimensional questionnaires • HRQOL results were congruent with survival outcomes in 2[40,215] of 4 studies (both positive in 1,[215] both negative in 1[40]); congruent with menopausal symptoms (hot flashes) in 1[69]; discordant with NK activity[126] and tumor response[212] in 1 each • HRQOL outcomes were the primary determinant of treatment decisions in all but 1 study[215] (they supported survival benefits in that study)

BCS = breast-conserving surgery; CT = computerized tomography; DFS = disease-free survival; DUFSS = Duke University – University of North Carolina Social Support Questionnaire; IES = Impact of Events Scale; LASA Scales = Linear Analog Self-Assessment Scales; MAC = Mental Adjustment to Cancer Scale; MRI = magnetic resonance imaging; NK activity = natural killer cell activity; OS = overall survival; PACIS = Perceived Adjustment to Chronic Illness Scale; SIP = Sickness Impact Profile; STAI = State–Trait Anxiety Inventory; TTF = time to treatment failure; TTP = time to progression; XRT = radiation treatment.

of systemic adjuvant therapy used at least one multidimensional HRQOL instrument.

In general, the administration of chemotherapy or of more aggressive chemotherapy was associated with a poorer HRQOL compared to administration of hormonal interventions or less aggressive chemotherapy. However, these effects were often transient.[104,184,199] Important heterogeneity in HRQOL outcomes was seen within trials – over time, between subscales, and even with the approach used in the statistical analysis. For example, one trial[198] comparing goserelin to goserelin plus tamoxifen to tamoxifen to no treatment identified some aspects of HRQOL to be worse with goserelin, others to be worse with tamoxifen, and some to be similar regardless of treatment given. Two trials[109,199] yielded HRQOL results that differed with the instrument (BCQ or Q-TWIST, essentially a utility-based measurement) or analytic approach used (e.g., summary measures versus area under the curve). Additionally, the short-term HRQOL outcomes that have been reported were not always congruent with recurrence or survival outcomes (the former often reflecting transiently greater toxicity of more aggressive, and more effective, treatments). HRQOL outcomes reflected toxicity in all three chemotherapy trials that reported toxicity.

Because the ultimate goal of adjuvant treatment is to improve long-term survival, short-term toxicity is often considered an acceptable price to pay to reach this goal. As a result, unless treatments are shown to have equivalent effects on recurrence and survival, it is unlikely that transient deleterious effects of treatment on HRQOL will influence treatment decisions. Whether long-term HRQOL effects (e.g., cognitive impairment, sequelae of early menopause) would alter selection of treatments associated with longer survival is open to question – documentation of these long-term HRQOL effects after completion of adjuvant therapy is an area of active research. When results of these studies become available, this question will need to be addressed. To date, measurement of short-term HRQOL has not had an important influence on treatment selection in the adjuvant setting.

Treatment of advanced disease

The metastatic disease setting provided the largest single group of studies that measured HRQOL. A range of HRQOL instruments was used, the most common being the EORTC QLQ-C30 and the RSCL. Reporting of HRQOL outcomes in some of these studies was very brief.[e.g.,62,113]

Although differences in HRQOL and/or psychosocial outcomes were identified between study arms in most studies, these differences were usually not present for all items and/or subscales, and in some studies[e.g.,63,113,114,119,200] differences for some scales were in the opposite direction to differences for other scales, making interpretation difficult. There was no consistent pattern of domains influenced by treatment – pain, physical, psychological, social, interpersonal, and symptom scales or items all yielded significant results in different studies. Differences in HRQOL scores were often seen at one point in time and not at others.[e.g.,62,63,119] Several studies reporting no significant HRQOL effects were small in size[e.g.,201,206] or commented that power was inadequate.[e.g.,59] Low statistical power and use of instruments that were not sensitive to change or that did not include domains likely to be influenced by the interventions being studied may have contributed to some of the non-significant HRQOL results in these studies. In almost half of the studies (N = 8 of 18) that reported toxicity, HRQOL measurement did not reflect significant differences in toxicity between the treatments being studied. There was only moderate concordance between HRQOL effects and measures of tumor response or survival, with beneficial HRQOL effects being identified in the absence of response, or survival effects and vice-versa.

In the metastatic setting, the goal of treatment has traditionally been palliation of symptoms. The introduction of promising chemotherapeutic and hormonal agents in the last five to ten years has led to studies in which survival effects are also postulated. However, HRQOL outcomes in metastatic trials have had little influence to date on treatment selection in clinical practice. Medical outcomes, including tumor response, disease progression, survival, and toxicity, led to decisions regarding optimal treatment that were not influenced by HRQOL measurement in all but two studies. In both of these studies, medical outcomes were equivalent. In one,[61] doxorubicin administered every three weeks was associated with less psychological distress than when it was administered weekly. Although the simpler logistics of every three-week (as opposed to weekly) treatment would likely have led to its selection as the preferred treatment, the HRQOL results provided additional support for this selection. In a second study[62] comparing anastrozole and megestrol acetate, competing toxicity profiles were identified. Although reduced weight gain (a major problem with megestrol acetate) in patients receiving anastrozole was probably sufficient to select the preferred treatment, documentation of enhanced physical and psychological functioning (measured by the RSCL) in patients on anastrozole provided further support for this treatment.

Thus, careful measurements of toxicity, coupled with measures of tumor response and/or survival, are likely to be sufficient to make recommendations about optimal treatment in trials in metastatic breast cancer. Should two treatments be shown to be equivalent in response and/or survival and competing toxicities, then overall HRQOL measurement may contribute to selecting the preferable treatment. However, HRQOL assessment could probably be deferred to a follow-up trial in the rare situations in which this is an issue.

Symptom control and follow-up

The literature search identified eight trials of drug therapy for symptom control/supportive care that included HRQOL outcomes.[51,53,111,151,207–209] Four studies of chemotherapy-associated nausea[51,53,151] used standard HRQOL instruments, including the RSCL, HADS, and FLIC. All but one[151] reported enhanced HRQOL with ondansetron, a treatment that was also shown to reduce nausea and emesis as recorded in daily diaries. The remaining study,[151] which evaluated alprazolam versus placebo, identified no HRQOL effects using several instruments

including the HADS. The use of bisphosphonates in breast cancer metastatic to bone was evaluated in three additional studies.[111,207,208] All reported marked improvements in a variety of medical outcomes (including fracture rate, need for palliative radiation, hypercalcemia, and pain) in women receiving bisphosphonates, but only one[207] reported HRQOL to be improved. This study used a novel instrument that had been developed specifically for the trial. A final study in this group[209] examined the use of clonidine versus placebo for tamoxifen-induced hot flashes and found an improvement in overall HRQOL (measured on a 10-point scale) and hot flashes (recorded in a daily diary) when clonidine was used.

Measurement of HRQOL using multidimensional instruments did not increase the information above and beyond traditional medical outcomes in providing a basis for selecting optimal treatment in any of these randomized trials of symptom control (Table 5.5). However, use of very focused, often study-specific, measures of symptoms (e.g., pain and nausea diaries) made important contributions. It was disappointing to note that multidimensional HRQOL instruments failed to identify beneficial effects of bisphosphonates that were readily apparent when measures of symptoms or biomedical outcomes (e.g., fractures) were used.[111,208] These results suggest that studies of symptom control might best be conducted using instruments that focus on the symptoms being studied, rather than on general HRQOL.

Three follow-up studies were identified.[103,173,210] None identified significant effects of the intervention(s) being studied on medical outcomes or HRQOL. As a result, the role of HRQOL measurement in this situation cannot be assessed. Further research in this area is clearly needed.

Psychosocial interventions

A total of 20 psychosocial intervention trials in breast cancer were identified – 13 in the adjuvant setting,[124,126,135,154,166,169,211–213,216–219] 6 in metastatic disease,[16,40,177,178,214,220] and 1 in symptom control.[69] In the adjuvant setting, the interventions included support groups,[126,154,169] individual counseling,[124,211,218] relaxation training,[166,212] telephone counseling or screening,[135,213] couple counseling,[217] and peer discussion or education.[219] The POMS was the most commonly used instrument (6 studies). Seven adjuvant studies used multidimensional HRQOL instruments (FACT-B, FLIC, RSCL, MOS, CARES, SF-36); only two reported medical outcomes: immune parameters[126] and clinical or pathologic response to therapy.[212]

Nine of these adjuvant studies identified psychosocial benefits.[124,126,154,166,211,212,216,218,219] In all nine of these studies, benefits were identified using targeted psychosocial questionnaires (e.g., POMS). Only two[211,219] of the six studies that used a multidimensional instrument (FLIC, SF-36) reported improved overall HRQOL. Two studies reported at least one medical outcome,[126,212] and no significant effects were identified. These observations suggest that beneficial effects of psychosocial interventions in the adjuvant setting often occur in specific psychosocial attributes that are best identified using questionnaires that focus on psychological or emotional domains.

Six psychosocial intervention trials in metastatic breast cancer were identified.[16,40,177,178,214,220] All but one[220] included a group intervention, although the specific nature of the interventions varied across studies. All used the POMS, and some also used other psychological questionnaires. All studies but one[40] identified beneficial effects of the interventions using unidimensional psychosocial questionnaires. No HRQOL benefits were identified in either of the two studies[40,214] that used multidimensional HRQOL instruments. Although Spiegel identified a survival benefit for supportive-expressive group therapy (along with improved pain and mood),[16,215] three additional trials,[178,214,222] two of which identified psychological benefits,[178,214] failed to replicate these survival effects. As with trials conducted in other settings, there was frequent within-study variability, significant benefits being identified on some instruments/subscales, but not others. This variability reflects the importance of selecting instruments

that measure attributes most likely to be influenced by the intervention being studied and emphasizes the need to develop approaches to handling this heterogeneity in interpreting study results.

One report[69] examined the use of a comprehensive menopausal assessment in healthy breast cancer survivors. Beneficial effects were identified using subscales of both the CARES and SF-36, consistent with improved menopausal symptoms on a symptom scale.

In general, the psychosocial interventions evaluated in these reports resulted in enhanced psychosocial functioning, and these enhancements in psychosocial functioning were key determinants of optimal treatment selection. However, improvements were often identified with one psychosocial instrument, but not others, or in one subscale of one psychosocial instrument but not in others, at times making interpretation of results difficult. These studies were less likely to include multidimensional HRQOL measures, and when they did, significant effects were rarely identified. Thus, it is important to tailor the selection of instruments in psychosocial intervention studies to the specific intervention being evaluated to ensure that outcomes likely to be influenced by the intervention are captured, and not to rely only on generic or general cancer HRQOL instruments to identify therapeutic benefits.

Discussion

Potential added benefits of HRQOL measurement beyond that obtained using medical outcomes

Measurement of HRQOL in randomized trials increases burden on study participants, enhances trial complexity, and is time-consuming and expensive. Although there is general consensus that HRQOL measurements increase the comprehensiveness of clinical trial outcomes and enhance understanding of treatment effects, the contribution of HRQOL measurement beyond medical outcomes measures (e.g., response, survival, toxicity) remains an area of continuing debate.

One of the contributions of HRQOL measurement is its role in the selection of optimal treatments in the context of randomized trials. In the previous section, this potential contribution was addressed in a range of settings. In situations where medical outcomes are equivalent, such as the use of BCS in primary management of breast cancer, HRQOL measurements may play an important role in clinical decision-making. Similarly, when psychosocial interventions are evaluated, HRQOL and psychosocial outcomes may be the only outcomes influenced, making their measurement extremely important. In contrast, in the metastatic setting when treatment toxicity is substantial and medical outcomes may differ, traditional biomedical outcomes measures alone may provide sufficient information to make decisions about the relative benefits of different treatments. In this situation, formal HRQOL measurements may not affect this decision-making process unless medical outcomes are equivalent. In the adjuvant setting in breast cancer, where improvement in survival is the primary goal, toxicity or transient effects on HRQOL may not influence decisions regarding optimal treatment. Assessing long-term HRQOL effects of these treatments is an area of active, and essential, research.

Thus, there appear to be situations in which HRQOL measurements play important roles in selecting optimal treatments and situations in which they have little influence. As with all clinical trial outcomes, there may be subgroups of patients within trials who experience different HRQOL outcomes from those seen in the overall study population, for example, the elderly or the seriously ill. In one trial in metastatic breast cancer, women whose tumors responded to treatment were shown to have enhanced HRQOL.[203] Similarly, patients enrolled in trials may differ from all patients with the illness under investigation, for example, the elderly, those with comorbid illness, and the psychologically ill may be less likely to be enrolled. Hence, the observations and conclusions made in clinical trials may not be fully generalizable to all women with breast cancer. Although important, these concerns cannot be addressed using available data, and they should be the focus of future research. Such investigations may require the use of non-randomized study designs to capture a broader spectrum of patients.

HRQOL measurement may also make important contributions beyond the selection of optimal treatment in the context of randomized clinical trials. These contributions include a description of the experience of patients in a variety of situations, including during active treatment, during long-term survivorship, or at the end of life. This descriptive information may help individual patients (and their physicians) make individual decisions about potential treatments and life plans. It may also facilitate comparisons across groups of patients and with healthy individuals; these comparisons may be particularly useful when examining issues relating to long-term survivorship. HRQOL may also provide prognostic information beyond that obtained from biomedical variables. A prognostic effect of HRQOL (physical well-being, mood, appetite, coping, pain) has been demonstrated in metastatic breast cancer, such that poor HRQOL is associated with poor biomedical outcomes.[63,223,224] Coping style and depression have also been shown to predict outcomes in early-stage breast cancer.[155] It is possible HRQOL measurement may also help to identify individuals at greater risk of certain toxicities, so that alternate treatments can be recommended or interventions to reduce toxicity can be implemented. Finally, HRQOL data may be used by policy makers and third-party payers to contribute to decisions about policy or reimbursement. This use may involve the application of data obtained using generic HRQOL instruments and may also involve measurement of preference-based utilities, an approach that is not discussed here, but is the standard in economic evaluations. Alternatively, it may involve the collection of HRQOL data outside of the clinical trials setting. This may be particularly important in populations such as the elderly that do not routinely participate in randomized trials.

Although these other contributions of HRQOL are of enormous potential value, they were not a focus of this discussion of randomized trials because the information needed for these other purposes can often be obtained more expeditiously (and less expensively) using non-randomized designs. As noted above, simple utility-based measures of preference may be preferred for formal economic evaluation and decision analyses, although global HRQOL measurements have also been used. Convenience samples of patients or inception cohorts may be most appropriate for descriptive or prognostic studies, respectively. These samples can often be recruited rapidly and may lead to more generalizable results than those obtained in randomized trials. Regardless of the study design or ultimate use of the HRQOL data, careful selection of instruments is needed to ensure that the desired information is captured. As found in this review of randomized trials, selection of targeted instruments rather than more general questionnaires may be advisable. This observation would be equally relevant in studies using other designs.

Recommendations and future research needs

This chapter has provided a comprehensive review of the breadth and scope of work to date examining HRQOL outcomes in breast cancer clinical trials. A number of issues have been addressed: the fundamental aspects of measurement, questions of divergence and convergence of instruments and their domains, the relative strengths and weaknesses of the most frequently used instruments, the effects of cancer treatment on HRQOL based on clinical trial data, and the extent to which HRQOL data contribute additional information (beyond standard medical outcomes) to the selection of optimal treatment in randomized clinical trials. Potential contributions of HRQOL measurement in clinical and health policy settings were also discussed. With more than a quarter of a century of work in this area, much has been accomplished; however, more needs to be done.

Some limitations to the work accomplished so far relate to the general under-funding of this type of research, such that relatively few studies have been done using the same patient samples, instruments,

research questions, and interventions. Instrument development and primary psychometric evaluation studies, in general, are not given high priority in peer review; thus, these types of methodological studies (e.g., head-to-head comparisons of the different instruments) are sparse. As a result, there is a lack of cross-talk or equivalency evaluations among instruments, such that the translation from physical functioning scores on one measure to the next is not always easily accomplished. While some work is underway in this area, more needs to be done. Underfunding may also have led to small sample sizes and low power in some studies (e.g., small convenience samples).

Lack of funding and research priority are major problems in randomized clinical treatment trials where investigators have long struggled to have HRQOL given the same emphasis as disease outcomes. With the exception of the clinical trials sponsored by the National Cancer Institute of Canada, the European Organization for Research and Treatment of Cancer, and some pharmaceutical companies, investigators in the US cooperative groups have had to make case-by-case arguments for the inclusion of HRQOL endpoints in trials, as HRQOL measurement is seen as too resource intensive compared to the clinical components of the study.[225] In addition, assessment batteries in these trials are often extremely short, primarily due to perceived patient and staff burden as well as analytic challenges in dealing with missing data.[226] The general cancer measures, even with their breast-specific modules (e.g., FACT-B, EORTC QLQ-BR-23), may not have sufficient sensitivity and breadth to detect trial-specific HRQOL outcomes. If more condition or treatment-specific items are not included in these clinical trial batteries, then the important HRQOL outcomes of treatment may go undetected. For example, in an observational study of women in the first year after breast cancer,[33] an extensive assessment battery was used to examine the HRQOL outcomes in women receiving mastectomy or breast-conserving surgery. Only because the CARES examined 32 specific subdomains of HRQOL was it apparent that there was any difference in HRQOL for these two treatments. Physical, psychosocial, and sexual functioning did not differ. However, the body image and clothing subscales of the CARES showed significant differences in the expected direction favoring breast conservation.[33] The authors of this study concluded that, while loss of the breast is an important issue for women, their concerns about mortality and the other toxicities of treatment (e.g., radiation, chemotherapy) dominate the broad dimensions of HRQOL, and that, without a condition-specific measure related to loss of the breast, the impact of surgical treatment would not have been detected. A parallel example comes from the Breast Cancer Prevention Trial HRQOL study;[227,228] no differences in HRQOL would have been detected between women receiving tamoxifen or placebo had a trial-specific symptom checklist not been used in the study.

There is a need for development of targeted instruments that contain items or scales that measure areas likely to be affected by breast cancer or its treatment that are not captured by general measures of HRQOL. Examples include menopausal symptoms or cognitive functioning in trials of adjuvant therapy or studies of long-term survivors and body image (including arm symptoms) in trials of primary therapy. This need could be addressed through the development of specific modules or by the addition of a small number of items (with appropriate validation) to existing questionnaires. Notably, treatment effects on social functioning were rarely identified using available HRQOL instruments, either because the treatments studied did not affect this domain or because this domain is poorly measured using available instruments.

As discussed above, instruments should be shown to be sensitive to clinically important changes in the domains they measure if they are to be used in clinical trials. This requirement demands agreement on what a clinically important change is (an area of active research that is discussed in Chapter 19 by Osoba in this volume)[229] and scaling that is sufficiently fine that it is possible to identify an effect of that magnitude. It is also essential that sample size be calculated for HRQOL outcomes (and not just medical outcomes); these calculations should incorporate anticipated differences and variability in HRQOL outcomes.

Additional research should address several general methodological and/or statistical issues that arise from the incorporation of HRQOL measurement into research of any type. Examples of these issues include instrument selection (which one, how many), timing of measurements (how often, for what period of time), reconciliation of multiple HRQOL outcomes (convergence and divergence of results obtained from different instruments/subscales at different times), statistical analysis (multiple testing, use of summary statistics and measures, handling of missing data, sample size calculations), and interpretation of results (medical outcomes versus HRQOL, hierarchy of HRQOL outcomes, clinically meaningful differences). Much of this fundamental research is underway. It should be undertaken alongside work on the development and validation of specific instruments.

This review was valuable in that it identified certain areas of inquiry where adding an assessment of HRQOL to randomized clinical trials contributes very little to decision-making about treatment alternatives, for example, comparing adjuvant drug treatments for breast cancer. The reason for this result may be the lack of precision of the currently available instruments (i.e., the measures are too coarse to detect the differences that matter to patients) or failure of existing instruments to capture important domains (e.g., cognitive functioning); however, it may also be that HRQOL outcomes are of secondary importance when medical outcomes are significantly affected by treatment. It is clear that when treatments are medically superior, most patients will desire such therapy, even if there may be an increase in short-term toxicity. (An opposing paradigm is probably operational in the setting of prevention,[5,228] where even when a treatment is superior, healthy or high-risk individuals are risk averse and any toxicity is unacceptable.) However, if treatments have equivalent medical outcomes, then differences in toxicity and HRQOL may be important. Perhaps HRQOL measures should only be included in randomized treatment trials when medical equivalency of treatments is likely. Differences in HRQOL may then be a primary outcome. An exception may occur when economic evaluations are planned; however, in this situation, utility measurements, rather than multidimensional HRQOL measurement, may be most useful.

Assessments of psychosocial interventions, which have often demonstrated measurable HRQOL outcomes in the absence of medical effects, are an example of studies where HRQOL may be a primary outcome. These studies have often used very detailed psychosocial assessments and have not relied on general cancer or breast cancer-specific multidimensional HRQOL tools (e.g., FACT, EORTC QLQ-C30, FLIC). To the extent that specific dimensions of HRQOL are targeted in these interventions, then appropriate instruments known to be responsive to change in those dimensions can be chosen. These types of intervention studies will probably continue to use measures that are drawn from psychology rather than from the HRQOL measurement arena, and incorporation of such measures is essential to identifying the beneficial effects of the interventions. To some extent, psychosocial intervention trials have had more resources to conduct the intervention and collect outcomes data from individual patients, making detailed evaluation of HRQOL more feasible. Whether the HRQOL outcomes in biomedical intervention trials would have been more compelling with more detailed assessments is an open question that is worthy of investigation.

In making decisions about inclusion of HRQOL endpoints in clinical trials, increased trial complexity, respondent burden, and cost should be balanced against the expected gain in additional knowledge, so that resources for HRQOL measurement (dollars, personnel) can be allocated to those trials in which benefits are likely to be greatest. This review provides little support for the routine incorporation of HRQOL in all clinical trials in breast cancer; however, there may be other settings in which HRQOL measurement plays an important role. These settings include description of patient experience, examination of prognostic effects, and health policy decision making.

One area that is increasingly of interest is the long-term late effects associated with adjuvant therapy, since more complex and intensive therapies are being given to patients with very small tumors whose likelihood of long-term survival is high.[230] In studying these areas, investigators may not use randomized controlled trial designs, opting instead for observational designs that provide descriptive information about HRQOL. These types of studies could also be attached to large randomized controlled trials and, in this way, specific treatments and doses can be evaluated for their late effects.

These findings also raise the question of whether treatment should be considered an important predictor of HRQOL and whether other theoretical models might be considered. There is a large body of observational research in breast cancer patients and survivors[33,68,79,231–233] that suggests type of breast surgery is not a significant predictor of major group differences in HRQOL. That being said, this does not mean that, for an individual woman, the type of surgery she has received may not play a substantial role in her assessment of HRQOL. As Fallowfield suggests, it is being offered the choice of therapy that probably plays the most important role in adaptation to surgery.[232] As for examinations of different types of treatments (e.g., radiation, chemotherapy, hormonal therapy), there are emerging data that different treatments have different outcomes for women. For example, in two separate analyses from a large cohort of breast cancer survivors assessed at two points in time, chemotherapy had deleterious effects on sexual functioning.[70,234] More recently, any form of adjuvant therapy in early-stage breast cancer patients was shown to lead to poorer long-term physical health as measured by the physical component scale of the MOS SF-36.[70] The results from these well-funded, hypothesis-driven research studies emphasize the importance of a comprehensive assessment approach that includes condition-specific measures along with broad-based measures of HRQOL. However, the importance of other non-treatment related factors such as income, comorbidity, emotional well-being, and social support should not be underestimated when predicting global HRQOL, as recently demonstrated by Ganz et al.[70]

Across North America, Europe, Australia, New Zealand, and elsewhere, there are many trials that will soon report their treatment and HRQOL results. At that point in time, firm conclusions may be made about the added value (or lack thereof) of including HRQOL assessments in treatment trials designed to identify optimal treatment. In the meantime, findings of this review suggest that caution should be used when initiating new HRQOL studies with breast cancer patients unless treatment equivalency is an expectation, especially in the adjuvant setting, or unless the HRQOL questions target unique or specific issues that can only be assessed through patient self-report. Investigators should address the methodological and descriptive research priorities discussed above while these ongoing clinical trials are maturing, so that the outcomes of these research endeavors can be used, in conjunction with results of the randomized controlled trials, to inform future HRQOL research, both in the setting of clinical trials and in other research areas.

REFERENCES

1 Jemal, A., Tiwari, R. C., Murray, T. et al. (2004). Cancer statistics, 2004. CA: Cancer Journal for Clinicians 54:8–29.

2 Howe, H. L., Wingo, P. A., Thun, M. J. et al. (2001). Annual report to the nation on the status of cancer (1973 through 1998), featuring cancers with recent increasing trends. Journal of the National Cancer Institute 93:824–42.

3 Yancik, R., Ries, L. G., Yates, J. W. (1989). Breast cancer in aging women. A population-based study of contrasts in stage, surgery, and survival. Cancer 63:976–81.

4 Yancik, R. (1997). Epidemiology of cancer in the elderly. Current status and projections for the future. Rays 22:3–9.

5 Fisher, B., Costantino, J. P., Wickerham, D. L., Redmond, C. K. et al. (1998). Tamoxifen for prevention of breast cancer: report of the National Surgical Adjuvant Breast and Bowel Project P-1 Study. Journal of the National Cancer Institute 90:1371–88.

6 National Institutes of Health (1990). Early stage breast cancer. Consensus Statement 8:1–19.

7 National Institutes of Health (2001). National Institutes of Health Consensus Development Conference Statement: Adjuvant Therapy for Breast Cancer, November 1–3, 2000. Journal of the National Cancer Institute 93:979–89.

8 Early Breast Cancer Trialists' Collaborative Group. (1998). Tamoxifen for early breast cancer: an overview of the randomised trials. Lancet 351:1451–67.

9 Early Breast Cancer Trialists' Collaborative Group. (1998). Polychemotherapy for early breast cancer: an overview of the randomised trials. Lancet 352:930–42.

10 Shapiro, C. L., Recht, A. (2001). Side effects of adjuvant treatment of breast cancer. New England Journal of Medicine 344:1997–2008.

11 Priestman, T. J., Baum, M. (1976). Evaluation of quality of life in patients receiving treatment for advanced breast cancer. Lancet 1:899–900.

12 Selby, P. J., Chapman, J. A., Etazadi-Amoli, J. et al. (1984). The development of a method for assessing the quality of life of cancer patients. British Journal of Cancer 50:13–22.

13 Schag, C. C., Heinrich, R. L., Ganz, P. A. (1983). Cancer inventory of problem situations: an instrument for assessing cancer patients' rehabilitation needs. Journal of Psychosocial Oncology 1:11–24.

14 Schipper, H., Clinch, J., McMurray, A. et al. (1984). Measuring the quality of life of cancer patients: the Functional Living Index-Cancer: development and validation. Journal of Clinical Oncology 2:472–83.

15 Schag, C. A., Heinrich, R. L. (1990). Development of a comprehensive quality of life measurement tool: CARES. Oncology 4:135–8.

16 Spiegel, D., Bloom, J. R., Yalom, I. (1981). Group support for patients with metastatic cancer. A randomized prospective outcome study. Archives of General Psychiatry 38:527–33.

17 Ganz, P. A., Coscarelli, A., Fred, C. et al. (1996). Breast cancer survivors: psychosocial concerns and quality of life. Breast Cancer Research and Treatment 38:183–99.

18 Meyerowitz, B. E. (1980). Psychosocial correlates of breast cancer and its treatments. Psychological Bulletin 87:108–31.

19 McNair, P. M., Lorr, M., Droppelman, L. EDITS Manual for Profile of Mood States. (1981). San Diego: Educational and Industrial Testing Service.

20 Radloff, L. S. (1977). The CES-D Scale: A self-report depression scale for research in the general population. Applied Psychological Measurement 1:385–401.

21 Coates, A., Gebski, V., Bishop, J. F. et al. (1987). Improving the quality of life during chemotherapy for advanced breast cancer. A comparison of intermittent and continuous treatment strategies. New England Journal of Medicine 317:1490–5.

22 Aaronson, N. K., Ahmedzai, S., Bergman, B. et al., for the EORTC Study Group on Quality of Life. (1993). The

European Organization for Research and Treatment of Cancer QLQ-C30: a quality-of-life instrument for use in international clinical trials in oncology. *Journal of the National Cancer Institute* **85**:365–76.

23 Cella, D. F., Tulsky, D. S., Gray, G. *et al.* (1993). The Functional Assessment of Cancer Therapy scale: development and validation of the general measure. *Journal of Clinical Oncology* **11**:570–9.

24 Schag, C. A., Heinrich, R. L., Aadland, R. L. *et al.* (1990). Assessing problems of cancer patients: psychometric properties of the cancer inventory of problem situations. *Health Psychology* **9**:83–102.

25 Ganz, P. A., Schag, C. A., Lee, J. J. *et al.* (1992). The CARES: a generic measure of health-related quality of life for patients with cancer. *Quality of Life Research* **1**:19–29.

26 Schag, C. A., Ganz, P. A., Heinrich, R. L. (1991). Cancer Rehabilitation Evaluation System – short form (CARES-SF). A cancer specific rehabilitation and quality of life instrument. *Cancer* **68**:1406–13.

27 Levine, M. N., Guyatt, G. H., Gent, M. *et al.* (1988). Quality of life in stage II breast cancer: an instrument for clinical trials. *Journal of Clinical Oncology* **6**:1798–1810.

28 Sprangers, M. A., Groenvold, M., Arraras, J. I. *et al.* (1996). The European Organization for Research and Treatment of Cancer breast cancer-specific quality-of-life questionnaire module: first results from a three-country field study. *Journal of Clinical Oncology* **14**:2756–68.

29 Brady, M. J., Cella, D. F., Mo, F. *et al.* (1997). Reliability and validity of the Functional Assessment of Cancer Therapy-Breast quality-of-life instrument. *Journal of Clinical Oncology* **15**:974–86.

30 National Institutes of Health (1985). Consensus conference. Adjuvant chemotherapy for breast cancer. *Journal of the American Medical Association* **254**:3461–3.

31 Feeny, this volume, Chapter 4.

32 Erickson, this volume, Chapter 3.

33 Ganz, P. A., Schag, A. C., Lee, J. J. *et al.* (1992). Breast conservation versus mastectomy. Is there a difference in psychological adjustment or quality of life in the year after surgery? *Cancer* **69**:1729–38.

34 Ganz, P. A., Schag, C. A., Cheng, H. L. (1990). Assessing the quality of life – a study in newly-diagnosed breast cancer patients. *Journal of Clinical Epidemiology* **43**:75–86.

35 Schag, C. A., Ganz, P. A., Polinsky, M. L. *et al.* (1993). Characteristics of women at risk for psychosocial distress in the year after breast cancer. *Journal of Clinical Oncology* **11**:783–93.

36 Lindley, C., Vasa, S., Sawyer, W. T. *et al.* (1998). Quality of life and preferences for treatment following systemic adjuvant therapy for early-stage breast cancer. *Journal of Clinical Oncology* **16**:1380–7.

37 Ingham, J., Seidman, A., Yao, T. J. *et al.* (1996). An exploratory study of frequent pain measurement in a cancer clinical trial. *Quality of Life Research* **5**:503–7.

38 Seidman, A. D., Portenoy, R., Yao, T. J. *et al.* (1995). Quality of life in phase II trials: a study of methodology and predictive value in patients with advanced breast cancer treated with paclitaxel plus granulocyte colony-stimulating factor. *Journal of the National Cancer Institute* **87**: 1316–22.

39 Chu, L., Sutton, L. M., Peterson, B. L. *et al.* (1996). Continuous infusion 5-fluorouracil as first-line therapy for metastatic breast cancer. *Journal of Infusional Chemotherapy* **6**:211–6.

40 Edmonds, C. V., Lockwood, G. A., Cunningham, A. J. (1999). Psychological response to long-term group therapy: a randomized trial with metastatic breast cancer patients. *Psycho-Oncology.* **8**:74–91.

41 Goss, P. E. (1998). Pre-clinical and clinical review of vorozole, a new third generation aromatase inhibitor. *Breast Cancer Research and Treatment* **49** (Suppl. 1):S59–65.

42 Kornblith, A. B., Hollis, D. R., Zuckerman, E. *et al.* (1993). Effect of megestrol acetate on quality of life in a dose-response trial in women with advanced breast cancer. The Cancer and Leukemia Group B. *Journal of Clinical Oncology* **11**:2081–9.

43 Riley, B. B., Perna, R., Tate, D. G. *et al.* (1998). Types of spiritual well-being among persons with chronic illness: their relation to various forms of quality of life. *Archives of Physical Medicine and Rehabilitation* **79**:258–64.

44 Tate, D. G., Riley, B. B., Perna, R. *et al.* (1997). Quality of life issues among women with physical disabilities or breast cancer. *Archives of Physical Medicine and Rehabilitation* **78**:S18–25.

45 Winer, E. P., Lindley, C., Hardee, M. *et al.* (1999). Quality of life in patients surviving at least 12 months following high dose chemotherapy with autologous bone marrow support. *Psycho-Oncology* **8**:167–76.

46 De Haes, J. C. J. M., Pruyn, J. F. A., van Knippenberg, F. C. E., klachtenlijst voor kankerpatienten, eerste ervaringen. (1983). *Netherlands Tijdschrift voor de Psychologie en Haar Grensgebieden* **38**:403.

47 Watson, M., Law, M., Maguire, G. P. *et al.* (1992). Further development of a quality of life measure for cancer patients: The Rotterdam Symptom Checklist (Revised). *Psycho-Oncology* **1**:35–44.

48 Bosnjak, S., Radulovic, S., Neskovic-Konstantinovic, Z. *et al.* (2000). Patient statement of satisfaction with antiemetic

treatment is related to quality of life. *American Journal of Clinical Oncology* **23**:575–8.

49 Hall, A., A'Hern, R., Fallowfield, L. (1999). Are we using appropriate self-report questionnaires for detecting anxiety and depression in women with early breast cancer? *European Journal of Cancer* **35**:79–85.

50 Jansen, S. J., Stiggelbout, A. M., Nooij, M. A. *et al.* (2000). Response shift in quality of life measurement in early-stage breast cancer patients undergoing radiotherapy. *Quality of Life Research* **9**:603–15.

51 Clavel, M., Soukop, M., Greenstreet, Y. L. (1993). Improved control of emesis and quality of life with ondansetron in breast cancer. *Oncology* **50**:180–5.

52 de Haes, J. C., Olschewski, M. (1998). Quality of life assessment in a cross-cultural context: use of the Rotterdam Symptom Checklist in a multinational randomised trial comparing CMF and Zoladex (Goserlin) treatment in early breast cancer. *Annals of Oncology* **9**:745–50.

53 Soukop, M., McQuade, B., Hunter, E. *et al.* (1992). Ondansetron compared with metoclopramide in the control of emesis and quality of life during repeated chemotherapy for breast cancer. *Oncology* **49**:295–304.

54 Goldberg, J. A., Scott, R. N., Davidson, P. M. *et al.* (1992). Psychological morbidity in the first year after breast surgery. *European Journal of Surgical Oncology* **18**:327–31.

55 Kiebert, G. M., Hanneke, J., de Haes, C. J. *et al.* (1990). Effect of peri-operative chemotherapy on the quality of life of patients with early breast cancer. *European Journal of Cancer* **26**:1038–42.

56 Fulton, C. L. (1997). The physical and psychological symptoms experienced by patients with metastatic breast cancer before death. *European Journal of Cancer Care (England)* **6**:262–6.

57 Hopwood, P., Howell, A., Maguire, P. (1991). Psychiatric morbidity in patients with advanced cancer of the breast: prevalence measured by two self-rating questionnaires. *British Journal of Cancer* **64**:349–52.

58 Ramirez, A. J., Towlson, K. E., Leaning, M. S. *et al.* (1998). Do patients with advanced breast cancer benefit from chemotherapy? *British Journal of Cancer* **78**:1488–94.

59 Harper-Wynne, C., English, J., Meyer, L. *et al.* (1999). Randomized trial to compare the efficacy and toxicity of cyclophosphamide, methotrexate and 5-fluorouracil (CMF) with methotrexate mitoxantrone (MM) in advanced carcinoma of the breast. *British Journal of Cancer* **81**:316–22.

60 Joensuu, H., Holli, K., Heikkinen, M. *et al.* (1998). Combination chemotherapy versus single-agent therapy as first- and second-line treatment in metastatic breast cancer: a prospective randomized trial. *Journal of Clinical Oncology* **16**:3720–30.

61 Richards, M. A., Hopwood, P., Ramirez, A. J. *et al.* (1992). Doxorubicin in advanced breast cancer: influence of schedule on response, survival and quality of life. *European Journal of Cancer* **28A**:1023–8.

62 Buzdar, A. U., Jones, S. E., Vogel, C. L. *et al.* (1997). A phase III trial comparing anastrozole (1 and 10 milligrams), a potent and selective aromatase inhibitor, with megestrol acetate in postmenopausal women with advanced breast carcinoma. Arimidex Study Group. *Cancer* **79**:730–9.

63 Kramer, J. A., Curran, D., Piccart, M. *et al.* (2000). Randomised trial of paclitaxel versus doxorubicin as first-line chemotherapy for advanced breast cancer: quality of life evaluation using the EORTC QLQ-C30 and the Rotterdam symptom checklist. *European Journal of Cancer* **36**:1488–97.

64 Hopwood, P., Howell, A., Maguire, P. (1991). Screening for psychiatric morbidity in patients with advanced breast cancer: validation of two self-report questionnaires. *British Journal of Cancer* **64**:353–6.

65 Paci, E. (1992). Assessment of validity and clinical application of an Italian version of the Rotterdam Symptom Checklist. *Quality of Life Research* **1**:129–34.

66 Steginga, S., Occhipinti, S., Wilson, K. *et al.* (1998). Domains of distress: the experience of breast cancer in Australia. *Oncology Nursing Forum* **25**:1063–70.

67 Ganz, P. A., Schag, C. C., Polinsky, M. L. *et al.* (1987). Rehabilitation needs and breast cancer: the first month after primary therapy. *Breast Cancer Research and Treatment* **10**:243–53.

68 Ganz, P. A., Rowland, J. H., Desmond, K. *et al.* (1998). Life after breast cancer: understanding women's health-related quality of life and sexual functioning. *Journal of Clinical Oncology* **16**:501–14.

69 Ganz, P. A., Greendale, G. A., Petersen, L. *et al.* (2000). Managing menopausal symptoms in breast cancer survivors: results of a randomized controlled trial. *Journal of the National Cancer Institute* **92**:1054–64.

70 Ganz, P. A., Desmond, K. A., Leedham, B. *et al.* (2002). Quality of life in long-term, disease-free survivors of breast cancer: a follow-up study. *Journal of the National Cancer Institute* **94**:39–49.

71 Ganz, P. A., Lee, J. J., Sim, M. S. *et al.* (1992). Exploring the influence of multiple variables on the relationship of age to quality of life in women with breast cancer. *Journal of Clinical Epidemiology* **45**:473–85.

72 Ganz, P. A., Hirji, K., Sim, M. S. *et al.* (1993). Predicting psychosocial risk in patients with breast cancer. *Medical Care* **31**:419–31.

73 Frost, M. H., Arvizu, R. D., Jayakumar, S. *et al.* (1999). A multidisciplinary healthcare delivery model for women with breast cancer: patient satisfaction and physical and psychosocial adjustment. *Oncology Nursing Forum* **26**: 1673–80.

74 Wyatt, G. K., Friedman, L. L. (1998). Physical and psychosocial outcomes of midlife and older women following surgery and adjuvant therapy for breast cancer. *Oncology Nursing Forum* **25**:761–8.

75 Rustoen, T., Moum, T., Wiklund, I. *et al.* (1999). Quality of life in newly diagnosed cancer patients. *Journal of Advanced Nursing* **29**:490–8.

76 Shimozuma, K., Ganz, P. A., Petersen, L. *et al.* (1999). Quality of life in the first year after breast cancer surgery: rehabilitation needs and patterns of recovery. *Breast Cancer Research and Treatment* **56**:45–57.

77 Rustoen, T., Wiklund, I., Hanestad, B. R. *et al.* (1998). Nursing intervention to increase hope and quality of life in newly diagnosed cancer patients. *Cancer Nursing* **21**:235–45.

78 Ganz, P. A., Rowland, J. H., Meyerowitz, B. E. *et al.* (1998). Impact of different adjuvant therapy strategies on quality of life in breast cancer survivors. *Recent Results Cancer Research* **152**:396–411.

79 Rowland, J. H., Desmond, K. A., Meyerowitz, B. E. *et al.* (2000). Role of breast reconstructive surgery in physical and emotional outcomes among breast cancer survivors. *Journal of the National Cancer Institute* **92**:1422–9.

80 Ashing-Giwa, K., Ganz, P. A., Petersen, L. (1999). Quality of life of African-American and white long term breast carcinoma survivors. *Cancer* **85**:418–26.

81 Frost, M. H., Suman, V. J., Rummans, T. A. *et al.* (2000). Physical, psychological and social well-being of women with breast cancer: the influence of disease phase. *Psycho-Oncology* **9**:221–31.

82 Aaronson, N. K., Ahmedzai, S., Bullinger, M. *et al.* (1987). The EORTC core quality of life questionnaire: Interim results of an international field study. In *Effect of Cancer on Quality of Life*, ed. D. Osoba, pp. 185–203. Boston: Yale University Press.

83 Aaronson, N. K., Cull, A., Kaasa, S. *et al.* (1994). The European Organization for Research and Treatment of Cancer (EORTC) modular approach to quality of life assessment in oncology. *International Journal of Mental Health* **23**:75–96.

84 Kaasa, S., Bjordal, K., Aaronson, N. *et al.* (1995). The EORTC core quality of life questionnaire (QLQ-C30): validity and reliability when analysed with patients treated with palliative radiotherapy. *European Journal of Cancer* **31A**:2260–3.

85 Osoba, D., Zee, B., Pater, J. *et al.* (1994). Psychometric properties and responsiveness of the EORTC Quality of Life Questionnaire (QLQ-C30) in patients with breast, ovarian and lung cancer. *Quality of Life Research* **3**:353–64.

86 Niezgoda, H. E., Pater, J. L. (1993). A validation study of the domains of the core EORTC quality of life questionnaire. *Quality of Life Research* **2**:319–25.

87 McLachlan, S. A., Devins, G. M., Goodwin, P. J. (1999). Factor analysis of the psychosocial items of the EORTC QLQ-C30 in metastatic breast cancer patients participating in a psychosocial intervention study. *Quality of Life Research* **8**:311–17.

88 Chie, W. C., Huang, C. S., Chen, J. H. *et al.* (1999). Measurement of the quality of life during different clinical phases of breast cancer. *Journal of Formosan Medical Association* **98**:254–60.

89 Taenzer, P. A., Speca, M., Atkinson, M. J. *et al.* (1997). Computerized quality-of-life screening in an oncology clinic. *Cancer Practice* **5**:168–75.

90 Carlsson, M., Hamrin, E. (1996). Measurement of quality of life in women with breast cancer. Development of a Life Satisfaction Questionnaire (LSQ-32) and a comparison with the EORTC QLQ-C30. *Quality of Life Research* **5**:265–74.

91 Mercier, M., Bonneterre, J., Schraub, S. *et al.* (1998). The development of a French version of a questionnaire on the quality of life in cancerology (Functional Living Index-Cancer: FLIC). *Bulletin du Cancer* **85**:180–6.

92 King, M. T., Dobson, A. J., Harnett, P. R. (1996). A comparison of two quality-of-life questionnaires for cancer clinical trials: the functional living index–cancer (FLIC) and the quality of life questionnaire core module (QLQ-C30). *Journal of Clinical Epidemiology* **49**:21–9.

93 McLachlan, S. A., Devins, G. M., Goodwin, P. J. (1998). Validation of the European Organization for Research and Treatment of Cancer Quality of Life Questionnaire (QLQ-C30) as a measure of psychosocial function in breast cancer patients. *European Journal of Cancer* **34**:510–17.

94 McLachlan, S. A., Pintilie, M., Tannock, I. F. (1999). Third line chemotherapy in patients with metastatic breast cancer: an evaluation of quality of life and cost. *Breast Cancer Research and Treatment* **54**:213–23.

95 Osoba, D., Rodrigues, G., Myles, J. *et al.* (1998). Interpreting the significance of changes in health-related quality-of-life scores. *Journal of Clinical Oncology* **16**:139–44.

96 Wilson, K. A., Dowling, A. J., Abdolell, M. *et al.* (2000). Perception of quality of life by patients, partners and treating physicians. *Quality of Life Research* **9**:1041–52.

97 Apolone, G., Filiberti, A., Cifani, S. *et al.* (1998). Evaluation of the EORTC QLQ-C30 questionnaire: a comparison with SF-36 Health Survey in a cohort of Italian long-survival cancer patients. *Annals of Oncology* **9**:549–57.

98 Kemmler, G., Holzner, B., Kopp, M. *et al.* (1999). Comparison of two quality-of-life instruments for cancer patients: the Functional Assessment of Cancer Therapy–General and the European Organization for Research and Treatment of Cancer Quality of Life Questionnaire-C30. *Journal of Clinical Oncology* **17**:2932–40.

99 Montazeri, A., Harirchi, I., Vahdani, M. *et al.* (2000). The EORTC breast cancer-specific quality of life questionnaire (EORTC QLQ-BR23): translation and validation study of the Iranian version. *Quality of Life Research* **9**:177–84.

100 Klee, M., Groenvold, M., Machin, D. (1997). Quality of life of Danish women: population-based norms of the EORTC QLQ-C30. *Quality of Life Research* **6**:27–34.

101 Macquart-Moulin, G., Viens, P., Palangie, T. *et al.* (2000). High-dose sequential chemotherapy with recombinant granulocyte colony- stimulating factor and repeated stem-cell support for inflammatory breast cancer patients: does impact on quality of life jeopardize feasibility and acceptability of treatment? *Journal of Clinical Oncology* **18**: 754–64.

102 King, M. T., Kenny, P., Shiell, A. *et al.* (2000). Quality of life three months and one year after first treatment for early stage breast cancer: influence of treatment and patient characteristics. *Quality of Life Research* **9**:789–800.

103 Grunfeld, E., Mant, D., Yudkin, P. *et al.* (1996). Routine follow up of breast cancer in primary care: randomised trial. *British Medical Journal* **313**:665–9.

104 van Dam, F. S., Schagen, S. B., Muller, M. J. *et al.* (1998). Impairment of cognitive function in women receiving adjuvant treatment for high-risk breast cancer: high-dose versus standard-dose chemotherapy. *Journal of the National Cancer Institute* **90**:210–18.

105 Cohen, L., Hack, T. F., de Moor, C. *et al.* (2000). The effects of type of surgery and time on psychological adjustment in women after breast cancer treatment. *Annals of Surgical Oncology* **7**:427–34.

106 Kornblith, A. B., Herndon, J. E., Zuckerman, E. *et al.* (2001). Social support as a buffer to the psychological impact of stressful life events in women with breast cancer. *Cancer* **91**:443–54.

107 Kramer, J. A., Curran, D., Piccart, M. *et al.* (2000). Identification and interpretation of clinical and quality of life prognostic factors for survival and response to treatment in first-line chemotherapy in advanced breast cancer. *European Journal of Cancer* **36**:1498–506.

108 Pater, J. L., Zee, B., Palmer, M. *et al.* (1997). Fatigue in patients with cancer: results with National Cancer Institute of Canada Clinical Trials Group studies employing the EORTC QLQ-C30. *Supportive Care in Cancer* **5**:410–13.

109 Curran, D., Aaronson, N., Standaert, B. *et al.* (2000). Summary measures and statistics in the analysis of quality of life data: an example from an EORTC-NCIC-SAKK locally advanced breast cancer study. *European Journal of Cancer* **36**:834–44.

110 Geels, P., Eisenhauer, E., Bezjak, A. *et al.* (2000). Palliative effect of chemotherapy: objective tumor response is associated with symptom improvement in patients with metastatic breast cancer. *Journal of Clinical Oncology* **18**:2395–405.

111 Kristensen, B., Ejlertsen, B., Groenvold, M. *et al.* (1999). Oral clodronate in breast cancer patients with bone metastases: a randomized study. *Journal of Internal Medicine* **246**:67–74.

112 Osoba, D., Burchmore, M. (1999). Health-related quality of life in women with metastatic breast cancer treated with trastuzumab (Herceptin). *Seminars in Oncology* **26**:84–8.

113 Kaufmann, M., Bajetta, E., Dirix, L. Y. *et al.* (2000). Exemestane is superior to megestrol acetate after tamoxifen failure in postmenopausal women with advanced breast cancer: results of a phase III randomized double-blind trial. The Exemestane Study Group. *Journal of Clinical Oncology* **18**:1399–411.

114 Nabholtz, J. M., Senn, H. J., Bezwoda, W. R. *et al.* and 304 Study Group (1999). Prospective randomized trial of docetaxel versus mitomycin plus vinblastine in patients with metastatic breast cancer progressing despite previous anthracycline-containing chemotherapy. 304 Study Group. *Journal of Clinical Oncology* **17**:1413–24.

115 Norris, B., Pritchard, K. I., James, K. *et al.* (2000). Phase III comparative study of vinorelbine combined with doxorubicin versus doxorubicin alone in disseminated metastatic/recurrent breast cancer: National Cancer Institute of Canada Clinical Trials Group Study MA8. *Journal of Clinical Oncology* **18**:2385–94.

116 Hack, T. F., Cohen, L., Katz, J. *et al.* (1999). Physical and psychological morbidity after axillary lymph node dissection for breast cancer. *Journal of Clinical Oncology* **17**:143–9.

117 Kissane, D. W., Clarke, D. M., Ikin, J. *et al.* (1998). Psychological morbidity and quality of life in Australian women with early-stage breast cancer: a cross-sectional survey [see comments]. *Medical Journal of Australia* **169**:192–6.

118 Holzner, B., Kemmler, G., Kopp, M. *et al.* (2001). Quality of life in breast cancer patients – not enough attention for long-term survivors? *Psychosomatics* **42**:117–23.

119 Hakamies-Blomqvist, L., Luoma, M., Sjostrom, J. et al. (2000). Quality of life in patients with metastatic breast cancer receiving either docetaxel or sequential methotrexate and 5-fluorouracil. A multicentre randomised phase III trial by the Scandinavian breast group. *European Journal of Cancer* **36**:1411–17.

120 Joly, F., Espie, M., Marty, M., Heron, J. F. et al. (2000). Long-term quality of life in premenopausal women with node-negative localized breast cancer treated with or without adjuvant chemotherapy. *British Journal of Cancer* **83**:577–82.

121 Stanton, A. L., Danoff-Burg, S., Cameron, C. L. et al. (2000). Emotionally expressive coping predicts psychological and physical adjustment to breast cancer. *Journal of Consulting and Clinical Psychology* **68**:875–82.

122 Dow, K. H., Ferrell, B. R., Leigh, S. et al. (1996). An evaluation of the quality of life among long-term survivors of breast cancer. *Breast Cancer Research and Treatment* **39**:261–73.

123 Wenzel, L. B., Fairclough, D. L., Brady, M. J. et al. (1999). Age-related differences in the quality of life of breast carcinoma patients after treatment. *Cancer* **86**:1768–74.

124 Ritz, L. J., Nissen, M. J., Swenson, K. K. et al. (2000). Effects of advanced nursing care on quality of life and cost outcomes of women diagnosed with breast cancer. *Oncology Nursing Forum* **27**:923–32.

125 Nissen, M. J., Swenson, K. K., Ritz, L. J. et al. (2001). Quality of life after breast carcinoma surgery: a comparison of three surgical procedures. *Cancer* **91**:1238–46.

126 Richardson, M. A., Post-White, J., Grimm, E. A. et al. (1997). Coping, life attitudes, and immune responses to imagery and group support after breast cancer treatment. *Alternative Therapies in Health and Medicine* **3**:62–70.

127 Ware, J. E., Jr., Sherbourne, C. D. (1992). The MOS 36-item short-form health survey (SF-36). I. Conceptual framework and item selection. *Medical Care* **30**:473–83.

128 McHorney, C. A., Ware, J. E., Jr., Raczek, A. E. (1993). The MOS 36-Item Short-Form Health Survey (SF-36): II. Psychometric and clinical tests of validity in measuring physical and mental health constructs. *Medical Care* **31**: 247–63.

129 McHorney, C. A., Ware, J. E., Jr., Lu, J. F. et al. (1994). The MOS 36-item Short-Form Health Survey (SF-36): III. Tests of data quality, scaling assumptions, and reliability across diverse patient groups. *Medical Care* **32**:40–66.

130 Ganz, P. A., Greendale, G. A., Kahn, B. et al. (1999). Are older breast carcinoma survivors willing to take hormone replacement therapy? *Cancer* **86**:814–20.

131 Stein, K. D., Jacobsen, P. B., Hann, D. M. et al. (2000). Impact of hot flashes on quality of life among postmenopausal women being treated for breast cancer. *Journal of Pain and Symptom Management* **19**:436–45.

132 Burstein, H. J., Gelber, S., Guadagnoli, E. et al. (1999). Use of alternative medicine by women with early-stage breast cancer. *New England Journal of Medicine* **340**:1733–9.

133 Bloom, J. R., Stewart, S. L., Johnston, M., Banks, P. (1998). Intrusiveness of illness and quality of life in young women with breast cancer. *Psycho-Oncology* **7**:89–100.

134 Velanovich, V., Szymanski, W. (1999). Quality of life of breast cancer patients with lymphedema. *American Journal of Surgery* **177**:184.

135 Maunsell, E., Brisson, J., Deschenes, L. et al. (1996). Randomized trial of a psychologic distress screening program after breast cancer: effects on quality of life. *Journal of Clinical Oncology* **14**:2747–55.

136 Bower, J. E., Ganz, P. A., Desmond, K. A. et al. (2000). Fatigue in breast cancer survivors: occurrence, correlates, and impact on quality of life. *Journal of Clinical Oncology* **18**:743–53.

137 Broeckel, J. A., Jacobsen, P. B., Balducci, L. et al. (2000). Quality of life after adjuvant chemotherapy for breast cancer. *Breast Cancer Research and Treatment* **62**:141–50.

138 Andrykowski, M. A., Curran, S. L., Studts, J. L. et al. (1996). Psychosocial adjustment and quality of life in women with breast cancer and benign breast problems: a controlled comparison. *Journal of Clinical Epidemiology* **49**:827–34.

139 Jacobsen, P. B., Widows, M. R., Hann, D. M. et al. (1998). Posttraumatic stress disorder symptoms after bone marrow transplantation for breast cancer. *Psychosomatic Medicine* **60**:366–71.

140 Hann, D. M., Jacobsen, P. B., Martin, S. C. et al. (1997). Quality of life following bone marrow transplantation for breast cancer: a comparative study. *Bone Marrow Transplantation* **19**:257–64.

141 Wapnir, I. L., Cody, R. P., Greco, R. S. (1999). Subtle differences in quality of life after breast cancer surgery. *Annals of Surgical Oncology* **6**:359–66.

142 Stearns, V., Isaacs, C., Rowland, J. et al. (2000). A pilot trial assessing the efficacy of paroxetine hydrochloride (Paxil) in controlling hot flashes in breast cancer survivors. *Annals of Oncology* **11**:17–22.

143 Hann, D. M., Jacobsen, P. B., Azzarello, L. M. et al. (1998). Measurement of fatigue in cancer patients: development and validation of the Fatigue Symptom Inventory. *Quality of Life Research* **7**:301–10.

144 Dorval, M., Maunsell, E., Deschenes, L. et al. (1998). Long-term quality of life after breast cancer: comparison of 8-year survivors with population controls. *Journal of Clinical Oncology* **16**:487–94.

145 McCaul, K. D., Sandgren, A. K., King, B. *et al.* (1999). Coping and adjustment to breast cancer. *Psycho-Oncology* **8**: 230–6.

146 Carpenter, J. S., Andrykowski, M. A., Cordova, M. *et al.* (1998). Hot flashes in postmenopausal women treated for breast carcinoma: prevalence, severity, correlates, management, and relation to quality of life. *Cancer* **82**:1682–91.

147 Cordova, M. J., Andrykowski, M. A., Kenady, D. E. *et al.* (1995). Frequency and correlates of posttraumatic-stress-disorder-like symptoms after treatment for breast cancer. *Journal of Consulting and Clinical Psychology* **63**:981–6.

148 Zigmond, A. S., Snaith, R. P. (1983). The hospital anxiety and depression scale. *Acta Psychiatrica Scandinavica* **67**: 361–70.

149 Groenvold, M., Fayers, P. M., Sprangers, M. A. *et al.* (1999). Anxiety and depression in breast cancer patients at low risk of recurrence compared with the general population: a valid comparison? *Journal of Clinical Epidemiology* **52**: 523–30.

150 Watson, M., Greer, S., Rowden, L. *et al.* (1991). Relationships between emotional control, adjustment to cancer and depression and anxiety in breast cancer patients. *Psychological Medicine* **21**:51–7.

151 Razavi, D., Delvaux, N., Farvacques, C. *et al.* (1993). Prevention of adjustment disorders and anticipatory nausea secondary to adjuvant chemotherapy: a double-blind, placebo-controlled study assessing the usefulness of alprazolam. *Journal of Clinical Oncology* **11**:1384–90.

152 Wallace, L. M., Priestman, S. G., Dunn, J. A. *et al.* (1993). The quality of life of early breast cancer patients treated by two different radiotherapy regimens. *Clinical Oncology (Royal College of Radiologists)* **5**:228–33.

153 Spiegel, D., Morrow, G. R., Classen, C. *et al.* (1999). Group psychotherapy for recently diagnosed breast cancer patients: a multicenter feasibility study. *Psycho-Oncology* **8**:482–93.

154 Fukui, S., Kugaya, A., Okamura, H. *et al.* (2000). A psychosocial group intervention for Japanese women with primary breast carcinoma. *Cancer* **89**:1026–36.

155 Watson, M., Haviland, J. S., Greer, S. *et al.* (1999). Influence of psychological response on survival in breast cancer: a population-based cohort study. *Lancet* **354**:1331–6.

156 Millar, K., Jelicic, M., Bonke, B. *et al.* (1995). Assessment of preoperative anxiety: comparison of measures in patients awaiting surgery for breast cancer. *British Journal of Anesthesia* **74**:180–3.

157 Brezden, C. B., Phillips, K. A., Abdolell, M. *et al.* (2000). Cognitive function in breast cancer patients receiving adjuvant chemotherapy. *Journal of Clinical Oncology* **18**:2695–701.

158 Cimprich, B. (1999). Pretreatment symptom distress in women newly diagnosed with breast cancer. *Cancer Nursing* **22**:185–94.

159 Graydon, J. E. (1994). Women with breast cancer: their quality of life following a course of radiation therapy. *Journal of Advanced Nursing* **19**:617–22.

160 Miaskowski, C., Dibble, S. L. (1995). The problem of pain in outpatients with breast cancer. *Oncology Nursing Forum* **22**:791–7.

161 Romsaas, E. P., Malec, J. F., Javenkoski, B. R. *et al.* (1986). Psychological distress among women with breast problems. *Cancer* **57**:890–5.

162 Wolberg, W. H., Tanner, M. A., Romsaas, E. P. *et al.* (1987). Factors influencing options in primary breast cancer treatment. *Journal of Clinical Oncology* **5**:68–74.

163 Levy, S. M., Herberman, R. B., Lee, J. K. *et al.* (1989). Breast conservation versus mastectomy: distress sequelae as a function of choice. *Journal of Clinical Oncology* **7**: 367–75.

164 Schwartz, A. L. (1999). Fatigue mediates the effects of exercise on quality of life. *Quality of Life Research* **8**:529–38.

165 Swain, S. M., Rowland, J., Weinfurt, K. *et al.* (1996). Intensive outpatient adjuvant therapy for breast cancer: results of dose escalation and quality of life. *Journal of Clinical Oncology* **14**:1565–72.

166 Bridge, L. R., Benson, P., Pietroni, P. C. *et al.* (1988). Relaxation and imagery in the treatment of breast cancer. *British Medical Journal* **297**:1169–72.

167 Pozo, C., Carver, C. S., Noriega, V. *et al.* (1992). Effects of mastectomy versus lumpectomy on emotional adjustment to breast cancer: a prospective study of the first year postsurgery. *Journal of Clinical Oncology* **10**:1292–8.

168 Wolberg, W. H., Romsaas, E. P., Tanner, M. A. *et al.* (1989). Psychosexual adaptation to breast cancer surgery. *Cancer* **63**:1645–55.

169 Bultz, B. D., Speca, M., Brasher, P. M. *et al.* (2000). A randomized controlled trial of a brief psychoeducational support group for partners of early stage breast cancer patients. *Psycho-Oncology* **9**:303–13.

170 McQuellon, R. P., Craven, B., Russell, G. B. *et al.* (1996). Quality of life in breast cancer patients before and after autologous bone marrow transplantation. *Bone Marrow Transplantation* **18**:579–84.

171 Broeckel, J. A., Jacobsen, P. B., Horton, J. *et al.* (1998). Characteristics and correlates of fatigue after adjuvant chemotherapy for breast cancer. *Journal of Clinical Oncology* **16**: 1689–96.

172 Levy, S. M., Haynes, L. T., Herberman, R. B. *et al.* (1992). Mastectomy versus breast conservation surgery: mental

health effects at long-term follow-up. *Health Psychology* 11: 349–54.

173 Interdisciplinary Group for Cancer Care Evaluation (GIVIO). Impact of follow-up testing on survival and health-related quality of life in breast cancer patients. A multicenter randomized controlled trial. (1994). *Journal of the American Medical Association* 271:1587–92.

174 Classen, C., Koopman, C., Angell, K. *et al.* (1996). Coping styles associated with psychological adjustment to advanced breast cancer. *Health Psychology* 15:434–7.

175 Koopman, C., Hermanson, K., Diamond, S. *et al.* (1998). Social support, life stress, pain and emotional adjustment to advanced breast cancer. *Psycho-Oncology* 7: 101–11.

176 Ahles, T. A., Tope, D. M., Furstenberg, C. *et al.* (1996). Psychologic and neuropsychologic impact of autologous bone marrow transplantation. *Journal of Clinical Oncology* 14:1457–62.

177 Classen, C., Butler, L. D., Koopman, C. *et al.* (2001). Supportive-expressive group therapy and distress in patients with metastatic breast cancer: a randomized clinical intervention trial. *Archives of General Psychiatry* 58: 494–501.

178 Edelman, S., Bell, D. R., Kidman, A. D. (1999). A group cognitive behaviour therapy programme with metastatic breast cancer patients. *Psycho-Oncology* 8:295–305.

179 Tannock, I. F., Boyd, N. F., DeBoer, G. *et al.* (1988). A randomized trial of two dose levels of cyclophosphamide, methotrexate, and fluorouracil chemotherapy for patients with metastatic breast cancer. *Journal of Clinical Oncology* 6:1377–87.

180 Butow, P., Coates, A., Dunn, S. *et al.* (1991). On the receiving end. IV: Validation of quality of life indicators. *Annals of Oncology* 2:597–603.

181 Hurny, C., Bernhard, J., Gelber, R. D. *et al.* (1992). Quality of life measures for patients receiving adjuvant therapy for breast cancer: an international trial. The International Breast Cancer Study Group. *European Journal of Cancer* 28:118–24.

182 Hurny, C., Bernhard, J., Bacchi, M. *et al.* (1993). The Perceived Adjustment to Chronic Illness Scale (PACIS): a global indicator of coping for operable breast cancer patients in clinical trials. Swiss Group for Clinical Cancer Research (SAKK) and the International Breast Cancer Study Group (IBCSG). *Supportive Care in Cancer* 1:200–8.

183 Whelan, T. J., Levine, M., Julian, J. *et al.* (2000). The effects of radiation therapy on quality of life of women with breast carcinoma: results of a randomized trial. Ontario Clinical Oncology Group. *Cancer* 88:2260–6.

184 Levine, M. N., Bramwell, V. H., Pritchard, K. I. *et al.* (1998). Randomized trial of intensive cyclophosphamide, epirubicin, and fluorouracil chemotherapy compared with cyclophosphamide, methotrexate, and fluorouracil in premenopausal women with node-positive breast cancer. National Cancer Institute of Canada Clinical Trials Group. *Journal of Clinical Oncology* 16:2651–8.

185 Fetting, J. H., Gray, R., Fairclough, D. L. *et al.* (1998). Sixteen-week multidrug regimen versus cyclophosphamide, doxorubicin, and fluorouracil as adjuvant therapy for node-positive, receptor-negative breast cancer: an Intergroup study. *Journal of Clinical Oncology* 16:2382–91.

186 Bernhard, J., Hurny, C., Coates, A. S. *et al.* (1997). Quality of life assessment in patients receiving adjuvant therapy for breast cancer: the IBCSG approach. The International Breast Cancer Study Group [published erratum appears in *Ann Oncol* (1998) 9(2):231]. *Annals of Oncology* 8:825–35.

187 Coates, A. S., Hurny, C., Peterson, H. F. *et al.* (2000). Quality-of-life scores predict outcome in metastatic but not early breast cancer. International Breast Cancer Study Group. *Journal of Clinical Oncology* 18:3768–74.

188 Bull, A. A., Meyerowitz, B. E., Hart, S. *et al.* (1999). Quality of life in women with recurrent breast cancer. *Breast Cancer Research and Treatment* 54:47–57.

189 Litwin, M. S., Hays, R. D., Fink, A. *et al.* (1995). Quality-of-life outcomes in men treated for localized prostate cancer. *Journal of the American Medical Association* 273: 129–35.

190 Guyatt, G. H., Kirshner, B., Jaeschke, R. (1992). Measuring health status: what are the necessary measurement properties? *Journal of Clinical Epidemiology* 45:1341–5.

191 Goodwin, P. J., Black, J. T., Bordeleau, L. J. *et al.* (2003). Health-related quality of life measurement in randomized clinical trials in breast cancer – taking stock. *Journal of the National Cancer Institute* 95:263–81.

192 Poulsen, B., Graversen, H. P., Beckmann, J. *et al.* (1997). A comparative study of post-operative psychosocial function in women with primary operable breast cancer randomized to breast conservation therapy or mastectomy. *European Journal of Surgical Oncology* 23:327–34.

193 Curran, D., van Dongen, J. P., Aaronson, N. K. *et al.* (1998). Quality of life of early-stage breast cancer patients treated with radical mastectomy or breast-conserving procedures: results of EORTC Trial 10801. The European Organization for Research and Treatment of Cancer (EORTC), Breast Cancer Co-operative Group (BCCG). *European Journal of Cancer* 34:307–14.

194 de Haes, J. C., van Oostrom, M. A., Welvaart, K. (1986). The effect of radical and conserving surgery on the quality of

life of early breast cancer patients. *European Journal of Surgical Oncology* **12**:337–42.

195 Kemeny, M. M., Wellisch, D. K., Schain, W. S. (1988). Psychosocial outcome in a randomized surgical trial for treatment of primary breast cancer. *Cancer* **62**:1231–7.

196 Bates, T., Riley, D. L., Houghton, J. *et al.* (1991). Breast cancer in elderly women: a Cancer Research Campaign trial comparing treatment with tamoxifen and optimal surgery with tamoxifen alone. The Elderly Breast Cancer Working Party. *British Journal of Surgery* **78**:591–4.

197 Hurny, C., Bernhard, J., Coates, A. S. *et al.* (1996). Impact of adjuvant therapy on quality of life in women with node-positive operable breast cancer. International Breast Cancer Study Group [published erratum appears in *Lancet* (1997) **350**(9073):298]. *Lancet* **347**:1279–84.

198 Nystedt, M., Berglund, G., Bolund, C. *et al.* (2000). Randomized trial of adjuvant tamoxifen and/or goserelin in premenopausal breast cancer – self-rated physiological effects and symptoms. *Acta Oncologica* **39**:959–68.

199 Fairclough, D. L., Fetting, J. H., Cella, D. *et al.* (1999). Quality of life and quality adjusted survival for breast cancer patients receiving adjuvant therapy. Eastern Cooperative Oncology Group (ECOG). *Quality of Life Research* **8**:723–31.

200 Fraser, S. C., Dobbs, H. J., Ebbs, S. R. *et al.* (1993). Combination or mild single agent chemotherapy for advanced breast cancer? CMF vs epirubicin measuring quality of life. *British Journal of Cancer* **67**:402–6.

201 Kloke, O., Klaassen, U., Oberhoff, C. *et al.* (1999). Maintenance treatment with medroxyprogesterone acetate in patients with advanced breast cancer responding to chemotherapy: results of a randomized trial. Essen Breast Cancer Study Group. *Breast Cancer Research and Treatment* **55**:51–9.

202 Buzdar, A., Douma, J., Davidson, N. *et al.* (2001). Phase III, multicenter, double-blind, randomized study of Letrozole, an aromatase inhibitor, for advanced breast cancer versus megestrol acetate. *Journal of Clinical Oncology* **19**: 3357–66.

203 Goss, P. E., Winer, E. P., Tannock, I. F. *et al.* (1999). Randomized phase III trial comparing the new potent and selective third-generation aromatase inhibitor vorozole with megestrol acetate in postmenopausal advanced breast cancer patients. North American Vorozole Study Group. *Journal of Clinical Oncology* **17**:52–63.

204 Bertsch, L. A., Donaldson, G. (1995). Quality of life analyses from vinorelbine (Navelbine) clinical trials of women with metastatic breast cancer. *Seminars in Oncology* **22**: 45–53.

205 Stewart, D. J., Evans, W. K., Shepherd, F. A. *et al.* (1997). Cyclophosphamide and fluorouracil combined with mitoxantrone versus doxorubicin for breast cancer: superiority of doxorubicin. *Journal of Clinical Oncology* **15**:1897–905.

206 Riccardi, A., Tinelli, C., Brugnatelli, S. *et al.* (2000). Doubling of the epirubicin dosage within the 5-fluorouracil, epirubicin and cyclophosphamide regimen: a prospective, randomized, multicentric study on antitumor effect and quality of life in advanced breast cancer. *International Journal of Oncology* **16**:769–76.

207 Holten-Verzantvoort, A. T., Zwinderman, A. H., Aaronson, N. K. *et al.* (1991). The effect of supportive pamidronate treatment on aspects of quality of life of patients with advanced breast cancer. *European Journal of Cancer* **27**:544–9.

208 Hultborn, R., Gundersen, S., Ryden, S. *et al.* (1996). Efficacy of pamidronate in breast cancer with bone metastases: a randomized double-blind placebo controlled multicenter study. *Acta Oncologica* **35** (Suppl. 5):73–4.

209 Pandya, K. J., Raubertas, R. F., Flynn, P. J. *et al.* (2000). Oral clonidine in postmenopausal patients with breast cancer experiencing tamoxifen-induced hot flashes: a University of Rochester Cancer Center Community Clinical Oncology Program study. *Annals of Internal Medicine* **132**: 788–93.

210 Dixon, A. K., Wheeler, T. K., Lomas, D. J. *et al.* (1993). Computed tomography or magnetic resonance imaging for axillary symptoms following treatment of breast carcinoma? A randomized trial. *Clinical Radiology* **48**: 371–6.

211 Marchioro, G., Azzarello, G., Checchin, F. *et al.* (1996). The impact of a psychological intervention on quality of life in non-metastatic breast cancer. *European Journal of Cancer* **32A**:1612–15.

212 Walker, L. G., Walker, M. B., Ogston, K. *et al.* (1999). Psychological, clinical and pathological effects of relaxation training and guided imagery during primary chemotherapy. *British Journal of Cancer* **80**:262–8.

213 Sandgren, A. K., McCaul, K. D., King, B. *et al.* (2000). Telephone therapy for patients with breast cancer. *Oncology Nursing Forum* **27**:683–8.

214 Goodwin, P. J., Leszcz, M., Ennis, M. *et al.* (2001). The effect of group psychosocial support on survival in metastatic breast cancer. *New England Journal of Medicine* **345**: 1719–26.

215 Spiegel, D., Bloom, J. R., Kraemer, H. C. *et al.* (1989). Effect of psychosocial treatment on survival of patients with metastatic breast cancer. *Lancet* **2**:888–91.

216 Fogarty, L. A., Curbow, B. A., Wingard, J. R. *et al.* (1999). Can 40 seconds of compassion reduce patient anxiety? *Journal of Clinical Oncology* **17**:371–9.

217 Christensen, D. N. (1983). Postmastectomy couple counseling: an outcome study of a structured treatment protocol. *Journal of Sex and Marital Therapy* **9**:266–75.

218 Wengström, Y., Häggmark, C., Strander, H. *et al.* (1999). Effects of a nursing intervention on subjective distress, side effects and quality of life of breast cancer patients receiving curative radiation. *Acta Oncologica* **38**:763–70.

219 Helgeson, V. S., Cohen, S. (2001). Long-term effects of educational and peer discussion group interventions on adjustment to breast cancer. *Health Psychology* **20**:387–92.

220 Arathuzik, D. (1994). Effects of cognitive-behavioral strategies on pain in cancer patients. *Cancer Nursing* **17**: 207–14.

221 Bordeleau, L., Szalai, J. P., Goodwin, P. J. *et al.* (2002). Quality of life (QOL) and psychosocial support in women with metastatic breast cancer (MBC): results of a multicenter randomized trial. *Proceedings of the American Society of Clinical Oncology* **21**: A1424.

222 Cunningham, A. J., Edmonds, C. V., Jenkins, G. P. *et al.* (1998). A randomized controlled trial of the effects of group psychological therapy on survival in women with metastatic breast cancer. *Psycho-Oncology* **7**:508–17.

223 Coates, A., Gebski, V., Signorini, D. *et al.* (1992). Prognostic value of quality-of-life scores during chemotherapy for advanced breast cancer. Australian New Zealand Breast Cancer Trials Group. *Journal of Clinical Oncology* **10**: 1833–8.

224 Simes, R. J., Coates, A. S. (2001). Patient preferences for adjuvant chemotherapy of early breast cancer: how much benefit is needed? *Journal of the National Cancer Institute Monographs* **30**:146–52.

225 Moinpour, C. M. (1996). Costs of quality-of-life research in Southwest Oncology Group trials. *Journal of the National Cancer Institute Monographs* **20**:11–16.

226 Bernhard, J., Cella, D. F., Coates, A. S. *et al.* (1998). Missing quality of life data in cancer clinical trials: serious problems and challenges. *Statistics in Medicine* **17**:517–32.

227 Ganz, P. A., Day, R., Ware, J. E., Jr. *et al.* (1995). Baseline quality-of-life assessment in the National Surgical Adjuvant Breast and Bowel Project Breast Cancer Prevention Trial. *Journal of the National Cancer Institute* **87**: 1372–82.

228 Day, R., Ganz, P. A., Costantino, J. P. *et al.* (1999). Health-related quality of life and tamoxifen in breast cancer prevention: a report from the National Surgical Adjuvant Breast and Bowel Project P-1 Study. *Journal of Clinical Oncology* **17**:2659–69.

229 Osoba, this volume, Chapter 19.

230 Lippman, M. E., Hayes, D. F. (2001). Adjuvant therapy for all patients with breast cancer? *Journal of the National Cancer Institute* **93**:80–2.

231 Kiebert, G. M., de Haes, J. C., van de Velde, C. J. (1991). The impact of breast-conserving treatment and mastectomy on the quality of life of early-stage breast cancer patients: a review. *Journal of Clinical Oncology* **9**:1059–70.

232 Fallowfield, L. (1997). Offering choice of surgical treatment to women with breast cancer. *Patient Education and Counseling* **30**:209–14.

233 Moyer, A. (1997). Psychosocial outcomes of breast-conserving surgery versus mastectomy: a meta-analytic review [published erratum appears in *Health Psychology* 1997 **16**(5):442]. *Health Psychology* **16**:284–98.

234 Ganz, P. A., Desmond, K. A., Belin, T. R. *et al.* (1999). Predictors of sexual health in women after a breast cancer diagnosis. *Journal of Clinical Oncology* **17**:2371–80.

6

Measuring quality of life in prostate cancer: progress and challenges

Mark S. Litwin, M.D., M.P.H.[1] **and James A. Talcott, M.D., S.M.**[2]

[1]University of California at Los Angeles, Los Angeles, CA
[2]Massachusetts General Hospital, Boston, MA

Introduction

The potential for health-related quality of life (HRQOL) assessment to edify prostate cancer research and improve patient care is exceptional, but its application is recent and evolving rapidly. While breast cancer patients have been subject to HRQOL evaluation since the early 1980s,[1] sophisticated studies of prostate cancer patient-reported HRQOL began appearing only a decade ago.[2] The goal of this chapter is to survey the published record of HRQOL studies in prostate cancer, describe the most commonly used instruments and how they have performed, as well as some recently described instruments, and to sketch some potentially useful future research directions.

Continuum of care

The diagnosis and management of prostate cancer, the most common non-cutaneous malignancy and the second leading cause of cancer death in American men,[3] are uniquely controversial among human malignancies. Many groups advocate forcefully for widespread screening of asymptomatic men with the prostate-specific antigen (PSA), while many others argue just as strongly for restraint. Once diagnosed, prostate cancer may be managed with qualitatively different treatment modalities or initial observation ("watchful waiting"), but the virtual absence of data from randomized clinical trials makes the treatment decision-making process frustrating for patients, while physicians often struggle to provide the most helpful advice. The clinical management of recurrent cancer is also subject to controversy which parallels that for early disease: PSA technology allows identification of tumor progression years before symptoms of cancer emerge, if ever, and the toxicity of treatment options at that stage is important and increasingly evident. For patients with advanced hormone-refractory prostate cancer, most treatments have limited efficacy, while documenting symptomatic palliation is paramount.

Prevention and screening

It is unknown whether primary prevention of prostate cancer is possible, although epidemiological associations with dietary risk factors are emerging. A chemoprevention trial with 18 000 patients using finasteride, a 5-alpha reductase inhibitor, the Prostate Cancer Prevention Trial (PCPT), which evaluated HRQOL prospectively,[4] has terminated early after showing a decreased incidence of low-grade tumors, but an increase in high-grade tumors.[5]

Prostate cancer screening – measurement of the serum PSA level and palpation of the prostate by digital rectal examination (DRE) – has the potential to cause anxiety, discomfort, and medical complications.[6–9] Patients with abnormal findings, usually an elevated PSA, undergo transrectal ultrasonography and tissue sampling through prostate needle biopsies. A negative biopsy provides welcome but incomplete reassurance, since the imperfect sensitivity of systematic prostate sampling allows for future biopsies if PSA elevation persists. While results that diagnose a malignancy that would otherwise have remained undetected are unwelcome, the information justifies the screening process for many, if not most, men.

As such, the value of screening is intensely controversial.[4,5,10,11] Despite the absence of definitive evidence of benefit,[12] and in conflict with the recommendations of many preventive medicine organizations, prostate cancer screening is occurring with great frequency and at significant cost to health care systems throughout the world.[13] In the early 1990s, a dramatic increase in PSA screening doubled the reported incidence of prostate cancer, sharply reduced the median age at diagnosis, and both strengthened the rationale for treatment of younger patients and significantly prolonged the clinical natural history. The more frequent diagnosis and prolonged natural history rapidly increased the prevalence of the disease to an estimated 1.4 million men in 1999. Most of these men have undergone treatment and experience long-term treatment-related symptoms.[10,11,14]

Quality-of-life measurement is central to the screening and treatment controversy: if treatment-related impairments could be sufficiently reduced, mitigated by rehabilitative treatments, or shown not to reduce quality of life, medical (versus economic) arguments against screening would largely dissolve, pending definitive randomized trials. Two large randomized trials of PSA screening are currently underway, the European Randomized Study of Screening for Prostate Cancer[15] and the US Prostate, Lung, Colon and Ovary trial (PLCO).[16] Initial results of these studies are expected in 2007 at the earliest, with additional follow-up potentially necessary to compensate for lost power because of noncompliance and contamination (screening in control patients).

Treatment

Early stage prostate cancer may be managed expectantly (i.e., "watchful waiting") or with potentially curative local treatments, including radical prostatectomy, external beam irradiation, interstitial seed implants (brachytherapy), and in selected patients, cryotherapy. The local treatments have distinctive patterns of urinary, bowel, and sexual dysfunction, while expectant management entails potential anxiety about the progression of untreated cancer. Recent technical modifications to primary therapies include nerve-sparing radical prostatectomy, offering potential post-surgical potency; conformal external beam radiation, improving ratios of tumor to normal tissue irradiation; and percutaneous, ultrasound-guided brachytherapy, significantly shortening the period of treatment and acute convalescence.

Use of androgen deprivation therapy (ADT) is increasing rapidly with the more frequent diagnosis of prostate cancer and informally expanding indications for its use, often despite little if any supporting data. It is increasingly often used in primary treatment alone or in combination with other treatments, especially radiotherapy.[17] Another common scenario for ADT use is a minimal PSA rise in serial testing in follow-up after primary therapy, detecting recurrence years before metastasis will become apparent or symptomatic.[18]

Changes in treatment have occurred in advanced prostate cancer as well. Advanced stage prostate cancer, including asymptomatic metastatic cancer, may be managed expectantly, with medical or surgical ADT, or when hormone-refractory with other anti-androgenic therapy, cytotoxic chemotherapy, or other novel systemic therapy. At both the hormone-sensitive and hormone-refractory stages, quality-of-life assessment adds importance to efficacy measures such as survival and changes in tumor size. While causing less acute and obvious toxicity than the cytotoxic agents used to treat most other advanced cancers, ADT produces an increasingly well-documented array of short- and long-term complications, including vasomotor instability ("hot flashes"), bone mineral loss, changes in body composition, and fatigue.[19,20] While the increased use of ADT in these settings may prolong life, similar to hormonal manipulation of breast cancer, the rapid expansion of ADT is of uncertain value in many settings where use is common. An underappreciated source of increased costs for treating prostate cancer is "indication creep" in the use of ADT to more patients without documented bone metastases in the rapidly increasing population of prostate cancer survivors. The financial burden of prostate cancer on the American public has grown substantially,[14] due to both the increased use of active treatment and to the increased use of ADT,[21] which now accounts for about one-third of Medicare expenditures for treating prostate cancer.[22] The extraordinary cost of ADT treatment, combined with the high and rapidly increasing prevalence of diagnosed and treated prostate cancer, make a more thorough evaluation of ADT essential. Documenting the impact of adverse changes in quality of life will be central in determining the result.

Conventional cytotoxic chemotherapy has a limited role in palliative treatment of men with androgen-insensitive metastatic prostate cancer.[23,24] In this setting, quality-of-life outcomes are paramount; reduction of the dominant symptom, pain, is the primary endpoint. Improved quality of life without a survival benefit justified FDA approval for one regimen, mitoxantrone and prednisone;[24] a marginally efficacious agent, suramin, has been largely abandoned because of treatment toxicity.[25,26] Quality-of-life evaluation will be central to the rapidly expanding evaluation of new agents in this setting.

Survivorship

Quality of life is a critical issue for prostate cancer survivors. Once prostate cancer is diagnosed and treated, a patient's life is necessarily and permanently altered. Even if he is thought to be cured, his level of functioning may be diminished, and he may sustain specific side effects of local and systemic treatments, such as impotence, urinary incontinence, bowel dysfunction, urethral strictures, or decreased libido. He may also suffer negative psychosocial and economic consequences from having cancer. Conversely, many men anecdotally report that the cancer experience adds new meaning to their lives and enriches their perspectives and insights. Evaluating the net impact of these potentially conflicting effects on the long course of

most patients' lives largely determines the long-term assessment of which treatment choice is best.

End of life

The extended period without cancer-related symptoms but with important disease-specific symptoms distinguishes outcomes measurement for clinically localized and advanced or recurrent but hormone-responsive prostate cancer from that of other common malignancies. However, the patient's experience of hormone-refractory advanced prostate cancer resembles that of other advanced cancers for which curative or effective palliative treatments are largely unavailable. The most prominent symptom for prostate cancer patients nearing the end of life is pain, usually from bone metastases, including vertebral metastases potentially causing spinal cord compression. However, other symptoms of end-stage malignancy such as fatigue, anorexia, and nausea (commonly assessed in cancer-specific quality-of-life instruments, as discussed below) are also frequent.[12–14,21,22,27–30]

Role of health-related quality of life (HRQOL)

HRQOL encompasses a broad range of human experience, including functioning and subjective responses to illness, as well as physical, emotional, and social well-being.[31–33] To assess the impact of prostate cancer and its treatments fully, quality-of-life measurement must address a wide spectrum of the components of well-being. However, in the rather brief history of HRQOL measurement in prostate cancer, nearly all attention has been devoted to specific areas of function or symptoms, along with how much the functional deficits or symptoms bother patients, with little assessment of how these problems affect diverse aspects of men's lives.

In broad terms, HRQOL may be conceived as the quotient of an individual's actual health status over the health status he or she expects to have, given the circumstances. For example, to the degree that a prostate cancer patient's erectile dysfunction is expected, not bothersome, and not intrusive into his life or self-image, it does not affect his HRQOL. Conversely, a patient whose expectations and interest in erectile function are high may perceive even a modest decrement as very harmful.[34]

The traditional efficacy endpoint for cancer treatment, survival, remains salient for prostate cancer, especially metastatic cancer. Survival is of less practical use for early stage prostate cancer, which for most men does not cause mortality, even if untreated. Because of the long expected survival time, even modest changes in HRQOL may have a large cumulative impact. Hence, treatment modalities for localized tumors without differences in survival efficacy may produce qualitatively different profiles of enduring treatment-related complications.

Localized treatment modalities likely improve survival for some patients with early prostate cancer. More than three-fourths of men with prostate cancer die of another cause, and many who die of prostate cancer have occult metastases unaffected by local therapy at diagnosis. Therefore, for most men with early prostate cancer, survival is unaffected by treatment, leaving quality of life the definitive outcome. Despite the use of surrogates for mortality available earlier, such as rising PSA, conclusive evidence of survival benefits for early prostate cancer treatments probably requires post-treatment observation of at least a decade, while stable estimates of long-term changes in treatment-related function may appear within a year or two of treatment. The recently published results from the Scandinavian trial of surgery versus observation, for example, show no overall survival benefit, despite a suggestive trend after a median of 6.2 years of follow-up and despite a two-fold difference in cause-specific survival after surgery.[35] The accompanying quality-of-life survey documented important treatment-related changes an average of 1.5 years after treatment.[36]

Treatment alternatives for advanced prostate cancer vary little in their impact on survival. However, marginally efficacious agents may importantly improve critical symptoms such as pain from bone metastases for patients with hormone-refractory disease. Alternate strategies for asymptomatic patients with progression of hormone-sensitive disease, including ADT, anti-androgens, and observation may differ substantially in outcomes affecting quality of life, such as erectile function, fatigue, loss of muscle mass, and bone mineral loss.

Hence, HRQOL is a critical outcome for men with prostate cancer and will remain so, particularly until the appearance of evidence that available treatments prolong survival. Even when treatments with important adverse effects offer modest survival benefit, patients must balance the often competing goals of quantity and quality of life. In summary, quality-of-life considerations may be decisive in medical decision-making for many men with prostate cancer.[31–34,37]

Methods

Literature search strategy

The strategy used to identify potentially relevant articles was designed to maximize the sensitivity and specificity of the search; it was initially conducted in 1999 and then updated in 2001. English-language articles published from 1990 through 2001 were included. MeSH headings included quality of life, survival analysis, health status indicators, activities of daily living, decision support techniques, costs and cost analysis, health services research, quality of health care, outcome and process assessment, and others. To identify additional, more recent clinical studies using particular HRQOL instruments, the Science Citation Index was also used.

Each retrieved article was reviewed by one of the authors. Full-length research articles were included in the overview if they presented original data on any patient-centered outcome (including costs or survival alone) for men with prostate cancer; review papers were excluded. Decision-analytic and preference-based papers[38,39] were excluded in favor of patient-reported outcomes. Because randomized data are largely unavailable for patients with early prostate cancer, attention was focused on the extensive use of HRQOL in observational studies, with special emphasis on studies using complete validated instruments.

Results

Measurement of HRQOL in prostate cancer

The addition of health-related quality of life to survival as an outcome measure enhances the value of clinical research and may be decisive at several treatment decision-making points in the long natural history of the disease. Generic HRQOL instruments are used to compare pretreatment status and outcomes across different populations and interventions, while disease-targeted scales focus on cancer- and prostate cancer-specific issues.[40]

For patients with prostate cancer, HRQOL may be affected in a variety of ways. Correspondingly, the instruments used to evaluate HRQOL differ in their intended breadth and specificity, from general (or generic) measures that facilitate comparisons with individuals with other diseases or with the general population,[41,42] to general cancer measures that facilitate comparisons across tumor sites,[43-46] to prostate cancer-specific measures that focus expressly on the impact of this particular cancer.[47-50] As for other tumors, symptom- or domain-specific measures may provide crucial information in some settings. For example, for many patients with advanced metastatic prostate cancer, patient quality of life is dominated by painful bone lesions, making assessment of changes in pain the central HRQOL issue.[24]

Investigators have used a three-part approach to compare outcomes in patients who have undergone various treatments for their localized prostate cancer with each other, with patients who have different forms of cancer,[51] and with patients who do not have cancer. The impact of HRQOL measurement on clinical decision-making has been limited by the paucity of randomized trials comparing primary treatment modalities for patients with early prostate cancer with unbiased comparisons of treatment outcomes. Recently, some such trials have emerged for primary treatment[35,36,52,53] and for psychosocial or supportive care interventions.[54,55] Observational trials are subject to bias and confounding by treatment received. That is especially true for early prostate cancer, whose strong specialty-dependent physician biases[56,57] have largely blocked development of and recruitment to randomized trials. The plentiful observational trials, which are more representative and thus more generalizable than randomized trials, have provided important insights into real-world scenarios of prostate cancer treatment. Adjustment for age, comorbidity, race, socioeconomic status, education, insurance coverage, and other variables may partially address the impact of confounding by treatment choice. However, residual confounding resists such adjustment. Patient populations undergoing surgical treatment, for example, have higher SF-36 scores than patients undergoing radiation therapy, those managed expectantly, or even age-matched volunteers without prostate cancer. This underscores the dangers of unadjusted comparisons of treatment groups, even at the same medical center during the same time period. This concern is particularly relevant if patients' baseline functional status, usually the most powerful predictor of outcome, is unknown, as in post-treatment, cross-sectional assessments.

While issues of comparability also apply to traditional outcomes such as survival, generic HRQOL instruments were designed to compare the physical and mental health states of patient populations and have well-established population-based norms.[42,58,59] Therefore, these instruments can be used to identify differences between patient populations as surrogates for comorbidity and non-prostate cancer survival. In contrast, in patients with metastatic prostate cancer, assessment of HRQOL has been used more extensively and occasionally decisively in randomized trials.[24,52,60-65] Although patients with prostate cancer have been assessed using instruments that broadly measure general HRQOL, until recently, disease-specific scales have not been widely used in this population. Prostate cancer and its treatments may directly affect sexual, urinary, and bowel function; hence, most disease-specific quality-of-life instruments contain sexual, urinary, and bowel scales focused on symptoms or functional deficits in these areas. Reduced function varies in its subjective impact on patients' lives. This impact, or bother, has been distinguished from dysfunction in the literature, and most instruments include items to assess it.[66] Most men with early prostate cancer have no symptoms from cancer, although obstructive urinary symptoms most commonly attributed to benign prostatic hyperplasia are highly prevalent in older men. Therefore prostate cancer-specific instruments focus on treatment-related symptoms.

Sexual dysfunction is the most commonly reported complication of treatment for prostate cancer and is a paradigmatic symptom: all prostate cancer-specific HRQOL instruments measure it. Some men with significant sexual dysfunction are minimally bothered by it, while others with only mild dysfunction may be miserable. Erectile dysfunction precluding intercourse does not prevent satisfaction from other sexual activities. So while sexual function and bother are undeniably linked, they are independent domains and must be measured separately.

However, this additional dimension, the impact of dysfunction perceived by patients on their lives, is complex and challenging to assess. For example, the degree of dysfunction patients report is inherently correlated with the intensity of their feelings about the symptom. Therefore, simply asking patients to report the severity of and bother from their symptoms may add little to the self-report of function alone.[67] Attempts to assess the disparate impacts of sexual dysfunction[68] and other treatment-related dysfunction on complex dimensions of men's lives are beginning to appear.[69]

Even when both dysfunction and its impact on men's lives are validly assessed, the relationship may evolve over time as men accommodate to their dysfunction or their life circumstances change. Furthermore, some men suffer from erectile dysfunction not as a direct result of prostate cancer treatment but because of age or comorbidity that predates the cancer and its treatment.

Urinary function may be affected by both the expanding intraprostatic cancer mass, especially obstructive symptoms, and by treatment. Dysfunction may be manifest primarily as obstruction, irritation, or incontinence; in practice, the first two

symptom groups may be difficult to distinguish. Irritative and obstructive symptoms are common in older men and may be the dominant urinary symptoms, especially shortly after brachytherapy. Urinary incontinence after treatment may be long-lasting. It may be measured by patient reports of the circumstances, frequency, and quantity of leaked urine, or by the frequency of pad use. However, these measures may be inexact. As for sexual dysfunction, the organic dysfunction and the distress caused by incontinence may diverge, both *ab initio* or over time.[70,71] For some men with significant dysfunction, distress may be mitigated because of satisfactory control of constant dripping with a pad or device or because of the expectation of improved function. For others with even mild dysfunction, an occasional unexpected squirt may cause social embarrassment and humiliation that is psychologically damaging.

Assessment of bowel symptoms, including diarrhea, rectal urgency, tenesmus, rectal bleeding, and others is also essential, especially for patients who undergo radiation therapy. Like urinary symptoms, bowel dysfunction may be highly disruptive in some men's lives, and the time course and severity of specific bowel symptoms may diverge.

The focus of prostate cancer-specific HRQOL measurement has been expanded by both changes in the treatment practice, such as the expansion of ADT into primary treatment of early prostate cancer, and by awareness of previously underappreciated effects of treatment, such as fatigue associated with ADT.[72] This evolution is expected to continue.

Commonly used HRQOL measures in prostate cancer

Outcomes measurement in prostate cancer can be usefully grouped into generic measures of HRQOL, general cancer measures, prostate cancer-specific measures, and symptom-specific scales, although the domains of instruments in these categories may overlap (Table 6.1). Generic HRQOL measures assess both physical and mental health broadly. General cancer domains assess symptoms commonly arising from cancer and its treatment, especially systemic

Table 6.1. Key instruments used in HRQOL research in prostate cancer

Construct	General Quality of Life	Psychological State		Pain	Cancer Related Quality of Life					
	SF-36	POMS	HADS	BPI	EORTC QLQ-C30	FACT-G	CARES	FLIC	RSCL	QLI
Physical functioning	10				5	2	4		4	2
Role – physical	5				2	3	7	4	4	
Mental health										
Psychological distress/adjustment	3				4	7	5	4	8	
– Anxiety		9	7							1
– Depression		15	7							1
– Anger-hostility		12								
– Anxiety re cancer, treatment							4	2		
– Anxiety in medical situations							8			
Psychological well-being	2									
Role – emotional	3					2	2			
Social	2				2	6	14	2		
Energy/fatigue	4	15			3	1	3		2	
Cognitive		7			2		3			
Sleep					1	1	1		2	
Pain	2			15	2	1	4	3	1	
General health/global QOL	4				2	6		2		1
Health change	1									
Urinary (general)										
Urinary obstruction/irritation										
Urinary incontinence										
Bowel symptoms										
Sexual interest/function/ attractiveness						1	14		1	
Nausea/vomiting					2	2	6	2	2	
Hair loss							1			
Weight loss							2			
Appetite/taste/dry mouth/swallowing					1		3		1	
Other GI symptoms					2		1		3	
Shortness of breath					1				1	
Hormone ablation symptoms										
Other physical symptoms							6		8	
Medical interaction						2	11			
Patient compliance							4			
Relationship with partner							18			
Family relationships										1
Interaction with children							3			
Dating problems							5			
Employment concerns							7			
Hardship due to cancer (self)					1		3	1		
Hardship (family)							2			
Not scored		7								
TOTAL items	36	65	14	15	30	34	139	22	38	6

Table 6.1. (*cont.*)

| | Number of items included for each construct | | | | | | | | | | | |
| | Prostate Cancer Specific Quality of Life | | | | | | | | | Sexual Scales | | Obstruction/ BPH |
Construct	UCLA-PCI	EPIC	PROS QOLI	Clark & Talcott	Clark *et al.*	Dale *et al.*	FACT -P	Borghede *et al.*	Giesler *et al.*	IIEF	BSFI	AUA/ IPSS
Physical functioning			1									
Mental health												
– Prostate cancer decision-making					5							
– Regret					5			1				
– Depression		2	1									
– Cancer concern					7			3				
– Health concern					8							
Energy/fatigue		2	1									
Pain			1				3					
General health/global QOL			1									
Urinary												
Urinary (general)	2	1	1		5	3			9			
Urinary obstruction/ irritation		7		10	8	2	4					6
Urinary incontinence	4	4		4	3	2		1	5			1
Bowel symptoms	5	14	1	10		12	1	8	16			
Sexuality												
Sexual interest	1	2				2	1	3		2	2	
Sexual function	6	7		5		4	1	2	4	7	4	
Sexual satisfaction	2	4			11	4		1	11	6	5	
Gender identity					8			1				
Hormone ablation symptoms		4						1				
Hair loss					1							
Weight loss					2							
Appetite/taste/dry mouth/swallowing			1				1					
Other physical symptoms							1					
Relationship with partner					3							
Family relationships			1									
TOTAL items	20	50	9	29	55	35	12	19	52	15	11	7

effects. Prostate cancer-specific measures also assess cancer- and treatment-related effects, but focus on areas specifically related to prostate cancer. Specific symptom scales usually target areas of function highly salient in particular settings, such as pain or fatigue. The currently available HRQOL instruments include an assortment of validated tools that perform well across disease stages and clinically relevant domains (Table 6.2). The choice of an instrument, then, is largely based on the content relevance of its items in a given sample.

In this review, we focus primarily on studies using complete, validated instruments assessing more than one domain or symptom group. However, we acknowledge that this approach may obscure valid and appropriate use of scales taken from instruments for specialized assessments and to reduce respondent burden, such as the National Cancer Institute's Prostate Cancer Outcomes Study;[73] useful results from instruments without complete psychometric data published at the time of this writing;[36] and symptom-specific instruments highly relevant to some clinical situations.[24]

We found the most commonly used non-prostate, cancer-specific HRQOL instruments used in prostate cancer are those used elsewhere in oncology.[74] However, their use in prostate cancer is relatively recent and is evolving in response to the cancer's unique characteristics. These include the prolonged period in which cancer-specific symptoms are uncommon while treatment-specific symptoms predominate, the slow pace of symptomatic progression, and the paucity of clearly efficacious systemic treatments for patients with hormone-refractory advanced cancer. As a result, use of some established instruments, such as the SF-36, has become more constrained with experience, and the development of prostate cancer-specific instruments is evolving rapidly. We describe their performance in prostate cancer populations below. We have abstracted representative values for the most commonly used instruments in prostate cancer populations (Table 6.3).

Commonly used generic measures of HRQOL in prostate cancer include the RAND Medical Outcomes Study Short Form Health Survey (SF-36),[75] the Profile of Mood States (POMS),[42] and the Hospital Anxiety and Depression Scale (HADS).[59] These measures are robust, particularly the SF-36, with extensive validation, published population norms, extensive use in cancer populations, and multiple translations available. To reduce respondent burden, shorter versions, the SF-12[76] and the Brief POMS,[77] have been developed, but there is little reported use of these in prostate cancer studies so far.

We found 24 references using the SF-36 in prostate cancer,[9,37,48,55,64,72,78–95] including validation studies.[47,48,87,95] Studies in patients with early prostate cancer documented small or largely transient changes in the first 1–2 years after treatment for early disease,[9,79,82,83,85,86,90,91] usually confined to a subset of its eight domains. Another found that lower-income patients had lower global HRQOL and deficits on 4 of 8 prostate cancer-specific scales before treatment.[78] In patients with metastatic prostate cancer this instrument, or its subscales, can distinguish between patients with hormone-sensitive and hormone-refractory prostate cancer[37] and document the decline in HRQOL in patients with metastatic prostate cancer as cancer progresses.[92,94] Studies not distinguishing early and advanced prostate cancer found that patients with prostate cancer have higher functioning than those with lung cancer[93] and may be indistinguishable from the normal population.[94] In brief, the SF-36 is helpful in some settings. While it is not sensitive to treatment-related changes in patients with localized prostate cancer, especially over relatively short observational periods, the SF-36 helps to characterize patient populations, identify important early changes within specific domains that may increase over time or deserve future investigation, and document important changes in patients with advanced disease for whom disease progression often corresponds with important functional declines.[81,96,97]

Psychological distress is an important component of quality of life in prostate cancer populations as elsewhere in oncology. As a result, the POMS[39,72,98,99] and HADS[100,101] have been used in prostate cancer populations. Here, too, measures of distress may increase transiently in some men prior to diagnostic

Table 6.2a. Description and psychometric properties of prostate cancer specific questionnaires

Instrument name	Supplement to the EORTC QLQ-C30[116]	Functional Assessment of Cancer Therapy-General (FACT-G); Functional Assessment of Cancer Therapy – Prostate (FACT-P)[122]
Purpose for which developed	A prostate cancer-specific questionnaire to be used in conjunction with the EORTC QLQ-C30.	To measure the general and unique HRQOL of patients diagnosed with prostate cancer. Includes FACT-General plus prostate cancer-specific module.
Length	19 items. Time frame: present symptoms.	39 items: 27 FACT-G, 12 PCS. Time frame: past 7 days.
Administration time	Not reported.	10 minutes.
Domains included	Bowel symptoms (8 items), urinary incontinence (1), urinary irritation or blockage (4), sexual function or interest symptoms (4), hormone symptoms (1).	Physical Well-Being (7 items), Emotional Well-Being (5), Social Well-Being (7), Functional Well-Being (7), Relationship with Doctor (2), Prostate Cancer (12), Weight (1), Appetite (1), Pain (3), Emotional Role (1), Urinary (3), Bowel (1), Sexual Function (1).
Scoring	4-point Likert scale ("not at all, a little, quite a bit, very much"). Scores are re-scaled to a 0 to 100 scale, with higher scores representing better health.	0 to 4 Likert scale ("not at all, a little bit, somewhat, quite a bit, very much"). Global score, FACT-G score, subscale scores. Scores are re-scaled to a 0 to 100 scale, with higher scores representing better health.
Validated modes of administration	Self-administered mail.	Self-administered or interview format.
Validated translations/ Cultural adaptations	Swedish.	Chinese, Czech, Danish, Dutch, English, Finnish, Flemish, French (Canada, France, Belgium), German (Germany, Austria, Switzerland), Greek, Hebrew, Hungarian, Italian, Japanese, Norwegian, Polish, Portuguese, Russian, Spanish, Swedish, Turkish.
Evidence of reliability (internal consistency, test-retest, other)	Reliability and validity tested in 1,138 unselected Swedish patients. Internal consistency was measured using Cronbach's alpha: sexuality scales (0.92), urinary scales (0.76), and bowel scales (0.66).	Reliability tested in 96 patients visiting the Prostate & Urology Center at the University of Chicago Hospitals. Cronbach's alpha was calculated for the following scales: physical well-being (0.64), social/family well-being (0.71), relationship with doctor (0.84), emotional well-being (0.75), functional well-being (0.83), FACT-G (0.87), and prostate cancer subscale (0.69).
Evidence of validity (content, construct, criterion-related)	Content of the prostate module developed by G. Borghede with the input of two oncologists and two urologists. Multitrait factor analysis supported all scales.	Content: The prostate cancer subscale items were developed with input from 8 patients with prostate cancer and 8 oncology professionals, including medical oncologists, surgical oncologists, radiation oncologists, and advanced practice nurses.
Evidence of responsiveness/sensitivity to change	No formal demonstration.	Patients were given a performance status rating (PSR, Zubrod) by investigators. Those patients with improved or unchanged PSR also had higher scores for physical well-being, functional well-being, prostate cancer subscale, and FACT-P compared to patients with worsened PSR. Falling PSA showed a significant difference compared to rising PSA in the FACT-G, prostate cancer subscale, and FACT-P. The FACT-P differentiates patients across disease stage.
Interpretability (availability of normative data, clinically meaningful difference)	No formal demonstration.	No formal demonstration.

Table 6.2b. Description and psychometric properties of prostate cancer specific questionnaires

Instrument name	Expanded Prostate Index Composite (EPIC)[48]	UCLA Prostate Cancer Index (UCLA-PCI)[47]
Purpose for which developed	To create a more comprehensive assessment of prostate cancer-related HRQOL by expanding the UCLA-PCI.	To measure multidimensional HRQOL in patients with prostate cancer. This prostate cancer-specific module is typically administered with the SF-36.
Length	50 items. Time frame: past 4 weeks.	20 items. Time frame: past 4 weeks.
Administration time	Not reported.	10 minutes.
Domains included	Bowel symptoms (14 items), urinary symptoms (12), sexual function or interest symptoms (13), hormone symptoms (11).	Urinary function (5), sexual function (8), bowel function (4), urinary bother (1), sexual bother (1), bowel bother (1).
Scoring	0 to 4 Likert scale for single items and multi-item scales. Scale scores transformed linearly to a 0 to 100 scale, with higher scores representing better HRQOL.	3, 4, and 5 point Likert scales. Scales transformed linearly to a 0 to 100 scale.
Validated modes of administration	Self-administered mail.	Self-administered mail.
Validated translations/ Cultural adaptations	English (US).	English, Spanish, Dutch, French, Japanese.
Evidence of reliability (internal consistency, test-retest, other)	Reliability and validity tested in 252 American patients with equal representation of patients treated with radical prostatectomy, external beam radiation, and brachytherapy. In each domain, Cronbach's alpha $\geq$.82, with retest reliability of r $\geq$.80. Internal consistency of EPIC scores was confirmed in non-whites through separate analysis of 59 non-white participants, Cronbach's alpha $\geq$.74 for each summary score.	Reliability and validity tested in 255 patients with prostate cancer and a comparison group of 273 individuals without prostate cancer. Internal: Cronbach's alpha for urinary function = 0.87, alpha for sexual function = 0.93, alpha for bowel function = 0.65. Test-retest: product-moment, intraclass correlations, 4 weeks apart, urinary function r = 0.93, 0.92; sexual function r = 0.92, 0.92; bowel function r = 0.79, 0.77; urinary bother r = 0.66, 0.66; sexual bother r = 0.70, 0.70; bowel bother = 0.77, 0.77. Missing data: 2.5% missing responses.
Evidence of validity (content, construct, criterion-related)	Content: UCLA-PCI was expanded to the EPIC with guidance from a cohort of experts including patients, urologic oncologists, radiation oncologists, survey researchers, and prostate cancer nurses; a literature review was also performed. EPIC urinary function and bother scales were correlated at r = 0.69, bowel function and bother at 0.87, and sexual function and bother at 0.64.	Content: Four focus groups of prostate cancer patients and spouses facilitated by a trained moderator identified and developed items within three primary domains of concern for dysfunction and bother: urinary, bowel, and sexual. Exploratory factor analysis and multitrait scaling analysis of responses factored into final item selection. Multitrait scaling analysis supported the three domains (urinary, sexual, bowel). Function and bother correlated substantially: urinary (r = 0.71), sexual (0.73), and bowel (0.65).

Table 6.2b. (*cont.*)

Instrument name	Expanded Prostate Index Composite (EPIC)[48]	UCLA Prostate Cancer Index (UCLA-PCI)[47]
Evidence of validity (*cont'd*)	Construct: EPIC correlation to the FACT-P scales in the urinary, bowel, sexual, and hormonal domains were 0.58, 0.51, 0.44, and 0.61, respectively. EPIC correlation to the AUA-SI urinary scale was 0.77.	SF-36 scales correlations: Correlations for urinary function ranged from 0.17 (bodily pain) to 0.29 (emotional well-being). Correlations for urinary bother ranged from 0.19 (emotional well-being) to 0.33 (energy/fatigue). Correlations for sexual function ranged from 0.19 (emotional well-being) to 0.42 (general health perceptions) and correlations for sexual bother ranged from 0.10 (emotional well-being) to 0.28 (general health perceptions). Correlations for bowel function ranged from 0.27 (role limitations due to emotional health problems) to 0.37 (general health perceptions), and correlations for bowel bother ranged from 0.28 (role limitations due to emotional health problems) to 0.37 (social function, energy/fatigue). CARES-SF correlation: Allowing for the reversal of scales, the sexual function correlation was 0.43.
Evidence of responsiveness/ Sensitivity to change	No formal demonstration.	Responsiveness has not been formally demonstrated. However, longitudinal data have been published.
Interpretability (availability of normative data, clinically meaningful difference)	No formal demonstration.	The clinical significance of score differences has not been formally assessed in prostate cancer populations. However, results of the instrument in age-matched non-prostate cancer populations have been reported.

Table 6.2c. Description and psychometric properties of prostate cancer specific questionnaires

Instrument name	Prostate Cancer Specific Quality of Life Instrument (PROSQOLI)[49]	Clark and Talcott[67]
Purpose for which developed	To create a measure of HRQOL to be an outcome measure for clinical trials in advanced hormone-resistant prostate cancer.	To develop indexes of urinary, bowel, and sexual function, and related distress.
Length	10 items. Timeframe: past 24 hours.	29 items. Timeframe: In the past week for urinary, bowel, and related distress items. In the past 4 weeks for sexual function items.
Administration time	Not reported.	Not reported.
Domains included	Pain (2), physical activity (1), fatigue (1), appetite (1), constipation (1), family/ marriage relationships (1), mood (1), urinary function (1), and overall well-being (1).	Symptom domains include urinary incontinence (3), urinary obstruction/irritation (5), bowel dysfunction (6), and sexual dysfunction (5). Symptom related distress domains include urinary incontinence (1), urinary obstruction/irritation (5), and bowel distress (4).

Table 6.2c. (*cont.*)

Instrument name	Prostate Cancer Specific Quality of Life Instrument (PROSQOLI)[49]	Clark and Talcott[67]
Scoring	9 items on a linear analog scale, and one item on a Likert scale from 0 to 5. Linear analog scale items are rescaled to a 0 to 100 scale.	All items are on a 4 or 5 point Likert scale. Items are rescaled to a 0 to 100 scale, with higher scores representing greater dysfunction or distress.
Validated modes of administration	Self-administered.	Self administered.
Validated translations/ Cultural adaptations	English (Canada).	English (US).
Evidence of reliability (internal consistency, test-retest, other)	Reliability and validity tested in a randomized trial of 161 patients with HRPC at 10 Canadian institutions, where patients were randomized to receive treatment with either intravenous mitoxantrone every 3 weeks plus daily oral prednisone, or daily oral prednisone alone. Most patients answered all the questions; the lowest response rate for an individual question was 157/161 for the marriage/family relationships question.	Reliability was tested with 94 prostatectomy patients and 90 radiotherapy patients from clinics in the greater Boston area who filled out questionnaires at baseline, a 3-month post-treatment follow-up, and a 12-month follow-up. Internal consistency of symptom indexes was strong for urinary incontinence (Cronbach's alpha = 0.86), bowel function (0.80), and sexual function (0.92), while internal consistency was moderate for urinary obstruction/irritation (0.65). Missing data on most items ranged from less than 1% to 9%. Two items pertaining to ejaculation and orgasm adapted from the MOS scale drew limited response.
Evidence of validity (content, construct, criterion-related)	Content: Developed and tested in two single-arm studies. Construct: Correlations between the PROSQOLI and the QLQ-C30/QLM-P14 were as follows: appetite (r = 0.80), constipation (0.66), mood (0.63), pain (0.59), fatigue (0.49), physical activity (0.46), overall well-being (0.45), passing urine (0.44), and family/marriage relationships (0.11).	Contents for the symptom-function indexes were based on the AUA Symptom Index for benign prostatic hyperplasia and the BPH-impact scale. Scales for symptom related distress were constructed as a parallel set of questions asking whether each symptom had been a problem. Substantial correlations between symptom indexes and corresponding levels of distress were found, in agreement with the findings of Barry *et al.* (AUA/IPSS) and with factor analysis reported by Litwin *et al.* (UCLA PCI).
Evidence of responsiveness/ Sensitivity to change	No formal demonstration.	Urinary incontinence and sexual function indexes were highly responsive to prostatectomy, while bowel indexes were highly responsive to radiotherapy. Indexes documented the initial impact of prostate resection and radiation and subsequent improvement between 3 and 12 months after treatment.
Interpretability (availability of normative data, clinically meaningful difference)	No formal demonstration.	No formal demonstration.

Table 6.2d. Description and psychometric properties of prostate cancer specific questionnaires

Instrument name	Dale et al.[50]	Clark et al.[135]
Purpose for which developed	To develop a clinically useful questionnaire to assess health-related quality of life in patients undergoing external beam radiation for prostate cancer.	To construct patient-centered measures of the outcomes of treatment for early prostate cancer.
Length	35 items. Timeframe: past week.	55 items. Timeframe: present.
Administration time	Not reported.	Not reported.
Domains included	Urinary function (12 items), sexual function (9 items), and bowel function (11 items), with one additional bother question in each dimension. Two distinct domains were identified within each dimension.	For all men: urinary control (8), sexual intimacy (7), sexual confidence (4), marital affection (3), masculine self esteem (8), health worry (6), PSA concern (2). For prostate cancer patients only: cancer control (5), quality of treatment decision making (5), regret of treatment choice (5), and cancer-related outlook (2).
Scoring	All items are on a 4 to 6 point Likert scale.	All items on a Likert scale.
Validated modes of administration	Self administered.	Self administered.
Validated translations/ Cultural adaptations	English (US).	English (US).
Evidence of reliability (internal consistency, test-retest, other)	Reliability and validity were tested in 150 patients referred for radiotherapy treatment of localized prostate cancer.\n\nInternal consistency was measured for each domain: daily bowel function (Cronbach's alpha = 0.80), bowel urgency (0.71), urinary urgency (0.81), urinary stream (0.74), sexual interest/satisfaction (0.95), and impotence (0.63).	Reliability tested with 749 patients, of which about half did not have prostate cancer and half did. Patients were not selected for particular treatments, though they were asked to provide information about their treatment.\n\nCronbach's alpha was between 0.77 and 0.93 for all scales except for the two-item measure of PSA concern among prostate cancer patients.
Evidence of validity (content, construct, criterion-related)	Content development was not reported.\n\nMost convergence correlations were greater than 0.40. The only exception (painful bowel movements) did not correlate with scales outside its own dimension.\n\nDivergence correlations showed that no item from a scale of a dimension was more highly correlated with a scale in a separate dimension.\n\nStudy population was 90% black due to referral patterns.	Content: Scales were developed using themes and categorized text from focus groups of recently diagnosed (in the last 12 to 24 months, regardless of treatment) prostate cancer patients. Focus groups were mediated by a sociologist and a medical oncologist.\n\nMasculinity and the Mental Component Summary of the SF-12 correlated at r = 0.55.\n\nInterscale correlations were lower than 0.42 with the exceptions of health worry with cancer control (0.65), and masculine self-image with sexual intimacy (0.51), with health worry (-0.56), and with cancer control (0.51).
Evidence of responsiveness/ Sensitivity to Change	Most patients had clinical Stage B and grade 2 tumors, but those with either Stage A or grade 1 disease had lower dysfunction scores, and those with Stage C tumors had higher scores, indicating worse quality of life.	No formal demonstration.
Interpretability (availability of normative data, clinically meaningful difference)	No formal demonstration.	No formal demonstration.

Table 6.2e. Description and psychometric properties of prostate cancer specific questionnaires

Instrument name	Giesler et al.[134]
Purpose for which developed	To create a comprehensive, multi-scale quality-of-life instrument that can be tailored to the needs of the clinician/investigator in multiple settings.
Length	52 items. Timeframe: past 4 weeks.
Administration time	15 minutes.
Domains included	Urinary function (5), urinary role activity limitations (5), urinary bother (4), sexual function (7), sexual role activity limitations (5), sexual bother (5), bowel function (7), bowel role activity limitations (5), bowel bother (4), and cancer worry (4).
Scoring	52 Likert-type items, ranging from a 3-point scale to a 6-point scale.
	Items were linearly transformed to a 0 to 100 scale, with higher scores denoting better outcomes.
Validated modes of administration	Self-administered.
Validated translations/ Cultural adaptations	English (US).
Evidence of reliability (internal consistency, test-retest, other)	Reliability and validity were tested in a group of 300 patients diagnosed with localized prostate cancer. Test-retest reliability was evaluated with an additional group of 200 patients.
	Internal consistency, measured by Cronbach's alpha, was reported for urinary function (0.89), urinary limitations (0.81), urinary bother (0.89), sexual function (0.90), sexual limitations (0.70), sexual bother (0.87), bowel function (0.70), bowel limitations (0.88), bowel bother (0.90), and cancer worry (0.80).
	Test-retest: product moment, intra-class correlations. Urinary function (0.92, 0.92), urinary limitations (0.86, 0,86), urinary bother (0.92, 0.92), sexual function (0.91, 0.91), sexual limitations (0.86, 0.86), sexual bother (0.87, 0.87), bowel function (0.72, 0.72), bowel limitations (0.68, 0.63), bowel bother (0.68, 0.68), and cancer worry (0.60, 0.59).
Evidence of validity (content, construct, criterion-related)	Content was developed by the authors with consideration to the literature and to the limitations of other prostate cancer-specific quality of life instruments.
	Convergent and discriminant validity were confirmed by the product-moment correlations. Scales within the same organ system area tended to converge, while scales of different content areas tended to diverge.
	The function scales and bother scales correlated highly with the UCLA-PCI scales for all three organ system areas: urinary ($r = 0.94$, 0.90), sexual (0.95, 0.75), and bowel (0.92, 0.93). The limitations scales did not correlate strongly with either the function or bowel scales of the organ system for the UCLA-PCI.
	All scales, except for urinary function, correlate significantly with PANAS-N, the negative affect assessment of the global quality of life instrument.
Evidence of responsiveness/ Sensitivity to change	No formal demonstration.
Interpretability (availability of normative data, clinically meaningful difference)	No formal demonstration.

Table 6.3. Representative scores for five commonly used HRQOL instruments in prostate cancer

	EORTC QLQ-C30					
Author	Borghede and Sullivan, 1996[109] Sweden	Borghede et al., 1997[116] Sweden			Albertsen et al., 1997[37] United States	
Disease Phase	Primary	Primary and Metastatic		Metastatic	Metastatic	Metastatic
Patient Group	Post-radiation	Age 55–59*	Age 75–79*	LHRH agonist, post-treatment	Remission	Progression
Domain						
Physical	88.8	87.7	73.9	73.1	82.3	72.5
Role	91.9	74.4	71.7	71.3	72.5	71.7
Emotional	85.6	76.9	82.3	79.0	81.4	76.9
Cognitive	87.5	88.5	79.2	79.3	84.7	84.0
Social	85.5	79.5	80.6	77.7	80.3	74.2
Global QOL	75.0	68.6	67.4	65.7	70.3	58.3
Fatigue	21.7	22.2	33.6	35.3	26.3	39.4
Nausea/vomiting	2.3	5.1	3.5	4.4	5.3	10.1
Pain	12.5	17.9	17.9	19.6	18.3	33.6
Dyspnea	16.7	23.1	29.6	29.6	20.0	18.9
Sleep disturbance	14.5	20.5	20.0	22.6	25.0	31.4
Appetite loss	1.9	7.7	6.0	6.5	4.5	26.4
Constipation	7.3	2.6	13.8	14.5	16.7	27.0
Diarrhea	20.8	7.7	5.4	5.6	11.1	9.6
Financial problems	3.4	15.4	4.7	8.7	15.6	25.0
Sexuality	54.5	82.7	74.6	86.4	Not reported**	Not reported**
Urinary symptoms	5.5	11.3	15.9	16.9	Not reported**	Not reported**
Bowel symptoms	24.9	Not reported	Not reported	Not reported	Not reported	Not reported

Mean scores, scales = 0–100

* Age groups are subsets of large study

** This study used other scales to assess these symptoms

Table 6.3. (cont.)

Author	Esper et al., 1997[122] United States	Lee et al., 2001[123] United States						Litwin et al., 1995[88] United States		
Disease Phase	All phases	Primary	Primary	Primary	Primary	Primary	Primary	Primary	Primary	Primary
Patient Group	Pre- and post-treatment	Pre-brachytherapy	12-month post-brachytherapy	Pre-prostatectomy	12-month post-prostatectomy	Pre-EBRT	12-months post-EBRT	Post-prostatectomy	Post-radiation	Observation
Domain										
Physical well-being	26.2	25.9	25.3	26.3	26.3	25.2	25.1	25.4	24.9	25.2
Emotional well-being	15.5	20.8	22.3	17.9	21.7	20.7	21.9	16.6	17.3	16.6
Social well-being	23.5	23.0	22.7	24.4	22.8	23.6	23.1	21.6	21.6	21.1
Functional well-being	21.6	23.3	24.1	23.6	23.3	22.9	23.2	20.9	21.2	20.7
Relationship with doctor	6.5	7.7	7.8	7.7	7.7	7.5	7.7	6.5	6.5	6.3
FACT-G total	93.6	100.7	102.2	99.8	101.9	99.9	101.0	91	91.5	89.5
Prostate Cancer Subscale	36.9	37.7	36.3	38.5	38.6	37.2	35.8	Not reported*	Not reported*	Not reported*
FACT-P total	130.5	138.4	138.5	138.3	140.4	137.1	136.9	Not reported*	Not reported*	Not reported*

Mean scores, 0–100 scale

* Only the FACT-G was used in this study

Table 6.3. (cont.)

SF-36

Domain	Bacon et al., 2002[80] United States Primary Post-treatment	Pietrow et al., 2001[149] United States Primary Post-prostatectomy, no PSA recurrence	Pietrow et al., 2001[149] United States Primary Post prostatectomy, PSA recurrence	Lubeck et al., 1999[90] United States Primary 2 years post-prostatectomy	Lubeck et al., 1999[90] United States Primary 2 years post-radiation	Lubeck et al., 1999[90] United States Primary 2 years post-hormones	Lubeck et al., 1999[90] United States Primary 2 years post-observation	Albertsen et al., 1997[37] United States Metastatic Remission	Albertsen et al., 1997[37] United States Metastatic Progression
Physical functioning	87.0	85	80	85.8	65.1	72.6	70.8	62.3	54.5
Role – physical	80.5	77	70	72.3	55.4	75.8	62.8	53.6	49.5
Role – emotional	87.0	86	76	84.4	75.8	83.4	72.5	71.8	59.1
Energy/fatigue	67.8	66	61	70.9	54.1	58.3	57.1	60.1	49.8
Emotional well-being	82.8	81	82	86.0	77.6	80.3	75.9	78.9	71.6
Social functioning	90.2	88	84	88.8	76.9	83.9	77.9	80.4	66.5
Pain	82.2	84	78	84.4	73.8	79.0	76.1	73.5	60.5
General health	76.8	71	65	74.6	53.9	64.2	53.8	60.8	53.4
Health change	Not reported	Not reported	Not reported	60.2	47.3	53.1	46.4	Not reported	Not reported

Mean scores, 0 to 100 scale

Table 6.3. (cont.)

UCLA-PCI

Author	Bacon et al., 2002[80] United States	Litwin et al., 1998[47] United States	Pietrow et al., 2001[149] United States		Davis et al., 2001[83] United States		
Disease Phase	Primary	All phases	Primary	Primary	Primary	Primary	Primary
Patient Group	Post-treatment		Post-prostatectomy, no PSA recurrence	Post-prostatectomy, PSA recurrence	Post-prostatectomy	Post-radiation	Post-brachytherapy
Domain							
Urinary function (5)	81.7	83.8	71	67	69.3	85.8	85.7
Sexual function (8)	29.4	38.5	26	15	50.8	23.4	30.5
Bowel function (4)	84.3	84.4	87	84	85.7	76.5	82.3
Urinary bother (1)	81.4	79.4	75	71	75.5	82.0	75.2
Sexual bother (1)	49.1	36.3	35	28	27.1	38.9	38.9
Bowel bother (1)	82.8	83.1	88	84	84.0	70.9	78.6

Mean scores, 0–100 scale

EPIC

Author	Wei et al., 2000[48] United States
Disease Phase	All phases
Patient Group	Ages 28–86; 46% white, 51% black
Domain	
Urinary function (5)	86.5
Urinary bother (7)	75.8
Sexual function (9)	29.5
Sexual bother (4)	41.1
Bowel function (7)	87.9
Bowel bother (7)	85.3
Hormonal function (5)	84.0
Hormonal bother (6)	88.7

Mean scores, 0–100 scale

biopsy[39] and after initial local therapy.[72, 100] Little distress is evident a year or more after treatment,[98–100] although fatigue may indicate high levels of distress.[101]

The EORTC Quality of Life Core Questionnaire (QLQ-C30)[43] is a general cancer instrument used in clinical trials, especially in Europe. Its 30 items assess physical, role, cognitive, emotional, and social function, three specific symptoms associated with cancer and its treatment (fatigue, pain, and nausea/vomiting), global health, and quality of life. It is designed as a core instrument for a modular approach to measuring quality of life in patients with various cancer diagnoses. Its construct validity has been demonstrated in prostate cancer patients: it distinguishes patients with hormone-responsive and hormone-refractory prostate cancer.[37] It is responsive to change, although much more so in patients with advanced disease. Its overall agreement with the Functional Assessment of Cancer Therapy–General (FACT-G) (see below) is moderate, with little overlap in its social and cognitive domains.[102] We found 26 citations for this instrument in both localized and metastatic prostate cancer.[5,37,49,52,53,62,63,65,91,92,99–101,103–115] Like generic measures, this instrument has found small or transient changes in 1–2 year follow-up after initial therapy for early prostate cancer.[91] In longer follow-up (median 58.5 months) of a small randomized trial of ADT combined with radical prostatectomy or external beam radiation therapy, improved quality-of-life benefit for the radiation arm, despite a survival trend in favor of surgery, was found.[52] In randomized trials in metastatic prostate cancer, the EORTC QLQ-C30 documented HRQOL deterioration in patients with newly diagnosed poor prognosis M1 prostate cancer who received mitomycin-C chemotherapy after orchiectomy[63] and in patients with hormone-refractory prostate cancer who received flutamide versus prednisone.[62] In a randomized trial of epoetin beta versus transfusion support, no difference in quality of life was found, although the instrument documented improvement for all patients with an increase in hemoglobin of more than 20 g/l.[60] It was also

used to anchor validation studies of two new prostate cancer-specific instruments[5, 106] and to provide quality-of-life values for a Q-TWiST analysis of an EORTC study of goserelin acetate with and without flutamide.[107]

A new 19-item prostate cancer-specific supplement to the EORTC instrument assesses urinary, bowel, and sexual symptoms, domains common to all prostate cancer-specific instruments, and an item assessing the impact of hormone ablation. The prostate-specific module has been shown to have good test-retest and internal consistency reliability, as well as content, criterion, and construct validity, in men with both localized[109, 116] and metastatic[37] prostate cancer. No benefit was found for megestrol acetate in patients with hormone-refractory prostate cancer,[117] and in a non-randomized trial, decreased quality of life was found for men with asymptomatic metastatic prostate cancer who chose ADT rather than deferring therapy.[118]

The FACT-G[44] is a well-validated 27-item instrument developed and widely used in the United States. Like the EORTC QLQ-C30, it is designed for use with modules for specific cancers. It measures social/family well-being and relationship with doctor as well as physical, emotional, and functional well-being. As noted above, it converges with the EORTC QLQ-C30 in some but not all dimensions. Internal consistency, convergent/divergent validity, and responsiveness are well-documented in cancer patients. We found 9 citations in prostate cancer patients.[48,65,88,92,104,110,119–121] In cross-sectional studies, similar outcomes were found for previously treated surgery and radiation therapy patients[119] and for observation patients and non-cancer controls.[88] However, other studies found lower quality of life among patients who also received external beam radiation therapy and brachytherapy compared to patients who underwent either modality alone[104] and patients who underwent salvage radiation therapy versus radical prostatectomy for locally recurrent prostate cancer.[121] A 12-item prostate cancer-specific module (FACT-P) is available as a supplement to the FACT-G. The FACT-P items assess weight, appetite, pain, and emotional role in addition to urinary, bowel, and sexual function.[122] Its use of single items for some domains and a single summary score emphasizes brevity over robustness and richness of the data set. We found 8 citations.[48,101,110,121,123–126] The FACT-P documented transient changes that disappeared by 12 months after treatment for early prostate cancer[101,126] and distinguished treatment groups who underwent salvage therapy for local recurrence[121] It was used to document criterion validity for the EPIC prostate cancer-specific instrument (see below).[48]

Other scales commonly used in cancer patients, including the Functional Living Index-Cancer (FLIC),[46] the Quality of Life Index (QL-Index),[45] and the Rotterdam Symptom Checklist (RSCL),[127] have also been used in men with prostate cancer (Table 6.1).

The most commonly used instruments that examine prostate-specific domains are noted in Tables 6.1 and 6.2. While they overlap, they vary in the domains assessed, their optimal circumstances for use, and the extent of their use in prostate cancer populations.

Prostate cancer-specific instruments have proliferated (Tables 6.1 and 6.2). We found that the UCLA Prostate Cancer Index (UCLA PCI)[47,88] developed by Litwin and colleagues, which assesses sexual, urinary, and bowel dysfunction and bother, or distress, is the most widely cited prostate-cancer-specific instrument.[9,70,71,78–80,82,83,87,89,90,94,128–130] It was used in an early and influential comparison of treatment groups for early prostate cancer.[62] The UCLA PCI has been semantically, culturally, and psychometrically validated beyond English, in Spanish,[131] French, Dutch, and Japanese, joining the cancer-specific module for the EORTC QLQ-C30 and the FACT-P. Its urinary function scale assesses incontinence and irritation but not obstruction. It does not specifically address domains associated with advanced disease, such as metastatic bony pain, nausea, vomiting, or weight loss. Although its disease-specific domains are best suited for examining HRQOL changes following treatment for localized disease, the UCLA PCI characterizes men treated for prostate cancer of all stages.[47,87,94]

Other instruments assess similar domains, although several distinguish between urinary incontinence, obstruction, and irritation, despite the lack of specificity of most urinary symptoms.[48,50,67,109,132] Later prostate cancer-specific instruments added new domains, including symptoms of ADT[48,109] and medical regret.[69,133] The Expanded Prostate Cancer Index Composite (EPIC)[48] includes items on painful or difficult urination and rectal or urinary bleeding. These symptoms, commonly encountered by prostate cancer patients, are not measured by the UCLA PCI. The EPIC also includes a domain regarding hormonal symptoms, such as hot flashes, relevant to the growing group of asymptomatic patients receiving ADT. A number of studies have demonstrated that symptom severity and bother ratings are highly correlated [50,67] and suggest that more specific indicators of the impact of self-reported symptoms on HRQOL are needed. The observation that fear of cancer recurrence motivates many treatment decisions has led to a measure for regret about treatment choices.[133,134] Several other instruments assessing disease- and treatment-specific symptoms have recently undergone psychometric testing, but their use so far has been limited (Table 6.1).[49,50,67,109,122,134,135]

In part because of their relatively recent development, the prostate cancer-specific instruments have psychometric properties that are less thoroughly established than the general measures (Table 6.2). All instruments included here have demonstrated internal consistency and content validity in prostate cancer populations, but only a few have been shown to be responsive to change over time. Minimally important group differences in HRQOL scores have not been well established for any disease-specific measure. In fact, that large functional deficits identified by prostate cancer-specific instruments,[85,90] especially in brief follow-up, are not associated with significant decline in robust measures of HRQOL such as the SF-36, has been used to challenge the importance of these prostate cancer-specific deficits to patients.

Measurement of sexual function has tended to follow that of the Massachusetts Male Aging Study directed by McKinlay;[136,137] more recent scales include the Brief Male Sexual Function Inventory[138] and the International Index of Erectile Function (IIEF).[139]

The American Urological Association's International Prostate Symptom Score (IPSS), a widely used measure to assess urinary obstructive symptoms in men with benign prostatic hyperplasia (BPH), has also been used in the setting of prostate cancer, since radiation, especially brachytherapy, acutely increases urinary obstruction.

Measures of specific symptoms other than sexual and urinary function have been useful in certain settings, such as advanced, hormone-refractory prostate cancer in which measures of pain may be used to assess palliative treatments.[24,60–65,140] One important study used several complementary measures of pain to assess the palliative benefit of mitoxantrone for patients with symptomatic metastatic prostate cancer.[24] Because pain is the dominant symptom for these men, its documented reduction resulted in mitoxantrone's approval by the United States Food and Drug Administration for this indication.

Discussion

Added value of HRQOL assessments

Prostate cancer differs from other common cancers in several ways that enhance the importance of measuring quality-of-life outcomes. Definitive efficacy benefits of the primary treatment modalities in early prostate cancer using traditional survival endpoints are largely unavailable. Available data, including a recent randomized trial in early prostate cancer,[35] suggest that survival benefits from various interventions for both early and advanced prostate cancer may be small enough that their anticipated cumulative impact over time will make HRQOL remain relevant to patient decision making. For early cancer, surgery, two alternative radiation therapy techniques, and initial observation are widely used options, and for some patients the currently disfavored options of ADT and cryotherapy may be considered. For advanced hormone-responsive cancer, surgical and medical castration differ little in measured outcomes but may be experienced very differently because of changes to body image. For hormone-refractory prostate cancer, alternative treatments differ little in efficacy measured by survival, but differences in HRQOL outcomes may denote important palliative benefits or serve as an early indicator of improved efficacy.

The specific organ systems affected and their time course vary by treatment. For example, several studies have documented that sexual function declines early after radical prostatectomy but improves subsequently, while radiation therapy results in slower but ongoing declines.[70,88] Documenting these changes may influence patient treatment choice and facilitate adaptation to complications. Patients vary in how much functional deficits bother them and the impact may change over time.[8] Characterizing groups for whom functional losses are disproportionately important or unimportant may help match patients and treatments, thus improving patient outcomes. Valid measures of prostate cancer-specific outcomes provide both a means of comparing competing established treatments and evaluating techniques altered to reduce treatment-related toxicity, although the latter has been used infrequently.[128,141]

HRQOL endpoints have also been incorporated into studies assessing treatment efficacy.[24,36,64] In all, only a few longitudinal studies in prostate cancer have relied upon validated HRQOL measures as key endpoints (Table 6.4). As additional domains of HRQOL are identified, the value of measuring HRQOL endpoints increases further. Depiction of the fundamental elements in quality of life for men with prostate cancer requires study of their perceptions of function, symptoms, and other aspects of their health and how it affects their daily activities. Physical and emotional well-being form the cornerstone of this approach, but research also extends to anxiety, fatigue, and depression. Interpretation of these outcomes may require measuring other factors affecting the response to illness, such as rapport

Table 6.4. Use of HRQOL instruments in longitudinal clinical studies in prostate cancer

	n	Primary Instruments Used (NOTE: Some studies used >1 instrument)					
		EORTC QLQ-C30	FACT-G	FACT-P	BPI	SF-36	Other
Local Treatment	5	1	0	1	0	0	4
• Primary treatment[36,52,53]	3	1	0	1	0	0	2
• Psychosocial intervention[54,55]	2	0	0	0	0	0	2
Metastatic	7	4	1	0	1	1	3
• Anti-cancer therapy[24,61–64,140]	6	3	1	0	1	1	3
• Supportive care[60]	1	1	0	0	0	0	0
Total (Local Treatment + Metastatic)	12	5	1	1	1	1	7

with the physician, the availability of a spouse, partner, or another close confidant, and social interactions.

As noted above, prostate cancer-specific instruments document much larger changes than generic measures of HRQOL. Additional research is required to understand the implications of this apparent discrepancy between significant functional losses in intimate bodily functioning and stable global HRQOL scores. Potential resolution of these conflicting results could arise from demonstrating that one measurement approach is preferred, from designing generic measures with greater responsiveness or from improved understanding of the factors resulting in individual and population variation in these outcomes measures and their subjective impact. Beyond measuring outcomes, broader HRQOL measures, along with typical demographic and clinical characteristics, help characterize and distinguish treatment groups, further accenting pretreatment differences that could influence the interpretation and generalization of outcomes.

The most useful research initiatives rely on established HRQOL instruments with proven records of statistical reliability and validity. Quality of life can have many different definitions and interpretations, but its measurement must adhere strictly to psychometric science.

Performance of HRQOL measures in observational studies and clinical trials

Few randomized controlled trials of prostate cancer treatments have included methodologically rigorous HRQOL assessments, especially for early cancer. Medical specialists who treat early prostate cancer strongly prefer the treatment modality they provide,[56,57] reducing enthusiasm for randomized trials. The "either-or" choice of primary treatment modality for prostate cancer, in contrast to breast cancer for which two surgical treatments (modified radical mastectomy versus breast-conserving surgery) compete, increases the economic stakes of such a trial. Important randomized trials have been initiated, but slow accrual raises concerns about potential erosion of study power. One of these, the Prostate Cancer Intervention Versus Observation (PIVOT) trial,[142] includes prospective quality-of-life measurement. A recently published interim analysis of the Scandinavian trial[35] comparing radical prostatectomy to observation was accompanied by the results of a survey early in the study using a novel disease-specific instrument.[36] Nonetheless, the HRQOL impact of early prostate cancer treatment modalities has been almost exclusively gleaned from cross-sectional and longitudinal observational studies, which limit conclusions.

Table 6.5. Patient-reported outcomes compared with clinical measures in prostate cancer studies

Phase of Disease	Number of Studies	Most Commonly Used Patient-Reported Outcome Measures (#)	Most Commonly Used Clinical Measures	Key Observations: Comments on the Value Provided by Patient-Reported Outcomes
Primary treatment	Numerous	• UCLA PCI (14)	• Not performed	• Impairments in the sexual, urinary, and bowel domains of HRQOL after treatment for early stage prostate cancer are more common than previous estimates based on physician assessments
				• Global measures of HRQOL may be little changed despite profound disease- or treatment-specific effects
				• The association between organ-specific dysfunction and bother is variable and unstable
				• The time course of treatment-related dysfunction varies over time and by treatment modality
				• All aspects of HRQOL are inherently very personal and, hence, contribute differently to the many choices that men make along the prostate cancer disease trajectory
				• Measures of psychological stress were useful outcomes for non-medical interventions
Advanced disease	7	• EORTC QLQ-C30 (4) • Pain scales • Toxicity	• Survival • Performance Status	• Of the studies identifying significant HRQOL benefit, 1[24] found a parallel benefit in TTP/TTF and 3[61–63] did not
				• Most studies found no or a small difference in survival; conclusions were based on HRQOL differences if any
				• Conclusions were strengthened when more general quality of life instruments showed changes parallel with prostate cancer-specific instruments

Recent trials of medical adjuvant and advanced cancer treatments incorporate HRQOL,[61,62,117] occasionally decisively.[24,64] In addition, the Prostate Cancer Prevention Trial also measures global HRQOL (SF-36), urinary obstructive symptoms, and sexual function.[4]

Several important lessons have emerged from studies based on patient-reported quality-of-life outcomes using validated instruments (Table 6.5).

First, impairments in the sexual, urinary, and bowel domains of HRQOL after treatment for early stage prostate cancer are more common than previously believed. Reports of observational studies using patient-reported, disease-specific quality-of-life instruments strongly suggest that previous reports from treating physicians on the consequences of active treatment may have been overly optimistic for the general population,[2,13,70,88,141,143–145] an impression subsequently confirmed.[89] The less favorable results may have altered patient treatment choices. Between 1983 and 1989, prostatectomy rates increased threefold in SEER areas,[28] and almost six-fold between 1984 and 1990 among Medicare beneficiaries.[29] With the subsequently declining incidence of prostate cancer diagnosis as PSA screening achieved near-saturation in American men over age 50, prostatectomy rates fell between 1992 and 1996 but were offset by an increase in brachytherapy procedures.[30] For brachytherapy, the sparse initial reports of outcomes were largely favorable but addressed only short-term results.[102,111,121,122]

Second, global measures of HRQOL may be little changed despite profound disease- or treatment-specific effects.[82,85,123] In particular, global assessments of physical function, emotional well-being, and social functioning are often largely unaffected, despite substantial decrements in sexual, urinary, and bowel domains, especially shortly after surgery or radiation.[85] This result requires further exploration. The patient's distinction between cancer and treatment effects could distort patient responses to bother items. Further, a more wide-ranging assessment of the impact of symptoms on patients' lives may uncover impacts invisible to items focused strictly on the frequency or severity of specific symptoms.

Third, the association between organ-specific dysfunction and bother is variable and unstable. Patients may simultaneously report substantial dysfunction but little bother or the reverse, and the discordance can widen or shrink with changed circumstances.[9] Patient expectations that symptoms may improve and adaptation to adverse changes may reduce perceived functional impairment or reduce bother. In contrast, a belief that further improvement is unlikely or the diagnosis of advanced or recurrent cancer may decrease patient tolerance of stable dysfunction.[88,146–150] The problem of unstable patient assessment of clinical states pervades outcomes measurement, especially in attempts to adjust survival outcomes for quality of life.

Fourth, the organ systems affected and the time course of treatment-related dysfunction vary over time and by treatment modality. Sexual function and urinary incontinence after prostatectomy and bowel function after radiation tend to suffer initially and then improve, while sexual function after radiation deteriorates progressively over time. Urinary incontinence after radical prostatectomy improves slowly if at all beyond the first year after surgery, and sexual function declines for at least two years after radiation therapy.[70,71,88]

Fifth, all aspects of HRQOL are inherently very personal and hence contribute differently to the many choices that men make along the prostate cancer disease trajectory. Close collaboration between patients and their physicians, explicitly discussing expected quality-of-life outcomes and patient values, is required for optimal treatment decision-making.

Relative strengths and weaknesses of the commonly used measures

Generic, general cancer, and prostate cancer-specific quality-of-life instruments are commonly administered in combination to assess a broader range of domains than a single instrument would allow. Measures of overall health-related quality of life, such as the SF-36 or the Functional Living Index-Cancer (FLIC), and a measure of mental health or moods, such as the Profile of Mood States (POMS) or the RAND Mental Health Index, document the physical and mental health status of the study sample. This characterization allows comparison with population norms or with patients suffering from other chronic diseases.[84] Comparison of various patient groups with men with prostate cancer may allow investigators both to further validate the generic instruments in this population and to assess the construct validity of the prostate cancer-specific instruments. That is, the administration of generic and general cancer instruments to disease-specific populations, such as prostate cancer patients, builds further evidence for the generalizability of data gathered with those instruments. Likewise, the administration of prostate cancer-specific measures alongside more established ones may reveal new constructs or dimensions of health-related quality of life unique to this population.

The population norms arising from the widespread use of the generic measures, especially the SF-36, can be used to characterize particular patient populations, producing robust measures of the overall health of patient populations (Table 6.3). These comparisons allow dissimilar populations to be identified; for early prostate cancer, for example, patients undergoing radical prostatectomy tend to be both younger and healthier than those who receive external beam radiation therapy. Age differences are easy to quantify, but with the SF-36 this can also be accomplished for overall health status for which age is a rough and potentially misleading surrogate. Specific measures of disease comorbidity, including the Charlson Index and the Index of Coexistent Disease (ICED), may accomplish similar goals more efficiently, but they require additional information from medical records that can be difficult and expensive to obtain. The greatest limitation of generic measures is their limited responsiveness to clinical change. When the impact of a disease or treatment is confined to a small number of bodily functions, change may be difficult to demonstrate. Several groups have reported that significant a priori deterioration of functions likely to affect quality of life, such as sexual, urinary, or bowel function, correlate poorly with changes in the SF-36 or its subscales.

General cancer measures such as the EORTC QLQ-C30 and the FACT-G measure global HRQOL domains as well as symptoms commonly affected by cancer and its therapy, including fatigue and malaise specific symptoms such as pain, shortness of breath and nausea, psychological functioning, impact on the family, and relationship with medical caregivers. These measures are particularly useful in patients with advanced cancer, for whom multiple symptoms are common. But they are not as sensitive to the impact of early disease when performance status is excellent despite specific defects in urinary, bowel, or sexual function. In low-income

patients with metastatic prostate cancer, simultaneous administration of the EORTC QLQ-C30, the FACT-G, and the Quality of Life Index (QLI) revealed that the QLQ-C30 and FACT-G converged in emotional, physical, and role/functional dimensions but not social function.[65]

Prostate cancer- or treatment-specific instruments measure clinically important outcomes not assessed by other measures, particularly urinary, bowel, and sexual function. Several disease-specific instruments have been published, differing somewhat in coverage of additional domains, validation approach, how function and "bother" measurements are combined, and format. While additional domains have been incorporated (such as the impact of castration into the EPIC) and domains further broken into sub-domains (such as the distinction between urinary incontinence and obstruction/irritation), the correlation between corresponding scales has been striking, implying that all instruments successfully measure the key functional domains well.[134]

Because they measure inherently different constructs of quality of life, disease-specific and generic or cancer-specific measures may diverge or reinforce one another (Table 6.5). Cancer- and symptom-specific instruments showed parallel changes, reinforcing the clinical benefit of palliative mitoxantrone and prednisone in symptomatic metastatic prostate cancer;[24] parallel changes in emotional functioning enhanced the bowel benefit of placebo over flutamide in surgically castrated men with asymptomatic metastatic prostate cancer.[64]

By assessing bother explicitly, several prostate cancer-specific instruments such as the UCLA PCI attempt to assess both dysfunction and its subjective impact. However, the relation between dysfunction and bother may be difficult to characterize and report. Patient reports of the magnitude of their symptoms (function) correlate strongly with the magnitude of subjective impact of those symptoms (bother), eroding the distinction.[50,67] Symptom summary scales provide an indication of the extent to which pathophysiological changes result in subjective functional outcomes. However, reporting both bother and function items may complicate interpretation by attempting to combine symptom severity with the patient's subjective reaction to the symptom. This distinction is conceptually difficult to maintain, although there are examples of patients reporting similar symptom severity but differing strikingly in their response to the symptoms, as measured in a bother item. This divergence increases overall variability of the scale score, and, because characteristics of patients in a given study may particularly affect bother reports, may limit the generalizability of study findings to other populations. One approach to unifying these disparate domains into relevant profiles has been to try to identify specific situations in which a treatment-related dysfunction (or concerns about cancer control arising from expectant management) has an impact on men's lives. For example, a patient with urinary incontinence may have very specific social difficulties, such as self-consciousness about odors, reluctance to travel because of the need to attend to absorptive pads, or occupational limitations because long-lasting activities must be interrupted frequently.[135] Also, development and use of more broadly focused but carefully targeted measures may document a more significant impact of treatment-related symptoms, their relative unimportance compared to the desire to optimally control cancer, or establish the irrelevance of one or both to men's concept of their HRQOL.

Conclusions

While substantial progress in assessing health-related quality of life in men with prostate cancer has been achieved in recent years, important issues remain unresolved. These issues involve choosing specific instruments and methodological approaches for measuring and reporting quality of life, identifying situations in which quality of life matters most, and fitting quality of life into the question of treatment choice. The importance of HRQOL is due, in part, to the fact that the paramount issue for most patients, preventing death from cancer, is usually remote, both chronologically and statistically.

Measures and reports of quality of life in prostate cancer are inconsistent. Formal comparisons between the UCLA PCI, the EPIC, and the instrument of Giesler et al.[134] indicate that those instruments assess the accepted core prostate-cancer specific domains (sexual, urinary, and bowel function) similarly and well. However, instruments are not interchangeable. While consistent results using different instruments in different treatment groups drawn from different populations reinforce one another, the reasons for conflicting results are less clear when instruments vary between studies. Converging on a single instrument may be premature and disadvantageous, but it would be useful to compare the instruments formally to identify any clinically important differences.

Available instruments may not collect all the information needed to understand HRQOL in prostate cancer. Additional domains, such as fatigue and the various effects of castration and other hormonal manipulations, will enhance understanding of functional changes due to prostate cancer and its treatment. Further, little has been done to assess the impact of changes in function on men's lives overall.

Research is needed to understand, ascertain, and convey the clinical importance of the changes measured. Unless the meaning of numerical changes can be communicated to patients in relevant terms, their value in decision-making will be limited. Analogous to a medical student's growing understanding of blood pressure measurements, meaning adheres to numerical scales only through extensive clinical exposure to patients with varying values and to clinically relevant thresholds. Few clinicians and far fewer patients currently comprehend the meaning of numerical changes in HRQOL scales for prostate cancer. However, progress is being made; many urologists have a growing appreciation for numerical IPSS scores measured in patients with obstructive voiding symptoms. Improved attention to measuring clinically meaningful differences through formal calibration studies[151–153] and to presenting results will enhance the interpretability and application of HRQOL findings.

Until randomized trials can be completed and analyzed, information from observational studies needs to be collected consistently to make approximate comparisons of the impacts of the primary treatments for early prostate cancer. The patient is the best judge of his own quality of life and should be the direct source of information reported. Meanwhile, the HRQOL impacts of prostate cancer and its treatments must be assessed using a strong evidence-based approach. Then, methods for communicating this information to individual patients must be assessed. If the overarching purpose of quality-of-life research is to improve quality of life for patients, then the myriad available technologies for making HRQOL data practical and user-friendly need to be explored. With better information on quality of life in addition to clinical outcomes and duration of survival, clinicians will be better able to evaluate new treatment modalities, educate patients, and counsel them individually on what to do when they are diagnosed with prostate cancer.

Acknowledgments

Cited articles were initially reviewed and abstracted by Patrick Chun, B.S., and Bevan Londergan, B.S.A.

REFERENCES

1 Ganz, Goodwin, this volume, chapter 5.

2 Flower, F. J., Jr., Barry, M. J., Lu-Yao, G. *et al.* (1993). Patient-reported complications and follow-up treatment after radical prostatectomy. The National Medicare Experience: 1988–1990 (updated June 1993). *Urology* **42**(6):622–9.

3 Jemal, A., Thomas, A., Murray, T. *et al.* (2002). Cancer statistics, 2002. *Ca: a Cancer Journal for Clinicians* **52**(1):23–47.

4 Moinpour, C. M., Lovato, L. C., Thompson, I. M., Jr. *et al.* (2000). Profile of men randomized to the prostate cancer prevention trial: baseline health-related quality of life, urinary and sexual functioning, and health behaviors. *Journal of Clinical Oncology* **18**(9):1942–53.

5 Thompson, I. M., Klein, E. A., Lippman, S. M. *et al.* (2003). Prevention of prostate cancer with finasteride:

U.S./European perspective. *European Urology* **44**: 650–5.

6 Cormier, L., Valeri, A., Azzouzi, R. *et al.* (2002). Worry and attitude of men in at-risk families for prostate cancer about genetic susceptibility and genetic testing. *Prostate* **51**(4):276–85.

7 Cormier, L., Guillemin, F., Valeri, A. *et al.* (2002). Impact of prostate cancer screening on health-related quality of life in at-risk families. *Urology* **59**(6):901–6.

8 Essink-Bot, M. L., de Koning, H. J., Nijs, H. G. *et al.* (1998). Short-term effects of population-based screening for prostate cancer on health-related quality of life. *Journal of the National Cancer Institute* **90**(12):925–31.

9 Smith, D. S., Carvalhal, G. F., Schneider, K. *et al.* (2000). Quality-of-life outcomes for men with prostate carcinoma detected by screening. *Cancer* **88**(6):1454–63.

10 Potosky, A. L., Miller, B. A., Albertsen, P. C. *et al.* (1995). The role of increasing detection in the rising incidence of prostate cancer. *Journal of the American Medical Association* **273**(7):548–52.

11 Potosky, A. L., Feuer, E. J., Levin, D. L. (2001). Impact of screening on incidence and mortality of prostate cancer in the United States. *Epidemiology Review* **23**(1):181–6.

12 Rietbergen, J. B., Schroder, F. H. (1998). Screening for prostate cancer – more questions than answers [see comments]. *Acta Oncologica* **37**(6):515–32.

13 Perkins, J. J., Sanson-Fisher, R. W., Clarke, S. J. *et al.* (1998). An exploration of screening practices for prostate cancer and the associated community expenditure. *British Journal of Urology* **82**(4):524–9.

14 Litwin, M. S., Pasta, D. J., Stoddard, M. L. *et al.* (1998). Epidemiological trends and financial outcomes in radical prostatectomy among Medicare beneficiaries, 1991 to 1993 [published erratum appears in *Journal of Urology* (1998) **160**(6 Pt 1):2164]. *Journal of Urology* **160**(2): 445–8.

15 Standaert, B., Denis, L. (1997). The European Randomized Study of Screening for Prostate Cancer: an update. *Cancer* **80**(9):1830–4

16 Gohagan, J. K., Prorok, P. C., Hayes, R. B. *et al.* (2000). The Prostate, Lung, Colorectal and Ovarian (PLCO) Cancer Screening Trial of the National Cancer Institute: history, organization, and status. *Controlled Clinical Trials* **21** (6 Suppl):251S–72S.

17 Potosky, A. L., Reeve, B. B., Clegg, L. X. *et al.* (2002). Quality of life following localized prostate cancer treated initially with androgen deprivation therapy or no therapy. *Journal of the National Cancer Institute* **94**(6):430–7.

18 Pound, C. R., Partin, A. W., Eisenberger, M. A. *et al.* (1999). Natural history of progression after PSA elevation following

radical prostatectomy. *Journal of the American Medical Association* **281**(17):1591–7.

19 Smith, M. R., Finkelstein, J. S., McGovern, F. J. *et al.* (2002). Changes in body composition during androgen deprivation therapy for prostate cancer. *Journal of Clinical Endocrinology and Metabolism* **87**(2):599–603.

20 Smith, M. R., McGovern, F. J., Zietman, A. L. *et al.* (2001). Pamidronate to prevent bone loss during androgen-deprivation therapy for prostate cancer. *New England Journal of Medicine* **345**(13):948–55.

21 Harlan, L., Brawley, O., Pommerenke, F. *et al.* (1995). Geographic, age, and racial variation in the treatment of local/regional carcinoma of the prostate. *Journal of Clinical Oncology* **13**(1):93–100.

22 Talcott, J. A. (2002). Androgen deprivation as primary treatment for early prostate cancer: should we "just do something"? *Journal of the National Cancer Institute* **94**(6):407–9.

23 Tannock, I., Gospodarowicz, M., Meakin, W. *et al.* (1989). Treatment of metastatic prostatic cancer with low-dose prednisone: evaluation of pain and quality of life as pragmatic indices of response. *Journal of Clinical Oncology* **7**(5): 590–7.

24 Tannock, I. F., Osoba, D., Stockler, M. R. *et al.* (1996). Chemotherapy with mitoxantrone plus prednisone or prednisone alone for symptomatic hormone-resistant prostate cancer: a Canadian randomized trial with palliative end points. *Journal of Clinical Oncology* **14**(6):1756–64.

25 Small, E. J., Halabi, S., Ratain, M. J. *et al.* (2002). Randomized study of three different doses of suramin administered with a fixed dosing schedule in patients with advanced prostate cancer: results of intergroup 0159, cancer and leukemia group B 9480. *Journal of Clinical Oncology* **20**(16):3369–75.

26 Hussain, M., Fisher, E. I., Petrylak, D. P. *et al.* (2000). Androgen deprivation and four courses of fixed-schedule suramin treatment in patients with newly diagnosed metastatic prostate cancer: A Southwest Oncology Group Study. *Journal of Clinical Oncology* **18**(5):1043–9.

27 Greenlee, R. T., Hill-Harmon, M. B., Murray, T. *et al.* (2001). Cancer statistics, 2001. *Ca: a Cancer Journal for Clinicians* **51**(1):15–36.

28 Lu-Yao, G. L., Greenberg, E. R. (1994). Changes in prostate cancer incidence and treatment in USA. *Lancet* **343**(8892):251–4.

29 Lu-Yao, G. L., McLerran, D., Wasson, J. *et al.* (1993). An assessment of radical prostatectomy. Time trends, geographic variation, and outcomes. The Prostate Patient Outcomes Research Team. *Journal of the American Medical Association* **269**(20):2633–6.

30 Bubolz, T., Wasson, J. H., Lu-Yao, G. *et al.* (2001). Treatments for prostate cancer in older men: 1984–1997. *Urology* **58**(6):977–82.

31 Osoba, D. (1991). *Measuring the Effect of Cancer on Quality of Life.* Boca Raton: CRC Press.

32 Patrick, D. L., Erickson, P. (1993). Assessing health-related quality of life for clinical decision-making. In *Quality of Life Assessment: Key Issues in the 1990's,* ed. S. R. Walker, R. M. Rosser, pp. 11–64. Dordrecht: Kluwer Academic Publishers.

33 World Health Organization (WHO) (1948). *Constitution of the World Health Organization, basic documents.* Geneva: WHO.

34 Fitzpatrick, J. M., Kirby, R. S., Krane, R. J. *et al.* (1998). Sexual dysfunction associated with the management of prostate cancer. *European Urology* **33**(6):513–22.

35 Holmberg, L., Bill-Axelson, A., Helgesen, F. *et al.* (2002). A randomized trial comparing radical prostatectomy with watchful waiting in early prostate cancer. *New England Journal of Medicine* **347**(11):781–9.

36 Steineck, G., Helgesen, F., Adolfsson, J. *et al.* (2002). Quality of life after radical prostatectomy or watchful waiting. *New England Journal of Medicine* **347**(11):790–6.

37 Albertsen, P. C., Aaronson, N. K., Muller, M. J. *et al.* (1997). Health-related quality of life among patients with metastatic prostate cancer. *Urology* **49**(2):207–16.

38 Krahn, M., Ritvo, P., Irvine, J. *et al.* (2000). Construction of the Patient-Oriented Prostate Utility Scale (PORPUS): a multi-attribute health state classification system for prostate cancer. *Journal of Clinical Epidemiology* **53**(9):920–30.

39 Perczek, R. E., Burke, M. A., Carver, C. S. *et al.* (2002). Facing a prostate cancer diagnosis: who is at risk for increased distress? *Cancer* **94**(11):2923–9.

40 Patrick, D. L., Deyo, R. A. (1989). Generic and disease-specific measures in assessing health status and quality of life. *Medical Care* **27**(3 Suppl):S217–32.

41 McHorney, C. A., Ware, J. E., Jr., Raczek, A. E. (1993). The MOS 36-Item Short-Form Health Survey (SF-36): II. Psychometric and clinical tests of validity in measuring physical and mental health constructs. *Medical Care* **31**(3):247–63.

42 McNair, D. M., Lorr, M., Droppleman, L. F. (1981). *Profile of Mood States* (2nd edn.) San Diego: Educational and Industrial Testing Service.

43 Aaronson, N. K., Ahmedzai, S., Bergman, B. *et al.* (1993). The European Organization for Research and Treatment of Cancer QLQ-C30: a quality-of-life instrument for use in international clinical trials in oncology. *Journal of the National Cancer Institute* **85**(5):365–76.

44 Cella, D. F., Tulsky, D. S., Gray, G. *et al.* (1993). The Functional Assessment of Cancer Therapy scale: development

and validation of the general measure. *Journal of Clinical Oncology* **11**(3):570–9.

45 Spitzer, W. O., Dobson, A. J., Hall, J. *et al.* (1981). Measuring the quality of life of cancer patients: a concise QL-index for use by physicians. *Journal of Chronic Diseases* **34**(12):585–97.

46 Schipper, H., Clinch, J., McMurray, A. *et al.* (1984). Measuring the quality of life of cancer patients: the Functional Living Index-Cancer: development and validation. *Journal of Clinical Oncology* **2**(5):472–83.

47 Litwin, M. S., Hays, R. D., Fink, A. *et al.* (1998). The UCLA Prostate Cancer Index: development, reliability, and validity of a health-related quality of life measure. *Medical Care* **36**(7):1002–12.

48 Wei, J. T., Dunn, R. L., Litwin, M. S. *et al.* (2000). Development and validation of the expanded prostate cancer index composite (EPIC) for comprehensive assessment of health-related quality of life in men with prostate cancer. *Urology* **56**(6):899–905.

49 Stockler, M. R., Osoba, D., Corey, P. *et al.* (1999). Convergent discriminative and predictive validity of the Prostate Cancer Specific Quality of Life Instrument (PROSQOLI) assessment and comparison with analogous scales from the EORTC QLQ-C30 and a trial-specific module. European Organisation for Research and Treatment of Cancer. Core Quality of Life Questionnaire. *Journal of Clinical Epidemiology* **52**(7):653–66.

50 Dale, W., Campbell, T., Ignacio, L. *et al.* (1999). Self-assessed health-related quality of life in men being treated for prostate cancer with radiotherapy: instrument validation and its relation to patient-assessed bother of symptoms. *Urology* **53**(2):359–66.

51 Ganz, P. A., Schag, C. A., Lee, J. J. *et al.* (1992). The CARES: a generic measure of health-related quality of life for patients with cancer. *Quality of Life Research* **1**(1):19–29.

52 Akakura, K., Isaka, S., Akimoto, S. *et al.* (1999). Long-term results of a randomized trial for the treatment of Stages B2 and C prostate cancer: radical prostatectomy versus external beam radiation therapy with a common endocrine therapy in both modalities. *Urology* **54**(2):313–18.

53 Fransson, P., Damber, J. E., Tomic, R. *et al.* (2001). Quality of life and symptoms in a randomized trial of radiotherapy versus deferred treatment of localized prostate carcinoma. *Cancer* **92**(12):3111–19.

54 Auvinen, A., Vornanen, T., Tammela, T. L. *et al.* (2001). A randomized trial of the choice of treatment in prostate cancer: design and baseline characteristics. *BJU International* **88**(7):708–15.

55 Rosenberg, H. J., Rosenberg, S. D., Ernstoff, M. S. *et al.* (2002). Expressive disclosure and health outcomes in a prostate cancer population. *International Journal of Psychiatry in Medicine* **32**(1):37–53.

56 Moore, M. J., O'Sullivan, B., Tannock, I. F. (1988). How expert physicians would wish to be treated if they had genitourinary cancer. *Journal of Clinical Oncology* **6**(11):1736–45.

57 Fowler, F. J., Jr., McNaughton Collins, M., Albertsen, P. C. *et al.* (2000). Comparison of recommendations by urologists and radiation oncologists for treatment of clinically localized prostate cancer. *Journal of the American Medical Association* **283**(24):3217–22.

58 McHorney, C. A., Ware, J. E., Jr., Lu, J. F. *et al.* (1994). The MOS 36-item Short-Form Health Survey (SF-36): III. Tests of data quality, scaling assumptions, and reliability across diverse patient groups. *Medical Care* **32**(1):40–66.

59 Zigmond, A. S., Snaith, R. P. (1983). The hospital anxiety and depression scale. *Acta Psychiatrica Scandinavica* **67**(6):361–70.

60 Johansson, J. E., Wersall, P., Brandberg, Y. *et al.* (2001). Efficacy of epoetin beta on hemoglobin, quality of life, and transfusion needs in patients with anemia due to hormone-refractory prostate cancer – a randomized study. *Scandinavian Journal of Neurology and Nephrology* **35**(4): 288–94.

61 Boccardo, F., Rubagotti, A., Barichello, M. *et al.* (1999). Bicalutamide monotherapy versus flutamide plus goserelin in prostate cancer patients: results of an Italian Prostate Cancer Project study. *Journal of Clinical Oncology* **17**(7):2027–38.

62 Fossa, S. D., Slee, P. H., Brausi, M. *et al.* (2001). Flutamide versus prednisone in patients with prostate cancer symptomatically progressing after androgen-ablative therapy: a phase III study of the European Organization for Research and Treatment of Cancer Genitourinary Group. *Journal of Clinical Oncology* **19**(1):62–71.

63 Fossa, S. D., Curran, D., Aaronson, N. K. *et al.* (2000). Quality of life of patients with newly diagnosed poor prognosis M1 prostate cancer undergoing orchiectomy without or with mitomycin C. Results from the EORTC Phase-III trial 30893. *European Urology* **37**(5):541–51.

64 Moinpour, C. M., Savage, M. J., Troxel, A. *et al.* (1998). Quality of life in advanced prostate cancer: results of a randomized therapeutic trial. *Journal of the National Cancer Institute* **90**(20):1537–44.

65 Sharp, L. K., Knight, S. J., Nadler, R. *et al.* (1999). Quality of life in low-income patients with metastatic prostate cancer: divergent and convergent validity of three instruments. *Quality of Life Research* **8**(5):461–70.

66 Jacobsen, S. J., Girman, C. J., Guess, H. A. *et al.* (1993). Natural history of prostatism: factors associated with discordance between frequency and bother of urinary symptoms. *Urology* **42**(6):663–71.

67 Clark, J. A., Talcott, J. A. (2001). Symptom indexes to assess outcomes of treatment for early prostate cancer. *Medical Care* **39**(10):1118–30.

68 Bokhour, B. G., Clark, J. A., Inui, T. S. *et al.* (2001). Sexuality after treatment for early prostate cancer: exploring the meanings of "erectile dysfunction." *Journal of General Internal Medicine* **16**(10):649–55.

69 Clark, J. A., Wray, N., Brody, B. *et al.* (1997). Dimensions of quality of life expressed by men treated for metastatic prostate cancer. *Social Science and Medicine* **45**(8):1299–309.

70 Talcott, J. A., Manola, J., Clark, J. A. *et al.* (2003). Time course and predictors of symptoms after primary prostate cancer therapy. *Journal of Clinical Oncology* **21**:3979–86.

71 Litwin, M. S., Flanders, S. C., Pasta, D. J. *et al.* (1999). Sexual function and bother after radical prostatectomy or radiation for prostate cancer: multivariate quality-of-life analysis from CaPSURE. Cancer of the Prostate Strategic Urologic Research Endeavor. *Urology* **54**(3):503–8.

72 Beard, C. J., Propert, K. J., Rieker, P. P. *et al.* (1997). Complications after treatment with external-beam irradiation in early-stage prostate cancer patients: a prospective multi-institutional outcomes study. *Journal of Clinical Oncology* **15**(1):223–9.

73 Potosky, A. L., Harlan, L. C., Stanford, J. L. *et al.* (1999). Prostate cancer practice patterns and quality of life: the Prostate Cancer Outcomes Study. *Journal of the National Cancer Institute* **91**(20):1719–24.

74 Erickson, this volume, Chapter 3.

75 Ware, J. E., Jr., Sherbourne, C. D. (1992). The MOS 36-item short-form health survey (SF-36). I. Conceptual framework and item selection. *Medical Care* **30**(6):473–83.

76 Ware, J., Jr., Kosinski, M., Keller, S. D. (1996). A 12-Item Short-Form Health Survey: construction of scales and preliminary tests of reliability and validity. *Medical Care* **34**(3):220–33.

77 Cella, D. F., Jacobsen, P. B., Orav, E. J. *et al.* (1987). A brief POMS measure of distress for cancer patients. *Journal of Chronic Diseases* **40**(10):939–42.

78 Penson, D. F., Stoddard, M. L., Pasta, D. J. *et al.* (2001). The association between socioeconomic status, health insurance coverage, and quality of life in men with prostate cancer. *Journal of Clinical Epidemiology* **54**(4):350–8.

79 Eton, D. T., Lepore, S. J., Helgeson, V. S. (2001). Early quality of life in patients with localized prostate carcinoma: an examination of treatment-related, demographic, and psychosocial factors. *Cancer* **92**(6):1451–9.

80 Bacon, C. G., Giovannucci, E., Testa, M. *et al.* (2002). The association of treatment-related symptoms with quality-of-life outcomes for localized prostate carcinoma patients. *Cancer* **94**(3):862–71.

81 Litwin, M. S., Lubeck, D. P., Stoddard, M. L. *et al.* (2001). Quality of life before death for men with prostate cancer: results from the CaPSURE database. *Journal of Urology* **165**(3):871–5.

82 Schapira, M. M., Lawrence, W. F., Katz, D. A. *et al.* (2001). Effect of treatment on quality of life among men with clinically localized prostate cancer. *Medical Care* **39**(3):243–53.

83 Davis, J. W., Kuban, D. A., Lynch, D. F. *et al.* (2001). Quality of life after treatment for localized prostate cancer: differences based on treatment modality. *Journal of Urology* **166**(3):947–52.

84 Schlenk, E. A., Erlen, J. A., Dunbar-Jacob, J. *et al.* (1998). Health-related quality of life in chronic disorders: a comparison across studies using the MOS SF-36. *Quality of Life Research* **7**(1):57–65.

85 Clark, J. A., Rieker, P., Propert, K. J. *et al.* (1999). Changes in quality of life following treatment for early prostate cancer. *Urology* **53**(1):161–8.

86 Potosky, A. L., Legler, J., Albertsen, P. C. *et al.* (2000). Health outcomes after prostatectomy or radiotherapy for prostate cancer: results from the Prostate Cancer Outcomes Study. *Journal of the National Cancer Institute* **92**(19):1582–92.

87 Lubeck, D. P., Litwin, M. S., Henning, J. M. *et al.* (1997). Measurement of health-related quality of life in men with prostate cancer: the CaPSURE database. *Quality of Life Research* **6**(5):385–92.

88 Litwin, M. S., Hays, R. D., Fink, A. *et al.* (1995). Quality-of-life outcomes in men treated for localized prostate cancer. *Journal of the American Medical Association* **273**(2):129–35.

89 Litwin, M. S., Lubeck, D. P., Henning, J. M. *et al.* (1998). Differences in urologist and patient assessments of health related quality of life in men with prostate cancer: results of the CaPSURE database. *Journal of Urology* **159**(6):1988–92.

90 Lubeck, D. P., Litwin, M. S., Henning, J. M. *et al.* (1999). Changes in health-related quality of life in the first year after treatment for prostate cancer: results from CaPSURE. *Urology* **53**(1):180–6.

91 Janda, M., Gerstner, N., Obermair, A. *et al.* (2000). Quality of life changes during conformal radiation therapy for prostate carcinoma. *Cancer* **89**(6):1322–8.

92 Kim, S. P., Bennett, C. L., Chan, C. *et al.* (1999). QOL and outcomes research in prostate cancer patients with low socioeconomic status. *Oncology (Huntington)* **13**(6):823–38.

93 Kurtz, M. E., Kurtz, J. C., Stommel, M. *et al.* (1997). Loss of physical functioning among geriatric cancer patients:

relationships to cancer site, treatment, comorbidity and age. *European Journal of Cancer* **33**(14):2352–8.

94 Litwin, M. S., Shpall, A. I., Dorey, F. *et al.* (1998). Quality-of-life outcomes in long-term survivors of advanced prostate cancer. *American Journal of Clinical Oncology* **21**(4):327–32.

95 Stier, D. M., Greenfield, S., Lubeck, D. P. *et al.* (1999). Quantifying comorbidity in a disease-specific cohort: adaptation of the total illness burden index to prostate cancer. *Urology* **54**(3):424–9.

96 Melmed, G. Y., Kwan, L., Reid, K. *et al.* (2002). Quality of life at the end of life: trends in patients with metastatic prostate cancer. *Urology* **59**(1):103–9.

97 Wei, J. T., Dunn, R. L., Sandler, H. M. *et al.* (2002). Comprehensive comparison of health-related quality of life after contemporary therapies for localized prostate cancer. *Journal of Clinical Oncology* **20**(2):557–66.

98 Lim, A. J., Brandon, A. H., Fiedler, J. *et al.* (1995). Quality of life: radical prostatectomy versus radiation therapy for prostate cancer. *Journal of Urology* **154**(4):1420–5.

99 Braslis, K. G., Santa-Cruz, C., Brickman, A. L. (1995). Quality of life 12 months after radical prostatectomy. *British Journal of Urology* **75**(1):48–53.

100 Bisson, J. I., Chubb, H. L., Bennett, S. *et al.* (2002). The prevalence and predictors of psychological distress in patients with early localized prostate cancer. *British Journal of Urology International* **90**(1):56–61.

101 Stone, P., Hardy, J., Huddart, R. *et al.* (2000). Fatigue in patients with prostate cancer receiving hormone therapy. *European Journal of Cancer* **36**(9):1134–41.

102 Kemmler, G., Holzner, B., Kopp, M. *et al.* (1999). Comparison of two quality-of-life instruments for cancer patients: The Functional Assessment of Cancer Therapy-General and the European Organization for Research and Treatment of Cancer Quality of Life Questionnaire-C30. *Journal of Clinical Oncology* **17**(9):2932–40.

103 Fossa, S. D., Woehre, H., Kurth, K. H. *et al.* (1997). Influence of urological morbidity on quality of life in patients with prostate cancer. *European Urology* **31**(Suppl. 3):3–8.

104 Krupski, T., Petroni, G. R., Bissonette, E. A. *et al.* (2000). Quality-of-life comparison of radical prostatectomy and interstitial brachytherapy in the treatment of clinically localized prostate cancer. *Urology* **55**(5):736–42.

105 Lilleby, W., Fossa, S. D., Waehre, H. R. (1999). Long-term morbidity and quality of life in patients with localized prostate cancer undergoing definitive radiotherapy or radical prostatectomy. *International Journal of Radiation Oncology, Biology, and Physics* **43**(4):735–43.

106 Ben-Tovim, D., Dougherty, M. L., Stapleton, A. M. *et al.* (2002). Coping with prostate cancer: a quantitative analysis using a new instrument, the centre for clinical excellence in urological research coping with cancer instrument. *Urology* **59**(3):383–8.

107 Rosendahl, I., Kiebert, G. M., Curran, D. *et al.* (1999). Quality-adjusted survival (Q-TWiST) analysis of EORTC trial 30853: comparing goserelin acetate and flutamide with bilateral orchiectomy in patients with metastatic prostate cancer. European Organization for Research and Treatment of Cancer. *Prostate* **38**(2):100–9.

108 Wang, H., Huang, E., Dale, W. *et al.* (2000). Self-assessed health-related quality of life in men who have completed radiotherapy for prostate cancer: instrument validation and its relation to patient-assessed bother of symptoms. *International Journal of Cancer* **90**(3):163–72.

109 Borghede, G., Sullivan, M. (1996). Measurement of quality of life in localized prostatic cancer patients treated with radiotherapy. Development of a prostate cancer-specific module supplementing the EORTC QLQ-C30. *Quality of Life Research* **5**(2):212–22.

110 Knight, S. J., Chmiel, J. S., Kuzel, T. *et al.* (1998). Quality of life in metastatic prostate cancer among men of lower socioeconomic status: feasibility and criterion related validity of 3 measures. *Journal of Urology* **160**(5):1765–9.

111 Wilson, K. A., Dowling, A. J., Abdolell, M. *et al.* (2000). Perception of quality of life by patients, partners and treating physicians. *Quality of Life Research* **9**(9):1041–52.

112 Curran, D., Fossa, S., Aaronson, N. *et al.* (1997). Baseline quality of life of patients with advanced prostate cancer. European Organization for Research and Treatment of Cancer (EORTC), Genito-Urinary Tract Cancer Cooperative Group (GUT-CCG). *European Journal of Cancer* **33**(11):1809–14.

113 Joly, F., Brune, D., Couette, J. E. *et al.* (1998). Health-related quality of life and sequelae in patients treated with brachytherapy and external beam irradiation for localized prostate cancer. *Annals of Oncology* **9**(7):751–7.

114 Moore, M. J., Osoba, D., Murphy, K. *et al.* (1994). Use of palliative end points to evaluate the effects of mitoxantrone and low-dose prednisone in patients with hormonally resistant prostate cancer. *Journal of Clinical Oncology* **12**(4):689–94.

115 Fossa, S. D. (1994). Quality of life after palliative radiotherapy in patients with hormone-resistant prostate cancer: single institution experience. *British Journal of Urology* **74**(3):345–51.

116 Borghede, G., Karlsson, J., Sullivan, M. (1997). Quality of life in patients with prostatic cancer: results from a Swedish population study. *Journal of Urology* **158**(4):1477–85.

117 Dawson, N. A., Conaway, M., Halabi, S. *et al.* (2000). A randomized study comparing standard versus moderately high dose megestrol acetate for patients with advanced prostate carcinoma: cancer and leukemia group B study 9181. *Cancer* **88**(4):825–34.

118 Herr, H. W., O'Sullivan, M. (2000). Quality of life of asymptomatic men with nonmetastatic prostate cancer on androgen deprivation therapy. *Journal of Urology* **163**(6):1743–6.

119 Shrader-Bogen, C. L., Kjellberg, J. L., McPherson, C. P. *et al.* (1997). Quality of life and treatment outcomes: prostate carcinoma patients' perspectives after prostatectomy or radiation therapy. *Cancer* **79**(10):1977–86.

120 Heathcote, P. S., Mactaggart, P. N., Boston, R. J. *et al.* (1998). Health-related quality of life in Australian men remaining disease-free after radical prostatectomy. *Medical Journal of Australia* **168**(10):483–6.

121 Tefilli, M. V., Gheiler, E. L., Tiguert, R. *et al.* (1998). Quality of life in patients undergoing salvage procedures for locally recurrent prostate cancer. *Journal of Surgical Oncology* **69**(3):156–61.

122 Esper, P., Mo, F., Chodak, G. *et al.* (1997). Measuring quality of life in men with prostate cancer using the functional assessment of cancer therapy-prostate instrument. *Urology* **50**(6):920–8.

123 Lee, W. R., Hall, M. C., McQuellon, R. P. *et al.* (2001). A prospective quality-of-life study in men with clinically localized prostate carcinoma treated with radical prostatectomy, external beam radiotherapy, or interstitial brachytherapy. *International Journal of Radiation Oncology, Biology, and Physics* **51**(3):614–23.

124 Lee, W. R., McQuellon, R. P., Case, L. D. *et al.* (1999). Early quality of life assessment in men treated with permanent source interstitial brachytherapy for clinically localized prostate cancer. *Journal of Urology* **162**(2): 403–6.

125 Robinson, J. W., Saliken, J. C., Donnelly, B. J. *et al.* (1999). Quality-of-life outcomes for men treated with cryosurgery for localized prostate carcinoma. *Cancer* **86**(9):1793–801.

126 Monga, U., Kerrigan, A. J., Thornby, J. *et al.* (1999). Prospective study of fatigue in localized prostate cancer patients undergoing radiotherapy. *Radiation Oncology Investigations* **7**(3):178–85.

127 de Haes, J. C., van Knippenberg, F. C., Neijt, J. P. (1990). Measuring psychological and physical distress in cancer patients: structure and application of the Rotterdam Symptom Checklist. *British Journal of Cancer* **62**(6): 1034–8.

128 Gralnek, D., Wessells, H., Cui, H. *et al.* (2000). Differences in sexual function and quality of life after nerve sparing and nonnerve sparing radical retropubic prostatectomy. *Journal of Urology* **163**(4):1166–70.

129 Krongrad, A., Litwin, M. S., Lai, H. *et al.* (1998). Dimensions of quality of life in prostate cancer. *Journal of Urology* **160**(3 Pt 1):807–10.

130 Johnstone, P. A., Gray, C., Powell, C. R. (2000). Quality of life in T1-3N0 prostate cancer patients treated with radiation therapy with minimum 10-year follow-up. *International Journal of Radiation Oncology, Biology, and Physics* **46**(4):833–8.

131 Krongrad, A., Perczek, R. E., Burke, M. A. *et al.* (1997). Reliability of Spanish translations of select urological quality of life instruments. *Journal of Urology* **158**(2):493–6.

132 Barry, M. J., Fowler, F. J., Jr., O'Leary, M. P. *et al.* (1992). The American Urological Association symptom index for benign prostatic hyperplasia. The Measurement Committee of the American Urological Association. *Journal of Urology* **148**(5):1549–64.

133 Clark, J. A., Wray, N. P., Ashton, C. M. (2001). Living with treatment decisions: regrets and quality of life among men treated for metastatic prostate cancer. *Journal of Clinical Oncology* **19**(1):72–80.

134 Giesler, R. B., Miles, B. J., Cowen, M. E. *et al.* (2000). Assessing quality of life in men with clinically localized prostate cancer: development of a new instrument for use in multiple settings. *Quality of Life Research* **9**(6):645–65.

135 Clark, J. A., Bokhour, B. G., Inui, T. S. *et al.* (2003). Measuring patients' perceptions of the outcomes of treatment for early prostate cancer. *Medical Care* **41**: 923–36.

136 Gray, A., Feldman, H. A., McKinlay, J. B. *et al.* (1991). Age, disease, and changing sex hormone levels in middle-aged men: results of the Massachusetts Male Aging Study. *Journal of Clinical Endocrinology and Metabolism* **73**(5): 1016–25.

137 Feldman, H. A., Goldstein, I., Hatzichristou, D. G. *et al.* (1994). Impotence and its medical and psychosocial correlates: results of the Massachusetts Male Aging Study. *Journal of Urology* **151**(1):54–61.

138 O'Leary, M. P., Fowler, F. J., Lenderking, W. R. *et al.* (1995). A brief male sexual function inventory for urology [see comments]. *Urology* **46**(5):697–706.

139 Rosen, R. C., Riley, A., Wagner, G. *et al.* The international index of erectile function (IIEF): a multidimensional scale for assessment of erectile dysfunction. *Urology* **49**(6):822–30.

140 Small, E. J., Meyer, M., Marshall, M. E. *et al.* (2000). Suramin therapy for patients with symptomatic hormone-refractory prostate cancer: results of a randomized phase III trial comparing suramin plus hydrocortisone to placebo

plus hydrocortisone. *Journal of Clinical Oncology* **18**(7): 1440–50.

141 Seo, P. H., D'Amico, A. V., Clark, J. A. *et al.* (2004). Assessing a prostate cancer brachy therapy technique using early patient-reported symptoms: a potential early indicator for technology assessment? *Clinical Prostate Cancer* **3**:38–42.

142 Wilt, T. J., Brawer, M. K. (1994). The Prostate Cancer Intervention Versus Observation Trial: a randomized trial comparing radical prostatectomy versus expectant management for the treatment of clinically localized prostate cancer. *Journal of Urology* **152** (5 Pt 2):1910–14.

143 Fowler, F. J., Jr., Barry, M. J., Lu-Yao, G. *et al.* (1996). Outcomes of external-beam radiation therapy for prostate cancer: a study of Medicare beneficiaries in three surveillance, epidemiology, and end results areas. *Journal of Clinical Oncology* **14**(8):2258–65.

144 Talcott, J. A., Rieker, P., Clark, J. A. *et al.* (1998). Patient-reported symptoms after primary therapy for early prostate cancer: results of a prospective cohort study. *Journal of Clinical Urology* **16**(1):275–83.

145 Hamilton, A. S., Stanford, J. L., Gilliland, F. D. *et al.* (2001). Health outcomes after external-beam radiation therapy for clinically localized prostate cancer: results from the Prostate Cancer Outcomes Study. *Journal of Clinical Oncology* **19**(9):2517–26.

146 Walsh, P. C., Marschke, P., Ricker, D. *et al.* Patient-reported urinary continence and sexual function after anatomic radical prostatectomy. *Urology* **55**(1):58– 61.

147 Litwin, M. S., Melmed, G. Y., Nakazon, T. (2001). Life after radical prostatectomy: a longitudinal study. *Journal of Urology* **166**(2):587–92.

148 Hanlon, A. L., Watkins Bruner, D., Peter, R. *et al.* (2002). Quality of life study in prostate cancer patients treated with three-dimensional conformal radiation therapy: comparing late bowel and bladder quality of life symptoms to that of the normal population. *International Journal of Radiation Oncology, Biology, and Physics* **49**(1):51–9.

149 Pietrow, P. K., Parekh, D. J., Smith, J. A., Jr. *et al.* (2001). Health related quality of life assessment after radical prostatectomy in men with prostate specific antigen only recurrence. *Journal of Urology* **166**(6):2286–90.

150 Hagedoorn, M., Sneeuw, K. C., Aaronson, N. K. (2002). Changes in physical functioning and quality of life in patients with cancer: response shift and relative evaluation of one's condition. *Journal of Clinical Epidemiology* **55**(2):176–83.

151 Sloan, J. A., Cella, D., Frost, M. *et al.* (2002). Assessing clinical significance in measuring oncology patient quality of life: introduction to the symposium, content overview, and definition of terms. *Mayo Clinic Proceedings* **77**(4):367–70.

152 Guyatt, G. H., Osoba, D., Wu, A. W. *et al.* (2002). Methods to explain the clinical significance of health status measures. *Mayo Clinic Proceedings* **77**(4):371–83.

153 Cella, D., Bullinger, M., Scott, C. *et al.* Group vs individual approaches to understanding the clinical significance of differences or changes in quality of life. *Mayo Clinic Proceedings* **77**(4):384–92.

7

The science of quality-of-life measurement in lung cancer

Craig C. Earle, M.D., M.Sc. and Jane C. Weeks, M.D., M.Sc.

Dana-Farber Cancer Institute, Boston, MA

Introduction

Lung cancer is the leading cause of cancer death in the US.[1] Non-small-cell lung cancer (NSCLC) (squamous, adenocarcinoma, and large cell carcinoma) is responsible for about 75% of these cases, while small cell lung cancer (SCLC) accounts for the other 25%. Most patients present with incurable disease at the time of diagnosis and, because of early hematogenous spread, even those presenting with "early" stage disease will usually eventually develop incurable metastases.[2] The five-year survival rate for all lung cancer patients is only 15% and has not improved significantly over the last 30 years.[3]

Surgery is the only treatment modality that can consistently cure a small number of patients with early NSCLC, although radiation can be curative in some limited circumstances. Chemotherapy may contribute in an adjuvant or neoadjuvant role, but it is mostly used as a palliative therapy for advanced disease. SCLC, on the other hand, is more chemosensitive and can be cured in a minority of patients with chemotherapy and radiation. Nevertheless, most patients relapse and die within one year of diagnosis.[2]

Treatments for all stages and histologies of lung cancer are difficult, expensive, and come with nontrivial toxicity. Because the prognosis is almost uniformly poor despite intervention, many of these therapies are controversial. At presentation, over 80% of lung cancer patients report disease-related symptoms, most commonly cough and dyspnea, as well as systemic effects like fatigue and anorexia and high degrees of psychological distress.[4] Consequently, in addition to survival and response outcomes, information about treatment effects on health-related quality of life (HRQOL) is crucial for rational clinical decision making.

Methods

A computerized literature search was done centrally at the National Library of Medicine. It was designed to look for Medical Subject Headings (MeSH) relevant to HRQOL research in lung cancer, published between January 1990 and December 2001, restricted to English-language articles, and with on-line abstracts. Personal reprints and reference lists were also reviewed. All abstracts were examined and relevant articles were retrieved. Papers were subsequently excluded if they were found to be reviews, editorials, or opinion pieces. Studies that claimed to measure HRQOL but did so without an instrument (i.e., relying on the general impressions of the physicians), or that measured only performance status, were excluded. Predetermined data elements were abstracted and entered immediately into an electronic database. These elements included the intervention studied; measurement instruments used; study design and perspective; years of data collection; sample size; stages and histology of lung cancer in the study population; percent female subjects; percent non-white subjects; average age of the patients; biomedical outcomes; the phase of care being addressed by the study; whether the sample size was based on an a priori power calculation; whether confidence limits were presented around measured estimates; and a short description of the study findings. Some of these data items required subjective interpretation, which were taken as much as possible from the authors' peer-reviewed conclusions about the results. Database manipulation and descriptive analyses were carried out using the Statistical Analysis Software (SAS), version 8.01 for Windows (SAS Institute Inc., Cary NC, 1999).

The literature search yielded 419 articles, of which 117 were deemed appropriate for retrieval and review on the basis of the abstract. Of these, 9 were excluded: 5 were reviews[5–9] and 4 did not have any true outcomes component.[10–13] Thus, there were 108 studies dealing primarily with HRQOL measurement in lung cancer.

Results

Literature search

There has been an accelerating rise in the number of HRQOL studies published each year over the course of the decade. Fully one-quarter of the studies (27 studies) were primarily methodological in nature. Most studies focused on NSCLC (58 studies, 54%), although a significant number examined both histologies (33 studies, 31%). Seventeen studies (16%) looked at SCLC. Almost half of the studies (52 studies, 48%) examined patients with all stages of disease, and another 44 papers (41%) were restricted to the study of advanced, incurable cancer, leaving just 9% (10 studies) dealing with potentially curable disease. One study assessed HRQOL in lung cancer survivors.

A prospective cohort design was most common, being used in 52 (48%) of publications, followed by HRQOL companions alongside randomized controlled trials (RCTs) (29 studies, 27%). Seventeen studies (16%) were carried out prospectively alongside phase I or II trials. Eight papers (7%) were cross-sectional, and there was one paper using both retrospective cohort and case-control designs.

Most studies came from the United States (32 studies, 30%), followed by the United Kingdom (19 studies, 18%), Italy (8 studies, 7%), and Canada (7 studies, 6%). Six studies were carried out in more than one country. The average sample size was 202 patients, ranging from 11 to 2300, the latter being a methodological study looking at accrual rates in randomized trials.[14] The mean age of patients in lung cancer HRQOL studies was 62 years, and 30% of patients were women. There were three studies, all from the same author, that examined HRQOL issues in cohorts made up exclusively of women.[15–17] Only 17 articles (16%) commented on the racial makeup of their study population; all were US-based. Of those publications that did report a racial distribution, an average of 15% of patients were non-white (range 1–38%). Levels of comorbidity were generally not recorded. One study examined HRQOL based on physician assessment.[18] Fifty-seven percent presented HRQOL estimates with some indication of variability (confidence intervals, standard deviation, etc.).

Instruments/measures

Over half of the studies used more than one HRQOL instrument. Forty-one percent used 2, and 13% used 3 or more, for an average of 1.7 instruments per study. When two or more scales were used in the same study, it was usually as complementary instruments in a clinical trial. Although generally not paired for methodological reasons, the different instruments tended to show convergent results. The European Organization for Research and Treatment of Cancer Quality of Life Questionnaire (EORTC QLQ-C30), used either alone or with its lung cancer subscale, the LC13, clearly dominates the literature, being used in 39 (36%) studies (Table 7.1), especially in more recent studies. The next most commonly used scales were the Rotterdam Symptom Checklist (RSCL) and the Hospital Anxiety and Depression Scale (HADS), which were often used together in British Medical Research Council (MRC) studies in the early 1990s along with the MRC daily diary card. These instruments are not lung cancer-specific, however. The EORTC QLQ-C30 is emerging as the most commonly used HRQOL instrument in lung cancer, in part

Table 7.1. The most frequently used instruments for quality of life assessment in lung cancer (n = 108 studies)

Measure	No.	(%)
EORTC QLQ-C30	39	(36)
EORTC QLQ-LC13	19	(18)
Rotterdam Symptom Checklist (RSCL)	13	(12)
Hospital Anxiety and Depression Scale (HADS)	12	(11)
Lung Cancer Symptom Scale (LCSS)	9	(8)
Linear Analogue Self-Assessment (LASA)	8	(8)
MRC Daily Diary Card	7	(6)
Functional Living Index – Cancer (FLIC)	6	(6)
FACT-G and –L	5	(5)
Spitzer Index	4	(4)

EORTC-LC13: European Organization for Research and Treatment of Cancer Lung Cancer 13 item module; EORTC QLQ-C30: EORTC Quality of Life Questionnaire 30 item core instrument; FACT-G: Functional Assessment of Cancer Therapy – General instrument; FACT-L: FACT lung cancer module.

because of the MRC's decision to switch from the RSCL and HADS to the EORTC scale as a required component of all of its sponsored trials. United States studies tended to use the domestically developed Lung Cancer Symptom Scale (LCSS) or Functional Assessment of Cancer Therapy with its lung cancer subscale (FACT-L). In 6 studies, the investigators developed unique, unvalidated instruments to measure HRQOL. The generic and general cancer instruments are described in more detail in the chapter by Erickson in this volume.[19]

The three lung cancer-specific instruments in common use, the EORTC-LC13, the FACT-L, and the LCSS, are all meant to be self-administered, although the LCSS has an optional observer component. It is also recommended that the LCSS initially be given as a face-to-face interview to familiarize patients with the visual analogue scale (VAS). However, in different studies, these measures have been administered in a variety of ways,[14] including being sent to physicians to fill out,[20] administered by computer,[21] or being only partially administered[22–26] or scored.[27,28] Partial administration was sometimes done to focus on global HRQOL questions (such as questions 29 and 30 of the EORTC QLQ-C30). All three of these instruments have undergone fairly extensive field testing, and they appear to have acceptable psychometric properties.[6,29,30] They have never been empirically compared head-to-head in one study, however.

EORTC QLQ-LC13

The EORTC QLQ-C30 consists of 30 questions in Likert and numerical analogue scale (NAS) formats,[31] covering the week leading up to its administration (Table 7.2). Prior versions also had yes/no questions, but these have been removed in the most recent edition. The LC13 adds 13 questions.[32–34] The core instrument combined with the lung cancer subscale is estimated to take about 11 minutes to complete.[35] At the time of this writing, it has been translated into 23 major languages.

Because the lung cancer module, the LC13, was the first disease-specific module of the EORTC system, much of the early psychometric validation was carried out in lung cancer patients.[36–40] However, there has been only one publication dealing specifically with the reliability and validity of the lung cancer subscale.[32] This study reported on an international effort that began with 883 lung cancer patients of all stages and histologies who completed the questionnaire before starting chemotherapy and/or radiation. A total of 735 patients completed at least one follow-up questionnaire during treatment. Internal consistency was evaluated by comparing items hypothesized to track together as a scale. The dyspnea scale, in particular, was found to be very reliable with a Cronbach's alpha coefficient greater than 0.80 in several analyses. A reliable pain scale could not be identified, however. The LC13 was found to be adequately responsive to change, able to detect modulations in the expected direction as patients' symptoms and performance status improved or as they experienced treatment-related toxicity. Interrater reliability has not been assessed.

The content validity of the EORTC-LC13 was established solely by a "project group,"[32] consisting of health care professionals and research methodologists from the many countries represented in the

Table 7.2. Lung cancer-specific measures of HRQOL

	EORTC QLQ-LC13	FACT- L	LCSS
Purpose for Which Developed	Site-specific module of a generic cancer instrument, measuring HRQOL in the past week for clinical studies.	Site-specific module of a generic instrument for patients with chronic illness, measuring HRQOL in the past week for clinical studies.	Site-specific instrument only, measuring HRQOL in the past 24 hours for clinical studies.
Length	17 items	7 items (Likert, NAS)	9 items + 6 optional observer items (VAS)
Administration Time	11–12 minutes (including EORTC QLQ-C30)	10 minutes (including FACT-G)	5–8 minutes; 3–5 minutes after demonstration. Observer scale: 2 minutes
Domains Included	Symptoms (anorexia, fatigue, cough, dyspnea, pain, and hemoptysis) and toxicities (hair loss, dysphagia, stomatitis, neuropathy, nausea, vomiting, constipation, diarrhea, and insomnia)	Symptoms (anorexia, fatigue, cough, dyspnea, and pain) and some toxicities (weight loss, dysphagia, cognition)	Symptoms only (anorexia, fatigue, cough, dyspnea, pain, and hemoptysis)
Scoring	Likert and NAS items. Scales are scored as the mean of the item scores which can be re-scaled to 0–100. Total scores are not recommended.	Subscale scores added to obtain a total score. Alternative "Trial Outcome Index" (TOI) is the sum of the Physical and Functional subscales of the generic instrument and the Lung Cancer Subscale.	Aggregate score is the sum of all items.
Validated Modes of Administration	Designed for patient self-administration	Designed for patient self-administration, but has been used in interview format	Face-to-face interview initially for demonstration of VAS with a simple example question related to the weather, then self-administered. Telephone interview acceptable once patient is familiar with the VAS
Validated Translations/Cultural Adaptations	Arabic, Chinese, Taiwanese, Czech, Danish, Dutch, English, Finnish, French, German, Greek, Hebrew, Hungarian, Italian, Japanese, Norwegian, Polish, Portuguese, Russian, Slovakian, Spanish, Swedish, Turkish	Chinese-Simplified, Chinese-Traditional, Czech, Danish, Dutch, English, Finnish, French, German, Greek, Hungarian, Italian, Japanese, Norwegian, Polish, Portuguese, Russian, Spanish, Swedish, Thai	Afrikaans, Chinese, Dutch, English, Estonian, Finnish, French, German, Lithuanian, Malay, Portuguese, Spanish
Evidence of Reliability (internal consistency, test-retest, other)	Internal consistency alphas 0.53–0.83.[32] Multi-item dyspnea scale had good reliability (alpha > 0.80).[32] Pain scale reliability was poor, however (alpha 0.53–0.54)[32]	Internal consistency alpha 0.68.[43] TOI even more reliable (alpha 0.89)[43]	Internal consistency alpha 0.82.[48] Test-retest with 1-hour interval prior to treatment for 52 patients (Pearson r > 0.75 for all items).[46] Repeated interrater agreement 95% to 100% for 21 raters at 8 centers[46]

Table 7.2. (*cont.*)

	EORTC QLQ-LC13	FACT- L	LCSS
Evidence of Validity (content, construct, criterion-related)	Construct validity: able to discriminate patients by disease stage and performance status (N = 883).[32] Correlations (0.19–0.73) with WHO toxicity scales (N = 883)[32]	Content validity: items rated by 30 lung cancer patients.[43] Construct validity: correlation coefficient of 0.60 with the Functional Living Index – Cancer (FLIC), as well as the General FACT instrument	Content validity: 96% agreement among 24 physicians, 28 nurses, and 121 patients on items.[46] Construct validity: able to discriminate groups with different performance status, good convergence (r = 0.77) with the Brief Symptom Inventory (n = 207).[47] Criterion validity: correlations of 0.47–0.67 with a variety of HRQOL instruments (n = 207)[48]
Evidence of Responsiveness/ Sensitivity to Change	Symptoms decreased and toxicity scores increased during treatment (n = 883)[32]	Sensitivity to change in performance status over 2 months in 41 patients (P = .03)[43]	Able to detect improvement in symptoms following intervention in 144 patients[47]
Interpretability (availability of normative data, clinically meaningful difference)	Normative data available on 883 patients;[32] clinically meaningful difference not explicitly defined	Normative data available on 116 patients;[43] a 2 point change is considered to be a clinically meaningful difference	Normative data available on 673 patients;[49] clinically meaningful difference not explicitly defined

EORTC-LC13: European Organization for Research and Treatment of Cancer Lung Cancer 13 item module; FACT-L: Functional Assessment of Cancer Therapy – lung cancer module; LCSS: Lung Cancer Symptom Scale; NAS: Numeric Analogue Scale; VAS: Visual Analogue Scale

EORTC.[29] Construct validity was demonstrated by using the instrument to distinguish between subgroups of patients expected to be in different HRQOL states, such as those of different performance status, toxicity ratings (measured with WHO toxicity grading), or undergoing different modalities of treatment. It was also able to discriminate between stages of disease, but not as well as it could distinguish performance status. The investigators found that the LC13 added important information not captured by the QLQ-C30. Dyspnea, hemoptysis, dysphagia, and pain in the thoracic region explained significant amounts of the variance in global HRQOL, as measured by the core instrument. Toxicity items such as peripheral neuropathy from chemotherapy and dysphagia, which may occur either as an effect of radiotherapy or from the underlying disease, also contributed significantly to the variance in HRQOL. This paper provided normative data (scores of typical lung cancer patients) for the instrument as well.

Criterion-related validity, based on a comparison of the instrument to other validated HRQOL "gold standards" external to the scale, has not been formally assessed for the LC13.

FACT-L

The FACT-G[41] consists of 34 questions, 28 of which are scored, while the FACT-L[42] currently adds 7 questions (Table 7.2). The FACT-L previously had 9 questions, but items about hair loss and regret for smoking were removed in 1995, a change that increased the internal consistency of the scale. It also uses Likert and NAS formats to ask questions about HRQOL in the week leading up to its administration. It has been assessed at a Grade 6–7 reading level and has been translated into at least 20 major languages. Like the EORTC instrument, at 10 minutes, it can sometimes be fairly burdensome in this very ill population. As a result, some investigators have combined the Physical and Functional scales with the lung cancer module to form a shorter 21-item "Trial Outcome Index."[43,44]

The lung cancer module of the FACT has also only been evaluated in one methodological publication.[43] In this study, 116 patients with all stages and histologies of lung cancer were given both the FACT-G and FACT-L. A subset of 41 patients was tested again at 2 months to evaluate sensitivity to change. The scale was found to be internally consistent, especially after dropping the items of hair loss and regret for smoking, and was sensitive to changes in performance status. This paper also provides normative data for the FACT-L scale.

The FACT boasts well-documented content validity. It was developed using patient input as well as that of medical professionals for item generation and review. As a result, it emphasizes social and emotional well-being, making it, its developers argue, more multidimensional in scope than other instruments. Construct and criterion-related validity were assessed by the simultaneous administration of the Brief Profile of Mood States with a patient-completed performance status questionnaire, and the Functional Living Index – Cancer (FLIC) scale, respectively. All instruments were highly statistically significantly correlated (p < .001). Furthermore, the information provided by the FACT-L appears to be complementary to that provided by the FACT-G, not redundant. In the studies we examined, the FACT-G and FACT-L were always used together. Moreover, in the only instance in which a lung cancer-specific HRQOL instrument has been used in a clinical study (outside of validation exercises) in conjunction with another instrument, the FACT-L showed convergent results with the UNISCALE in a Phase II chemotherapy trial.[45]

LCSS

The LCSS is a lung cancer-specific instrument only, with no general cancer component.[46–50] It focuses exclusively on the symptoms of lung cancer and does not attempt to assess the toxicity of treatment (Table 7.2). Its advantage is its simplicity. It is rated at a Grade 2 level of comprehension, consists only of 9 visual analogue scales (VAS) and 6 optional items for an observer to fill out, and asks about HRQOL in the previous 24 hours.[51] It takes 5–8 minutes to complete initially for demonstration of the VAS, but only 3–5 minutes for subsequent administrations. The observer scale for health professionals takes 2 minutes to complete. The LCSS has been translated into at least 39 languages and sub-languages at the time of this writing.[51]

Of the three lung cancer-specific HRQOL instruments, the LCSS has the most published literature documenting its psychometric properties. Its internal consistency is good, with a Cronbach's alpha coefficient of 0.82 measured among 207 NSCLC patients. Interrater reliability was very high, with mean kappa statistics of well over 90%.[46] Test-retest reliability examined over a 1-hour interval prior to receiving therapy was also high (r > 0.75, p < .01 for all items). It has been found to be sensitive to change on repeat administration in a clinical trial[47,52] and sensitive to changes along the full health-illness continuum.[48]

The LCSS is based on a conceptual model in which the physical and functional dimensions are the main determinants of a patient's HRQOL. Indeed, of the three lung cancer-specific HRQOL instruments, the LCSS is the only one to have its construct validity empirically tested using a model. As expected, these two dimensions explain nearly half of the variability in overall HRQOL.[47] Content validity has also been confirmed by a mean of 96% agreement with the content of the items in a survey of 52 oncology nurses and physicians and 121 patients (including both NSCLC and SCLC patients).[46] Construct validity has also been successfully supported by correlating the LCSS with performance status and by showing convergence between the patient and observer components.[46] Finally, criterion-related validity was supported by high correlation coefficients between the individual items of the LCSS and the following gold standard measures: the American Thoracic Society (ATS) and McGill Pain questionnaires, Profile of Mood States (POMS), and the Sickness Impact Profile (SIP), thus showing the LCSS to be a valid instrument for measuring HRQOL.[48] Normative data for the LCSS were reported for 673 clinic patients and 63 inpatients with NSCLC.[49]

Findings of lung cancer HRQOL studies

In observational studies that did not compare different interventions head-to-head, HRQOL differences over time with intervention could be detected in all studies of surgery[20,40,53] and radiotherapy.[22,54-56] In observational studies of patients receiving chemotherapy, HRQOL changes were found in 65% of studies,[23,45,52,57-64] but not detected in 35%.[28,65-69] Fatigue and malaise were often important drivers of overall HRQOL scores.[4,56,70,71] It was commonly noted that the toxicity of chemotherapy treatment was counterbalanced by decreased tumor-related symptoms.[5,23,61,72] Other interesting findings included the observation that health care professionals underestimate HRQOL compared to patient self-reports,[73] that HRQOL can improve even with only stable, non-responding disease,[59] and that HRQOL can change rapidly in lung cancer patients and so should be measured frequently (at least every 3–4 weeks) to get an accurate picture of the disease course.[74] Missing data due to patient deterioration was frequently cited as a technical problem, often resulting in compliance of around 50% or less.[27,28,57,63,65,69,72,75-79] Simple diary cards have been reported to have better completion rates.[39,80]

HRQOL differences were detected more often in studies comparing intervention with no intervention than in studies that compared two interventions. For example, both of the randomized controlled trials (RCTs) comparing radiotherapy with no radiotherapy indicated negative HRQOL effects with treatment, even when survival appeared to improve.[39,81] Only one[82] of the two RCTs[83] comparing different radiotherapy strategies found an improvement in symptoms. Similarly, seven of eight RCTs comparing chemotherapy with supportive care alone found that chemotherapy improved HRQOL,[26,27,72,84-87] the other one finding at least trends toward improvement in some subscales, with no overall decrement.[88] In contrast, only slightly more than half[24,78-80,89-93] of the 16 randomized studies[44,94-99] that compared different chemotherapeutic regimens were able to detect a difference in HRQOL endpoints. In intervention studies, the EORTC instrument found differences between the treatment groups 78% of the time, the FACT 60%, LCSS 100%, MRC daily diary card 100%, and the RSCL 50%, suggesting that symptom measures may be more sensitive to detecting differences between treatments. There were no significant differences in the sample sizes of studies that did and did not detect differences in quality of life.

Value added

Studies reporting both HRQOL and more conventional clinical endpoints, including response, survival, toxicity, and performance status, provide an opportunity to determine how often and in what settings HRQOL represents "value added." In intervention studies, formal HRQOL assessment is sometimes included as an endpoint along with survival, response, time to progression, symptom control, and toxicity (Table 7.3). The operational definition of value added used in this analysis was that HRQOL data provided information beyond that of the traditional biomedical outcomes and influenced the overall conclusions of the study.

Curative treatment

In the curative phase of lung cancer treatment, HRQOL is currently used to determine whether the toxicity of therapy is acceptable when weighed against the benefits in terms of disease control. For example, surgery is associated with an initial decrease in HRQOL that usually returns to near baseline levels within several months.[20,40,53] Similarly, radiotherapy can improve survival with mild[83] or only transient decreased HRQOL.[81] These results are interesting but are unlikely to affect practice, as cure is the overwhelming goal of treatment almost at any cost. However, when more successful treatments are developed, as is the case currently for testicular cancer and Hodgkin's disease, it will be crucial to study

Table 7.3. Concordance between biomedical outcomes and HRQOL measures in intervention studies

Phase of Study	# Studies	Most common HRQOL Measures (#)	Biomedical Outcomes (#)	Key Observations
Potentially curative therapy	2	• POMS (1) • RSCL + HADS (1)	• OS (2) • Tox (2)	• Two randomized radiation trials: One found that adding RT to chemotherapy in limited SCLC improved survival at the expense of transiently decreased HRQOL.[81] The other found that CHART improved survival over standard RT in localized unresectable NSCLC with no significant decrement in HRQOL.[83]
Non-curative interventions A) non-randomized	18	• EORTC QLQ-C30 (7) • With LC13 (5) • FACT G & L (4) • LCSS (2)	• RR (16) • Sx (7) • OS (3) • TTP (1) • Tox (1)	• Of 16 trials with RR as an endpoint, 14 showed significant activity, while 2 did not. Despite this, one of those without activity demonstrated an improvement in HRQOL,[100] while the other did not.[65] Three interventions with important response rates demonstrated a worsening of HRQOL.[45,58,60] Six showed improvement,[57,59,61,62,64,76] while 5 found no difference.[28,63,66,68,69] • Of the 7 trials reporting symptoms, 6 showed improvement with treatment, while one found worsening symptoms.[58] This latter trial also demonstrated decreased HRQOL. Of the other 6, 2 found improved symptoms that were not detectable in overall HRQOL scores (one used the EORTC QLQ-C30[63] while the other used the Therapy Impact Questionnaire[69]), and 4 saw improvement in both symptoms and HRQOL.[38,54,57,100] • HRQOL improved in all 3 of the trials with OS as an endpoint. In two trials, HRQOL was found to be an important predictor of improved survival.[59,62] The third found improved HRQOL, but when compared to historical controls, no benefit from chemotherapy in survival or time to progression.[100] • The trial that found unacceptable toxicity also demonstrated a decrease in HRQOL.[45]
Non-curative interventions B) randomized (i) treatment vs no treatment	8	• EORTC QLQ-C30 (6) • With LC13 (4) • RSCL (3)	• OS (8) • RR (6) • Tox (6) • Sx (4) • TTP (4)	• Seven trials, all comparing chemotherapy to supportive care alone, found improved survival. Five of these also found improved HRQOL,[26,27,72,86,87] while 2 found no difference.[84,85] The one trial that did not find a survival difference did detect improved HRQOL, however.[88] • As would be expected, all trials reporting response rates demonstrated activity compared to supportive care alone. Five of these also showed better HRQOL,[26,72,84,86,87] while the other found no improvement.[88]

Table 7.3. (*cont.*)

Phase of Study	# Studies	Most common HRQOL Measures (#)	Biomedical Outcomes (#)	Key Observations
				• Similarly, the 6 studies reported finding toxicity in the intervention arm to (subjectively) a greater[26,72,88] or lesser[84,86,87] extent.
				• The 4 studies reporting symptoms all found an improvement and were all associated with better HRQOL.[72,85–87]
				• TTP was reported improved over supportive care in 4 studies. Three also found improved HRQOL[27,86,87] while one did not.[88]
Non-curative interventions B) randomized (ii) comparison of alternative treatments	16	• EORTC QLQ-C30 (6) • With LC13 (5) • RSCL (2) • MRC (3) • LASA (2) • FACT G & L (1) • LCSS (1)	• OS (16) • RR (14) • Tox (13) • TTP (11) • Sx (9)	• Differences in survival were detected in 8 of the 16 trials. One of these showed conflicting results, with improved survival for patients undergoing more intensive RT for locally advanced NSCLC, but worse HRQOL compared to a less intense treatment.[82] Two studies were concordant, with survival and HRQOL benefits both favoring the same treatment group.[89,92] Five found a difference in survival but no difference in HRQOL.[24,44,94–96] Of 8 studies that were null for survival, 2 had worse HRQOL,[78,80] 2 found no difference,[97,98] and 4 demonstrated an improvement in HRQOL for one of the arms.[79,90,93,118]
				• Response and TTP were always concordant with HRQOL, with the arm with the higher response rate or longer TTP showing either the same or better HRQOL. TTP tracked with OS results in 8/11 cases.[44,78,79,89,93,95,97,118] In 2, a survival advantage did not correspond to a longer TTP,[94,96] and in one study[98] a longer TTP did not translate into improved OS, although the response rate was higher.
				• Nine of 13 studies reporting toxicity found differences between arms. Two of these were discordant, in which the arm with greater toxicity had better HRQOL.[89,92] In both of these cases, improved HRQOL corresponded to improved RR. In 4 cases, the least toxic intervention had better HRQOL,[78,79,93,118] and in 3, the more toxic regimen's effects were mitigated by benefits resulting in no HRQOL difference between the arms.[24,44,94]
				• Symptom improvement was always associated with HRQOL that was the same or better than the comparator.

EORTC-LC13: European Organization for Research and Treatment of Cancer Lung Cancer 13 item module; EORTC QLQ-C30: EORTC Quality of Life Questionnaire 30 item core instrument; FACT-G: Functional Assessment of Cancer Therapy – General instrument; FACT-L: FACT lung cancer module; HADS: Hospital Anxiety and Depression Scale; HRQOL: health-related quality of life; LASA: Linear Analogue Self-Assessment; LCSS: Lung Cancer Symptom Scale; MRC: British Medical Research Council daily diary card; OS: overall survival; POMS: Profile of Mood States; RSCL: Rotterdam Symptom Checklist; RR: response rate; Sx: symptoms; Tox: toxicity; TTP: time to progression.

their HRQOL effects in order to minimize both short-term and long-term sequelae of cancer therapy without compromising survival.

Non-randomized studies

For incurable disease, development of new drugs and drug combinations initially proceeds stepwise through non-randomized phase I and II studies. Objective response is usually the primary outcome, but several of these trials have included HRQOL as a secondary endpoint with a goal of evaluating palliation. Active regimens often can improve or at least not worsen overall HRQOL, but some particularly toxic therapies can have high anti-tumor activity but worsen overall HRQOL.[45,58,60] Conversely, a treatment judged to be without important tumor activity can improve HRQOL.[100] Measures of specific symptoms are usually concordant with HRQOL measures. For example, symptom improvement usually leads to improved HRQOL, unless toxicity from the treatment counterbalances the beneficial effects.[63,69]

Because there is not a comparison group, it is difficult to determine whether the survival, time to progression, or toxicity levels reported in a phase I or II study have any meaning unless they are extreme, as is sometimes the case when a regimen has unacceptable toxicity.[45] While conventional toxicity grading is offered as the primary evidence for tolerability of the regimens, the inclusion of HRQOL endpoints provides a unique opportunity to obtain the patient's perspective on toxicity. For example, if patients' summary HRQOL scores are stable or improve over the course of treatment,[66,68] or rates of significant distress on patient self-reported toxicity measures are low,[13,58] it lends support to claims that a new regimen is well tolerated.

An important question that is not well answered by this literature is the relationship between tumor response and HRQOL improvement. One would hypothesize that this relationship would vary by treatment, with response to less toxic regimens more likely to translate into actual palliation. However, despite the fact that response rates are virtually always reported for each treatment group, none of the papers reviewed explicitly evaluated how well tumor response translated into symptomatic palliation.

Randomized studies

Randomized studies provide an appropriate control group for comparison of outcomes. However, when an intervention is being compared to supportive care alone, response and toxicity are still difficult to interpret. In these instances, HRQOL is an important secondary endpoint to help determine the balance between these often competing effects. In cases where a survival difference is not found, HRQOL effects could be the determining factor when choosing a course of treatment.[88]

Randomized trials comparing alternative interventions provide the best opportunity to examine the concordance between biomedical and HRQOL endpoints. As Table 7.3 indicates, there can be discordance between HRQOL results and survival[82] or toxicity.[89,92] In this particular subset of studies, longer time to progression and improved symptoms with one treatment translated into HRQOL measurements that were at least as good if not better than those of the comparator. However, there were several examples in which the counterbalancing toxicity resulted in an equivalent rather than superior HRQOL result.[44,94] Although it is unusual for HRQOL to conflict with the results of biomedical outcomes, it does not correlate perfectly with any single measure and, therefore, does provide added value; the balance between symptom improvement and toxicity, or the effects of delayed progression that is summarized in most HRQOL measures, cannot be consistently predicted by any of the other biomedical endpoints. Whether it is worth the time and expense required to obtain this information must be evaluated for each research situation, however.

Analytic concerns

Missing data continues to be a major challenge in HRQOL research. This problem is especially applicable to lung cancer, as the patients are often too sick to complete surveys and usually experience a rapid deterioration.[52] The effects of aggressive treatment can contribute to this phenomenon as well. Consequently, censoring is "informative," resulting in misleading analyses in which the average HRQOL can appear to increase over time as only healthier patients remain.[52] Several studies in this review found that only about half of the patients had more than a baseline evaluation,[27,28,57,63,65,69,72,75–79] making repeated measures analyses, and even comparisons of the proportions of patients who improved versus worsened, impossible. Some analysts have tried to impute missing data,[52] but this approach is difficult when there is only one measurement from a patient and the specific trajectory of HRQOL is uncertain. Others have tried to limit the analysis to those with complete data;[77] however, this may not be valid, as it assumes uninformative censoring. As a result, some researchers have turned to looking at other measures, such as performance status,[34] to estimate missing HRQOL data. More discussion of the effects of missing data can be found in the chapter by Fairclough in this volume.[101]

Because of the short survival of lung cancer patients, the handling of death presents another analytic challenge. HRQOL can be assessed at fixed time points or at the time of median survival, but such approaches will lead to overestimates since the patients who die before that time, and who consequently likely had worse HRQOL, will not be included. Some researchers have calculated an area under the survival curve, adjusted for HRQOL, to come up with an average daily HRQOL estimate by, for example, assigning death a value of 0.[52,102,103] However, patients have rated some health states pertinent to lung cancer, such as having constant pain, as being worse than death.[104]

Discussion

This review has found a substantial body of work assessing the HRQOL of patients with lung cancer, although less than exists for other cancer sites such as breast or prostate cancer. The quality of these studies varied widely, however, ranging from rigorous methodological evaluations to the use of unvalidated, investigator-developed HRQOL questionnaires in intervention trials. A priori consideration of probable analytical and statistical issues like sample size and missing data was uncommon. It is comforting to see, however, that minority patients, the elderly, and women were relatively well represented in lung cancer HRQOL studies. Lung cancer is a disease of the elderly and is more common in several minority groups, such as African Americans. Furthermore, lung cancer is increasing in women, while the incidence in men has leveled off and begun to decrease. By addressing the effects of socioeconomic status, literacy, and culture among these groups of patients, researchers have the opportunity to explore issues of equity and justice in these patients' access to care and the quality of the care they receive.

Clearly, HRQOL assessment is an essential tool in characterizing the experience of disease and survivorship and in identifying the service needs of patients throughout the cancer disease trajectory. Given the natural history of lung cancer, it is not surprising that the literature in this area is less extensive than it is for breast cancer or prostate cancer. Nonetheless, HRQOL measurement has been used to document that a high proportion of newly diagnosed patients experience significant anxiety and depression,[25,105] that pain and depression are prevalent and underdiagnosed among patients with inoperable disease,[106–109] and that survivors of lung cancer have significant rehabilitation problems.[110] Perhaps the most compelling evidence that HRQOL assessment adds value to clinical measures, however, is the consistent observation that baseline HRQOL is an important independent predictor of response and survival.[60,62,76,111–116] This makes it an important consideration when interpreting the results of clinical trials, or when assessing the expectations of treatment results in practice.

Unlike other diseases where there are technologies suitable for assessment in several distinct phases of care (screening, primary and adjuvant therapy, follow-up, and survivorship), HRQOL research in lung cancer, by virtue of the disease's poor prognosis, is largely focused on non-curative treatments like palliative chemotherapy. Since palliation, almost by definition, is an outcome that must be measured through patient self-report, HRQOL is a crucial end-point for most lung cancer trials. But, because the patients are so ill, HRQOL assessment in lung cancer is plagued by problems of drop-out and low response rates. This situation creates important analytic problems due to missing data that sometimes are insurmountable.[20,65]

The three lung cancer-specific HRQOL instruments, the EORTC-LC13, the FACT-L, and the LCSS, all have their own strengths and weaknesses in different situations. The EORTC scale focuses on disease-related symptoms and treatment-related toxicity. As a result, its psychometric properties are felt to be especially good in situations where patients are relatively ill. It is limited in this application, though, as its length and complexity may make it difficult to administer to the sickest patients. This measure is unique in including a question about the perceived financial impact of the disease, however.

Conversely, with its focus on psychosocial issues, the FACT may be best in situations where patients are not as ill. It does not have as comprehensive an assessment of symptoms as the other two lung cancer-specific instruments and, therefore, has been most successful in monitoring patients receiving supportive care rather than aggressive anti-cancer treatment. Interestingly, hair loss was a toxicity found not to be important in evaluations of both the FACT and EORTC instruments, likely because patients expect hair loss and realize that it will be transient. Consequently, the FACT dropped the hair loss item from its questionnaire. A question about regret for smoking was also dropped. This question can cause considerable distress in lung cancer patients who may already feel guilt about developing a self-imposed disease. Relatedly, the developers of the FACT-G replaced "I worry about dying" with "I worry that my condition will worsen."[30] Like the EORTC QLQ-C30 with its LC13 submodule, the FACT-L suffers from longer than ideal length, sometimes exacerbating problems of missing data in this already ill population.

The LCSS does not address toxicity of treatment. The developers see this omission as an advantage, however, as treatments, and hence the side effects of treatment, may change over time. Further, the LCSS only minimally assesses psychosocial effects. Though shorter, simpler, and possibly more sensitive to change, the LCSS's lack of a general component makes it difficult to compare across disease sites. Moreover, administrators must ensure that respondents adequately understand the VAS. It is the scale of choice, however, when trying to reduce respondent burden and limit the attrition in ill patients. Its focus on symptoms rather than toxicity makes it especially appropriate for trials in which "clinical benefit"[117] is being used as an outcome measure, rather than overall HRQOL. As such, it is surely one of the most well-validated measures available in oncology.

The field of HRQOL research in general has seen significant methodological development over the past decade. As a result, there are several existing measures applicable to lung cancer patients that have undergone extensive evaluation. There is little reason to create new ad hoc instruments, the results of which are difficult to interpret across studies. Future research should focus on comparing the existing lung cancer-specific instruments, not to decide which is "best," but rather to refine understanding of which scale might perform best with a given research aim in a particular patient population, intervention, or mode of administration, including the use of proxy respondents to minimize missing data. In fact, it may be optimal to move away from traditional fixed instruments, such as the FACT or EORTC measures, towards an approach where items from these scales are "banked" and selected individually based on the specific needs of a particular situation using computerized-adaptive testing and item response theory.

More work is also needed on the relationships among symptom measures, functional status scales, and global assessments of HRQOL to allow synthesis among or "cross-walking" between measures. This work should be goal-directed rather than exploratory, with those goals defined by the objectives of the common study paradigms. Given the availability of well-validated instruments, it is not unrealistic to think that over the next several years consensus on the optimal HRQOL measurement strategy could be achieved in each of the following settings: in randomized trials of curative and palliative therapies; characterizing the burden of illness and supportive care needs throughout the disease trajectory; and incorporating HRQOL considerations into cost-effectiveness analyses.

Acknowledgment

We would like to thank Candace Canto from the National Library of Medicine for assistance with the literature search.

REFERENCES

1 Greenlee, R. T., Murray, T., Bolden, S. *et al.* (2000). Cancer statistics, 2000. *Ca: Cancer Journal for Clinicians* **50**:7–33.

2 DeVita, V. T. Jr., Hellman, S., Rosenberg, S. A. (1993). *Cancer: Principles and Practice of Oncology.* Philadelphia, PA: J.B. Lippincott Co.

3 Reis, L. A. G., Kosary, C. L., Hankey, B. F. *et al.* (1999). *SEER Cancer Statistics Review, 1973–1996.* Bethesda, MD: National Cancer Institute.

4 Hopwood, P., Stephens, R. J. (1995). Symptoms at presentation for treatment in patients with lung cancer: implications for the evaluation of palliative treatment. *British Journal of Cancer* **71**:633–6.

5 Thatcher, N., Hopwood, P., Anderson, H. (1997). Improving quality of life in patients with non-small cell lung cancer: research experience with gemcitabine. *European Journal of Cancer* **33**:S8–13.

6 Hollen, P. J., Gralla, R. J. (1996). Comparison of instruments for measuring quality of life in patients with lung cancer. *Seminars in Oncology* **23**:31–40.

7 Hopwood, P. (1996). Quality of life assessment in chemotherapy trials for non-small cell lung cancer: are theory and practice significantly different? *Seminars in Oncology* **23**:60–4.

8 Manegold, C., Schwarz, R. (1996). Quality of life and supportive care in the treatment of NSCLC. *Chest* **109**:113S–14S.

9 Johnson, D. H. (2000). Evolution of cisplatin-based chemotherapy in non-small cell lung cancer: a historical perspective and the eastern cooperative oncology group experience. *Chest* **117**:133S–7S.

10 Chang, A. Y., Kim, K., Boucher, H. *et al.* (1998). A randomized phase II trial of echinomycin, trimetrexate, and cisplatin plus etoposide in patients with metastatic nonsmall cell lung carcinoma: an Eastern Cooperative Oncology Group Study (E1587). *Cancer* **82**:292–300.

11 Crawford, J., O'Rourke, M., Schiller, J. H. *et al.* (1996). Randomized trial of vinorelbine compared with fluorouracil plus leucovorin in patients with stage IV non-small-cell lung cancer. *Journal of Clinical Oncology* **14**:2774–84.

12 Li, B., Yu, J., Suntharalingam, M. *et al.* (2000). Comparison of three treatment options for single brain metastasis from lung cancer. *International Journal of Cancer* **90**:37–45.

13 White, S. C., Cheeseman, S., Thatcher, N. *et al.* (2000). Phase II study of oral topotecan in advanced non-small cell lung cancer. *Clinical Cancer Research* **6**:868–73.

14 Hopwood, P., Harvey, A., Davies, J. *et al.* (1998). Survey of the administration of quality of life (QL) questionnaires in three multicentre randomised trials in cancer. The Medical Research Council Lung Cancer Working Party the CHART Steering Committee. *European Journal of Cancer* **34**:49–57.

15 Sarna, L. (1993). Correlates of symptom distress in women with lung cancer. *Cancer Practice* **1**:21–8.

16 Sarna, L. (1993). Women with lung cancer: impact on quality of life. *Quality of Life Research* **2**:13–22.

17 Sarna, L., Brecht, M. L. (1997). Dimensions of symptom distress in women with advanced lung cancer: a factor analysis. *Heart Lung* **26**:23–30.

18 Movsas, B., Scott, C., Sause, W. *et al.* (1999). The benefit of treatment intensification is age and histology-dependent in patients with locally advanced non-small cell lung cancer (NSCLC): a quality-adjusted survival analysis of radiation therapy oncology group (RTOG) chemoradiation studies. *International Journal of Radiation Oncology, Biology, and Physics* **45**:1143–9.

19 Erickson, this volume, Chapter 3.

20 Hendriks, J., Van Schil, P., van Meerbeeck, J. *et al.* (1996). Short-term survival after major pulmonary resections for bronchogenic carcinoma. *Acta Chirurgica Belgica* **96**:273–9.

21 Taenzer, P., Bultz, B. D., Carlson, L. E. *et al.* (2000). Impact of computerized quality of life screening on physician behaviour and patient satisfaction in lung cancer outpatients. *Psycho-Oncology* **9**:203–13.

22 Lutz, S. T., Huang, D. T., Ferguson, C. L. *et al.* (1997). A retrospective quality of life analysis using the Lung Cancer Symptom Scale in patients treated with palliative radiotherapy for

advanced nonsmall cell lung cancer. *International Journal of Radiation Oncology, Biology, and Physics* **37**:117–22.

23 Bernhard, J., Hurny, C., Bacchi, M. *et al.* (1996). Initial prognostic factors in small-cell lung cancer patients predicting quality of life during chemotherapy. Swiss Group for Clinical Cancer Research (SAKK). *British Journal of Cancer* **74**:1660–7.

24 Joss, R. A., Alberto, P., Hurny, C. *et al.* (1995). Quality versus quantity of life in the treatment of patients with advanced small-cell lung cancer? A randomized phase III comparison of weekly carboplatin and teniposide versus cisplatin, adriamycin, etoposide alternating with cyclophosphamide, methotrexate, vincristine and lomustine. Swiss Group for Clinical Cancer Research (SAKK). *Annals of Oncology* **6**:41–8.

25 Montazeri, A., Milroy, R., Hole, D. *et al.* (1998). Anxiety and depression in patients with lung cancer before and after diagnosis: findings from a population in Glasgow, Scotland. *Journal of Epidemiology and Community Health* **52**:203–4.

26 Cullen, M. H., Billingham, L. J., Woodroffe, C. M. *et al.* (1999). Mitomycin, ifosfamide, and cisplatin in unresectable nonsmall-cell lung cancer: effects on survival and quality of life. *Journal of Clinical Oncology* **17**:3188–94.

27 Helsing, M., Bergman, B., Thaning, L. *et al.* (1998). Quality of life and survival in patients with advanced non-small cell lung cancer receiving supportive care plus chemotherapy with carboplatin and etoposide or supportive care only. A multicentre randomised phase III trial. Joint Lung Cancer Study Group. *European Journal of Cancer* **34**:1036–44.

28 Gridelli, C., Frontini, L., Perrone, F. *et al.* (2002). Gemcitabine plus vinorelbine in advanced non-small cell lung cancer: a phase II study of three different doses. Gem Vin Investigators. *British Journal of Cancer* **83**:707–14.

29 Aaronson, N. K., Cull, A. M., Kaasa, S., Sprangers, M. A. G. (1996). The European Organization for Research and Treatment of Cancer (EORTC) modular approach to quality of life assessment in oncology: an update. In *Quality of Life and Pharmacoeconomics in Clinical Trials* (2nd Edition), ed. B. Spilker, pp. 179–89. Philadelphia, PA: Lippincott-Raven.

30 Cella, D. F., Bonomi, A. E. (1996). The Functional Assessment of Cancer Therapy (FACT) and Functional Assessment of HIV Infection (FAHI) quality of life measurement system. In *Quality of Life and Pharmacoeconomics in Clinical Trials* (2nd Edition), ed. B. Spilker, pp. 203–14. Philadelphia, PA: Lippincott-Raven.

31 European Organization for Research and Treatment of Cancer. QLQ-C30 (core). http://www.eortc.be/home/qol/ Accessed September 10, 2004.

32 Bergman, B., Aaronson, N. K., Ahmedzai, S. *et al.* (1994). The EORTC QLQ-LC13: a modular supplement to the EORTC Core Quality of Life Questionnaire (QLQ-C30) for use in lung cancer clinical trials. EORTC Study Group on Quality of Life. *European Journal of Cancer* **30A**:635–42.

33 Bergman, B., Sullivan, M., Sorenson, S. (1992). Quality of life during chemotherapy for small cell lung cancer. II. A longitudinal study of the EORTC Core Quality of Life Questionnaire and comparison with the Sickness Impact Profile. *Acta Oncologica* **31**:19–28.

34 Herndon, J. E., Fleishman, S., Kosty, M. P. *et al.* (1997). A longitudinal study of quality of life in advanced non-small cell lung cancer: Cancer and Leukemia Group B (CALGB) 8931. *Controlled Clinical Trials* **18**:286–300.

35 Kosmidis, P. (1996). Quality of life as a new end point. *Chest* **109**:110S-2S.

36 Aaronson, N. K., Ahmedzai, S., Bergman, B. *et al.* (1993). The European Organization for Research and Treatment of Cancer QLQ-C30: a quality-of-life instrument for use in international clinical trials in oncology. *Journal of the National Cancer Institute* **85**:365–76.

37 Osoba, D., Zee, B., Pater, J. *et al.* (1994). Psychometric properties and responsiveness of the EORTC Quality of Life Questionnaire (QLQ-C30) in patients with breast, ovarian and lung cancer. *Quality of Life Research.* **3**:353–64.

38 Osoba, D., Murray, N., Gelmon, K. *et al.* (1994). Quality of life, appetite, and weight change in patients receiving dose-intensive chemotherapy. *Oncology (Huntington)* **8**:61–5.

39 Geddes, D. M., Dones, L., Hill, E. *et al.* (1990). Quality of life during chemotherapy for small cell lung cancer: assessment and use of a daily diary card in a randomized trial. *European Journal of Cancer* **26**:484–92.

40 Zieren, H. U., Muller, J. M., Hamberger, U. *et al.* (1996). Quality of life after surgical therapy of bronchogenic carcinoma. *European Journal of Cardiovascular Therapy* **10**:233–7.

41 Cella, D. F., Tulsky, D. S., Gray, G. S. B. *et al.* (1993). The Functional Assessment of Cancer Therapy Scale: development and validation of the general measure. *Journal of Clinical Oncology* **11**:570–9.

42 Cella, D. F., Tulsky, D. S., Gray, G. S. B. *et al.* Functional Assessment of Chronic Illness Therapy. http://www.facit.org. Accessed September 10, 2004.

43 Cella, D. F., Bonomi, A. E., Lloyd, S. R. *et al.* (1995). Reliability and validity of the Functional Assessment of Cancer Therapy-Lung (FACT-L) quality of life instrument. *Lung Cancer* **12**:199–220.

44 Bonomi, P., Kim, K., Fairclough, D. *et al.* (2000). Comparison of survival and quality of life in advanced non-small-cell lung cancer patients treated with two dose levels of

paclitaxel combined with cisplatin versus etoposide with cisplatin: results of an Eastern Cooperative Oncology Group trial. *Journal of Clinical Oncology* **18**:623–31.

45 Colon-Otero, G., Niedringhaus, R. D., Hillman, S. H. *et al.* (2001). A phase II trial of edatrexate, vinblastine, adriamycin, cisplastin, and filgrastim (EVAC/G-CSF) in patients with non-small-cell carcinoma of the lungs: a North Central Cancer Treatment Group Trial. *American Journal of Clinical Oncology* **24**:551–5.

46 Hollen, P. J., Gralla, R. J., Kris, M. G. *et al.* (1993). Quality of life assessment in individuals with lung cancer: testing the Lung Cancer Symptom Scale (LCSS). *European Journal of Cancer* **29A**(Suppl. 1):S51–8.

47 Hollen, P. J., Gralla, R. J., Kris, M. G. *et al.* (1994). Quality of life during clinical trials: conceptual model for the Lung Cancer Symptom Scale (LCSS). *Supportive Care in Cancer* **2**:213–22.

48 Hollen, P. J., Gralla, R. J., Kris, M. G. *et al.* (1994). Measurement of quality of life in patients with lung cancer in multicenter trials of new therapies. Psychometric assessment of the Lung Cancer Symptom Scale. *Cancer* **73**:2087–98.

49 Hollen, P. J., Gralla, R. J., Kris, M. G. *et al.* (1999). Normative data and trends in quality of life from the Lung Cancer Symptom Scale (LCSS). *Supportive Care in Cancer* **7**: 140–8.

50 Hollen, P. J., Gralla, R. J., Liepa, A. M. *et al.* (2001). Validation of a quality of life instrument for patients with pleural mesothelioma: Lung Cancer Symptom Scale. *Proceedings of the American Society for Clinical Onology* **20** (Abstract 1579).

51 Lung Cancer Symptom Scale. http://www.lcss-ql.com/. Accessed September 10, 2004.

52 Hollen, P. J., Gralla, R. J., Cox, C. *et al.* (1997). A dilemma in analysis: issues in the serial measurement of quality of life in patients with advanced lung cancer. *Lung Cancer* **18**:119–36.

53 Dales, R. E., Belanger, R., Shamji, F. M. *et al.* (1994). Quality-of-life following thoracotomy for lung cancer. *Journal of Clinical Epidemiology* **47**:1443–9.

54 Langendijk, J. A., ten Velde, G. P., Aaronson, N. K. *et al.* (2002). Quality of life after palliative radiotherapy in non-small cell lung cancer: a prospective study. *International Journal of Radiation Oncology, Biology, and Physics* **47**:149–55.

55 Schaafsma, J., Coy, P. (2000). Response of global quality of life to high-dose palliative radiotherapy for non-small-cell lung cancer. *International Journal of Radiation Oncology, Biology, and Physics* **47**:691–701.

56 Lutz, S., Norrell, R., Bertucio, C. *et al.* (2001). Symptom frequency and severity in patients with metastatic or locally recurrent lung cancer: a prospective study using the Lung Cancer Symptom Scale in a community hospital. *Journal of Palliative Medicine* **4**:157–65.

57 Hickish, T. F., Smith, I. E., Nicolson, M. C. *et al.* (1998). A pilot study of MVP (mitomycin-C, vinblastine and cisplatin) chemotherapy in small-cell lung cancer. *British Journal of Cancer* **77**:1966–70.

58 Shevlin, P. M., Muers, M. F., Peake, M. D. *et al.* (1998). Modified ICE study: a phase II study of an intensive, modified ICE regimen (ifosfamide, carboplatin and etoposide) in patients with better prognosis, small cell lung cancer. *Lung Cancer* **21**:115–26.

59 Frasci, G., Comella, P., Panza, N. *et al.* (1998). Carboplatin-oral etoposide personalized dosing in elderly non-small cell lung cancer patients. Gruppo Oncologico Cooperativo Sud-Italia. *European Journal of Cancer* **34**:1710–14.

60 Tester, W. J., Jin, P. Y., Reardon, D. H. *et al.* (1997). Phase II study of patients with metastatic nonsmall cell carcinoma of the lung treated with paclitaxel by 3-hour infusion. *Cancer* **79**:724–9.

61 Roychowdhury, D. F., Desai, P., Zhu, Y. W. (1997). Paclitaxel (3-hour infusion) followed by carboplatin (24 hours after paclitaxel): a phase II study in advanced non-small cell lung cancer. *Seminars in Oncology* **24**:S12.

62 Han, J. Y., Kim, H. K., Choi, B. G. *et al.* (1998). Quality of life (QOL) assessment of MIP (mitomycin, ifosfamide and cisplatin) chemotherapy in advanced non-small cell lung cancers (NSCLC). *Japanese Journal of Oncology* **28**:749–53.

63 Gridelli, C., Perrone, F., Gallo, C. *et al.* (1999). Single-agent gemcitabine' as second-line treatment in patients with advanced non small cell lung cancer (NSCLC): a phase II trial. *Anticancer Research* **19**:4535–8.

64 Kosmas, C., Tsavaris, N. B., Polyzos, A. *et al.* (2000). A phase II study of paclitaxel-ifosfamide-cisplatin combination in advanced nonsmall cell lung carcinoma. *Cancer* **89**:774–82.

65 Socinski, M. A., Steagall, A., Gillenwater, H. (1999). Second-line chemotherapy with 96-hour infusional paclitaxel in refractory non-small cell lung cancer: report of a phase II trial. *Cancer Investigation* **17**:181–8.

66 Pujol, J. L., Monnier, A., Berille, J. *et al.* (1994). Phase II study of nitrosourea fotemustine as single-drug chemotherapy in poor-prognosis non-small-cell lung cancer. *British Journal of Cancer* **69**:1136–40.

67 Maasilta, P. K., Rautonen, J. K., Mattson, M. T. *et al.* (1990). Quality of life assessment during chemotherapy for non-small cell lung cancer. *European Journal of Cancer* **26**:706–8.

68 Quantin, X., Riviere, A., Daures, J. P. *et al.* (2000). Phase I-II study of high dose epirubicin plus cisplatin in unresectable non-small-cell lung cancer: searching for the maximal

tolerated dose. *American Journal of Clinical Oncology* **23**:192–6.

69 Buccheri, G., Ferrigno, D. (2000). Vinorelbine in elderly patients with inoperable nonsmall cell lung carcinoma: a phase II study. *Cancer* **88**:2677–85.

70 Hurny, C., Bernhard, J., Joss, R. *et al.* (1993). "Fatigue and malaise" as a quality-of-life indicator in small-cell lung cancer patients. The Swiss Group for Clinical Cancer Research (SAKK). *Supportive Care in Cancer* **1**:316–20.

71 Tishelman, C., Degner, L. F., Mueller, B. (2000). Measuring symptom distress in patients with lung cancer. A pilot study of experienced intensity and importance of symptoms [published erratum appears in *Cancer Nursing* (2000)**23**(3):163]. *Cancer Nursing* **23**:82–90.

72 The Elderly Lung Cancer Vinorelbine Italian Study Group (1999). Effects of vinorelbine on quality of life and survival of elderly patients with advanced non-small-cell lung cancer. *Journal of the National Cancer Institute* **91**:66–72.

73 Regan, J., Yarnold, J., Jones, P. W. *et al.* (1991). Palliation and life quality in lung cancer: how good are clinicians at judging treatment outcome? *British Journal of Cancer* **64**:396–400.

74 Gralla, R. J., Hollen, P. J., Rittenberg, C. N. *et al.* (1999). Measuring quality of life (QL) in lung cancer clinical trials: Determining the frequency of QL assessment. *Proceedings of the American Society for Clinical Oncology* **18** (Abstract 2235).

75 Hurny, C., Bernhard, J., Joss, R. *et al.* (1992). Feasibility of quality of life assessment in a randomized phase III trial of small cell lung cancer – a lesson from the real world – the Swiss Group for Clinical Cancer Research SAKK. *Annals of Oncology* **3**:825–31.

76 Bergman, B., Sullivan, M., Sorenson, S. (1991). Quality of life during chemotherapy for small cell lung cancer. I. An evaluation with generic health measures. *Acta Oncologica* **30**:947–57.

77 Hopwood, P., Stephens, R. J., Machin, D. (1994). Approaches to the analysis of quality of life data: experiences gained from a medical research council lung cancer working party palliative chemotherapy trial. *Quality of Life Research* **3**:339–52.

78 Kosty, M. P., Fleishman, S. B., Herndon, J. E. *et al.* (1994). Cisplatin, vinblastine, and hydrazine sulfate in advanced, non-small- cell lung cancer: a randomized placebo-controlled, double-blind phase III study of the Cancer and Leukemia Group B. *Journal of Clinical Oncology* **12**:1113–20.

79 Giaccone, G., Splinter, T. A., Debruyne, C. *et al.* (1998). Randomized study of paclitaxel-cisplatin versus cisplatin-teniposide in patients with advanced non-small-cell lung cancer. The European Organization for Research and Treatment of Cancer Lung Cancer Cooperative Group. *Journal of Clinical Oncology* **16**:2133–41.

80 Earl, H. M., Rudd, R. M., Spiro, S. G. *et al.* (1991). A randomised trial of planned versus as required chemotherapy in small cell lung cancer: a Cancer Research Campaign trial. *British Journal of Cancer* **64**:566–72.

81 Ahles, T. A., Silberfarb, P. M., Rundle, A. C. *et al.* (1994). Quality of life in patients with limited small-cell carcinoma of the lung receiving chemotherapy with or without radiation therapy, for cancer and leukemia group B. *Psychotherapy and Psychosomatics* **62**:193–9.

82 Macbeth, F. R., Bolger, J. J., Hopwood, P. *et al.* (1996). Randomized trial of palliative two-fraction versus more intensive 13-fraction radiotherapy for patients with inoperable non-small cell lung cancer and good performance status. Medical Research Council Lung Cancer Working Party. *Clinical Oncology (Royal College of Radiology)* **8**:167–75.

83 Bailey, A. J., Parmar, M. K., Stephens, R. J. (1998). Patient-reported short-term and long-term physical and psychologic symptoms: results of the continuous hyperfractionated accelerated radiotherapy (CHART) randomized trial in non-small-cell lung cancer. CHART Steering Committee. *Journal of Clinical Oncology* **16**:3082–93.

84 Anderson, H., Hopwood, P., Stephens, R. J. *et al.* (2000). Gemcitabine plus best supportive care (BSC) vs BSC in inoperable non-small cell lung cancer–a randomized trial with quality of life as the primary outcome. UK NSCLC Gemcitabine Group. Non-Small Cell Lung Cancer. *British Journal of Cancer* **83**:447–53.

85 Agteresch, H. J., Dagnelie, P. C., van der Gaast, A. *et al.* (2000). Randomized clinical trial of adenosine 5'-triphosphate in patients with advanced non-small-cell lung cancer. *Journal of the National Cancer Institute* **92**:321–8.

86 Shepherd, F. A., Dancey, J., Ramlau, R. *et al.* (2000). Prospective randomized trial of docetaxel versus best supportive care in patients with non-small-cell lung cancer previously treated with platinum-based chemotherapy. *Journal of Clinical Oncology* **18**:2095–103.

87 Roszkowski, K., Pluzanska, A., Krzakowski, M. *et al.* (2000). A multicenter, randomized, phase III study of docetaxel plus best supportive care versus best supportive care in chemotherapy-naive patients with metastatic or non-resectable localized non-small cell lung cancer (NSCLC). *Lung Cancer* **27**:145–57.

88 Ranson, M., Davidson, N., Nicolson, M. *et al.* (2000). Randomized trial of paclitaxel plus supportive care versus supportive care for patients with advanced non-small-cell lung cancer. *Journal of the National Cancer Institute* **92**:1074–80.

89 Souhami, R. L., Spiro, S. G., Rudd, R. M. *et al.* (1997). Five-day oral etoposide treatment for advanced small-cell lung cancer: randomized comparison with intravenous chemotherapy. *Journal of National Cancer Institute* **89**:577–80.

90 Gower, N. H., Rudd, R. M., Ruiz de Elvra, M. C. *et al.* (1995). Assessment of 'quality of life' using a daily diary card in a randomised trial of chemotherapy in small-cell lung cancer. *Annals of Oncology* **6**:575–80.

91 Fayers, P. M., Bleehen, N. M., Girling, D. J. *et al.* (1991). Assessment of quality of life in small-cell lung cancer using a Daily Diary Card developed by the Medical Research Council Lung Cancer Working Party. *British Journal of Cancer* **64**:299–306.

92 Frasci, G., Lorusso, V., Panza, N. *et al.* (2000). Gemcitabine plus vinorelbine versus vinorelbine alone in elderly patients with advanced non-small-cell lung cancer. *Journal of Clinical Oncology* **18**:2529–36.

93 ten Bokkel, H., Bergman, B., Chemaissani, A. *et al.* (1999). Single-agent gemcitabine: an active and better tolerated alternative to standard cisplatin-based chemotherapy in locally advanced or metastatic non-small cell lung cancer. *Lung Cancer* **26**:85–94.

94 Rowland, K. M. J., Loprinzi, C. L., Shaw, E. G. *et al.* (1996). Randomized double-blind placebo-controlled trial of cisplatin and etoposide plus megestrol acetate/placebo in extensive-stage small-cell lung cancer: a North Central Cancer Treatment Group study. *Journal of Clinical Oncology* **14**:135–41.

95 Loprinzi, C. L., Goldberg, R. M., Su, J. Q. *et al.* (1994). Placebo-controlled trial of hydrazine sulfate in patients with newly diagnosed non-small-cell lung cancer. *Journal of Clinical Oncology* **12**:1126–9.

96 Thatcher, N., Girling, D. J., Hopwood, P. *et al.* (2000). Improving survival without reducing quality of life in small-cell lung cancer patients by increasing the dose-intensity of chemotherapy with granulocyte colony-stimulating factor support: results of a British Medical Research Council Multicenter Randomized Trial. Medical Research Council Lung Cancer Working Party. *Journal of Clinical Oncology* **18**:395–404.

97 Crino, L., Scagliotti, G. V., Ricci, S. *et al.* (1999). Gemcitabine and cisplatin versus mitomycin, ifosfamide, and cisplatin in advanced non-small-cell lung cancer: A randomized phase III study of the Italian Lung Cancer Project. *Journal of Clinical Oncology* **17**:3522–30.

98 Cardenal, F., Lopez-Cabrerizo, M. P., Anton, A. *et al.* (1999). Randomized phase III study of gemcitabine-cisplatin versus etoposide-cisplatin in the treatment of locally advanced or metastatic non-small-cell lung cancer. *Journal of Clinical Oncology* **17**:12–18.

99 Kosmidis, P., Mylonakis, N., Fountzilas, G. *et al.* (1997). Paclitaxel (175 mg/m2) plus carboplatin versus paclitaxel (225 mg/m2) plus carboplatin in non-small cell lung cancer: a randomized study. *Seminars in Oncology* **24**:S12.

100 Glimelius, B., Birgegard, G., Hoffman, K. *et al.* (1992). Improved care of patients with small cell lung cancer. Nutritional and quality of life aspects. *Acta Oncologica* **31**:823–31.

101 Fairclough, this volume, chapter 17.

102 Gelber, R. D., Goldhirsch, A., Cole, B. F. *et al.* (1996). A quality-adjusted time without symptoms or toxicity (Q-TWiST) analysis of adjuvant radiation therapy and chemotherapy for resectable rectal cancer. *Journal of the National Cancer Institute* **88**:1039–45.

103 Goldhirsch, A., Gelber, R. D., Simes, R. J. *et al.* (1989). Costs and benefits of adjuvant therapy in breast cancer: A quality-adjusted survival analysis. *Journal of Clinical Oncology* **7**:36–44.

104 Patrick, D. L., Starks, K. C., Cain, R. F. *et al.* (1994). Measuring preferences for health states worse than death. *Medical Decision Making* **14**:9–18.

105 Hyodo, I., Eguchi, K., Takigawa, N. *et al.* (1999). Psychological impact of informed consent in hospitalized cancer patients. A sequential study of anxiety and depression using the hospital anxiety and depression scale. *Supportive Care in Cancer* **7**:396–9.

106 Hopwood, P., Stephens, R. J. (2000). Depression in patients with lung cancer: prevalence and risk factors derived from quality-of-life data. *Journal of Clinical Oncology* **18**:893–903.

107 Faller, H., Bulzebruck, H., Drings, P. *et al.* (1999). Coping, distress, and survival among patients with lung cancer. *Archives of General Psychiatry* **56**:756–62.

108 McCarthy, E. P., Phillips, R. S., Zhong, Z. (2000). Dying with cancer: patients' function, symptoms, and care preferences as death approaches. *Journal of the American Geriatric Society* **48**:S110–21.

109 Claessens, M. T., Lynn, J., Zhong, Z. *et al.* (2000). Dying with lung cancer or chronic obstructive pulmonary disease: insights from SUPPORT. Study to Understand Prognoses and Preferences for Outcomes and Risks of Treatments. *Journal of the American Geriatric Society* **48**:S146–53.

110 Schag, C. A., Ganz, P. A., Wing, D. S. *et al.* (1994). Quality of life in adult survivors of lung, colon and prostate cancer. *Quality of Life Research* **3**:127–41.

111 Degner, L. F., Sloan, J. A. (1995). Symptom distress in newly diagnosed ambulatory cancer patients and as a predictor

of survival in lung cancer. *Journal of Pain and Symptom Management* **10**:423–31.

112 Ganz, P. A., Lee, J. J., Siau, J. (1991). Quality of life assessment. An independent prognostic variable for survival in lung cancer. *Cancer* **67**:3131–5.

113 Ruckdeschel, J. C., Piantadosi, S. (1994). Quality of life in lung cancer surgical adjuvant trials. *Chest* **106**:324S–8S.

114 Abratt, R., Viljoen, G. (1995). Assessment of quality of life by clinicians – experience of a practical method in lung cancer patients. *South African Medical Journal* **85**:896–8.

115 Buccheri, G. F., Ferrigno, D., Tamburini, M. *et al.* (1995). The patient's perception of his own quality of life might have an adjunctive prognostic significance in lung cancer. *Lung Cancer* **12**:45–58.

116 Langendijk, H., Aaronson, N. K., de Jong, J. M. *et al.* (2000). The prognostic impact of quality of life assessed with the EORTC QLQ-C30 in inoperable non-small cell lung carcinoma treated with radiotherapy. *Radiotherapy and Oncology* **255**:19–25.

117 Burris, H. A., Moore, M. J., Andersen, J. S. *et al.* (1997). Improvements in survival and clinical benefit with gemcitabine as first-line therapy for patients with advanced pancreas cancer: a randomized trial. *Journal of Clinical Oncology* **15**:2403–13.

118 Vansteenkiste, J. F., Vandebroek, J. E., Nackaerts, K. L. *et al.* (2001). Clinical-benefit response in advanced non-small-cell lung cancer: A multicentre prospective randomized phase II study of single agent gemcitabine versus cisplatin-vindesine. *Annals of Oncology* **12**:1221–30.

8

Treatment for colorectal cancer: impact on health-related quality of life

Carol M. Moinpour, Ph.D.[1] and Dawn Provenzale, M.D., M.S.[2]

[1]Fred Hutchinson Cancer Research Center, Seattle, WA
[2]Duke University Medical Center, Durham, NC

Introduction

Colorectal cancer (CRC) is the second leading cause of cancer death in the US each year. It is estimated that in 2002 there were 148 300 new cases and 56 600 deaths from CRC.[1] Direct evidence from randomized trials[2] and indirect evidence from case-control and cohort studies[3–5] suggest that screening affects 5-year survival. Specifically, screening can identify pre-cancerous lesions and prevent development of CRC or identify CRC in earlier stages (I and II) when it can be treated more effectively.[6] The relative 5-year survival rates for early-stage disease (I and II) and advanced disease have been estimated at 65%–90% and 9%, respectively.[7] Because most patients diagnosed with CRC have not undergone screening, most CRCs are diagnosed after local or regional spread, and nearly half of all patients so diagnosed will die from it.

Treatment for CRC is based on the stage and location of disease and includes surgery, chemotherapy, and/or radiation therapy. These modalities may be associated with substantial toxicity, including hair loss, profound nausea and vomiting, and fecal incontinence. Furthermore, therapy for CRC may result in the formation of a permanent or temporary stoma. All of these treatments may have side effects that have an important effect on health-related quality of life (HRQOL).

Treatment for colon cancer includes surgical resection for stage I and II disease, and surgery plus chemotherapy for stage III and selected patients with stage IV disease. Palliative care is provided to patients with unresectable disease. A National Cancer Institute (NCI) website summarizes current treatment for colon cancer.[6]

The initial approach to rectal cancer management is complete staging. Endorectal ultrasound is the standard method for assessing tumor stage. Where available, imaging techniques (e.g., CT or MRI) of the pelvis may also be useful in this evaluation. Surgical resection is used to treat T1 and T2 tumors, and surgery plus chemotherapy and radiation therapy are used to treat T3 and T4 tumors. Adjuvant chemotherapy and radiation therapy may be administered pre-operatively to decrease tumor size.[6]

The lifetime risk of developing CRC in the US is approximately 5.5%[7] with an equal risk in men and women. There has been an overall decrease in CRC incidence in the last decade, as well as a decrease in mortality.[6] However, there are racial disparities in both incidence and mortality, with blacks having higher CRC rates and deaths.[6] The reasons for this racial disparity are not known. Potential etiologies include differences in biology, tumor biology, access to care and screening, and treatment.

Given the overall trends in improved survival, HRQOL related to treatment and living with CRC becomes increasingly important. Therefore, research on the morbidity and toxicity associated with surgery and its potential for long-term effects (e.g., HRQOL impact of living with an ostomy) is critical. This paper will address the extent to which HRQOL has been included in randomized and non-randomized studies of CRC treatment (surgery, chemotherapy, and radiation).

Methods

A MEDLINE search was performed using the keywords colorectal cancer, quality of life, and treatment. Papers published between 1990 and 2001 that examined the effect of treatment for CRC and also included at least one HRQOL measure were reviewed. The following types of articles were excluded: (1) papers with a prevention, screening, or survivorship focus because these reviews are addressed by others in the Cancer Outcomes Measurement Working Group (COMWG, or "Working Group"); (2) studies with utility measures unless HRQOL data were presented along with the utility results; (3) published proceedings or meeting abstracts. The primary search generated 121 articles and was supplemented with papers cited in the original set (particularly with respect to citations for HRQOL measures). After applying the exclusion criteria, 44 papers were selected for review. From these articles, information on the development and psychometric performance of the HRQOL questionnaires specifically developed for use in CRC trials was abstracted.

Results of review

Commonly used HRQOL questionnaires in CRC treatment studies

The European Organization for Research and Treatment of Cancer (EORTC) Quality of Life Questionnaire-Core30 (QLQ-C30)[8] was used in 16 studies, and was the most frequently adopted HRQOL measure. A total of 25 other HRQOL measures (counting two cancer-specific modules separately from their respective core measures) were used in these studies, with as many as four questionnaires administered in a single study. In the studies we reviewed, there were several symptom questionnaires developed specifically for use in a CRC study, but the psychometric properties of these measures have not been fully documented. Examples include the Quality of Life and Well-being Questionnaire

used by Glimelius *et al.* involving a combination of items from two questionnaires;[9,10] a Specific Disease and Continence-Related Symptoms questionnaire[11] used by Renner *et al.*;[12] and a Symptom Checklist[13] used by Forsberg *et al.*[14]

Four general cancer questionnaires were used in two or more studies examined for this review: EORTC QLQ-C30;[8] Functional Living Index – Cancer (FLIC);[15,16] Rotterdam Symptom Checklist (RSCL);[17-20] and the Spitzer Quality of Life Index (QL-Index).[21] In addition, five generic health status and well-being measures were used in two or more studies examined for this review: EuroQoL Five Dimensional Index (EQ-5D);[22,23] Hospital Anxiety and Depression Scale (HADS);[24] Nottingham Health Profile (NHP);[25-27] Profile of Mood States (POMS);[28,29] and Sickness Impact Profile (SIP).[30,31] The generic and general cancer questionnaires are described in detail in Erickson's chapter in this book,[32] and specific reference to their performance in CRC patients is described below.

The relative strengths of these selected instruments are related to their ability to capture the concerns of patients with CRC. Many of the questionnaires found in the CRC HRQOL literature are either generic cancer HRQOL instruments (i.e., not specific for colorectal cancer such as the FLIC) or are generic health status measures (e.g., the SIP) with items that do not mention cancer at all. The generic instruments provide a broad overview of physical, psychological, social, and emotional function, and their results can be used to compare the quality of life of colorectal cancer patients with the quality of life of patients with other types of cancer. Generic questionnaires can also be used in CRC survivorship studies.

CRC-specific measures of treatment effects on HRQOL

Two CRC-specific modules combined with other "core" questionnaires were reviewed for this paper: (1) the EORTC QLQ-C30[8,33,34] has a newly developed CRC symptom module, the CR38,[35-39] which was used in one treatment study as an outcome measure; and (2) the Functional Assessment of Cancer Therapy-General (FACT-G)[40,41] has a recently developed CRC module, the FACT-C.[42,43] Although newly developed modules with few citations in the literature, these two modules have been included because of their potential usefulness for future research. Table 8.1 has detailed information on item content and psychometric properties for both modules.

EORTC QLQ-C30/CR38

The well-established measurement properties and normative database for cancer patients make the EORTC QLQ-C30 a reasonable choice for examining the effect of cancer treatment on HRQOL, particularly in randomized controlled trials of alternative chemotherapeutic agents.[8,33,34] Although the QLQ-C30 examines general, physical, emotional, and functional status, it may not capture specific concerns of CRC patients such as incontinence, having a stoma, diarrhea, and bowel obstruction. The colorectal cancer-specific module with 38 items, the QLQ-C30/CR38,[35–39] addresses these concerns more completely, but has only recently appeared in the literature in one clinical study[44] and one validation paper.[38] A more thorough evaluation of its clinical utility must await its further use in CRC clinical studies. The content of the EORTC's CRC module makes it extremely promising. Four functional scales address body image, sexuality, sexual enjoyment, and future perspective; seven symptom scales evaluate micturition/urination problems, gastrointestinal tract problems, chemotherapy side effects, defecation problems, stoma-related problems where relevant, male and female sexual problems, and weight loss. However, a number of the CR38's symptom scales had internal consistency reliabilities of less than the recommended benchmark of 0.70 for a scale of items measuring the same construct.[45] Specifically, the chemotherapy and gastrointestinal subscales, two important symptom areas for CRC, did not meet this criterion. The CR38 also failed to detect chemotherapy-related change as reported in the validation paper, but there were very few patients in the study undergoing chemotherapy.[38]

The developers of the CR38 module suggested that additional chemotherapy side effect items might need to be added to the "core" set of three items depending on the nature of the regimen used in a trial. The current set of items may not be comprehensive enough to address "late effects" of chemotherapy treatment. The CR38 does include other sets of symptom items that are completed only if they apply to the patient (e.g., defecation problems for patients with an intact sphincter and stoma-related problems for patients with a stoma). This skip pattern format for item content is difficult to avoid given the variety of treatment effects in CRC patients. However, the content and measurement properties of the stoma and non-stoma subscales are good and represent important symptom areas to address when evaluating CRC treatments.

Significant differences were not reported for CR38 subscale scores by Allal et al. in their non-randomized treatment study that included this CRC-specific questionnaire.[44] However, the study had insufficient power to detect HRQOL effects since only 23 patients completed HRQOL questionnaires. Sailer et al.[39] evaluated the use of the CR38 in a small pilot study with 23 patients. They concluded that chemotherapy and radiation side effects (relevant for advanced-stage disease) and sexual problems are over-emphasized, and that surgery-related side effects are under-emphasized. They suggested that anorectal function post-surgery for large bowel cancer is an important HRQOL area requiring more in-depth coverage in the questionnaire; for example, no questions are included about flatus, increased hygiene needs, skin irritation, need for pads, and need for medication post-surgery.

FACT-G/FACT-C

The FACT-G[40,41] functions as a core measure of HRQOL domains in cancer in a manner analogous to the EORTC QLQ-C30 questionnaire. Similar to the EORTC system, the modules containing different symptom and disease-/treatment-related concerns based on the disease site and/or cancer treatment can be used to supplement the core questionnaire. The FACT-G + Colorectal Cancer

Table 8.1. Colorectal cancer-specific HRQOL questionnaires

Name of Questionnaire	European Organization for Research and Treatment of Cancer (EORTC) Quality of Life Questionnaire-Core 30 (QLQ-C30)[8,33,34] Colorectal Cancer-Specific Module (CR38)[36,38,39]
Purpose for which developed	Colorectal Cancer-Specific Quality of Life Questionnaire Module (QLQ-C30 / CR38): The objective was to develop a module of symptom and side effect items specific to colorectal cancer and its treatment; the module could then be used in conjunction with the QLQ-C30 providing a comprehensive measure of HRQOL; the module covers a range of disease stages.[38]
Length	38 items
Administration time	10.3 minutes (S.D. = 5.6 minutes) in combination with the QLQ-C30[38]; 5 to 10 minutes each for QLQ-C30 and CR38[39]
Domains included	4 functional scales and single items: body image (3 items), sexuality (2 items), sexual enjoyment (1 item), and future perspective (1 item); and 7 symptom scales and single items: micturition/urination problems (3 items), gastrointestinal tract (5 items), chemotherapy side effects (3 items), defecation problems (patients with intact sphincters – 7 items), stoma-related problems (if has stoma – 9 items), male sexual problems (2 items), female sexual problems (if sexually active – 2 items), and weight loss (1 item). Time Frame: Past week.
Scoring	4-point Likert scale (not at all, a little, quite a bit, very much); one yes/no question re: having a stoma (one set of questions answered if yes, another if no). No items require reverse scoring. 0 to 100 scale with higher scores representing better HRQOL for the body image, sexual functioning, sexual enjoyment, and future perspective items; higher scores reflect worse functioning for the symptom scales and single items. No total score for the module at this time. The Manual includes information re: handling of missing items within scales.[33]
Validated modes of administration	Self-administration in the outpatient or hospital setting was examined in assessments 1 and 2 and determined to be feasible. At a 3rd assessment 3 months after the 2nd assessment, self-administration at the hospital, telephone interview, and mailed questionnaire modes of administration were compared with respect to test-retest reliability. No significant systematic differences across the 3 modes were detected. There were comparable intraclass correlation coefficients for the CR38 scales for the mail and telephone administration modes.[38]
Validated translations/cultural adaptations	CR38: Chinese, Chinese Taiwanese, Danish, Dutch, English, French, German, Italian, Norwegian, and Spanish. Finnish, Hungarian, Portuguese Brazilian, Romanian, Slovenian, and Swedish translations are in process.[38,99] Contact Karen West, Translation Coordinator: (kwe@eortc.be) or the EORTC website (http://www.eortc.be/home/qol/QLUactivities.htm) for information on available modules and translations.
Evidence of reliability (internal consistency, test-retest, other)	Sprangers et al.[38] reported coefficient alphas prior to treatment and during treatment (last day of 1st course of RT or 1st day of a subsequent cycle of chemotherapy). The following coefficient alphas were reported for multi-item scales for 2 time points and for all scales for test-retest reliability: body image scale (time 1 = .78, time 2 = .79, test-retest = .84); sexual function scale (time 1 = .86, time 2 = .87, test-retest = .92); sexual enjoyment (test-retest = .82); future perspective (test-retest = .53); micturition problems (time 1 = .63, time 2 = .72, test-retest = .79); gastrointestinal tract symptoms (time 1 = .61, time 2 = .49, test-retest = .78); chemotherapy side-effects (time 1 = .47, time 2 = .63, test-retest = .90); defecation problems (time 1 = .74, time 2 = .79, test-retest = .79); stoma-related problems (time 1 = .76, time 2 = .82, test-retest = .83); male sexual problems (time 1 = .83, time 2 = .91, test-retest = .79); female sexual problems (time 1 = .38, time 2 = .88, test-retest = .89); weight loss (test-retest = .55).

(cont.)

Table 8.1. (*cont.*)

Name of Questionnaire	European Organization for Research and Treatment of Cancer (EORTC) Quality of Life Questionnaire-Core 30 (QLQ-C30)[8,33,34] Colorectal Cancer-Specific Module (CR38)[36,38,39]
Evidence of validity (content, construct, criterion-related)	All data from Sprangers *et al.*[38] *Descriptive statistics*: Most CR38 subscales demonstrated the full range of possible scores and were reasonably symmetrical, but the body image scale was positively skewed. The symptom scales also showed good score range, but less normality than the function scores. The weight loss scale was negatively skewed and most of the others did not detect higher scores more indicative of severe problems. *Multitrait scaling*: With .40 as the criterion for correlation between an item and the rest of the scale items, only the chemotherapy side-effects scale totally failed this criterion at time 1, but had 67% of its items $\geq$ .40 at time 2. 60% of the items in the gastrointestinal scale correlated $\geq$ .4 at time 1, but the percentage dropped to 20% during treatment. Item discriminant validity was better for the body image (both time points), sexual function (both time points), micturition problems (better for time 1), defecation problems (better for time 2), and male sexual problems (better for time 2); other scales had item discriminant percentages ranging from 0% to 67%. *Known-groups comparisons*: At baseline, metastatic disease was associated with significantly worse scores for the future perspectives scale and gastrointestinal problems than earlier stage disease; patients with metastatic disease also reported significantly more chemotherapy side effects. The authors noted that one of the chemotherapy side effect items receiving high scores, dry mouth, was also a disease-related symptom. At baseline, worse gastrointestinal problems, chemotherapy side effects, and weight loss scores were significantly associated with poorer Karnofsky performance status ($<$ 70). For the during-treatment assessment, sexual functioning, gastrointestinal problems, chemotherapy side-effect problems, defecation problems, and weight loss were significantly associated with performance status. A third known-groups examination used use/non-use of a stoma at time 2 only; body image, micturition problems, and female sexual problems were significantly worse for patients with a stoma compared to patients with intact sphincters.
Evidence of responsiveness/ sensitivity to change	Using performance status as a basis for determining improvement, stability, and deterioration between baseline and during treatment assessment, there were significant changes in the future perspective, weight loss, micturition problems, and chemotherapy side effects scales. Treatment group (radiotherapy vs. chemotherapy) differences between baseline and the second assessment during treatment showed significant change for defecation problems, micturition problems, gastrointestinal problems; these changes were predicted to be worse for the radiotherapy group and were in the direction hypothesized. In addition, patients receiving radiotherapy reported significantly worse body image. The chemotherapy side effects scale did not detect significantly worse side effects for patients receiving chemotherapy, but there were only 3 patients in the chemotherapy treatment group.[38]
Interpretability (availability of normative data, clinically meaningful difference)	One problem was the inability of the chemotherapy side effects scale to detect chemotherapy-related change. The authors noted that three items might not be sufficient to address the scope of problems associated with chemotherapy. Although this scale and others of the set of symptom scales demonstrated less than desired levels of psychometric properties, the authors noted that a combination of the items based on clinical rationale can be defended (i.e., important to monitor from a clinical perspective) even in the face of less than desired psychometric properties. Given the recent development of this module, there are no published data re: clinical significance of score changes.[38]

Table 8.1. (*cont.*)

Name of Questionnaire	Functional Assessment of Chronic Illness Therapy (FACIT) Measurement System:[40,41] Colorectal Module (FACT -C) to be used with Functional Assessment of Cancer Therapy – General (FACT-G)[42,43]
Purpose for which developed	The colorectal module was developed to use with the FACT-G to measure the quality of life of patients with colorectal cancer. "It was designed for use in the research and clinical setting with colorectal cancer patients at all stages of the disease, and can be used to assess treatment effectiveness, compare/contrast QOL with other cancer groups (using the general subscales), and assess sensitivity of QOL to treatment effects and worsening physical condition" (p. 182).[42]
Length	34 items: 27 items from the FACT-G and 7 items from the colorectal cancer module
Administration time	FACT-C takes 5 to 10 minutes to complete when self-administered.
Domains included	FACT-G: Physical Well-being (7 items); Social/Family Well-being (7 items); Emotional Well-Being (6 items); Functional Well-Being (7 items) FACT-C: 4 domains in FACT-G; Additional Concerns/Colorectal Cancer Subscale (7 items)/Colorectal Cancer Subscale with 9 items (1 yes/no ostomy item + 2 items re: ostomy rated on "0" to "4" scale) TOI-PFC: Trial Outcome Index for Physical Well-Being, Functional Well-Being, and Colorectal Cancer Subscale (CCS) Time frame: Past 7 days
Scoring	5-point Likert scale (not at all, a little bit, somewhat, quite a bit, very much). 3 types of scores are provided for the 5 subscales, FACT-G, FACT-C, and TOI-PFC. Some items require reversal for scoring and all within a subscale or across all scales in FACT-G, FACT-C, and TOI-PFC are summed. The Manual provides a prorating procedure for handling missing items within scales. Standardized scores on a 0 to 100 scale are based on the Rasch rating scale model, with "0" reflecting the worst HRQOL and "100" reflecting the best HRQOL.
Validated modes of administration	Primary mode of administration is self-administration but can also be administered by interview.[41]
Validated translations/cultural adaptations	Translations of the FACT-C exist for Chinese-Traditional, Chinese-Simplified, Croatian, Czech, Danish, Dutch, English, Finnish, French, German, Greek, Hungarian, Italian, Japanese, Korean, Norwegian, Polish, Russian, Slovak, Spanish, Swedish and Tai. The translation and validation process is ongoing.[41,42] Contact Sonya Eremenco (s-eremenco@nwu.edu) or the FACIT website (www.facit.org) for updated information.
Evidence of reliability (internal consistency, test-retest, other)	Data from Cella, 1997[41] and Ward *et al.*, 1999[42] *Advanced CRC Patient Sample* (n = 60). Coefficient alpha reliability: Physical Well-Being (.80); Social/Family Well-Being (.71); Emotional Well-Being (.75); Functional Well-Being (.79); FACT-G (.88); Colorectal Cancer Subscale/7 items (.76); FACT-C total score (.91); TOI-PFC (.89). *English Sample with* CRC, *Mixed Stages* (n = 63): Physical Well-Being (.76); Social/Family Well-Being (.56); Emotional Well-Being (.63); Functional Well-Being (.82); FACT-G (.84); Colorectal Cancer Subscale/7 items (.63); FACT-C total score (.87); TOI-PFC (.87). *Spanish Sample with* CRC, *Mixed Stages* (n = 93): Physical Well-Being (.80); Social/Family Well-Being (.56); Emotional Well-Being (.64); Functional Well-Being (.86); FACT-G (.89); Colorectal Cancer Subscale/7 items (.62); FACT-C total score (.88); Trial Outcome Index for Physical Well-Being, Functional Well-Being, and Colorectal Cancer Subscale (TOI-PFC) (.87). *Spanish Sample with Ostomy Appliance, Mixed Stages* (n = 29/93): Physical Well-Being (.71); Social/Family Well-Being (.56); Emotional Well-Being (.56); Functional Well-Being (.84); FACT-G (.86); Colorectal Cancer Subscale/7 items (.47); Colorectal Cancer Subscale/9 items [2 ostomy items] (.61); FACT-C total score (.85); Trial Outcome Index for Physical Well-Being, Functional Well-Being, and Colorectal Cancer Subscale (TOI-PFC) (.81).

(*cont.*)

Table 8.1. (*cont.*)

Name of Questionnaire	Functional Assessment of Chronic Illness Therapy (FACIT) Measurement System:[40,41] Colorectal Module (FACT -C) to be used with Functional Assessment of Cancer Therapy – General (FACT-G)[42,43]
Evidence of validity (content, construct, criterion-related)	Data from Cella, 1997[41] and Ward *et al.*, 1999[42] *Convergent and divergent validity*: Interscale correlations and FACT-C correlations with POMS in expected directions. [42] *Known groups*: FACT-C discriminated groups of patients based on performance status and extent of disease in expected directions (differences were more consistently significant for Spanish samples).
Evidence of responsiveness/ sensitivity to change	Advanced disease CRC sample: Significant overall (MANOVA, p = .001) change in FACT subscales based on change in performance status categories (patient ratings) of worse vs. same/better. Univariate analyses for all subscales and total scores (FACT-G, FACT-C, TOI-PFC) significant for all except the Colorectal Cancer Subscale disease module (p = .609). Spanish CRC sample: Significant overall (MANOVA, p = .003) change in FACT subscales based on change in 3 performance status categories (patient ratings) of worse vs. same vs. improved. Univariate analyses for all subscales and total scores (FACT-G, FACT-C, TOI-PFC) significant for all except the Emotional Well-being subscale (p = .407).[42]
Interpretability (availability of normative data, clinically meaningful difference)	Effect sizes (both standardized mean difference and standardized response mean) calculated for advanced-stage disease CRC patients for 2 performance status categories, worse vs. same/better.[41,42] Authors suggest use of 9-item Colorectal Cancer Subscale because its measurement properties were similar to those of the 7-item module, and it is important to be able to describe HRQOL for patients with and without ostomy appliances.[42]

Subscale (CCS) module comprise the total score for the FACT-C.[42] The FACT-G's CCS module includes questions that are less chemotherapy specific; therefore, it appears to be a reasonable measure for colorectal cancer patients in general. Given its seven-item length, its sensitivity to the impacts of chemotherapy and surgery remains to be documented. The nine-item version of the CCS includes two items addressing care of and embarrassment about an ostomy appliance. Internal consistency reliability improved for the CCS when the nine-item version was used with patients who had ostomy appliances (from coefficient alpha of .47 to .61).[42]

Courneya *et al.*[43] examined colorectal survivors before, during, and after treatment; these data showed the sensitivity of FACT subscales to the cancer and treatment experience and associations with exercise behavior. FACT-C scores were significantly lower for the functional and CCS subscales relative to the other FACT subscales. Patients who had been regular exercisers, but who stopped exercise during

and after treatment, reported the lowest HRQOL scores.[43] Both the EORTC CR38 and the FACT-C appear promising for measuring HRQOL in patients with CRC, but their value as outcomes measures in clinical studies has yet to be demonstrated. In general, there is insufficient information to judge to what extent these disease-specific instruments can successfully capture the social and functional implications of symptoms such as diarrhea, incontinence, fear of odors, and having an ostomy that subgroups of colorectal cancer patients may experience. The importance of these symptoms and their impact on general functioning was raised in the CRC focus groups conducted as part of this Working Group project (see below).

HRQOL measurement issues

The questionnaires used in the studies reviewed for this paper vary in terms of validity, reliability, and responsiveness. Papers documenting the measurement properties of the two CRC modules highlighted in this chapter have only recently appeared in the literature, and properties such as responsiveness are not well studied at this time. Although general cancer instruments allow comparisons of the HRQOL of CRC patients with that of patients treated for other cancers (e.g., lung, breast, prostate), the results from the CRC-specific measures may provide information specific to the concerns of this group of patients. Whether the CRC-specific modules improve on the information obtained with either generic health status or general cancer measures in monitoring patient status over time and evaluating patient-reported benefits associated with treatment remains to be seen.

Most studies with HRQOL outcome measures evaluated alternative chemotherapy regimens and were generally conducted in patients with advanced-stage disease. There were few studies that provided strong support for the covariance of HRQOL and clinical outcomes such as survival, disease free survival, and response. In general, the HRQOL instruments were unable to discriminate between those patients who had better versus worse clinical outcomes. When treatment arm differences were found, they usually were associated with one or two HRQOL domains and/or specific time periods. It was difficult to gauge the degree to which overall patient functioning was affected. The measures were not consistently sensitive to change over time or to known side effects of chemotherapy. However, as will be discussed below, there were serious design and analysis problems with many of these studies, such that the failure to detect impacts of treatment on HRQOL cannot be convincingly attributed to questionnaire sensitivity or to a lack of differences between the treatment regimens.

Impact of CRC treatment on HRQOL

Table 8.2 provides a summary of the most commonly used HRQOL measures and how their performance compares to the clinical measures used in the studies reviewed. The studies are categorized as mixed treatments and treatment for metastatic disease.

Mixed treatments

Eleven papers reported results of medical interventions with diverse patient groups; the samples included patients with different cancer sites, stages of disease, and treatments (primary, adjuvant, and metastatic disease treatments as well as treatments characterized as palliative). Only two studies[46,47] were clinical trials, and only 5 out of 11 included both clinical and HRQOL assessments.

Three studies used the EORTC QLQ-C30 as well as clinical indicators. In two of these studies, HRQOL and clinical measures showed similar results, and HRQOL outcomes contributed no significant new information. One study[44] suggested no differences according to treatment (sphincter-sparing surgery versus the standard procedure, abdominoperineal resection) in either clinical or HRQOL outcomes, but the sample size, particularly for the HRQOL measures, was very small. A randomized study[46] found no differences between arms for either physician-rated toxicity measures or HRQOL, and HRQOL did not change over time. The third study[48] found that HRQOL covaried with stage of disease and cancer site categories as expected. However, patient-reported outcomes provided additional information about treatment effects by suggesting that, although the addition of preoperative radiation therapy reduced physical and role function, some HRQOL domains improved over time. In this study, HRQOL data enhanced the clinical findings.

Two studies used the Nottingham Health Profile[12,49] to examine impacts of surgery on HRQOL. Whynes et al.[49] reported only HRQOL outcomes, and found that two symptoms predicted early versus late stage disease. Renner et al.[12] included both physician- and patient-rated measures of continence. Findings indicated more incontinence and lower subjective quality of health for the coloanal anastomosis (CAA) group, compared to the other two surgery groups. The HRQOL data led the authors to conclude that while sphincter

Table 8.2. Treatment and disease stage by HRQOL and clinical assessments

Phase of Study	# Studies	Most Commonly Used Patient-Reported Outcome Measures	Most Commonly Used Clinical Measures (# Studies)	Key Observations and Comments on the Value Provided by Patient-Oriented Outcomes
Mixed Treatment: Primary, Adjuvant, Metastatic/ Palliative	11	*EORTC QLQ-C30*[8] Study Citations[44,46,48] *Nottingham Health Profile*[25-27] Study Citations[12,49] *Others* (6): * *Quality of Life Index-Radiation Therapy (QLI-RT)*[51] Study citation[51] * *Functional Assessment of Cancer Therapy-General (FACT-G)*[40] Study citation[52] * *Profile of Mood States (POMS)*[28,29] * *Beck Depression Inventory (BDI)*[100] * *Enforced Social Dependency*[101,102] Study citation[50] * *Linear Analogue Self-Assessment (LASA)*[103,104] Study citation[47] * *SF-36*[54,105-107] Study citation[53] * *Health Index*[14,55] * *Symptom Checklist*[13] * *Sense of Coherence [SOC] Scale*[56] Study-specific Questionnaire, multi-item visual analogue scale using VAS format[14] Single-item VAS measure of general health[14] Study citation[14]	Toxicity (2) Survival/recurrence (6) Disease free survival (1) Confirmation of disease status (2) Surgeries performed (2) Symptoms and complications (2) No clinical measures (6)	Mixed Treatments: 11 studies included patients with different cancer sites, or different stage of disease, and/or different treatments (primary, adjuvant, treatment for metastatic disease, or palliative). All of these studies used a multi-dimensional measure. Five studies reported both clinical and patient reported outcome measures. Six described only patient reported outcomes.[14,47-48,50-52] Two studies were randomized[46,47] while nine were not.[12,14,44,48-53] Six studies examined the effect of surgery on HRQOL.[12,14,44,48-50] These studies found no differences or minimal effects of surgery on HRQOL, with both improvements and deterioration reported. Three additional non-randomized studies found minimal effects of CRC treatment on patient HRQOL or minimal differences between CRC patients and other groups.[51-53] Many studies had small sample sizes and substantial loss to follow-up.
Treatment for Metastatic Disease	29	*Rotterdam Symptom Checklist*[17,18,19,20] Study citations[61,72-77] *Spitzer Quality of Life Index*[21] Study citations[79,80]	Overall survival (29) Progression free survival/time to progression (21)	29 studies included HRQOL measures in the treatment for metastatic disease; all studies also included overall survival. Thirteen of the 24 randomized trials for advanced-stage disease found no

Table 8.2. (*cont.*)

Phase of Study	# Studies	Most Commonly Used Patient-Reported Outcome Measures (# Studies)	Most Commonly Used Clinical Measures (# Studies)	Key Observations and Comments on the Value Provided by Patient-Oriented Outcomes
		Functional Living Index[15,16] Study citations[81–83] *EORTC QLQ-C30*[8,33,34] Study citations[57–59,62–71] *Hospital Anxiety and Depression Scale*[24] Study citations[61,72,73,75,76] *Sickness Impact Profile*[30,31] Study citations[61,73,75] *EuroQoL*[22,23] Study citations[71,74] *Others*(3): * *LASA*[103,104] Study citation[78]	Survival with good or bad HRQOL (6) Response/size of metastases (30) Complications and toxicities (18)	significant HRQOL differences between treatment arms. Eleven of the 24 trials reported at least one significant treatment arm difference in a HRQOL outcome, often at one of the earlier time points during the assessment schedule.
			Quality adjusted life years (1) Performance status (1) Others (4) LASA[103,104] Study citation[78] Quality of Life Questionnaire (Interview)[10]/Psychosocial Well-being Scale[9,10] Study citation[61] Southwest Oncology Group Quality of Life Questionnaire[86,87] Study citation[87] Multi-Attribute Health Status (MAHS) Classification[88] Study citation[60]	Five non-randomized studies were conducted in patients with advanced-stage CRC: two small studies (n = 35 and n = 26) reported no significant differences;[57,58] another (n = 44) reported no change in HRQOL scores over the treatment period;[59] one (n = 80) noted HRQOL improvement with disease stabilization and HRQOL deterioration with disease progression[60] and in the fifth study (n = 35), the Sickness Impact Profile compared to the Rotterdam Symptom Checklist and the Hospital Anxiety and Depression Scale detected much more deterioration in one treatment arm.[61]

salvage techniques such as the CAA procedure could substitute for a permanent colostomy, this technique was not free of fecal incontinence problems and negative effects that translated into perceived poor health status. In these reports, the HRQOL outcomes enhanced the clinical findings.

Findings from six studies were somewhat difficult to synthesize since they failed to include clinical outcomes or utilized less common patient-reported outcome measures. One study[51] used a disease-specific measure for patients who were undergoing radiation therapy for CRC versus other cancers. Findings indicated that HRQOL was similar across disease groups, and that a small decrement in HRQOL at week three returned to baseline by the end of follow-up. One study used the FACT-G[52] and found no significant changes in pre- and post-treatment assessments for any of the four FACT-G functional scales. Barsevick et al.[50] used three measures to examine pre- and post-operative HRQOL and found that depressive symptoms, having an ostomy, and adjuvant treatment predicted functional dependence at three months post-operatively. The authors suggested that patient-report measures provided a useful method for detecting depression both pre-treatment and pre-discharge.

Findings from Bernhard et al.[47] supported a "re-framing effect." Specifically, HRQOL ratings were lower pre-operatively than post-operatively, and also before toxic adjuvant therapy than during treatment. These findings suggest that patient perceptions of what was meant by "good HRQOL" changed over the course of their experience with cancer treatment. Findings from Anthony et al.[53] also supported "reframing." In this study, the SF-36 Physical Component and Health Perception scores favored two groups[54] of CRC patients (both treated with surgery, one group receiving adjuvant treatment as well), when compared to patients treated surgically for benign colonic disease. Forsberg et al.[14] used four HRQOL scales to describe the HRQOL of patients receiving surgery for rectal, colon, or stomach cancer pre- and post-surgery. Patients reported improvements in pain and bowel symptoms, but said their sleep, energy, and mobility deteriorated post-surgery. These investigators felt that two of the four scales, Health Index[55] and Sense of Coherence Scale,[56] were particularly useful in screening patients for potential adjustment problems and preparing nursing care plans.

Treatment for metastatic disease

Twenty-nine studies evaluated treatment for advanced-stage CRC. Of the 29 studies, 13 used the EORTC QLQ-C30,[8] seven the RSCL,[19] and five the HADS.[24] Thirteen of the 24 randomized trials for advanced-stage disease found no significant HRQOL differences between treatment arms. Eleven of 24 trials reported at least one significant treatment arm difference in a HRQOL outcome, often at one of the earlier time points in the assessment schedule. Five non-randomized studies were reported: two studies (N = 35 and N = 26) reported no significant differences;[57,58] another (N = 44) reported no change in HRQOL scores over the treatment period;[59] one study (N = 80) noted HRQOL improvement with disease stabilization and HRQOL deterioration with disease progression;[60] and in the fifth study (N = 35), the SIP, compared to the RSCL and the HADS, was able to detect patient deterioration over the survival period.[61]

Thirteen studies (three non-randomized) used the EORTC QLQ-C30. In 12 of these studies,[57–59,62–70] the HRQOL data were consistent with the clinical data, usually because there was no significant decrease in HRQOL and/or the treatment arms did not differ with respect to HRQOL. The authors viewed no difference in HRQOL as support for equivalence, and no significant deterioration as support for a patient benefit (i.e., new treatment does no harm). In six studies,[57–59,62,66,67] patient-reported outcomes were consistent with the finding of either no clinical benefit or marginal clinical support for the experimental treatment. In three studies,[63,67,70] the patient-reported outcomes enhanced the clinical outcomes. In the remaining studies, conclusions were based on clinical outcomes. The paper by Norum et al.[71] was difficult to compare with other studies using the QLQ-C30 because it was a cost-effectiveness study. The authors concluded that, considering HRQOL data, adjuvant chemotherapy for CRC was cost-effective only if the improvement in 5-year survival conferred by the new treatment was at least 5%.

All seven studies that used the RSCL[61,72-77] reported HRQOL results that were consistent with the clinical results. In only one trial did both these results not support the experimental arm;[76] in this study, IFNα did not improve clinical parameters and negatively affected HRQOL. The other six trials concluded that the HRQOL data provided support for the new therapies because the new treatments sustained HRQOL over time, and/or HRQOL did not significantly differ for the compared regimens. Fordy et al.[61] noted that the finding of better HRQOL data reported by two other studies[72,75] suggested that earlier hepatic arterial floxuridine infusion (HAI) treatment allowed for both better survival and more sustained HRQOL. An example of non-consistent effects on HRQOL was reported in a comparison of 5-FU + folinic acid (FU-FA) versus continuous infusion 5-FU alone (FUcont); patients on the FUcont arm reported significantly better global HRQOL at four months, but not at two or six months.[78] In a trial comparing 5-FU versus irinotecan, patients receiving irinotecan took significantly longer to have a 50% decrease in the global EORTC QLQ-C30 score (i.e., a worsening of the HRQOL measure), but patients on this arm reported significantly more nausea/vomiting, diarrhea, and concern about finances than did patients on the 5-FU arm.[70] In the studies by Allen-Mersh et al.[72] and Earlam et al.,[75] the HRQOL data enhanced the conclusions of the study. In the other five studies, conclusions were generally based on clinical outcomes.

Five studies used the HADS.[61,72,73,75,76] In all studies, patient-reported outcomes and clinical outcomes were in general agreement. However, only one study reported significant differences for the HADS scores.[75] Three reports[61,72,75] found some support for clinical efficacy, but inconsistent support for better HADS depression or anxiety scores. The Fordy et al.[61] study had one arm, a small sample (N = 35), and data were presented descriptively. Another

study[73] found no differences in either clinical or HADS outcomes for the two treatment arms, while Seymour et al.[76] reported worse clinical outcomes in the experimental arm (IFNα), but no differences in HADS scores by arm. Conclusions in these studies were based on clinical outcomes.

Of the two studies that used the Spitzer Quality of Life Index, one found that both HRQOL and clinical outcomes data indicated that the experimental regimen was not efficacious.[79] The other study[80] reported on two trials, both involving Tauromustine (TCNU), with only marginal clinical benefit in one trial (time to progression); HRQOL was decreased in both studies, and the Spitzer Quality of Life Index predicted survival. The HRQOL data played a much more prominent role in all sections of the Loprinzi[79] manuscript, while the Smyth paper[80] did not provide much detail and discussion related to the HRQOL findings. The conclusions in this paper appeared to be based on the clinical outcomes.

Of the three studies that used the FLIC,[81-83] two[81,83] found that the FLIC results were consistent with clinical outcomes: there were no treatment arm differences in either clinical or FLIC outcomes. Thus, the patient-reported data did not provide additional information. However, Sullivan[83] suggested that while measures like the FLIC may not be helpful for evaluating treatment efficacy, they may be more useful in monitoring patient progress and in documenting achievement of palliation (i.e., through maintenance of stable HRQOL). Scheithauer[82] found that the chemotherapy arm led to significantly better overall survival and time to progression, but FLIC scores did not differ significantly. There were some signs of more improvement in the chemotherapy arm, but the difference was not significant. The authors concluded that chemotherapy confers a beneficial survival effect, and for symptomatic patients, a beneficial HRQOL effect. The conclusions of the study were based largely on the clinical outcomes.

Two studies used the SIP. Fordy et al.[61] found marginal support for clinical efficacy, but the study had one treatment group with a small sample size and HRQOL outcomes were presented descriptively.

In this study, the SIP detected more compromised HRQOL than the RSCL and HADS. For example, for 35 patients receiving HAI, 25 lived with significant HRQOL deficits; their SIP Profile score was abnormal for 44% of the time they survived.[61] In the second study,[75] both the chemotherapy regimen and HAI had longer survival with abnormal SIP scores when compared to the symptom control arm. The authors concluded that the two treatment arms were similar in survival but HAI had better sustained HRQOL.

Two studies used a version of the EuroQoL (EQ-5D). In one study,[74] two clinical outcomes did not differ by arm, while time to progression favored the experimental regimen (raltitrexed); three EQ-5D items favored raltitrexed early on, but found no differences over time. Therefore, in general, clinical and EQ-5D outcomes were consistent in not showing superiority for the experimental regimen. In this study, the negative early EQ-5D results for the comparator arm were consistent with the RSCL and toxicity findings. The authors concluded the two regimens had comparable clinical and HRQOL outcomes, and that the convenience associated with administration of raltitrexed supported its future use. In the second study,[71] clinical outcomes were not reported. Since this was a decision analytic model, it was not possible to evaluate the degree to which clinical and HRQOL findings were consistent.

Finally, four studies[60,78,84–86] used a HRQOL measure not reported in any of the other studies reviewed here. Caudry et al.[78] found a significant transient improvement in HRQOL using the Linear Analogue Assessment Scale, favoring continuous infusion of 5-FU over 5-FU combined with folinic acid; otherwise, the two arms did not differ. The study demonstrated clinical benefit for the continuous infusion arm, and the authors noted HRQOL was preserved with this regimen (i.e., not worsened). Glimelius et al.[84] used a psychosocial well being scale[9] and a quality-of-life interview.[10] Clinical outcomes did not differ, and HRQOL was reported in terms of patient improvement, stability, and deterioration, using a criterion of 20% change. Whether there were HRQOL differences by treatment arm was not clear from the published report. Leichman et al.[85] summarized the clinical findings for a seven-arm trial in which there were no significant clinical differences, but two arms with better survival times were selected for a follow-up trial; HRQOL data were reported separately.[86] HRQOL information from the seven-arm trial did not influence this decision because substantial missing HRQOL data complicated and delayed analysis of these data; longitudinal analyses were considered inappropriate.[86] The Southwest Oncology Group Quality of Life Questionnaire was used to measure patient-reported outcomes.[86,87] A study by Henry et al.[60] used the Multiattribute Health Status (MAHS)[88] classification (which later became known as the Health Utilities Index) in a non-randomized trial for second line chemotherapy of any type. Five health states were defined using clinical measures. MAHS scores were similar for responders and stable patients, but scores were worse for patients who deteriorated. The HRQOL measure correlated with disease state and response to treatment.

Across this body of literature, HRQOL conclusions should be qualified because of a number of methodological weaknesses in many of the studies. These include: (1) severe missing data problems in follow-up assessments, such as insufficient information about follow-up sample sizes, inappropriate analysis, and thus compromised conclusions regarding HRQOL stability;[70,81,83] (2) insufficient presentation and discussion of HRQOL findings;[59,73,77,80,81] (3) comparison of regimens from different treatment trials;[75] and (4) small or less than ideal sample size.[44,61,72–75,77,82]

Qualitative findings

To support the COMWG review project, focus groups were conducted with cancer patients and survivors.[89] However, only two patients with colorectal cancer currently undergoing treatment for their disease participated in the single focus group addressing impacts of CRC treatment on patient HRQOL. Both of these patients were female and were receiving chemotherapy treatment, steroids, and antidepressant medications at the time of the focus groups; one has a colostomy. The impact of treatment mentioned by the two women is described below; however, due to small numbers, only personal narration of possible treatment impacts can be provided.

The two women reported that their physical functioning (particularly fatigue) was affected during treatment; they also noted problems with memory (referring to "chemo brain"). Emotional functioning issues were mentioned, as well; their need for antidepressant medications provides evidence of problems in this HRQOL domain. The women mentioned impacts on their social functioning, although both were very active in multiple support groups, attending these meetings frequently. Changes in the dynamics of relationships with family and friends presented real concerns; the woman with a colostomy faced more physical problems that embarrassed her and limited her social activities.

Sixteen survivors of CRC participated in two groups (nine women in one group and seven men in the other). Although these individuals were not currently undergoing treatment for CRC, they reported long-term dietary problems and limitations on social functioning associated with surgery. Survivor HRQOL is described in more detail in the Zebrack and Cella chapter in this volume.[90] It remains to be seen whether the social dysfunction reported by these survivors can be documented for patients undergoing treatment and for those in the early post-treatment phase of recovery.

Discussion

Value-added provided by inclusion of HRQOL outcomes

This review of the use of HRQOL outcome measures in randomized and non-randomized studies of the treatment of CRC might suggest that HRQOL measures added very little to the information provided by clinical measures in these studies. The vast majority of studies found little change over time in HRQOL and minimal differences in HRQOL based on CRC treatment received. Investigators reported

such results as positive, noting that the new treatment maintained HRQOL and/or was equivalent to that reported for standard therapy. Several studies did report either significant effects of treatment for CRC on HRQOL[63,64,76] or change over time in both arms.[83] One study showed time to deterioration in global HRQOL significantly favored the irinotecan arm, but also reported significantly worse symptom scores for this arm.[70] HRQOL data were often not presented in detail or, in some cases, not at all. An example of the latter was the study by Smyth *et al.*,[80] which noted ". . . a more profound decrease in the index [Spitzer QL-Index] in the TCNU treated patients than in either of the reference groups" (pp. 948–49). However, no data were presented to support this summary of results.

It would be premature to conclude that HRQOL outcomes tend to remain stable over time or show minimal effects of treatment, because many of the studies were flawed in two related ways. First, initial sample sizes were quite small, leading to reduced power to detect HRQOL effects should they exist. Second, the authors usually failed to note the extent of drop-out they observed in submission of HRQOL questionnaires over time. These design and reporting problems affect conclusions that can be drawn from the HRQOL data, particularly when the studies are evaluating the treatment for patients with advanced-stage disease. Non-ignorable missing data are usually associated with a bias in favor of the remaining patients, who are generally healthier. This type of bias occurs for advanced disease when the reason for missing data is associated with the outcome of interest (i.e., HRQOL status).[91] The authors of a randomized trial who reported their HRQOL findings for an advanced-stage CRC randomized trial addressed this problem explicitly;[86] longitudinal analyses were rejected because of the bias created by substantial missing data.

The authors of most of the CRC studies reviewed for this chapter did not report how many forms were missing at follow-up assessments and did not examine the extent to which these forms were missing due to death or deteriorating health status. In the context of substantial non-ignorable missing data, it becomes impossible to interpret the HRQOL findings unless they have been analyzed with techniques designed to account (in some way) for non-ignorable missing data; pattern mixture models represent one such technique.[92]

Investigators who want to include HRQOL outcome measures in CRC studies should examine and report the extent of missing data and the reasons for such missing data. If the treatment study is to be conducted with advanced-stage disease patients, it is critical for clinicians to involve a statistician familiar with techniques to examine longitudinal HRQOL data where missing follow-up forms are expected. For more information on issues related to missing data, see Chapter 17 by Fairclough in this volume.[93]

Performance of the HRQOL measures: relative strengths and weaknesses

A critique of HRQOL questionnaires is not meaningful if it occurs in isolation from the missing data problem just discussed. If sample sizes are small to begin with and there are poor submission rates for follow-up assessments, even questionnaires with stellar measurement properties will fail to detect treatment arm differences and change over time. The EORTC QLQ-C30 (core)[8] HRQOL questionnaire was used the most frequently in the studies reviewed for this paper, but this general cancer instrument was not particularly better than other questionnaires at detecting significant treatment arm differences or change over time. We also cannot conclude that generic measures were less sensitive than cancer-specific measures since the SIP,[30,31] a generic, non-cancer measure, performed better than the RSCL,[19] a general cancer measure, in one study[61] and detected significant positive differences for one treatment arm in another study.[75] Many HRQOL researchers believe that the current pool of questionnaires is sufficient for evaluating the effects of cancer treatment. Development and validation of a new questionnaire is a lengthy and resource-intensive process. However, more experience with the newly developed CRC-specific measures[38,42] is required to evaluate

the value of their targeted symptom assessment for measuring the impact of CRC treatment on patient HRQOL.

Sprangers et al.[94] reviewed the literature for studies of HRQOL in patients with and without a stoma. Both groups of patients were concerned about the frequency of bowel movements, but stoma patients, compared to non-stoma patients, reported more restrictions of social activities post-treatment, more emotional distress, and more sexual function problems. Sprangers et al.[94] suggested the importance of including HRQOL measures in trials comparing colostomy versus ultralow anastomosis.

Our review found one study that suggested no differences in HRQOL between those with sphincter-preserving surgery and those with colostomy.[44] However, another study reported that those who had coloanal anastomosis had lower HRQOL scores than those with an anterior resection,[12] and another study found that having an ostomy predicted dependency at three months post-operatively.[50]

No studies in this review, particularly those involving surgical treatment, reported significant group-related or change-over-time impacts of treatment on social functioning. The reports of compromised social function from two women who were currently receiving CRC treatment, along with insights provided by the Sprangers et al.[94] review, suggest that current HRQOL measures may not be sufficiently sensitive to impacts of treatment on social function. Perhaps there is a need for a re-evaluation of social function subscales of existing questionnaires and new methods research for this HRQOL domain. See reviews by Sprangers[36] for additional summaries of assessing HRQOL in CRC studies, and Camilleri-Brennan and Steele[95] regarding the impact of treatment for rectal cancer on HRQOL.

Wils et al.[96] discussed the distinction between HRQOL measures to detect improvement in patient status when treated with first-line regimens for metastatic disease versus detection of stability and delay in HRQOL deterioration. These two contexts could define strategies for patient follow-up with monitoring for late effects, and they suggested identifying "signal" symptoms such as pain, performance status, or weight. We might add the more global HRQOL domain of social functioning to a set of "signal" outcomes, as well as fatigue and patient-reported treatment-related side effects. Wils *et al.*[96] noted that current questionnaires used in CRC trials (and described in this paper) have tended to find minimal differences in HRQOL by treatment arm. They suggest that the availability of CRC modules for measures such as the QLQ-C30[8] and the FACT-G[40] may increase the sensitivity of these questionnaires for detecting important differences among individuals with different stages of disease who undergo different types of treatment (surgery with curative intent, palliative chemotherapy, and radiation therapy).

Other investigators have addressed criteria such as stability and time to deterioration in HRQOL when determining patient benefit.[97,98] A number of studies included in Table 8.2 concluded that the intervention of interest was associated with a patient benefit because the intervention did not cause a deterioration of patient HRQOL relative to the comparator regimen. HRQOL measures offer a number of ways of documenting such criteria.

Finally, these clinical papers rarely discussed or presented evidence in support of the psychometric properties of the HRQOL measures they selected. Many of these questionnaires have documentation of validity, reliability, and responsiveness (see Table 8.1 and Chapter 3 by Erickson in this volume).[32] To interpret and apply the findings of these clinical studies appropriately, the researcher or clinician needs to have ready access to this psychometric information, either as a summary in the clinical article itself or a reference to source documents.

Clinical implications

How then can the results of this review be used in the clinical setting? Measurement of HRQOL can guide clinical decision making in the following circumstances: (1) to involve patients in their medical care decision-making, particularly when there is a choice among multiple, clinically effective strategies or when one is treating patients with asymptomatic or mildly symptomatic disease; (2) when choosing between therapies for which there is only a small difference in survival between treatments; (3) when there are trade-offs between toxicity, survival, and costs; and (4) to improve detection of psychosocial impairments in patients with medical disease.

These circumstances are encountered throughout the phases of colorectal cancer treatment. For patients with early-stage disease who will undergo surgery, results of HRQOL measurement can be used to inform individuals about the potential outcomes of surgery, including a temporary or permanent ostomy, incontinence, body odors, change in body image, and potential isolation from friends and family. In addition, as outlined by the COMWG's focus groups, there may be substantial psychosocial effects after surgery that may require additional therapy and that may be identified by HRQOL measures. For those with advanced disease who will require adjuvant chemotherapy, results of HRQOL measures from clinical trials of the various agents can be used to inform individuals about potential side effects including hair loss, weight loss, neuropathy, and others. In the adjuvant setting, the trade-offs between survival and toxicity may be primary concerns, or there may be multiple clinically effective agents, and information about their effects on HRQOL can guide clinical decisions. For those with metastatic disease, the decision about whether to undergo chemotherapy may be influenced by the toxicities and their effects on HRQOL.

In addition, the integration of HRQOL measures into planned and existing clinical trials provides the opportunity to inform future decision-making for patients considering chemotherapy. HRQOL measures can provide information on the efficacy of interventions in other settings as well. Third-party payers typically seek information from randomized controlled trials to assist in decisions regarding coverage and benefits. For agents that have an equivalent impact on survival, recurrence, or disease-free survival, differences in HRQOL outcomes can aid the payer in choosing between alternative regimens. The payer can also use information on HRQOL as a "benchmark" to track patient outcomes and the quality of care provided, given the known outcomes from clinical trials.

The HRQOL instruments discussed in this chapter are primarily general cancer measures.[8,15,19,24] They have been used in a variety of settings but have been primarily applied in the setting of clinical trials of chemotherapeutic agents for advanced or metastatic disease. From a clinical perspective, most of these instruments are short, with completion times of 10–12 minutes and, in general, can be completed by the patient without assistance. Exceptions are the SIP,[30,31] requiring about 20–30 minutes to complete, and the FLIC's[15,16] modified linear analog scale that may be difficult for some patients. These general cancer measures provide a broad overview of physical, role, cognitive, social, and emotional function, and general quality of life. The results can be used to compare the quality of life of colorectal cancer patients with the quality of life of patients with other cancers.

The limitation of the general cancer measures is that they might not capture the specific concerns of colorectal cancer patients outlined above. Specifically, they do not address issues of incontinence, body odor, or changes in appetite and bowel habits that occur as a result of surgery and/or chemotherapy or radiation therapy. The two newer measures, the EORTC QLQ-C30 CR38[38] and the FACT-C,[42] are instruments that contain a general cancer component but have colorectal cancer-specific modules attached to them.

The EORTC QLQ-C30/CR38[38] addresses concerns about body image; sexual function; symptoms related to the urinary tract; specific gastrointestinal symptoms such as abdominal pain, belching, flatulence, incontinence, diarrhea, and constipation; and specific concerns for patients with ostomies including fear of noise, odor, leakage, and changes in body image related to having a stoma. In addition, there are specific questions about chemotherapy-related side effects for those undergoing this therapy. Although this measure appears to capture the many concerns of colorectal cancer patients, it has been used widely only in the last two years, and its

role in clinical decision-making across all phases of colorectal cancer care is yet to be determined.

The FACT-C,[42] the colorectal cancer module of the general FACT, addresses specific concerns of colorectal cancer patients, including abdominal symptoms, appetite and digestion, incontinence, weight loss, and ostomy-related issues. There are no chemotherapy-specific questions in this instrument, but the questions appear to address the major concerns of colorectal cancer patients and of the colorectal cancer survivors from the NCI-sponsored focus group. The FACT-C also shows promise as an overall measure of HRQOL of colorectal cancer patients, but it, like the EORTC QLQ-C30/CR38, has been recently released, and information on its performance in the clinical setting is limited.

How can the information on the results of HRQOL measurement in CRC patients in the clinical situations outlined above be used? For patients with early-stage disease, there are few data on HRQOL. This review identified a total of six studies related to surgery[14,44,48–51] and found two studies reporting either no differences in HRQOL based on surgery type or conflicting results, with the remaining four studies showing a mix of improvement and deterioration depending on the HRQOL domain. Thus, there is little HRQOL information upon which to base discussions of potential outcomes when advising patients who will undergo surgery. This phase of care, primary treatment, is the area of colorectal cancer treatment about which the least is known. Ironically, it is these patients who live the longest and, as the focus groups suggested, are often troubled by symptoms that are not addressed by the measures that are commonly used. There is a role for applying the colorectal cancer-specific instruments[38,42] to this group, either in randomized trials of surgical techniques (e.g., sphincter preserving surgery) or in the observational setting by following post-surgical patients over time to determine both the short- and long-term effects on HRQOL. Additional attention to symptoms that are expressed by the patient but may not be included in even the newer instruments is important, such as cognitive impairment related to chemotherapy and dietary changes necessitated by surgery and radiation therapy. Finally, the majority of the HRQOL measures have been applied to patients with advanced disease, typically those undergoing chemotherapy in the setting of randomized trials. Slightly less than half of these studies (11/24) reported at least one significant difference in treatment arms during at least one point in the study. This information suggests that, in fact, there are differences in HRQOL effects of these chemotherapeutic agents, which may be captured to a greater or lesser degree by the existing instruments. Again, there is a role for broader application of the newer, colorectal cancer-specific measures in this setting to help inform decisions for therapies which may have minimal differences in survival, or decisions about therapies for which there are therapeutic trade-offs between toxicity and survival. Careful attention to additional clinical symptoms in this group, particularly when new therapies are used and there are little data about their expected clinical effects and toxicities, is warranted.

In summary, measurement of HRQOL effects of colorectal cancer treatment is in its early phase. Although HRQOL instruments have been included in clinical trials for the past decade, the results to date may reflect the lack of specificity of the most widely used instruments, which in turn could interfere with their ability to capture concerns of patients with colorectal cancer that may have a profound impact on HRQOL. Faulty study designs have also played a role.

Recommendations and future research needs

The current HRQOL database for the impact of CRC treatment on patient functioning is still insufficient to support a departure from a more comprehensive measurement strategy that includes the basic HRQOL domains of emotional, physical, and social functioning as well as disease- and treatment-related symptoms. This need for complete coverage is partially due to design and analysis problems reflected in the previous HRQOL studies in CRC. Ideally, in the future, certain domains could be targeted for assessment in specific treatment settings because enough information would be available for certain domains in specific treatment settings. Targeted assessments would decrease both patient burden and the resources required to add the HRQOL outcomes to the trial or study. Attempts to detect improvement in status or stability in the palliative treatment context require questionnaires sensitive to change; in this context, symptom measures may be more sensitive, but that must be documented. The social function domain may well require the development of new, more sensitive measures to detect levels of discomfort expressed by CRC patients in the focus groups and observed by clinicians. Thus, the disease-specific measures, the EORTC QLQ-CR38 and the FACT-C, should be applied in patients across the disease spectrum, from early to metastatic disease, in order to identify gaps in these measures for capturing the concerns of the patients in each stage and for targeting assessments to specific groups. Particular attention should be given to developing measures that more completely address the post-operative changes that occur, for example in the area of diet, social, and sexual function.

Finally, studies should report complete sample size information at all HRQOL assessment points, and clearly define the groups under study regarding phase of care (primary, adjuvant, palliative) and the presence or absence of an ostomy. Evaluation of the reasons for missing forms in HRQOL data should be undertaken, and standardized methodology for handling missing data should be part of the statistical methods used in CRC studies.

Acknowledgments

The authors would like to acknowledge the assistance of Lauren Crowley in conducting the database search, obtaining articles, maintaining the reference list, and helping organize the studies for presentation in table format and Crystal Bernstein for abstracting the articles. We would also like to acknowledge Teresa Day for her assistance with some of the same tasks and for her preparation of this manuscript.

REFERENCES

1 National Cancer Institute. Colorectal Screening. http://www.cancer.gov/cancerinfo/pdq/screening/colorectal/healthprofessional. Last accessed September 11, 2004.

2 Mandel, J. S., Bond, J. H., Church, T. R. *et al.* (1993). Reducing mortality from colorectal cancer by screening for fecal occult blood. Minnesota Colon Cancer Control Study. *New England Journal of Medicine* **328**:1365–71.

3 Selby, J. V., Friedman, G. D., Quesenberry, Jr., C. P. *et al.* (1992). A case-control study of screening sigmoidoscopy and mortality from colorectal cancer. *New England Journal of Medicine* **326**:653–7.

4 Newcomb, P. A., Norfleet, R. G., Storer, B. E. *et al.* (1992). Screening sigmoidoscopy and colorectal cancer mortality. *Journal of the National Cancer Institute* **84**:1572–5.

5 Muller, A. D., Sonnenberg, A. (1995). Protection by endoscopy against death from colorectal cancer. *Archives of Internal Medicine* **155**:1741–8.

6 National Cancer Institute. Colon cancer treatment. http://www.cancer.gov/cancerinfo/pdq/treatment/colon. Last accessed September 11, 2004.

7 Ries, L. A. G., Eisner, M. P., Kosary, C. L. *et al.* (eds). (2002). *SEER Cancer Statistics Review, 1973–1999.* Bethesda, MD: National Cancer Institute, http://seer.cancer.gov/csr/1973_1999. Accessed September 11, 2004.

8 Aaronson, N. K., Ahmedzai, S., Bergman, B. *et al.* (1993). The European Organization for Research and Treatment of Cancer QLQ-C30: A quality-of-life instrument for use in international clinical trials in oncology. *Journal of the National Cancer Institute* **85**:365–76.

9 Kaasa, S., Mastekaasa, A., Stokke, I. *et al.* (1988). Validation of a quality of life questionnaire for use in clinical trials for treatment of patients with inoperable lung cancer. *European Journal of Cancer and Clinical Oncology* **24**:691–701.

10 Glimelius, B., Hoffman, K., Olafsdottir, M. *et al.* (1989). Quality of life during cytostatic therapy for advanced symptomatic colorectal carcinoma: a randomized comparison of two regimens. *European Journal of Cancer and Clinical Oncology* **25**:829–35.

11 Adang, E. M., Engel, G. L., Konsten, J. *et al.* (1993). Quality of life after dynamic graciloplasty for fecal incontinence: first results. *Thoracic Surgery* **8**:122–4.

12 Renner, K., Rosen, H. R., Novi, G. *et al.* (1999). Quality of life after surgery for rectal cancer: do we still need a permanent colostomy? *Diseases of the Colon and Rectum* **42**:1160–7.

13 Björvell, H., Hylander, B. (1989). Functional status and personality in patients on chronic dialysis. *Journal of Internal Medicine* **226**:319–24.

14 Forsberg, C., Bjorvell, H., Cedermark, B. (1996). Well-being and its relation to coping ability in patients with colo-rectal and gastric cancer before and after surgery. *Scandinavian Journal of Caring Science* **10**:35–44.

15 Schipper, H., Clinch, J., McMurray, A. *et al.* (1984). Measuring the quality of life of cancer patients: The Functional Living Index-Cancer: Development and validation. *Journal of Clinical Oncology* **2**:472–83.

16 Morrow, G. R., Lindke, J., Black, P. (1992). Measurement of quality of life in patients: psychometric analyses of the Functional Living Index-Cancer (FLIC). *Quality of Life Research* **1**:287–96.

17 de Haes, J. C. J. M., van Oostrom, M. A., Welvaart, K. (1986). The effect of radical and conserving surgery on the quality of life of early breast cancer patients. *European Journal of Surgical Oncology* **12**:337–42.

18 de Haes, J. C. J. M., Raatgever, J. W., van der Burg, M. E. L. *et al.* (1987). Evaluation of the quality of life of patients with advanced ovarian cancer treated with combination chemotherapy. In *The Quality of Life of Cancer Patients*, ed. N. K. Aaronson, J. Beckman, pp. 215–26. New York: Raven Press.

19 de Haes, J. C. J. M., van Knippenberg, F. C. E., Neijt, J. P. (1990). Measuring psychological and physical distress in cancer patients: structure and application of the Rotterdam Symptom Checklist. *British Journal of Cancer* **62**:1034–38.

20 de Haes, J. C. J. M., Olschewski, M. (1998). Quality of life assessment in a cross-cultural context: use of the Rotterdam Symptom Checklist in a multinational randomised trial comparing CMF and Zoladex (Goserlin) treatment in early breast cancer. *Annals of Oncology* **9**:745–50.

21 Spitzer, W. O., Dobson, A. J., Hall, J. *et al.* (1983). Measuring the quality of life of cancer patients. A concise QL- Index for use by physicians. *Journal of Chronic Disease* **34**:585–97.

22 EuroQoL Group (1990). EuroQoL – a new facility for the measurement of health-related quality of life. *Health Policy* **16**:199–208.

23 Kind, P. (1996). The EuroQoL instrument: an index of health-related quality of life. In *Quality of Life and Pharmacoeconomics in Clinical Trials* (2nd Edn), ed. B. Spilker, pp. 191–201. Philadelphia, PA: Lippincott-Raven.

24 Zigmund, A. S., Snaith, R. P. (1983). The Hospital Anxiety and Depression Scale. *Acta Psychiatrica Scandinavica* **67**:361–70.

25 Hunt, S. M., McEwen, J., McKenna, S. P. (1986). *Measuring Health Status.* London: Croom Helm.

26 Hunt, S. M., McKenna, S. P. (1991). *The Nottingham Health Profile User's Manual.* Manchester: Galen Research and Consultancy.

27 McEwen, J., McKenna, S. P. (1996). Nottingham Health Profile. In *Quality of Life and Pharmacoeconomics in Clinical Trials* (2nd Edition), ed. B. Spilker, pp. 281–86. Philadelphia, PA: Lippincott-Raven.

28 Lorr, M., McNair, D. M. (1982). *Profile of Mood States: Bi-polar Form.* San Diego: Educational and Industrial Testing Service.

29 Shacham, S. (1983). A shortened version of the Profile of Mood States. *Journal of Personality Assessment* **47**:305–6.

30 Bergner, M., Bobbitt, R. A., Carter, W. B. *et al.* (1981). The Sickness Impact Profile: development and final revision of a health status measure. *Medical Care* **19**:787–805.

31 Damiano, A. M. (1996). The Sickness Impact Profile. In *Quality of Life and Pharmacoeconomics in Clinical Trials* (2nd Edition), ed. B. Spilker, pp. 347–54. Philadelphia, PA: Lippincott-Raven.

32 Erickson, this volume, Chapter 3.

33 Fayers, P., Aaronson, N., Bjordal, K. *et al.*, on behalf of the EORTC Quality of Life Group. (2001). *EORTC QLQ-C30 Scoring Manual* (3rd Edition). Brussels: EORTC.

34 Fayers, P., Weeden, S., Curran, D. (1998). EORTC QLQ-C30 Reference Values. Brussels: EORTC Study Group on Quality of Life.

35 Sprangers, M. A., Cull, A., Bjordal, K. *et al.*, for the EORTC Study Group on Quality of Life (1993). The European Organization for Research and Treatment of Cancer approach to quality of life assessment: Guidelines for developing modules. *Quality of Life Research* **2**:287–95.

36 Sprangers, M. A. G. (1999). Quality-of-life assessment in colorectal cancer patients: evaluation of cancer therapies. *Seminars in Oncology* **26**:691–6.

37 Aaronson, N. K., Cull, A. M., Kaasa, S. *et al.* (1996). The European Organization for Research and Treatment of Cancer (EORTC) Modular Approach to Quality of Life Assessment in Oncology: An update. In *Quality of Life and Pharmacoeconomics in Clinical Trials* (2nd Edition), ed. B. Spilker, pp. 179–89. Philadelphia, PA: Lippincott-Raven.

38 Sprangers, M. A. G., te Velde, A., Aaronson, N. K. on behalf of the European Organization for Research and Treatment of Cancer Study Group on Quality of Life (1999). The construction of the EORTC colorectal cancer-specific quality of life questionnaire module (QLQ-CR38). *European Journal of Cancer* **35**:238–47.

39 Sailer, M., Debus, E. S., Fuchs, K.-H. (2000). How useful is the EORTC QLQ-CR38 in the pre- and post-operative evaluation of patients with rectal cancer? *Quality of Life Research Newsletter* **25**:13–14.

40 Cella, D. F., Tulsky, D. S., Gray, G. *et al.* (1993). The Functional Assessment of Cancer Therapy scale: development and validation of the general measure. *Journal of Clinical Oncology* **11**:570–9.

41 Cella, D. (1997). *FACIT Manual. Manual of the Functional Assessment of Chronic Illness Therapy (FACIT) Measurement System. Version 4.* Evanston, IL: Center on Outcomes, Research and Education (CORE).

42 Ward, W. L., Hahn, E. A., Mo, F. *et al.* (1999). Reliability and validity of the Functional Assessment of Cancer Therapy-Colorectal (FACT-C) quality of life instrument. *Quality of Life Research* **8**:181–95.

43 Courneya, K. S., Friedenreich, C. M. (1997). Relationship between exercise pattern across the cancer experience and current quality of life in colorectal cancer survivors. *Journal of Alternative and Complementary Medicine* **3**:215–26.

44 Allal, A. S., Bieri, S., Peloni, A. *et al.* (2002). Sphincter-sparing surgery after preoperative radiotherapy for low rectal cancers: feasibility, oncologic results and quality of life outcomes. *British Journal of Cancer* **82**:1131–7.

45 Cronbach, L. J. (1951). Coefficient alpha and the internal structure of tests. *Psychometrika* **16**:297–334.

46 Borras, J. M., Sanchez-Hernandez, A., Navarro, M. *et al.* (2001). Compliance, satisfaction, and quality of life of patients with colorectal cancer receiving home chemotherapy or outpatient treatment: a randomised controlled trial. *British Medical Journal* **322**:1–5.

47 Bernhard, J., Hürny, C., Maibach, R., Herrmann, R. *et al.*, for the Swiss Group for Clinical Cancer Research (SAKK). (1999). Quality of life as subjective experience: reframing of perception in patients with colon cancer undergoing radical resection with or without adjuvant chemotherapy. *Annals of Oncology* **10**:775–82.

48 Ulander, K., Jeppsson, B., Grahn, G. (1997). Quality of life and independence in activities of daily living preoperatively and at follow-up in patients with colorectal cancer. *Supportive Care in Cancer* **5**:402–9.

49 Whynes, D. K., Neilson, A. R. (1997). Symptoms before and after surgery for colorectal cancer. *Quality of Life Research* **6**:61–6.

50 Barsevick, A. M., Pasacreta, J., Orsi, A. (1995). Psychological distress and functional dependence in colorectal cancer patients. *Cancer Practice* **3**:105–10.

51 Padilla, G. V., Grant, M. M., Lipsett, J. *et al.* (1992). Health quality of life and colorectal cancer. *Cancer* **70**:1450–6.

52 Scieszka, M., Zielinski, M., Machalski, M. *et al.* (2000). Quality of life in cancer patients treated by chemotherapy. *Neoplasma* **47**:396–9.

53 Anthony, T., Jones, C., Antoine, J. *et al.* (2001). The effect of treatment for colorectal cancer on long-term health-related quality of life. *Annals of Surgical Oncology* **8**:44–9.

54 McHorney, C. A., Ware, Jr., J. E., Raczek, A. E. (1993). The MOS 36-item Short-Form Health Survey (SF-36): II. Psychometric and clinical tests of validity in measuring physical and mental health constructs. *Medical Care* **31**:247–63.

55 Langius, A., Björvell, H., Antonovsky, A. (1992). The Sense of Coherence concept and its relation to personality traits in Swedish samples. *Scandinavian Journal of Caring Science* **6**:165–71.

56 Antonovsky, A. (1987). *Unraveling the Mystery of Health: How People Manage Stress and Stay Well.* San Francisco, CA: Jossey-Bass Publishers.

57 Garufi, C., Brienza, S., Pugliese, P. *et al.* (2000). Overcoming resistance to chronomodulated 5-fluorouracil and folinic acid by the addition of chronomodulated oxaliplatin in advanced colorectal cancer patients. *Anticancer Drugs* **11**:495–501.

58 Garufi, C., Dogliotti, L., D'Attino, R. M. *et al.* (2001). Irinotecan and chronomodulated infusion of 5-fluorouracil and folinic acid in the treatment of patients with advanced colorectal carcinoma: a phase I study. *Cancer* **91**:712–20.

59 Hauns, B., Häring, B., Köhler, S. *et al.* (2001). Phase II study of combined 5 fluorouracil/*Ginkgo biloba* extract (GBE 761 ONC) therapy in 5-fluorouracil pretreated patients with advanced colorectal cancer. *Phytotherapy Research* **15**:34–8.

60 Henry, B., Becouarn, Y., Aussage, P. (1999). Clinical benefits of stabilization with second line chemotherapy in patients with metastatic colorectal cancer. *Oncology Hematology* **32**:145–54.

61 Fordy, C., Glover, C., Davies, M. M. *et al.* (1998). Hepatic arterial floxuridine as second-line treatment for systemic fluorouracil-resistant colorectal liver metastases. *British Journal of Cancer* **78**:1058–60.

62 Cunningham, D., Zalcberg, J. R., Rath, U. *et al.* (1996). Final results of a randomised trial comparing 'Tomudex' (raltitrexed) with 5-fluorouracil plus leucovorin in advanced colorectal cancer. "Tomudex" Colorectal Cancer Study Group. *Annals of Oncology* **7**:961–5.

63 Cunningham, D., Glimelius, B. on behalf of the V301 Study Group. (1999). A phase III study of irinotecan (CPT-11) versus best supportive care in patients with metastatic colorectal cancer who have failed 5-fluorouracil therapy. V301 Study Group. *Seminars in Oncology* **26**:6–12.

64 de Gramont, A., Figer, A., Seymour, M. *et al.* (2000). Leucovorin and fluorouracil with or without oxaliplatin as first-line treatment in advanced colorectal cancer. *Journal of Clinical Oncology* **18**:2938–47.

65 Douillard, J. Y., Cunningham, D., Roth, A. D. *et al.* (2000). Irinotecan combined with fluorouracil compared with fluorouracil alone as first-line treatment for metastatic colorectal cancer: a multicentre randomised trial. *Lancet* **355**:1041–7.

66 Hill, M., Norman, A., Cunningham, D. *et al.* (1995). Impact of protracted venous infusion fluorouracil with or without interferon alfa-2b on tumor response, survival, and quality of life in advanced colorectal cancer. *Journal of Clinical Oncology* **13**:2317–23.

67 Ross, P., Norman, A., Cunningham, D. *et al.* (1997). A prospective randomised trial of protracted venous infusion 5-fluorouracil with or without mitomycin C in advanced colorectal cancer. *Annals of Oncology* **8**:995–1001.

68 Rougier, P., Van Cutsem, E., Bajetta, E. *et al.* (1998). Randomised trial of irinotecan versus fluorouracil by continuous infusion after fluorouracil failure in patients with metastatic colorectal cancer. *Lancet* **352**:1407–12.

69 Saltz, L. B., Cox, J. V., Blanke, C. *et al.* (2000). Irinotecan plus fluorouracil and leucovorin for metastatic colorectal cancer. Irinotecan Study Group. *New England Journal of Medicine* **343**:905–14.

70 Van Cutsem, E., Blijham, G. H. on behalf of the V302 Study Group. (1999). Irinotecan versus infusional 5-fluorouracil: a phase III study in metastatic colorectal cancer following failure on first-line 5-fluorouracil. *Seminars in Oncology* **26**:13–20.

71 Norum, J., Vonen, B., Olsen, J. A. *et al.* (1997). Adjuvant chemotherapy (5-fluorouracil and levamisole) in Dukes' B and C colorectal carcinoma: a cost-effectiveness analysis. *Annals of Oncology* **8**:65–70.

72 Allen-Mersh, T. G., Earlam, S., Fordy, C. *et al.* (1994). Quality of life and survival with continuous hepatic-artery floxuridine infusion for colorectal liver metastases. *Lancet* **344**:1255–60.

73 Allen-Mersh, T. G., Glover, C., Fordy, C. *et al.* (2000). Randomized trial of regional plus systemic fluorinated pyrimidine compared with systemic fluorinated pyrimidine in treatment of colorectal liver metastases. *European Journal of Surgical Oncology* **26**:468–73.

74 Cocconi, G., Cunningham, D., Van Cutsem, E. *et al.* (1998). Open, randomized, multicenter trial of raltitrexed versus fluorouracil plus high-dose leucovorin in patients with advanced colorectal cancer. Tomudex Colorectal Cancer Study Group. *Journal of Clinical Oncology* **16**:2943–52.

75 Earlam, S., Glover, C., Davies, M. *et al.* (1997). Effect of regional and systemic fluorinated pyrimidine chemotherapy on quality of life in colorectal liver metastasis patients. *Journal of Clinical Oncology* **15**:2022–9.

76 Seymour, M. T., Slevin, M. L., Kerr, D. J. *et al.* (1996). Randomized trial assessing the addition of interferon alpha-2a to fluorouracil and leucovorin in advanced colorectal cancer. Colorectal Cancer Working Party of the United Kingdom Medical Research Council. *Journal of Clinical Oncology* **14**:2280–8.

77 Sobrero, A., Zaniboni, A., Frassineti, G. L. *et al.* (2000). Schedule specific biochemical modulations of 5-fluorouracil in advanced colorectal cancer: A randomized study. GISCAD, IOR and collaborating centers. *Annals of Oncology* **11**:1413–20.

78 Caudry, M., Bonnel, C., Floquet, A. *et al.* (1995). A randomized study of bolus fluorouracil plus folinic acid versus 21-day fluorouracil infusion alone or in association with cyclophosphamide and mitomycin C in advanced colorectal carcinoma. *American Journal of Clinical Oncology* **18**:118–25.

79 Loprinizi, C. L., Juross, S. A., O'Fallon, J. R. *et al.* (1994). Randomized placebo-controlled evaluation of hydrazine sulfate in patients with advanced colorectal cancer. *Journal of Clinical Oncology* **12**:1121–5.

80 Smyth, J. F., Hardcastle, J. D., Denton, G. *et al.* (1995). Two phase III trials of tauromustine (TCNU) in advanced colorectal cancer. *Annals of Oncology* **6**:948–9.

81 Laufman, L. R., Bukowski, R. M., Collier, M. A. *et al.* (1993). A randomized, double-blind trial of fluorouracil plus placebo versus fluorouracil plus oral leucovorin in patients with metastatic colorectal cancer. *Journal of Clinical Oncology* **11**:1888–93.

82 Scheithauer, W., Rosen, H., Kornek, G.-V. *et al.* (1993). Randomized comparison of combination 4 chemotherapy plus supportive care with supportive care alone in patients with metastatic colorectal cancer. *British Medical Journal* **306**:752–5.

83 Sullivan, B. A., McKinnis, R., Laufman, L. R. (1995). Quality of life in patients with metastatic colorectal cancer receiving chemotherapy: a randomized, double-blind trial comparing 5-FU versus 5-FU with leucovorin. *Pharmacotherapy* **15**:600–7.

84 Glimelius, B., Hoffman, K., Graf, W. *et al.* (1994). Quality of life during chemotherapy in patients with symptomatic advanced colorectal cancer. *Cancer* **73**:556–62.

85 Leichman, C. G., Fleming, T. R., Muggia, F. M. *et al.* (1995). Phase II study of fluorouracil and its modulation in advanced colorectal cancer: a Southwest Oncology Group study. *Journal of Clinical Oncology* **13**:1303–11.

86 Moinpour, C. M., Triplett, J. S., McKnight, B. *et al.* (2000). Challenges posed by non-random missing quality of life data in an advanced-stage colorectal cancer clinical trial. *Psycho-Oncology* **9**:340–54.

87 Moinpour, C. M., Savage, M., Hayden, K. A. *et al.* (1995). Quality of Life Assessment in Cancer Clinical Trials. In *Quality of Life in Behavioral Medicine Research*, ed. J. E. Dimsdale, A. Braun, pp. 79–95. Hillsdale, NJ: Lawrence Erlbaum Associates.

88 Feeny, D., Furlong, W., Boyle, M. *et al.* (1995). Multi-attribute health status classification systems: Health Utilities Index. *Pharmacoeconomics* **7**:490–502.

89 Tobin, E. (2001). *Report on Focus Group Research*. Conducted for NCI's COMWG with cancer patients and survivors by Cancer Care Strategies. September, 2001. Completed under contract to the National Cancer Institute by E. Tobin.

90 Zebrack, Cella, this volume, Chapter 11.

91 Bernhard, J., Cella, D. F., Coates, A. S. *et al.* (1998). Missing quality of life data in cancer clinical trials: serious problems and challenges. *Statistics in Medicine* **17**:517–32.

92 Hogan, J. W., Laird, N. M. (1997). Mixture models for the joint distribution of repeated measures and event times. *Statistics in Medicine* **16**:239–57.

93 Fairclough, this volume, Chapter 17.

94 Sprangers, M. A. G., Taal, B. G., Aaronson, N. K. *et al.* (1995). Quality of life in colorectal cancer. Stoma vs. nonstoma patients. *Diseases of the Colon and Rectum* **38**:361–9.

95 Camilleri-Brennan, J., Steele, R. J. C. (1998). Quality of life after treatment for rectal cancer. *British Journal of Surgery* **85**:1036–43.

96 Wils, J., Sahmoud, T., Sobrero, A. *et al.* (1998). Evaluation of clinical efficacy of new medical treatments in advanced colorectal cancer. Results of a workshop organized by the EORTC GITCCG. *Tumori* **84**:335–47.

97 Sobrero, A., Belvedere, O., Ramello, M. *et al.* (2001). Endpoints of medical treatment of colorectal cancer. *Tumori* **87**(Suppl. 1):S63–4.

98 Allen, M., Cunningham, D., Schmitt, C. (1998). The importance of stabilization as an endpoint in the treatment of metastatic colorectal carcinoma: recent quality of life studies. *Anti-Cancer Drugs* **9**:783–90.

99 Cull, A., Groenvold, M., on behalf of the EORTC Quality of Life Study Group. (1998). *EORTC Quality of Life Study Group Translation Procedure*. ISBN: 2-930064-15–3. Brussels: EORTC.

100 Beck, A. T., Steer, R. A. (1987). *Beck Depression Inventory (BDI) Manual*. San Antonio: Harcourt Brace Jovanovich.

101 Benoliel, J. Q., McCorkle, R., Young, K. (1983). The development of a social dependency scale. *Research in Nursing and Health* **3**:3–10.

102 McCorkle, R. M., Benoliel, J. Q., Donaldson, G. *et al.* (1989). A randomized clinical trial of home nursing care for lung cancer patients. *Cancer* **57**:358–64.

103 Priestman, T., Baum, M. (1976). Evaluation of quality of life in patients receiving treatment for advanced breast cancer. *Lancet* **24**:899–900.

104 Coates, A., Gebski, V., Bishop, J. F. *et al.* (1987). Improving the quality of life during chemotherapy for advanced breast cancer. *New England Journal of Medicine* **317**: 1633–7.

105 Ware, Jr., J. E., Sherbourne, C. D. (1992). The MOS 36-item short-form health survey (SF-36). I. Conceptual framework and item selection. *Medical Care* **30**:473–83.

106 McHorney, C. A., Ware, Jr., J. E., Lu, J. F. R., Sherbourne, C. D. (1994). The MOS 36-item Short-Form Health Survey (SF-36): III. Tests of data quality, scaling assumptions, and reliability across diverse patient groups. *Medical Care* **32**:40–66.

107 Ware, Jr., J. E., Snow, K. K., Kosinski, M. *et al.* (1993). *SF-36 Health Survey Manual and Interpretation Guide*. Boston, MA: New England Medical Center, The Health Institute.

9

Instruments to measure the specific health impact of surgery, radiation, and chemotherapy on cancer patients

Michael J. Barry, M.D.[1] and Janet E. Dancey, M.D.[2]

[1] Massachusetts General Hospital, Boston, MA
[2] National Cancer Institute, Bethesda, MD

Introduction

Surgery, radiation, and chemotherapy are used to cure, to prolong life, and to palliate symptoms of cancer patients. These treatments can have complicated effects on the patients who receive them. Their therapeutic effects on the cancers are intended to preserve or improve health status over time. However, these therapies can cause short-term and long-term adverse effects that result in deterioration in health status.[1-3] Prescribing these treatments requires a careful assessment of the risks and benefits of the proposed therapy by both the treating physician and patient. In situations where the benefits are curing the disease and the risks are minimal, treatment decisions are straightforward. Conversely, in situations where benefits are marginal, such as modest improvements in survival or palliation of symptoms, and the risks include treatment-related morbidity, treatment decisions are more difficult. If the fundamental question to be addressed by health care professionals and patients before prescribing treatment is "Does the toxicity and/or the inconvenience of the proposed treatment justify the expected gain?" then providing data on the impact of therapy on patient health from carefully conducted clinical studies, using robust instruments designed to assess impact of treatment-related morbidities specifically, could provide useful information. The purpose of this chapter is to review the treatment-specific instruments that have been developed and discuss their potential role in assessing the impact of therapy on cancer patients.

When early-stage cancers are treated with curative intent, patients often are not experiencing any impact of the cancer in the physical domain, although impact on the mental and emotional domains of health may certainly affect functioning. Attempted curative surgery or radiation in these circumstances may prolong life and prevent future cancer-related deteriorations in health status, but often only at the cost of side effects that may dominate the health status of the patient in the near term.[4,5] Examples of such circumstances would be radical prostatectomy or radiotherapy (external beam or brachytherapy) for the attempted curative treatment of clinically localized prostate cancer, and mastectomy or local excision plus radiotherapy for early-stage breast cancer. Similarly, chemotherapy may be prescribed either as the primary curative modality in a limited number of malignancies, such as lymphoma and small-cell lung carcinoma, or as adjuvant treatment after primary surgery and/or radiation. Adverse effects during treatment can impair the well-being of patients, and these ill effects may extend for a considerable period beyond the discontinuation of treatment.

Thus, surgery, radiation, and chemotherapy are invariably associated with immediate adverse effects on patient health during the peri-treatment period. There may even be a small risk of death attributable to these treatment modalities. The immediate impact of surgery includes the effects on a patient's life of going through the surgical experience, as well as the effects directly attributable to surgical wounds and recuperation. These effects can include postoperative pain, anesthetic complications, wound infection, medical complications, and restricted activity during recovery. Radiation can cause acute and chronic morbidities due to inflammation and subsequent fibrosis of tissues within the radiation fields. Patients may experience multiple adverse effects due to chemotherapy depending on the drugs that are administered; however, alopecia, myelosuppression, nausea, vomiting, stomatitis, diarrhea, and fatigue are among the most common and consistent side effects. Regardless of the treatment modality they receive, patients may experience fear, loss of independence, and financial hardship.

Patients are also at risk of experiencing chronic problems from treatment. Longer-term side effects usually reflect either damage to or removal of the target tissue and surrounding normal tissues. For example, removal of a cancerous breast may have a significant psychological impact and result in physical discomfort, while removal of a section of colon containing a cancer may result in changes in the pattern of bowel movements that may be viewed as problematic from the patient's perspective. When men with prostate cancer undergo radical prostatectomy, damage to the nearby bladder neck or neurovascular bundles can cause incontinence or erectile dysfunction. Radiation therapy to the prostate also has the potential to cause these side effects and may cause bowel dysfunction as well due to irradiation of adjacent sections of the rectum. The recent suggestion that radiation to the chest area may be associated with the late development of coronary artery disease illustrates that some late radiation toxicity to nearby tissues may be subtle and unexpected.[6] Chemotherapy may cause alopecia, stomatitis, diarrhea, and other systemic toxicities throughout the several months of treatment. In addition to these acute effects, chemotherapy may cause persistent toxicity to distant organs such as neuropathy and cardiac dysfunction, as well as increase the risk of localized chronic fibrosis when administered concurrently with radiation. Obviously, both acute and chronic effects can potentially adversely affect

physical, emotional, social, and financial well-being. However, measuring the impact of these treatment modalities on patient health-related quality of life (HRQOL) is difficult, as it requires the development of robust instruments that assess health status that are treatment specific. For patients, separating the impact of the cancer itself from the impact of the treatment may be particularly challenging.

The purpose of this review is to enumerate and describe health status measurement tools that have been used *specifically* to measure the total health impact of surgery, radiation, and chemotherapy on cancer patients regardless of the primary site. Instruments that broadly measure the health status of cancer patients, integrating treatment and cancer effects, are not the focus of this review, nor are instruments developed to measure the impact of treatment that is specific to a single primary cancer. These latter types of instruments are reviewed in other chapters.

Role of surgery, radiation, and chemotherapy in the treatment of breast, colorectal, lung, and prostate cancers

Breast cancer

According to the National Cancer Institute's Physician Data Query database for health professionals,[7] total mastectomy or breast-conserving surgery, often combined with adjuvant hormonal or chemotherapy or radiation, are potentially curative primary treatment options for women with ductal carcinoma in situ, or invasive stage I, II, and IIIA breast cancer. After total mastectomy, postoperative chest wall and regional lymph node irradiation may be given to selected women at high risk for local-regional failure (for example, women with four or more involved axillary nodes). Adjuvant radiation therapy is routinely given to women with invasive breast cancer who undergo breast-conserving surgery. Additional surgery may be performed for breast reconstruction. For more advanced stage IV/metastatic breast cancer, or for women with recurrent disease after primary treatment, surgery is used selectively for palliation; for example, a mastectomy may be performed for a fungating, uncomfortable breast mass. Radiation therapy may also be used palliatively, particularly for metastatic deposits causing, or about to cause, problems. Chemotherapy and/or hormone treatment may be given after primary surgery and radiation for localized or locally advanced disease, or as primary treatment to prolong survival and palliate symptoms of patients with metastatic disease. Chemotherapy may also be prescribed prior to surgery and radiation to downstage patients with locally advanced disease to allow breast-conserving surgery.

Colorectal cancer

Wide open surgical resection of the cancerous segment of the large intestine and regional nodes is the mainstay of therapy for stage I, II, and III colorectal cancer.[8] Adjuvant chemotherapy is used for stage III cancers and is under investigation for stage II disease. Radiation, with or without chemotherapy preoperatively and with chemotherapy postoperatively, is often prescribed to reduce the risk of local recurrence. Most patients with stage IV/metastatic disease receive chemotherapy to extend survival modestly and to palliate symptoms. For selected patients with recurrent/metastatic disease, surgery may be performed to treat or prevent local complications such as bleeding or obstruction or to resect isolated metastases for cure. Radiation therapy is used for palliative treatment of metastases, much as described for breast cancer. A special issue with rectal cancer treatment may be the need for abdomenoperineal resection with colostomy for lesions too distal to allow a conventional or colo-anal anastamosis.[9]

Lung cancer

For non-small-cell lung cancer, surgical resection for attempted cure is the mainstay of therapy for patients with stage I and II disease.[10] In general, radiation therapy, in combination with chemotherapy, is commonly used in patients with locally advanced disease. Many patients with non-small-cell lung cancer are destined to develop recurrent disease, regardless of primary treatment. For stage IV/metastatic or recurrent disease, surgery and radiation are generally used for palliation of symptoms due to localized tumor deposits. Chemotherapy may provide a modest extension of life and amelioration of disease-related symptoms.

For small-cell lung cancer, chemotherapy is the most common treatment.[11] Radiation therapy directed to the chest may be used for some patients with limited stage disease. Prophylactic cranial irradiation may also be considered for patients with a good initial response to chemotherapy. As for the other cancer sites, radiation may also be used in selective cases for treating or preventing complications secondary to other metastases.

Prostate cancer

Surgery or radiation therapy (either external beam or brachytherapy) is commonly attempted for stage I and II disease.[12] The same treatments are used for stage III disease, often in combination with hormonal therapy (androgen deprivation). Patients with stage IV/metastatic prostate cancer are usually treated with androgen deprivation. Hormone refractory patients may receive palliative benefit from chemotherapy. Once again, surgery and radiation may be used for palliative treatment of focal metastatic deposits, particularly bone and spinal metastases.

Methods

The goal of this review was to identify instruments developed specifically to measure the impact of surgery, radiotherapy, and chemotherapy on the health and functioning of cancer patients, regardless of primary tumor site. Instruments designed to assess treatment effects comprehensively, rather than those designed to assess effects on individual domains such as fatigue[13-16] or body image,[17] were the foci of this analysis.

To investigate the domains of HRQOL affected by treatment for cancer, focus groups were conducted with patients currently undergoing cancer treatment. These focus groups were supplemented with information from the literature. In addition, a literature search was performed to identify instruments commonly used to assess these treatment effects on HRQOL regardless of tumor site.

The literature search was performed using PubMed, the National Library of Medicine's medical literature search engine. The final search strategy was formulated after reviewing the Medical Subject Headings (MeSH) provided by the National Library of Medicine and after performing many preliminary, more broadly defined searches that resulted in the retrieval of thousands of articles; the vast majority of these were not relevant to this review. The final search strategy was designed to capture, with acceptable sensitivity and specificity, methodological references describing the development of instruments measuring HRQOL and other outcomes after surgery, radiotherapy, or chemotherapy for cancer, without capturing every paper describing a study that simply used a given questionnaire. The first search focused on surgery and radiation and used the following terms: neoplasms (MeSH term) AND surgery (MeSH term or Subheading) OR radiotherapy (MeSH term or Subheading) AND psychometrics (MeSH term) OR questionnaires (MeSH term). The search was conducted in all years and languages and retrieved 923 references. One of the authors reviewed the titles and abstracts, and all papers that seemed possibly relevant were retrieved (N = 30). A similar search strategy using the MeSH term or subheading "chemotherapy" was performed and retrieved 239 abstracts. The search was repeated without restrictions on the search terms and retrieved 1129 abstracts. One of the authors reviewed all titles and abstracts and relevant full-text papers were retrieved (N = 21). The references from these papers,

additional papers in the authors' files, and articles identified through supplemental searches were also reviewed for relevant citations.

Results

Domains of HRQOL affected by therapy for cancer: focus group findings

Of the various focus groups conducted as part of the Cancer Outcomes Measurement Working Group's (COMWG) research, the ones most likely to elicit themes about the impact of surgery and radiation were two "generic" groups representing a total of 16 men and women, most (but not all) of whom had been treated for breast or prostate cancer. The breast cancer patients had been treated with mastectomy or breast-conserving surgery plus radiation, while the prostate cancer patients had been treated with radical prostatectomy, external beam radiotherapy, or brachytherapy. Thus, patients who had experienced either surgery or radiation therapy were reasonably well-represented in these groups, and some participants had had both treatments.

Treatment-specific concerns affecting physical, emotional, and social domains of HRQOL were identified. In the physical domain, some participants identified surgery-related pain and radiation-related fatigue as important issues. Breast cancer patients also mentioned functional problems with the arm ipsilateral to their mastectomy and node dissection, as well as problems with sleep due to post-surgical discomfort. Among the many issues that were identified as adversely affecting emotional well-being, most involved the impact of the cancer diagnosis and prognosis rather than its treatment with surgery or radiation, although treatments were viewed as a constant reminder of the cancer. Social impacts of surgery included changes in body image after mastectomy and sexual dysfunction after prostate cancer treatment.

Many participants described their interactions with health professionals around treatment as problematic. Participants viewed cancer treatment to be fragmented and clinicians to be insensitive at times. While participants may have been projecting their difficulties in coping with the uncertainty of treatment outcome onto their clinicians, participants clearly expressed their view that the impact of treatments cannot be separated from the effects of environment and social setting in which the treatments are delivered.

The focus groups conducted with patients with specific types of cancer identified many of the same issues. However, the breast cancer focus group participants also reported a distorted body image after mastectomy, not only related to the removal of the breast but also their general appearance during treatment. Some survivors noted long-term discomfort or numbness in the arm after lumpectomy or mastectomy. Radiation appeared to cause fewer problems than surgery or chemotherapy early on, but some survivors noted fatigue long after radiotherapy. Prostate cancer patients emphasized problems with both sexual function and continence after radical prostatectomy. Some colorectal cancer patients mentioned problems with colostomies, such as an unpleasant smell, dietary intolerances, and the need to alter lifestyle. Many colorectal cancer survivors mentioned difficulties with dietary intolerances and bowel habits years after surgery, even without a colostomy. Colorectal cancer survivors who had radiation were dealing with problems such as strictures, lower urinary tract symptoms, and leg weakness.

The focus groups were not specifically designed to identify the impact of chemotherapy on health; however, subjects in the COMWG breast cancer focus group reported feeling confined or controlled by their chemotherapy regimens. Sexual dysfunction long after chemotherapy and longstanding menopausal symptoms on tamoxifen were also an issue for some women, as were short-term symptoms such as nausea, vomiting, fatigue, and alopecia related to chemotherapy. Prostate cancer patients discussed the adverse effects of androgen deprivation, particularly weakness and fatigue, but also vasomotor instability and gynecomastia. Lung cancer patients primarily discussed nausea, vomiting, dehydration, and weight changes; as many had received both radiation and chemotherapy at the same time, attribution of these symptoms between the two treatments was often uncertain. Colorectal cancer patients who had received chemotherapy noted nausea, diarrhea, alopecia, skin changes, and memory loss.

Researchers assessing the impact of chemotherapy in specific patient cohorts have also identified many of the same concerns and issues raised by the focus group participants. For example, results from studies assessing the effects of adjuvant chemotherapy on the health of women following their surgery and radiation for localized breast cancer, when compared to healthy women without cancer, indicated that the chemotherapy group had poorer physical functioning, more problems with work or other daily activities, more bodily pain, worse general health, poorer vitality, and worse social and cognitive functioning.[18–22] Two large-scale clinical trials found that adjuvant chemotherapy had a measurable effect on health-related quality of life. But contrary to expectations, this effect was transient and minor compared with the effect of patients' adjustment and coping after diagnosis and surgery.[23–25] Interestingly, selected trials of chemotherapy regimens in patients with metastatic colon,[26–28] prostate,[29] lung,[30–31] and breast cancers,[32–34] have reported favorable treatment effects on disease-related symptoms and physical, emotional, and functional domains, suggesting that treatment-related toxicity is not as concerning as disease-related effects to patients' well-being.

Differentiating between cancer-related symptoms, acute side effects, chronic side effects, and symptoms not related to cancer can often be difficult because cancer, treatment, and other life issues interact to influence the assessment of health parameters in a complex manner. Thus, the contributions of disease and treatment modality often cannot easily be separated out from each other and from unrelated effects on health.[35] This problem of attribution is a key issue in considering the value of treatment-specific instruments.

Instruments for measuring the health impact of surgery, radiation, or chemotherapy for cancer: toxicity criteria

The first efforts to describe systematically the side effects of cancer treatment on patients were a number of scales developed for non-experimental and experimental studies of the outcomes of radiation therapy. The first toxicity criteria, developed in the late 1970s through collaboration between the Radiation Therapy Oncology Group (RTOG) and European Organization for Research and Treatment of Cancer (EORTC), were the Late Morbidity Scoring Criteria.[5] In 1985, a complementary set of criteria for early toxicity of radiotherapy was developed by RTOG, the Acute Radiation Morbidity Scoring Criteria.[5] Both sets of criteria categorize toxicity to individual organ systems (14 for the early effects, 17 for the late effects) by severity using a five-point scale ranging from 0 (no effect) to 5 (death directly related to treatment).

Similar efforts to standardize the categorization of cancer treatment toxicity led to the development of Common Toxicity Criteria through the US National Cancer Institute (NCI) in the early 1980s, by the World Health Organization (WHO), and by the National Cancer Institute of Canada Clinical Trials Group (NCIC-CTG).[36] All three groups sought to categorize organ-specific toxicities, such as hematologic, gastrointestinal, and peripheral nerve toxicities as well as treatment-related pain, on scales of 0 to 4, with higher grades indicating worse toxicities. The criteria differ in the number of toxicities or domains and the specific definitions of grades for individual toxicities.

In 1995, working groups from RTOG and EORTC collaborated to develop a new scoring system for late toxicities of radiotherapy, resulting in the Late Effects of Normal Tissues/Subjective-Objective Management Analytic (LENT/SOMA) scales.[37–38] These scales are designed to use information from multiple sources, including patient reports, clinical exams, required treatments, and testing, to grade late toxicities. Within each organ system, toxicity is graded on one or more of the SOMA axes into one of four ordered categories from grades 1 to 4. For example, in the LENT/SOMA bladder scale, subjective hematuria grades range from occasional to refractory, objective grades range from microscopic with normal hemoglobin to refractory with more than a 20% decrease in hemoglobin, and management grades range from iron therapy to surgical intervention.

Most recently, NCI led an effort to revise and expand its earlier Common Toxicity Criteria and to merge the assessment of the acute toxicities of all cancer treatment modalities into one scoring system.[39] This ambitious system grades more than 260 individual adverse events from 0 to 4. The grading rests on descriptions of individual toxicities that approximate what is considered to be mild, moderate, severe, and life threatening by a consensus of medical experts. A grade of 0 indicates the toxicity is absent, and a grade of 4 indicates that the event is life threatening. The full range of the scale is not used for toxicities that are not severe. For example, the score for allergic rhinitis ranges from 0 (none) to 2 (moderate, requiring treatment), while the score for edema ranges from 0 (none) to 4 (anasarca).

As these toxicity criteria were developed by consensus to standardize the categorization, and thus facilitate the reporting of adverse effects of cancer treatments across clinical studies, there is, unsurprisingly, little published documentation regarding individual or comparative reliability and validity of the criteria. Some exceptions include a comparison of the WHO toxicity criteria and the NCI Common Toxicity Criteria for measuring nausea and vomiting secondary to chemotherapy by Franklin and colleagues,[40] an assessment of the inter-rater reliability of the NCIC-CTG and World Health Organization toxicity criteria by Brundage and colleagues,[36] and a correlation of the LENT/SOMA and RTOG/EORTC late effects scoring systems for the bladder and rectal domains among women undergoing radiotherapy for gynecologic malignancies by Anacak and colleagues.[41]

These toxicity criteria offer a standardization of classifying and reporting the severity of acute and delayed treatment effects on various "parts" of patients. Of note, the classification of severity was developed from a medical rather than patient-oriented perspective using "objective" criteria. For example, grade 3 diarrhea (severe) is defined by the number of bowel movements in a day rather than by the subjective distress caused by the toxicity. In addition, by categorizing treatment effects by organ system, the toxicity criteria do not offer a composite view of how treatments affect cancer patients' health and functioning.[42] Moreover, the toxicity criteria are based on the occurrence of the toxicity but not its duration. One would anticipate that increased severity, duration, and number of treatment toxicities would correlate with greater degrees of impairment in overall health and function, but research to support this hypothesis is scant. Lastly, the toxicity criteria are designed to be applied by health providers rather than patients. The literature search did not find comparisons of symptom reporting from the health provider and patient perspectives; however, one might reasonably expect discordance between these two approaches.

Efforts to quantify the severity of treatment-related toxicity more from the patient's perspective have led to the development of two instruments designed for patient self-report of acute side effects of chemotherapy and radiation. The precursor instrument, the Oncology Treatment Toxicity Assessment Tool (OTTAT), was initially described by Youngblood and colleagues in 1994.[43] Respondents are asked to score 37 possible side effects (such as "loss of appetite," "shortness of breath," "headache," and "difficulty concentrating") on a scale with five ordered categories (0 = none, 1 = mild, 2 = moderate, 3 = severe, 4 = intolerable). A total score is derived by summing the scores. In a validation study that included chemotherapy and radiotherapy patients, the instrument was reported to have a Cronbach's alpha measure of internal consistency reliability of 0.88 and a strong and significant correlation with a more global cancer-specific quality-of-life measure.

In two follow-up papers, the precursor instrument was reduced into a shorter, 25-item Therapy-Related Symptom Checklist (TRSC) (Figure 9.1) using principal components analysis. In a validation study, again

including both chemotherapy and radiotherapy patients, the TRSC scores correlated very strongly with scores on the parent instrument and moderately but significantly inversely with subjects' Karnofsky Performance Index scores. Moreover, internal consistency reliability was preserved, and the item scores could be used to discriminate between chemotherapy and radiotherapy patients.[44]

Munro and Potter have also published a computer-based symptom checklist that can be completed by patients undergoing radiotherapy.[45] Respondents rate how much they are troubled by 26 symptoms on a linear analog scale, regardless of primary cancer site (though additional short cancer site-specific modules are added). A limited psychometric assessment documented significant correlations between some subscales and more general health status measures, as well as responsiveness to patients' changing status as therapy progressed to completion.

These latter symptom checklists are unique in terms of both their focus on the impact of chemotherapy and radiotherapy (though not surgery) from the patient's perspective and from the psychometric data, at least partially supporting their reliability and validity. The literature searches found no papers examining the role of general, non-cancer-specific symptom questionnaires for measuring the impact of cancer treatment.

Measurement of the HRQOL impact of surgery for cancer

The literature search found no instruments specifically designed to measure the effect of cancer surgery on health status.

Measurement of the HRQOL impact of radiation therapy for cancer

The literature search identified one instrument specifically used to measure the total impact of radiation therapy on health and functioning for cancer patients, regardless of primary tumor site: the Quality of Life-Radiation Therapy Instrument

PLEASE CHECK THE *PROBLEMS* YOU HAVE *HAD IMMEDIATELY AFTER AND SINCE YOUR LAST TREATMENT.* PLEASE *CIRCLE* HOW SEVERE IT WAS ACCORDING TO THE FOLLOWING SCALE:
0 = none   1 = mild   2 = moderate   3 = severe   4 = very severe

EXAMPLE	Degree of severity				
Pain	0	1	2	3	4
Taste change	0	1	2	3	4
Loss of appetite	0	1	2	3	4
Nausea	0	1	2	3	4
Vomiting	0	1	2	3	4
Weight loss	0	1	2	3	4
Sore mouth	0	1	2	3	4
Cough	0	1	2	3	4
Sore throat	0	1	2	3	4
Difficulty swallowing	0	1	2	3	4
Jaw pain	0	1	2	3	4
Shortness of breath	0	1	2	3	4
Numbness in fingers and/or toes	0	1	2	3	4
Feeling sluggish	0	1	2	3	4
Depression	0	1	2	3	4
Difficulty concentrating	0	1	2	3	4
Fever	0	1	2	3	4
Bruising	0	1	2	3	4
Hair loss	0	1	2	3	4
Skin changes	0	1	2	3	4
Soreness in vein where chemotherapy was given	0	1	2	3	4
Difficulty sleeping	0	1	2	3	4
Pain	0	1	2	3	4
Decreased interest in sexual activity	0	1	2	3	4
Constipation	0	1	2	3	4
Other problems (please list)					
_____	0	1	2	3	4
_____	0	1	2	3	4

Figure 9.1. The Therapy-Related Symptom Checklist (TRSC), [44] reprinted with permission from Elsevier Science: Williams, P. D., Ducey, K. A., Sears, A. M. *et al.* (2001). Treatment type and symptom severity among oncology patients by self-report. *International Journal of Nursing Studies* **38**: 359–67.

(QOL-RTI).[46,47] The original QOL-RTI addressed domains of function (9 items), emotion (7 items), family/socioeconomic situation (6 items), and overall quality of life (2 items). In a small validation study (N = 19), the Cronbach's alpha statistic for the instrument was 0.87, and the one-week test-retest correlation coefficient was 0.79. Scores on the QOL-RTI also correlated with scores on the Ferrans and Powers Quality of Life Index, providing some evidence of construct validity.[46] A head-and-neck module for the QOL-RTI has also been published and validation data provided.[47] The current version of the QOL-RTI, including an additional question added more recently by the authors, is provided in Figure 9.2.

Measurement of the HRQOL impact of chemotherapy for cancer

In addition to the OTTAT/TRSC instrument developed for assessing the effects of radiation and chemotherapy, there have been publications reporting on three other instruments developed to assess chemotherapy effects and one subscale to be used with the Functional Assessment of Cancer Therapy general questionnaire (FACT-G) to assess the effects of endocrine therapy.

The Chemotherapy Symptom Assessment Scale (C-SAS) is a 24-item scale designed for the routine assessment of symptoms and side effects

QUALITY OF LIFE -RADIATION THERAPY INSTRUMENT (QOL-RTI)

Please circle the number on the line to indicate how you felt relating to each statement during the past week.
BE SURE TO CIRCLE A NUMBER ON EVERY LINE EVEN IF YOU ARE NOT SURE OF YOUR ANSWER.

1. My appearance is about the same as before I was diagnosed as having cancer.
2. I have my normal appetite.
3. I enjoy good food.
4. I am bothered by nausea.
5. I feel tired.
6. My cancer treatments frighten me.
7. I worry about my bills.
8. I feel cheerful.
9. I have skin discomfort in the treatment area.
10. I feel hopeful about my future.
11. I feel discouraged.
12. I look forward to seeing my friends and family.
13. My health care is interfering with my job, going to school, or other activities.
14. I look forward to getting out and doing things.
15. I feel satisfied with my life.
16. I receive support from the staff giving me my cancer treatments.
17. I receive support from my family and friends.
18. I receive support from my relationship with God/a "Supreme Being".
19. My illness interferes with my ability to take care of myself.
20. In general, I would say my health is good.
21. I feel in control of my life.

Response frame for questions 1-21:

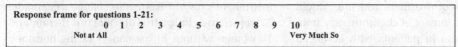
```
        0   1   2   3   4   5   6   7   8   9   10
      Not at All                              Very Much So
```

The following choices are worded a little differently than the previous questions. The pain question goes from Not at all to Worst Possible instead of Very Much So and the sexual activity and sleep at night questions go from Not At All to Normal For Me.

22. I experience pain.

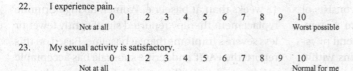
```
        0   1   2   3   4   5   6   7   8   9   10
      Not at all                              Worst possible
```

23. My sexual activity is satisfactory.
```
        0   1   2   3   4   5   6   7   8   9   10
      Not at all                              Normal for me
```

24. I sleep at night.
```
        0   1   2   3   4   5   6   7   8   9   10
      Not at all                              Normal for me
```

25. On a scale from 0 to 10 please rate your overall quality of life during the past week with 0 being a very poor quality of life and 10 being a very good quality of life.
```
        0   1   2   3   4   5   6   7   8   9   10
      Very poor                               Very good
```

Figure 9.2. The Quality of Life-Radiation Therapy Instrument (QOL-RTI).[46] Used with permission: Johnson, D. J., Casey, L., Noriega, B. (1994). A pilot study of patient quality of life during radiation therapy treatment. *Quality of Life Research* **3**: 267–72.

experienced by patients receiving cytotoxic chemotherapy in outpatient facilities.[48] The C-SAS is designed to assess the prevalence and characteristics of a symptom and the degree to which it causes distress or impairs health. Unfortunately, the instrument has undergone limited psychometric evaluation; thus, it lacks evidence of reliability and sensitivity to change.

The Japanese Quality of Life Research Group developed the Quality of Life Questionnaire for Cancer Patients Treated with Anticancer Drugs (QOL-ACD).[49] This instrument has 22 questions, which sort into four major categories (daily activities, physical condition, social activities, and mental and psychological status) that are graded on a five-point scale. Internal consistency, construct validity by inter-scale correlations, and concurrent validity with the State-Trait Anxiety Inventory, Self-Rating Depression Scale, and Karnofsky Performance Status were assessed. The internal consistency within domains was good, with Cronbach's alpha coefficients of 0.70 or greater for all domains except psychological status, which was 0.58. Reliability was verified for the final 22-question form using test-retest procedures, and it demonstrated acceptable stability. Although psychometric assessment has not been extensive, the instrument appears to be valid and reliable. Of note, although this instrument was developed for patients receiving chemotherapy, the items within the domains included in the instrument may be influenced by cancer or treatment and, thus, would not differentiate the impact of chemotherapy from the impact of disease in patients with advanced cancer.

The Worthing Chemotherapy Questionnaire is another patient self-report instrument to document side effects of chemotherapy.[50] The tool consists of 75 items covering six domains: digestive system, mouth and nose, skin and hair, eyes, general physical health, and moods and feelings. Items within each grouping ask about the degree of discomfort. The severity of each side effect is rated using a five-point score of 0 (not experienced the side effect at all) to 4 (extremely bad). The instrument has been evaluated for content validity, construct validity, and for test-retest reliability. For the latter evaluation, the weighted kappas ranged from 0.51 to 1.00 (median = 0.88) and were not found to be dependent on respondents' age, gender, treatment regimen, or diagnosis.

Only one instrument developed to measure the side effects and putative benefits of hormonal treatments given in breast cancer was identified from the literature search. Fallowfield and colleagues developed an 18-item endocrine subscale to accompany a standardized cancer quality of life measure, the Functional Assessment of Cancer Therapy (FACT).[51] Alpha coefficients for all subscales demonstrated good internal consistency (range = 0.65–0.87). Test-retest reliability of the subscale indicated good stability ($r = 0.93$, $p < 0.001$). The most frequently reported symptoms were loss of sexual interest, weight gain, and hot flushes. Significant differences were found between treatment groups for hot flushes and vaginal dryness. Hot flushes were more common in both adjuvant chemotherapy treatment groups and in patients with advanced breast cancer taking tamoxifen. Least likely to experience hot flushes were women who were not on endocrine therapy, with only 3 out of 41(7%) endorsing this item ($p = 0.004$). Vaginal dryness varied significantly according to treatment ($p < .01$), with 11 patients (26.2%) receiving adjuvant chemotherapy most likely to report dryness, followed by 5 patients (18.5%) receiving megestrol acetate, and 2 patients (6.1%) receiving anastrozole. Two assessments of the instrument's responsiveness to change were made: 32 women in a clinical trial of endocrine therapy and 18 women without breast cancer taking hormone replacement therapy completed the FACT endocrine subscale at baseline, 4, 8, and 12 weeks. Trial patients reported significantly more symptoms at 8 and 12 weeks than at baseline. Women taking hormone replacement therapy reported significantly fewer or less severe symptoms than at baseline. Based on this report, the FACT endocrine subscale has acceptable validity and reliability and is sensitive to change, making it suitable for clinical trials of endocrine therapy.[51]

Discussion

Although many cancer-specific HRQOL measures, such as the FACT-G[35] and the EORTC QLQ-C30[52] (as well as the cancer site-specific modules that complement these general instruments), have items addressing common treatment-related concerns, these questionnaires do not specifically focus on treatment effects. The lack of emphasis on assessing the side effects of therapy in general questionnaires may lead to an inaccurate estimation of the distress and discomfort therapy imposes on patients.

This perceived shortcoming of cancer-specific questionnaires may be overcome through the use of treatment-specific measures.

The literature search conducted for this review found no instruments developed specifically to capture the impact of surgery on health and functioning, one instrument designed to do so for radiotherapy, three for chemotherapy, and one for endocrine therapy. These instruments should be regarded as having been only partially validated and not having been widely used. There are a number of toxicity criteria, essentially symptom severity inventories, available for cancer treatments. However, once again, the reliability and validity of these instruments, despite considerable face validity, is unclear.

Whether this dearth of instruments is actually a problem is even less clear. Although there are some commonalities to the experience of surgery and radiotherapy for breast and prostate cancer, there are also many differences. A generic measure of the impact of radiation or surgery would likely miss important aspects of each treatment from the perspective of the men and women undergoing them. Similarly, while many chemotherapy drugs cause similar toxicities, the type, frequency, and severity of the adverse effects can be quite different depending on which agents are prescribed for a particular cancer, and the tolerance of these adverse effects may depend on stage of disease. Some treatments may have very different profiles of impact on patients' lives than standard cancer surgery, radiotherapy, or chemotherapy. Examples might include bone marrow transplantation for breast cancer or cryosurgery for prostate cancer. In these circumstances, treatment-specific measures may be particularly important for assessing the full range of the novel treatment's impact on patients' HRQOL.

Besides the narrow focus of treatment-specific instruments, which are assessing treatment-related effects on health but may be missing cancer-related concerns, there is an additional concern that these instruments may not correctly identify changes in patients' health due to treatment effects. Implicit in the use of these instruments is the assumption that patients can accurately attribute the effects on

their health and functioning resulting from their treatment rather than their cancer. For some early-stage cancers and some domains of health, e.g., physical functioning, such attributions may indeed be possible. In the setting of localized disease that can be removed by surgery or treated by radiation, there are few if any physical symptoms of the cancer once it has been treated and, thus, adverse effects experienced by patients can more readily be attributed to treatment. However, for patients with more advanced cancers, it may be quite difficult to separate treatment effects from cancer effects in domains like physical and emotional health, fatigue, and pain.

In addition to the overlapping adverse effects of treatment and disease that may limit the value of using treatment-specific instruments in patients with advanced disease, the potential benefits of treatment may be missed if instruments are designed to assess only specific adverse effects of treatment. Patients with metastatic disease may experience immediate, although temporary, relief of cancer-related symptoms, and this benefit may offset or exceed the inconvenience and discomfort of treatment-related toxicity. In this situation, focusing on measuring the impact of treatment-related adverse effects might be an inadequate assessment of the impact of therapy on health, as the immediate benefit of ameliorating cancer-related symptoms is not being captured. Arguably, to assess the impact of treatment on patient health in the setting of metastatic disease adequately requires measuring the effects of the therapeutic intervention on cancer-specific symptoms, treatment-related toxicity, and broader domains of HRQOL. Focusing exclusively on symptom improvement or treatment side effects will not provide a comprehensive understanding of the overall burden or benefit of therapy to patients.

Thus, instruments designed to assess the adverse effects of treatment on health in a generic fashion will not necessarily capture the impact of cancer-specific concerns or even cancer-specific treatment effects that may be important to individual patients. Unlike treatment-specific health status measures, cancer-specific instruments are often designed to capture the impact of disease and its therapy on patient health and functioning. In addition, general cancer measures like the FACT-G and EORTC QLQ-C30 can further focus on the impact of therapies through the use of validated subscales or modules devised to assess the concerns particular to a stage of cancer and treatment regimen. Interestingly, a number of clinical trials have used these cancer-specific questionnaires to assess different treatment inventions, usually new chemotherapy drugs or drug combinations, but few have shown significant differences in health domains for patients receiving different treatments despite differences in survival or in frequency and severity of toxicity experienced by patients.[26-34]

The lack of measurable differences in therapeutic effects using these instruments may be due to a number of factors. First, the general cancer measures may lack sensitivity as, without their cancer site-specific submodules, the general instruments have few tumor-specific or treatment-specific items. Second, the timing of the administration of the questionnaire may have been after the effects had resolved. Third, poor compliance in completing questions may result in loss of power to detect differences. Finally, patients may not perceive differences in health or treatment-related adverse effects or benefits, despite differences documented using toxicity criteria or modest differences in survival.

By far the most widely used instruments to categorize treatment-related adverse effects are the toxicity criteria. Despite limited data on their validity and reliability, toxicity criteria, by providing standardized categories and definitions of severity, are quite helpful for comparing treatments in clinical trials. Moreover, information on the likelihood of short-term and long-term adverse effects of various treatments can help patients choose among them, particularly when the candidate treatments have very different side-effect profiles and similar outcomes in terms of cancer control. Such choices include mastectomy versus lumpectomy and radiation for early-stage breast cancer, and radical prostatectomy versus radiotherapy for early-stage prostate cancer. In these circumstances, prospective patients may prefer data on the probabilities of various side effects of different degrees of severity; they can then apply their own values and preferences to the treatment choice.

While toxicity criteria allow for the generation of information on the frequency and severity of symptoms attributable to treatment, they do not provide information on degree of discomfort or distress imposed by these symptoms on the patients. The severity of individual toxicities has been defined by the consensus opinion of physicians, and toxicity criteria are applied in studies by health professionals. This lack of patient-oriented perspective is unfortunate, as it is unlikely that all toxicities of the same grade have equivalent impact on patients' health. Grade 3 toxicities are considered to be severe; however, grade 3 neutropenia is unlikely to have an appreciable effect on patients' perception of their health, while grade 3 diarrhea may be distressing and restrict function for fear of being incontinent. Grade 3 vomiting may be tolerable if transient, while grade 3 neuropathy may be debilitating, particularly if protracted or irreversible. Similarly, multiple toxicities of lesser severity experienced by a patient may cause greater discomfort or disability than fewer toxicities of greater severity. Unfortunately, there has been little research done to date on evaluating the burden of treatment effects from the patients' perspective, or on the influences of factors such as type, duration, and number of toxicities on patient well-being.

In conclusion, an extensive search uncovered few validated instruments to measure specifically the impact of radiotherapy and chemotherapy on cancer patients' health and functioning; no such instruments were found for cancer surgery. Treatment-specific instruments may provide more information on the perceived burden of treatment than is provided currently by toxicity criteria because they are patient-oriented. However, these instruments may lack the ability to differentiate treatment from disease-related effects on health and, by focusing exclusively on treatment, may not assess the impact of disease-specific concerns of importance to cancer patients. As the COMWG-sponsored focus groups indicated, a number of issues which patients mentioned as important are not well represented in current questionnaires. Further research is recommended to determine how items related to treatment impact should be included in cancer site-specific HRQOL modules being developed for the major cancer HRQOL instruments. One approach might be to develop treatment-specific "submodules" for the cancer site-specific modules, which would only require completion by patients who had undergone that particular treatment. The marginal value of such additional submodules could be assessed in terms of their "face validity" to patients and their ability to enhance prediction of overall HRQOL among cancer patients.

Acknowledgments

The authors wish to thank Jean-Francois Caubet and Elizabeth Walker-Corkery for their assistance in preparing this report.

REFERENCES

1 Donovan, K., Sanson-Fisher, R., Redman, S. (1989). Measuring quality of life in cancer patients. *Journal of Clinical Oncology* **7**:959–68.

2 Scott, C. B. (1998). Issues in quality of life assessment during cancer therapy. *Seminars in Radiation Oncology* **8**: 5–9.

3 Carlsson, M., Strang, P., Bjurstrom, C. (2000). Treatment modality affects long-term quality of life in gynaecological cancer. *Anticancer Research* **20**(1B):563–8.

4 Langenhoff, B. S., Krabbe, P. F., Wobbes, T. *et al.* (2001). Quality of life as an outcome measure in surgical oncology. *British Journal of Surgery* **88**:643–52.

5 Cox, J., Stetz, J., Pajak, T. (1995). Toxicity criteria of the radiation therapy oncology group (RTOG) and the European Organization for Research and Treatment of Cancer (EORTC). *International Journal of Radiation Oncology, Biology, and Physics* **31**:1341–6.

6 Paszat, L., Mackillop, W., Groome, P. *et al.* (1998). Mortality from myocardial infarction after adjuvant radiotherapy for breast cancer in the surveillance, epidemiology, and end-results cancer registries. *Journal of Clinical Epidemiology* **16**:2625–31.

7 National Cancer Institute (2001). CancerNet PDQ Cancer Information Summary. Breast Cancer Treatment (for health professionals). http://www.cancer.gov/cancerinfo/ pdq/treatment/breast/healthprofessional. Last accessed September 11, 2004.

8 National Cancer Institute (2001). CancerNet PDQ Cancer Information Summary. Colon Cancer Treatment (for health professionals). http://www.cancer.gov/cancerinfo/ pdq/treatment/colon/healthprofessional. Last accessed September 11, 2004.

9 National Cancer Institute (2001). CancerNet PDQ Cancer Information Summary. Rectal Cancer Treatment (for health professionals). http://www.cancer.gov/cancerinfo/ pdq/treatment/rectal/healthprofessional. Last accessed September 11, 2004.

10 National Cancer Institute (2001). CancerNet PDQ Cancer Information Summary. Non-small Cell Lung Cancer Treatment (for health professionals). http://www.cancer. gov/cancerinfo/pdq/treatment/non-small-cell-lung/ healthprofessional. Last accessed September 11, 2004.

11 National Cancer Institute (2002). CancerNet PDQ Cancer Information Summary. Small Cell Lung Cancer Treatment (for health professionals). http://www. cancer.gov/cancerinfo/pdq/treatment/small-cell-lung/ healthprofessional. Last accessed September 11, 2004.

12 National Cancer Institute (2001). CancerNet PDQ Cancer Information Summary. Prostate Cancer Treatment (for health professionals). http://www.cancer.gov/cancerinfo/ pdq/treatment/prostate/healthprofessional. Last accessed September 11, 2004.

13 Smets, E. M., Garssen, B., Bonke, B. *et al.* (1995). The Multidimensional Fatigue Inventory (MFI) psychometric qualities of an instrument to assess fatigue. *Journal of Psychosomatic Research* **39**:315–25.

14 Smets, E. M., Garssen, B., Cull, A. *et al.* (1996). Application of the multidimensional fatigue inventory (MFI-20) in cancer patients receiving radiotherapy. *British Journal of Cancer* **73**:241–5.

15 Smets, E. M., Visser, M. R., Garssen, B. *et al.* (1998). Understanding the level of fatigue in cancer patients undergoing radiotherapy. *Journal of Psychosomatic Research* **45**:277–93.

16 Ahsberg, E., Furst, C. J. (2001). Dimensions of fatigue during radiotherapy – an application of the Swedish Occupational Fatigue Inventory (SOFI) on cancer patients. *Acta Oncologia* **40**:37–43.

17 Hopwood, P. (1993). The assessment of body image in cancer patients. *European Journal of Cancer* **29A**:276–81.

18 Klee, M. C., King, M. T., Machin, D. *et al.* (2000). A clinical model for quality of life assessment in cancer patients receiving chemotherapy. *Annals of Oncology* **11**(1):23–30.

19 Broecke, J. A., Jacobsen, P. B., Balducci, L. *et al.* (2000). Quality of life after adjuvant chemotherapy for breast cancer. *Breast Cancer Research and Treatment* **62**(2):141–50.

20 van Dam, F. S., Schagen, S. B., Muller, M. J. *et al.* (1998). Impairment of cognitive function in women receiving adjuvant treatment for high-risk breast cancer: high-dose versus standard-dose chemotherapy. *Journal of the National Cancer Institute* **90**:210–18.

21 Schagen, S. B., van Dam, F. S., Muller, M. J. *et al.* (1999). Cognitive deficits after postoperative adjuvant chemotherapy for breast carcinoma. *Cancer* **85**:640–50.

22 Brezden, C. B., Phillips, K. A., Abdolell, M.(2000). Cognitive function in breast cancer patients receiving adjuvant chemotherapy. *Journal of Clinical Oncology* **18**:2695–701.

23 Hurny, C., Bernhard, J., Coates A. (1998). Quality of life assessment in the International Breast Cancer Study Group: past, present, and future. *Recent Results in Cancer Research* **152**:390–5.

24 Hurny, C., Bernhard, J., Coates, A. S. *et al.* (1996). Impact of adjuvant therapy on quality of life in women with node-positive operable breast cancer. International Breast Cancer Study Group. *Lancet* **347**:1279–84.

25 Fairclough, D. L., Fetting, J. H., Cella, D. *et al.* (1999). Quality of life and quality adjusted survival for breast cancer patients receiving adjuvant therapy. Eastern Cooperative Oncology Group (ECOG). *Quality of Life Research* **8**:723–31.

26 Douillard, J. Y., Cunningham, D., Roth, A. D. *et al.* (2000). Irinotecan combined with fluorouracil compared with fluorouracil alone as first-line treatment for metastatic colorectal cancer: a multicentre randomised trial. *Lancet* **355**(9209):1041–7.

27 Cunningham, D., Pyrhonen, S., James, R. D. *et al.* (1998). Randomised trial of irinotecan plus supportive care versus supportive care alone after fluorouracil failure for patients with metastatic colorectal cancer. *Lancet* **352**(9138):1413–18.

28 Rougier, P., Van Cutsem, E., Bajetta, E. *et al.* (1998). Randomised trial of irinotecan versus fluorouracil by continuous infusion after fluorouracil failure in patients with metastatic colorectal cancer. *Lancet* **352**(9138):1407–12.

29 Osoba, D., Tannock, I. F., Ernst, D. S. *et al.* (1999). Health-related quality of life in men with metastatic prostate cancer treated with prednisone alone or mitoxantrone and prednisone. *Journal of Clinical Oncology* **17**:1654–63.

30 Cullen, M. H., Billingham, L. J., Woodroffe, C. M. *et al.* (1999). Mitomycin, ifosfamide, and cisplatin in unresectable non-small-cell lung cancer: effects on survival and quality of life. *Journal of Clinical Oncology* **17**:3188–94.

31 Shepherd, F. A., Dancey, J., Ramlau, R. *et al.* (2000). Prospective randomized trial of docetaxel versus best supportive care in patients with non-small-cell lung cancer previously treated with platinum-based chemotherapy. *Journal of Clinical Oncology* **18**:2095–103.

32 Hakamies-Blomqvist, L., Luoma, M., Sjostrom, J. *et al.* (2000). Quality of life in patients with metastatic breast cancer receiving either docetaxel or sequential methotrexate and 5-fluorouracil. A multicentre randomised phase III trial by the Scandinavian breast group. *European Journal of Cancer* **36**:1411–17.

33 Kramer, J. A., Curran, D., Piccart, M. *et al.* (2000). Randomised trial of paclitaxel versus doxorubicin as first-line chemotherapy for advanced breast cancer: quality of life evaluation using the EORTC QLQ-C30 and the Rotterdam symptom checklist. *European Journal of Cancer* **36**:1488–97.

34 Harper-Wynne, C., English, J., Meyer, L. *et al.* (1999). Randomized trial to compare the efficacy and toxicity of cyclophosphamide, methotrexate and 5-fluorouracil (CMF) with methotrexate mitoxantrone (MM) in advanced carcinoma of the breast. *British Journal of Cancer* **81**:316–22.

35 Cella, D., Tulsky, D., Gray, G. *et al.* (1993). The Functional Assessment of Cancer Therapy Scale: Development and validation of the general measure. *Journal of Clinical Oncology* **11**:570–9.

36 Brundage, M., Pater, J., Zee, B. (1993). Assessing the reliability of two toxicity scales: implications for interpreting toxicity data. *Journal of the National Cancer Institute* **85**:1138–48.

37 Pavy, J. J., Denekamp, J., Letschert, J. *et al.* (1995). Late effects toxicity scoring: the SOMA Scale. *International Journal of Radiation Oncology, Biology, and Physics* **31**:1043–7.

38 Rubin, P., Constine, L., Fajardo, L. *et al.* (1995). Overview: Late effects of normal tissues (LENT) scoring system. *International Journal of Radiation Oncology, Biology, and Physics* **31**:1041–2.

39 Trotti, A., Byhardt, R., Stetz, J. *et al.* (2000). Common toxicity criteria: Version 2.0. An improved reference for grading the acute effects of cancer treatment: Impact on radiotherapy. *International Journal of Radiation Oncology, Biology, and Physics* **47**:13–47.

40 Franklin, H., Simonetti, G., Dubbelman, A. *et al.* (1994). Toxicity grading systems. A comparison between the WHO scoring system and the Common Toxicity Criteria when used for nausea and vomiting. *Annals of Oncology* **5**:113–17.

41 Anacak, Y., Yalman, D., Ozsaran, Z. *et al.* (2001). Late radiation effects to the rectum and bladder in gynecologic cancer patients: the comparison of LENT/SOMA and RTOG/EORTC late-effects scoring systems. *International Journal of Radiation Oncology, Biology, and Physics* **50**:1107–12.

42 Bruner, D., Wasserman, T. (1995). The impact on quality of life by radiation late effects. *International Journal of Radiation Oncology, Biology, and Physics* **31**:1353–5.

43 Youngblood, M., Williams, P. D., Eyles, H. *et al.* (1994). A comparison of two methods of assessing cancer therapy-related symptoms. *Cancer Nursing* **17**:37–44.

44 Williams, P. D., Ducey, K. A., Sears, A. M. *et al.* (2001). Treatment type and symptom severity among oncology patients by self-report. *International Journal of Nursing Studies* **38**:359–67.

45 Munro, A. J., Potter, S. (1996). A quantitative approach to the distress caused by symptoms in patients treated with radical radiotherapy. *British Journal of Cancer* **74**:640–7.

46 Johnson, D. J., Casey, L., Noriega, B. (1994). A pilot study of patient quality of life during radiation therapy treatment. *Quality of Life Research* **3**:267–72.

47 Trotti, A., Johnson, D. J., Gwede, C. *et al.* (1998). Development of a head and neck companion module for the quality of life-radiation therapy instrument (QOL-RTI). *International Journal of Radiation Oncology, Biology, and Physics* **42**: 257–61.

48 Brown, V., Sitzia, J., Richardson, A. *et al.* (2001). The development of the Chemotherapy Symptom Assessment Scale (C-SAS): a scale for the routine clinical assessment of the symptom experiences of patients receiving cytotoxic chemotherapy. *International Journal of Nursing Studies* **38**(5):497–510.

49 Kurihara, M., Shimizu, H., Tsuboi, K. *et al.* (1999). Development of quality of life questionnaire in Japan: quality of life assessment of cancer patients receiving chemotherapy. *Psycho-Oncology* **8**(4):355–63.

50 Sitzia, J., Dikken, C., Hughes, J. (1997). Psychometric evaluation of a questionnaire to document side-effects of chemotherapy. *Journal of Advanced Nursing* **25**(5):999–1007.

51 Fallowfield, L. J., Leaity, S. K., Howell, A. *et al.* (1999). Assessment of quality of life in women undergoing hormonal therapy for breast cancer: validation of an endocrine symptom subscale for the FACT-B. *Breast Cancer Research and Treatment* **55**(2):189–99.

52 Aaronson, N., Ahmedzai, S., Bergman, B. *et al.* (1993). The European Organization for Research and Treatment of Cancer QLQ-C30: a quality-of-life instrument for use in international clinical trials in oncology. *Journal of the National Cancer Institute* **85**:365–76.

10

Short-term outcomes of chemoprevention, genetic susceptibility testing, and screening interventions: What are they? How are they measured? When should they be measured?

Jeanne S. Mandelblatt, M.D., M.P.H.[1] **and Joe V. Selby, M.D., M.P.H.**[2]

[1]Georgetown University, Washington, DC

[2]Kaiser-Permanente Medical Care Program, Oakland, CA

Introduction

Cancer is a frequent and serious illness with major impact on the quantity and quality of life. For several common cancers, preventive measures and periodic screening can reduce the risk for cancer incidence or, through early detection, lower morbidity and mortality from incident cancers. More recently, genetic testing has been introduced to screen for cancer susceptibility mutations. Presumably, the benefits of screening and early detection are accompanied by net improvements in the quality of life for persons in whom cancers are prevented or detected early. However, both prevention efforts and screening also have the potential to influence quality of life more subtly, either positively or negatively, for the large majority of asymptomatic individuals who would never have developed the cancer.

Faced with an increasing number of effective prevention and screening strategies and technologies, individual patients, health care systems, and policy analysts need accurate assessments of quality-of-life outcomes to inform shared decision making and to conduct relevant decision and cost-effectiveness analyses.[1–4] However, there has been little research on short-term effects on quality of life, which may be the predominant effects of chemopreventive or screening interventions.

In this chapter, short-term outcomes are defined, a framework for understanding and measuring these outcomes presented, the quality-of-life domains most relevant to cancer prevention and screening activities explored, the existing literature and tools currently employed to measure outcomes reviewed, methodological challenges highlighted, and recommendations for future studies made. This review is intended to support ongoing efforts to preserve and improve the quality of life for populations in whom effective preventive and screening services are indicated.

This discussion focuses on prevention and early detection activities conducted within the context of medical care, including chemoprevention; screening for breast, cervical, colorectal, and prostate cancers; and genetic testing and counseling. These cancers were selected because there is a body of literature on the short-term impact associated with their prevention, genetic testing, or early detection. Other preventive interventions, such as smoking cessation, exercise, weight loss, and dietary changes, have short-term as well as long-term effects on cancer incidence and mortality. However, the initiation of these behaviors largely occurs outside of the medical care system, and a thorough consideration of this literature is beyond the scope of this chapter.

Definition of short-term outcomes

Outcomes of care are the net effects of the health care structure and processes operating on the health and well-being of individuals and populations.[5] Unlike patients requiring treatment for cancer, persons considering cancer screening, genetic testing, or primary chemoprevention are asymptomatic individuals without diagnoses of cancer. These persons may be at greater than average risk (e.g., women considering tamoxifen for breast cancer prevention; persons considering colonoscopy for colorectal cancer screening), but their health status has not been directly affected by the illness in question. Hence, prevention and screening interventions should convey minimal risk, especially for rare long-term consequences such as mortality or irreversible decrements in health status (e.g., colon perforation during colonoscopy or endometrial cancer from taking tamoxifen).

This review covers the subset of transient outcomes that may affect many or all persons who take up a screening or prevention activity. These outcomes are "short-term effects," meaning changes in health status or quality of life occurring within the period from several days immediately before a preventive or early detection activity is initiated to no more than 6 months beyond the end of the intervention. Implicit in this definition is the assumption that these outcomes are reversible and do not persist to become long-term health outcomes.

Framework

Preferences for, the act of deciding to participate in, and subsequent participation in chemopreventive, genetic testing, or screening activities comprise a multistage process (Table 10.1). The decision to undergo or engage in the activity can generate a variety of short-term changes in aspects of quality of life. Preparation for screening tests may involve steps that cause transient discomfort or embarrassment. Having a screening test or taking a chemopreventive agent may also be associated with short-term effects on health and well-being.

Table 10.1. Framework of the processes of prevention or screening care that affect short-term outcomes

Activity	Events	Duration
Chemoprevention	Invitation to participate	Days to weeks
	Taking study agent	Weeks to years
	Follow-up	Years
Genetic Testing	Invitation to participate	Days to weeks
	Counseling and testing	Days
	Getting results	Days to weeks
	Post-testing behavior	Years
Screening		
True negative	Invitation to screening	Days to weeks
	Have screening test	One day
	Receive negative result	Days to weeks
False positive	Invitation to screening	Days to weeks
	Have screening test	One day
	Receive positive result- recall for more testing	Days to weeks
	No evidence of cancer	Months
True positive	Invitation to screening	Days to weeks
	Have screening test	One day
	Receive positive result- recall for more testing	Days to weeks
	Diagnosed and treated with cancer	Years
False negative	Invitation to screening	Days to weeks
	Have screening test	One day
	Receive negative result	Days to weeks
	Cancer discovered with symptoms or at next screen	Months to years

Adapted from Johnston, Brown, Gerard et al.[6]

For screening tests, the usual result is either a test that is negative for any abnormalities or known genetic mutations, or else positive for lesions requiring some further diagnostic follow-up, or for a mutation conferring high cancer risk. Individuals receiving a negative result may either be truly disease free ("true negative") or have a lesion (or mutation) that was undetected by the screening test (a "false negative" or a genetic "indeterminate"). Since these types of negative results are indistinguishable in the short term, the short-term outcomes from all negative tests are included in one group. Persons with false negative tests may eventually experience cancer incidence or mortality with long-term effects, which may be regarded as efficacy estimates and are not considered here. Among individuals with a positive test, some will subsequently be diagnosed with cancer ("true positive") while others will prove to be disease free ("false positive"). The proportions of each are determined by test characteristics (sensitivity and specificity). Outcomes for individuals *with* cancer are analyzed elsewhere in the book.

The short-term outcomes following from the events in these sequences are primarily experiential, including psychological effects (e.g., anxiety, distress, or possibly reassurance), physiological effects (e.g., side effects of treatments, typical pain associated with procedures, and atypical effects in the case of complications), and satisfaction effects. Personality, social support, the quality of patient-provider communication, and the individual's underlying risk status may, in turn, moderate each of these effects.

The choice of the appropriate measure(s) of such short-term outcomes will depend on the research question and the intended uses of the data. For instance, if the objective were a thorough comparison of the effectiveness and cost-effectiveness of two technologies for use in population screening or prevention, then general health status measures as well as indices for assessing all possible side effects would be needed. For evaluation of a specific intervention that aims to reduce psychological distress associated with screening or genetic testing, a psychological tool may be sufficient. Other uses of short-term outcomes data range from shared decision making in individual provider-patient encounters to research on how short-term outcomes affect future behaviors, such as continued screening, in populations. In each section that follows, a tabular summary of commonly used instruments is provided.

Methods

A comprehensive literature review was performed to describe and evaluate potential short-term outcomes following from drugs, tests, and devices designed to prevent or detect cancer early or to identify genetic mutations conferring cancer risk. OVID and PUBMED mechanisms were used to search MEDLINE for English language articles on breast, cervical, colorectal, and prostate cancers and chemoprevention, genetic testing, or screening published between January 1, 1985 and December 31, 2001. While the Cancer Outcomes Measurement Working Group (COMWG) is focused on lung, breast, prostate, and colorectal cancers, the cancer types included in this review were selected to focus on cancer sites that had proven chemoprevention modalities, known genetic susceptibility mutations, and/or early detection tests. The search strategy used the subject terms "breast neoplasms," "cervix neoplasms," "colorectal neoplasms," or "prostate neoplasms" with the subject terms "mass screening," "genetics," "testing and counseling," "prevention," and "chemoprevention." Studies were selected if they included key or text words of "outcomes," "short-term outcomes," "psychological outcomes," "distress," "adverse effects," "well-being," "health status," "anxiety," "depression," or "quality of life." Studies conducted outside the United States or Western Europe were excluded due to concerns about comparability of health care systems, attitudes, and culture. Non-peer-reviewed journal articles, reviews, letters, and case studies were also excluded. Additionally, because computerized searches are known to identify only a portion of relevant articles,[7] a backward search was conducted using the bibliographies of published studies, books, and reviews to identify other relevant current published articles and key studies from the period prior to 1985.

Chemoprevention

The possibility of altering the molecular processes involved in carcinogenesis to prevent the occurrence of cancer has received a great deal of attention in recent years.[8] Many classes of potentially protective agents, both naturally occurring and pharmaceutical, are under evaluation in phase I, II, and III trials.[9] The diversity of these chemopreventive

Table 10.2. Instruments used to measure short-term outcomes of chemoprevention for breast, prostate, colorectal, or cervical cancer

Instrument/Tool and Source	Cancer Site	No. of Studies Using Tools	Citations
Medical Outcomes	Breast	1	Ganz et al.[12]
Study SF-36[13]	Prostate	1	Moinpour et al.[10]
General Health Questionnaire – 30[14]	Breast	1	Fallowfield et al.[11]
Spielberger State/Trait Anxiety Inventory[15]	Breast	1	Fallowfield et al.[11]
Multidimensional Health Locus of Control[16]	Breast	1	Fallowfield et al.[11]
CES-D[17]	Breast	1	Ganz et al.[12]
American Urological Association Symptom Index (AUASI)[18,19]	Prostate	1	Moinpour et al.[10]
Medical Outcomes Study Sexual	Breast	1	Ganz et al.[12]
Problems Scale[20]	Prostate	1	Moinpour et al.[10]
Sexual Activity Scale[21]	Breast	1	Fallowfield et al.[11]
Women's Health Questionnaire[22]	Breast	1	Strickler et al.[23]
Sexual Activity Scale[24]	Prostate	1	Moinpour et al.[10]

agents suggests that effects on quality of life will vary. Measurement of health-related quality of life (HRQOL) is being incorporated increasingly into these trials.[10–12] Some chemopreventive agents used in high-risk individuals confer low but measurable risks for long-term morbidity (e.g., an increased risk of endometrial cancer with tamoxifen), but this review focuses on the more frequent, reversible short-term influences. In measuring HRQOL effects of chemoprevention, careful attention must be paid to assessing any known or suspected effects of the agent. However, it is also advisable to cast a broad net by looking for changes in general mental and physical health status that could be mediated by unsuspected effects of the agent. The tools used to study the effects of chemoprevention are summarized in Table 10.2.

Effects of engaging in chemoprevention on HRQOL

The act of taking a chemopreventive agent may affect one's sense of well-being, positively or negatively, independent of any direct effects of the specific agent, but there is little useful data on this question. In a survey of participants in a one-year colorectal

cancer chemoprevention trial, respondents identified the possibility of reducing their risk for cancer as a major benefit of trial participation.[25] Participants in two large chemoprevention trials, the Breast Cancer Prevention Trial (BCPT)[12] and the Prostate Cancer Prevention Trial (PCPT),[10] scored substantially higher than community samples on general measures of physical and mental health functioning at baseline – differences attributed to selection criteria for study entry. In longitudinal analyses of the BCPT, there was no indication of improvement over time in measures of depression or physical or mental health functioning that might indicate a general benefit of participation.[26]

Neither the BCPT nor the PCPT included specific measures of anxiety, which might be heightened at baseline, given the high-risk status of invited participants, and possibly affected by the opportunity to initiate a chemoprevention regimen. Thirlaway et al.[27] found higher levels of anxiety in women with a positive family history for breast cancer compared to those without. However, among high-risk women, those who were participating in a British tamoxifen chemoprevention trial reported lower levels of anxiety. In fact, their anxiety levels were similar to levels of women without a family history.

Anxiety was specifically measured over time in two small British tamoxifen chemoprevention trials.[11] Anxiety levels did not change from baseline over the course of the studies in either intervention or control groups.

Because efficacy trials involve unproven agents and randomization to an uncertain treatment status, they are not ideal for assessing the effects of taking proven chemopreventive agents on general health and well-being. Prospective or cross-sectional observational studies in general populations may provide more useful information.

Chemoprevention of breast cancer

The most notable achievements of chemoprevention to date are for breast cancer. Selective estrogen receptor modulators (SERMs) have been shown convincingly to lower risk for breast cancer incidence in high-risk women.[28,29] Tamoxifen, the first SERM to be evaluated, reduced breast cancer incidence by 49% in more than 11 000 women in the BCPT.[29] Tamoxifen was also suspected of increasing risk for several complications, including uterine cancer, deep venous thrombosis, stroke, hot flashes, menstrual irregularities, and vaginal discharge. Given these various adverse effects, the BCPT carefully assessed subjective HRQOL at baseline and serially throughout the study.[12] Attention was paid to both general physical and mental health function, using the MOS SF-36[13,20,30] and the Center for Epidemiologic Studies-Depression Scale (CES-D)[31,32] and to specific known or suspected side effects of tamoxifen, using a 43-item symptom checklist and the MOS Sexual Problems Scale.[20]

In the report of findings at 36 months follow-up, no differences in either the depression scale or in general measures of physical or mental health function were found between tamoxifen and placebo groups.[26] However, a number of gynecologic symptoms were reported more frequently in women receiving tamoxifen. Symptom differences appeared shortly after the study began and persisted without further increase through 36 months. In addition, women on tamoxifen were somewhat more likely to report lack of sexual interest, difficulty becoming sexually aroused, and having orgasm as "definite or serious" problems.

Two small British chemoprevention trials of tamoxifen[11] measured anxiety using the Spielberger State/Trait Anxiety Inventory.[15] Although anxiety levels varied within participants over time, no trend was observed in either group over the five years of follow-up, and tamoxifen-treated subjects did not differ at any time from those on placebo. These smaller trials were consistent with the BCPT in showing no treatment-related effects on measures of depression.

A second SERM, raloxifene, was reported to lower breast cancer incidence by 76% in the Multiple Outcomes of Raloxifene Evaluation (MORE) Trial.[28] The side effect profile of raloxifene is generally similar to tamoxifen, except that raloxifene has a lower risk of uterine cancer. Unfortunately, no formal assessment of HRQOL has been reported from the MORE trial. In a smaller trial, Strickler et al.[23] measured changes in HRQOL in postmenopausal women randomized to raloxifene, estrogen, or placebo. Quality of life was assessed at baseline and 12 months using the Women's Health Questionnaire,[22] a multidimensional instrument designed and validated for peri- and postmenopausal women. No differences between groups were found for several aspects of general health status, including depression, concentration, memory, sexual behavior, sleep problems, or perceived attractiveness. Estrogen users had a reduction in vasomotor symptoms while raloxifene users did not; however, raloxifene was associated with greater improvement in anxiety/fear scores than for other groups.

A large randomized trial comparing tamoxifen with raloxifene (STAR) is currently enrolling 22 000 postmenopausal women.[33] The primary aim of the study is to determine if either of these agents is superior in reducing the incidence of invasive breast cancer. Secondary aims include in situ breast cancer and endometrial cancer, ischemic heart disease, fractures, toxicity and side effects, and quality of life. The HRQOL assessment is similar to that used in the BCPT, including use of the SF-36 and similar symptom indices. Because the sample size is so large,

HRQOL is being assessed only in a subgroup of 2000 women.

Adverse event profiles of tamoxifen and raloxifene restrict their use to patients at high risk for breast cancer.[34] As newer and lower risk agents appear,[35] evaluation of short-term outcomes, both symptoms and psychological effects, will be even more important.

Chemoprevention of prostate cancer

The first major chemoprevention trial for prostate cancer, the PCPT,[36] is evaluating an anti-androgenic agent, finasteride. Unlike the anti-estrogenic compounds, tamoxifen and raloxifene, finasteride has a remarkably benign side-effect profile. Large trials conducted in men with benign prostatic hyperplasia indicate that essentially the only noteworthy side effects are a very modest decrease in some aspects of sexual functioning and increased breast tenderness.[37] These symptoms also appear to decrease over time.

The PCPT enrolled and randomized more than 18 000 men between 1994 and 1996. Trial results are expected in 2004. HRQOL is assessed at baseline and annually during the trial.[10] General health and functional status are assessed with the MOS SF-36. Specific treatment-related effects are assessed using the American Urological Association's Symptom Index,[18,19] the MOS Sexual Problems Scale,[20] and a Sexual Activity Scale adapted from previous trials of benign prostatic hyperplasia.[24] In baseline comparisons,[10] participants were found to be highly educated, primarily white, and with healthy lifestyles. Scores on seven of the eight scales of the SF-36 were higher than for general population samples. Disease-specific symptom scores were also slightly below population norms. No longitudinal data have been published to date.

A distinct chemopreventive approach to prostate cancer will evaluate the trace mineral selenium and vitamin E, alone and in combination.[38,39] The Selenium and Vitamin E Cancer Prevention Trial (SELECT) aims to enroll and randomize more than 32 000 men to study the effect of these two agents on the clinical incidence of prostate cancer. A secondary objective is assessment of quality of life in a subgroup of 9200 subjects. General health status will be measured with the physical and mental component scores of the Veterans' SF-36 (SF-36V), which is a modification of the SF-36 intended to increase the precision and discriminatory validity of the instrument's role functioning scales when administered to a predominantly older, male population.[40] Population norms for this scale will be available shortly. No patient-reported symptom survey is planned in SELECT.

Chemoprevention of colorectal cancer

Several chemopreventive approaches have been studied for colorectal cancer,[41] including aspirin[42] and other non-steroidal anti-inflammatory agents (NSAIDS).[43] If these agents prove to be efficacious in preventing adenomatous polyps in high-risk groups, larger trials will be needed in average-risk populations. Some studies suggest that protection by NSAIDS does not occur until 20 years of regular use and that the effect disappears promptly when use is terminated. With prolonged use, the potential for adverse gastrointestinal effects, including bleeding and pain, may be substantial. Studies to date have not formally assessed HRQOL, but conclusions for average-risk patients may ultimately require data on short-term outcomes related to gastrointestinal symptoms.

Dietary calcium has also been associated in some studies with a lower risk for colorectal cancer. In the largest positive trial,[44] the only HRQOL assessment was reporting of gastrointestinal side effects or treatment termination due to perceived side effects. Outcome did not differ by treatment group, and 80% of each group were still taking their assigned medication regularly at 4 years.

Chemoprevention of cervical cancer

It is now widely accepted that human papilloma virus (HPV) is the primary etiologic agent for cervical cancer.[45] Strategies of testing specifically for HPV in conjunction with Pap smear screening are currently being evaluated. Once a strategy is selected, chemo-preventive approaches to eradicating HPV may prove efficacious. However, no trials of chemopreventive agents for cervical cancer are currently underway in this country.

Genetic testing

The past decade has witnessed the first identification of genes that predispose to cancer and the testing for these predictive genetic markers.[46] Despite these scientific advances, there is a paucity of data on the short-term psychological effects of undergoing counseling and testing for cancer genetic mutations.[47] In this review, testing for mutations in the BRCA1 and 2 genes is used as an example. These genes confer high risk of breast and ovarian (and other) cancers, have a large body of data available on testing outcomes, and involve a cancer with proven early detection effectiveness (breast).

Undergoing counseling or testing for high-risk genetic mutations may affect not only individuals but also their families and even future unborn generations.[48] Having information about a genetic susceptibility to cancer can lead to short-term psychological changes, increases or decreases in cancer risk perceptions, alterations in cancer surveillance or prevention behaviors, and even prophylactic surgery to remove the at-risk organ (e.g., bilateral mastectomy).[49,50] Finally, information from genetic testing may have an impact on insurability and job prospects.[51] Instruments used to evaluate the impact of genetic testing are numerous and are highlighted in Table 10.3.

Attendance at genetic counseling and testing clinics has generally been noted to alleviate worry and/or decrease depression, partly due to provision of more accurate information on cancer risk to individuals with inappropriate perceptions of very high risks.[52,84] Among those testing negative, significant decreases in distress,[59] worry,[52,80] anxiety,[85] perceived cancer risk,[59,80] depression,[60] and role impairment[61] have been reported, although some

still over-estimate their cancer risk,[52] and a few report a sense of guilt about a negative result when other family members are affected.[50,65,86]

Among those testing positive, some women note disturbed family relationships and/or have expressed guilt over passing on a mutation to their offspring.[81] In one small study in Canada, Ritvo *et al.* noted that post-counseling levels of depression were moderated by self-perceived risk of cancer, where those who thought themselves at low risk had low levels of depression, while those who over-estimated their risk were significantly more depressed.[52] Interestingly, depression levels were not associated with actual risk level discussed during the counseling sessions but were moderated by dispositional optimism.[52] In other studies, pre-test distress has been noted to be the strongest predictor of post-test distress, independent of test result.[53,60,61,63,85] Levels of distress also appear to be moderated by pre-testing expectations about the effects of testing.[71]

Some groups have noted increases in short-term distress related to notification of positive mutation status,[53] but other researchers failed to find such effects.[59,65,85] Absence of an increase in anxiety or distress may, in part, reflect the removal of uncertainty,[87] the success of the counseling programs,[60,61,71] effective coping styles,[53,56,58,88] or effects of social supports.[48] Differences in post-test levels of anxiety or depression between persons testing positive and those testing negative appear to be due to decreases among those testing negative, especially among persons with high baseline anxiety, rather than to increased distress among those who tested positive.[53,60,61,63] Interestingly, women at high risk of mutations who show high levels of stress but decline testing and counseling have been noted to have a higher risk of depression than women who decide to be tested.[61]

The effects of having a genetic test on subsequent surveillance behavior are not clear. Lerman *et al.*[46] reported that testing positive for a high-risk mutation for breast cancer led to significantly higher rates of routine screening mammography one year later. Nevertheless, as many as one-third failed to

Table 10.3. Instruments used to measure short-term outcomes of genetic testing and counseling for breast and ovarian cancer susceptibility mutations

Instrument/Tool and Source	No. of Studies Using Tool	Citations
Spielberger State/Trait Anxiety Inventory[15]	3	Smith et al.[48]
		Ritvo et al.[52]
		Tercyak et al.[53]
		Hatcher et al.[54]
Profile of Mood States[55]	1	Schwartz et al.[56]
Perceptions of Risk [57,58]	1	Schwartz et al.[56]
		Schwartz et al.[59]
CES-D[17]	3	Ritvo et al.[52]
		Lerman et al.[60]
		Lerman et al.[61]
Hospital Anxiety and Depression Scale (HADS)[62]	1	Lodder et al.[63]
Self-Rating Depression Scale[64]	1	Wagner et al.[65]
Coping Test[66]	1	Hatcher et al.[54]
Body Image Scale[67]	1	Hatcher et al.[54]
(Hopkins) Symptom Checklist (25 or 90 items)[68–70]	3	Schwartz et al.[59]
		Dorval et al.[71]
		Coyne et al.[72]
Brief Symptom Inventory (53 items)[69]	1	Dorval et al.[71]
Miller Behavioral Style Scale[73]	1	Tercyak et al.[53]
Life Orientation Test[74]	1	Ritvo et al.[52]
Revised Impact of Events Scale/ Impact of Events Scale[75]	4	Lerman et al.[46]
		Smith et al.[48]
		Schwartz et al.[56]
		Schwartz et al.[59]
		Lodder et al.[63]
		Grilli et al.[76]
Risk Perception Questionnaire[49]	1	Hatcher et al.[54]
General Health Questionnaire – 28[77]	1	Hatcher et al.[54]
Sexual Activity Questionnaire[21]	1	Hatcher et al.[54]
Medical Outcomes Study SF-36[30]	1	Lerman et al.[60]
Medical Outcomes Study – Social Support Scale[78]	1	Ritvo et al.[52]
Medical Outcomes Study – Sexual Function Scales[20]	1	Lerman et al.[60]
Structured Clinical Psychiatric Interview – Present State Examination[79]	1	Coyne et al.[72]
Developed for Study	6	Evans et al.[49]
		Coyne et al.[72]
		Plon et al.[80]
		Metcalfe et al.[81]
		Frost et al.[82]
		Payne et al.[83]
Open-ended Questions	2	Lodder et al.[63]
		Metcalfe et al.[81]
		Frost et al.[82]

obtain mammography and only about 10% sought ovarian cancer screening. Others have also reported that mutation carriers increase their screening use.[81] Women testing negative for mutations were found to maintain high rates of recommended screening over two years in a single study.[80] The possibility that anxiety/worry could be a barrier to screening in some mutation carriers has also been suggested.[89–91] Prior inappropriately high rates of screening among women who test negative represent a possible selection bias in understanding post-test behaviors. Lack of measurement sensitivity for explanatory variables such as anxiety or unmeasured personality factors may also explain discordant results. Future studies in this important area must carefully characterize tested populations in terms of baseline risk, personality, pre-test screening behaviors, and levels of anxiety during follow-up.

Another possible response to having a positive genetic test may be prophylactic surgery. While such surgery may have psychological benefits for some women,[54,82] up to one-quarter of women testing positive who choose bilateral prophylactic mastectomy report psychological distress or dissatisfaction with their decision.[82,83] Overall, these limited studies suggest that there are short-term psychological and role disturbances associated with genetic testing. No data were found on the short-term effects of testing on health and mental care use, missed work days, satisfaction with care, the quality of provider-client communication, or on patient preferences or utilities for short-term effects.

Screening

As mass screening for various cancers continues to increase, attention is being drawn to possible unintended consequences of screening, such as potential adverse physiological[92] and psychological effects[93,94,95] and opportunity costs. Public campaigns as well as one-on-one counseling by health care providers can increase the receipt of screening but may also induce some worry about cancer.[96,97] For some screening tests (e.g., colonoscopy or sigmoidoscopy), both preparation for testing and the procedure itself may cause temporary discomfort or embarrassment.[98] For those who test positive, including false positives, there may be anxiety and distress related to being recalled for additional diagnostic procedures and waiting for results. Thus, standard psychological and HRQOL tools have been used to measure consequences of the screening process; in some cases, investigators have developed new instruments to attempt to capture some of the less tangible aspects of undergoing screening (Table 10.4).

Colorectal cancer

Colorectal cancer screening recommendations were codified only in the late 1990s. Thus, at present, there is little literature on colorectal screening determinants[179] and even less data on short-term effects on HRQOL. Given the nature of colorectal cancer screening tests, it is possible that the profile of short-term effects will vary from those reported for breast and cervical cancer screening. For colonoscopy, there is considerably more time involved in pre-test preparation, undergoing the test itself, and post-test recovery[158] than for cervical or breast cancer screening testing. Colonoscopy also entails a small risk of major complications (e.g., colonic perforation) not seen with other cancer site-specific screening tests. In common with other modalities, studies of short-term sequelae associated with colorectal screening have noted concerns about worry, distress, embarrassment, fear, anxiety, and pain associated with the test, particularly in anticipation of the test.[158,171,172,174] These effects often turn out to be less intense than anticipated. One study failed to find higher anxiety or depression among participants in a screening trial compared to controls.[119] In the only study of patients with false screening results, those with a false positive result were twice as likely to report distress as those with negative results.[171]

Since reactions to screening tests may vary by gender[170] and both men and women are screened, future explorations of short-term outcomes of colorectal cancer screening are particularly important.

Table 10.4. Instruments used to measure short-term outcomes of screening

Instrument/Tool and Source	Cancer Site	No. of Studies Using Tool	Citations
Psychosocial Effects of Abnormal Pap Smears Questionnaire (PEAPS-Q)[99]	Cervix	1	Bennett [100]
Anxiety Screening Questionnaire[170]	Cervix	1	Wolfe et al.[101]
Spielberger State/Trait Anxiety Inventory[15]	Colorectal	3	Tomaino-Brunner et al.[102]
			Nugent et al.[103]
			Gath et al. [104]
	Cervix	3	Somerset et al.[105]
			Palmer et al.[106]
			Marteau et al.[107]
	Breast	5	Aro et al.[97]
			Aro et al. [98]
			Sutton et al.[108]
			Brett et al.[109]
			Ong et al.[110]
	Prostate	1	Essink-Bot et al.[111]
Perceptions of Risk[57]	Breast	1	Diefenbach et al.[112]
CES-D[17]	Breast	2	Aro et al.[97]
			Andrykowski et al.[113]
Hospital Anxiety and Depression Scale (HADS)[62]	Breast	4	Lampic et al.[114]
			Bull et al.[115]
			Scaf-Klomp et al.[116]
			Gilbert et al.[117]
	Cervix	1	Bell et al.[118]
	Colorectal	1	Thiis-Evensen et al.[119]
Beck Depression Scale[120]	Cervix	1	Gath et al.[104]
	Breast	3	Aro et al.[97]
			Aro et al.[98]
			Northouse et al.[121]
Leeds Depression and Anxiety Scale[122]	Cervix	1	Gath et al.[104]
Profile of Mood States (POMS)[55]	Breast	2	Andrykowski et al.[113]
			Steggles et al.[123]
	Prostate	1	Taylor et al.[124]
Positive and Negative Affect Scale (PANAS)[125]	Breast	1	Andrykowski et al.[113]
	Cervix	1	Lauver et al.[126]
Mood Adjective Check List (mood)[127]	Breast	1	Lidbrink et al.[92]
Taylor Manifest Anxiety Scale[128]	Breast	1	Kash et al.[90]
Cancer-Related Anxiety and Helplessness Scale[129]	Breast	1	Kash et al.[90]
Coping Test[66]	Breast	1	Lidbrink et al.[92]

(cont.)

Table 10.4. (*cont.*)

Instrument/Tool and Source	Cancer Site	No. of Studies Using Tool	Citations
Coping Styles[130]	Cervix	1	Bell *et al.*[118]
Rosenberg Self-Esteem Scale[131]	Cervix	1	Bell *et al.*[118]
Maudsley Personality Inventory[132]	Cervix	1	Bell *et al.*[118]
Brief Symptom Inventory[69]	Breast	2	Northouse *et al.*[121]
Hopkins Symptom Checklist (somatic complaints)[68]	Breast	1	Scaf-Klomp *et al.*[116]
Miller Behavioral Style Scale[73]	Cervix	1	Miller *et al.*[134]
Dispositional Optimism[74]	Breast	1	Deiner *et al.*[135]
Smilkstein Stress Scale[136]	Breast	1	Northouse *et al.*[121]
Impact of Events Scale [75]	Cervix	2	Palmer *et al.*[106] Miller *et al.*[134]
	Breast	1	Kash *et al.*[90]
	Prostate	1	Taylor *et al.*[124]
Fear of Cancer Scale[137]	Breast	1	Scaf-Klomp *et al.*[116]
Perceived Health Questionnaire (global HRQOL)[113]	Breast	1	Andrykowski *et al.*[113]
Locus of Health Control[16,138]	Cervix	1	Palmer *et al.*[106]
	Breast	1	Aro *et al.*[97]
Illness Attitudes Scale[139]	Breast	1	Aro *et al.*[97]
Health Questionnaire (7 items – stress related feelings and symptoms)[140]	Breast	1	Gilbert *et al.*[117]
General Health Questionnaire – 28[77]	Cervix	1	Gath *et al.*[104]
	Breast	7	Sutton *et al.*[108] Scaf-Klomp *et al.*[116] Gilbert *et al.*[117] Dean *et al.*[141] Ellman *et al.*[142]
	Colorectal	1	Thiis-Evensen *et al.*[119]
Psychological Consequences Questionnaire – (thoughts about breast cancer)[143]	Breast	6	Olsson *et al.*[95] Brett *et al.*[109] Ong *et al.*[110] Steggles *et al.*[123] Lowe *et al.*[144]
Cooper's Coping Scale of Social Adjustment[133]	Cervix	2	Gath *et al.*[104] Bell *et al.*[118]
Dyadic Adjustment Scale[145]	Cervix	1	Gath *et al.*[104]
	Breast	1	Northouse *et al.*[121]
Eysenck Personality Inventory[146]	Cervix	1	Gath *et al.*[104]
Uncertainty in Illness Scale[147]	Cervix	1	Lauver *et al.*[126]
	Breast	1	Northouse *et al.*[121]
Mental Health Inventory[148]	Cervix	1	Lerman *et al.*[149]

Table 10.4. (*cont.*)

Instrument/Tool and Source	Cancer Site	No. of Studies Using Tool	Citations
Breast Cancer Specific Beliefs[150–152]	Breast	1	Aro *et al.*[97]
Medical Outcomes Study SF-36[30]	Breast	1	Andrykowski *et al.*[113]
	Prostate	2	Essink-Bot *et al.*[111] Naughton *et al.*[153]
EuroQol 5D[154]	Prostate	1	Essink-Bot *et al.*[111]
Physiological Parameters	Breast	1	Lidbrink *et al.*[92]
Clinical Psychiatric Interview – Present State Examination[79]	Cervix	1	Gath *et al.*[104]
	Breast	1	Dean *et al.*[141]
Decision Analysis Model	Prostate	1	Volk *et al.*[155]
Time Trade-Off[156]	Breast	1	Johnston *et al.*[6] Gram *et al.*[157]
	Colorectal	1	Dominitz *et al.*[158]
Linear Rating Scale	Breast	1	de Haes *et al*[159]
Developed for Study	Cervix	7	Nugent *et al.*[103] Lauver *et al.*[126] Lerman *et al.*[149] Orbell *et al.*[160] Wilson *et al.*[161] Paskett *et al.*[162] Reelick *et al.*[163]
	Breast	8	Lerman *et al.*[149] Gram *et al.*[157] Pisano *et al.*[164] Pisano *et al.*[165] Gram *et al.*[166] Schwartz *et al.*[167] Benedict *et al.*[168] Lindfors *et al.*[169]
	Colorectal	3	Lindholm *et al.*[170] Mant *et al.*[171] Winawer *et al.*[172] Drossman *et al.*[173] McCarthy *et al.*[174]
	Prostate	4	Essink-Bot *et al.*[111] Naughton *et al.*[153] Pedersen *et al.*[175] Myers *et al.*[176]
Open-Ended Questions	Cervix	6	Nugent *et al.*[103] Somerset *et al.*[105] Scaf-Klomp *et al.*[116] Lauver *et al.*[126] Reelick *et al.*[163] Lauver *et al.*[177] Quilliam[178]
	Breast	1	Pisano *et al.*[165]
	Colorectal	1	Drossman *et al.*[173]

Identification of common domains that cut across all cancer sites as well as cancer site-specific domains would be valuable.

Prostate cancer

Evaluation of routine screening for prostate cancer is still underway in trials in the United States and Europe (e.g.,[180,181]) and consistent professional guidelines for prostate cancer are not yet available. Hence, there is little literature on the effects of participating in screening or of having a false positive prostate cancer screening test and fewer reports of the effects of abnormal screening results on future screening behavior.

In a study from the Netherlands, men who underwent prostate cancer screening had comparable levels of physical, psychological, and social functioning and anxiety as population controls not participating in screening.[111] However, the instruments used (the SF-36 and the EQ-5D) may not have been sufficiently sensitive to detect small short-term effects. A higher predisposition to anxiety was a strong predictor of experiencing screening-related anxiety. Any anxiety related to false positive tests appeared to be transient. Some distress was noted in another study among 13% of men undergoing prostate cancer screening.[175] Levels of distress have also been noted to vary by levels of perceived risk.[124] Many men (~40%) experience anxiety[175] and discomfort associated with digital rectal examination of the prostate or transrectal sonography (~30%),[111] but transrectal biopsies do not appear to affect emotional well-being, physical role functioning, or return to work.[153]

Myers and colleagues[176] asked US black men about their intentions to be screened and, if screened positive, to have a biopsy. They found that intentions to have a biopsy were negatively related to barriers such as worry about cancer. Volk and colleagues have also suggested that men's spouses[155] may influence prostate screening behaviors.

If prostate cancer screening is not shown ultimately to increase life expectancy, screening will have serious adverse longer-term consequences, including early labeling and potential overtreatment for cancer, and living with treatment-related side effects[182] for a greater number of years than would have occurred in the absence of screening.[111,183] Alternatively, if screening is shown to reduce mortality, then further research will be needed to delineate the full spectrum of short-term screening outcomes.

Breast and cervical cancer

Negative screening results

No data were found that suggest increased anxiety associated with undergoing screening and receiving a negative mammography or Pap smear result.[94,108,123,140–142,166,184] Most individuals receiving negative results experience considerable relief at not having cancer[185] and show lower anxiety levels than those in the general population who have not undergone screening.[116] However, one study has suggested that negative screening results may lead some individuals to believe unrealistically that they cannot get cancer,[94] which can lead to failure to return for subsequent examinations.

False positive screening results

Cancer is a rare disease and screening tests are less than perfect in their ability to separate those with disease from those who are cancer-free. As mass screening increases, more and more individuals will be falsely labeled as potentially having cancer.[186–189] As many as 35% to 56% of women who begin mammography screening at age 50 will have a false positive test over ten years of screening; even higher false positive rates will be observed for younger women.[190,191]

Although some individuals may be willing to accept high rates of false positive tests,[167] on a population basis, abnormal screening tests are likely to have a large short-term impact on health and well-being[6] and on health care utilization and costs.[192] Previous work has identified a number of domains, particularly psychosocial spheres of function, that are affected during the interval from notification of an abnormal mammogram or Pap smear to determination that cancer is absent. Affected domains are extremely similar for Pap smear and mammography and include short-term distress,[90,109,110,121,142,149,163,193] fear and worry about having or getting cancer,[144,177] intrusive thoughts about cancer including anxiety,[99,103,107,108,114–118,151,166,184,194,195] mood changes,[126,149,157] sense of uncertainty,[126] disturbances in family, social, and/or sexual roles,[99,106,118,121,149,196,197] increase in perceived risk of cancer,[198] a sense of "bodily betrayal" or having a post-biopsy scar,[199] behavioral symptoms such as crying, sleep disturbance, and irritability,[116,149,200] concerns about future reproduction,[126,201] and, very rarely, possible suicide.[202] In some studies, having a family history of cancer has been noted to increase anxiety levels during this interval.[117]

These effects, when found, are generally transient (e.g.,[104,114,116,117,142,144,163,203]), have no effect on endocrine and immunological function,[192] and are inversely related to the time from abnormal notification to resolution as normal.[114] However, in some studies, these experiences, including anxiety[107] and an increased sense of susceptibility to cancer,[98,116] have been noted to persist for 6 months or even longer after an abnormal test result.[95,98,109,110,116,157,184,198] As with genetic testing, levels of adverse psychological effects or symptoms following receipt of an abnormal mammogram or Pap smear vary by individuals' inherent coping styles,[95,134,177] educational level,[95] degree of compliance with, or timeliness of resolution of the false positive[149] and severity of the result.[149]

Short-term experiences following mammography or Pap smear have been linked inconsistently to future screening behaviors.[200] Several researchers have noted that persons having false positive results are less likely to return to routine screening schedules and more likely to delay follow up after current or future abnormal screens.[91,162,204,205] However, others have observed that individuals with false positive results have similar[160] or higher compliance rates with future screening[168,193,198,206,207] or excessive practice of self-examinations.[98,206,208] Some of these apparent inconsistencies may be related to the observations that low to moderate levels of anxiety and worry increase breast and/or cervical cancer screening use, while pathologically high levels apparently lead to low screening rates.[89,149,209] The variability in the effects of short-term distress on future actions may also be a result of interactions of distress with levels of perceived cancer risk.

Short-term outcomes measurement

Determining the short-term impact of chemoprevention, genetic testing and counseling, or screening on quality of life is complex for several reasons. There is a diverse range of possible outcomes, from transient anxiety, discomfort, or minor side effects of chemopreventive agents, to the impact of receiving a cancer diagnosis. The duration of HRQOL effects may be highly variable across individuals and interventions. Most target populations will be initially asymptomatic so that prevention and screening frequently imposes upfront cost with the promise of (yet unseen) benefits downstream. Moreover, in part because the area of inquiry is relatively new, there are a lack of measurement standards.[6] To date, most studies measuring short-term outcomes have focused on psychological states (anxiety, depression), symptoms, or general health status at one or more discrete points in time. Most investigations have used previously validated, reliable non-cancer instruments. Many researchers also add cancer-specific measures, such as perceived cancer risk or symptom indices, appropriate to the intervention. None of the studies identified measured satisfaction or the quality of provider-client communication. One report examined workdays lost, but other economic outcomes were not evaluated. Only one study has specifically measured preferences, or utilities, for short-term outcomes using time trade-off methods, and none used standard gamble, linear rating scale, or willingness-to-pay methods.

The measurement approach will vary depending on the research question and intended use of results. Measurement of psychological states and symptoms may be sufficient for informing patients contemplating use of a chemopreventive agent or screening test or for studying the effects of short-term psychological change on future health behaviors. If the question under study involves assessment or comparison of costs, harms, and benefits of a program, use of preference (utility)-based health status instruments or direct assessment of preferences will be needed so that quality-adjusted life-years (QALYs) can be calculated.[210,211] In general, researchers should assess both general and symptom-specific health status using instruments that have been previously validated in populations similar to that under investigation; have established population norms; are reliable and reproducible; represent a minimal patient burden; and are practical from a research perspective.

As mentioned previously, studying participants in blinded efficacy trials is not sufficient for assessing the general impact of chemoprevention. Trial participants understand both the uncertainty of whether the intervention is effective and, in blinded studies, the additional uncertainty as to whether they are receiving the active agent or placebo. The impact of these preventive or early detection interventions on HRQOL should ultimately be evaluated after efficacy is known, using observational methods in representative samples of the target population.

Several generic methodological flaws have been common among the studies completed to date. With rare exception, (e.g.,[95,98]) studies have been conducted in self-selected convenience samples of individuals attending a specific practice or clinic or in healthy volunteers. Low response rates in many chemoprevention and screening studies make it difficult to generalize findings to target populations. Failure to measure and control for baseline personality and psychological traits is particularly troublesome. In considering distress after receipt of a false positive screening result, all but four studies[98,114,117,144] failed to control for pre-screening level of distress, anxiety, depression, and/or symptoms, although baseline distress has been shown to be the single strongest predictor of distress after the resolution of an abnormal mammogram.[95] An alternative means of controlling for population characteristics and psychological symptoms is the use of a concurrent control group. Several studies (e.g.,[198,212]) have examined individuals screened in the same time period who had normal results or comparable populations who had not undergone screening.[157,212] The utility of an unscreened control group drawn from the same target population was underscored by findings of Scaf-Klomp et al., who found that differences in distress between women with false positive mammograms and those with normal results were largely attributable to the lower-than-average rates of distress seen in association with relief experienced by the group who screened negative, compared to their age-matched unscreened counterparts in the general population.[116]

Many studies have failed to measure or control for factors likely to confound or interact with the relationship between process and outcome under study. In particular, none of the studies was designed to detect differences in effect by age, race, language, gender, or other important subgroups defined by personality factors, such as coping and information seeking styles. Several researchers have noted that these traits can interact with stress to affect short-term outcomes (e.g.,[95,134,177]).

Several methodological issues are specific to measuring short-term outcomes. The sensitivity of instruments generally used for chronic states in detecting short-term changes is largely unexplored. The timing of assessment is particularly important in capturing short-term effects. For instance, patients report greater decrements in quality of life associated with emesis during chemotherapy when instruments are administered at the same time as the maximal emesis, while decrements are rated as being less severe just one to two weeks later.[213] Measuring preferences for use in a summary measure such as QALYs can be problematic because these transient effects must be measured on the same scale as that used for chronic states, usually a zero to one interval scale.[214] Methods such as "chaining" or "cascading" have been applied to this problem. In these techniques, the worst short-term effect is valued relative to death (zero), and then outcomes rated as being better than the worst are converted relative to this lower value.[214] However, the choice of death as the anchor may induce unintended framing effects and has not been well validated.[6] Further, valuing health states, using either time trade-off, standard gamble, or linear rating scales, may be influenced by cognitive abilities, past experiences, age, non-health values, or other factors.[215] Willingness-to-pay methods may also be influenced by financial status. Finally, it is unclear whether people value "bad" health states more highly (i.e., as more tolerable) if they are seen as transient versus chronic.[216] Thus, it has been suggested that the usefulness of preference measures for short-term outcomes would be enhanced by interpretation within the context of qualitative analyses.[6]

Summary and recommendations

This chapter has focused on short-term effects of screening and chemoprevention in asymptomatic populations. Patients and health care systems will increasingly be faced with options or choices for preventing or detecting common cancers. Competing strategies that offer roughly equivalent risks and benefits in terms of reduction in cancer incidence or death may nevertheless differ in subtler effects on short-term quality of life. Alternatively, one strategy may confer greater clinical benefit but be accompanied by greater adverse effects on HRQOL. The individual patient's personal preferences and personality may amplify these differences. In these situations, accurate, representative information on short-term outcomes may be useful for comparing

two or more strategies aimed at the same cancer. Adoption of a standard battery of instruments would facilitate such comparisons. More research is needed to achieve a consensus on the optimal minimal data set that would be applicable to most questions and populations under evaluation.

From the health care system or policy analyst's perspective, careful patient-reported quality-of-life assessments from clinical trials and population samples will be needed to conduct quantitative assessments of the costs and benefits of competing strategies. Before these data can be input, however, responses must be translated into a quantitative currency. Patient utility (or disutility) is that currency. Utilities quantify the overall value or loss of value associated with specific symptoms or functional impairments.[210,217] Measurement of utilities is difficult and time consuming and is often not feasible in the context of large clinical trials. Once effects on quality of life for screening or chemoprevention are identified, additional research is needed to assess the value or importance of these decrements for representative patients. In this context, special attention must be paid to the baseline risk status of patients. However, before investing substantial resources in measuring utilities for short-term health states, the analyst should assess, *via* sensitivity analyses, whether different values would affect conclusions about overall effectiveness or cost-effectiveness.

Many of the study results reported in this chapter can be questioned for their representativeness of the general population. Selection criteria for participation in clinical trials often exclude persons with poorer baseline quality of life and those at greatest risk for experiencing adverse effects of the intervention. As with medical therapy, there is a need for carefully conducted, population-based observational studies to evaluate the impact of screening, genetic testing, and chemoprevention in populations that more broadly represent those who will ultimately be encouraged to take up the activity.

Based on results to date, there seems little reason to expect that most screening and chemopreventive interventions will have detectable effects on general health status measures such as the SF-36. Future studies should continue to develop and use sensitive methods for detecting short-term effects on psychological characteristics and on symptoms. Careful attention to baseline characteristics, using pre-intervention measurements, control groups, or both, and attention to timing of measurement will help to identify these short-term effects.

The art and science of defining and measuring short-term outcomes is at a very elementary level. The work necessary to standardize measurement of short-term outcomes will need to be considered within the overall context of HRQOL research needs and national cancer program priorities.

REFERENCES

1 Strain, J. J. (1990). The evolution of quality of life evaluations in cancer therapy. *Oncology* **4**:22–7.

2 Heithoff, K. A. (1990). *Effectiveness and Outcomes in Health Care: Proceedings of an Invitational Conference by the Institute of Medicine, Division of Health Care Services.* Washington, DC: National Academy Press.

3 Holland, J. C. (1986). *Assessment of Quality of Life and Cancer Treatment.* Brookline, MA: Cancer and Leukemia Group B (CALGB).

4 Mandelblatt, J., Armetta, C., Yabroff, Y. *et al.* (2004). A descriptive review of the literature on breast cancer outcomes:1990–2000. *Journal of the National Cancer Institute*, in press.

5 Patrick, D. L., Erickson, P. (1993). *Health Status and Health Policy: Quality of Life in Health Care Evaluation and Resource Allocation.* New York, NY: Oxford University Press.

6 Johnston, K., Brown, J., Gerard, K. *et al.* (1998). Valuing temporary and chronic health states associated with breast screening. *Social Science and Medicine* **47**(2): 213–22.

7 Dickersin, K. (1994). Identifying relevant studies for systematic reviews. *British Medical Journal* **309**:1286–91.

8 Greenwald, P. (2001). From carcinogenesis to clinical interventions for cancer prevention. *Toxicology* **166**:37–45.

9 Osborne, M., Boyle, P., Lipkin, M. (1997). Cancer prevention. *Lancet* **2**(Suppl.):27–30.

10 Moinpour, C., Lovato, L., Thompson, I., Ware J. *et al.* (2000). Profile of men randomized to the prostate cancer prevention trial: baseline health-related quality of life, urinary and sexual functioning and health behaviors. *Journal of Clinical Oncology* **18**(1942):1953.

11 Fallowfield, L., Fleissig, A., Edwards, R. *et al.* (2001). Tamoxifen for the prevention of breast cancer: psychosocial impact on women participating in two randomized controlled trials. *Journal of Clinical Oncology* **19**(7): 1885–92.

12 Ganz, P. A., Day, R., Ware, J. E. *et al.* (1995). Base-line quality-of-life assessment in the National Surgical Adjuvant Breast and Bowel Project Breast Cancer Prevention Trial. *Journal of the National Cancer Institute* **87**(18):1372–82.

13 Stewart, A. L., Ware, J. E. (eds) (1992). *Measuring Functioning and Well-Being: The Medical Outcomes Study Approach.* Durham, NC: Duke University Press.

14 Goldberg, D. P., Hillier, V. F. (1979) A scaled version of the General Health Questionnaire. *Psychology Medicine* **9**(1):139–45.

15 Spielberger, C. D. (1983). *Manual for the State-Trait Anxiety Inventory STAI (form Y) "Self evaluation questionnaire."* Palo Alto, CA: Consulting Psychologists Press.

16 Wallston, K. A. (1978). Development of the Multidimensional Health Locus of Control (MHLC) Scales. *Health Education Monograph* **6**(2):160–70.

17 Andresen, E. M., Malmgren, J. A., Carter, W. B. *et al.* Screening of depression in well older adults: evaluation of a short form of the CES-D (Center for Epidemiologic Studies Depression Scale). *American Journal of Preventive Medicine* **10**:77–84.

18 Barry, M. J. (1995). Measuring disease-specific health status in men with benign prostatic hyperplasia. Measurement Committee of the American Urological Association. *Medical Care* **33**(4(Suppl.)):AS145–55.

19 Barry, M. J., Fowler, F. J., O'Leary, M. P. *et al.* (1992). The American Urological Association symptom index for benign prostatic hyperplasia. The Measurement Committee of the American Urological Association. *Journal of Urology* **148**(5):1549–57.

20 Sherbourne, C. D. (1992). Social functioning: sexual problems measures. In *Measuring Functioning and Well-being: The Medical Outcomes Study Approach*, eds. A. L. Stewart, J. E. Ware, Jr., pp. 194–204. Durham, NC: Duke University Press.

21 Thirlaway, K. (1996). The Sexual Activity Questionnaire: a measure of women's sexual functioning. *Quality of Life Research* **5**(1):81–90.

22 Hunter, M. (1992). The Women's Health Questionnaire. A measure of mid-aged women's perceptions of their

emotional and physical health. *Psychology and Health* **7**: 15–54.

23 Strickler, R. (2000). Raloxifene and estrogen effects on quality of life in healthy postmenopausal women: a placebo-controlled randomized trial. *Obstetrics and Gynecology* **96**(3):359–65.

24 Epstein, R. S., Deverka, P. A., Chute, C. G. *et al.* (1992). Validation of new quality of life questionnaire for benign prostatic hyperplasia. *Journal of Clinical Epidemiology* **45**: 1431–45.

25 Hudmon, K., Lover, R., Chamberlain, R. (1999). Perceived benefits and barriers to participation in a phase I/II colon cancer prevention trial. *Journal of Cancer Education* **14**: 83–7.

26 Day, R., Ganz, P. A., Costantino, J. P. *et al.* (1999). Health-related quality of life and tamoxifen in breast cancer prevention: a report from the National Surgical Adjuvant Breast and Bowel Project P-1 Study. *Journal of Clinical Oncology* **17**(9):2659–69.

27 Thirlaway, K., Fallowfield, L., Cuzick, J. (1996). Anxiety in women "at risk" of developing breast cancer. *British Journal of Cancer* **73**:1422–4.

28 Cummings, S. R., Eckert, S., Krueger, K. A. *et al.* (1999). The effect of raloxifene on risk of breast cancer in post-menopausal women: results from the MORE randomized trial. Multiple Outcomes of Raloxifene Evaluation. *Journal of the American Medical Association* **281**(23): 2189–97.

29 Fisher, B., Costantino, J. P., Wickerham, D. L. *et al.* (1998). Tamoxifen for prevention of breast cancer: report of the National Surgical Adjuvant Breast and Bowel Project P-1 Study. *Journal of the National Cancer Institute* **90**(18): 1371–88.

30 Ware, J. E., Jr., Sherbourne, C. D. (1992). The MOS 36-item short-form health survey (SF-36): Conceptual framework and item selection. *Medical Care* **30**(6):473–81.

31 Roberts, R. E., Vernon, S. W. (1983). The center for epidemiologic studies depression scale: Its use in a community sample. *American Journal of Psychiatry* **140**(1):41–6.

32 Radloff, L. S. (1977). The CES-D Scale: a self-report depression scale for research in the general population. *Applied Psychological Measurement* **1**:385–401.

33 Dunn, B. K., Ford, L. G. (2001). From adjuvant therapy to breast cancer prevention: BCPT and STAR. *Breast Journal* **7**(3):144–57.

34 Levine, M., Moutquin, J. M., Walton, R. *et al.* (2001). Chemoprevention of breast cancer. A joint guideline from the Canadian Task Force on Preventive Health Care and the Canadian Breast Cancer Initiative's Steering Committee on Clinical Practice Guidelines for the Care and Treatment of Breast Cancer. *Canadian Medical Association Journal* **164**(12):1681–90.

35 Fabian, C. J. (2001). Breast cancer chemoprevention: beyond tamoxifen. *Breast Cancer Research* **3**(2):99–103.

36 Thompson, I. M. J., Kouril, M., Klein, E. A. *et al.* (2001). The prostate cancer prevention trial: current status and lessons learned. *Urology* **57**(4 (Suppl.)):230–4.

37 Kaplan, S., Garvin, D., Gilhooly, P. *et al.* (2000). Impact of baseline symptom severity on future risk of benign prostatic hyperplasia-related outcomes and long-term response to finasteride. *Urology* **56**(4):610–16.

38 Clark, L. C., Dalkin, B., Krongrad, A. *et al.* (1998). Decreased incidence of prostate cancer with selenium supplementation: results of a double-blind cancer prevention trial. *British Journal of Urology* **81**:730–4.

39 Clark, L. C., Combs, G. F., Turnbull, B. W. *et al.* (1996). Effects of selenium supplementation for cancer prevention in patients with carcinoma of the skin. A randomized controlled trial. Nutritional Prevention of Cancer Study Group. *Journal of the American Medical Association* **276**: 1957–63.

40 Kazis, L. E., Ren, X. S., Lee, A. *et al.* (1999). Health status in VA patients: results from the Veterans Health Study. *American Journal of Medical Quality* **14**(1):28–38.

41 Baron, J. A. (2000). Nonsteroidal anti-inflammatory drugs and cancer prevention. *Annual Review of Medicine* **51**: 511–23.

42 Kune, G. A. (1988). Colorectal cancer risk, chronic illnesses, operations, and medications: case control results from the Melbourne Colorectal Cancer Study. *Cancer Research* **48**(15):4399–404.

43 Clapper, M. L. (2001). Chemoprevention of colorectal cancer. *Current Opinion in Oncology* **13**:307–13.

44 Baron, J. A. (1999). Calcium supplements for the prevention of colorectal adenomas. Calcium Polyp Prevention Study Group. *American College of Physicians Journal Club* **131**(2):39.

45 Schiffman, M. H., Bauer, H. M., Hoover, R. N. *et al.* (1993). Epidemiologic evidence showing that human papillomavirus infection causes most cervical intraepithelial neoplasia. *Journal of the National Cancer Institute* **85**: 958–64.

46 Lerman, C., Hughes, C., Croyle, R. T. *et al.* (2000). Prophylactic surgery decisions and surveillance practices one year following BRCA1/2 testing. *Preventive Medicine* **31**(1): 75–80.

47 Freyer, G., Dazord, A., Schlumberger, M. *et al.* (1999). Psychosocial impact of genetic testing in familial

medullary-thyroid carcinoma: a multicentric pilot-evaluation. *Annals of Oncology* **10**(1):87–95.

48 Smith, K. R., West, J. A., Croyle, R. T. *et al.* (1999). Familial context of genetic testing for cancer susceptibility: moderating effect of siblings' test results on psychological distress one to two weeks after BRCA1 mutation testing. *Cancer Epidemiology, Biomarkers and Prevention* **8**(4 Pt 2): 385–92.

49 Evans, D. G., Blair, V., Greenhalgh, R. *et al.* (1994). The impact of genetic counselling on risk perception in women with a family history of breast cancer. *British Journal of Cancer* **70**(5):934–8.

50 Biesecker, B. B., Boehnke, M., Calzone, K. *et al.* (1993). Genetic counseling for families with inherited susceptibility to breast and ovarian cancer. *Journal of the American Medical Association* **269**(15):1970–4.

51 Billings, P. B. J. (1992). Genetic testing in the workplace: a view from the USA. *Trends in Genetics* **6**:198–202.

52 Ritvo, P., Robinson, G., Irvine, J. *et al.* (2000). Psychological adjustment to familial genetic risk assessment: differences in two longitudinal samples. *Patient Education and Counseling* **40**(2):163–72.

53 Tercyak, K. P., Lerman, C., Peshkin, B. N. *et al.* (2001). Effects of coping style and BRCA1 and BRCA2 test results on anxiety among women participating in genetic counseling and testing for breast and ovarian cancer risk. *Health Psychology* **20**(3):217–22.

54 Hatcher, M. B., Fallowfield, L., A'Hern, R. (2001). The psychosocial impact of bilateral prophylactic mastectomy: prospective study using questionnaires and semistructured interviews. *British Medical Journal* **322**(7278): 76.

55 McNair, P. M., Lorr, M., Droppelman, L. (1971). *EITS Manual for the Profile of Mood States*. San Diego, CA: Educational and Industrial Testing Service.

56 Schwartz, M. D., Lerman, C., Miller, S. M. *et al.* (1995). Coping disposition, perceived risk, and psychological distress among women at increased risk for ovarian cancer. *Health Psychology* **14**(3):232–5.

57 Diefenbach, M. A. (1993). Scales for assessing perceptions of health hazard susceptibility. *Health Education and Research* **8**(2):181–92.

58 Audrain, J., Rimer, B., Cella, D. *et al.* (1998). Genetic counseling and testing for breast-ovarian cancer susceptibility: what do women want? *Journal of Clinical Oncology* **16**(1):133–8.

59 Schwartz, M. D., Peshkin, B. N., Hughes. C. *et al.* (2002). The impact of BRCA1/BRCA2 mutation testing on psychological distress in a clinic-based sample. *Journal of Clinical Oncology* **20**(2):514–20.

60 Lerman, C., Narod, S., Schulman, K. *et al.* (1996). BRCA1 testing in families with hereditary breast-ovarian cancer. A prospective study of patient decision making and outcomes. *Journal of the American Medical Association* **275**(24):1885–92.

61 Lerman, C., Hughes, C., Lemon, S. J. *et al.* (1998). What you don't know can hurt you: adverse psychologic effects in members of BRCA1-linked and BRCA2-linked families who decline genetic testing. *Journal of Clinical Oncology* **16**(5):1650–4.

62 Zigmond, A. S., Snaith, R. P. (1983). The hospital anxiety and depression scale. *Acta Psychiatrica Scandanavica* **67**: 361–70.

63 Lodder, L., Frets, P. G., Trijsburg, R. W. *et al.* (2001). Psychological impact of receiving a BRCA1/BRCA2 test result. *American Journal of Medical Genetics* **98**(1):15–24.

64 Zung, W. W., King, R. E. (1983). Identification and treatment of masked depression in a general medical practice. *Journal of Clinical Psychiatry* **44**(10):365–8.

65 Wagner, T. M., Moslinger, R., Langbauer, G. *et al.* (2000). Attitude towards prophylactic surgery and effects of genetic counselling in families with BRCA mutations. Austrian Hereditary Breast and Ovarian Cancer Group. *British Journal of Cancer* **82**(7):1249–53.

66 Folkman, S. (1980). An analysis of coping in a middle-aged community sample. *Journal of Health and Social Behavior* **21**(3):219–39.

67 Hopwood, P. (2001). A body image scale for use with cancer patients. *European Journal of Cancer* **37**(2):189–97.

68 Derogatis, L. R., Lipman, R. S., Rickels, K. *et al.* (1974). The Hopkins symptoms checklist (HSCL): a measure of primary symptom dimensions. *Psychological Measurements in Psychopharmacology* **7**:79–110.

69 Derogatis, L. R., Melisaratos, N. (1983). The Brief Sympton Inventory: an introductory report. *Psychological Medicine* **13**(3):595–605.

70 Derogatis, L. R. (1977). *SCL-90 Administration scoring and procedures. Manual-I to the (revised) version.* Baltimore, MD: Johns Hopkins University School of Medicine.

71 Dorval, M., Patenaude, A. F., Schneider, K. A. *et al.* (2000). Anticipated versus actual emotional reactions to disclosure of results of genetic tests for cancer susceptibility: findings from p53 and BRCA1 testing programs. *Journal of Clinical Oncology* **18**(10):2135–42.

72 Coyne, J. C., Benazon, N. R., Gaba, C. G. *et al.* (2000). Distress and psychiatric morbidity among women from high-risk

breast and ovarian cancer families. *Journal of Consulting Clinical Psychiatry* **68**(5):864–74.

73 Miller, S. M. (1987). Monitoring and blunting: validation of a questionnaire to assess styles of information seeking under threat. *Journal of Personality and Social Psychology* **52**:345–53.

74 Scheier, M. F., Carver, C. S. (1985). Optimism, coping, and health: assessment and implications of generalized outcome expectancies. *Health Psychology* **4**(3): 219–47.

75 Horowitz, M., Wilner, N., Alvarez, W. (1979). Impact of Event Scale: a measure of subjective stress. *Psychosomatic Medicine* **41**(3):209–18.

76 Grilli, R., Mainini, F., Penna, A. *et al.* (1993). Inappropriate Halsted mastectomy and patient volume in Italian hospitals. *American Journal of Public Health* **83**(12): 1762–4.

77 Goldberg, D. P., Williams, P. (1988). *A Users Guide to the General Health Questionnaire*. Windsor: NFER-Nelson.

78 Sherbourne, C. D., Stewart, A. L. (1991). The MOS Social Support Survey. *Social Sciences and Medicine* **32**:705–15.

79 First, M. B., Spitzer, R. L., Gibbon, M. *et al.* (1995). *Structured Clinical Interview for DSM–IV Axis I Disorders – Patient Edition* (SCID-I-P, Version 2.0). New York: Biometrics Research Dept., New York State Psychiatric Institute.

80 Plon, S. E., Peterson, L. E., Friedman, L. C. *et al.* (2000). Mammography behavior after receiving a negative BRCA1 mutation test result in the Ashkenazim: a community-based study. *Genetics in Medicine* **2**(6):307–11.

81 Metcalfe, K. A., Liede, A., Hoodfar, E. *et al.* (2000). An evaluation of needs of female BRCA1 and BRCA2 carriers undergoing genetic counselling. *Journal of Medical Genetics* **37**(11):866–74.

82 Frost, M. H., Schaid, D. J., Sellers, T. A. *et al.* (2000). Long-term satisfaction and psychological and social function following bilateral prophylactic mastectomy. *Journal of the American Medical Association* **284**(3):319–24.

83 Payne, D. K., Biggs, C., Tran, K. N. *et al.* (2000). Women's regrets after bilateral prophylactic mastectomy. *Annals of Surgical Oncology* **7**(2):150–4.

84 Collins, V., Halliday, J., Warren, R. *et al.* (2000). Cancer worries, risk perceptions and associations with interest in DNA testing and clinic satisfaction in a familial colorectal cancer clinic. *Clinical Genetics* **58**(6):460–8.

85 Croyle, R. T., Smith, K. R., Botkin, J. R. *et al.* (1997). Psychological responses to BRCA1 mutation testing: preliminary findings. *Health Psychology* **16**(1):63–72.

86 Lynch, H. T., Lynch, J., Conway, T. *et al.* (1994). Psychological aspects of monitoring high risk women for breast cancer. *Cancer* **74**(3 Suppl.):1184–92.

87 Lynch, H. T., Watson, P., Tinley, S. *et al.* (1999). An update on DNA-based BRCA1/BRCA2 genetic counseling in hereditary breast cancer. *Cancer Genetics and Cytogenetics* **109**(2):91–8.

88 Women's use of coping strategies while waiting for genetic testing results (2000). Poster session presented at the annual meeting of the American Society of Preventive Oncology. Bethesda, MD.

89 Lerman, C., Schwartz, M. (1993). Adherence and psychological adjustment among women at high risk for breast cancer. *Breast Cancer Research and Treatment* **28**(2):145–55.

90 Kash, K. M., Holland, J. C., Halper, M. S. *et al.* (1992). Psychological distress and surveillance behaviors of women with a family history of breast cancer. *Journal of the National Cancer Institute* **84**(1):24–30.

91 Lerman, C., Caputo, C., Brody, D. (1990). Factors associated with inadequate cervical cancer screening among lower income primary care patients. *Journal of the American Board of Family Practice* **3**(3):151–6.

92 Lidbrink, E., Levi, L., Pettersson, I. *et al.* (1995). Single-view screening mammography: psychological, endocrine and immunological effects of recalling for a complete three-view examination. *European Journal of Cancer* **31A**(6): 932–3.

93 Lazarus, R. S. (1974). Psychological stress and coping in adaptation and illness. *International Journal of Psychiatry and Medicine* **5**(4):321–33.

94 Wardle, J., Pope, R. (1992). The psychological costs of screening for cancer. *Journal of Psychosomatic Research* **36**(7):609–24.

95 Olsson, P., Armelius, K., Nordahl, G. *et al.* (1999). Women with false positive screening mammograms: how do they cope? *Journal of Medical Screening* **6**(2):89–93.

96 Skrabanek, P. (1985). False premises and false promises of breast cancer screening. *Lancet* **2**(8450):316–20.

97 Aro, A. R., Pilvikki Absetz, S., van Elderen, T. M. *et al.* (2000). False-positive findings in mammography screening induces short-term distress – breast cancer-specific concern prevails longer. *European Journal of Cancer* **36**(9):1089–97.

98 Aro, A. R., Absetz-Ylostalo, P., Eerola, T. *et al.* (1996). Pain and discomfort during mammography. *European Journal of Cancer* **32A**(10):1674–9.

99 Bennetts, A., Irwig, L., Oldenburg, B. *et al.* (1995). PEAPS-Q: A questionnaire to measure the psychosocial effects of

having an abnormal pap smear. Psychosocial Effects of Abnormal Pap Smears Questionnaire. *Journal of Clinical Epidemiology* **48**(10):1235–43.

100 Bennett, A. K. (1995). Overview of 1995 PIAA Breast Cancer Study. *Missouri Medicine* **92**(10):624–6.

101 Wolfe, C., Doherty, I., Raju, K. S. *et al.* (1992). First steps in the development of an information and counselling service for women with an abnormal smear result. *European Journal of Obstetrics, Gynecology and Reproductive Biology* **45**(3): 201–6.

102 Tomaino-Brunner, C., Freda, M. C., Damus, K. *et al.* (1998). Can precolposcopy education increase knowledge and decrease anxiety? *Journal of Obstetrics, Gynecology and Neonatal Nursing* **27**(6):636–45.

103 Nugent, L. S., Tamlyn-Leaman, K., Isa, N. *et al.* (1993). Anxiety and the colposcopy experience. *Clinical Nursing Research* **2**(3):267–77.

104 Gath, D. H., Hallam, N., Mynors-Wallis, L. *et al.* (1995). Emotional reactions in women attending a UK colposcopy clinic. *Journal of Epidemiology and Community Health* **49**(1): 79–83.

105 Somerset, M. (1998). Intervening to reduce anxiety for women with mild dyskaryosis: do we know what works and why? *Journal of Advanced Nursing* **28**(3):563–70.

106 Palmer, A. G., Tucker, S., Warren, R. *et al.* (1993). Understanding women's responses to treatment for cervical intra-epithelial neoplasia. *British Journal of Clinical Psychology* **32**(Pt 1):101–12.

107 Marteau, T. M. (1990). Screening in practice: reducing the psychological costs. *British Medical Journal* **301**(6742): 26–8.

108 Sutton, S., Saidi, G., Bickler, G. *et al.* (1995). Does routine screening for breast cancer raise anxiety? Results from a three wave prospective study in England. *Journal of Epidemiology and Community Health* **49**(4):413–18.

109 Brett, J., Austoker, J., Ong, G. (1998). Do women who undergo further investigation for breast screening suffer adverse psychological consequences? A multi-centre follow-up study comparing different breast screening result groups five months after their last breast screening appointment. *Journal of Public Health Medicine* **20**(4):396–403.

110 Ong, G., Austoker, J., Brett, J. (1997). Breast screening: adverse psychological consequences one month after placing women on early recall because of a diagnostic uncertainty. A multicentre study. *Journal of Medical Screening* **4**(3):158–68.

111 Essink-Bot, M. L., de Koning, H. J., Nijs, H. G. *et al.* (1998). Short-term effects of population-based screening

for prostate cancer on health-related quality of life. *Journal of the National Cancer Institute* **90**(12):925–31.

112 Diefenbach, M. A. (1999). Specific worry about breast cancer predicts mammography use in women at risk for breast and ovarian cancer. *Health Psychology* **18**(5):532–6.

113 Andrykowski, M. A., Curran, S. L., Studts, J. L. *et al.* (1996). Psychosocial adjustment and quality of life in women with breast cancer and benign breast problems: a controlled comparison. *Journal of Clinical Epidemiology* **49**(8):827–34.

114 Lampic, C., Thurfjell, E., Bergh, J. *et al.* (2001). Short- and long-term anxiety and depression in women recalled after breast cancer screening. *European Journal of Cancer* **37**(4):463–9.

115 Bull, A., Mountney, L., Sanderson, H. (1991). Stage distribution of breast cancer: a basis for the evaluation of breast screening programmes. *British Journal of Radiology* **64**(762):516–19.

116 Scaf-Klomp, W., Sanderman, R., van de Wiel, H. B. *et al.* (1997). Distressed or relieved? Psychological side effects of breast cancer screening in The Netherlands. *Journal of Epidemiology and Community Health* **51**(6):705–10.

117 Gilbert, F. J., Cordiner, C. M., Affleck, I. R. *et al.* (1998). Breast screening: the psychological sequelae of false-positive recall in women with and without a family history of breast cancer. *European Journal of Cancer* **34**(13): 2010–14.

118 Bell, S., Porter, M., Kitchener, H. *et al.* (1995). Psychological response to cervical screening. *Preventive Medicine* **24**(6):610–16.

119 Thiis-Evensen, E., Wilhelmsen, I., Hoff, G. S. *et al.* (1999). The psychologic effect of attending a screening program for colorectal polyps. *Scandinavian Journal of Gastroenterology* **34**(1):103–9.

120 Beck, A. T., Steer, R. A. (1993). *Beck Depression Inventory Manual.* San Antonio, TX: Harcourt Brace.

121 Northouse, L. L., Jeffs, M., Cracchiolo-Caraway, A. *et al.* (1995). Emotional distress reported by women and husbands prior to a breast biopsy. *Nursing Research* **44**(4): 196–201.

122 Snaith, R. P. (1976). The Leeds scales for the self-assessment of anxiety and depression. *British Journal of Psychiatry* **128**:156–65.

123 Steggles, S., Lightfoot, N., Sellick, S. M. (1998). Psychological distress associated with organized breast cancer screening. *Cancer Prevention and Control* **2**(5):213–20.

124 Taylor, K. L., DiPlacido, J., Redd, W. H. *et al.* (1999). Demographics, family histories, and psychological

characteristics of prostate carcinoma screening participants. *Cancer* **85**(6):1305–12.

125 Watson, D., Clark, L. A., Tellegen, A. (1988). Development and validation of brief measures of positive and negative affect: the PANAS scales. *Journal of Personality and Social Psychiatry* **54**(6):1063–70.

126 Lauver, D. R., Kruse, K., Baggot, A. (1999). Women's uncertainties, coping, and moods regarding abnormal Papanicolaou results. *Journal of Womens Health and Gender-Based Medicine* **8**(8):1103–12.

127 Sjoberg, L. (1979). The measurement of mood. *Scandinavian Journal of Psychology* **20**(1):1–18.

128 Taylor, J. A. (1953). A personality scale of manifest anxiety. *Journal of Abnormal Social Psychology* **48**:285–90.

129 Kerner, J. F., Yedidia, M., Padgett, D. *et al.* (2003). Realizing the promise of breast cancer screening: clinical follow-up after abnormal screening among black women. *Preventive Medicine* **37**:92–101.

130 Billings, A. G. (1981). The role of coping responses and social resources in attenuating the stress of life events. *Journal of Behavioral Medicine* **4**(2):139–57.

131 Rosenberg, M. (1965). *Society and the Adolescent Self Image.* Princeton, NJ: Princeton University Press.

132 Abi Rafi, A. (1965). The Maudsley Personality INVENTORY: a cross-cultural study. *British Journal of Social and Clinical Psychology* **4**(4):266–8.

133 Cooper, P., Osborn, M., Gath, D. H. (1982). Evaluation of a modified self-report measure of social adjustment. *British Journal of Psychiatry* **141**:68–75.

134 Miller, S. M., Roussi, P., Altman, D. *et al.* (1994). Effects of coping style on psychological reactions of low-income, minority women to colposcopy. *Journal of Reproductive Medicine* **39**(9):711–18.

135 Deiner, E., Emmons, R., Larsen, R., Griffin, S. (1985). The satisfaction with life scale. *Journal of Personality Assessment* **49**:71–5.

136 Smilkstein, G., Zimlich, R. (1990). *A stress scale validation study. An instrument for psychosocial stressor assessment.* New York, NY: Oxford University Press.

137 Boer, H. *Psychosocial effects of breast cancer screening.* University of Twente 1993. Dissertation.

138 Lau, R. R., Jr. (1981). Refinements in the measurement of health-specific locus-of-control beliefs. *Medical Care* **19**(11):1147–58.

139 Kellner, R. (1987). Psychological measurements in somatization and abnormal illness behavior. *Advances in Psychosomatic Medicine* **17**:101–18.

140 Walker, L. G., Cordiner, C., Gilbert, F. J. (1994). How distressing is attendance for routine breast screening. *Psycho-Oncology* **3**:299–304.

141 Dean, C., Roberts, M. M., French, K. *et al.* (1986). Psychiatric morbidity after screening for breast cancer. *Journal of Epidemiology and Community Health* **40**(1):71–5.

142 Ellman, R., Angeli, N., Christians, A. *et al.* (1989). Psychiatric morbidity associated with screening for breast cancer. *British Journal of Cancer* **60**(5):781–4.

143 Cockburn, J., De Luise, T., Hurley, S. *et al.* (1992). Development and validation of the PCQ: a questionnaire to measure the psychological consequences of screening mammography. *Social Science and Medicine* **34**(10):1129–34.

144 Lowe, J. B., Balanda, K. P., Del Mar, C. *et al.* (1999). Psychologic distress in women with abnormal findings in mass mammography screening. *Cancer* **85**(5):1114–18.

145 Spanier, G. B. (1976). Measuring dyadic adjustment: new scales for assessing the quality of marriage and similar dyads. *Journal of Marriage and Family* **38**:15–28.

146 Eysenck, H. J., Eysenck, S. B. G. (1963). *The Eysenck Personality Inventory.* London: University of London Press.

147 Mishel, M. H. (1981). The measurement of uncertainty in illness. *Nursing Research* **30**(5):258–63.

148 Veit, C. T., Ware, J. E., Jr. (1983). The structure of psychological distress and well-being in general populations. *Journal of Consulting Clinical Psychology* **51**:730–42.

149 Lerman, C., Miller, S. M., Scarborough, R. *et al.* (1991). Adverse psychologic consequences of positive cytologic cervical screening. *American Journal of Obstetrics and Gynecology* **165**(3):658–62.

150 Stillman, M. J. (1977). Women's health beliefs about breast cancer and breast self-examination. *Nursing Research* **26**(2):121–7.

151 Fallowfield, L. J., Rodway, A., Baum, M. (1990). What are the psychological factors influencing attendance, non-attendance and re-attendance at a breast cancer screening centre. *Journal of the Royal Society of Medicine* **83**(9):547–551.

152 Slenker, S. E., Grant, M. C. (1989). Attitudes, beliefs, and knowledge about mammography among women over forty years of age. *Journal of Cancer Education* **4**(1):61–5.

153 Naughton, C. K. (2001). Impact of transrectal ultrasound guided prostate biopsy on quality of life: a prospective randomized trial comparing 6 versus 12 cores. *Journal of Urology* **165**(1):100–3.

154 EuroQOL Group. (1990). EuroQol – a new facility for the measurement of health related quality of life. *Health Policy* **16**:199–208.

155 Volk, R. J., Cantor, S. B., Spann, S. J. *et al.* (1997). Preferences of husbands and wives for prostate cancer screening. *Archives of Family Medicine* **6**(1):72–6.

156 Torrance, G. W. (1987). Utility approach to measuring health-related quality of life. *Journal of Chronic Disease* **40**:593–600.

157 Gram, I. T., Lund, E., Slenker, S. E. (1990). Quality of life following a false positive mammogram. *British Journal of Cancer* **62**(6):1018–22.

158 Dominitz, J. A., Provenzale, D. (1997). Patient preferences and quality of life associated with colorectal cancer screening. *American Journal of Gastroenterology* **92**(12):2171–8.

159 de Haes, J. C., de Koning, H. J., van Oortmarssen, G. J. *et al.* (1991). The impact of a breast cancer screening programme on quality-adjusted life-years. *International Journal of Cancer* **49**(s):538–44.

160 Orbell, S. (1996). Cognition and affect after cervical screening: the role of previous test outcome and personal obligation in future uptake expectations. *Social Science and Medicine* **43**(8):1237–43.

161 Wilson, J. D., Hines, B. (2000). Nurse counselling for women with abnormal cervical cytology improves colposcopy and cytology follow up attendance rates. *Sexually Transmitted Infections* **76**(4):322.

162 Paskett, E. D., Carter, W. B., Chu, J. *et al.* (1990). Compliance behavior in women with abnormal Pap smears. Developing and testing a decision model. *Medical Care* **28**(7): 643–56.

163 Reelick, N. F., de Haes, W. F., Schuurman, J. H. (1984). Psychological side-effects of the mass screening on cervical cancer. *Social Science and Medicine* **18**(12):1089–93.

164 Pisano, E. D., Earp, J., Schell, M. *et al.* (1998). Screening behavior of women after a false-positive mammogram. *Radiology* **208**(1):245–9.

165 Pisano, E. D., Earp, J. A., Gallant, T. L. (1998). Screening mammography behavior after a false positive mammogram. *Cancer Detection and Prevention* **22**(2):161–7.

166 Gram, I. T., Slenker, S. E. (1992). Cancer anxiety and attitudes toward mammography among screening attenders, nonattenders, and women never invited. *American Journal of Public Health* **82**(2):249–51.

167 Schwartz, L., Woloshin, S., Sox, H. *et al.* (2000). US women's attitudes to false-positive mammography results and detection of ductal carcinoma in situ: cross-sectional survey. *Original Research* **173**:307–9.

168 Benedict, S., Williams, R. D., Baron, P. L. (1994). The effect of benign breast biopsy on subsequent breast cancer detection practices. *Oncology Nursing Forum* **21**(9):1467–75.

169 Lindfors, K. K., O'Connor, J., Parker, R. A. (2001). False-positive screening mammograms: effect of immediate versus later work-up on patient stress. *Radiology* **218**(1): 247–253.

170 Lindholm, E., Berglund, B., Kewenter, J. *et al.* (1997). Worry associated with screening for colorectal carcinomas. *Scandinavian Journal of Gastroenterology* **32**(3):238–45.

171 Mant, D., Fitzpatrick, R., Hogg, A. *et al.* (1990). Experiences of patients with false positive results from colorectal cancer screening. *British Journal of General Practice* **40**(339): 423–5.

172 Winawer, S. J., Miller, C., Lightdale, C. *et al.* (1987). Patient response to sigmoidoscopy. a randomized, controlled trial of rigid and flexible sigmoidoscopy. *Cancer* **60**(8): 1905–8.

173 Drossman, D. A., Brandt, L. J., Sears, C. *et al.* (1996). A preliminary study of patients' concerns related to GI endoscopy. *American Journal of Gastroenterology* **91**(2):287–91.

174 McCarthy, B. D., Moskowitz, M. A. (1993). Screening flexible sigmoidoscopy: patient attitudes and compliance. *Journal of General Internal Medicine* **8**(3):120–5.

175 Pedersen, K. V., Carlsson, P., Varenhorst, E. *et al.* (1990). Screening for carcinoma of the prostate by digital rectal examination in a randomly selected population. *British Medical Journal* **300**(6731):1041–4.

176 Myers, R. E., Hyslop, T., Wolf, T. A. *et al.* (2000). African-American men and intention to adhere to recommended follow-up for an abnormal prostate cancer early detection examination result. *Urology* **55**(5): 716–20.

177 Lauver, D., Rubin, M. (1991). Women's concerns about abnormal Papanicolaou test results. *Journal of Obstetrics, Gynecology, and Neonatal Nursing* **20**(2):154–9.

178 Quilliam, S. (1989). Emotional aspects of positive smears. *Health Visit* **62**(10):308–9.

179 Wardle, J., Sutton, S., Williamson, S. *et al.* (2000). Psychosocial influences on older adults' interest in participating in bowel cancer screening. *Preventive Medicine* **31**(4): 323–34.

180 Auvinen, A. (1996). Prospective evaluation plan for randomised trials of prostate cancer screening. The International Prostate Cancer Screening Trial Evaluation Group. *Journal of Medical Screening* **3**(2): 97–104.

181 Kramer, B. S. (1993). Prostate cancer screening: what we know and what we need to know. *Annals of Internal Medicine* **119**(9):914–23.

182 Carvalhal, G. F., Smith, D. C., Ramos, C. *et al.* (1999). Correlates of dissatisfaction with treatment in patients with

prostate cancer diagnosed through screening. *Journal of Urology* **162**(1):113–18.

183 Stewart-Brown, S. F. A. (1997). Screening could seriously damage your health. *British Medical Journal* **1314**(7080):533–4.

184 Cockburn, J., Staples, M., Hurley, S. F. *et al.* (1994). Psychological consequences of screening mammography. *Journal of Medical Screening* **1**(1):7–12.

185 Gerard, K., Salkeld, G., Hall, J. (1990). Counting the costs of mammography screening: first year results from the Sydney study. *Medical Journal of Australia* **152**(9):466–71.

186 Rimer, B. K., Bluman, L. G. (1997). The psychosocial consequences of mammography. *Journal of the National Cancer Institute Monographs* **22**:131–8.

187 Fletcher, S. W. (1999). False-positive screening mammograms: good news, but more to do. *Annals of Internal Medicine* **131**(1):60–2.

188 Sickles, E. A. (1991). Periodic mammographic follow-up of probably benign lesions: results in 3,184 consecutive cases. *Radiology* **179**(2):463–8.

189 Breen, N., Wagener, D. K., Brown, M. L. *et al.* (2001). Progress in cancer screening over a decade: results of cancer screening from the 1987, 1992, and 1998 National Health Interview Surveys. *Journal of the National Cancer Institute* **93**(22):1704–13.

190 Olivotto, I. A., Kan, L., Coldman, A. J. (1998). False positive rate of screening mammography. *New England Journal of Medicine* **339**(8):560.

191 Elmore, J. G., Barton, M. B., Moceri, V. M. *et al.* (1998). Ten-year risk of false positive screening mammograms and clinical breast examinations. *New England Journal of Medicine* **338**(16):1089–96.

192 Lidbrink, E., Elfving, J., Frisell, J. *et al.* (1996). Neglected aspects of false positive findings of mammography in breast cancer screening: analysis of false positive cases from the Stockholm trial. *British Medical Journal* **312**(7026):273–6.

193 Lipkus, I. M., Halabi, S., Strigo, T. S. *et al.* (2000). The impact of abnormal mammograms on psychosocial outcomes and subsequent screening. *Psycho-Oncology* **9**(5):402–10.

194 Veit, C. T., Ware, J. E., Jr. (1983). The structure of psychological distress and well-being in general populations. *Journal of Consulting Clinical Psychology* **51**(5):730–42.

195 Fallowfield, L. (1990). *The Quality of Life: The Missing Measurement in Health Care.* New York, NY: Oxford University Press.

196 Mould, T. A., Rodgers, M. E., Singer, A. (1995). The psychological reaction of women to a colposcopy clinic. *British Journal of Obstetrics and Gynecology* **102**(5):428–9.

197 Campion, M. J., Brown, J. R., McCance, D. J. *et al.* (1988). Psychosexual trauma of an abnormal cervical smear. *British Journal of Obstetrics and Gynecology* **95**(2):175–81.

198 Pisano, E. D. (1998). Screening behavior of women after a false-positive mammogram. *Radiology* **208**(1):245–9.

199 Miller, A. B. (1993). Canadian National Breast Screening Study: public health implications. *Canadian Journal of Public Health* **84**(1):14–16.

200 Lerman, C. E. (1993). Psychosocial impact of cancer screening. *Oncology (Huntington)* **7**(4):67–72.

201 Gotay, C. C. (1984). The experience of cancer during early and advanced stages: the views of patients and their mates. *Social Science and Medicine* **18**(7):605–13.

202 Weil, J. G. (1997). Positive findings of mammography may lead to suicide. *British Medical Journal* **314**(7082):754–5.

203 Fentiman, I. S. (1988). Pensive women, painful vigils: consequences of delay in assessment of mammographic abnormalities. *Lancet* **1**(8593):1041–2.

204 McCarthy, B. D. (1997). Screening mammography use: the importance of a population perspective. *American Journal of Preventive Medicine* **12**(2):91–5.

205 Kerner, J. F., Mandelblatt, J. S., Silliman, R. A. *et al.* (2001). Screening mammography and breast cancer treatment patterns in older women. *Breast Cancer Research and Treatment* **69**(1):81–91.

206 Burman, M. L. (1999). Effect of false-positive mammograms on interval breast cancer screening in a health maintenance organization. *Annals of Internal Medicine* **131**(1):1–6.

207 Stidley, C. A., Tollestrup, K., Frost, F. *et al.* (2001). Mammography utilization after a benign breast biopsy among Hispanic and non-Hispanic women. *Cancer* **91**(9):1716–23.

208 Bull, A. R., Campbell, M. J. (1991). Assessment of the psychological impact of a breast screening programme. *British Journal of Radiology* **64**(762):510–15.

209 McCaul, K. D., Schroeder, D. M., Reid, P. A. (1996). Breast cancer worry and screening: some prospective data. *Health Psychology* **15**(6):430–3.

210 Feeny, this volume, Chapter 4.

211 Gold, M. R., Siegel, J. E., Russell, L. B. *et al.* (1996). *Cost-Effectiveness in Health and Medicine.* New York, NY: Oxford University Press.

212 Olsson, P., Armelius, K., Nordahl, G. (1999). Women with false positive screening mammograms: how do they cope? *Journal of Medical Screening* **6**(2):89–93.

213 Pater, J., Osoba, D., Zee, B. *et al.* (1998). Effects of altering the time of administration and the time frame of quality of life assessments in clinical trials: an example using the EORTC QLQ-C30 in a large anti-emetic trial. *Quality of Life Research* **7**(3):273–8.

214 Katz, S. (1963). Studies of illness in the aged. The index of ADL: a standardized measure of biological and psychological function. *Journal of the American Medical Association* **185**:914–19.

215 Llewellyn-Thomas, H., Sutherland, H. J., Tibshirani, R. *et al.* (1982). The measurement of patients' values in medicine. *Medical Decision Making* **2**(4):449–62.

216 Nord, E., Pinto, J. L., Richardson, J. *et al.* (1999). Incorporating societal concerns for fairness in numerical valuations of health programmes. *Health Economics* **8**(1): 25–39.

217 Dolan, P., Gudex, C. (1995). Time preference, duration and health state valuations. *Health Economics* **4**(4):289–99.

218 Torrance, G. W. (1976). Toward a utility theory foundation for health status index models. *Health Services Research* **11**:349–69.

11

Evaluating quality of life in cancer survivors

Brad Zebrack, Ph.D., MSW[1] and David Cella, Ph.D.[2]

[1]University of Southern California, Los Angeles, CA
[2]Northwestern University, Evanston, IL

Introduction

Currently, about 1.27 million new cancer cases are diagnosed each year, and 60% of all persons diagnosed with cancer are expected to be alive at least five years from the time of their diagnosis. Furthermore, the US death rate for all cancers combined has been declining since 1990, so annual growth in the number of individuals living with or beyond cancer is expected. Today, there are approximately 9 million cancer survivors in the US.[1] Based upon 1996–1997 population estimates from the US Bureau of the Census, this represents approximately 3% of the entire population. Some of these individuals can be considered cured, while others still have evidence of active disease. Of the 9 million individuals living with a cancer history, over 1 million were diagnosed more than 20 years ago.

While these statistics indicate increased length of survival for individuals diagnosed with cancer, they give no indication of the quality of life:

Regardless of the type of cancer or the extent of survival, all persons diagnosed with cancer must manage the enduring and complex ways in which cancer transforms the self and everyday life. (p. 239)[2]

Understanding how individuals who are cancer survivors manage the impact of cancer and experience the transformation of their lives is critical for health care professionals committed to assisting cancer patients and survivors in their recovery, for payers of health care, and for those engaged in policy regarding health insurance, employment, and disability-related rights of these many survivors.

Beginning in the early 1980s, and owing to prior advances in achieving curative therapies for some pediatric and adult cancers, interest in the long-term impact of cancer has grown steadily.[3,4] Existing studies document the late and delayed physical and psychosocial sequelae and changes associated with cancer and its treatment in adults, but these studies are limited in several ways. First, the average length of follow-up among research participants rarely exceeds ten years, thereby limiting understanding of cancer's impact on "very long-term" survivors. Second, methods tend to examine negative outcomes, and yet good evidence accrued over 20 years of research suggests there are important positive outcomes that, if studied more carefully with regard to their basis, could promote the positive health of cancer survivors. Third, insufficient attention is given to the age and life stage of the survivor, so the impact of factors associated with human development across the life span remains essentially unknown. Fourth, there are very few comprehensive (i.e., multidimensional) studies of survivorship that cover the spectrum of physical, mental, and social well-being. Fifth, studies tend to be retrospective and cross-sectional in design, without regard to external factors such as health care delivery and coverage for cancer survivors, thereby limiting the ability to apply conclusions about this population to the development and implementation of an effective health care delivery system. Finally, most studies have ignored the impact that comorbidity and other physical and mental health problems, both those related to and those independent of the cancer history, have upon the health of cancer survivors.

In their comprehensive review, Gotay and Muraoka[5] conclude:

> The quality of life reported by survivors varies a great deal, making it impossible at this time to come to firm conclusions about the magnitude and nature of long-term consequences for cancer survivors. It seems clear, however, that considerable numbers of survivors continue to experience negative effects of cancer and/or treatment on their daily lives, resulting in decrements in quality of life, well beyond the completion of therapy. (p. 664)

An emerging body of research has contributed to the understanding of cancer survivorship by documenting positive outcomes and perceived benefits among long-term cancer survivors.[6-11] These studies suggest that quality of life may be enhanced, rather than diminished, by the experience of having faced a potentially fatal disease, undergone toxic and/or painful treatment, and survived. New approaches to assess both positive and negative aspects of quality of life have recently been developed and are beginning to be incorporated into quality-of-life studies. These approaches assess constructs such as positive change,[6,12-14] positive outcomes or benefits,[7,15-18] posttraumatic growth or stress-related growth,[19-21] and thriving.[22-26]

The purpose of this report is to summarize current knowledge of the health-related quality of life (HRQOL) in survivors of breast, colorectal, lung, and prostate cancer and recommend future research directions that address current methodologic limitations. Special emphasis is placed on the evaluation of instruments that have been used to assess survivors of these cancers. By reviewing the state of the science of measuring HRQOL in cancer survivors, one can identify areas where future research on HRQOL in general, and measurement in particular, can help move the field forward.

Methods

Literature search strategy

An exhaustive literature search of MEDLINE/HealthStar was conducted to identify investigative reports and reviews dating from 1990 through 2001. Some key articles published prior to 1990 also were included. Keywords searched included: lung cancer, prostate cancer, breast cancer, colorectal cancer, quality of life, cancer survivors, and survivorship. The review was limited to studies that included breast, colorectal, lung, and/or prostate cancer survivors because these are the four cancers being studied by the Cancer Outcomes Measurement Working Group (COMWG). Some articles that were familiar to the investigators, but did not turn up on the search, were also included.

For this report, a "cancer survivor" is defined as an individual off-treatment, regardless of length of time, with no indication of current or active disease. In the case of lung and prostate cancer, this definition requires some clarification. Because so many people are diagnosed with lung cancer in advanced stages, most patients never meet this definition, yet they may live for a considerable period of time in a state of self-identified survivorship. With prostate cancer, an increasing number of men are being informed of biochemical (prostate specific antigen) recurrence after definitive treatment but are otherwise healthy and living as disease-free survivors. Thus, the definition of "survivor" was extended to also include persons alive after initial therapy for prostate or lung cancer has been completed.

Data abstraction techniques

Articles were abstracted and summarized by entering article titles and authors into a database, along with pertinent information from the study. This information included study design, sample size, measures used, reports on reliability and validity of the measures in cancer survivors, and HRQOL outcomes.

Description of studies included in analysis

The studies reviewed here include both homogenous samples of breast, colorectal, lung, or prostate cancer survivors and heterogenous samples in which these survivor groups were included. Reviewed studies include those evaluating cancer therapies longitudinally, as well as cohort studies of cancer survivors with retrospective accounting of therapy.

There were 42 articles reporting or addressing HRQOL outcomes in homogenous samples of breast cancer survivors. In prostate cancer, there was one review, 27 empirical studies of men with localized disease, 13 empirical studies of men with advanced disease, and 11 empirical studies of men with the full range of disease stage. In colorectal cancer, there were 10 empirical studies; in lung cancer, there were 3 literature reviews and 35 empirical studies. Finally, there were 19 empirical studies of HRQOL in heterogenous samples that included breast, prostate, colorectal, and/or lung cancer survivors.

Results

Survivorship and HRQOL

As reported in the literature, long-term survivors describe a range of both positive and negative outcomes that they attribute to their cancer. These late effects are divided into four major domains of quality of life: physical, mental, social, and spiritual/existential (Table 11.1).

Although categorized into various domains, the physical, psychological, social, and existential effects of cancer and its treatment are interrelated. Quantitative studies have tended to reveal significant and moderately strong relationships among various quality of life domains;[27] survivors studied qualitatively often report that many of the physical effects have psychological and social ramifications. For instance, urinary incontinence can be a troublesome problem for both male and female cancer survivors. This problem, while not life threatening, may be of sufficient magnitude to interfere with social

and recreational activities for survivors. Pain, physical discomfort, and fatigue are other commonly reported physical late effects that have direct psychological and social implications. Furthermore, infertility remains a vexing problem for many young adult survivors and has the potential to create distress as they age and enter into long-term intimate relationships.

Long-term survivors describe a range of physical, mental, social, and spiritual concerns that often are attributed to their cancer. However, it is not always clear which reported changes are age-related versus cancer-related. For example, the problem of unilateral arm edema after breast surgery is readily attributed to cancer treatment, while other problems such as fatigue, diminished strength, or lack of sexual interest may or may not be related to cancer, especially among people with comorbid conditions.

In contrast to physical effects, many of the mental, social, and existential issues discussed by survivors seem directly linked to the cancer experience. Many survivors describe their worries and concerns about their health (including a cancer recurrence), as well as a heightened sense of vulnerability associated with being a survivor – a sense that their bodies may have let them down and that good health habits and behaviors did not protect them. This perspective, however, has both positive and negative implications, such as living life to the fullest and enjoying each moment or being paralyzed and unable to make future plans or save money for the future.

Women with a history of breast cancer are the largest group of female cancer survivors (NCI Office of Cancer Survivorship)[28] and account for the largest proportion of cancer survivor studies. Overall, HRQOL outcomes in this sub-group of survivors are mixed. Some studies suggest that breast cancer survivors experience reduced HRQOL,[29] are at increased risks for psychological distress,[30] or experience ongoing problems years after the completion of treatment. These problems include dissatisfaction in intimate relationships and sex,[31,32] anxiety, depression or mood impairment,[32,33] fears or thoughts of disease recurrence,[33–35] uncertainty,[33,34] pain,

Table 11.1. Commonly reported late effects of cancer treatment

Physical	*Psychological*
Body changes: scars, disfigurement, amputation	Concerns about the future, death
Cardiorespiratory symptoms	Sadness and symptoms of depression and post-traumatic stress
Co-morbid conditions	Feelings of gratitude and good fortune
Fatigue or decreased energy	Health worries and hypervigilance, including anxiety about
Immune dysfunction	physician appointments, recurrence
Infertility	Inability to make plans
Lymphedema	Enhanced self-esteem, mastery
Osteoporosis/fractures	Uncertainty and vulnerability
Pain, neuropathy, numbness	Cognitive problems
Premature menopause and menopausal symptoms	
Second cancers	
Sexual dysfunction, pain during sex	
Changes in sexual activity, more nonsexual intimacy	
Skin sensitivity to UV radiation	
Urinary/bowel incontinence, discomfort, and inconvenience	
Weight gain	
Social	*Spiritual/Existential*
Affinity and altruism	Appreciation of life
Alienation and isolation	Changed or new orientation to time and future
Comparison with peers	Changed values and goals
Concerns about small children's welfare and risks for cancer	Concerns about death and dying, particularly regarding pain
Social relationship changes	during death
Socioeconomic concerns: health insurance and "job lock,"	Religious convictions strengthened or challenged
employment problems and discrimination, return to school,	Sense of purpose
financial impact	

discomfort, and/or fatigue,[33,34,36–38] and problems with work.[39]

In contrast, other HRQOL and breast cancer survivor studies indicate that most survivors report high levels of functioning and HRQOL after treatment[31,38,40] and more favorable HRQOL when compared to various comparison groups.[41] Some have significantly lower distress scores than comparison groups.[42] Furthermore, in the aggregate, breast cancer survivors report very good health,[35] general life satisfaction,[35] altruism,[43] and a sense of hope and positive changes attributable to having overcome cancer.[34,41,43,44]

Survivors of lung cancer report a host of problems in physical, psychological, and social domains. Declines in physical and functional areas of HRQOL

are common.[45,46] Of particular concern are lung cancer-specific symptoms such as pain, dyspnea, coughing, sleep disturbance, appetite, and weight loss. While chemotherapy and radiotherapy do ease many of these problems and prolong survival times, both can result in debilitating side effects such as fatigue, cognitive dysfunction, nausea/vomiting, and alopecia.[47–53] While most survivors of lung cancer do not develop serious psychological disorders, rates of emotional distress (i.e., anxiey and depression) tend to be higher than those of other cancer patients.[45] For long-term survivors, difficulties in working and disruptions in daily living and social activities are persistent problems.[45,54]

Survivors of prostate cancer typically have different problems depending upon stage of disease at diagnosis and the type of therapy received.[55] Most survivors of localized disease treated curatively with either surgery (radical prostatectomy) or radiation will experience problems in three disease-specific domains: urinary, sexual, and bowel function. Urinary and sexual problems are the worst in men treated with prostatectomy, but occur to a lesser extent in men treated with radiation.[56–59] Radiation-treated men often report the greatest problems in bowel function.[59–62] For most men, these disease-specific problems dissipate significantly within a year of treatment.[57,63,64]

In survivors of advanced disease, a greater number of problems exist in the general domains of HRQOL.[55] While significant sexual problems exist in men with advanced disease, these problems are reported to be only moderately distressing.[65,66] Urinary and bowel problems are less prevalent in men with advanced disease.[65–67] What appears more troublesome are the deficits in general domains of HRQOL such as pain, fatigue, social, and emotional well-being.[66–70] Men treated hormonally with either surgical or medical castration often experience these problems in the year after treatment. The use of anti-androgens, a less aggressive form of hormonal therapy, results in a better HRQOL profile than castration.[71–73] However, it may not be an option for all men, especially those with rapidly progressing disease.[55]

Relatively little has been reported with regard to distinct HRQOL outcomes for survivors of colorectal malignancies. Issues of concern appear to be associated with the stage and location of the cancer at the time of diagnosis, and include problems with social interaction and cognition, fear of cancer recurrence, pain, fatigue, problems or changes in bowel habits, sexual dysfunction, and decreased physical functioning.[74–76] Individuals who achieve a long-term remission from colorectal carcinoma may experience a relatively high quality of life, yet also report continuing pain and deficits in functional and social well-being, particularly for those of low socioeconomic status.[77]

Because of the various effects that cancer can have on survivors, assessment of HRQOL is important.

Below, the measures that have been commonly used to assess HRQOL in survivor populations are described and evaluated in terms of their performance among cancer survivors.

Measures commonly used to assess HRQOL in cancer survivors

In this section, the measures and methods used to assess HRQOL in long-term survivors of breast, colorectal, lung, and prostate cancer are summarized and evaluated. The review focuses on the commonly used measures as well as measures and approaches that appear to have the greatest potential for advancing HRQOL assessment in survivors. The more commonly used and promising of the instruments applied to the cancer survivor population are summarized in Table 11.2.

Quality-of-life measures designed specifically for cancer patients, as well as generic measures of quality of life, have been administered in studies of both heterogenous samples of off-treatment cancer survivors and homogenous samples of off-treatment survivors diagnosed with a similar cancer. The most well-established generic HRQOL measure used in survivor populations is the Medical Outcomes Study 36-Item Short Form Health Survey,[78] also known as the SF-36, derived from the Medical Outcomes Study of the 1970s.[79] HRQOL measures used in survivors having a cancer-specific focus include the Cancer Rehabilitation Evaluation System (CARES),[80,81] the EORTC QLQ-C30,[82] the Ferrans-Powers HRQOL-Cancer Version,[83] the Functional Assessment of Cancer Therapy (FACT) Measurement System,[84] and the Functional Living Index-Cancer (FLIC).[85] In addition, two questionnaires have been developed specifically for off-treatment cancer survivors: the Long-Term Quality of Life (LTQL) Scale[27] and the Quality of Life – Cancer Survivors (QOL-CS).[3] Finally, there have been many unidimensional instruments used in cancer survivor studies to evaluate individual components or dimensions of HRQOL, such as mental well-being. Instruments to measure single symptoms or other single dimensions of HRQOL were not included in this review. Exceptions were made for

Table 11.2. Summary of Instruments Commonly Used in Survivorship Studies

Instrument	References	Psychometric data
Measures Commonly Used to Assess HRQOL in Cancer Survivors		
Medical Outcomes Study (MOS) short forms: SF-36, SF-20, SF-12	Litwin et al.[56] Moinpour et al.[67] Mangione et al.[105]	*Reliability* Test-retest: 0.78 and greater Internal consistency: 0.78–0.93 *Validity* – Sensitive to changes in function over time – Criterion-related: Distinguishes between treatment groups and clinical status (i.e., progression vs. remission); Distinguishes between age and ethnic groups – Concurrent: Subscale scores are associated with global health
Cancer Rehabilitation Evaluation System – Short Form (CARES-SF)	Litwin et al.[56] Schag et al.[107] Herr et al.[152]	*Reliability* Alpha: 0.74 and greater *Validity* – Negative associations with number of co-morbid conditions
EORTC Quality of Life Questionnaire – Core 30 (QLQ-C30) and disease-specific modules	Anderson et al.[117] Borghede et al.[183] Albertsen et al.[68] Crino et al.[118] Joly et al.[112] Janda et al.[98] Giaccone et al.[184] Helsing et al.[50] Langendijk et al.[119] Sneeuw et al.[115]	*Reliability* Internal consistency: 0.65–0.92 Test-retest: 0.68 and greater *Validity* – Sensitive to changes in function over time – Criterion-related: Distinguishes between clinical status groups (i.e., progression vs. remission; treatment responders vs. non-responders; performance status levels; curative vs. palliative patients); Scores associated with clinical response to treatment – Concurrent: Fatigue subscale associated with global QOL; Changes in respiratory symptoms associated with changes in QLQ scores
Ferrans & Powers QOL Index	Yarbro & Ferrans[62]	*Reliability* Alpha: 0.95 *Validity* – Convergent: Scores correlate with life satisfaction – Known-groups: Score differences based upon pain, depression, and coping ability
Functional Assessment of Cancer Therapy (FACT) and disease-specific subscales	Litwin et al.[56] Shrader-Bogen et al.[59] Cella et al.[84,136] Bonomi et al.[137] Esper et al.[70] Lee et al.[132] Dow et al.[127] Ferrell et al.[128] Holzner et al.[29]	*Reliability* Test-retest: r = 0.92 Internal consistency: 0.56–0.89 *Validity* – Known-groups: Distinguishes between clinically distinct groups (localized vs. advanced patients); Sensitive to changes in performance status – Sensitive to changes in function over time – Criterion-related: High levels of dyspnea associated with worse FACT-L scores – Concurrent: Associated with scores on the Brief POMS and FLIC – Discriminant: Low association with social desirability

Table 11.2. (*cont.*)

Instrument	References	Psychometric data
Functional Living Index Cancer (FLIC)	Lim et al.[61] Cassileth et al.[69] Thongprasert[53] Thongprasert et al.[143]	*Reliability* Internal consistency: 0.78–0.83 *Validity* – Sensitive to changes in function over time – Criterion-related: Distinguishes between treatment groups; Associated with Karnofsky Performance Status rating – Convergent: Associated with Spitzer QOL index scores
Long-Term Quality of Life (LTQL)	Wyatt & Friedman[27] Kurtz et al.[108]	*Reliability* Internal consistency: 0.65–0.89 *Validity* – Construct: Factor analysis-generated scales
Quality of Life-Cancer Survivors (QOL-CS)	Dow et al.[127] Ferrell et al.[3,33,34,144] Whedon et al.[145]	*Reliability* Test-retest: 0.81–0.90 Internal consistency 0.71–0.93 *Validity* – Concurrent: Correlates with comparable FACT-G subscales and total score – Known groups: Survivor scores were higher than active disease; Those living alone had lower scores – Construct: Factor-derived scoring for physical, social, and fear of recurrence
Brief Symptom Inventory (BSI)	Zabora et al.[185] Cella & Tross[7]	*Reliability* Alpha: 0.71–0.85 Test-retest: 0.68–0.91 *Validity* – Convergent: Correlates r = 0.92 to 0.98 with the SCL-90 – Criterion-related: Sensitive to differences in psychological distress across diagnostic groups
Center for Epidemiologic Studies Depression (CES-D)	Radloff[148]	*Reliability* Test-retest: 0.51–0.67 Internal consistency: 0.84–0.90 *Validity* – Known-groups: Scores discriminate psychiatric inpatients from general population sample – Criterion-related: Scores correlate with clinician ratings of depression both before and after treatment; Scores correlate with the occurrence of negative events – Concurrent: Correlates with other scales of depressive symptomatology (Lubin, Bradburn Negative Affect, Bradburn Balance) – Discriminant: Correlates negatively with positive affect scales (Bradburn Positive Affect); Low correlations with Marlowe-Crowne Social Desirability – Sensitivity to Change: Sensitive to improvements after treatment

(*cont.*)

Table 11.2. (*cont.*)

Instrument	References	Psychometric data
Impact of Event Scale (IES)	Cella & Tross[7] Herr et al.[152]	*Reliability* Alpha: 0.74 and above
Mental Adjustment to Cancer Scale (MAC)	Watson et al.[153] Schwartz et al.[186]	*Reliability* Internal consistency: 0.65–0.84 in UK sample; 0.51–0.83 in US sample *Validity* – Factorial: For UK sample, scales include "fighting spirit," "helplessness/hopelessness," "fatalism," "avoidance," and "anxious preoccupation;" Intercorrelations between subscales; For US sample, scales include "vigilant participation," "hopelessness," "positive reframing/present oriented," and "belief in the importance of a positive attitude" – Concurrent: Scales correlated with other measures of anxiety and depression (HADS) – Convergent: Spousal ratings correlated highly with those of patients
Profile of Mood States (POMS)	Beard et al.[93] Cassileth et al.[69]	*Validity* – Sensitive to changes in function over time – Criterion-related: Distinguishes between treatment groups
Psychological Adjustment to Illness Scale (PAIS & PAIS-SR [self-report])	Derogatis & Lopez[158] Merluzzi & Martinez-Sanchez[187]	*Reliability* Internal consistency: 0.12–0.93 Inter-rater: 0.56–0.86 *Validity* – Factorial: Scales included "health care orientation," "vocational environment," "domestic environment," "sexual relationships," "extended family," "social environment," and "psychological distress;" Intercorrelations between subscales and between subscales and total score; In a sample of mixed cancer patients (N = 502), the following scales emerged: "health care orientation," "job and household duties," "sexual relationship," "help from others," "relationships with partner and family," "psychological distress," and "social and leisure activities" – Convergent: Scores correlated highly with the Global Adjustment to Illness Scale, SCL-90-R General Severity Index, Affect Balance Scale, and Patient's Attitudes Information & Expectancies Scale; In a sample of mixed cancer patients, scores correlated with the Sickness Impact Profile, the Mental Health Index, and the COPE scale – Predictive: Sensitive to differences between patients screened positive vs. negative for lung cancer

Other Measures to Assess HRQOL in Cancer Survivors

Instrument	References	Psychometric data
Nottingham Health Profile (NHP)	Joly et al.[112] Whynes & Neilson[188]	*Validity* – Criterion-related: Distinguishes between on-treatment and off-treatment groups – -Identified symptoms which improve in colorectal cancer survivors after successful treatment

Table 11.2. (*cont.*)

Instrument	References	Psychometric data
Activities of Daily Living (ADL) Instrumental Activities of Daily Living (IADL)	Katz[189] Ulander et al.[76]	Focus is on physical functioning; Correlates with other generic measures of physical functioning, but less sensitive among most survivor populations due to ceiling effects
Spitzer Quality of Life Index (QLI)	Thongprasert[53] Thongprasert et al.[143]	*Reliability* Alpha: 0.78–0.83 *Validity* – Sensitive to changes in function over time – Convergent: Associated with FLIC scores – Criterion-related: Associated with Karnofsky Performance Status rating
Rotterdam Symptom Checklist (RSCL)	Gregor et al.[49] Ranson et al.[190] Souhami et al.[191] Stiggelbout et al.[91] Whynes & Neilsen[188]	*Validity* – Criterion-related: Distinguishes between treatment groups – Identified problematic symptoms extending into survivorship, and those which improve in colorectal cancer survivors
Policy Analysis Institute Questionnaire	Chodak et al.[71] Iversen et al.[72]	*Reliability* Alpha: 0.74–0.96 *Validity* – Sensitive to changes in function over time – Criterion-related: Distinguishes between treatment groups – Convergent: Correlates highly with general health perceptions
Affect Balance Scale (ABS)	Bradburn[192] Bradburn & Caplovitz[193] Greaves-Otte et al.[194]	Measure of positive and negative affect; Also yields a single measure of psychological well-being; Allows comparison of mood of cancer survivors to general population norms
Hospital Anxiety & Depression Scale (HADS)	Zigmond & Snaith[195] Gregor et al.[49] Hopwood & Stephens[54] Okuyama et al.[196] Olweny et al.[160] Ringdal & Ringdal[122] and others	*Validity* – Criterion-related: Depression scale associated with greater functional impairment and symptom burden; Higher scores on depression associated with poorer performance status
Cancer Worry Scale	Lerman et al.[197] Anderson & Urban[87]	*Validity* – Concurrent: Correlated with other more general measures of HRQOL
Post-Traumatic Stress Disorder (PTSD) Checklist – Civilian (PCL-C)	Weathers et al.[198] Andrykowski & Cordova[199] Cordova et al.[89] Cordova et al.[200] Smith et al.[201]	*Validity* – Concurrent: Correlated with more general measures of HRQOL (e.g., SF-36), with symptom inventories (e.g., BSI-53, and with the IES – Criterion-related: predicts PTSD diagnosis by formal criteria
Dyadic Adjustment Scale (DAS)	Spanier[202] Ganz et al.[88]	*Validity* Known groups: Distinguishes couples with marital discord post diagnosis and treatment of cancer

(*cont.*)

Table 11.2. (*cont.*)

Instrument	References	Psychometric data
UCLA Prostate Cancer Index	Brandeis *et al.*[94] Eton *et al.*[96] Litwin *et al.*[56,63,66,203] Litwin & McGuigan[63] Lubeck *et al.*[57,100] Schapira *et al.*[104]	*Reliability* Test-retest: 0.66–0.93 Alpha: 0.65–0.93 *Validity* – Sensitive to changes in function over time – Criterion-related: Distinguishes between treatment groups; Distinguishes among age and ethnic groups – Convergent: Scores correlated with existing scales
Fowler Prostate Cancer Outcomes Assessment	Fowler *et al.*[60]	*Validity* – Sensitive to changes in function over time – Criterion-related: Distinguishes between treatment groups
PCOS Prostate Index	Potosky *et al.*[103] Stanford *et al.*[64]	*Validity* – Sensitive to changes in function over time – Criterion-related: Distinguishes between treatment groups, clinical categories, and demographic groups (i.e., age, ethnicity)
SWOG Prostate Outcomes Questionnaire	Moinpour *et al.*[67] Clark *et al.*[95]	*Validity* – Sensitive to changes in function over time – Criterion-related: Distinguishes between treatment groups
International Prostate Symptom Score (IPSS)	Lee *et al.*[132] Fossa *et al.*[113]	*Validity* – Sensitive to changes in function over time – Convergent: Associated with QLQ-C30 global QOL score
Prostate Cancer Treatment Outcome Questionnaire	Shrader-Bogen *et al.*[59]	*Reliability* Test-retest: r = 0.91 *Validity* – Criterion-related: Distinguishes between treatment groups

some promising measures evaluating specific issues of survivorship.

The measures are described in more detail below, and their psychometric properties are summarized in Table 11.2. For summaries of the generic and general cancer measures (e.g., SF-36, Nottingham Health Profile) see Chapter 3 by Erickson in this volume;[86] however, their use in survivorship populations is summarized here.

Medical Outcomes Study 36-Item Short Form Health Survey (SF-36)

The SF-36 has been used in interventional, cross-sectional, and longitudinal studies involving healthy and clinical populations, including cancer survivors.[41,87,88] Abbreviated versions (MOS-20) and subscales extracted from the SF-36 have been used in studies examining HRQOL and its correlates.[36,89–92] The scale is a standardized, general measure of health status with available normative data, allowing for normative comparisons. The SF-36 has been used in studies of many prostate cancer survivors,[56,58,63,66–68,93–104] and in one known study of lung cancer survivors.[105] Its performance psychometrically rivals that in general population cohorts as well as outpatient samples in general medical and specialty practices, including oncology treatment (see Erickson for details of SF-36 performance beyond cancer survivors).[86]

Cancer Rehabilitation Evaluation System (CARES)

The CARES has been used with breast cancer survivors,[38,41,80,106,107] prostate cancer survivors,[56,107] heterogeneous groups of survivors,[108] and studies specifically focused on ethnic minorities.[109,110] In these studies, the CARES performed well, again comparably to studies of patients on-treatment.

European Organization for Research and Treatment of Cancer Quality of Life Questionnaire – Core 30 (EORTC QLQ-C30)

Results from the QLQ-C30 have been reported in investigations of breast cancer survivors,[29,111,112] colorectal cancer survivors,[76] and prostate cancer survivors.[65,98,112–116] Lung cancer survivor utilization studies include Anderson et al.,[117] Crino et al.,[118] Fossella et al.,[47] Gatzemeier et al.,[48] Helsing et al.,[50] Langendijk et al.,[119] Langendijk et al.,[52] Langendijk et al.,[120] Roszkowski et al.,[121] and a follow-up study of mixed diagnosis survivors 3–4 years post-diagnosis.[122] Its performance in survivors is comparable to that in on-treatment patients.

Ferrans-Powers HRQOL-Cancer Version

This instrument has been administered to breast cancer survivors and heterogeneous samples of survivors in descriptive studies[43,123,124] and studies examining the relationship of psychological distress and HRQOL.[125]

Functional Assessment of Cancer Therapy (FACT)

The FACT-G(eneral) and its disease-specific subscales have been used in several studies of cancer survivors. For example, some investigators have used the FACT-G or versions adapted for specific sub-groups, like the FACT-B for breast cancer survivors and the FACT-C for colorectal carcinoma survivors, in descriptive studies to characterize the population.[29,37,77,126] Others have used it to examine the validity of other measures.[127,128] The FACT also has been used as an outcome variable in investigations of predictor variables (e.g., exercise, coping) hypothesized to be associated with quality of life.[129–131] The FACT has been used with prostate cancer survivors[56,59,70,132–135] and with lung cancer survivors.[136–140] As with the others, the FACT questionnaires perform in cancer survivors in a way comparable to its performance with patients on-treatment.

The FACIT is an extension of the FACT Measurement System that has the 27-item FACT-G questionnaire as its foundation. It has been validated with individuals with HIV, Parkinson's disease, and multiple sclerosis, and includes assessment of symptoms or issues common across many chronic conditions, such as fatigue and spiritual well-being. The available pool of FACIT items includes over 400 questions, some of which are translated into over 40 languages. For example, it has been used to measure the association of HRQOL with spiritual well-being (as measured by the Spiritual Well-Being subscale of the FACIT) in breast cancer survivors.[141,142]

Functional Living Index-Cancer (FLIC)

Although there appears to be a replicable factor structure, multidimensional scoring was never developed formally; thus, the usefulness of the FLIC in cancer survivors is largely unknown, although it has been used to some extent with prostate cancer survivors[61,69] and lung cancer survivors.[53,143]

Long-Term Quality of Life (LTQL)

The LTQL assessment conceptualizes HRQOL of long-term cancer survivors as a multidimensional interaction of life domains, stressing the importance of spiritual/philosophical issues, social support, and behavioral health changes, while minimizing the past physical events of cancer. The instrument consists of scales assessing somatic concerns, health habits, social/emotional support giving, and philosophical/spiritual view. Results from administrations of the LTQL have been reported in a homogenous sample of breast cancer survivors[27] and a heterogenous sample consisting of breast, colorectal, and other cancer survivors.[108]

Quality of Life-Cancer Survivors (QOL-CS)

The QOL-CS was modeled after HRQOL instruments developed at the City of Hope National Medical Center to assess HRQOL in patients receiving radiation therapy, chemotherapy, or bone marrow transplant. The QOL-CS evolved from these earlier studies and assesses issues and concerns relevant to cancer survivors. Results have been reported in homogenous samples of breast cancer survivors[33,127,144] as well as in mixed samples of survivors.[3,145]

Brief Symptom Inventory-53 (BSI-53)

Derived from the larger, 90-item Symptom Checklist (SCL-90), the BSI contains 53 items addressing 9 symptom dimensions: somatization, obsessive-compulsive, interpersonal sensitivity, depression, anxiety, hostility, phobic anxiety, paranoid ideation, and psychoticism.[146] Subscale and global scores are calculated to determine levels of psychological distress in respondents. The BSI reportedly separates the emotional aspects of psychological distress from the physical aspects, thereby helping to distinguish psychological symptoms from disease- or treatment-related effects. The BSI scale has been used extensively with cancer patients, and results in breast cancer survivors[92] and heterogeneous samples of survivors[7,147] have been reported.

Center for Epidemiologic Studies-Depression (CES-D)

This 20-item self-report questionnaire is designed to assess depressive symptomatology in the general population.[148] It is widely used across many health care and epidemiological studies and has been, for example, incorporated with good results in breast cancer survivor studies.[36,88]

Impact of Event Scale (IES)

The IES is a measure of current subjective distress that has been used in evaluating stress reactions after traumatic and life-threatening events.[149] A shortened version has been found to reliably assess the two most commonly reported responses to stressful events: experiences of intrusive thoughts related to the event, and conscious avoidance of ideas and feelings about the event.[150] The IES has been applied in studies evaluating the psychological impact of diagnosis and stress reactions among cancer survivors.[7,89,151] Some investigators have focused on intrusive thoughts for its symptomatic relevance to diagnoses of post-traumatic stress disorder.[92] Post-traumatic stress responses are a commonly reported problem of survivorship, so instruments such as the IES (used also with prostate cancer survivors by Herr et al.[152]), as well as the Post-Traumatic Growth Inventory (PTGI),[21] are useful to have available.

Mental Adjustment to Cancer (MAC) Scale

This scale assesses psychological adjustment styles of fighting spirit, fatalism, helpless/hopeless, anxious preoccupation, and cognitive avoidance.[153] Survivor studies include administration of an abbreviated version to examine the association between HRQOL, spiritual well-being, and adjustment.[141] Results using the full version were reported in a six-year follow-up study on psychosocial morbidity in long-term survivors.[147]

Profile of Mood States (POMS)

The POMS is a standardized instrument to assess mood. It comprises 6 subscales (tension-anxiety, depression-dejection, anger-hostility, vigor-activity, fatigue-inertia, and confusion-bewilderment), and a total score indicating overall mood disturbance.[154] The POMS has been used to study psychological aspects/distress in numerous cancer survivor studies.[38,41,69,90,93,131,142,155] The fatigue-inertia and vigor-activity subscales also have been used as a measure of physical well-being in cancer survivors.[156]

Psychological Adjustment to Illness Scale (PAIS)

This instrument consists of seven subscales, including vocational environment, domestic environment, sexual relationship, social environment, and psychological distress.[157,158] The PAIS has been used as a measure of "psychosocial function" in several survivor studies (e.g., Bekkers *et al.*,[159] Olweny *et al.*, 1993[160]). Reliability and validity appear to be comparable to that seen in cancer patients receiving active treatment.

Qualitative approaches to evaluating HRQOL

Qualitative investigations of HRQOL include broad approaches and questions aimed at identifying and describing survivors' experiences and changes in their lives after cancer.[7,10,44,144,161–172] Some studies have been more focused on specific issues such as the impact of treatment-induced effects like menopause[173] and work-related problems.[39]

Some investigators have used qualitative approaches for determining content areas that have contributed to the design of new quantitative measures.[27,174] Some of the most extensive work in this area has been conducted by Ferrell and colleagues at the City of Hope[128,175,176] and includes efforts to validate themes assessed in long-term survivor studies.[177]

Discussion

How assessing HRQOL in cancer survivors adds value

Evaluations of cancer survivors' health-related quality of life provide detailed and comprehensive information about individuals' perceptions of the harms and benefits associated with being diagnosed with and treated for cancer. HRQOL should be assessed as a multidimensional construct, in contrast to the historical (pre-1980) practice of evaluating survivors' medical and psychosocial outcomes using traditional clinical assessment (e.g., symptom inventories or checklists, depression or psychological distress scales). This practice can elucidate instances in which a situation or condition in one quality-of-life domain is associated with, and perhaps even causes, a problem in another. Understanding these interdependencies and potential causal relationships can lead to the identification of survivor needs and the subsequent design and development of supportive interventions. Quality-of-life assessments in survivors also can assist in determining the most efficacious and cost-effective times to implement interventions that may prevent long-term negative sequelae and promote long-term adjustment and physical health.

Performance of the HRQOL instruments in the survivorship studies

There has been substantial debate about both meaning and measurement approaches in quality-of-life studies of cancer patients and survivors.[155,178,179] Even when meaning has been clear, measurement, sampling, and sample size have varied from study to study. Some investigators have used psychometric instruments standardized on "normal" populations, while others have developed (and, to some extent, "normed") instruments on cancer patients. Still others have used qualitative approaches, which have allowed for new insights into relatively understudied areas of cancer survivorship.

The benefit of using standardized measures is the ability to compare results to other (healthy and patient) population norms and to compare on-treatment HRQOL to post-treatment HRQOL (i.e., to measure change from the active treatment period). These more general measures also allow one to detect the impact of co-morbidities, providing a "total picture" of the individual in a context outside cancer in particular. One drawback of these generic approaches is that they may not detect subtle, or survivor-specific issues; instead, they reflect an amalgam of cancer and cancer treatment effects with other factors. Furthermore, generic health status questionnaires tend to over-emphasize physical health at the expense of multidimensional issues that emerge during off-treatment survivorship.

The use of measures that have been developed for generic or cancer treatment populations in cancer survivors has been explored. The most promising of these measures include the EORTC and FACT questionnaires, as they have been validated in non-cancer populations and include many language translations. However, in some cases, investigators report the psychometric properties of the instrument as derived from patient populations or normative groups and then *assume* the measure's reliability and validity in a survivor population. Testing the reliability and validity of these measures in off-treatment survivors is an important avenue for future research. Evidence from the literature, however, indicates that these instruments perform comparably in cancer patients on and off active therapy. The primary drawback of "on-treatment" and generic instruments is their lack of coverage of some of the "survivor-emergent" issues such as post-traumatic personal growth, chronic physical compromise, and fear of recurrence.

Two instruments to date have been designed specifically for measuring quality of life in cancer survivors, and their developers have detailed a rigorous process for establishing their reliability and validity. Specifically, both the LTQL and QOL-CS evolved out of systematic evaluations of long-term cancer survivors via iterative procedures involving focus groups and interviews to identify salient HRQOL issues and concerns. Their strengths lie in their comprehensive coverage of psychosocial issues that are relevant to survivorship. These two instruments distinguish themselves from the commonly used generic and general cancer instruments in that they have item content covering areas reported to be of specific relevance to cancer survivors. This distinction, while relevant from a content validity standpoint, should not imply that commonly used generic and general cancer instruments are invalid among cancer survivors. Rather, survivor-specific measures complement standardized measures by recognizing

emerging themes such as fear of recurrence, existential or spiritual well-being, and health maintenance behaviors. However, these survivor-specific instruments do not currently allow one to record changes in self-reported health status as cancer patients move from active treatment into survivorship. They also do not permit comparisons to healthy, non-cancer populations, to other cohorts, or to normative data. In other words, across the list of candidate instruments for studying cancer survivorship, each has its advantages and disadvantages that can be weighed when considering one's choice.

Dimension-specific approaches focus on single domains, often in the area of mental well-being. As such, they tend to possess good psychometric characteristics because they employ multi-item scales to evaluate relatively narrow constructs, and because they have often been previously validated in other populations. Thus, they offset their lack of breadth with depth and responsiveness to differences or changes in the measured domain. However, in addition to lacking comprehensive coverage, they tend to focus on pathology rather than adaptation or growth. Therefore, these instruments have a role in the screening and diagnosis of domain-specific problems and in the evaluation of domain-targeted prevention and treatment interventions, but they do not capture the full scale of psychological and adaptive reactions experienced and expressed by cancer survivors.

Qualitative approaches tend to contribute critical new and unexpected information in the study of any important phenomenon. Therefore, they are of greatest benefit when little is already known about the subject matter. Since cancer survivorship as a formal area of study is, for the most part, only about 20 years old, past qualitative research has been very important and helpful in uncovering issues such as fear of recurrence, spiritual/existential well-being, post-traumatic growth, aspects of social well-being, and delayed onset of medical effects. Qualitative approaches to assessing HRQOL in cancer survivors have uncovered aspects of the survivorship experience that are not fully addressed by instruments originally designed primarily for patients in active treatment. Some investigators caution that certain items may not be relevant.[112,180]

Qualitative research will continue to be important in the study of culture-specific issues, response to changes in prevailing therapies, and site-specific sequelae of prostate, breast, lung, and colorectal cancer treatments. It also has the potential to uncover the extent to which cancer survivors adjust over time, attribute meaning to their experience, and express current and ongoing needs as they grow older and confront issues and tasks associated with different developmental stages. Qualitative approaches do not, however, enable one to estimate the prevalence or causes of a given problem, which compromises intervention and policy planning.

Further research required to develop a state-of-the-art measurement model

It is important to note that evaluating and interpreting survivors' self-reports and attributions about cancer's effects may be problematic when trying to distinguish aging effects from cancer effects. Thus, attributions introduce a potential for confounding when trying to evaluate survivors' "health-related" or "cancer-related" quality of life. In this regard, the availability of normative data becomes important.

Although many survivors are happy to be alive, they are often saddened by lost potential (e.g., becoming a biological parent) or limited physical and/or social functioning. Survivors articulate and report both positive and negative outcomes associated with their experience; therefore, quality-of-life evaluations need to tease out the sadness/sense of loss aspects from the sense of gratitude and personal growth. This can be understood as the "Paradox of Cancer Survivorship." A good measurement instrument will capture both sides of the paradox: the physical losses, the anxiety, and the sadness *and* the sense of enhanced appreciation for life and sense of meaning or purpose driven by the experience. To quote one cancer survivor studied by Cella and Tross[7]: "I wouldn't wish cancer on my worst enemy, and yet I'm a better person for having had it." This paradox is at the core of the survivor's experience.

Given the existence of hundreds of HRQOL instruments designed to assess many dimensions, debate continues regarding the meaning of quality of life, its theoretical utility, and thus its validity in clinical studies and other areas of psychosocial research. There is still uncertainty as to whether existing standardized instruments and deductive approaches used to assess quality of life for cancer survivors are adequate for fully understanding the impact that having had cancer has had and will have on a person's life. On the other hand, several well-validated and commonly used questionnaires have performed well in studies in which respondents are no longer taking therapy for active disease. The MOS SF-36, for example, is as valid in measuring physical functioning and general mental well-being in cancer survivors as it is in cancer patients receiving therapy, persons with other medical conditions, or the healthy population. Similarly, but even more targeted to cancer-specific issues, the EORTC QLQ-C30 plus its modules, or FACT with its site-specific subscales, do not lose their established psychometric properties after patients are rendered disease-free. Thus, they can and should be used with confidence in cancer survivors, especially in longitudinal survivorship studies. Adjustments to a small number of items that may lose their relevance to some respondents after treatment completion may be needed.

Another consideration in the use and reporting of commonly used measures is that the language in reports of HRQOL in cancer survivors often is unclear with regard to when a situation, condition, or phenomenon is an element of quality of life and when it is a factor that affects or influences quality of life. Some investigators discuss the interdependency of physical, social, and/or psychological well-being, which contributes to the confusion of clarifying what quality of life is. Often there is not a distinction between what quality of life is and the variables that influence it. Fayers and Machin[181] have attempted to reconcile this by referring to symptoms of disease and treatment as "causal" variables and to health and functional status as "indicator" variables. Similarly, Wilson and Cleary[182] have offered a useful explanatory model disputing the relationship between disease symptoms and HRQOL as mediated by individual (personality) and clinical (treatment, etc.) characteristics.

Understanding the individual's perspective is critical for understanding quality of life. Because relatively little is known about the experience of very long-term (>10 years) survivors, an optimal approach to evaluating quality of life in long-term survivors involves multiple methods that utilize self-report measures and intensive face-to-face conversations with survivors. In this way, investigators will achieve a greater understanding of the meanings and interpretations that individuals attribute to the experiences that make up the quality of their lives. This will position the National Cancer Institute and other interested organizations to intervene with effective cancer survivorship policy and research directions.

REFERENCES

1 Jemal, A., Thomas, A., Murray, T. *et al.* (2002). Cancer Statistics, 2002. *CA: Cancer Journal for Clinicians* **52**:23–47.

2 Clark, E. J., Stovall, E. L. (1996). Advocacy: the cornerstone of cancer survivorship. *Cancer Practice* **4**:239–44.

3 Ferrell, B. R., Dow, K. H., Grant, M. (1995). Measurement of the quality of life in cancer survivors. *Quality of Life Research* **4**:523–31.

4 Tross, S., Holland, J. (1990). Psychological sequelae in cancer survivors. In *Handbook of Psycho-oncology*, ed. J. C. Holland, J. H. Rowland, Chapter 7. New York, NY: Oxford University Press.

5 Gotay, C. C., Muraoka, M. Y. (1998). Quality of life in long-term survivors of adult-onset cancers. *Journal of the National Cancer Institute* **90**:656–67.

6 Andrykowski, M., Brady, M. J., Hunt, J. W. (1993). Positive psychosocial adjustment in potential bone marrow transplant recipients: Cancer as a psychosocial transition. *Psycho-Oncology* **2**:261–76.

7 Cella, D. F., Tross, S. (1986). Psychological adjustment to survival from Hodgkin's disease. *Journal of Consulting and Clinical Psychology* **54**:616–22.

8 Collins, R. L., Taylor, S. E., Skokan, L. A. (1990). A better world or a shattered vision? Changes in life perspectives following victimization. *Social Cognition* **8**:263–85.

9 Fromm, K., Andrykowski, M. A., Hunt, J. (1996). Positive and negative psychosocial sequelae of bone marrow transplantation: implications for quality of life assessment. *Journal of Behavioral Medicine* **19**:221–40.

10 Wilson, S. E., Andersen, M. R., Meischke, H. (2000). Meeting the needs of rural breast cancer survivors: What still needs to be done? *Journal of Women's Health and Gender-Based Medicine* **9**:667–77.

11 Zebrack, B. J. (2000). Quality of life in long-term survivors of leukemia and lymphoma. *Journal of Psychosocial Oncology* **18**:39–59.

12 Curbow, B., Somerfield, M. R., Baker, F. *et al.* (1993). Personal changes, dispositional optimism, and psychological adjustment to bone marrow transplantation. *Journal of Behavioral Medicine* **16**:423–43.

13 McMillen, J. C., Fisher, R. H. (1998). The perceived benefit scales: Measuring perceived positive life changes after negative events. *Social Work Research* **22**:173–87.

14 Miller, W. R., C'deBaca, J. (1994). Quantum change: toward a psychology of transformation. In *Can Personality Change?* ed. T. F. Heatherton, J. L. Weinberger, pp. 253–81. Washington, DC: American Psychological Association.

15 Affleck, G., Tennen, H. (1996). Construing benefits from adversity: adaptational significance and dispositional underpinnings. *Journal of Personality* **64**:899–922.

16 Allswede, J. S. (1991). *Perceptions of personal change reported by people with leukemia or lymphoma.* Unpublished doctoral dissertation, University of Michigan, Ann Arbor, MI.

17 Davis, S. H., Chesler, M. A., Chesney, B. (1990). Coping with cancer: life changes reported by patients and significant others dealing with leukemia and lymphoma. In *The Working Paper Series*, #427. Ann Arbor, MI: Center for Research on Social Organization, University of Michigan.

18 Taylor, S. E., Lichtman, R. R., Wood, J. V. (1984). Attributions, beliefs about control, and adjustment to breast cancer. *Journal of Personality and Social Psychology* **46**:489–502.

19 O'Leary, V., Alday, C. S., Ickovics, J. R. (1998). Models of Life Change in Posttraumatic Growth. In *Models of Life Change and Posttraumatic Growth*, eds. V. O'Leary, C. S. Alday, J. R. Ickovics, pp. 127–51. Mahwah, NJ: Lawrence Erlbaum Publishers.

20 Park, C. L., Cohen, L. H., Murch, R. L. (1996). Assessment and prediction of stress-related growth. *Journal of Personality* **64**:71–105.

21 Tedeschi, R. G., Calhoun, L. G. (1996). The Posttraumatic Growth Inventory: measuring the positive legacy of trauma. *Journal of Traumatic Stress* **9**:455–71.

22 Carver, C. S. (1998). Resilience and thriving: issues, models, and linkages. *Journal of Social Issues* **54**:245–66.

23 Cohen, L. H., Cimbolic, K., Armeli, S. R. (1998). Quantitative assessment of thriving. *Journal of Social Issues* **54**:323–35.

24 Dow, K. H. (1990). The enduring seasons in survival. *Oncology Nursing Forum* **17**:511–16.

25 Massey, S., Cameron, A., Ouellette, S. *et al.* (1998). Qualitative approaches in the study of thriving: what can be learned? *Journal of Social Issues* **54**:337–55.

26 Park, C. L. (1998). Stress-related growth and thriving through coping: the roles of personality and cognitive processes. *Journal of Social Issues* **54**:267–77.

27 Wyatt, G. K., Friedman, L. L. (1996). Development and testing of a quality of life model for long-term female cancer survivors. *Quality of Life Research* **5**:387–94.

28 National Cancer Institute Office of Cancer Survivorship. Prevalence by Cancer Site. Available at http://cancercontrol.cancer.gov/ocs/. Last accessed September 11, 2004.

29 Holzner, B., Kemmler, G., Kopp, M. *et al.* (2001). Quality of life in breast cancer patients – not enough attention for long-term survivors? *Psychosomatics* **42**:117–23.

30 Saleeba, A., Weitzner, M. A., Meyers, C. A. (1996). Subclinical psychological distress in long-term survivors of breast cancer: a preliminary communication. *Journal of Psychosocial Oncology* **14**:83–93.

31 Dorval, M., Maunsell, E., Deschenes, L. *et al.* (1998). Long-term quality of life after breast cancer: comparison of 8-year survivors with population controls. *Journal of Clinical Oncology* **16**:487–94.

32 Omne-Ponten, M., Holmberg, L., Sjoden, P. O. (1994). Psychosocial adjustment among women with breast cancer stages I and II: six-year follow-up of consecutive patients. *Journal of Clinical Oncology* **12**:1778–82.

33 Ferrell, B. R., Grant, M., Funk, B. *et al.* (1998). Quality of life in breast cancer. Part II: Psychological and spiritual well-being. *Cancer Nursing* **21**:1–9.

34 Ferrell, B. R., Grant, M., Funk, B. *et al.* (1996). Quality of life in breast cancer. *Cancer Practice* **4**:331–40.

35 Halttunen, A., Hietanen, P., Jallinoja, P. *et al.* (1992). Getting free of breast cancer. An eight-year perspective of the relapse-free patients. *Acta Oncologica* **31**:307–10.

36 Bower, J. E., Ganz, P. A., Desmond, K. A. *et al.* (2000). Fatigue in breast cancer survivors: occurrence, correlates, and impact on quality of life. *Journal of Clinical Oncology* **18**:743–53.

37 Northouse, L. L., Caffey, M., Deichelbohrer, L. *et al.* (1999). The quality of life of African American women with breast cancer. *Research in Nursing and Health* **22**:449–60.

38 Shimozuma, K., Ganz, P. A., Petersen, L. *et al.* (1999). Quality of life in the first year after breast cancer surgery: rehabilitation needs and patterns of recovery. *Breast Cancer Research and Treatment* **56**:45–57.

39 Maunsell, E., Brisson, C., Dubois, L. *et al.* (1999). Work problems after breast cancer: an exploratory qualitative study. *Psycho-Oncology* **8**:467–73.

40 Ganz, P. A., Desmond, K. A., Leedham B. *et al.* (2002). Quality of life in long-term, disease-free survivors of breast cancer: a follow-up study. *Journal of the National Cancer Institute* **94**:39–49.

41 Ganz, P. A., Coscarelli, A., Fred, C. *et al.* (1996). Breast cancer survivors: psychosocial concerns and quality of life. *Breast Cancer Research and Treatment* **38**:183–99.

42 Vinokur, A. D., Threatt, B. A., Caplan, R. D. *et al.* (1989). Physical and psychosocial functioning and adjustment to breast cancer. Long-term follow-up of a screening population. *Cancer* **63**:394–405.

43 Lee, C. O. (1997). Quality of life and breast cancer survivors. Psychosocial and treatment issues. *Cancer Practice* **5**:309–16.

44 Carpenter, J. S., Brockopp, D. Y., Andrykowski, M. A. (1999). Self-transformation as a factor in the self-esteem and well-being of breast cancer survivors. *Journal of Advanced Nursing* **29**:1402–11.

45 Sarna, L. (1998). Lung cancer. In *Psycho-oncology*, ed. J. C. Holland, pp. 340–8. New York: Oxford University Press.

46 Montazeri, A., Gillis, C. R., McEwen, J. (1998). Quality of life in patients with lung cancer: a review of literature from 1970 to 1995. *Chest* **113**:467–81.

47 Fossella, F., DeVore, R., Kerr, R. *et al.* (2000). Randomized phase III trial of docetaxel versus vinorelbine or ifosfamide in patients with advanced non-small cell lung cancer previously treated with platinum-containing chemotherapy regimens. *Journal of Clinical Oncology* **18**:2354–62.

48 Gatzemeier, U., von Pawel, J., Gottfried, M. *et al.* (2000). Phase III comparative study of high-dose cisplatin versus a combination of paclitaxel and cisplatin in patients with advanced non-small-cell lung cancer. *Journal of Clinical Oncology* **18**:3390–9.

49 Gregor, A., Cull, A., Stephens, R. *et al.* (1997). Prophylactic cranial irradiation is indicated following complete response to induction therapy in small cell lung cancer: results of a multicenter randomized trial. *European Journal of Cancer* **33**:1752–8.

50 Helsing, M., Bergman, B., Thaning, L. *et al.* (1998). Quality of life and survival in patients with advanced non-small cell lung cancer receiving supportive care plus chemotherapy with carboplatin and etoposide or supportive care only. A

multicentre randomized phase III trial. *European Journal of Cancer* **34**:1036–44.

51 Herndon, J. E., Fleishman, S., Kosty, M. P. *et al.* (1997). A longitudinal study of quality of life in advanced non-small cell lung cancer: Cancer and Leukemia Group B (CALGB) 8931. *Controlled Clinical Trials* **18**:286–300.

52 Langendijk, J., Aaronson, N., ten Velde, G. *et al.* (2000). Pretreatment quality of life of inoperable non-small cell lung cancer patients referred for primary radiotherapy. *Acta Oncologica* **39**:949–58.

53 Thongprasert, S. (1998). Lung cancer and quality of life. *Australia and New Zealand Journal of Medicine* **28**:397–9.

54 Hopwood, P., Stephens, R. (2000). Depression in patients with lung cancer: prevalence and risk factors derived from quality-of-life data. *Journal of Clinical Oncology* **18**: 893–903.

55 Eton, D. T., Lepore, S. J. (2002). Prostate cancer and health-related quality of life: a review of the literature. *Psycho-Oncology* **11**:307–26.

56 Litwin, M. S., Hays, R. D., Fink, A. *et al.* (1995). Quality-of-life outcomes in men treated for localized prostate cancer. *Journal of the American Medical Association* **273**:129–35.

57 Lubeck, D. P., Litwin, M. S., Henning, J. M. *et al.* (1999). Changes in health-related quality of life in the first year after treatment for prostate cancer: results from CaPSURE. *Urology* **53**:180–6.

58 Potosky, A., Legler, J., Albertsen, P. *et al.* (2000). Health outcomes after prostatectomy or radiotherapy for prostate cancer: results from the Prostate Cancer Outcomes Study. *Journal of the National Cancer Institute* **92**:1582–92.

59 Shrader-Bogen, C. L., Kjellberg, J. L., McPherson, C. P. *et al.* (1997). Quality of life and treatment outcomes: prostate carcinoma patients' perspectives after prostatectomy or radiation therapy. *Cancer* **79**:1977–86.

60 Fowler, Jr., F. J., Barry, M. J., Lu-Yao, G. *et al.* (1996). Outcomes of external-beam radiation therapy for prostate cancer: a study of Medicare beneficiaries in three Surveillance, Epidemiology, and End Results areas. *Journal of Clinical Oncology* **14**:2258–65.

61 Lim, A. J., Brandon, A. H., Fiedler, J. *et al.* (1995). Quality of life: radical prostatectomy versus radiation therapy for prostate cancer. *The Journal of Urology* **154**:1420–5.

62 Yarbro, C. H., Ferrans, C. E. (1998). Quality of life of patients with prostate cancer treated with surgery or radiation therapy. *Oncology Nursing Forum* **25**:685–93.

63 Litwin, M. S., McGuigan, K. A., Shpall, A. I. *et al.* (1999). Recovery of health related quality of life in the year after radical prostatectomy: early experience. *Journal of Urology* **161**:515–19.

64 Stanford, J. L., Feng, Z., Hamilton, A. S. *et al.* (2000). Urinary and sexual function after radical prostatectomy for clinically localized prostate cancer: the Prostate Cancer Outcomes Study. *Journal of the American Medical Association* **283**:354–60.

65 Da Silva, F. C., Fossa, S. D., Aaronson, N. K. *et al.* (1996). The quality of life of patients with newly diagnosed M1 prostate cancer: experience with EORTC clinical trial 30853. *European Journal of Cancer* **32A**:72–7.

66 Litwin, M. S., Shpall, A. I., Dorey, F. *et al.* (1998). Quality-of-life outcomes in long-term survivors of advanced prostate cancer. *American Journal of Clinical Oncology* **21**: 327–32.

67 Moinpour, C. M., Savage, M. J., Troxel, A. *et al.* (1998). Quality of life in advanced prostate cancer: results of a randomized therapeutic trial. *Journal of the National Cancer Institute* **90**:1537–44.

68 Albertsen, P. C., Aaronson, N. K., Muller, M. J. *et al.* (1997). Health-related quality of life among patients with metastatic prostate cancer. *Urology* **49**:207–16.

69 Cassileth, B. R., Soloway, M. S., Vogelzang, N. J. *et al.* (1992). Quality of life and psychosocial status in stage D prostate cancer. Zoladex Prostate Cancer Study Group. *Quality of Life Research* **1**:323–9.

70 Esper, P., Mo, F., Chodak, G. *et al.* (1997). Measuring quality of life in men with prostate cancer using the Functional Assessment of Cancer Therapy-Prostate instrument. *Urology* **50**:920–8.

71 Chodak, G., Sharifi, R., Kasimis, B. *et al.* (1995). Single-agent therapy with bicalutamide: a comparison with medical or surgical castration in the treatment of advanced prostate carcinoma. *Urology* **46**:849–55.

72 Iversen, P., Tyrrell, C. J., Kaisary, A. V. *et al.* (1998). Casodex (bicalutamide) 150-mg monotherapy compared with castration in patients with previously untreated nonmetastatic prostate cancer: results from two multicenter randomized trials at a median follow-up of 4 years. *Urology* **51**:389–96.

73 Tyrrell, C. J., Kaisary, A. V., Iversen, P. *et al.* (1998). A randomised comparison of 'Casodex' (bicalutamide) 150 mg monotherapy versus castration in the treatment of metastatic and locally advanced prostate cancer. *European Urology* **33**:447–56.

74 Mannaerts, G. H., Schijven, M. P., Hendrikx, A. *et al.* (2001). Urologic and sexual morbidity following multimodality treatment for locally advanced primary and locally recurrent rectal cancer. *European Journal of Surgical Oncology* **27**:265–72.

75 Ness, R. M., Holmes. A., Klein, R. *et al.* (1998). Outcome states of colorectal cancer: identification and description

using patient focus groups. *American Journal of Gastroenterology* **93**:1491–7.

76 Ulander, K., Jeppsson, B., Grahn, G. (1997). Quality of life and independence in activities of daily living preoperatively and at follow-up in patients with colorectal cancer. *Supportive Care in Cancer* **5**:402–9.

77 Ramsey, S. D., Andersen, M. R., Etzioni, R. *et al.* (2000). Quality of life in survivors of colorectal carcinoma. *Cancer* **88**:1294–1303.

78 Hays, R. D., Sherbourne, C. D., Mazel, R. M. (1993). The RAND 36-Item Health Survey 1.0. *Health Economics* **2**: 217–27.

79 Ware, J. E., Sherbourne, C. D. (1992). A 36-item Short Form Health Survey (SF-36): I. Conceptual framework and item selection. *Medical Care* **30**:473–83.

80 Ganz, P. A., Schag, C. A., Lee, J. J. *et al.* (1992). The CARES: a generic measure of health-related quality of life for cancer patients. *Quality of Life Research* **1**:19–29.

81 Schag, C. A., Ganz, P. A., Heinrich R. L. (1991). Cancer Rehabilitation Evaluation System–Short Form (CARES-SF). A cancer specific rehabilitation and quality of life instrument. *Cancer* **68**:1406–13.

82 Aaronson, N. K., Ahmedzai, S., Bergman, B. (1993). The European Organization for Research and Treatment of Cancer QLQ-C30: a quality of life instrument for use in international trials in oncology. *Journal of the National Cancer Institute* **85**:365–76.

83 Ferrans, C. E., Power, M. J. (1995). Quality of life index: development and psychometric properties. *Annals of Nursing Science* **8**:15–24.

84 Cella, D. F., Tulsky, D. S. (1993). Quality of life in cancer: definition, purpose, and method of measurement. *Cancer Investigation* **11**:327–36.

85 Schipper, H., Clinch, J., McMurray, A. *et al.* (1984). Measuring the quality of life of cancer patients: The Functional Living Index-Cancer: Development and validation. *Journal of Clinical Oncology* **2**:472–83.

86 Erickson, this volume, Chapter 3.

87 Andersen, M. R., Urban, N. (1999). Involvement in decision-making and breast cancer survivor quality of life. *Annals of Behavioral Medicine* **21**:201–9.

88 Ganz, P. A., Rowland, J. H., Desmond, K. *et al.* (1998). Life after breast cancer: understanding women's health-related quality of life and sexual functioning. *Journal of Clinical Oncology* **16**:501–14.

89 Cordova, M. J., Andrykowski, M. A., Kenady, D. E. *et al.* (1995). Frequency and correlates of posttraumatic stress disorder like symptoms after treatment for breast cancer. *Journal of Consulting and Clinical Psychology* **63**:981–6.

90 Polinsky, M. L. (1994). Functional status of long-term breast cancer survivors: demonstrating chronicity. *Health and Social Work* **19**:165–73.

91 Stiggelbout, A. M., de Haes, J. C. J. M., Vree, R. *et al.* (1997). Follow-up of colorectal cancer patients: quality of life and attitudes toward follow-up. *British Journal of Cancer* **75**:914–20.

92 Vickberg, S. M. J., Bovbjerg, D. H., DuHamel, K. N. *et al.* (2000). Intrusive thoughts and psychological distress among breast cancer survivors: global meaning as a possible protective factor. *Behavioral Medicine* **25**:152–60.

93 Beard, C. J., Propert, K. J., Rieker, P. P. *et al.* (1997). Complications after treatment with external-beam irradiation in early-stage prostate cancer patients: a prospective multi-institutional outcomes study. *Journal of Clinical Oncology* **15**:223–9.

94 Brandeis, J., Litwin, M., Burnison, M., Reiter, R. (2000). Quality of life outcomes after brachytherapy for early stage prostate cancer. *Journal of Urology* **163**:851–7.

95 Clark, J. A., Rieker, P., Propert, K. J. *et al.* (1999). Changes in quality of life following treatment for early prostate cancer. *Urology* **53**:161–8.

96 Eton, D., Lepore, S., Helgeson, V. (2001). Early quality of life in localized prostate carcinoma: treatment-related, demographic, and psychosocial factors. *Cancer* **92**:1451–9.

97 Hamilton, A., Stanford, J., Gilliland, F. *et al.* (2001). Health outcomes after external-beam radiation therapy for clinically localized prostate cancer: results from the Prostate Cancer Outcomes Study. *Journal of Clinical Oncology* **19**:2517–26.

98 Janda, M., Gerstner, N., Obermair, A. *et al.* (2000). Quality of life changes during conformal radiation therapy for prostate carcinoma. *Cancer* **89**:1322–8.

99 Litwin, M., McGuigan, K. (1999). Accuracy of recall in health-related quality-of-life assessment among men treated for prostate cancer. *Journal of Clinical Oncology* **17**: 2882–8.

100 Lubeck, D., Grossfeld, G., Carroll, P. (2001). The effect of androgen deprivation therapy on health-related quality of life in men with prostate cancer. *Urology* **58**:94–100.

101 Madalinska, J., Essink-Bot, M., de Koning, H. *et al.* (2001). Health-related quality-of-life effects of radical prostatectomy and primary radiotherapy for screen-detected or clinically diagnosed localized prostate cancer. *Journal of Clinical Oncology* **19**:1619–28.

102 Penson, D., Stoddard, M., Pasta, D. *et al.* (2001). The association between socioeconomic status, health insurance coverage, and quality of life in men with prostate cancer. *Journal of Clinical Epidemiology* **54**:350–8.

103 Potosky, A., Knopf, K., Clegg, L. *et al.* (2001). Quality-of-life outcomes after primary androgen deprivation therapy: results from the Prostate Cancer Outcomes Study. *Journal of Clinical Oncology* **19**:3750–7.

104 Schapira, M., Lawrence, W., Katz, D., McAuliffe, T., Nattinger, A. (2001). Effect of treatment on quality of life among men with clinically localized prostate cancer. *Medical Care* **39**:243–53.

105 Mangione, C. M., Goldman, L., Orav, J. *et al.* (1997). Health-related quality of life after elective surgery: measurement of longitudinal changes. *Journal of General Internal Medicine* **12**:686–97.

106 Ganz, P. A., Hirji, K., Sim, M. *et al.* (1993). Predicting psychosocial risk in patients with breast cancer. *Medical Care* **31**:419–31.

107 Schag, C. A., Ganz, P. A., Wing, D. S. *et al.* (1994). Quality of life in adult survivors of lung, colon and prostate cancer. *Quality of Life Research* **3**:127–41.

108 Kurtz, M. E., Wyatt, G., Kurtz, J. C. (1995). Psychological and sexual well-being, philosophical/spiritual views, and health habits of long-term cancer survivors. *Health Care Women International* **16**:253–62.

109 Ashing-Giwa, K., Ganz, P. A., Petersen, L. (1999). Quality of life of African-American and White long-term breast carcinoma survivors. *Cancer* **85**:418–26.

110 Canales, S., Ganz, P. A., Coscarelli, C. A. (1995). Translation and validation of quality of life instrument for Hispanic American cancer patients: methodological considerations. *Quality of Life Research* **4**:3–11.

111 Cousson-Gelie, F. (2000). Breast cancer, coping and quality of life: a semi-prospective study. *European Review of Applied Psychology* **50**:315–20.

112 Joly, F., Espie, M., Marty, M. *et al.* (2000). Long-term quality of life in premenopausal women with node-negative localized breast cancer treated with or without adjuvant chemotherapy. *British Journal of Cancer* **83**:577–82.

113 Fossa, S. D., Woehre, H., Kurth, K. H. *et al.* (1997). Influence of urological morbidity on quality of life in patients with prostate cancer. *European Urology* **31**:3–8.

114 Moore, M. J., Osoba, D., Murphy, K. *et al.* (1994). Use of palliative end points to evaluate the effects of mitoxantrone and low-dose prednisone in patients with hormonally resistant prostate cancer. *Journal of Clinical Oncology* **12**:689–94.

115 Sneeuw, K., Albertsen, P., Aaronson, N. (2001). Comparison of patient and spouse assessments of health related quality of life in men with metastatic prostate cancer. *Journal of Urology* **165**:478–82.

116 Stockler, M. R., Osoba, D., Goodwin, P. *et al.* (1998). Responsiveness to change in health-related quality of life in a randomized clinical trial: a comparison of the Prostate Cancer Specific Quality of Life Instrument (PROSQOLI) with analogous scales from the EORTC QLQ-C30 and a trial specific module. European Organization for Research and Treatment of Cancer. *Journal of Clinical Epidemiology* **51**:137–45.

117 Anderson, H., Hopwood, P., Stephens, R. *et al.* (2000). Gemcitabine plus best supportive care (BSC) vs BSC in inoperable non-small cell lung cancer – a randomized trial with quality of life as the primary outcome. *British Journal of Cancer* **83**:447–53.

118 Crino, L., Scagliotti, G., Ricci, S. *et al.* (1999). Gemcitabine and cisplatin versus mitomycin, ifosfamide, and cisplatin in advanced non-small-cell lung cancer: A randomized phase III study of the Italian Lung Cancer Project. *Journal of Clinical Oncology* **17**:3522–30.

119 Langendijk, H., Aaronson, N., de Jong, J. *et al.* (2000). The prognostic impact of quality of life assessed with the EORTC QLQ-C30 in inoperable non-small cell lung carcinoma treated with radiotherapy. *Radiotherapy and Oncology* **55**:19–25.

120 Langendijk, J., ten Velde, G., Aaronson, N. *et al.* (2000). Quality of life after palliative radiotherapy in non-small cell lung cancer: a prospective study. *International Journal of Radiation Oncology, Biology, and Physics* **47**:149–55.

121 Roskowski, K., Pluzanska, A., Krzakowski, M. *et al.* (2000). A multicenter, randomized, phase III study of docetaxel plus best supportive care versus best supportive care in chemotherapy-I patients with metastatic or non-resectable localized non-small cell lung cancer (NSCLC). *Lung Cancer* **27**:145–57.

122 Ringdal, G. I., Ringdal, K. (2000). A follow-up study of the quality of life in cancer patients with different prognoses. *Quality of Life Research* **9**:65–73.

123 Pedro, L. W. (2001). Quality of life for long-term survivors of cancer. *Cancer Nursing* **24**:1–11.

124 Sammarco, A. (2001). Perceived social support, uncertainty, and quality of life of younger breast cancer survivors. *Cancer Nursing* **24**:212–19.

125 Weitzner, M. A., Meyers, C. A., Stuebing, K. K. *et al.* (1997). Relationship between quality of life and mood in long-term survivors of breast cancer treated with mastectomy. *Supportive Care in Cancer* **5**:241–8.

126 Ramsey, S. D., Berry, K., Moinpour, C. *et al.* (2002). Quality of life in long term survivors of colorectal cancer. *American Journal of Gastroenterology* **97**:1128–34.

127 Dow, K. H., Ferrell, B. R., Leigh, S. *et al.* (1996). An evaluation of the quality of life among long-term survivors of breast cancer. *Breast Cancer Research and Treatment* **39**:261–73.

128 Ferrell, B. R., Dow, K. H., Leigh, S. *et al.* (1995). Quality of life in long-term cancer survivors. *Oncology Nursing Forum* **22**:915–22.

129 Courneya, K. S., Friedenreich, C. M. (1997). Relationship between exercise pattern across the cancer experience and current quality of life in colorectal cancer survivors. *Journal of Alternative and Complementary Medicine* **3**:215–26.

130 Courneya, K. S., Friedenreich, C. M. (1997). Relationship between exercise during treatment and current quality of life among survivors of breast cancer. *Journal of Psychosocial Oncology* **15**:35–57.

131 Stanton, A. L., Danoff-Burg, S., Cameron, C. L. *et al.* (2000). Emotional expressive coping predicts psychological and physical adjustment to breast cancer. *Journal of Consulting and Clinical Psychology* **68**:875–82.

132 Lee, W., McQuellon, R., Case, D. *et al.* (1999). Early quality of life assessment in men treated with permanent source interstitial brachytherapy for clinically localized prostate cancer. *Journal of Urology* **162**:403–6.

133 Monga, U., Kerrigan, A., Thornby, J. *et al.* (1999). Prospective study of fatigue in localized prostate cancer patients undergoing radiotherapy. *Radiation and Environmental Biophysics* **7**:178–85.

134 Robinson, J., Saliken, J., Donnelly, B. *et al.* (1999). Quality-of-life outcomes for men treated with cryosurgery for localized prostate carcinoma. *Cancer* **86**:1793–801.

135 Tefilli, M. V., Gheiler, E. L., Tiguert, R. *et al.* (1998). Quality of life in patients undergoing salvage procedures for locally recurrent prostate cancer. *Journal of Surgical Oncology* **69**:156–61.

136 Cella, D. F. (1995). Measuring quality of life in palliative care. *Seminars in Oncology* **22**:73–81.

137 Bonomi, P., Kim, K. M., Fairclough, D. *et al.* (2000). Comparison of survival and quality of life in advanced non-small-cell lung cancer patients treated with two dose levels of paclitaxel combined with cisplatin versus etoposide with cisplatin: results of an Eastern Cooperative Oncology Group trial. *Journal of Clinical Oncology* **18**:623–31.

138 Kelly, K., Crowley, J., Bunn, P. *et al.* (2001). Randomized phase III trial of paclitaxel plus carboplatin versus vinorelbine plus cisplatin in the treatment of patients with advanced non-small-cell lung cancer: a Southwest Oncology Group Trial. *Journal of Clinical Oncology* **19**:3210–18.

139 Schiller, J., Adak, S., Cella, D. *et al.* (2001). Topotecan versus observation after cisplatin plus etoposide in extensive-stage small-cell lung cancer: E7593 – A phase III trial of the Eastern Cooperative Oncology Group. *Journal of Clinical Oncology* **19**:2114–22.

140 Smith, E., Hann, D., Ahles, T. *et al.* (2001). Dyspnea, anxiety, body consciousness, and quality of life in patients with lung cancer. *Journal of Pain Symptom Management* **21**:323–9.

141 Cotton, S. P., Levine, E. G., Fitzpatrick, C. M., Dold, K. H., Targ, E. (1999). Exploring the relationships among spiritual well-being, quality of life, and psychological adjustment in women with breast cancer. *Psycho-Oncology* **8**:429–38.

142 Shapiro, S. L., Lopez, A. M., Schwartz, G. E. *et al.* (2001). Quality of life and breast cancer: relationship to psychosocial variables. *Journal of Clinical Psychology* **57**:501–19.

143 Thongprasert, S., Sanguanmitra, P., Juthapan, W. *et al.* (1999). Relationship between quality of life and clinical outcomes in advanced non-small cell lung cancer: best supportive care (BSC) versus BSC plus chemotherapy. *Lung Cancer* **24**:17–24.

144 Ferrell, B. R., Grant, M., Funk, B. *et al.* (1997). Quality of life in breast cancer. Part I: Physical and social well-being. *Cancer Nursing* **20**:398–408.

145 Whedon, M., Stearns, D., Mills, L. E. (1995). Quality of life of long-term adult survivors of autologous bone marrow transplantation. *Oncology Nursing Forum* **22**:1527–35.

146 Derogatis, L. R., Spence, P. (1982). *The Brief Symptom Inventory (BSI) Administration, Scoring and Procedures Manual – I.* Baltimore, MD: Clinical Psychometric Research.

147 Grassi, L., Rosti, G. (1996). Psychosocial morbidity and adjustment to illness among long-term cancer survivors. *Psychosomatics* **37**:523–32.

148 Radloff, L. (1977). The CES-D Scale: A self-report depression scale for research in the general population. *Applied Psychological Measurement* **1**:385–401.

149 Horowitz, M., Wilner, N., Alvarez, W. (1979). Impact of event scale: a measure of subjective stress. *Psychosomatic Medicine* **41**:209–18.

150 Zilberg, N. J., Weiss, D. S., Horowitz, M. J. (1982). Impact of event scale: a cross-validation study and some empirical evidence supporting a conceptual model of stress response syndromes. *Journal of Consulting Clinical Psychology* **50**:407–14.

151 McBride, C. M., Clipp, E., Peterson, B. L. *et al.* (2000). Psychological impact of diagnosis and risk reduction among cancer survivors. *Psycho-Oncology* **9**:418–27.

152 Herr, H. W., Kornblith, A. B., Ofman, U. (1993). A comparison of the quality of life of patients with metastatic prostate cancer who received or did not receive hormonal therapy. *Cancer* **71**:1143–50.

153 Watson, M., Greer, J. Y., Inayat, Q. *et al.* (1988). Development of a questionnaire measure of adjustment to cancer: the MAC scale. *Psychology Medicine* **18**:203–9.

154 McNair, D. M., Lorr, M., Droppleman, L. F. (1971). EITS manual for the Profile of Mood States. San Diego, CA: Educational & Industrial Testing Service 1971/1981.

155 Mast, M. E. (1995). Definition and measurement of quality of life in oncology nursing research: review and theoretical implications. *Oncology Nursing Forum* **22**:957–64.

156 Schwartz, A. L. (1999). Fatigue mediates the effects of exercise on quality of life. *Quality of Life Research* **8**:529–38.

157 Derogatis, L. R. (1986). The psychosocial adjustment to illness scale (PAIS). *Journal of Psychosomatic Research* **30**: 77–91.

158 Derogatis, L., Lopez, M. (1983). *The Psychosocial Adjustment to Illness Scale (PAIS& PAIS-SR): Administration, Scoring, & Procedures Manual I.* Baltimore, MD: Clinical Psychometric Research.

159 Bekkers, M. J. T. M., van Knippenberg, F. C. E., van Dulmen, A. M. *et al.* (1997). Survival and psychosocial adjustment to stoma surgery and nonstoma bowel resection: a 4-year follow-up. *Journal of Psychosomatic Research* **42**:235–44.

160 Olweny, C. L., Juttner, C. A., Rofe, P. *et al.* (1993). Long-term effects of cancer treatment and consequences of cure: cancer survivors enjoy quality of life similar to their neighbours. *European Journal of Cancer* **29A**:826–30.

161 Carter, B. J. (1993). Long-term survivors of breast cancer. A qualitative descriptive study. *Cancer Nursing* **16**:354–61.

162 Dunn, J., Steginga, S. K. (2000). Young women's experience of breast cancer: defining young and identifying concerns. *Psycho-Oncology* **9**:137–46.

163 Ferrell, B. R., Grant, M. M., Funk, B. *et al.* (1997). Quality of life in breast cancer survivors as identified by focus groups. *Psycho-Oncology* **6**:13–23.

164 Ferrell, B. R., Grant, M. M., Funk, B. M. *et al.* (1998). Quality of life in breast cancer survivors: implications for developing support services. *Oncology Nursing Forum* **25**:887–95.

165 Fredette, S. L. (1995). Breast cancer survivors: concerns and coping. *Cancer Nursing* **18**:35–46.

166 Ganz, P. A., Zebrack, B. (2001). Long-term impact of cancer therapy in adults. In *American Society of Clinical Oncology Educational Book, 37th Annual Meeting of the American Society of Clinical Oncologists*, ed. C. Perry. Alexandria, VA.

167 Langelier, K. M., Sullivan, C. F. (1998). Breast talk in breast cancer narratives. *Qualitative Health Research* **8**:76–94.

168 Loescher, L. J., Clark, L., Atwood, J. R. *et al.* (1990). The impact of the cancer experience on long-term survivors. *Oncology Nursing Forum* **17**:223–9.

169 Pelusi, J. (1997). The lived experience of surviving breast cancer. *Oncology Nursing Forum* **24**:1343–53.

170 Taylor, E. J. (2000). Transformation of tragedy among women surviving breast cancer. *Oncology Nursing Forum* **27**:781–8.

171 Utley, R. (1999). The evolving meaning of cancer for long-term survivors of breast cancer. *Oncology Nursing Forum* **26**:1519–23.

172 Wyatt, G., Kurtz, M. E., Liken, M. (1993). Breast cancer survivors: An exploration of quality of life issues. *Cancer Nursing* **16**:440–8.

173 Davis, C. S., Zinkand, J. E., Fitch, M. I. (2000). Cancer treatment induced menopause: meaning for breast and gynecological cancer survivors. *Cancer Oncology Nursing Journal* **10**:14–21.

174 Ferrans, C. E. (1994). Quality of life through the eyes of survivors of breast cancer. *Oncology Nursing Forum* **21**: 1645–51.

175 Ferrell, B. R., Grant, M., Schmidt, G. *et al.* (1992). The meaning of quality of life for bone marrow transplant survivors. Part 1: The impact of bone marrow transplant on quality of life. *Cancer Nursing* **15**:153–60.

176 Ferrell, B. R., Grant, M., Schmidt, G. M. *et al.* (1992). The meaning of quality of life for bone marrow transplant survivors. Part 2: Improving quality of life for bone marrow transplant survivors. *Cancer Nursing* **15**:247–53.

177 Dow, K. H., Ferrell, B. R., Haberman, M. R. *et al.* (1999). The meaning of quality of life in cancer survivorship. *Oncology Nursing Forum* **26**:519–28.

178 Clark, E. (1993). The linkage of research and practice in oncology. *Advances in Medical Psychotherapy* **6**: 215–26.

179 Somerfield, M., Curbow, B. (1992). Methodological issues and research strategies in the study of coping with cancer. *Social Science and Medicine* **34**:1203–16.

180 Zebrack, B. J., Chesler, M. A. (2001). A psychometric analysis of the Quality of Life-Cancer Survivors (QOL-CS) in survivors of childhood cancer. *Quality of Life Research* **10**:319–29.

181 Fayers, P. M., Machin, D. (2000*). Quality of Life: Assessment, Analysis and Interpretation.* Chichester: John Wiley & Sons.

182 Wilson, I. B., Cleary, P. D. (1995). Linking clinical variables with health-related quality of life. A conceptual model of patient outcomes. *Journal of the American Medical Association* **273**:59–65.

183 Borghede, G., Karlsson, J., Sullivan, M. (1997). Quality of life in patients with prostatic cancer: results from a Swedish population study. *Journal of Urology* **158**:1477–85.

184 Giaccone, G., Splinter, T., Debruyne, C. *et al.* (1998). Randomized study of paclitaxel-cisplatin versus cisplatin-teniposide in patients with advanced non-small-cell lung cancer. *Journal of Clinical Oncology* **16**:2133–41.

185 Zabora, J., Brintzenhofeszoc, K., Curbow, B. *et al.* (2001). The prevalence of psychological distress by cancer site. *Psycho-Oncology* **10**:19–28.

186 Schwartz, C., Daltroy, L., Brandt, U. *et al.* (1992). A psychometric analysis of the Mental Adjustment to Cancer Scale. *Psychological Medicine* **22**:203–10.

187 Merluzzi, T., Martinez-Sanchez, M. (1997). Factor structure of the Psychological Adjustment to Illness Scale (Self-Report) for persons with cancer. *Psychological Assessment* **9**:269–76.

188 Whynes, D. K., Neilson, A. R. (1997). Symptoms before and after surgery for colorectal cancer. *Quality of Life Research* **6**:61–6.

189 Katz, S. (1963). Studies of illness in the aged – the Index of ADL: a standardized measure of biological and psychosocial function. *Journal of the American Medical Association* **185**:914–19.

190 Ranson, M., Davidson, N., Nicolson, M. *et al.* (2000). Randomized trial of paclitaxel plus supportive care versus supportive care for patients with advanced non-small-cell lung cancer. *Journal of the National Cancer Institute* **92**:1074–80.

191 Souhami, R., Spiro, S., Rudd, R. *et al.* (1997). Five-day oral etoposide treatment for advanced small-cell lung cancer: randomized comparison with intravenous chemotherapy. *Journal of the National Cancer Institute* **89**:577–80.

192 Bradburn, N. M. (1969). *The Structure of Psychological Well-being.* Chicago, IL: Aldine.

193 Bradburn, N. M., Caplovitz, D. (1965). *Reports on Happiness: A Pilot Study of Behavior Related to Mental Health.* Chicago, IL: Aldine.

194 Greaves-Otte, J. G. W., Greaves, J., Kruyt, P. M. *et al.* (1991). Problems at social re-integration of long-term cancer survivors. *European Journal of Cancer* **27**:178–81.

195 Zigmond, A. S., Snaith, R. P. (1983). The hospital anxiety and depression scale. *Acta Psychiatrica Scandinavica* **67**:361–70.

196 Okuyama, T., Tanaka, K., Akechi, T. *et al.* (2001). Fatigue in ambulatory patients with advanced lung cancer: prevalence, correlated factors, and screening. *Journal of Pain Symptom Management* **22**:554–64.

197 Lerman, C., Trock, B., Rimer, B. *et al.* (1991). Psychological and behavioral implications of abnormal mammograms. *Annals of Internal Medicine* **114**:657–61.

198 Weathers, F. W., Huska, J. A., Keane, T. M. (1991). *The PTSD Checklist-Civilian Version (PCL-C).* Boston, MA: National Center for PTSD/Boston VA Medical Center.

199 Andrykowski, M. A., Cordova, M. J. (1998). Factors associated with PTSD symptoms following treatment for breast cancer: test of the Andersen Model. *Journal of Traumatic Stress* **11**:189–203.

200 Cordova, M. J., Studts, J. L., Hann, D. M. *et al.* (2000). Symptom structure of PTSD following breast cancer. *Journal of Traumatic Stress* **13**:301–19.

201 Smith, M. Y., Redd, W., DuHamel, K. *et al.* (1999). Validation of the PTSD Checklist-Civilian Version in survivors of bone marrow transplantation. *Journal of Traumatic Stress* **12**:485–99.

202 Spanier, G. B. (1976). Measuring dyadic adjustment: New scales for assessing the quality of marriage and similar dyads. *Journal of Marriage and the Family* **38**:15–28.

203 Litwin, M., Lubeck, D., Stoddard, M. *et al.* (2001). Quality of life before death for men with prostate cancer: results from the CaPSURE database. *Journal of Urology* **165**:871–5.

12

Assessing health-related quality of life at end of life

Betty R. Ferrell, Ph.D., F.A.A.N.*

City of Hope Medical Center, Duarte, CA

Assessment of health-related quality of life (HRQOL) at end of life (EOL) can be quite challenging. However, understanding how treatment affects HRQOL during the terminal phases of care is critical to providing the quality of cancer care called for by the National Cancer Policy Board (NCPB) of the Institute of Medicine.[1] The stage at diagnosis, disease progression, and personal and social factors make cancer care at the end of life extraordinarily complex. Inevitably, as one approaches death, symptoms are dynamic and change in an unpredictable fashion, requiring rapid modifications in medications and other therapies. At this time, assessment of HRQOL, as well as patient management, are formidable tasks.

In studying terminally ill populations, it is important to articulate what is meant by palliative and "end of life" care. The World Health Organization (WHO) defines palliative care as the "active total care of patients whose disease is not responsive to curative treatments."[2] The NCPB has adopted the WHO definition of palliative care, but it also notes that palliative care should begin at the time of cancer diagnosis and extend through the course of the disease to the time of death. While palliative care and EOL care are often seen as equivalent, some make the distinction that EOL care is focused only on the terminal stage, whereas palliative care may extend throughout the disease trajectory. For purposes of this paper, palliative care and EOL care will be used interchangeably, per the WHO definition. Specifically, this chapter focuses on HRQOL assessment in patients in the terminal phases of care for whom curative treatment is no longer an option. It is important to note that, while some have equated HRQOL at EOL with palliation of symptoms and a "peaceful death," this is an oversimplification. In fact, HRQOL at EOL is a complex, multidimensional construct that includes all the aspects of patients' physical and mental well-being as they approach death.

Importance of HRQOL at the end of life

With improved cancer treatments, the quantity of life is increasingly being extended. As a result, patients may face a longer illness trajectory as their disease progresses and enters a terminal phase. During the final phase of disease, the primary emphases of both home care and hospice programs are symptom management and quality of life. Researchers have argued in recent years that both quantity and quality of life must be assessed beginning at diagnosis and extending through this final phase of care. However, while "quantity" of life is easily measured, "quality" of life is far more difficult to define and assess. This may partially explain why investigations of HRQOL at the end of life are sparse.[3–5] Nevertheless, in several research venues, including the palliative surgery literature, improved HRQOL has been invoked as an indicator of treatment or intervention "success."[6] Even for patients with limited time remaining, there can be quality of life, and studies that assess HRQOL in EOL can help promote improved care for patients as they approach death.

Historically, HRQOL and its measurement were linked with assessment of physical symptoms; it was assumed that there was an absolute inverse relationship between physical symptoms and HRQOL.[7,8] This notion was the basis for much of the initial, rudimentary research in this area. Although symptoms are subjective experiences, many studies assumed that physical symptoms, and a decrease in them, are easily quantifiable with "objective" measures.[9-15] As such, physical symptoms became the most widely researched area of terminal care,[16,17] with the main focus on pain and fatigue.

The management of one symptom in particular – pain – has recently received a great deal of attention. Initiatives include new standards developed by the Joint Commission on Accreditation of Healthcare Organizations (JCAHO) and evidence-based practice guidelines developed through the Agency for Healthcare Research and Quality (AHRQ) and the National Comprehensive Cancer Network (NCCN). In addition, WHO, NCCN/American Cancer Society, and the American Pain Society have each developed guidelines for managing cancer pain.[18-22] Interestingly, many of the published guidelines, carefully crafted by many experts from multiple disciplines, have limited content on care at the end of life. Evidence suggests that symptom relief continues to be a major problem in health care and at end of life in particular.

Many studies on pain and physical symptoms demonstrate the strong link between physical complications and multiple domains of HRQOL, including functional status, emotional well-being, psychosocial functioning, and spirituality/existentialism.[23-28] The impact that physical symptoms have on a person's HRQOL, regardless of age, communication ability, cognitive status, ethnicity, culture, or type of cancer, has been well-documented.[1,5,9,29-32] In fact, Morris and colleagues[33,34] describe pain as the key component of quality of life. While other researchers might not place such a primary emphasis on pain, few would dispute the impact of pain and symptom management on HRQOL at the end of life.

The importance of HRQOL at EOL is well recognized, but studies of patients in the terminal phase of care have been hampered by the chal-

lenges associated with assessing HRQOL at this point in the disease trajectory. Specifically, a combination of ethical dilemmas, system barriers, family misunderstanding, the dynamic status of the patient, and the appropriateness of proxy responses can be obstacles to research in these terminal patients. In addition, there is continued debate over how to validate instruments in such populations. For instance, test-retest assessments may be inappropriate in fragile patients due to their constantly changing status and may be impossible as patients die. In addition, the instruments that require respondent input or response (e.g., HRQOL measures) often depend on the patient's physical ability, or on family willingness to answer for the patient. The use of family members as respondents on behalf of patients, i.e., as their proxies, raises methodological challenges and questions of validity.

Family members, who frequently serve as informal caregivers, may also be asked to assess the impact of the patient's cancer and its treatment on their own HRQOL and that of others in the family unit. The patient's loved ones commonly experience physical and emotional distress, and a number of researchers have revealed the dramatic impact of caregiving for the terminally ill on the individual, the family, social networks, communities, and the health care system.[26,35-42] For more information on HRQOL in informal caregivers, see Chapter 16 by Snyder in this volume.[43]

Domains of HRQOL affected at EOL

Cancer patients in the terminal phase may experience effects on their physical, psychological, social, and spiritual well-being, as described below. Because of the multidimensional nature of HRQOL, unidimensional measures cannot provide a complete assessment of impact. For example, to measure the effects of depression from terminal cancer in isolation would likely miss the influence that depression has on satisfaction with care, social withdrawal, relationships and communication, spirituality, and physical symptoms. Thus, in HRQOL assessment, it is important to consider both the full range of HRQOL domains and how they relate to one another.

Physical well-being

Physical well-being has received an enormous amount of attention, likely due to the general goal of medicine to "cure" or resolve symptoms or disease. Aspects of physical well-being critical at the EOL include: (1) functional ability; (2) strength/fatigue; (3) sleep and rest; (4) nausea; (5) appetite; (6) constipation; and (7) pain.[5,9,16,23,29,44-47]

Psychological well-being

A substantial body of literature documents the psychological, psychiatric, and neuropsychological effects of cancer, particularly in advanced disease.[48-53] Moreover, research has shown that patients may experience a wide range of psychological symptoms including adjustment disorders, depression, and anxiety disorders. Cancer treatments and medications may cause serious neurotic and psychotic symptoms, and neuropsychiatric effects may result from metabolic disturbances.[51,54-56] Psychological problems may become especially exacerbated with impending death.[45]

Social well-being

The social realm is, by its very nature, affected by environmental factors. As such, social aspects of HRQOL may undergo considerable changes as the patient's health deteriorates at EOL. The impacts on social well-being include: (1) caregiver burden; (2) roles and relationships; (3) affection/sexual function; and (4) appearance. While little research has been conducted in the areas of affection/sexual function and appearance, there is a growing body of literature on caregiver burden and roles and relationships. Much of that research has been conducted in the context of home care with retrospective assessment of the family member.[27,38,57,58] This research

has indicated a need for additional studies of patients and their families during terminal care. Important social issues requiring further assessment are life closure and redefinition of family roles.[59-62]

Spiritual well-being

Since the 1970s, the contributions of spirituality in medicine have been increasingly recognized,[63-68] although its role in palliative medicine has been only tacitly accepted.[69,70] For the most part, the link between spirituality and HRQOL in EOL has been a result of the evidence, support, and advocacy of the nurses, hospice professionals, and faith communities.[66,70-73] Life's end, or the threat of it, often results in a search for meaning, comfort, and hope.[65,71,74] While the direct link between spirituality and HRQOL at EOL has not undergone extensive study, research is needed in this area.

The following section reviews the HRQOL instruments whose performance has been evaluated within the context of end of life.

HRQOL instruments frequently used at EOL

Increased interest in patient-oriented assessments has led to the investigation and development of various HRQOL measures. By 1993, there were 170 different HRQOL instruments being actively used in research and clinical settings for various chronic and life-threatening illnesses, although there is limited evidence regarding the use of these instruments in palliative care.[22] Although most of these tools were not designed for terminally ill populations and may not be appropriate in this context, some instruments may be adapted for EOL care, and a few have been developed specifically for palliative care populations.

Teno and colleagues have developed the TIME (Toolkit of Instruments to Measure End of life care) project to evaluate the properties of various instruments used in EOL care assessment. This chapter focuses on single instruments rather than batteries of tools and emphasizes scales especially relevant for the last month of life. Research has demonstrated that the final month is when cancer patients experience the greatest symptom burden, dynamic interaction among symptoms, and the most rapid decline in function.[75-79]

Funded by the Robert Wood Johnson Foundation, Teno and colleagues reviewed HRQOL instruments for use at EOL and developed a comprehensive website of their findings.[78] Specifically, they searched the MEDLINE database for terms that addressed measurement, instrument, quality of life, and terminal care or palliative care.[78] They found a total of 131 scientific articles published between 1983 and 2000. From those articles, they identified 41 potential instruments, only some of which were judged applicable for an EOL cancer population.

The various instruments used to assess HRQOL at EOL include the Brief Hospice Inventory (BHI);[80] City of Hope Quality of Life Scale (COH-QOLS); Edmonton Symptom Assessment Scale (ESAS); European Organization for Research and Treatment of Cancer (EORTC QLQ-C30);[81] EuroQol Quality of Life Scale (EuroQol); Functional Assessment of Cancer Therapy (FACT-G);[24] Ferrans and Powers Quality of Life Index;[82] Functional Living Index-Cancer (FLIC);[83] Hospice Quality of Life Index-Revised;[84] LEIPAD (World Health Organization project acronym derived from the first two of the three most involved universities: LEIden-the Netherlands, PADua-Italy, and Helsinki-Finland);[2] McGill Quality of Life Questionnaire (MQOL);[85,86] Medical Outcomes Study Short Form Health Survey (SF-36);[87] Memorial Symptom Assessment Scale (MSAS); Missoula-VITAS Quality of Life Index (MVQOLI);[88,89] National Hospice Study Quality of Life Scale;[90] Quality of Life Index;[91] Quality of Well-Being Scale;[92] Sickness Impact Profile;[93] Southwest Oncology Group Quality of Life Questionnaire;[94] and Spitzer QL-Index.[95]

Of these, the instruments that have been shown to be most relevant for EOL settings are the BHI, MVQOLI, MQOL, ESAS, COH-QOLS, and MSAS. Each is described in more detail below, and a summary of their properties is found in Table 12.1. In addition,

the EORTC and FACT instruments and their applications in end-of-life care research are described briefly; more information on these cancer general HRQOL measures can be found in Chapter 3 by Erickson in this volume.[96] A description and discussion of the preference-based measures (EuroQol and Quality of Well-Being Scale) can be found in Chapter 4 by Feeny in this volume.[97]

Brief Hospice Inventory

The Brief Hospice Inventory (BHI)[80] was developed by the Utah VistaCare Hospice physicians, staff, and collaborators. The main objective of creating the instrument was to assess the perceptions of patients and their caregivers on a wide variety of symptoms and general quality-of-life items, with the notion that the patient's perspective on her own HRQOL is an important element in assessing outcomes.[80,98] The BHI is a 17-item instrument that assesses physical and psychological symptoms, patients' perceptions of hospice care, and patients' rating of overall QOL. The instrument uses a visual analogue scale (VAS) format. Physical symptoms that are assessed include pain, tiredness, nausea, loss of appetite, and dyspnea/shortness of breath. The psychological symptoms domain consists of depression, anxiety, and distress related to changes in self-care ability. Patients' perceptions of hospice care are assessed through overall symptom management, sense of being cared for, and the helpfulness of hospice care. Quality-of-life issues are assessed by items that address comfort, feelings of life as a gift versus a burden, sense of HRQOL, satisfaction with relationships, meaning of life, and fulfillment of previously identified goals for the preceding week.

To develop the BHI, the authors used information from previous researchers who asserted that a large group of items assessing common physical and psychological symptoms may be more useful, particularly for tracking clinical changes that result from various treatments and interventions.[80,99] As such, the BHI has been shown to be a valid and reliable tool to examine key outcome variables during discrete time intervals after admission to hospice. The

Table 12.1. Instruments in end-of-life care

	Brief Hospice Inventory	Missoula-VITAS QOL Index
Purpose for which developed	Developed to assess the perceptions of patients and caregivers on symptoms and general HRQOL in Hospice/EOL.[80,98]	Designed to measure HRQOL of patients with advanced, incurable diseases. The VITAS weights each HRQOL dimension according to patient-reported importance and subjective language.[88,89]
Length & item format	17 items in a visual analogue (0–10) format.	27 items; each item on 5-point scale with two opposing agree/disagree response anchors.
Administration time	Approximately 15 minutes.	No available data.
Domains included	Physical (pain, tiredness, nausea, loss of appetite, dyspnea) and psychological symptoms (depression, anxiety, distress related to changes in self-care ability).	Symptoms, Function, Interpersonal, Well-being, and Transcendence.
Scoring	Individual scores for items and a total score.	Weighted dimension scores can be presented graphically; the score is translated into a number 0 to 30 which facilitates analysis of aggregate group data.
Practical issues	Useful to examine key outcome variables in discrete time intervals after admission to hospice; can be completed by either patient or caregiver; brevity of the instrument useful in EOL and frail;[107] may be used in an interactive voice response system at home.	The MVQOLI does not seem to place an undue burden on patients. Its weighting system allows patients and clinicians to identify dimensions of HRQOL that necessitate intervention, making it useful in clinical settings. Has been acceptable to dying patients.
Validated modes of administration	Administered in self-report or oral format or completed by caregiver.	Designed as a patient-reported measure. No information is available on whether completing it with assistance influences reliability or validity.
Validated translations/Cultural adaptations	To date, only English version is available; tested only on an older Caucasian sample.	Patients of various educational levels and religious backgrounds have been able to complete the MVQOLI; mostly tested in Caucasian samples and no available information on cross-cultural assessment.
Evidence of reliability (internal consistency, test-retest)	*Internal Consistency*: In a 145 patient sample, alpha coefficient ranges from 0.84–0.91 for symptom subscale and 0.92–0.95 for HRQOL subscale. For Caregiver BHI, alpha coefficient ranges from 0.86–0.92 for symptom and 0.92–0.95 for HRQOL subscale. *Test-retest*: Test-retest reliability of 0.58–0.63 when evaluating correlation coefficients for each scale separately at weeks 1 and 2; low test-retest finding may be a result of vagaries of symptoms with impending death.	*Internal Consistency*: Alpha coefficient shown to be 0.77 for overall tool. *Test-retest*: No test-retest evaluation has been conducted for the MVQOLI.

(*cont.*)

Table 12.1. (*cont.*)

	Brief Hospice Inventory	**Missoula-VITAS QOL Index**
Evidence of validity (content, construct, criterion-related)	*Content*: Based on clinical and research experience of health care staff who emphasized that patients' perspective on their own HRQOL should be incorporated into outcome assessment. The BHI combines measures of what patients identify as the most common physical and psychological symptoms and items related to general HRQOL. *Construct*: Principal axis rotation with direct obliman rotation and acceptable eigenvalues confirmed a 2 factor solution model.[80]	*Content*: Assessed by hospice professionals who reviewed the instrument and found 77% accuracy rate in the instrument's ability to correctly assign items to their intended dimensions. *Concurrent*: Tested against the MQOLS-CA2 demonstrating a Pearson's correlation coefficient of 0.43. *Construct*: Examined with both convergent and divergent constructs. For convergence, the MVQOLI dimensions score was compared with the overall HRQOL item, revealing a Pearson's correlation coefficient of 0.43. For divergence, the MVQOLI score was compared with the KPS (Karnofsky Performance Scale), demonstrating a Pearson's correlation coefficient of 0.18.
Evidence of responsiveness/Sensitivity to change	Initial evaluation demonstrated sensitivity to vagaries of multiple symptom changes in terminally ill and repeated measures of VAS have been shown to guide hospice staff in understanding pertinent changes.[80]	Evidence reveals high compliance by patients who know they are dying. The weighting system seems to be sensitive to changes in HRQOL dimensions necessitating intervention.
Interpretability (availability of normative data, clinically meaningful difference)	Normative data only on 145 older Caucasian hospice patients. Limited generalizability to younger, minority, or HIV/AIDS populations. Clinically meaningful difference in VAS scales have been documented but BHI allows for patient determination of meaningful outcome.	Limited normative data with Caucasian patients who know they are dying and know the goal of treatment is palliative. Testing with non-hospice, non-Caucasian patients with variety of terminal diagnoses and moving global HRQOL item to front of the tool may provide more clinically meaningful information about differences. Weighted aggregate may be useful in providing such information as well.
	McGill QOL Questionnaire	**Edmonton Symptom Assessment Scale**
Purpose for which developed	Designed to measure HRQOL of people at all stages of a life threatening illness. MQOL was created to overcome shortcomings in traditional measures used to assess patients with life threatening illness.[8,98]	Developed for terminally ill patients in a palliative care setting.[105,136]
Length & item format	16 items plus a single item global scale each on a 0–10 scale with anchors at opposing ends.	9 items along 100mm (0–100) Visual Analogue Scales.
Administration time	Between 10 and 30 minutes.	Approximately 10 minutes or less.
Domains included	5 domains plus a single Global Index: physical well-being, physical symptoms, psychological, existential, and support.	9 individual symptom scales: pain, anxiety, nausea, depression, anxiety, drowsiness, appetite, shortness of breath, sense of well-being.

(*cont.*)

Table 12.1. (*cont.*)

	McGill QOL Questionnaire	Edmonton Symptom Assessment Scale
Scoring	Each of the 5 domains is scored as a separate subscale. An overall index score can be calculated from the means of the 5 subscales. The single global HRQOL is included as a validity variable but can be used with the overall MQOL and subscale scores.	Each item is scored individually from 0–100. Once collected, the data are transferred to a symptom assessment graph.
Practical issues	MQOL has been useful to providers in a clinical setting and has been preferred by nurses over the Hospice QOL Index.[135] MQOL can be administered by reading aloud, which affords greater completion rates and less burden on the dying patient.	Assessment is conducted twice a day. Collected information is graphed and records assessments up to 21 days on one page.
Validated modes of administration	Designed as a patient self-report measure but can be either self-completed or read aloud by staff. Testing of the MQOL showed that the mode of administration was not correlated with MQOL scores.	Self-administered report but if patients are unable to complete the form, health care staff may assist without affecting results.
Validated translations/Cultural adaptations	The MQOL has been developed simultaneously in English and French although most literature comes from English speaking samples. No other information is available on other cultural adaptations.	ESAS is available in English. No information is available on validated translations or efforts for cultural adaptations.
Evidence of reliability (internal consistency, test-retest)	*Internal Consistency*: Alpha coefficients were shown to be as follows: psychological symptoms = 0.81; physical symptoms = 0.62. Physical well-being did not load strongly with physical symptoms and has been rewritten to more accurately reflect that domain; existential = 0.79 and support = 0.74; total scale = 0.83. *Test-retest*: Tested among oncology patients and intra-class correlation coefficients were found to be in the medium range.[85]	*Internal Consistency*: Overall Cronbach's alpha coefficient was 0.79. *Test-retest*: Spearman correlation coefficients for the summary ESAS distress measure were 0.86 at 2 days and 0.45 at 1 week. All ESAS items were significantly correlated at 2 days, but at 1 week, this was only true for pain, activity, depression, shortness of breath, and ESAS distress.[135] Single-item VAS scores were significantly correlated at 1 day (0.43, p < .04) but not at 1 week.
Evidence of validity (content, construct, criterion-related)	*Content*: based on evaluation of shortcomings of other traditional HRQOL measures and designed to evaluate subscale and item ability to assess overall status and discrete symptoms. *Construct*: Demonstrated through analysis of patterns of correlations with items from the Spitzer QOL Index[95] and the MQOL's single-item overall HRQOL rating (measured before and after completion of the full questionnaire). Strongest validity found with single item HRQOL measure. Correlation with the single-item HRQOL	*Content*: Based on determination by medical experts in oncology and in relation to other instruments assessing symptoms and HRQOL in cancer patients. *Construct*: Demonstrated by comparison of the ESAS items and distress score with corresponding items from the MSAS and FACT-G. *Criterion*: Shown by comparison with Karnofsky Performance Scale (KPS) and with validated subscales from the FACT and MSAS. All the items on the ESAS as well as the summary distress score,

(*cont.*)

Table 12.1. (*cont.*)

	McGill QOL Questionnaire	Edmonton Symptom Assessment Scale
Evidence of validity (*cont'd*)	was highest with MQOL total (0.66), then physical well being (0.59), existential (0.53), psychological symptoms (0.44), support (0.41), and physical symptoms (0.21). The single item measure was validated as an overall HRQOL indicator.	correlated significantly with the KPS with P value of < 0.001. The highest correlation was with the item ESAS distress (−0.56), followed by activity (−0.46), appetite (−0.45), well being (−0.42), pain (−0.40), nausea (−0.32), depression (-0.30), shortness of breath (−0.30), and anxiety (−0.15). Concurrent validity was demonstrated by comparison with ESAS items and distress score with corresponding items from MSAS and with FACT. Significant correlation coefficients (p < 0.0001) were obtained when correlating the ESAS summary distress measure against summary scores from the MSAS with coefficients of 0.72 for the MSAS scale, 0.73 for the Global Distress Index, 0.74 for physical symptom scale, and 0.56 for the psychological symptom subscale. The ESAS distress score correlated most with the FACT physical well-being subscale (−0.75), sum HRQOL (−0.69), functional well-being (−0.63), and emotional well-being (−0.52), and social/family well-being (−0.25).
Evidence of responsiveness/ Sensitivity to change	Responsiveness to change tests show the MQOL tool score and its subscales are able to detect change between good, average, and bad days. The MQOL can be used to measure impact of interventions on self-rated type of day. Effect sizes of differences between types of days for MQOL total, MQOL single item, and subscales are largest for differences between good and bad days. Effects sizes are also large for differences between bad and average days.	Graphical representation of VAS scores indicates responsiveness. Scaling on a 100mmVAS makes the ESAS more sensitive to slight changes than a 10mm scale. In a study of 101 palliative care patients, few subjects refused participation.
Interpretability (availability of normative data, clinically meaningful difference)	MQOL has been used in patients with advanced cancer, patients with cancer at any stage, HIV-positive outpatients, palliative care inpatients, and hospice patients. Both the subscales and the overall score can range from 0 to 10, facilitating the identification of clinically meaningful changes in specific domains and those that need attention.	Normative data come from a study of 101 patients in a palliative care unit.[105] Additional normative data came from a prospective study of 240 patients with a cancer diagnosis. The ESAS is used primarily for symptom assessment rather than comprehensive view of HRQOL. Initially validated in a non-hospice population. It has been found to provide clinically meaningful information specific to palliative care.
	City of Hope Quality of Life Scale	**Memorial Symptom Assessment Scale**
Purpose for which developed	COH QOLS was developed for cancer patients at various stages of the disease to determine overall HRQOL and within discrete dimensions.[28, 106, 115]	Developed to measure the prevalence, characteristics, and distress of a diverse group of common symptoms in seriously ill individuals.[99]

(*cont.*)

Table 12.1. (*cont.*)

	City of Hope Quality of Life Scale	Memorial Symptom Assessment Scale
Length and item format	41-item ordinal scale	32 items determined to be highly prevalent symptoms.
Administration time	Approximately 20–30 minutes	Approximately 20–30 minutes.
Domains included	4 Domains found to be the most pertinent in cancer: physical, psychological, social, and spiritual well being.	3 Domains with subscales: (1) psychological state (MSAS-PSYCH); (2) high frequency physical symptoms (MSAS-PHYS related to pain and pain treatment and a subgroup related to gastrointestinal distress); and (3) low frequency symptoms. Another brief subscale is used as a measure of "global distress index."
Scoring	Each item is based on an ordinal scale 0 to 10 with descriptive anchors at opposing ends.	Global Distress Index is the combination of 10 items including frequency of emotional symptoms and distress items from pain and treatment. The GDI is the average of the frequency of 4 prevalent psychological symptoms and the distress associated with 6 prevalent physical symptoms. MSAS-PHYS is the average frequency, severity, and distress associated with 12 prevalent physical symptoms. MSAS-PSYCH is the average of 6 prevalent psychological symptoms. The total MSAS is the average of 32 items; each symptom score is the average of its dimensions. The intended level of measurement is ordinal.
Practical issues	This instrument can be used in research and in clinical practice. It can be administered either by mail or in person. Initial development of the instrument was for surviving cancer patients; a shortened version is being evaluated specifically for palliative care.	The MSAS can be self-administered or interviewer administered. The 10-item Global Distress Index can be used alone if global symptom distress is the only characteristic of interest.
Validated modes of administration	The COH-QOLS is a self-report measure. If need be, items can be read aloud to the patient.	The MSAS is in a self-report format and is acceptable to be verbally presented by an interviewer.
Validated translations/Cultural adaptations	English and Spanish versions have been validated.	English version has been validated. A Short version with one-third the items has been validated to accommodate waning status of terminally ill.[137] MSAS has also been validated for children ages 7–12.[138]
Evidence of reliability (internal consistency, test-retest)	*Internal Consistency*: Cronbach's alpha coefficient of 0.93 overall. Subscale alphas ranged from 0.71 for spiritual well-being, 0.77 for physical, 0.81 for social, and 0.89 for psychological.	*Internal consistency*: Cronbach's alpha coefficient was found to be high for high prevalence symptoms and psychological state subscales (0.88 and 0.83, respectively). Internal consistency for the pain

(cont.)

Table 12.1. (*cont.*)

	City of Hope Quality of Life Scale	Memorial Symptom Assessment Scale
	Test-retest: Overall test-retest reliability was 0.89 with subscales of physical (0.88), psychological (0.88), social (0.81), and spiritual (0,90).	subgroup was also high (0.87) and moderate for gastrointestinal distress (0.75). For low prevalence symptoms, internal consistency was low (0.58). Reproducibility was not addressed.
Evidence of validity (content, construct, criterion-related)	*Content*: Based on a panel of HRQOL researchers and nurses with expertise in oncology. *Construct*: Stepwise multiple regression determined factors most predictive of overall HRQOL in cancer. 17 variables accounted for 91% of the variance. Pearson's correlations were used to estimate relationships between QOLS subscales and subscales on the FACT-G. There was moderate to strong correlation between associated scales including QOLS Physical to FACT Physical (0.74), QOLS Psychological to FACT Emotional (0.78), QOLS Social to FACT Social (0.44). Overall QOLS correlation with FACT-G was 0.78.	*Content*: Researchers determined a battery of measures that independently evaluate phenomena related to HRQOL. *Construct*: The authors tested construct validity by comparing MSAS scores in populations that varied clinically. Predictions that inpatients would have higher symptom distress than outpatients were confirmed. The correlation between mean severity scores and mean frequency scores across symptoms was $r = 0.80$; the correlation between mean severity scores and mean distress scores was $r = 0.70$; and the correlation between mean frequency scores and mean distress scores was $r = 0.43$. Pairwise correlation was calculated, revealing an average correlation of $r = 0.65$ (range 0.27–0.80) for severity and frequency; an average correlation of $r = 0.67$ (range 0.43–0.87) for severity and distress; and an average correlation of $r = 0.55$ (range 0.21–0.77) for frequency and distress. Canonical correlation findings suggested that the distress measure was the single most informative dimension. Validation measures were correlated with total MSAS scores, single dimensions of severity, frequency, and distress and major symptom groups averaged across all three dimensions. Highly significant association was found between the MSAS and MSAS subscales and the validation measures.
Evidence of responsiveness/Sensitivity to change	Responsiveness on the QOLS has been found to be very good on first assessment and averaging 73% in test-retest situations. Items within the 4 domain subscales have been found to be sensitive to symptom changes including their influence on overall HRQOL.	The MSAS was used as an outcome measure for quality of life in a study of quality of life in advanced breast cancer patients receiving chemotherapy.[110] Longitudinal data were analyzed associating tumor response to changes in quality of life scores throughout the course of treatment. MSAS was also used to assess symptoms as a component of a study of quality of life as an outcome in cancer clinical trials.[111]
Interpretability (availability of normative data, clinically meaningful difference)	Normative data analysis was conducted on 686 cancer survivors. A shortened version for use in palliative care is being evaluated.	MSAS has been utilized in AIDS patients and cancer patients. The 10-item Global Distress Index was considered to be the most clinically useful subscale as it is easy to interpret and can be used alone.

brevity of the instrument (17 items) and the 0–10 numerical rating VAS make it fairly easy to use in a frail population, such as the terminally ill. That it can be completed by a caregiver offers another advantage for acquiring accurate and useful information of symptoms and HRQOL at the end of life.

Missoula-VITAS Quality of Life Index

The Missoula-VITAS Quality of Life Index (MVQOLI)[88,89] was designed to measure HRQOL in patients with advanced, incurable illnesses. As such, the target population for this instrument consists of persons who are aware both of their terminal status and that the goal of care is palliative. The instrument's scoring system weights each HRQOL dimension according to patient-reported importance, and the subjective language is geared toward measuring a patient's experience over the course of illness.

The MVQOLI is a 27-item, self-report instrument that addresses five dimensions of HRQOL in addition to a global item. Each item is structured as a five-point scale with opposing response anchors on each end. The five dimensions are symptoms, function, interpersonal, well-being, and transcendence. They were identified by a literature review and informal interviews with hospice professionals, patients, and family members. The MVQOLI has been used primarily in cancer but also in end-stage lung disease and end-stage heart disease. The weighted dimension scores can be used to produce graphic representations to aid patient-physician communication, guide care planning, and identify HRQOL dimensions that require intervention. The total score is translated into a positive number (between 0 and 30) that facilitates analysis of aggregate group data, making it a useful tool with frail populations in clinical settings. The MVQOLI has good psychometric properties, and it appears to be acceptable to dying patients.

McGill Quality of Life Questionnaire

The McGill Quality of Life Questionnaire (MQOL, Revised)[85,86] was designed to measure HRQOL in persons at all stages of a life-threatening illness, from diagnosis to cure or death. The goal of creating the instrument was to overcome some of the shortcomings of traditional measures used to assess patients with life-threatening illnesses. The MQOL assesses general domains applicable to all patients, balances physical and non-physical aspects of HRQOL, includes both positive and negative influences on HRQOL, and even incorporates the existential domain. It is useful to highlight the inclusion of the existential domain in the MQOL since some other instruments neglect or negate the importance of that dimension in HRQOL. According to the authors of the MQOL, within the existential domain of the MQOL, they aim to capture: concerns regarding death (existential obliteration); freedom (the absence of external structure); isolation (the "unbridgeable gap" separating self from all else); and the question of meaning ("the dilemma of meaning-seeking creatures who recognize the possibility of the cosmos without meaning").[100–103] The authors capture these dimensions of the domain with questions addressing subjective perception of life as worthwhile, control over life, viewing a day in life as a burden or a gift, feeling the world has been an "impersonal unfeeling place" or caring and responsive to one's needs and one's overall sense of feeling supported in life.[85]

The MQOL is a patient-reported instrument that employs 16 items plus a single-item global scale, each with a 2-day timeframe. Five domains (physical well-being, physical symptoms, psychological, existential, and support) were identified through principal components analysis, and each of the domains is scored as a separate subscale. An overall index score can be calculated from the means of the five subscales. The single-item global HRQOL scale is included as a validity variable but also can be used in conjunction with the overall MQOL and subscale scores. The instrument was designed to be generic in nature to maintain brevity and to assure applicability to all patients. The instrument has demonstrated sound psychometric properties.

The MQOL has been used with patients with advanced cancer, patients with cancer at any stage, HIV-positive outpatients, palliative care inpatients, and hospice patients. The instrument offers a balanced assessment of both physical and non-physical domains, as well as both positive and negative factors associated with HRQOL. The MQOL appears to be a valid measure that is acceptable to patients, even those in the final few weeks of life,[104] and the instrument has been shown to be useful for quality improvement efforts in a clinical setting.

Edmonton Symptom Assessment System

The Edmonton Symptom Assessment System (ESAS)[105] consists of nine 100 mm visual analog scales for pain, activity, nausea, depression, anxiety, drowsiness, appetite, shortness of breath, and sensation of well-being. The instrument was designed for symptom assessment twice a day. Once collected, information from the ESAS can be transferred to a symptom assessment graph that records the assessments for up to 21 days on one page, providing a graphical representation indicating changes.

The ESAS was developed for terminally ill patients in a palliative care setting, and Bruera and colleagues[105] found patients to be amenable to participating in the studies using this questionnaire; few refused to complete the form. If patients are physically unable to complete the form, health care staff or caregivers may assist them, and evidence suggests that the results are not affected. While the ESAS assesses major symptoms that are important in EOL care and that have been shown to affect HRQOL, this instrument is used primarily for symptom assessment rather than a comprehensive view of overall HRQOL. Nevertheless, it has been shown to be a valid tool in EOL populations.

City of Hope Quality of Life Scale

The City of Hope (COH) Quality of Life Scale (QOLS) is a 41-item ordinal scale that measures the HRQOL of cancer patients and was developed through research at COH.[36,106,107] This tool can be useful in clinical practice as well as for research and is validated for mail and in-person administration. A His-

panic version of this questionnaire is available.[108,109] The QOLS has been used in many different settings with cancer patients, and a shortened version for use in palliative care is currently being evaluated. The COH-QOLS has demonstrated strong psychometric properties.

Memorial Symptom Assessment Scale

The Memorial Symptom Assessment Scale (MSAS) is a validated multidimensional scale developed to measure the prevalence, characteristics, and distress of common symptoms of the seriously ill.[99] It assesses three domains: (1) psychological state, which can be divided into an emotional symptom subgroup and a concentration subgroup; (2) high frequency physical symptoms, which can be divided into a subgroup related to pain and pain treatment and a subgroup related to gastrointestinal distress; and (3) low frequency symptoms. The authors also sought to develop a brief subscale that could be used as a measure of global symptom distress. The combination of 10 items including emotional symptoms and distress items from pain and treatment is termed the MSAS Global Distress Index.

The MSAS has been used as a HRQOL measure in a study of advanced breast cancer patients receiving chemotherapy[110] and in cancer clinical trials.[111] Despite longitudinal studies through disease treatment, little has been done to evaluate its use specifically within EOL care outcomes. Notably, the 10-item Global Distress Index (GDI) was considered to be the most clinically useful subscale. The MSAS can be self- or interviewer-administered. Its brevity and ease of use are advantages, but its limited use in terminally ill populations and its limited assessment of overall HRQOL are weaknesses.

EORTC system

The EORTC (European Organization for Research and Treatment of Cancer) Study Group on Quality of Life has developed a family of questionnaires to measure the HRQOL of cancer patients participating in clinical trials.[81,112] The EORTC approach includes a core instrument (QLQ-C30) that addresses issues relevant to all cancer patients and supplemental modules specific to various types of cancer or tumor location.[113] To date, 11 disease-specific modules have been developed. Several additional modules are under development, including a "Palliative Care" module that is in the preliminary stages of investigation.

FACT/FACIT system

Cella and colleagues developed the FACT/FACIT family of instruments based on the original FACT (Functional Assessment of Cancer Therapy).[24,114] They are known as the "FACIT family of instruments," and they assess the HRQOL of people living with chronic and life limiting illnesses. Although there is not a FACT module specific for EOL research, using the FACT in patients with terminal illnesses and in palliative care settings has been considered.[44]

Discussion

An ideal measurement tool for HRQOL assessment at EOL needs to consider the interaction of the four domains (physical, psychological, social, and spiritual).[23,26,28,115,116] There has been significant debate as to the appropriateness of EOL-specific HRQOL instruments compared to generic measures that can be used across disease stages and medical conditions.[116,117] In addition, researchers have spent enormous time debating the advantages and disadvantages of a single instrument versus a battery of tools that measure various domains of the HRQOL construct.[8] Another unresolved issue is the role of quantitative measures in a terminally ill population, for whom qualitative measures are more commonly applied. Despite these pending concerns, many experts agree that HRQOL assessment can play a vital role in EOL care and may help improve the quality of care for the terminally ill. Future studies of HRQOL and EOL need to address the specific methodological challenges of research at EOL, as well as assess HRQOL fully, rather than focusing exclusively on symptoms.

Moving away from narrow symptom focus

As previously noted, in recent years, there has been increased attention on HRQOL at EOL. As a result, there has been more interest in conducting research in this area. Contributing factors to the current emphasis on EOL include financial considerations by Medicare and various health care institutions and growing public attention to death and dying. Further, recent events related to physician-assisted suicide and federal legislation on EOL care have heightened the public's interest in palliative care,[75,118] issues related to patient and family participation in treatment decision making, and death. Moreover, professional organizations such as the American Society for Clinical Oncology and the American Cancer Society, as well as academic institutions, have examined various treatment outcomes for EOL.[3,18,119]

This new focus raises interesting questions about "endpoints" in EOL care, not only in terms of defining outcomes, but also regarding whom to assess and what items to measure. In the palliative care arena, most "outcomes research" has been conducted with family members after the death of the one for whom they cared.[26] Staff member interviews after death have yielded further subjective information. However, this research has been primarily aimed at determining "success" regarding palliation of specific symptoms, rather than providing a comprehensive view of the HRQOL and care of the terminally ill patients and their families. Recently, there has been a movement to consider the goals and outcomes of the care received as death approaches as determined by terminally ill patients themselves. This research may add an additional dimension to the understanding of what is important to consider when assessing HRQOL at EOL.

For years, the endpoints used in outcomes research have been focused on the goals and objectives of cancer care and on factors directly influenced by clinicians, rather than on other aspects of an individual's life, such as life satisfaction and sense of well-being. This is well illustrated in the surgery literature, where much of the outcomes research has been aimed at symptom resolution.[6]

As King and Hinds[8] note, even research that has included HRQOL endpoints has been linked directly to physical health-related outcomes. Historically in HRQOL research, subjective factors such as well-being were not necessarily considered health related unless they were linked to disease and treatment issues.[8] However, many researchers would argue that HRQOL is much more comprehensive, involving many interrelated personal and environmental factors going well beyond mere symptom improvement. A global approach to HRQOL assessment is particularly relevant in terminally ill populations, where the outcomes are much more complex, personal, and dynamic. Endpoints should include the subjective impression of the terminally ill person and his/her family across the multiple domains that are relevant.

While many instruments demonstrate strong psychometric properties (as reviewed earlier), they may have questionable content validity across the spectrum of HRQOL dimensions important at EOL. While the intent of the HRQOL instruments is parsimony, this brevity should not be at the expense of comprehensiveness and accuracy. Important symptoms, not only physical but also social, psychological, and spiritual, should be assessed. For instance, many of the instruments reviewed have few or no items that assess the spiritual domain. The instruments that do mention spirituality may not necessarily have adequate coverage to evaluate unique EOL concerns. In addition, several instruments focus heavily on specific physical symptoms. However, they may not focus enough on the most relevant symptoms, or may not address functional ability. For instance, the ESAS and MSAS essentially assess specific symptoms rather than comprehensive domains; in a sense, they are symptom checklists. Although they do form a composite view of a person's physical and emotional state with regard to HRQOL, they do not provide a global integrated assessment. The MVQOLI, the McGill QOL Questionnaire, and the COH-QOLS offer a comprehensive assessment of the four critical domains important to HRQOL at EOL. The Brief Hospice Inventory (BHI) provides a quick assessment of how physical symptoms affect the psychological

domain of HRQOL, but does not address spiritual or social issues. Nonetheless, the advantage of the BHI is that it has been validated for both self-report as well as for caregiver completion. The FACT and EORTC are excellent, well-validated tools, but they have been used primarily in clinical trials of curative treatment. The disease-specific modules that have been developed for certain cancer types may be advantageous for assessing the subtleties and unique HRQOL aspects of these cancers, but these modules (to date) do not provide the best evaluation of overall HRQOL at EOL.

Methodological considerations in EOL research

There are several important methodological considerations in EOL research, as discussed now.

Subject burden

The majority of current HRQOL instruments require patient stamina, fairly intact cognitive function, and adequate reading ability.[23] Recently, recognition of the respondent burden associated with such measures has led to the development of instruments that are more amenable to the vulnerable physical and cognitive states of terminally ill patients.[23,44,106,116,120] Also, some instruments not originally designed for EOL populations have been adapted to take into consideration the waning physical ability of seriously or terminally ill patients. The BHI, FACT, McGill QOL Questionnaire, and COH-QOLS are especially useful in frail populations.[24,28,44,80,85,106] Other tools, such as the ESAS and MSAS, present a brief checklist of symptoms rather than a comprehensive assessment.[99,105,116]

Institutional review boards and family members may feel that research in patients at the end of life presents undue burden on a vulnerable population, and they may also view such research as invading a private, emotional time and taking away from the limited time remaining. Additionally, constantly changing symptoms, leading to decreased physical functioning, can make assessment of HRQOL at EOL complicated. Investigators assert the need for quantitative research to develop standardized instruments that meet stringent psychometric criteria. However, at EOL, the clinical environment and patient characteristics, in addition to family dynamics and availability, make collection of data to validate such questionnaires very difficult.

Some researchers involve family members in gathering information, but that approach can add to the burden on caregivers. Both the BHI and the COH-QOLS have used family members effectively to assist with instrument completion. Nonetheless, subject burden presents an important barrier and may have precluded much of the research in EOL care. To move forward, funding agencies and reviewers need to consider the implications of respondent burden for research methods and designs that are appropriate in this field and to be open to innovative methodologies, including qualitative studies. Alternative approaches may be needed for the research to be viewed as meaningful to terminally ill patients and their families and for it to reflect their perspectives accurately.

Longitudinal designs

One of the greatest challenges in EOL research is conducting longitudinal studies. In a population at the EOL, this methodological concern is particularly noteworthy given attrition rates and the need to measure significant outcomes accurately. Attrition in a terminally ill population is often unpredictable, given the difficulty of determining the nature and course of dynamic symptoms coupled with the rapidity of disease progression. Increased symptoms, and approaching death, often render the patient unable to engage in formal assessments and interventions.[7,60,121]

While missing data due to morbidity and mortality occurs in many research settings, in this population, the reality of imminent death must be considered when developing the design, selecting the measurement instruments, and planning the analysis. This limitation may discourage some researchers from investigating the population at EOL. At the same time, it provides the potential for new statistical approaches and research designs.

Much recent longitudinal literature has involved family members. Initial data may be collected when the patients enter the terminal stage, then the outcome measures are reported by family members after the death of their loved one, and the study may continue through the bereavement period.[77,122–124] In fact, this trend has seemed to characterize EOL research in recent years.[5,7,26,36,47] However, the posthumous approach makes validation of the interventions, as well as the assessment, difficult. For instance, one could argue that assessment of intervention and outcome can be affected by the emotional poignancy associated with losing a loved one, as well as recall bias. These factors can substantially interfere with objective evaluation and veracity. Research has demonstrated that a negative situation coupled with strong emotional attachment can produce unfavorable recall, especially with regard to pain.[125–127]

The relevance of bias in assessments conducted after the patient's death is supported by studies in the hospice literature. Specifically, family members who have experienced the death of a loved one who had inadequate symptom management report negatively on the patient's treatment and care.[26,36,122,128,129] These family members also have increased psychological distress and prolonged and complicated bereavement. Thus, family member responses to posthumous questions regarding their loved one's death may present some reporting bias, and the degree of bias may be reflective of the extent to which the family members recall (and perceive) the patient's HRQOL at the end of life. For example, if the dying patient did have unsatisfactory care, leading to a deficit in HRQOL compared to what might have been – and if the family sees and reports that – they may be more likely to have negative recollection and subsequently overstate a deficit in HRQOL at EOL.

More research is needed into how to collect important intervention and treatment outcomes data without subjecting the patient to undue hardship and without requiring the family caregiver to disengage emotionally for the sake of objectivity. In addition, researchers planning a study at EOL need to consider carefully the design, measures, and methods used to capture the patient's perspective.

Barriers to EOL research

The limited number of reliable instruments specifically designed for terminally ill patients and the previous low level of public investment in EOL research have posed major barriers to advancing the research agenda in this population. While there is literature that provides insight into symptoms experienced at the EOL, there is very little information about the particular dying experiences, and overall HRQOL, experienced by the patient and their family. This lack of information hinders progress, and advancement cannot occur to any great extent without further investigation. Perhaps the recent increase in awareness and interest in EOL research will help address this barrier.

HRQOL in health services research at EOL

Cleeland[7] articulates the unique characteristics of HRQOL outcomes in health services research in EOL care versus such HRQOL investigation in chronic conditions generally. While HRQOL research is fairly advanced in other areas of medicine and has contributed significantly to clinical trials, there are important distinctions that must be considered in designing studies and defining outcomes in EOL research.

Qualitative versus quantitative methods

In EOL studies, patients report their symptoms, including pain, fatigue, bowel management, and other complications, and these are often recorded in a quantitative fashion. However, other domains of HRQOL may not always be able to be objectively measured, despite the penchant of researchers to develop quantitative measures and report findings numerically. Pursuing completely "objective" evaluations, such as with standardized, validated instruments, would be difficult and in some cases unwise in this population, given the intensely personal nature of death and dying. Moreover, quantitative assessment may make it difficult to define clinically relevant outcomes as determined by the patient.

Qualitative techniques, on the other hand, have been shown to be particularly valuable in identifying patient themes, and this method has seemed to be far less taxing to the patient and the caregiver.[8] While there may appear to be a chasm between qualitative and quantitative research methods, their use can be complementary, especially when the emphasis is on defining what is important, meaningful, and subjectively determined to be a successful outcome to the individual in light of the impending death.

Extensive work in qualitative research has found it to be highly effective in terms of revealing important themes, particularly at the EOL.[36,115] These qualitative findings have paved the way for inclusion of such elements into quantitative research and have also served to validate further the four key domains in HRQOL at EOL. Combining qualitative and quantitative techniques is a viable option and can be used to advance research with the dying. Moreover, qualitative analysis can shed light on the content validity of instruments designed for quantitative assessment.

Role for HRQOL outcomes in palliative care research

Assessment of HRQOL at EOL has an important role, but further methodological development is required to improve the state of the science. There is an important need to incorporate HRQOL outcomes in pain and symptom research to broaden the scope of understanding and to provide a more comprehensive perspective on care of the dying.[1,5,130] Cleeland[7] clearly defines the areas for further research in EOL and how these are interrelated naturally.

Notably, Cleeland draws the example of investigation and training conducted in cancer pain management as a model for research and evaluation in other areas of EOL care. For instance, he asserts that studies of the prevalence, severity, and treatment of pain, through descriptive research, can set a precedent for studying other areas of symptom management and EOL care. In essence, the prevalence and severity of various symptoms in patients throughout the disease course, particularly near the end of life, need to be carefully identified and studied. This includes the behavioral, economic, and social impact of the symptoms. He notes that there is an urgent need to learn more about how care for advanced disease is reimbursed. Moreover, Cleeland highlights that it is important to include longitudinal designs in such investigation so that changes in symptom patterns over time can be determined. In addition, clinicians and researchers need to identify the adequacy of care for the symptoms, including the identification of what factors are predictive of poor symptom management and poor EOL care, including the interrelationship between patient, clinician, and system factors. Cleeland notes the following specific areas of investigation: pain, anorexia and cachexia, cognitive failure (delirium, temporary or permanent cognitive impairment), dyspnea, fatigue, gastrointestinal symptoms (such as nausea and vomiting), psychiatric, and affective symptoms (including anxiety and depression). These areas should be included in any investigation of HRQOL and outcomes.

Importantly, Cleeland asserts that the same reasons for inadequate EOL care can apply to management of pain and other symptoms and can partially explain the dearth and challenges of research in this field. He notes that inadequately trained health care providers, low priority for this type of care, lack of patient demand for better care, and negative sanctions against aggressive pain management add to the complexity of advancing the research agenda in EOL care.[7] Heightening the awareness of these issues in the public domain, coupled with enhanced training and incentives for research in EOL care, may spawn a new era for increasing funding and investigation in this important area of life.

In addition, there is increasing emphasis on the importance of communication between health care providers and patients/families, as well as between patients/families and the health care system at EOL. There have been important improvements in training for physicians on how to communicate bad news about terminal illness and prognosis, but evidence of the impact of this improved communication on HRQOL is scant.[3,131]

Another area that should incorporate HRQOL measures is research on grief. There is a substantial literature on grief and bereavement, aside from the implications for overall HRQOL.[132,133] Some of these analyses offer insight into the dynamic and intense need of caregivers after the death of their loved one. However, there is limited information regarding how grief and bereavement affect HRQOL.

The 2001 NCPB report repeatedly asserts the importance of HRQOL in many dimensions of cancer care, with the underlying theme of how those domains and such care affect health systems and costs.[1] In other areas of medicine, outcomes studies grew out of the need for cost containment and quality improvement. The high costs of unmanaged pain and symptoms to communities and the health care system are well documented.[4,40,130,134] Information about HRQOL outcomes can shed additional light on the human costs of providing EOL care. These data can and should support outcomes research to improve the quality and abate the costs of end-of-life care, as well as to increase satisfaction among patients, caregivers, and health care providers.

REFERENCES

1 Foley, K. M., Gelband, H. (ed.) (2001). *Institute of Medicine and National Research Council: Improving Palliative Care for Cancer Summary and Recommendations*. Washington, DC: National Academy Press.

2 World Health Organization Division of Mental Health (1993). *WHO-QOL Study Protocol: The Development of the World Health Organization Quality of Life Assessment Instrument (MNG/PSF/93.9)*. Geneva, Switzerland: World Health Organization.

3 American Society of Clinical Oncology (1996). Outcomes of cancer treatment for technology assessment and cancer treatment guidelines. *Journal of Clinical Oncology* **14**: 671–9.

4 Franks, P. J., Salisbury, C., Bosanquet, N. *et al.* (2000). The level of need for palliative care: a systematic review of the literature. *Palliative Medicine* **14**(2):93–104.

5 Holland, J. C., Chertkov, L. (2001). Clinical practice guidelines for the management of psychosocial and physical symptoms of cancer. In *Institute of Medicine and National Research Council: Improving Palliative Care for Cancer Summary and Recommendations*, ed. K. M. Foley, H. Gelband, pp. 7-1–7-60. Washington, DC: National Academy Press.

6 McCahill, L., Ferrell, B. R., Virani, R. (2001). Improving cancer care at the end of life. *Lancet Oncology* **2**:103–8.

7 Cleeland, C. S. (2001). Cross-cutting research issues: a research agenda for reducing distress of patients with cancer. In *Institute of Medicine and National Research Council: Improving Palliative Care for Cancer Summary and Recommendations*, ed. K. M. Foley, H. Gelband, pp. 8-1–8-85. Washington, DC: National Academy Press.

8 King, C. R., Hinds, P. S. (1998). *Quality of Life from Nursing and Patient Perspectives: Theory, Research, Practice.* Sudbury, MA: Jones and Bartlett Publishers, Inc.

9 Breitbart, W., Payne, D. K. (1998). Pain. In *Psycho-Oncology*, ed. J. C. Holland, pp. 450–67. New York: Oxford University Press.

10 Cherny, N. (1998). Cancer pain: principles of assessment and syndromes. In *Principles and Practice of Supportive Oncology*, ed. A. Berger, R. K. Portenoy, D. E. Weissman, pp. 3–43. Philadelphia, PA: Lippincott-Raven Publishers.

11 Dean, G. E., Anderson, P. A. (2001). Fatigue. In *Textbook of Palliative Nursing*, ed. B. R. Ferrell, N. Coyle, pp. 91–100. New York: Oxford University Press.

12 Greenberg, D. B. (1998). Fatigue. In *Psycho-Oncology*, ed. J. C. Holland, pp. 485–93. New York: Oxford University Press.

13 Portenoy, R. K. (2000). Physical symptom management in the terminally ill. In *Handbook of Psychiatry in Palliative Medicine*, ed. H. M. Chochinov, W. Breitbart, pp. 99–129. New York: Oxford University Press.

14 Portenoy, R. K., Itri, L. M. (1999). Cancer-related fatigue: guidelines for evaluation and management. *Oncologist* **4**: 1–10.

15 Portenoy, R. K., Lesage, P. (1999). Management of cancer pain. *Lancet* **353**(9165):1695–700.

16 Berger, A. M., Portenoy, R. K., Weissman, D. E. (1998). *Principles and Practice of Supportive Oncology.* Philadelphia, PA: Lippincott-Raven Publishers.

17 Doyle, D., Hanks, G. W. C., MacDonald, E. (Ed.) (1998). *Oxford Textbook of Palliative Medicine*, (2nd edition). New York: Oxford University Press.

18 National Comprehensive Cancer Network and American Cancer Society (NCCN/ACS) (2001). *Patient Guidelines for the Treatment of Cancer Pain.* Atlanta, GA: American Cancer Society.

19 American Pain Society (APS) Quality Care Committee (1998). Quality improvement guidelines for the treatment of acute pain and cancer pain. *Journal of the American Medical Association* **274**:1874–80.

20 World Health Organization (1986). *Cancer Pain Relief.* Geneva, Switzerland: World Health Organization.

21 World Health Organization (1996). *Report of the WHO Expert Committee on Cancer Pain Relief and Active Supportive Care: Cancer Pain Relief with a Guide to Opioid Availability. Technical Series 804, 2nd edition.* Geneva: World Health Organization.

22 World Health Organization (1998). *Symptom Relief in Terminal Illness.* Geneva, Switzerland: World Health Organization.

23 Cella, D. F. (1998). Quality of life. In *Psycho-Oncology*, ed. J. C. Holland, pp. 1135–46. New York: Oxford University Press.

24 Cella, D. F., Tulsky, D. S., Gray, G. *et al.* (1993). The Functional Assessment of Cancer Therapy Scale: development and validation of the general measure. *Journal of Clinical Oncology* **11**:570–9.

25 Ferrell, B. R. (1996). Pain: how patients and families pay the price. In *Pain Treatment Centers at a Crossroads: A Practical and Conceptual Reappraisal. Progress in Pain Management, Vol. 7*, ed. M. J. M. Cohen, J. N. Campbell, pp. 229–37. Seattle, WA: International Association for the Study of Pain.

26 Ferrell, B. R. (1998). The family. In *Oxford Textbook of Palliative Medicine* (2nd edition), ed. D. Doyle, G. W. C. Hanks, N. MacDonald, pp. 909–17. New York: Oxford University Press.

27 Ferrell, B. R., Borneman, T. (1999). Pain and suffering at the end of life (EOL) for older patients and their families. *Generations* **XXIII**(1):12–17.

28 Ferrell, B. R., Wisdom, C., Schneider, C. (1989). Quality of life as an outcome variable in the management of cancer pain. *Cancer* **63**:2321–7.

29 Holland, J. C. (ed.) (1998). *Psycho-Oncology.* New York: Oxford University Press.

30 Die-Trill, M. (1998). The patient from a different culture. In *Psycho-Oncology*, ed. J. C. Holland, pp. 857–66. New York: Oxford University Press.

31 Die-Trill, M., Holland, J. C. (1993). Cross-cultural differences in the care of patients with cancer: A review. *General Hospital Psychiatry* **15**:21–30.

32 Payne, R. (2000). At the end of life, color still divides. *The Washington Post*, February 15, p. 15.

33 Morris, J. N., Mor, V., Goldberg, R. J., Sherwood, S., Greer, D. S., Hiris, J. (1986). The effect of treatment setting and patient characteristics on pain in terminal cancer patients: a report of the national hospice study. *Journal of Chronic Diseases* **39**(1):27–35.

34 Morris, J. N., Suissa, S., Sherwood, S., Wright, S. M., Gree, D. (1986). Last days: a study of the quality of life of terminally ill cancer patients. *Journal of Chronic Diseases* **39**(1):47–62.

35 Davies, B. (2001). Supporting families in palliative care. In *Textbook of Palliative Nursing*, ed. B. R. Ferrell, N. Coyle, pp. 363–73. New York: Oxford University Press.

36 Ferrell, B. R. (2001). Pain observed: the experience of pain from the family caregiver's perspective. *Clinics in Geriatric Medicine* **17**(3):595–609.

37 Ferrell, B. R., Rivera, L. M. (1995). Cancer pain: impact on elderly patients and their family caregivers. In *Chronic Pain in Old Age: An Integrated Biopsychosocial Perspective*, ed. R. Roy. Toronto: University of Toronto Press.

38 Ferrell, B. R., Rivera, L. M. (1997). Cancer pain education for patients. *Seminars in Oncology Nursing* **13**(1):42–8.

39 Emanuel, E. J., Fairclough, D. L., Slutsman, J., Emanuel, L. L. (2000). Understanding economic and other burdens of terminal illness: the experience of patients and their caregivers. *Annals of Internal Medicine* **132**(6):451–9.

40 Levine, C. (Ed.) (2000). *Always on Call: When Illness Turns Families into Caregivers*. New York: United Hospital Fund of New York.

41 O'Connell, L. J. (1996). Changing the culture of dying. A new awakening of spirituality in America heightens sensitivity to the needs of dying persons. *Health Progress* **77**(6):6–20.

42 Steinhauser, K. E., Christakis, N. A., Clipp, E. C., McNeilly, M., McIntyre, L., Tulsky, J. A. (2000). Factors considered important at the end of life by patients, family, physicians, and other care providers. *Journal of the American Medical Association* **284**(19):2476–82.

43 Snyder, this volume, Chapter 16, pp. 329–345.

44 Cella, D. F. (1995). Measuring quality of life in palliative care. *Seminars in Oncology* **22**(2 Suppl. 3):73–8.

45 Breitbart, W., Jaramillo, J. R., Chochinov, H. M. (1998). Palliative and terminal care. *Psycho-Oncology*, ed. J. C. Holland, pp. 437–49. New York: Oxford University Press.

46 Curt, G. A. (2000). Impact of fatigue on quality of life in oncology patients. *Seminars in Hematology* **37**(4 Suppl. l6):14–17.

47 Ferrell, B. R., Coyle, N. (2001). *Textbook of Palliative Nursing*. New York: Oxford University Press.

48 Breitbart, W. C., Cohen, K. R. (1998). Delirium. In *Psycho-Oncology*, ed. J. C. Holland, pp. 564–75. New York: Oxford University Press.

49 Bruera, E., Franco, J. J., Maltoni, M., Watanabe, S., and Suarez-Almazor, M. (1995). Changing pattern of agitated impaired mental status in patients with advanced cancer: association with cognitive monitoring, hydration, and opioid rotation. *Journal of Pain and Symptom Management* **10**:287–91.

50 Bruera, E., Miller, L., McCallion, J. *et al.* (1992). Cognitive failure in patients with terminal cancer: a prospective study. *Journal of Pain and Symptom Management* **7**(4):192–5.

51 Bruera, E., Neumann, C. M. (1998). Management of specific symptom complexes in patients receiving palliative care. *Canadian Medical Association Journal* **158**:1717–26.

52 Chochinov, H. M., Breitbart, W. (Ed.) (2000). *Handbook of Psychiatry in Palliative Medicine*. New York: Oxford University Press.

53 Walch, S. E., Ahles, T. A., Saykin, A. J. (1998). Neuropsychological impact of cancer and cancer treatment. In *Psycho-Oncology*, ed. J. C. Holland, pp. 500–8. New York: Oxford University Press.

54 Breitbart, W. C., Wein, S. E. (1998). *Metabolic Disorders and Neuropsychiatric Symptoms*. In *Psycho-Oncology*, ed. J. C. Holland, pp. 639–52. New York: Oxford University Press.

55 Passik, S. D., Breitbart, W. (1993). Psychiatric and psychological approaches to cancer pain. In *Management of Cancer Pain*, ed. E. Arbit, pp. 151–77. Mount Kisko, NY: Futura Publishing Company.

56 Pereira, J., Hanson, J., Bruera, E. (1997). The frequency and clinical course of cognitive impairment in patients with terminal cancer. *Cancer* **69**:835–41.

57 Ferrell, B. R., Grant, M., Rhiner, M., Padilla, G. V. (1992). Home care: maintaining quality of life for patient and family. *Oncology* **6**(2):136–40.

58 Ferrell, B. R., Grant, M., Chan, J., Ahn, C., Ferrell, B. A. (1995). The impact of cancer pain education on family caregivers of elderly patients. *Oncology Nursing Forum* **22**(8):1211–18.

59 Fox, B. H. (1998). Psychosocial factors in cancer incidence and prognosis. In *Psycho-Oncology*, ed. J. C. Holland, pp. 110–24. New York: Oxford University Press.

60 Gavrin, J., Chapman, C. R. (1995). Clinical management of dying patients. *Western Journal of Medicine* **163**(3):268–77.

61 Zabora, J., Brintzenhofeszoc, K., Curbow, B., Hooker, C., Piantadosa, S. (2001). The prevalence of psychological distress by cancer site. *Psycho-Oncology* **10**:9–28.

62 Zabora, J. R., Loscalzo, M. J. (1996). Comprehensive psychosocial programs: a prospective model of care. *Oncology Issues* **1**:14–18.

63 Benson, H. (1984). *Beyond the Relaxation Response*. New York: Times Books.

64 Benson, H. (1996). *Timeless Healing: The Power of Biology and Belief*. New York: Simon and Schuster.

65 Jenkins, R. A., Pargament, K. I. (1995). Religion and spirituality as resources for coping with cancer. *Journal of Psychosocial Oncology* **13** (1/2):51–74.

66 Johnston-Taylor, E. (2001). *Spiritual Care: Nursing Theory, Research, and Practice*. Upper Saddle River, NJ: Prentice Hall.

67 Larson, D. B., Greenwold-Molano, M. A. (1995). Are religion and spirituality clinically relevant in health care? *Mind/Body Medicine* **1**:147–57.

68 Matthews, D. A., Larson, D. B. (1995). *The Faith Factor: An Annotated Bibliography of Clinical Research on Spiritual Subjects, Volume 3*. Bethesda, MD: National Institute for Healthcare Management.

69 Koenig, H., Idler, E., Kasl, S. *et al.* (1999). Religion, spirituality, and medicine: a rebuttal to skeptics. *International Journal of Psychiatry in Medicine* **29**(2):123–31.

70 Pargament, K. A. (1997). *The Psychology of Religion and Coping*. New York: Guilford Press.

71 Johnston-Taylor, E. (2001). Spiritual Assessment. In *Textbook of Palliative Nursing*, ed. B. R. Ferrell, N. Coyle, pp. 397–406. New York: Oxford University Press.

72 Kemp, C. (2001). Spiritual Care Interventions. In *Textbook of Palliative Nursing*, ed. B. R. Ferrell, N. Coyle, pp. 407–14. New York: Oxford University Press.

73 Wenzl, C. (2001). The role of the nurse chaplain: a personal reflection. In *Textbook of Palliative Nursing*, ed. B. R. Ferrell, N. Coyle, pp. 425–34. New York: Oxford University Press.

74 Borneman, T., Brown-Slatzman, K. (2001). Meaning in illness. In *Textbook of Palliative Nursing*, ed. B. R. Ferrell, N. Coyle, pp. 415–24. New York: Oxford University Press.

75 Lynn, J. (2001). Serving patients who may die soon and their families: The role of hospice and other services. *Journal of the American Medical Association* **285**(7):925–32.

76 Field, M. J., Cassel, C. K. (Ed.) (1997). *Approaching Death: Improving Care at the End of Life*. Washington, DC: National Academy Press.

77 Lynn, J., Teno, J. M., Phillips, R. S. *et al.* (1997). Perceptions by family members of the dying experience of older and seriously ill patients. *Annals of Internal Medicine* **126**: 97–106.

78 Teno, J. (2000). *Toolkit of Instruments to Measure End of Life Care*. http://www.chcr.brown.edu/pcoc/. Last accessed on September 11, 2004.

79 Teno, J. (2001). Quality of care and quality indicators for end-of-life cancer care: hope for the best, yet prepare for the worst. In *Improving Palliative Care for Cancer: Summary and Recommendations*, ed. K. M. Foley and H. Gelband, pp. 3-1–3-49. Washington, DC: National Academy Press.

80 Guo, H., Fine, P. G., Mendoza, T. R., Cleeland, C. S. (2001). A preliminary study of the utility of the brief hospice inventory. *Journal of Pain and Symptom Management* **22**(2): 637–48.

81 Aaronson, N. K., Ahmedzai, S., Bergman, B. *et al.* (1993). The European Organization for Research and Treatment of Cancer QLQ-C30: a quality-of-life instrument for use in international clinical trials in oncology. *Journal of the National Cancer Institute* **85**:365–76.

82 Ferrans, C. E., Powers, M. J. (1985). Quality of Life Index: development and psychometric properties. *Advances in Nursing Science* **8**:5–24.

83 Finkelstein, D. M., Cassileth, B. R., Bonomi, P. D. *et al.* (1988). A pilot study of the functional living index-cancer (FLIC) scale for the assessment of quality of life for metastatic lung cancer patients. *American Journal of Clinical Oncology* **11**:630–3.

84 McMillan, S. C. (1996). Quality of life in hospice patients. *Oncology Nursing Forum* **22**:1401–9.

85 Cohen, S. R., Mount, B. M., Bruera, E. *et al.* (1997). Validity of the McGill Quality of Life Questionnaire in the palliative care setting: a multi-centre Canadian study demonstrating the importance of the existential domain. *Palliative Medicine* **11**:3–20.

86 Cohen, S. R., Mount, B. M., Strobel, M. G. *et al.* (1995). The McGill Quality of Life Questionnaire: a measure of quality of life appropriate for people with advanced disease. A preliminary study of validity and acceptability. *Palliative Medicine* **9**:207–19.

87 Ware, J. E., Sherbourne, C. D. (1992). The MOS 36-item short form health survey (SF-36): conceptual framework and item selection. *Medical Care* **30**(6):473–83.

88 Byock, I. R. (1995). *Missoula-VITAS Quality of Life Index: Version-25S*. Missoula, MT: VITAS Healthcare Corporation.

89 Byock, I., Merriman, M. P. (1998). Measuring quality of life for patients with terminal illness: the Missoula VITAS quality of life index. *Palliative Medicine* **12**:231–44.

90 Greer, D. S., Mor, V., Sherwood, S. *et al.* (1984). *National Hospice Study Final Report*. Providence, RI: Brown University.

91 Padilla, G. V., Presant, G., Grant, M. M. *et al.* (1983). Quality of life index for patients with cancer. *Research Nursing in Health* **6**:117–26.

92 Andresen, E. M., Rothenberg, B. M., Kaplan, R. M. (1998). Performance of a self-administered mailed version of the Quality of Well-Being (QWB-SA) questionnaire among older adults. *Medical Care* **36**:1349–60.

93 Bergner, M., Bobbitt, R., Carter, W. B., Gilson, B. S. (1981). The Sickness Impact Profile: development and final revision of a health status measure. *Medical Care* **19**(8):787–805.

94 Moinpour, C. M., Hutchinson, F., Hayden, K. *et al.* (1990). Quality of life assessment in Southwest Oncology Group trials. *Oncology* (*Huntington*) **4**:79–93.

95 Spitzer, W. O., Dobson, A. J., Hall, J. *et al.* (1981). Measuring the quality of life of cancer patients: a concise QL-index for use by physicians. *Journal of Chronic Diseases* **34**:585–97.

96 Erickson, this volume, Chapter 3.

97 Feeny, this volume, Chapter 4.

98 O'Boyle, C. A., Waldron, D. (1997). Quality of life issues in palliative medicine. *Journal of Neurology* **244** (Suppl. 4): S18–25.

99 Portenoy, R. K., Thaler, H. T., Kornblith, A. B. *et al.* (1994). The Memorial Symptom Assessment Scale: an instrument for the evaluation of symptom prevalence, characteristics, and distress. *European Journal of Cancer* **30A**:1326–36.

100 Cohen, S. R., Mount, B. M., Tomas, J. N., Mount, L. F. (1996). Existential well-being is an important determinant of quality of life. Evidence from the McGill Quality of Life Questionnaire. *Cancer* **77**:576–86.

101 O'Connor, A. P., Wicker, C. A., Germino, B. B. (1990). Understanding the cancer patient's search for meaning. *Cancer Nursing* **13**:167–75.

102 Reed, P. G. (1987). Spirituality and well being in terminally ill hospitalized adults. *Research Nursing in Health* **10**:335–44.

103 Yalom, I. D. (1980). *Existential Psychotherapy*. New York: Basic Books.

104 Tierney, R. M., Horton, S. M., Hannan, T. J., Tierney, W. M. (1998). Relationships between symptom relief, quality of life, and satisfaction with hospice care. *Palliative Medicine* **12**:333–44.

105 Bruera, E., Kuehn, N., Miller, M. J. *et al.* (1991). The Edmonton Symptom Assessment System (ESAS): A simple method for the assessment of palliative care patients. *Journal of Palliative Care* **7**:6–9.

106 Ferrell, B. R., Grant, M., Padilla, G., Vemuri, S., Rhiner, M. (1991). The experience of pain and perceptions of quality of life: validation of a conceptual model. *The Hospice Journal* **7**(3):9–24.

107 Ferrell, B. R., Dow, K. H., Grant, M. (1995). Measurement of the quality of life in cancer survivors. *Quality of Life Research* **4**:523–31.

108 Juarez, G., Ferrell, B. R., Borneman, T. (1998a). Influence of culture on cancer pain management in Hispanic patients (Part I). *Cancer Practice* **6**(Part 5):262.

109 Juarez, G., Ferrell, B. R., Borneman, T. (1998b). Perceptions of quality of life in Hispanic patients (Part II). *Cancer Practice* **6**(Part 6):318.

110 Seidman, A. D., Portenoy, R. K., Yao, T. J. *et al.* (1995). Quality of life in phase II trials: a study of methodology and predictive value in patients with advanced breast cancer treated with paclitaxel plus granulocyte colony-stimulating factor. *Journal of the National Cancer Institute* **87**:1316–22.

111 Ingham, J. M., Seidman, A., Yao, T.-J. *et al.* (1996). The importance of frequent pain measurement in a cancer clinical trial: a lesson for quality of life assessment. *Quality of Life Research* **5**:503–7.

112 Osoba, D., Zee, B., Pater, J. *et al.* (1994). Psychometric properties and responsiveness of the EORTC Quality of Life Questionnaire (QLQ-C30) in patients with breast, ovarian and lung cancer. *Quality of Life Research* **3**:353–64.

113 Osoba, D., Aaronson, N., Zee, B. *et al.* (1997). Modification of the EORTC QLQ-C30 (version 2.0) based on content validity and reliability testing in large samples of patients with cancer. The Study on Quality of Life of the EORTC and the Symptom Control and Quality of Life Committees of the NCI of Canada Clinical Trials Group. *Quality of Life Research* **6**:103–8.

114 Cella, D. F., Tulsky, D. S. (1990). Measuring quality of life today: Methodological aspects. *Oncology* **4**(5):29–38.

115 Ferrell, B. R. (1995). The impact of pain on quality of life: a decade of research. *Nursing Clinics of North America* **30**(4):609–24.

116 Spilker, B. (1996). *Quality of Life and Pharmacoeconomics in Clinical Trials* (2nd Edition). New York: Raven Press.

117 Frank-Stromborg, M., Olsen, S. J. (1997). *Instruments for Clinical Health-Care Research* (2nd Edition). Sudbury, MA: Jones and Bartlett Publishers.

118 Lynn, J., O'Mara, A. (2001). Reliable, high-quality, efficient end-of-life care for cancer patients: economic issues and barriers. In *Improving Palliative Care for Cancer: Summary and Recommendations,* ed. K. M. Foley, H. Gelband, pp. 2-1–2-45. Washington, DC: National Academy Press.

119 Holland, J. C. (1999). NCCN practice guidelines for the management of psychosocial distress. *Oncology* **13**(5A):113–47.

120 Cella, D. F., Bonimi, A. E. (1996). The Functional Assessment of Cancer Therapy (FACT) and Functional Assessment of HIV Infection (FAHI) quality of life measurement systems. In *Quality of Life and Pharmacoeconomics in Clinical Trials* (2nd Edition), ed. B. Spilker, pp. 203–14. New York: Raven Press.

121 Casarett, D., Ferrell, B. R., Kirschling, J. *et al.* (2001). NHPCO Task Force on Ethics of Hospice Participation in Research. *Journal of Palliative Medicine* **4**(4):441–9.

122 Baer, W. L., Hanson, J. C. (2000). Families perception of the added value of hospice in the nursing home. *Journal of American Geriatric Society* **48**(8):879–82.

123 McCorkle, R., Robinson, L., Nuameh, I., Lev, E., Benoliel, J. Q. (1998). The effects of home nursing care for patients during terminal illness on the bereaved's psychological distress. *Nursing Research* **47**(1):2–10.

124 Payne, S., Smith, P., Dean, S. (1999). Identifying the concerns of informal carers in palliative care. *Palliative Medicine* **13**(1):37–44.

125 Eich, E., Reeves, J. L., Jaeger, B., Graff-Radford, S. B. (1985). Memory for pain: relation between past and present intensity. *Pain* **23**:375–9.

126 Eich, E., Reeves, J. L., Katz, R. L. (1985). Anesthesia, amnesia, and the memory/awareness distinction. *Anesthesia and Analgesia* **64**:1143–8.

127 Jamison, R. N., Reeves, J. L., Salovey, P., Pearson, R. (1990). Symposium on pain memory: clinical and cognitive issues. *Proceedings of the Ninth Annual Meeting of the American Pain Society* **1**:1.

128 Aucoin-Gallant, G. (1999). Description of caregiver's educational needs and the degree of their dissatisfaction. *Canadian Oncology Nursing* **9**(4):165–7, 170–4.

129 Hickman, S. E., Tilden, V. P., Tolle, S. W. (2001). Family reports of dying patients' distress: the adaptation of a research tool to assess global symptom distress in the last week of life. *Journal of Pain and Symptom Management* **22**(1):565–74.

130 Ferrell, B. R., Grant, M. (2001). Nursing research. In *Textbook of Palliative Nursing*, ed. B. R. Ferrell, N. Coyle, pp. 701–12. New York: Oxford University Press.

131 American Medical Association (1998). *EPEC: Educating Physicians in End of Life Care*. Chicago, IL: American Medical Association.

132 Loscalzo, M. (1996). Psychological approaches to the management of pain in patients with advanced cancer. *Hematology/Oncology Clinics of North America* **10**(1):139–55.

133 Loscalzo, M., Jacobsen, P. B. (1990). Practical behavioral approaches to effective management of pain and distress. *Journal of Psychosocial Oncology* **8**(2/3):139–69.

134 Grant, M., Ferrell, B. R., Rivera, L., Lee, J. (1995). Unscheduled readmissions for uncontrolled symptoms: a health care challenge for nurses. *Nursing Clinics of North America* **30**(4):673–82.

135 Eischens, M. J., Elliott, B. A., Elliott, T. E. (1998). Two hospice quality of life surveys: a comparison. *American Journal of Hospice and Palliative Care* **15**(3):143–8.

136 Chang, V. T., Hwang, S. S., Feuerman, M. (2000). Validation of the Edmonton Symptom Assessment Scale. *Cancer* **88**(9):2164–71.

137 Chang, V. T., Hwang, S. S., Feuerman, M., Kasimis, B. S., Thaler, H. T. (2000). The Memorial Symptom Assessment Scale Short Form (MSAS-SF): reliability and validity. *Cancer* **89**(5):1163–71.

138 Collins, J. J., Devine, T. D., Dick, G. S. *et al.* (2002). The measurement of symptoms on young children with cancer. The validation of the Memorial Symptom Assessment Scale in children aged 7–12. *Journal of Pain and Symptom Management* **23**(1):10–16.

*   The author wishes to acknowledge the assistance of Barbara Hastie, Ph.D., in the preparation of this chapter.

13

Patient advocate perspective on health-related quality of life issues with prostate cancer survivors

(Col. Ret.) James E. Williams, Jr.

Intercultural Cancer Council, Camp Hill, PA

"Survivorship is the experience of living with, through or beyond cancer"[1]

Introduction

In the past 20 years, the use of prostate-specific antigen (PSA) testing to diagnose prostate cancer, and improved techniques for treating the disease, have resulted in a dramatic rise in the long-term survival rate of prostate cancer patients. Oncologists have focused on the narrow goal of shrinking (or removing) the tumor to increase the survival of cancer patients.[2] However, from the survivors' perspective, preserving health-related quality of life (HRQOL) is the most important consideration, even more than extending life and delaying the progression of disease.[3] It is important to keep in mind that prostate cancer is not just a disease with associated medical treatment. Beginning at the time of diagnosis and extending through treatment and beyond, survivors experience physical, emotional, and social impacts.

The purpose of this chapter is to provide the perspective of a prostate cancer survivor, based on my almost 11 years of activities as an advocate, activist, and facilitator who has observed survivors and their families in support group activities in local, regional, and national venues. The chapter tells the story, from the patient's perspective, of what it means to be a cancer survivor and the role HRQOL plays in the life of a survivor.

HRQOL from the survivor's perspective

A review of the literature reveals that, when surveyed about their HRQOL, most survivors and their clinicians focus on the physical symptoms and limitations imposed by cancer and its treatments.[4] For the most part, questionnaires examine organic dysfunction, e.g., the mechanics of an erection and urinary continence. There is considerable diversity in the methods being employed to measure outcomes, including both qualitative and quantitative studies. Given the differences between study methodologies, it is not surprising that reported quality of life varies. This inconsistency makes it difficult to draw firm conclusions about the magnitude and nature of the long-term consequences of prostate cancer for survivors.

Clearly, more data about all aspects of quality of life are needed to provide a more comprehensive and complete perspective on the needs of long-term cancer survivors. The full HRQOL effects include emotional responses and social interactions, as well as the physical impacts that accompany the course of the disease. For prostate cancer survivors, HRQOL concerns begin at the "Moment of Terror" when prostate cancer is diagnosed, and extend until the end of life. Each phase in the survivorship continuum is accompanied by different HRQOL considerations.

Diagnosis

The diagnosis of prostate cancer is particularly stressful. Men experience great anxiety and fear, as well as concern about deeply personal aspects of their manhood (e.g., sexuality). Sexuality includes the sexual response cycle that consists of four phases: desire, arousal, orgasm, and resolution,[5] and men may have concerns about any of these phases. The diagnosis period is a time of emotional immobilization for many men. They may find it very difficult to talk about what they are facing and the feelings that they are experiencing. Regardless of differences in sexual attitudes, practices, and preferences, a person has a lifetime need for intimacy, affection, social interaction, and touch.[6]

Treatment

The active treatment phase of care is an important time when there should be open communication between patients and their physicians. Many survivors claim they were active in the treatment decision process (this is what men are supposed to do). However, these men bring little knowledge of their condition to the health system, and they tend to depend heavily on their mates, health care providers, and the "word on the street" concerning their treatment options. Many men have been infrequent participants in health care decision-making up to this time, and depend heavily on others for information, coordination, and support concerning their health.

Despite the very common side effects that accompany prostate cancer and its treatments, many prostate cancer patients do not discuss with their physicians how treatment might affect their quality of life. For many men, HRQOL may be just as important as survival.[7]

Frequently, survivors claim their doctor did not fully discuss the potential side effects of treatment and, in many cases, they thought they were told that side effect issues were secondary to the cancer and would be discussed in detail after treatment completion. Further, prior to treatment, health professionals rarely pose in-depth questions to patients about their views of the importance of incontinence and impotence for their quality of life, and how these side effects may affect treatment choices. The main emphasis in these encounters is getting rid of the cancer; all other aspects of care can wait. Many feel they were rushed into a treatment decision. At the same time it must be acknowledged that these same men also admit to having a high degree of anxiety and to wanting the cancer removed as soon as possible.

Long-term survivorship

The long-term HRQOL impacts on prostate cancer survivors are of increasing importance as the number of survivors increases and the length of the survivorship period grows. Prior to the introduction of the PSA test, prostate cancer was an "old man disease." Life expectancy for many survivors was less than 10 years, and many men were diagnosed with metastatic disease. Today, that is no longer the case. In particular, the "younger" survivors (under age 55) attending support group meetings with their mates have tremendous anxiety and frustration in attempting to determine which treatments to pursue, or what they should do now that the side effects have set in after completion of a treatment protocol.

Currently, many men claim that little or no psychological support is given after treatment. So what do they do: "suck it up" like good boys and move on. The results of this strategy cause major depression in many, and great strain on the survivor's relationship with his mate, family, and friends.

In addition, although many survivors state publicly that they continue to enjoy life and feel hopeful about the future, my one-on-one discussions with them reflect a different attitude. It is not uncommon to learn that they have restless sleep all or most of the time, have trouble with depression, are concerned about the lack of a sex drive, and wonder when their cancer will return. However, when asked if they have discussed these matters with a physician, the answer is usually no. Open lines of communication between survivor and doctor are essential but, in many cases, do not exist. The perception in the survivor world is that there is little opportunity to address emotional and psychological well-being with their doctors. As a result, many men seek out support groups because, in their minds, this is the only environment available to them to express their concerns openly. One survivor said, "I needed to find someone immediately who knew my terror: someone I could talk with on a personal – rather than on a clinical level; someone who had been there – I needed to find a survivor."[8]

Potential contributions of HRQOL assessment

There appears to be a great void in the medical community regarding efforts to meet the needs of survivors of prostate cancer. Systematic assessment of HRQOL could help facilitate communication between patients and physicians regarding the implications of prostate cancer and its treatment.

However, in many cases, the HRQOL assessment tools used are introduced late or not at all in the treatment process. The "you don't ask – I won't tell" game begins early in the diagnosis process and is reinforced throughout the survivor's medical journey. When and if HRQOL assessment is introduced in the process, a communication pattern has been established in which little information is exchanged. Thus, ways to integrate these tools into the treatment *decision* process need to be explored. Involving other health professionals (e.g., psychologists, psychiatrists, marriage counselors) in the treatment team could help ensure that a holistic approach is used in the treatment process. These health professionals, in cooperation with the treating physicians, could assist in assessing HRQOL and in addressing deficits when found.

Recommendations

Based on my personal experience as a prostate cancer survivor and my interactions with other prostate cancer survivors and their mates through support groups, I have developed several recommendations about how HRQOL and other methods can be used to improve the quality of care.

First, there is a need to consider the individual's preferences when planning treatment. When making treatment decisions, men with prostate cancer may have different perspectives on the potential trade-offs between quantity and quality and may choose longer life over quality of life, or vice versa.

Second, there is a need to develop better measures of HRQOL for use in follow-up studies of survivors. The validity and reliability of these HRQOL instruments should be evaluated for different population groups, including different age groups, racial and ethnic groups, income levels, education levels, and occupations.

In particular, assessing HRQOL in men may pose specific challenges. The observation that, "men are from Mars and women are from Venus" correctly reflects that men and women are "emotionally" different. Thus, the assessment and interpretation of HRQOL must be approached differently in men and women. For example, most HRQOL instruments in use today were developed for the purpose of group comparisons (e.g., patients on one treatment compared to patients on another treatment). Many men are intimidated by a regimen of tests given by health professionals in white coats in a group environment in a hospital setting. This venue is not conducive to obtaining unbiased psychosocial information. Hence, the assessment of HRQOL in men with prostate cancer should be more individualized and personalized.

Third, because HRQOL issues will vary as men travel across the continuum of care, ongoing assessment is needed. HRQOL assessment should be incorporated into standard medical practice across the trajectory of care – from prevention through diagnosis to end of life. Further, changes in HRQOL should be assessed as men move from diagnosis, to treatment, to survivorship. Creating practice standards for follow-up visits after treatment that include assessment of both physical and mental well-being will help ensure that men's HRQOL concerns are addressed.

Fourth, there needs to be a recognition of the impact of prostate cancer on the men's mates and families. Their HRQOL should be assessed as well – to measure the impact on them and to help address deficits when found. This recommendation surely applies to virtually all other types of cancer as well.

Fifth, the need to create informed consumers is also very important. Funding is needed to improve patient education on the various aspects of prostate cancer care that are likely to influence HRQOL, including symptom management, psychosocial, legal, and practical issues.

Sixth, improving HRQOL hinges on providing adequate support services. Survivor support groups should be included in the mix of resources provided from diagnosis and across the continuum of care. While some health professionals believe prostate cancer support groups provide little or no quality supportive services, many men and their families give more credibility to peer counseling than to their health care providers. Closer liaison is necessary between prostate cancer support groups and health professionals. As an example, breast cancer peer counseling and breast cancer support groups are currently much better integrated into breast cancer care than is the case for prostate cancer.

Finally, studies that seek to measure the impact of prostate cancer should include control groups of age-matched men who do not have the disease and should assess the impact over time. This strategy will help control for changes that are due to age and not to the disease.

None of the above recommendations will be effective unless government health care programs and private insurers eliminate barriers to and ensure adequate funding for HRQOL assessments. The HRQOL tools must be incorporated into the total health care package from the day of the initial office visit to the primary care physician to the end of life.

REFERENCES

1 Leigh, S. (1996). Defining our destiny. In *Cancer Survivor's Almanac: Charting the Journey*, ed. B. A. Hoffman, pp. 261–71. Minneapolis, MN: Chronimed Publishing.

2 Schneider, M. (2002). Quality of life (Editorial). *CancerFutures*, March 2002, p. 1.

3 Leitman, R. (1995). Perspectives on prostate cancer treatments, awareness, attitudes and relationships. In *A Study of Patients and Urologists*, p. 3. Lewis Harris and Associates, July 31–August 17, 1995.

4 Zebrack, B. (2000). How you can achieve quality of life after a cancer diagnosis. *Coping*, March/April 2000, p.13.

5 Hughes, M. K. (1997). Sexuality issues of the cancer survivor. *Coping*, March/April: 51.

6 Hughes, M. K. (1996). Sexuality issues: keeping your cook. *Oncology Nursing Forum* **23** (10):1595–600.

7 D'Amico, A. V., Whittington, R., Malkowicz, S. B. *et al.* (1998). Biochemical outcome after radical prostatectomy, external beam radiation therapy, or interstitial radiation therapy for clinically localized prostate cancer. *Journal of the American Medical Association* **280** (11):969–74.

8 Leigh, S. A., Williams, J. E., Jr., Stoval, E. (1998). Survivorship: from the moment of diagnosis. *Cancer* **83** (Suppl. 8): 1710–13.

14

Measuring the patient's perspective on the interpersonal aspects of cancer care

Charles Darby

Agency for Healthcare Research and Quality, Rockville, MD

Introduction

This chapter provides a critical review of the literature on patient reports and evaluations of interpersonal aspects of cancer care as indicators of the quality of cancer care, which we will call "the patient's perspective." The rationale for placing the patient at the center of efforts to assess the quality of health care is well established: policy makers, health care providers, purchasers of care, and researchers are interested in what patients think. For example, the National Health Care Quality Report, to be published in 2003, will include the consumer's perspective as a key indicator of health care quality.[1]

Donabedian stated that "achieving and producing health and satisfaction, as defined for its individual members by a particular society or subculture is the ultimate validator of the quality of care." He saw that the patient's greatest contribution to measuring health care quality is assessing the interpersonal aspects of care.[2]

The specific justifications for the interest in the patient's perspective have changed somewhat over time. Originally, they were based on evidence that patients who are satisfied are more likely to comply with treatment regimens, provide relevant information to the health care provider, and return for care.[3–7] Thus, measuring the patient's perspective, particularly satisfaction, may be important to the health care provider from the standpoint of keeping the patient as a customer, because satisfied patients are more likely to stay with their doctors.[8] Patients who changed doctors say that the doctor's style and personality were the main reasons.[9] Health care practices use patient satisfaction data to choose between alternative methods of organizing and providing care, e.g., length of consulting arrangements for out-of-hours care.[10] In a survey of internists, 86% agreed that cancer patient judgments are important in assessing the quality of care, particularly for changing specific physician behaviors.[8]

Beyond improved processes and outcomes of care, consideration of the patient's perspective has gained an importance of its own. While some[11] have argued that information based on measures of satisfaction may merely reflect health gains because of the correlation between satisfaction and health care processes and outcomes, other researchers have asserted that patients play a role in defining what constitutes quality care by determining the values that should be associated with different outcomes.[9] Measuring the patient's perspective has become a major component of health care plan and provider accreditation systems, such as the National Committee for Quality Assurance (NCQA). The World Health Organization's recent World Health Report includes a measure of the patient's perspective, which it refers to as responsiveness, as a discrete component in its framework for assessing the performance of health systems of countries around the world.[12]

The growing interest in the patient's perspective led the National Cancer Institute (NCI) to include a critical evaluation of approaches for assessing the patient's perspective in its Cancer Outcomes

Measurement Working Group (COMWG) initiative, whose report is the basis for this book. We first consider areas where the patient's perspective is apt to be informative.

Patient perspective and categories of health care quality

When studying quality of care issues, it is useful to group the aspects of care into two main categories: technical and interpersonal. According to Donabedian, technical care is the application of the science and technology of medicine and the other health sciences to the management of a personal health problem, while interpersonal aspects of health care are the psychosocial components of the interaction between the health care provider and the patient. Interpersonal care also involves the interaction between the patient/consumer and the health care system, which is necessary to arrange for and receive care.[2]

In evaluating the quality of care in both its technical and interpersonal aspects, patients have been a source of information and assessment. Patients are seen as a source of information on technical care in situations where gaining access to medical records is costly, or when patients may have more up-to-date or accurate information. For example, whether a patient received a mammogram during a given period may be more accurately obtained from the patient as she may receive the mammogram from a number of different facilities. A check of a patient's medical record maintained by her health care provider may miss a mammogram given at a mobile mammography van at her workplace.

As this area of investigation has progressed, more emphasis has been placed on patient reports and evaluations of the interpersonal aspects of care. While patients are unlikely to have enough knowledge to assess many technical aspects of clinical care, they may be the best or, in some instances, the only source of information for interpersonal aspects of care. Research has generally focused on formal health care services, but the same approach could be applied to informal health care services, as long as these fit the definition of interpersonal aspects of care.

Such perspectives may be assessed through different kinds of questions. For example, health survey researchers may ask patients to *report* on the experience with care and/or to *evaluate* the care.

The *report* task asks patients to describe the interpersonal aspects of their care. For example, a respondent might be asked, "In the last 12 months, how often did doctors, nurses, or other health care providers explain things in a way you could understand? Would you say never, sometimes, usually, or always?" The *evaluation* task asks patients to consider the care they received and then give an opinion regarding its quality. Patient evaluations may take the form of *ratings* of the care received or expressions of *satisfaction* with care. For example, a *ratings* question is, "In the last 12 months, how would you rate doctors, nurses, and other health providers on how well they explained things to you in a way you could understand?" Responses could be indicated on a numerical (e.g., 0–10) or verbal (e.g., very good, good, bad, very bad) scale. *Satisfaction* could be measured by asking, "In the last 12 months, how satisfied were you with how well doctors, nurses, or other health care providers explained things in a way you could understand? Would you say very dissatisfied, dissatisfied, satisfied, or very satisfied?"

Both reports and evaluations of care rely on patient surveys; therefore, they are influenced by the patient's perception of the events that took place during the care experience. Getting a report or evaluation of care that is independent of the patient's perception is difficult or impossible. One could ask an expert in interpersonal aspects of care to observe a patient's health care experience and report on what occurred and then to evaluate what occurred. One approach involves a systematic analysis of the communication between the medical provider and patient. Known as "interaction analysis," this system seeks to quantify and explain the important elements of communication and considers both "task focused" and "socio-emotional" aspects of communication.[13] Regardless of the approach used, a better understanding of this communication is important given its influence on outcomes of care.[14]

Both reports and evaluation items are important to measuring the patient's perspective on the quality of care. Report items can be used to infer the quality of the interpersonal aspects of care from the distribution of responses across the never, sometimes, usually, and always response options. Properly constructed, the report item is made personal for the patient. For example, the patient is asked how often the doctor or nurse explained things *in a way she or he could understand*. Thus, patients with different levels of ability to understand can report on the quality of communication using a common framework. Ratings items ask the respondent for a direct evaluation of quality of care, e.g., was it good or poor. Satisfaction items ask for an evaluation in terms of how satisfied the respondent is with the care.

This chapter evaluates the published literature on both patient reports and evaluations of cancer care.

Methods

We explored issues surrounding the measurement of the perspectives of patients and their families on the quality of health care. We also identified surveys that might offer potential items, item sets, or entire questionnaires from which to develop a set of measures of these perspectives applicable to cancer care in particular. The focus of this chapter is on the patient's perspective, not to suggest that the perspective of family members regarding the quality of care is not important but, rather, because our literature review identified little work done on the family member's perspective. However, a series of instruments measuring the family member's perspective is summarized in Table 14.1 (along with other instruments).

Searches were conducted of the scientific literature from 1980–2002 in MEDLINE, PsychLit, and CINAHL. The search terms used were "patient satisfaction," "cancer," "instruments," "surveys,"
"questionnaires," "measures," and "scales." The search was not limited to studies of the four major cancer sites (breast, colorectal, lung, prostate) because instruments that relate to the measurement of patient and family perspectives in other cancers and diseases and general health care might prove useful. We sought articles to address all phases of the continuum of cancer care: prevention/screening, treatment, survivorship, and end of life. Articles that addressed topics reflected in the search terms, included a survey instrument, or addressed research directly relevant to surveying patients about their care were selected. A large number of articles were eliminated because they dealt with patients' reports of their quality of life or their satisfaction with their quality of life.

We also drew on personal knowledge of the Consumer Assessment of Health Plans (CAHPS®) survey, which was sponsored by the Agency for Healthcare Research and Quality (AHRQ) to provide consumers and purchasers with reliable and valid information to assess and choose among health plans.

Instruments found in the literature were abstracted using a standard template, which included the elements specified by NCI and additional elements added by the author.

Results of instrument review

A total of 90 survey instruments or families of instruments used to survey patients or their families about health care experiences in general, or about cancer care in particular, were identified. Not all articles reviewed included a survey instrument, e.g., some addressed the measurement of the patient's perspective in general. A number of characteristics were used to assess these instruments, including domains, response options, reliability, validity, sensitivity, reference period, cultural and language comparability, continuum of care, sites, and whether measures are general or cancer specific. A brief summary of the results is presented below. More detailed information on each instrument is presented in Table 14.1.

Table 14.1. Patient perspective questionnaires

Instrument name	FAMCARE Scale; F-Care Perceptions Scale; F-Care Expectations Scale[63]	Princess Margaret Hospital Patients Satisfaction with Doctor Questionnaire (PMH/PSQ-MD)[8]
Purpose for which developed	Measure family satisfaction with palliative care (3 questionnaires used in conjunction)	Measure patient satisfaction with physician
Length	FAMCARE Scale – 20 items; F-Care Perceptions Scale – 20 items; F-Care Expectations Scale – 16 items	41 items
Administration time	40 minutes	10 minutes
Domains included	Information giving; availability of care; psychological and physical care	Information exchange; interpersonal skills; quality of time; overall satisfaction
Response options and scoring	Very satisfied to very dissatisfied	Strongly agree, agree, disagree, strong/strongly disagree, does not apply
Validated modes of administration	Self-administered	Self-administered
Validated translations/cultural adaptations	NA	NA
Evidence of reliability (internal consistency, test-retest, other)	FAMCARE Scale: Internal consistency = 0.90–0.95; test-retest 0.91; F-Care Perceptions Scale: Internal consistency 0.86–0.90; F-Care Expectations Scale: Internal consistency = 0.88–0.95	Internal consistency (instrument) = 0.97; Domains = 0.88–0.92
Evidence of validity (content, construct, criterion-related)	NA	Correlation with similar measures = 0.005–0.86
Instrument name	**Worthington Chemotherapy Satisfaction Questionnaire (WCSQ)[64,65]**	**Comprehensive Assessment of Satisfaction with Care Questionnaire (CASC)[66,67]**
Purpose for which developed	Satisfaction with chemotherapy	Measure cancer patient's perception of quality of medical and nursing care
Length	47 items	61 items
Administration time	NA	20 minutes
Domains included	Accessibility; interpersonal aspects of care; technical aspects of care; patient information; multi-disciplinary team work; overall satisfaction	Technical quality; interpersonal communication skills; coordination of care; waiting time; continuity/availability of care; access; physical environment
Response options and scoring	Twenty-seven satisfaction items, using either Visual Analogue Scale (VAS) or a 5 point adjectival scale (low satisfaction – high satisfaction). Six "interpersonal nursing care" items assessed by VAS. Global satisfaction using 5 point adjectival scale (low satisfaction – high satisfaction). Overall satisfaction assessed by the single global item and by a composite score. Mean for items in each six composites calculated (1 = low satisfaction – 5 = high satisfaction). Minimum score = 6; maximum score = 30	Most of items rating on 5 point poor-excellent scale. Items evaluating patient wish for improvement use yes/no options manner

(cont.)

Table 14.1. (*cont.*)

Validated modes of administration	Self-administered	Self-administered
Validated translations/cultural adaptations	NA	French and Italian
Evidence of reliability (internal consistency, test–retest, other)	Internal consistency = 0.71–0.92	Internal consistency = 0.71–0.95
Evidence of validity (content, construct, criterion-related)	NA	NA
Instrument name	**Mammography Questionnaire**[68]	**Medical Care Attitude Scale (MCAS) – Versions for patient (MCAS – p), caretaker (MCAS – c), and post-bereavement (MCAS – b)**[29]
Purpose for which developed	Measure patient satisfaction with mammography services	Attitudes towards the medical care of chronically and terminally ill patient and their families
Length	24 items	42 items
Administration time	10 minutes	NA
Domains included	Convenience/accessibility and physical surroundings; staff's interpersonal skills; staff's perceived technical competence; physical and psychological discomfort; general satisfaction now; expected satisfaction later	Availability of care; continuity of care; physician availability; physician competence; personal qualities of physician; communication with physician; preference for home care; preference for patient and family involvement in treatment decisions; freedom from pain; pain control
Response options and scoring	5 point agree – disagree; Pain measured on 10 point vertically printed scale. Items summed and transcribed to 0 (least satisfied/most pain) to 100 (most satisfied/no pain)	Five point scale strongly agree (1) – strongly disagree (5)
Validated modes of administration	Self-administered	Interviewer administered
Validated translations/cultural adaptations	Norwegian	NA
Evidence of reliability (internal consistency, test-retest, other)	Internal consistency > than 0.5 for all dimensions, except structure; Test/Retest = 92%–97% of cases in 95% confidence interval	MCAS – p and MCAS – b by in person interview; MCAS – c self administered Internal consistency for patients 0.10–0.75. For caretakers 0.50–0.85
Evidence of Validity (content, construct, criterion-related)	Construct validity: There were differences in scale scores between groups that were expected to differ Convergent validity: All but 7 items correlated higher with own dimension than with other dimensions	Discriminant validity acceptable only for certain scales

Table 14.1. (*cont.*)

Instrument name	Picker Survey[61,62]	CAHPS Survey[28,56,69,70]
Purpose for which developed	Measure patient experience with hospital care	Measure consumers reports and ratings of health care experience
Length	3 questionnaires varying in length from 37–41 items	46 core items
Administration time	NA	20 minutes
Domains included	Information and education; emotional support; access; coordination of care	Patient – health provider communication; getting needed care; getting care quickly; interpersonal aspects of office staff
Response options and scoring	Yes/no; 5 point poor-excellent; yes, always – no; not at all organized – very organized; yes, completely–no	Never – always; no problem – big problem; 0–10. Composite scores on domains using equal weights on items
Validated modes of administration	Self-administered	Self-administered and telephone interview
Validated translations/cultural adaptations	NA	Spanish
Evidence of reliability (internal consistency, test-retest, other)	Internal consistency = 0.92–0.94	Internal consistency = 0.51–0.86 Health plan reliability = 0.82–0.96
Evidence of validity (content, construct, criterion-related)	NA	Correlation of global rating and willingness to recommend health plan = 0.75

Technical aspects of the questionnaires and surveys

Domains

Investigators agree that the patient's perspective on care includes multiple domains.[10,15–17] Patients can distinguish different components of care (e.g., provider communication and access) and may rate or report them differentially. They may be satisfied overall, but may be critical on selected domains.[18,19]

Weighting the importance of domains

To arrive at composites or global measures of the patient's perspective, it may be necessary to employ weights for the separate domains. Several approaches can be used, including strictly quantitative methods that take into account the contribution to variance of each composite to the overall score as well as methods that assess the importance of domains by survey respondents or some normative group.[20,21] Earlier work depended largely on health care practitioners indicating what was important to ask patients about their care.[22]

Only limited research specific to cancer patients has been reported. More research is needed on cancer patients' assessments of care because theirs may differ from those given by health care providers or patients with other diseases. Studies have shown that, compared to medical staff, cancer patients place greater emphasis on expressive or humanitarian aspects of care, as well as on specific instrumental aspects of care, such as staff being able to minimize the side effects of treatment. Several studies found that respondents did not easily distinguish between ranking the importance of the domains and rating their experience with them.[23–25] However, Gustafson and his colleagues have had success using critical incident and person-focused interviews to identify what is important to patients.[26] There is a need to study this area further, possibly using cognitive interviewing techniques, to understand better how respondents see these two tasks.

Response options

A variety of response option sets were used in the studies reviewed. These included visual analogue scale; scales with various verbal descriptors (e.g., strongly agree to strongly disagree; very satisfied to very dissatisfied; adjectival options; poor to excellent); scales with various numeric options (e.g., between 5 and 11 points) and dichotomous items (e.g., yes/no); and scales with varying frequency options (e.g., never-always). Ware and Hays found that the "poor-excellent" response set showed more response variability, and also was a better predictor of whether patients intended to return to the doctor in the future, would recommend the doctor to a friend, and would comply with medication. The scale was less skewed than the "very satisfied to very dissatisfied" scale.[27]

Investigators in the CAHPS project focused on development of reports and rating items and used cognitive testing extensively. In developing the survey instruments, they had difficulty with the "poor to excellent" scale, especially with its interpretation in Spanish. They chose a 0–10 response scale for ratings instead.[28]

The CAHPS surveys include a number of report items and a few overall rating items. Most of the CAHPS report items use the "never-always" response set. Cognitive testing showed respondents handled this form quite well.[28]

Reliability and validity

Most instruments reviewed were developed for use in only one or two research studies and not used again, serving just the narrow purpose of a particular study. These instruments were not pilot-tested and lacked reliability and validity data. Overall, of the studies reviewed to identify the 90 survey instruments, only 46% provided reliability data on the instruments and only 16% reported validity data.

Assessing sensitivity of measures

Very few studies assessed the ability of the instrument to detect differences between groups expected to differ, such as experimental and control groups. Since the ability of measures to distinguish among groups is of key importance, particularly in clinical trials, this issue needs further assessment.

Reference period

Surveys based on a single patient visit may miss changing views and expectations of people over time,[18] and any individual visit may be atypical.[28] In cancer care, each visit may be important in its own right, but this issue may not be as significant in other diseases. However, the reference period and use of measures over time require additional attention.

Respondents

Patients tend to report higher levels of patient satisfaction than family members do,[29] possibly because of different sets of priorities.[30] Development of separate items for patients and patients' families, and separate measures for patients and their families, are needed to address the family members' view of the patient's care and services provided to the family members.

Cultural and language differences

Assuring the comparability of measures of the patient perspective across cultures and language groups is an issue of growing concern.[31] Few of the surveys reviewed even acknowledged the issue, and little research has been conducted to assess the impact of these differences on survey results. (For a discussion of cross-cultural use of health-related quality of life assessments, see Chapter 20 by Aaronson in this volume.)[32]

Cancer specific versus general measures

It cannot be assumed that measures of the patient's perspective developed for evaluating either general health care or care for a disease other than cancer will be appropriate in cancer patients without carrying out cognitive and psychometric evaluation on samples of cancer patients. Even though some patient experiences may be common across many chronic illnesses (e.g., fatigue), the experience with treatment and organization of cancer care differs from that for other diseases. Also, cancer patients may have different needs and expectations about their care than patients with other chronic conditions.[8]

Continuum of care and cancer site

Careful consideration must be given to how well measures work across the continuum of care. Only with end-of-life care was this issue addressed to any extent in the literature. Components of survey instruments for end-of-life care are different than for general care. For example, caregivers more frequently are the respondents as patients are more likely to be too ill or confused to respond, and dying patients may refrain from criticizing providers because they are dependent upon them.[33]

It is apparent from our review that there are large gaps in the availability of any type of instrument for the four major cancer sites, but particularly in colorectal, lung, and prostate cancers. In terms of the continuum of care, there are few instruments for end-of-life care. In addition, there are few instruments for which family members are respondents. Few instruments specific to a site and continuum of care phase were available.

Challenges with patient evaluation measures

The literature addresses the difficulties in using patient *evaluations* for assessing health care quality; however, little research has been done on the degree to which patient *reports* on the quality of health care may share these same difficulties.

In looking at evaluations, investigators found that a patient's pre-treatment expectations, predispositions, and previous health care experiences may color her current perceptions of the quality of care. There is also a significant likelihood that ratings are differentially affected by patient characteristics and attributes that mediate (or filter) the respondent's evaluation of the events comprising the health care experience.

Influence of expectations, predispositions, and previous experiences

Most surveys designed to measure the patient's evaluation of care were developed without regard to any explicit underlying theory or conceptual framework.[34] When an effort has been made to explicate a framework, it has focused largely on the role that patients' expectations play in determining their evaluation of care.

However, a lack of clarity about the role of expectations continues to confuse the measurement and meaning of the results. The problem begins with the meaning of expectations. From an extensive literature review, de Silva identified four types of expectations:[35]

- Ideal – Aspirations, desires, preferred outcomes
- Predicted – Realistic, practical, anticipated outcomes
- Normative – Expectations that society sets as standards
- Unformed – No expectations can be assessed because a patient is unable or unwilling to express them.

Akao suggests a different configuration which includes "attractive needs," that is, expectations that people do not know they have. Therefore, individuals will not be dissatisfied if these unrecognized needs are not met.[36]

In a given study, investigators seldom define which of these types of expectations are being addressed. The variation in definitions is just the beginning of the complexity posed by the role of expectations. The theories that attempt to explain the influence of expectations on patient perspectives are many, varied, and sometimes contradictory.[11,30,34,35,37,38]

Given the varied definitions of expectations, it is probably not surprising that investigators disagree about whether expectations actually influence evaluation. Some investigators suggest that satisfaction is the degree to which expectations are met,[30,39–42] while others have found no evidence that the differences in satisfaction between patients could be explained reliably by differences in expectations and the degree to which they were met.[9,15,43–45] However, as there is little consistency in how expectations have been measured and studied, it is not clear whether the lack of consistent results is due to measurement problems or lack of influence of expectations.[9]

A related issue is the high levels of overall satisfaction with health care reported by patients. They report these high levels even when other measures indicate that the quality of care being rated is not high.[46, 47] A story about a patient who rated his satisfaction with care as "very high" might help to illustrate the point.

A patient, very worried by a family history of colon cancer, was referred to a clinic for a colonoscopy. After the procedure, he was sent home without first being told that the test had turned out positive. Assuming that he was all right, the patient felt relieved. Then, 10 days later his family doctor informed him of the positive test results. Later, when surveyed about his satisfaction with the clinic and the colonoscopy, he reported that he was "very satisfied" with the overall service, but "slightly dissatisfied" with the way the results were given.[48]

Global measures of patient satisfaction or ratings are most vulnerable to positive bias. Overall satisfaction and rating scores are generally so high that variance is restricted by a ceiling effect, which reduces the sensitivity of the measure for discovering differences between groups or changes over time.[16,49,50] When measures about specific aspects of quality of care are used, reported satisfaction levels are lower than with global measures.[51]

Investigators have offered a number of reasons to explain the high levels of satisfaction reported by patients:

- Patients' expectations are low, and they are satisfied when they focus on intent and effort of providers.[48,52]
- If patients have a negative experience, they may assume that the service being evaluated

was outside the health care provider's area of responsibility.[35,53]
- Patients take the blame if things do not work out.[18]
- Patients want doctors to like them, so they do not want to criticize them.[48]
- Patients need to justify the time and effort they have invested in treatment.[35]
- Patients are reluctant to express dissatisfaction and give socially desirable responses.[35]
- Patients may fear that they will get unfavorable treatment in the future if they complain or that the service might be discontinued.[35]
- Patients appreciate the interest shown in their satisfaction and that leads to a positive perception of the service.[35]

Patient characteristics that may influence evaluations

An individual's evaluation of the patient care experience may be mediated by her own life circumstances, as indexed by (and correlated with) such characteristics and attributes as education, income, age, gender, and race/ethnicity. This can raise difficult interpretive issues about the meaning, and thus validity and reliability, of these evaluations. For example, do poor people give higher ratings to their care because, over the years, their social and marketplace experiences have conditioned them to expect less? Questions of this type must be addressed if we are to determine the degree to which measured differences in the quality of the interpersonal aspects of health care are due to true differences in provider and system performance versus differences in (evaluation-affecting) attributes among the individuals doing the ratings.

The study of the relationship of satisfaction to sociodemographic variables has been characterized as "chaotic" because of contradictory results, possibly due to differences in the questions asked, timing, setting of care, and other factors.[9,54] Hall and Dornan[20] performed a meta-analysis of results from 110 patient satisfaction studies to assess the correlation between patient age, ethnicity, sex, social status, income, education, marital status, and family size, and patients' assessments of various aspects of medical care, including access, cost, overall quality of care, humanness of providers, competence of providers, bureaucracy, physical facilities, providers' attention to psychosocial problems, continuity of care, and outcomes of care. The overall conclusion was that sociodemographic variables are a minor predictor of patient satisfaction. The strongest correlation was with age; older people were more satisfied. Other weaker relationships showed persons who were married, had a higher social class (predominantly based on occupational status), or had less education were more satisfied with their care.[20] The CAHPS survey instruments, designed to measure consumers' reports and ratings of experience with health care providers and health plans, found older and less-educated persons evaluated their health plans and health care more positively, but also confirmed Hall and Dornan's findings that the amount of variance explained by these factors is small.[55] Hall and Dornan also concluded that self-reported health status is the strongest predictor of satisfaction,[20] and those with higher levels of self-reported health status are more satisfied. Their conclusions have been supported by the CAHPS survey.[55]

A patient's initial health status influences satisfaction with later medical care, such that a person with better initial health status experiences a greater positive change in satisfaction than someone in poorer health. This finding may stem from several factors. For example, doctors may react to sicker patients more negatively, leading to poor patient satisfaction. As well, patients in poor health may be generally less satisfied with other aspects of their lives, which may influence their satisfaction with their health care.[56] Persons who are emotionally sicker tend to be less satisfied with their care.[20]

Potential usefulness of patient reports

The preceding discussion illustrates many problems in relying solely on patient evaluation measures to represent patients' experience with care. However, the field of measurement of patients' perspectives on interpersonal aspects of health care has been evolving to address these shortcomings by including reports of the experience, as well as the evaluation, of care. The distinction between reports and evaluation has been discussed in the literature for some time.[17,45] Most recently, the CAHPS project team has developed surveys that include both reports on the experience of care, as well as some overall ratings of care. The project builds on the work done on patient satisfaction, while concentrating on a more direct approach to assessing quality.[57]

As described earlier, patient satisfaction items have generally tended to yield high levels of overall satisfaction with care that do not match with reports of experience or problems with care. There is some evidence that patients' reports reflect more negative assessments than do satisfaction items and may better reflect the actual care experience.[58]

Changes in the quality of health care perceived by patients may have direct effects on patient expectations. For example, if quality gets better, expectations may increase, resulting in little or no change in satisfaction even though quality has improved. The converse is also possible: lower quality may lead to lower expectations, with little to no change in satisfaction expressed by respondents, despite a change in quality of care. Report items, if less influenced by expectations, may more accurately reflect the changes taking place in quality of care.

Reports offer the potential to obtain data that are less influenced by respondent characteristics. Since reports and evaluations yield different information, the factors influencing them may be different. The investigation of the effects of respondent characteristics on reports and evaluations is in the early stages and has not demonstrated that these influences can be significantly reduced. However, the field is moving in this direction and shows promise.

There has been criticism of the reports approach, which has been sometimes referred to as "indirect measurement of patient satisfaction." It is argued that this type of indirect measurement blurs the distinction between satisfaction and its determinants, making the same items serve two purposes.[59] It is also argued that it is not possible to investigate the circumstances giving rise to satisfaction when measures of satisfaction employ items that also assess these circumstances.[60] Clearly, these issues require additional research. A first step is including measures of both reports and evaluations in both patients and family members in studies of cancer care. Such data will reflect what patients and family members experienced, as well as their evaluation of the experience.[51]

Recommended strategy

We recommend that:

- Surveys include both patient reports and ratings of care;
- To the degree possible, surveys include a subset of items that are common across cancer sites, the continuum of care, and type of respondent;
- Surveys selected as a starting point have strong scientific credentials and be adequately tested;
- Surveys selected have been widely used; and
- There be a mechanism established for the continued maintenance and expansion of the surveys.

The CAHPS project meets these requirements. The CAHPS surveys include a combination of reports and ratings, have a core set of items that are applicable across care settings, have been thoroughly tested, and have demonstrated high reliability and validity. The health plan version of CAHPS is accepted as the industry standard, and has been adopted by the National Committee for Quality Assurance (NCQA), the Centers for Medicare and Medicaid Services (CMS) and other Federal agencies. In 2002, data from CAHPS surveys were collected from health plans in which 120 000 000 Americans were enrolled. The CAHPS project is currently expanding the family of instruments to include measurement at the individual provider and hospital level. CAHPS is funded for an additional five years and provides a mechanism for continuing research and development on instruments for measuring the patient's perspective. AHRQ funds the ongoing maintenance and technical assistance for existing CAHPS surveys. The recommended strategy calls for drawing on the CAHPS approach, where feasible, for developing instruments that will

fill the gaps in measuring the patient's perspective on cancer care.

Content of questionnaires to measure patient perspectives

The CAHPS survey, with its common core set of items, is our recommended starting point for the development of a core set of items or domains for measuring the patient's perspective on cancer care. The majority of work has been done on measuring the patient's perspective on treatment, but less work has been done on measuring the patient's perspective on prevention, survivorship, and end-of-life care and the family member's perspective in all four phases of the continuum of care. Therefore, as measures are developed in these areas, work will begin at an earlier starting point.

When developing surveys in the areas of prevention, survivorship, end-of-life, and family member's perspective, it is recommended that development either begin. with surveys that possess attributes similar to those of the CAHPS surveys or that the development be guided by the same principles that were used in developing the CAHPS surveys. The goal is to provide surveys that include both patient reports and ratings that are scientifically sound and include a common core of items across cancer sites, the continuum of care, and type of respondent.

An initial starting point for a core set of items might include these domains:

- Communication/information giving
- Involvement in decision making
- Humanness (dignity, confidentiality, etc.)
- Getting needed care
- Continuity of care
- Rating(s) of care overall

Process for developing questionnaires to measure patient perspectives

Develop and refine domains

We recommend that qualitative research be initiated to help establish the domains and items deemed most important by patients and family members, and it is important that the research explore areas not previously included in satisfaction surveys. There has been recent success with critical incident and person-focused interviews to identify new areas of importance to patients and family members.[26]

Assemble and construct new items

New items will need to be developed to fill the gaps. As items are chosen and developed, we recommend that researchers utilize experience report items to ask about specific aspects of care and for overall rating of items.

Conduct cognitive testing

Cognitive testing may be the most important step in obtaining a thorough reading on how well respondents understand the items, particularly in areas where little testing has been done. Cognitive testing will allow exploration of the issues such as response sets, differences among respondents, continuum of care phases, and cancer sites, as well as language and cultural differences.

Conduct field testing

As part of field testing, it will be important to use a common reference period across cancer sites, care settings, and the continuum of care. The field testing will also provide the opportunity to evaluate the cultural and language comparability of instruments and to address issues such as mode effect and reports versus ratings. Field testing also needs to include evaluation of the sensitivity of the new measures.

Conduct longitudinal research

The collection of prospective assessments will allow us to study the dynamics that may change patients' and family members' reports and ratings over time, including an evaluation of the effect of changes such as in the patient's disease and symptom experience and length of relationship with the health care provider.

Conclusion

The field of assessing patient perspectives is entering a new paradigm. To date, much of the work has focused exclusively on patient ratings of satisfaction with their care, which are subject to considerable bias in self-report. New approaches, such as asking patients to report on the nature of what they have experienced during the care process, may provide valuable information and lead to improved cancer care.

REFERENCES

1 Agency for Healthcare Research and Quality National Healthcare Quality Report – Summary. Available at http://ahrq.gov/qual/nhqr03/nhqrsum03.htm. Last accessed on September 25, 2004.

2 Donabedian, A. (1966). Evaluating the quality of medical care. *Milbank Memorial Fund Quarterly: Health and Sociology* 4:166 .

3 Aharony, L., Strasser, S. (1993). Patient satisfaction: what we know about and what we still need to explore. *Medical Care Review* 50:49–79.

4 Borras, J. M., Sanchez-Hernandez, A., Navarro, M. *et al.* (2001). Compliance, satisfaction, and quality of life of patients with colorectal cancer receiving home chemotherapy or outpatient treatment: a randomized controlled trial. *British Medical Journal* 322:1–5.

5 Cassileth, B. R., Lusk, E. J., Walsh, W. P. *et al.* (1990). The satisfaction and psychosocial status of patients during treatment for cancer. *Journal of Psychosocial Oncology* 4: 47–57.

6 DiMatteo, M. R., Sherbourne, C. D., Hays, R. D. *et al.* (1993). Physicians' characteristics influence patients' adherence to medical treatment: results from the medical outcomes study. *Health Psychology* 12:93–102.

7 Gilson, L., Alilio, M., Heggenhougen, K. (1996). Community satisfaction with primary health care services: an evaluation undertaken in the Morogoro region of Tanzania. *Social Science and Medicine* 39:767–80.

8 Loblaw, D. A., Bezjak, A., Bunston, T. (1999). Development and testing of a visit-specific patient satisfaction questionnaire: the Princess Margaret Hospital satisfaction with doctor questionnaire. *Journal of Clinical Oncology* **17**: 1931–8.

9 Cleary, P. D., McNeil, B. J. (1988). Patient satisfaction as an indicator of quality care. *Inquiry* **25**:25–36.

10 Fitzpatrick, R. (1991). Surveys of patient satisfaction: I – Important general considerations. *British Medical Journal* **302**:887–9.

11 Haas, M. (1999). The relationship between expectations and satisfactions: a qualitative study of patients' experiences of surgery for gynecological cancer. *Blackwell Science Ltd* **2**: 51–60.

12 World Health Organization (2000). *The World Health Report 2000*. Geneva, Switzerland: World Health Organization.

13 Ong, L. M. L., de Haes, J. C. J. M., Hoos, A. M. *et al.* (1995). Doctor-patient communication: a review of the literature. *Social Science and Medicine* **40**:903–18.

14 Hall, J. A., Roter, D. L., Katz, N. R. (1988). Meta-analysis of correlates of provider behavior in medical encounters. *Medical Care* **26**:657.

15 Linder-Pelz, S., Struening, E. L. (1985). The multidimensionality of patient satisfaction with a clinic visit. *Journal of Community Health* **10**:42–54.

16 Sitzia, J., Wood, N. (1997). Patient satisfaction: a review of issues and concepts. *Social Science and Medicine* **45**: 1829–43.

17 Ware, J. E., Snyder, M. K., Wright, W. R. *et al.* (1983). Defining and measuring patient satisfaction with medical care. *Evaluation and Program Planning* **6**:247–63.

18 Avis, M., Bond, M., Arthur, A. (1997). Questioning patient satisfaction: an empirical investigation in two outpatient clinics. *Social Science and Medicine* **44**:85–92.

19 Williams, S. J., Calnan, M. (1991). Convergence and divergence: assessing criteria of consumer satisfaction across general practice, dental and hospital care settings. *Social Science and Medicine* **33**: 707–16.

20 Hall, J. A., Dornan, M. C. (1990). Patient sociodemographic characteristics as predictors of satisfaction with medical care: a meta-analysis. *Social Science and Medicine* **30**: 811–18.

21 Wiggers, J. H., Donovan, K. O., Redman, S. *et al.* (1990). Cancer patient satisfaction with care. *Cancer* **66**:610–16.

22 Cole, F. L., Mackey, T., Lindenberg, J. (1999). Quality improvement: psychometric evaluation of patient satisfaction with nurse practitioner care instrument. *Journal of the American Academy of Nurse Practitioners* **11**:471–5.

23 Widmark-Peterson, V., von Essen, L., Sjoden, P. O. (1998). Perceptions of caring: patients' and staff's association to CARE-Q behaviors. *Journal of Psychosocial Oncology* **16**:75–96.

24 Young, W. B., Minnick, A. F., Marcantonio, R. (1996). How wide is the gap in defining quality care? *Journal of Nursing Administration* **26**:15–20.

25 Attkisson, C. C., Roberts, R. E., Pascoe, G. C. (1983). The evaluation ranking scale: clarification of methodological and procedural issues. *Evaluation and Program Planning* **6**: 349–58.

26 Gustafson, D. H., Arora, N. J., Nelson, E. C., Boberg, E. W. (2001). Increasing understanding of patient needs during and after hospitalization. *Journal of Quality Improvement* **27**:81–92.

27 Ware, J. E., Hays, R. D. (1988). Methods for measuring patient satisfaction with specific medical encounters. *Medical Care* **26**:393–402.

28 Harris-Kojetin, L. D., Fowler, F. J., Brown, J. A. *et al.* (1999). The use of cognitive testing to develop and evaluate CAHPS 1.0 Core Survey items. *Medical Care* **37**: MS10–2.

29 McCusker, J. (1984). Development of scales to measure satisfaction and preferences regarding long-term and terminal care. *Medical Care* **22**:476–93.

30 Kristjanson, L. J., Leis, A., Koop, P. M. *et al.* (1997). Family members' care expectations, care perceptions, and satisfaction with advanced cancer care: results of a multi-site pilot study. *Journal of Palliative Care* **13**:5–13.

31 Hernandez, L., Chang, C. H., Cella, D. *et al.* (2000). Development and validation of the satisfaction with pharmacist scale. *Pharmacotherapy* **20**:837–43.

32 Aaronson, this volume, Chapter 20.

33 Fakhoury, W., McCarthy, M., Addington-Hall, J. (1996). Determinants of informal caregivers' satisfaction with services for dying cancer patients. *Social Science and Medicine* **42**:721–31.

34 Linder-Pelz, S. (1982). Toward a theory of patient satisfaction. *Social Science and Medicine* **16**:577–82.

35 de Silva, A. (2000). *A framework for measuring responsiveness. GPE Discussion Paper # 32*. Geneva, Switzerland: World Health Organization.

36 Gustafson, D. H., Otis-Taylor, J., Thompson, S. *et al.* (1993). Assessing the needs of breast cancer patients and their families. *Quality Management in Health Care* **2**:6–17.

37 Haas, M. (1999). A critique of patient satisfaction. *Health Information Management* **29**:9–13.

38 Linder-Pelz, S. (1982). Social psychological determinants of patient satisfaction: a test of five hypotheses. *Social Science and Medicine* **16**:583–9.

39 Knudtson, N. (2000). Patient satisfaction with nurse practitioner service in a rural setting. *Journal of the American Academy of Nurse Practitioners* **12**:405–12.

40 La Monica, E. L., Oberst, M. T., Madea, A. R. *et al.* (1986). Development of a patient satisfaction scale. *Research in Nursing and Health* **9**:43–50.

41 Miaskowski, C., Nichols, R., Brody, R. *et al.* (1994). Assessment of patient satisfaction utilizing the American Pain Society's quality assurance standards on acute and cancer-related pain. *U. S. Cancer Pain Relief Committee* **9**: 5–11.

42 McKinley, R. K., Roberts, C. (2001). Patient satisfaction with out of hours primary medical care. *Quality in Health Care* **10**:23–8.

43 Peck, B. M., Asch, D. A., Goold, S. D. *et al.* (2001). Measuring patient expectations: does the instrument affect satisfaction or expectations? *Medical Care* **39**:100–8.

44 Rogers, A., Saffron, K., Addington-Hall, J. (2000). 'All the services were excellent. It is when the human element comes in that things go wrong': Dissatisfaction with hospital care in the last year of life. *Journal of Advanced Nursing* **31**: 768–74.

45 Williams, B. (1994). Patient satisfaction: a valid concept? *Social Science and Medicine* **38**:509–16.

46 Thomas, L. H., Bond, S. (1996). Measuring patients' satisfaction with nursing: 1990–1994. *Journal of Advanced Nursing* **23**:747–56.

47 Oberst, M. (1984). Patients' perceptions of care: measurement of quality and satisfaction. *Cancer* **53**:2366–75.

48 Dougall, A., Russell, A., Rubin, G. *et al.* (2000). Rethinking patient satisfaction: patient experiences of an open access flexible sigmoidoscopy service. *Social Science* **50**: 53–63.

49 Grunfeld, E., Fitzpatrick, R., Mant, D. *et al.* (1999). Comparison of breast cancer patient satisfaction with follow-up in primary care vs. specialist care: results from a randomized controlled trial. *British Journal of General Practice* **49**: 705–10.

50 Pellino, T. A., Ward, S. E. (1998). Perceived control mediates the relationship between pain severity and patient satisfaction. *Journal of Pain and Symptom Management* **15**: 110–16.

51 Cleary, P. D. (1998). Satisfaction may not suffice! A commentary on 'A patient's perspective.' *International Journal of Technology Assessment in Health Care* **14**:35–7.

52 Ward, S. E., Gordon, D. (1994). Application of the American Pain Society quality assurance standards. *Pain* **56**:299–306.

53 Williams, B., Coyle, J., Healy, D. (1998). The meaning of patient satisfaction: an explanation of high reported levels. *Social Science and Medicine* **47**:351–9.

54 Carr-Hill, R. A. (1992). The measurement of patient satisfaction. *Journal of Public Health Medicine* **14**:236–49.

55 Zaslavsky, A. M., Zaborski, L., Ding, L. *et al.* (2001). Adjusting performance measures to ensure equitable plans comparison. *Health Care Financing Review* **22**:109–126.

56 Hall, J. A., Milburn, M. A., Epstein, A. M. (1993). A causal model of health status and satisfaction with medical care. *Medical Care* **31**:84–94.

57 Crofton, C., Lubalin, J. M., Darby, C. (1997). Foreword. *Medical Care.* **37**:MS 1–9.

58 Bernhart, M. H., Wiadnyana, I. G. P., Haryoko, W. *et al.* (1999). Patient satisfaction in developing countries. *Social Science and Medicine* **48**:989–96.

59 Fitzpatrick, R. (1991). Surveys of patient satisfaction: II – designing a questionnaire and conducting a survey. *British Medical Journal* **302**:1129–32.

60 McCracken, L. M., Klock, P. A., Mingay, D. J. *et al.* (1997). Assessment of satisfaction with treatment for chronic pain. *U.S. Cancer Pain Relief Committee* **14**:292–9.

61 Cleary, P. D., Edgman-Levitan, S., Roberts, M. *et al.* (1991). Patients evaluate their hospital care: a national survey. *Health Affairs* **10**:254–67.

62 Cleary, P. D., Edgman-Levitan, S., Mc Mullen, W. *et al.* (1992). The relationship between reported problems and patient summary evaluations of hospital care. *Quality Review Bulletin* **18**:53–9.

63 Medigovich, K., Porock, D., Kristjanson, L. J. *et al.* (1999). Predictors of family satisfaction with an Australian palliative home care service: a test of discrepancy theory. *Journal of Palliative Care* **15**:48–56.

64 Sitzia, J., Wood, N. (1999). Development and evaluation of a questionnaire to assess patient satisfaction with chemotherapy nursing care. *European Journal of Oncology Nursing* **3**:126–40.

65 Sitzia, J., Wood, N. (1998) Development and evaluation of a questionnaire to assess patient satisfaction with chemotherapy nursing care. *European Journal of Oncology Nursing* **2**:142–53.

66 Bredart, A., Razavi, D., Delvaux, N. *et al.* (1988). A comprehensive assessment of satisfaction with care for cancer patients. *Support Care Center* **6**:518–23.

67 Bredart, A., Razavi, D., Robertson, C. *et al.* (1999). A comprehensive assessment of satisfaction with care: preliminary psychometric analysis in an oncology institute in Italy. *Annals of Oncology* **10**:839–46.

68 Loeken, K., Steine, S., Sandvik, L. *et al.* (1997). A new instrument to measure patient satisfaction with mammography. *Medical Care* **35**:731–41.

67 Cleary, P. D., Edgman-Levitan, S., Roberts, M. *et al.* (1991). Patients evaluate their hospital care: a national survey. *Health Affairs* **10**:254–67.

69 Hays, R. D., Shaul, J. A., Williams, V. S. L. *et al.* (1997). Psychometric properties of the CAHPS survey measures. *Medical Care* (Suppl.) **37**: MS22–31.

70 Hargraves, J. L., Hays, R. D., Cleary, P. D. (2001). Psychometric properties of the Consumer Assessment of Health Plans (CAHPS) 2.0 Adult Core Survey. *Health Services Research* **38**(6 Part 1):1509–27.

15

Needs assessment in cancer

David H. Gustafson, Ph.D.

University of Wisconsin-Madison, Madison, WI

Introduction

The needs of a person facing a serious illness such as cancer are very complex. Maslow[1] argues that human needs arrange themselves in "hierarchies of pre-potency" such that the appearance of one depends upon prior satisfaction of more pre-potent needs. The most pre-potent of Maslow's needs are the physiological (e.g., maintaining homeostasis of oxygen, water). When these are not satisfied, as may be the case in a terminal cancer patient, no other needs are important. As long as those needs are satisfied, a patient or family member may be concerned about higher order needs such as the "safety" needs for predictability and orderliness that underlie the fear of the unknown often faced by newly diagnosed cancer patients. As long as these needs are met, one can hope that providers (as well as family and friends) will satisfy needs for affection and caring. And if these needs are met, one can seek to satisfy "esteem" needs such as the need for respect sought by many health care consumers today. Thus needs change as a patient's condition changes.

What are needs?

As discussed in Langley et al.,[2] Kano suggests that needs fall into three categories: expected, desired, and unexpected. And different types of needs have different effects on satisfaction. For instance, most patients and family members expect that they will be given the proper medication. Avoiding medication errors will not improve satisfaction, but making

errors could devastate satisfaction. In other cases, people desire, but may not expect, that a need will be satisfied. They may want a hospital to provide good food and parking. How well those desires are met will affect satisfaction. In still other cases, customers may not even hope that clinicians will meet certain needs because they see those needs as being the responsibility of another agency. For instance, patients may not see the physician as responsible for resolving family conflicts around caregiving. Hence not meeting these needs will not damage satisfaction. But if a physician were to help them meet that need, it could dramatically improve satisfaction with that health care provider.

No one fully understands his own or another person's needs. Patients may not realize that they need to deal with a slowly developing side effect from a medication because they do not recognize the connection. Also, persons' wants may be different from their needs. For instance, patients facing the end of life may not realize they need water. The symptom they may feel because of water deprivation may be fatigue. Hence they may want energy but need water. In still other cases, the things we want may not satisfy our underlying need.

Importance of needs assessment

Health care, including cancer care, is in the midst of a revolution driven by strong forces of cost containment and competition.[3] While economic pressures may be new to health care (and cancer care in particular), they are common in highly competitive industries where price reductions frequently occur simultaneously with performance improvements. In the future, cancer care providers will be expected to both improve performance and reduce costs; not as a one-time event but as a way of life. (P. Balden, Dartmouth Medical School, personal communication, 1998).

At the same time, because they feel that their needs do not drive provider behavior, a growing number of consumers are becoming more active in their care and, in some cases, migrating to alternatives such as complementary medicine and e-Health.[4] Many patients and caregivers do not even discuss their needs with their clinician and, when they do, they often omit important psychosocial concerns.[5–11] While some patients and caregivers do not share their needs because they believe that pain, grief, and suffering are inevitable with cancer, others believe that clinicians do not want to address those needs, in the absence of clinician inquiry or concern required to develop a meaningful dialog.[12–15] This growing alienation could be due to the aforementioned pressures to increase "productivity" or it could be a more fundamental problem: that the health system does not fully understand the needs of patients and their families.

Substantial evidence points to the damaging effects on suffering and health care costs of inadequately meeting needs, particularly needs for information and support.[16–22] Too many people suffer unnecessary pain and distress and face major impediments to good end-of-life care.[23–26] In fact, a large Institute of Medicine (IOM) study of seriously ill hospitalized patients documented substantial shortcomings in communication, treatment, and characteristics of death. In *Approaching Death*, the IOM[27] identified key patient needs, such as fears of abandonment and protracted death, and called for reliable, respectful care that promotes "norms of decency." The IOM report identified as a significant deficit the lack of data on patient and family needs, especially longitudinal data and data on needs of diverse populations.[28] Clearly, improvements are unlikely to occur without a much better

understanding of patient and family needs and the factors that influence them.

Needs assessments are designed to identify needs, measure their importance, and determine how well they are met. However, there are major obstacles to getting a complete picture. (1) Health care providers often overlook the needs of family members, possibly because they under-appreciate the role of the family in helping patients cope with cancer. In this paper, we will examine assessment of both patient and family needs. (2) Many assessments do not include a full set of patient and family needs. (3) With a few exceptions,[29] assessments do not document the changes in needs over time and/or tie those needs to key events that occur in patients' lives.[17,27,30–33] (4) Most needs assessments identify how well needs have been met (typically some variant of a Likert scale), but few offer guidance on *how* to meet the needs. (5) Strategies for measuring the importance of needs do not consider trade-offs among needs. (6) There is little understanding of how best to use needs assessment data to improve systems of care.

This paper will address those issues. But first, since a major focus of this book is on health-related quality of life (HRQOL), we will examine how needs assessment relates to HRQOL and to the associated concept of satisfaction. We will also address the complex relationships among needs themselves.

Distinction between needs, satisfaction, and HRQOL

Satisfaction surveys document how well a health care organization satisfies patient and family needs. HRQOL surveys capture how well the patient or family member is doing. Needs assessments provide raw material for satisfaction and HRQOL surveys, but are primarily aimed at guiding patient care planning while also contributing to program development, improvement, and evaluation. Satisfaction and HRQOL measures focus on *subsets* of patient/family needs. HRQOL surveys typically include needs that directly affect HRQOL (e.g., pain control or how much leakage is bothering a prostate cancer patient). They are less likely to include needs that indirectly affect HRQOL (e.g., keeping the family informed of the patient's progress).

Needs assessments measure the importance of needs and how well they are met, which is a concept related to, yet distinct from, satisfaction. Patients and families may be very satisfied with care received from a particular provider even though some very important needs go unmet, because they believe it is not possible, necessary, or appropriate for that provider to meet them. In this chapter, we will argue that it is very important for needs assessments to determine how well a broad range of needs are met regardless of who is responsible for meeting them.

HRQOL and satisfaction surveys are typically intended to provide a summary snapshot of the patient's health status and evaluation of the care process. Whether such data are collected as part of a clinical trial protocol, or by an observational study to monitor patient outcomes, or by providers to chart patient progress over time, there is typically a premium on administering a parsimonious set of survey items. On the other hand, needs assessments often will seek detailed data to advise on care planning or the design of new interventions. For instance, the following lists some caregiver needs that may arise if treatment stops working:

How to deal with anger. . . . . How to deal with grief. . . . . How to give the patient total focus & still keep my job. . . . . . Where do I get support. . . . . How can I stay strong & not panic. . . . . How to cook, pay bills, etc. . . . . How to prepare for death. . . . . When to tell others & how. . . . . How to assess previous life with patient. . . . . How to continue to have hope. . . . . How to figure out what patient wants. . . . . How to have fun while patient is dying and not feel guilty. . . . . Is there life after death?. . . . . How to know if I am doing the right things and doing them well. . . . . How to help the patient tell his life story. . . . . How to decide what goals to set. . . . . How to raise death issues (funeral plans). . . . What to talk about with the patient. . . . Whether to continue treatment. . . . . Whether to look for new treatments. . . . . Whether to seek non-traditional treatments. . . . . Whether to admit patient is dying.

While each need may be important, the entire list may be too detailed for a HRQOL or a satisfaction measure, or these needs may not be viewed as being

the responsibility of the entity collecting the satisfaction data.[34] In summary:

(1) A needs assessment pursues detail. It tries to capture information that will enable understanding of what it is like to be a person with "X" type cancer and what it is like to be that person's caregiver. Needs assessments can (and often do) include over 100 items. The needs assessment should examine how and why needs change over time. *In needs assessments, the key is to create a mutually exclusive and exhaustive set of needs precise enough to guide care planning and system improvement.* The main question addressed in needs assessment should be: "What is it like to be a person with this cancer or a family member of a person with the disease? Help us understand the details." In this context, "outcomes assessment in cancer" means, in effect, assessing the individual's needs to enhance the likelihood they can be met through appropriate services rendered within a more effective, efficient health care system.

(2) A satisfaction measure focuses on how well a particular provider organization satisfies a subset of those patient and caregiver needs. A satisfaction analysis might combine several needs into more global indicators. Its goal is to determine what would make a person recommend or return to a provider. A more innovative organization might conduct a satisfaction survey including needs a patient or family member might never expect the provider to address, thus identifying new opportunities to improve customer satisfaction. Still, the focus is on satisfaction with a health care organization's services and on asking, "What is it like to be our customer and how can we (the organization) improve the likelihood that you will return or recommend our service?"

(3) HRQOL is a more distal outcome that represents the summation and weighting of different needs into overall areas of well-being.[35] It employs a subset of needs directly affecting quality of life. The job of a HRQOL measure is to

determine how well a patient or family member is doing, given the presence of disease and the interventions undertaken. The scores on specific HRQOL dimensions might point the user to a more detailed set of needs. A HRQOL measure differs from satisfaction measures in that it is not limited to needs addressed by particular health care providers. Furthermore, since they might be applied frequently, HRQOL measures need to be relatively brief while at the same time representing many individual needs by a small set of domains, dimensions, or factors. Unlike needs assessment, HRQOL measures develop a limited number of summary statistics and focus less on individual elements. The key question asked is "How are you doing?"

Relationships among needs and between the concepts of need, satisfaction, and HRQOL

In developing needs assessments, it is important to understand how needs relate to each other, as well as how those interrelationships affect satisfaction and HRQOL. For instance, the way needs affect a patient or family's HRQOL is mediated by how well health care providers satisfy the need.

Consider this example: a patient does not have as much information as he wants about his prognosis. This uncertainty is making him anxious, thus having a negative impact on his HRQOL. He knows that he could obtain information about his prognosis from his physician, which could enhance his HRQOL and also his satisfaction with medical care. However, he wants to be a "good patient" and not bother his busy physician;[36] the thought that his physician might be annoyed by his questions also creates anxiety. Thus, the need to be a "good patient" conflicts with the need to get information about his condition, and each of these conflicting needs may have effects on both HRQOL and satisfaction. How could this dilemma be resolved? One possible resolution would be to change the image of a "good patient" through both patient and physician education, so that the prevailing perspective by both patients and physicians would be "A good patient is an informed patient, and providing information is the physician's responsibility." Another (and perhaps easier) solution to this conflict would be that someone other than the physician provides prognostic information; for example, an oncology nurse or oncology social worker. The interrelationships among needs and their effects on outcomes such as HRQOL and satisfaction are complex, have not been addressed in the literature to date, and are worthy of further consideration.

Review of needs assessment instruments related to cancer

A systematic search was conducted in MEDLINE (1966– Aug 2001) and CANCERLIT (1975– Aug 2001) to identify needs assessment instruments used to guide cancer care program design and intervention research. The search terms used, either singly or in combination, were "cancer," "patient need," "caregiver need," "audit measures," "instrument," "questionnaires," "survey," "assessment," and "outcome." While prostate, breast, colorectal, and lung cancers were the primary focus of the Cancer Outcomes Measurement Work Group (COMWG) activities, the search was not restricted according to cancer site since there might be instruments of interest developed for other cancers. Following the World Health Organization (WHO) assertion that needs of the family also should be addressed, instruments for assessing the needs of caregivers/families of cancer patients were also sought. The search produced 170 articles. Another 40 relevant articles were identified later.

Excluded from our analyses were instruments that (1) did not document how they were developed or tested,[37,38] (2) did not measure importance or satisfaction, and (3) measured satisfaction with specific health providers[39,40] (a subject addressed in Chapter 14 by Darby in this volume).[41] We did include instruments that studied the satisfaction of a broad set of needs derived from a health status perspective, and also instruments that studied one class of needs only, e.g., needs for information or for one type of cancer. Table 15.1 presents the 23 chosen instruments along with their intended application, number of items and dimensions, scoring format, item source, content and construct validity, internal consistency, reproducibility, responsiveness, and subject burden.

Analysis of instrument characteristics

The instruments analyzed focus on the needs of: any cancer patient (n = 10), patients with a specific type of cancer (n = 2), patients at a specific stage (n = 3), informal caregivers (n = 5), relatives (n = 1), and people during bereavement (n = 2). Sixteen are self-administered instruments. Seven are administered by clinician interview, although three of those claim that patients may be able to complete them. All but two are designed to be applicable to all cancers. Ten instruments are intended for all stages of cancer (but do not distinguish between stages in questions they ask), while 3 were for palliative care patients, and 2 for the bereavement period. The instruments varied in size, ranging from 12 to 144 items and from 1 to 8 domains. There is almost no consistency as to which domains are covered by the instruments. To illustrate this point, Table 15.2 lists the domains identified and in how many instruments each domain was used.

There was wide variation in how needs were identified. Target group interviews were most common (52% of instruments), followed by literature reviews (43%), expert input (43%), adaptations of other scales (39%), and theory (22%). We believe that lack of theory and customer involvement are significant and common deficits in developing needs assessments.[63] Of those conducting target group interviews, only one described in any detail how the interviews were conducted. We believe much more detail should be provided on how the items were identified because the items are the foundation upon which everything else in a needs assessment is based.

There was also a wide variation in the extent to which needs assessments were evaluated. Some test of internal consistency was reported for 91% of instruments. Construct validity was reported for 70%. Other important psychometric evaluations were less frequently reported. They include: completion time (56%), reproducibility (e.g., test re-test) (43%), responsiveness (e.g., ability to detect effects of an intervention) (26%), and reading level (13%).

Completion time ranged between 5 and 45 minutes. One way to reduce respondent burden might be to include only needs that are appropriate at each stage of disease. For instance, Gates et al.[44] administered the Cancer Patient Need Survey (CPNS) to both clinical cancer patients (n = 38) and hospice cancer patients (n = 28). They found that the two groups had significantly different needs for "help," "information," and "work" domains. Hospice patients were more likely to select "not applicable," which suggests that many CPNS needs were not appropriate to them. Item Response Theory (IRT) might be useful in tailoring current questionnaires to present needs that are relevant to particular populations.[64]

Five studies reported inter-rater reliability tests. Two instruments were clinician-administered. It makes sense to determine if different clinicians give similar ratings on the same patients. However, three examined extent of agreement among different patients. While this may be a useful way to identify the prevalence of needs across a customer group, such approaches to inter-rater reliability do not appear to provide an appropriate test of *instrument* reliability. It would be reasonable for a very good needs assessment to find wide variations among patients in the extent of their needs.

Five papers analyzed an instrument's ability to detect differences between patients or caregivers who reasonably should be expected to differ. Four of the six instruments that tested for responsiveness were sensitive enough to detect differences created by interventions.

Domains

In principle, there is nothing wrong with creating taxonomies of needs, especially if they offer a consistent organizing structure across different needs assessments. However, domains developed by different researchers often have very different organizing

Table 15.1. Selected instruments psychometric review

Instrument	Purpose and Administration	Items and Domains	Question Format	Item Source and Content Validity	Construct Validity	Internal Consistency	Reproducibility	Responsiveness	Burden
CARES[42] (Cancer Rehabilitation Evaluation System)	Find how cancer affects psychosocial, physical and behaviors. Patient completes.	93–132 items; 6 domains: physical, psychological, medical interaction, marital, sexual, miscellaneous.	Five-point scale plus "do you want help: yes/no?"	Literature. Interviews with patients and family. Expert review. Theoretical frame: competency-based model of coping.	Correlated with SCL-90, KPS, DAS. Good agreement with interviewers.	Domains: α ranged from 0.88 to 0.92.	Subscales: r = 0.84–0.95. 87% agreement; n = 71, time = 1 week.		Completion time: 10–45 min; Reading level N/A; Acceptability: most found it easy to use.
CARES-SF[43] (Cancer Rehabilitation Evaluation System-Short Form)	Shortens the CARES for use with clinical trials. Patient completes.	38–57 items; 5 domains: physical, psychological, medical interaction, marital, sexual.	Five-point scale plus "do you want help (yes/no)?"	Selected from the CARES by experts.	Correlated well with CARES, FLIC, KPS, DAS. Large sample sizes.	Domains: α ranged from 0.60 to 0.84.	Dimensions: r = 0.69–0.92; 81%–86% agreement; n = 120, time = 10 days.	Find physical, psychosocial change with time. Correlated with FLIC @ 1, 7, 14 months post-diagnosis.	Time N/A; Reading level N/A; Acceptability N/A.
CPNS[44] (Cancer Patient Need Survey)	Measures the importance of needs and the degree to which needs are met. Patient completes.	51 items; 5 domains: coping, help, information, work, and cancer shock.	"Importance": seven-point Likert scale; "how well met": seven-point Likert scale.	Interviews with nurses, patients, & caregivers using Objective Content Test and Q-sort method.		Overall: α = 0.91 Importance: 0.83–0.93; How well met: 0.79–0.95; Domain: α = 0.88 to 0.92.			Time: 2–45 min; Reading level N/A; Acceptability: reported no problems when used.
CPNQ[45] (Cancer Patient Need Questionnaire)	Assesses unmet needs of people with cancer. Patient completes.	71 items; 5 domains: psychological needs, health info, ADLs, patient care/support, interpersonal communication.	Five-point scale: "what is your level of need for help?"	Literature. Interviews. Expert review. Pilot test.	Discriminant validity: able to distinguish patients with different disease stages.	Domains: α ranged from 0.78 to 0.90.	Intercorrelation: all significant kappa >0.4; n = 124; time = 10–14 days.		Time: 20 min; Reading level: 4th or 5th grade; Acceptability: 25% non-completion rate.

Instrument	Purpose	Items and domains	Response format	Development	Validity	Reliability (domains)	Reliability (other)	Administration
SCNS[46] (Supportive Care Needs Survey)	Assesses impact of cancer on lives of cancer patients. Patient completes.	61 items; 5 domains: psychological needs, health information, physical/daily living needs, patient care and support, and sexuality	Five-point scale: "what is your level of need for help?"	Based on CPNQ. Expert review. Pilot test.		Domains: α ranged from 0.87 to 0.97.		Time: 20 min; Reading level: 5th grade; Acceptability: patients found it understandable, 35% non-completion.
HCS-PF[47] (Home Care Study-Patient Form)	Assesses attitudes of terminally and chronically ill patients toward medical care. Interview; patient may be able to complete.	33 items; 2 domains. *Satisfaction with:* care availability, care continuity, MD availability, MD competence, MD personality, MD communication, general satisfaction. *Preference:* home care, decision-making	Agreement with five-point Likert scale.	Based on scales by Zyranski and Ware. Pilot test.	Poor discriminant validity.	Domains: α ranged from 0.10–0.75.		Time: N/A; Reading level: N/A; Acceptability: N/A.
NEQ[48] (Need Evaluation Questionnaire)	Assess needs of hospitalized cancer patients in clinical setting. Patient completes.	23 items; 3 domains: helps diagnosis/prognosis, exam/treatment, communication and relations	Agreement with yes/no statement.	Interviews. Pilot tests.		Domain: α ranged from 0.69–0.81.	Cohen's kappa ranged from 0.54–0.94. Time = 1 week.	Time: 5 min; Reading level: N/A; Acceptability: 63% of patients OK; 24% incomplete; 3% missing data.

(cont.)

Table 15.1. (*cont.*)

Instrument	Purpose and Administration	Items and Domains	Question Format	Item Source and Content Validity	Construct Validity	Internal Consistency	Reproducibility	Responsiveness	Burden
PNAT[49] (Patient Needs Assessment Tool)	Screen cancer patients for physical & psychological functioning problems. Part of clinician interview.	16 items; 3 domains: physical, psychological, and social.	Five-item impairment scale for each area within domain.	Literature. Clinical experience.	Physical domain correlates with KPS; Psychological with GAIS, BSI MPAS, BDI; Social with ISEL.	Domains: α ranged from 0.85–0.94.	Interrater reliability: Friedman: 0.87, 0.76, 0.73; Spearman rank order: 0.59–0.98.		Time: 20–30 min.; Reading level: N/A; Acceptability: N/A.
DINA[50] (The Derdiarian Informational Needs Assessment)	Measures the informational needs of cancer patients. Interview.	144 items; 4 domains: disease, personal, family, and social relationship.	Check the need present and rate importance on 10-point scale.	Theory of information seeking. Needs and hierarchy of needs. Expert review.		Domains: α exceeded 0.9 for all domains.	80%–100% agreement found using McNemar test time = 15–20 min.	Detected difference between control group and experimental group.	Time: N/A; Reading Level N/A; Acceptability: N/A.
PINQ[51] (Patient Information Need Questionnaire)	Measures the information need among cancer patients for the improvement of clinical practice and research. Patient completes.	17 items; 2 domains: disease-oriented and information about access to help & solution.	Four-point scale.	Literature. Interviews.	Correlated with RSC, State-Anxiety Inventory & MMPI D-scale. Measurement invariance assessed with Hodgkins & breast cancer patients.	Domains: α ranged from 0.88–0.92; Inter-item correlation > 0.2.		Detected the changing needs of patients at three time points before and after first treatment.	Time: N/A; Reading level N/A; Acceptability: reasons to refuse include not wanting to be reminded of their illness, feeling too old, etc.
PCNA[52] (Prostate Cancer Needs Assessment)	Measures the importance and unmet needs of men with prostate cancer. Patient completes.	135 items; 3 domains: information, support, and care delivery.	Ten-point "Importance" scale. Ten-point "Extent Need Met" scale.	Literature. Interviews using Critical Incident Technique & Nominal Group. Expert review.	Correlated with overall satisfaction with care.	Agreement on classification by three researchers working independently.	r = 0.97, time = 2 weeks		Time: 43 min; Reading level: 7th grade; Acceptability: 11% non-completion.

Instrument	Purpose	Items/Domains	Scale	Development	Validity	Reliability (α)	Other reliability	Sensitivity	Practical
TINQ-BC[53] (Toronto Informational Needs Questionnaire-Breast Cancer)	Identify information needed by women with recent breast cancer diagnosis to deal with illness. Patient completes.	51 items; 5 domains: diagnosis, test, treatments, physical, psychosocial.	Five-point "Importance" scale.	Literature. Nurse opinions.	Correlated with the information scale of HOS.	Overall α = 0.97 Domains α ranged from 0.73 to 0.93; Correlation of subscales to total scale: 0.38–0.88			Time: 20 min; Reading level: N/A; Acceptability OK.
STAS[54] (Support Team Assessment Schedule)	Assess quality of palliative care of multi-disciplinary cancer support teams. Professional completes.	17 items; 8 domains: pain/symptom control, insight, psychosocial, family needs, home services, planning affairs, support of other professionals, communication.	Five-point Likert scale.	Literature. Clinical experience.	Correlated with patient & family score, Karnofsky score, Spitzer QOL Index. Support team scores correlate with patient and family scores.		Interrater reliability: 90% agreement except predictability.	Detected improvement in palliative care. Evaluated 2 palliative care support teams.	Time: 2 min. for existing patients, 5 min. new patients; Reading level: N/A; Acceptability: N/A.
PACA[55] (Palliative Care Assessment)	Assess effectiveness of hospital's palliative care program. Professional completes.	12 items; 3 domains: symptom control, insight, and future placement.	Four-point scale, except five-point scale for insight.	Interviews of patients.	Symptom scores correlated with McCorkle symptom distress scale.		Kappa ranged from 0.44–1.00	Sensitivity to detected statistically significant intervention effects.	Time: few min.; Reading level: N/A; Acceptability: N/A.
NEST[66] (The Needs Near the End-of-Life Care Screening Tool)	Measure experiences of end-of-life patients and possibly assess impact of interventions. Interview; patient completes if possible.	135 items; 8 domains: patient-MD relations, social connection, caregiving need, psychological distress, spirituality, personal acceptance, have purpose, clinician communication.	Five-point Likert scale.	Literature. Interviews and focus groups. Theory: frame for a good death. Symptom items from other scales. Pilot tests. Expert review.	Measurement invariance was assessed for demographic strata using CFA; 13-item IRT evaluated short form; 10 items work.	Domains: α ranged from 0.63–0.85 at baseline and 0.64–0.89 at follow up.			Time: N/A; Reading level N/A; Acceptability: 69.2% patients found interview helpful.

(cont.)

Table 15.1. (*cont.*)

Instrument	Purpose and Administration	Items and Domains	Question Format	Item Source and Content Validity	Construct Validity	Internal Consistency	Reproducibility	Responsiveness	Burden
FIN[57] (Family Inventory of Needs)	Measure needs of cancer patient's family and extent needs are met. Family completes.	20 items; 1 domain	Ten-point "importance" scale and met/unmet check.	Literature. Fulfillment theory. Items from original Critical Care Family Needs Inventory. Family review.	Correlated with FAMCARE.	Overall α for "importance" scale: 0.83.			Time: "short"; Reading level: N/A; Acceptability: N/A.
FIN-H[58] (Family Inventory of Needs-Husbands)	Measure information needs of husbands of women with breast cancer. Husband completes.	30 items; 5 domains: surgical care needs, communication with MD, family relations, diagnosis/treatment specifics, husband's involvement.	Five-point "Importance" subscale and three-point "Need Met" subscale.	Based on FIN. Pilot test.		Overall α ranged from 0.90–0.93; 73%–87% of items: item-total correlation 0.4–0.7.	Importance subscale: r = 0.82; Need Met subscale: r = 0.79; time: < 24 hrs		Time: 16–30 min; Reading level: N/A; Acceptability: 12 husbands refused to complete.
FAMCARE[59]	Measure family satisfaction with advanced cancer care. Family completes.	20 items; 4 domains: information giving, care availability, physical care, pain control, and 2 other items.	Five-point Likert "Satisfaction scale."	Interviews. Family ranking of items. Q-sort.	Correlated with McCusker and with overall satisfaction with care questions.	Overall α: 0.93; Domains: α ranged from 0.61–0.88.	r = 0.92, n = 23; time < 23 hrs		
HCNS (JW Hileman, University of Kansas, unpublished research) (Home Caregiver Need Survey)	Measures the importance and satisfaction of the needs of caregivers. Caregiver completes.	90 items; 6 domains: information, household, patient care, personal, spiritual, and psychological.	Seven-point "Importance" subscale and seven-point "Satisfaction" subscale.	Statements from patients and home caregivers. Expert evaluation. Theory: Lackey-Wingate model. Pilot test.	Psychological, patient care, personal and household domains correlated with KPS.	Overall α: 0.93, 0.98; Domains: α ranged from 0.85–0.97.		Detected changing caregiver needs at 3 time points.	Time: 30 min; Reading: 5th grade level; Acceptability: caregivers OK.

Instrument	Description	Items/Domains	Scale	Development	Validity	Reliability		Time/Reading level/Acceptability
HCS-CF[47] (Home Care Study–Caretaker Form)	Assess attitude of terminally and chronically ill caretakers toward medical care of their patients. Interview; patient may be able to complete.	42 items; 2 domains: *Satisfaction with care:* availability, continuity, MD availability, MD competence, MD personality, MD communication, general satisfaction. *Preference for:* home care, decision making.	Agreement with five-point Likert scale.	Based on scales by Zyranski and Ware. Pilot test.	Good discriminant validity.	Domains: α ranged from 0.50–0.85.		Time: N/A; Reading level: N/A; Acceptability: N/A.
ISNQ[60] (Information and Support Needs Questionnaire)	Assess information & support needs of women who have primary relative with breast cancer. Self-complete.	29 items; 2 domains: information and support.	Four-point "Importance" subscale and four-point "Need Met" subscale.	Literature. Interviews.		Domains: α ranged from 0.92–0.95.		Time: 37 min; Reading level: "middle" class; Acceptability: "several" reported it didn't apply.
ICG[61] (Inventory of Complicated Grief)	Assesses symptoms of complicated grief. Self-complete.	19 items; unidimensional.	Five-point frequency scale.		Correlated with BED, TRIG, GMS.	α = 0.94; item-total correlation >0.5.	r = 0.8; items = 18; time = 6 months.	Time: N/A; Reading level N/A; Acceptability: subjects stated it's tolerated.
RGEI[62] (The Revised Grief Experience Inventory)	A short practical tool to measure the grief experience. Self-complete.	22 items; 4 domains: existential, depression, tension/guilt, physical distress.	Six-point agreement scale.	Based on original GEI. Expert review. Theory: Parkes' grief construct.		Overall α: 0.93; Domains: α ranged from 0.72–0.87.		Time: N/A; Reading level N/A; Acceptability: 41.3% return rate.

Table 15.2. Number of cancer needs assessment instruments containing each domain name

Domain	No. of instruments	Domain	No. of instruments	Domain	No. of instruments
Pain	3	Social	5	Participation	3
Symptom Control	1	Communication	4	MD Interaction	5
Physical	2	Planning	1	MD Availability	2
Cancer Shock	1	Information	8	MD Competence	2
Psychological	8	Diagnostic Info	3	Patient Care	5
Psychosocial	2	Treatment Info	1	Care Continuity	2
Spiritual	2	Daily Living	2	Home Care	2
Insight	2	Work	1	Access to Care	2
Sexuality	4	Household	1	Financial	1
Personal	1	Activity Mgt	1	Help	2
Marital	2	Coping	1	Other	8
Family	3	Future Placement	1		

structures. Table 15.2 lists the frequency with which various domain names are found in the scales we examined. The number of domains reported in these scales ranges from 1–12, with 35 different domain names. Since all are cancer needs assessments, similarity in names would be expected. However, no domain name was used in a majority of instruments. Only two domain names (psychological and information) were used in even 8 of the 23 (35%) instruments, while only 3 domain names were used in 5 of the 23 (patient care, social, and interactions with physicians).

Furthermore, domains with similar names often contain items that are conceptually and operationally quite different. For example, consider the Patient Needs Assessment Tool (PNAT)[49] and Supportive Care Needs Survey (SCNS).[46] Both have Physical and Psychological domains. PNAT's Physical domain includes mobility, communication, alertness, and bowel-bladder function. None of these is included in SCNS's physical domain. SCNS's Physical domain contains pain, lack of energy, and feeling unwell, but none of these domains is found in the PNAT. Discomfort (one item within PNAT's Physical domain) lists fatigue, nausea, itch, and constipation as examples, but not Pain (the only discomfort-related item in SCNS). PNAT's Psychological domain contains history of psychological problems and attitude (e.g., hopelessness). Neither is part of the SCNS. The SCNS Psychological domain contains concerns about those close to the patient, but not found in the PNAT. Fear that the family will not be able to cope with caring for the patient is included in SCNS's Psychological domain, but in PNAT's Social domain. Differences are found in other domains as well.

These inconsistencies are not isolated cases. The 58-item Cancer Rehabilitation Evaluation System-Short Form (CARES-SF)[43] and the 68-item SCNS[46] were both designed to understand the impact of cancer on patients' lives. Both have Physical, Psychological, and Sexuality domains; CARES-SF adds Medical Interaction and Marital domains while the SCNS adds Health System and Information and Patient Care and Support. While the domains seem similar, there are substantial differences. The SCNS asks five questions about treatment environment (e.g., waits and delays); CARES-SF asks none. SCNS asks five questions on access to health services; CARES-SF asks one. SCNS asks ten questions related to clinician information and communication, while CARES-SF asks two. However, CARES-SF addresses four questions related to weight and nutrition; SCNS asks none. CARES-SF asks four questions about employment; SCNS asks none. And CARES-SF asks eight questions about sex and intimacy; SCNS asks three. Domains do not seem to produce conceptual or operational similarity and do not seem to provide a consistent organizing structure.

The most common measure of instrument cohesiveness reported in the needs assessments studies is how well items fit within domains. Twenty of the twenty-three instruments employ some kind of interclass correlation coefficient, and in nineteen of those cases, Cronbach's alpha is reported. We question the heavy reliance on Cronbach's alpha, given criticisms that have been leveled against this approach and the availability of a number of other domain fit indices.[65–67]

More importantly, we question why needs assessments use domains at all. Reducing scores to summary measures may not be as valuable in needs assessment as in other cancer outcomes measurement. The value of a needs assessment comes from understanding the importance of specific needs – not the development of summary scores to facilitate the comparisons of interventions or health plans, as often the case now with HRQOL or satisfaction measures, respectively. For example, developers have limited resources to allocate to creation of new e-Health programs. One should not spend the same resources on two needs with very different degrees of patient-perceived importance. Our research found that understanding what it will be like to have chemotherapy is a bigger unmet need for recently diagnosed breast cancer patients than is learning how to deal with unsupportive people. Knowing this, program developers might provide brief advice regarding the unsupportive-person need but create much more extensive offerings related to chemotherapy, for example, video clips of the chemotherapy process and of women talking about the experience, all tailored so the presentations involve culturally appropriate material. Moreover, the relative importance of the two needs might differ for different types of people. A person with low internal control might need more help in dealing with unsupportive people than help in understanding what chemotherapy would be like. Examining such refinements would call for even more precise analyses of specific needs, not information about domains.

We are concerned that reductionism can obscure the value of an intervention. One could argue that if the domain is a sensitive and appropriate measure of a concept, such obscurity should not occur. Unfortunately, many domains are too all-inclusive. Consider the "Physical" domain of the SCNS. An intervention could meet a patient's need for pain control, but not meet the need for more energy. Yet, one might conclude that an intervention has no effect on the physical domain if it was judged on the composite rather than the individual elements, because the effect on one item is washed out by the lack of effect on another. (This issue arises not infrequently in HRQOL studies as well.)

Certainly, there are challenges with single item analyses. However, the enormous increases in computing power make it practical to employ new approaches to data analyses that sidestep many of the restrictive assumptions of statistical analysis. For instance, one might use artificial intelligence to create mathematical operations that would explore all needs assessment items so that statistically based approaches to item reduction are no longer required. As a result, it might be possible to identify a set of needs-based rules that more effectively distinguish the effects of one intervention from another. It may also help us understand the relationships among needs as well as the relationships between those needs and other outcomes such as satisfaction and HRQOL. These data-mining approaches use search algorithms employing many algebraic operators to create a huge number of mathematical expressions and identify which performs best. For instance, one expression might be that if pain reaches a certain threshold and sleep is reduced below a certain number of hours then the patient will need help in making certain decisions. This approach can automatically fit and assess a wide variety of mathematical constructions including complex nonlinear algebraic expressions which make it unmatched as a knowledge discovery tool. Of course, like any statistical approach, it is important to use common sense in evaluating the merit of the resulting rules and to test the rules with an independent sample.

Observations on processes of developing and conducting a needs assessment

The literature analyzed here indicates that the methods used to identify and measure the importance of needs have not been widely addressed. These are issues of fundamental importance to the effectiveness of needs assessments and will be discussed below.

Needs identification

Needs identification is a very important step in needs assessments. No single person or group has a complete picture of the needs of cancer patients and their families. Provider, patient, and family perspectives of needs are each limited by their own world-view. For example, a doctor may understand a terminal cancer patient's medical needs, but not understand how important it is for a patient to understand what it will be like to die. Furthermore, providers may not fully appreciate how the family is affected by cancer and how important it is to meet family needs. A patient may want pain relief, but may not appreciate the importance of dealing with forgiveness before death. Family caregivers may want training in caregiving skills, but not appreciate the importance of taking time for themselves during caregiving. Therefore, a spectrum of people should be involved in needs identification, and people should be helped to identify needs they did not know they had.

Unfortunately, very little information is typically provided on how instrument developers went about identifying needs. While semi-structured interviews are frequently mentioned as a source, there is no description of what that actually means in those particular studies. Yet, the way one conducts these interviews or focus groups can influence what needs are identified. For instance, we believe that it is not sufficient to directly ask patients, caregivers, or providers what a patient or family needs because there are needs they may not be aware of until called to their attention. Below we discuss two approaches to identifying needs – the critical incident and person-focused techniques – that can lead to a more complete understanding of needs.

Critical incident technique[68]

This approach involves asking patients to think back to specific stages in their disease experience, and to critical incidents that stand out in their mind. For instance, a breast cancer patient might be asked to think back to the time when she first felt the lump, to when the surgeon said "I have bad news," to the choice of surgery, the surgery itself, the chemotherapy, radiation, recovery, and so forth. At each stage, patients (and family members) are asked to describe things that stand out in their minds: fears, frustrations, anxieties, and uncertainties. The researcher then examines the incidents to identify possible needs.

In one such interview, the patient (thinking about when the surgeon told her she had breast cancer) said the surgeon talked with her for over an hour, but that she remembered nothing. All she wanted was to go home. Such an interview suggests that one need was for time to pull herself together in a safe surrounding before taking the next steps. When asked to remember their recovery from surgery, many patients describe their surprises: that their expectations did not match reality. This example suggests that cancer patients need help visualizing what it will be like (for instance) to have a mastectomy. Different needs are identified using the critical incident technique than from direct questioning. Retrospection may interfere with accurate assessment of needs, given the challenges faced during times of stress. But this criticism can also be applied to other processes such as focus groups and semi-structured interviews. And like those techniques, the critical incident process can be used in current time by asking a person to describe what they are currently experiencing rather than being asked to only identify their current needs.

Person-focused techniques

Person-focused techniques also avoid asking patients directly about their needs. Rather, they ask the patient, "What is it like to be a woman (*not just a patient*) who had breast cancer," or ask the family member, "What it is like to be a partner of a woman with breast cancer?" (again not just the partner of a patient, but the partner of a person). The reason for this approach is that if one asks people to describe their experiences as patients, they are more likely to focus on medical care issues, rather than on other crucial issues that affect their wider being. Interviewees who are asked to think of themselves as persons (or as members of a family facing cancer), not patients (or family members), talk about issues in their lives that bother them deeply. They do not limit themselves to areas they believe to be the health care provider's responsibility. Once they address these broader issues, interviewees can later be asked "What is it like to be a patient?" or "What is it like to get health care from your provider?"

Critical incident and person-focused interviews widen one's understanding of people with cancer and their family. Without this wider perspective, providers and program developers risk addressing less important issues and ignoring more important ones.[63] This seems to be the case in cancer care.[27] Patients' fears of abandonment and protracted death seem to be justified, as well as their needs for reliable, respectful care, advance care planning that promotes "norms of decency" and reduction of pain and distress. However, attention to these needs often seems to be missing in cancer care.[23–26]

Factors influencing the importance of needs

To provide the right services at the right time to the right people, needs assessments must prioritize needs. Although some cancer needs assessments are designed for certain populations, most have been developed without considering how populations may vary. Ideally, a needs assessment would address: (1) the trade-offs patients or caregivers are willing to make between meeting different needs; (2) variation in needs among different patients or caregivers according to race, age, and other demographic factors;[69–71] and (3) changes over time in patient and caregiver needs during the progression of the disease and/or treatments.[71,72]

If a patient's condition deteriorates, needs change for patients, caregivers, and other family members. For instance, Mor and colleagues[29] found that the percentages of advanced cancer patients who expressed a need for assistance with personal care increased from 7% during chemotherapy to 16% just three to six months later. Yet, even though such changes have been documented for some time, few needs assessments actually investigate the changes over time and the causes of those changes.

Needs are influenced by the occurrence and timing of key events. These may include diagnosis, start of certain treatments, disease progression, learning that treatments are not working, onset of symptoms such as pain and dyspnea, changes in family roles, and the patient's need for help with activities of daily living. Table 15.3 illustrates how needs may emerge in conjunction with such events. The left column lists possible events. The remaining columns list needs (identified from critical incident interviews with caregivers) that may first appear when the event occurs.

Factors other than events such as personal preferences and life circumstances can also influence when a need becomes important enough to seek help for it. Some people tend to avoid conflict, while others prefer to confront it. Some people are coping with other issues that, for them, are more pressing than cancer (such as loss of a loved one or putting food on the table). Still others are more willing to accept death, while others hold out hope for miraculous cures.

As a result, the implementation of interventions should be modified according to the individual. For instance, it would be difficult to create a computer system with tailoring – that is, an informatics strategy whereby the computer collects data on users and then guides them to cancer information and support designed specifically for that situation – without understanding what needs individuals have at a particular time. Raising issues such as funeral planning at the wrong time can have a devastating impact on patient and family well-being. Program planners need to know the answers to questions such as: Is the family ready to think seriously about death? What factors influence when families are ready?

Unfortunately, little research has been conducted to understand when and why needs become more or less important. Answers to these questions are important for both clinical care and program

Table 15.3. A listing of needs faced by caregivers of patients with advanced cancer suggesting what events first initiate those needs

Events	Needs of patient and caregiver		
At diagnosis of advanced cancer	How to stay in touch with MDs and RNs. How to get RNs and MDs to listen to us. How to be validated by clinician • Receive respect • Be treated with dignity • Listen to information from family • Encourage family to ask questions • Give honest answers to questions • Include family in conversations • Give a sense of being partners • Being available to family	How to initiate info exchange with MD Understand prognosis How to keep family regularly informed • Project competence • Have positive attitude • Have family conference • Anticipate family needs • Orient family to new procedures • Keeping family informed • Interpret the facts • Explain the situation	How to get support from clinicians Guilt from bothering busy MD Getting honest updates re patient health How to deal with health system Reliving past deaths Know effects of Ca on the family How to help kids adjust to the cancer Deal with approach of widowhood How to manage stress How to get support from others Find someone to talk to re my feelings How to check truth of info provided
During treatment	Understand illness What care should patient get Who is coordinating treatment Accurately visualize treatment Know what symptoms to expect How to know if patient is getting good care How to care for the family How to maintain a normal family life Getting help beyond family and friends Able to show images of patient to family	Dealing with patients fatigue Patients physical needs and how to deal with them Patients psychological needs and how to deal with How to reassure patient Finding purposeful activities for patient Learn underlying reason for symptoms Know what to expect in the future How to deal with side effects of treatments/meds Someone else should be in charge Dealing with my fatigue and exhaustion	Know how to manage side effects How to be patient and tolerant Dealing with scheduling of drugs Dealing with sexual difficulties Are you giving care properly Meaning of symptoms that arise How to get sleep if worry patient will die What to expect in giving home care How to give injections Learning/teaching skills at discharge
Prior to MD visits	Finding transportation How to judge quality of care How to intervene if poor quality	Dealing with fear of treatment Fear of treatment ending Dealing with unpredictability of future	How to care for the family Dealing with fear re test results Finding child care
Told treatment isn't working	How to deal with anger How to deal with grief How to give patient total focus and keep job Where do I get support How can I stay strong and not panic Learning how to cook, pay bills, etc How to prepare for death When to tell others and how	Guilt of having fun while patient dies Is there life after death Will they have eternal life? How to know if caregiver is doing right How to help patient tell life story How to decide what goals to set How to raise death issues (funeral plans)	How to assess previous life with patient How to continue to have hope Whether to continue treatment Whether to look for new treatments Whether to seek non-traditional treatments Whether to admit they are dying How to figure out what patient wants

Table 15.3. (*cont.*)

Events	Needs of patient and caregiver		
Patient begins to suffer pain (reality hits patient will die)	How to relieve pain and distress What I can do to help with symptoms How to deal with feeling helpless How to deal with watching patient suffer How to find community resources Setting goals for rest of life Planning how to meet the goals What drugs to use Discussing suicide	What image to present (cheerful, sad) What should I talk about with patient How to keep support over long run How to still give hope Finding meaning in life Dealing with grief Conflict between religion and treatment Isolation from religious community Advance directives	How to update family MD on patient What treatments does patient want When to say its OK to go If and when to start hospice care Relationship with deity Concern with afterlife Loss of faith Worry about meaning of life How to get ritual needs met
Relationship problems arise	How to deal with personality changes Deal with patient as different person with drugs	Dealing with speeded agenda Dealing with guilt re old problems How to communicate with the patient	How to deal with finances How to do patient job and mine too
Roles must be changed	Where are the files, checkbooks, etc What key events to deal with How to take charge of care decisions	How to handle when patient stops working • Patient identity crisis • Loss of income • Loss of benefits • Loss of social supports	How to negotiate these changes with patient How to manage change to new roles How to set aside my other goals. How to help carry out these roles
Patient needs help with ADLs or daily functions (driving, cooking, cleaning)	What will it be like to die What will it be like with reduced activity If discuss death/hospice, am I giving up How to deal with the pity How to get skills to care for patient • How to give bowel care • How to give skin and wound care • How to ambulate/move patient • How to get proper nutrition to patient • How to prepare special foods	How to make patient comfortable Coping with the isolation Awful thoughts: I wish it would end What does suffering and death mean to: • My faith • See patient in heaven • Anger at God • How to be at peace How to deal with restrictions of own activities How to care for patient if caregiver gets sick	How to identify what patient needs How do we create space. Expert check to see if doing right How to get help giving physical care Coping with the odor Whether family should move in Whether to take a leave from work Whether to place patient in hospice/NH Whether to start family counseling Whether to initiate DNR orders
Big symptom (dypsnea, severe pain)	How to help patient breathe How to comfort patient What changes are patient's vs treatment's	No anger with patient; where to take emotions How to check up on patient How to cope with these symptoms	How to reduce these symptoms Likely HRQOL changes
Time just before death (death surround)	Know what to expect How to be sure you are there How to not be alone when death comes How to get help with last things	How to say goodbye to patient Where to die What to do if patients don't "die on time" Have physician say goodbye Whether to stop life support	How to get personal needs met Who will help with next steps Who to let know and how Family meet physician How to validate life of the patient

(*cont.*)

Table 15.3. (*cont.*)

Events	Needs of patient and caregiver		
Bereavement period	How to plan the funeral How to rehabilitate the family Dealing with problems with children How to regain normalcy	Changing relation with friends What to do with patient's stuff Taxes and other financial issues Dealing with phone calls to patient	Finding meaning in life What to do with time now Dealing with loneliness Deal with preoccupation with deceased
Establishing new identify (e.g. dating)	How to deal with disruption of old social ties Am I being faithful How to tell others I'm dating	If I call date by former partner's name Is it real or a rebound	How to date Am I being fair to the date Whether, when to date others

development. With a few exceptions, needs assessment research treats needs as equally important across time.[56,73,74]

Measuring importance of needs

There are many important needs; but, because providers, health care systems, and also patients and caregivers themselves face significant time and other resource constraints, it is important to understand the relative importance of these needs. In an ideal world, all needs would be ascertained and completely met. In the real world, it is important that the most compelling needs are identified and met to the extent possible. The question at hand, then, is how to measure the relative importance of needs and the perceived effectiveness of services to meet them.

Most cancer needs assessments ask patients or caregivers to rate importance directly. For instance, CARES-SF states "I find that frequency of sexual intercourse has decreased" and asks patients to document the extent to which that need applies to them ("not at all" to "very much") and to indicate whether they want help with the need. The SCNS lists "changes in sexual relationships" as a potential need and asks the respondent to indicate the extent to which the need is unmet (ranging from no need-not applicable to high need).

However, this approach to measuring importance does not consider potentially important trade-offs and interactions among needs. In actuality, patients

must trade-off increased nausea for the benefits of chemotherapy. That nausea may force patients to trade-off a good night's sleep, which may compromise their immune system. Some researchers suggest that direct rating of importance of needs without considering trade-offs may produce inaccurate importance scores.[75] Thus, direct weighting will not accurately indicate how to combine attributes to create better service.[76]

An alternative approach frequently used in satisfaction surveys is to obtain global satisfaction ratings for care (e.g., the extent to which patients would return to or recommend a health care organization) and to obtain ratings of satisfaction with specific services provided by the organization (e.g., caregiver training at patient discharge). The correlation coefficients between global and individual satisfaction scores are treated as measures of the importance of receiving the specific services. However, some studies[63] find little relationship between these derived importance scores and scores estimated directly. In a recent study,[52] 230 prostate cancer patients directly rated both importance and satisfaction of 135 needs and also provided a global rating of satisfaction with their care. Regression analysis derived the importance of items. The correlation between direct and derived weights was a notably small −0.0007.

Similarly, in cancer needs assessment, conjoint analysis would allow us to determine the individual's most salient needs *and* the combination(s) of services the individual deems most important in meeting those needs. To proceed, we first specify the candidate set of needs the individual might have, based either on previous consultations with the individual or by reference to the set of needs frequently noted by individuals with cancer. Because we may not be confident in advance of what these needs are, it may be prudent to select a fairly broad set, with the knowledge that a properly executed conjoint analysis will automatically provide feedback about which needs are relatively less salient (or simply not a "need" at all). Next, for the relevant set of needs, we specify possible alternative profiles of services capable of meeting those needs.

For example, the selected candidate needs in a given instance might be the following: controlling cancer pain, dealing with grief, and obtaining respite care. One profile of services in response to these needs could be: drugs for cancer pain, pastoral services to deal with grief, and a pamphlet on dealing with the guilt associated with seeking respite care. An alternative service profile might be: no narcotics for pain, no pastoral counseling, and a computer-based cognitive behavioral therapy program to help the caregiver work through her guilt about seeking respite care. In a given profile, each service is specified to be at a particular *level*, e.g., for the need "controlling cancer pain," the service "providing drugs for cancer pain" represents one level, and "no narcotics for pain" represents another. Note that for a given set of needs (like the three above), there may be numerous possible profiles of services (not just two).

To proceed with the analysis, the respondent is asked to rate each of the service profiles in terms of relative desirability, either providing a simple rank order of profiles or else a numerical score for each profile in turn; for example, the latter scoring could be done on a 0–1 scale, where 1 is the score for the very best, or most salient, service profile, and 0 is the score for the worst, or least salient. Rank ordering is typically easier for the individual, but numerical scores may provide more precise information about profile saliency. Either way, these holistic profile ratings by the individual then become the values of the dependent variable in a multiple regression model of the following general form:

$$\text{Profile Score} = b_1 X_{k1} + \cdots + b_n X_{jn} + \cdots \\ + c_k X_{ig} X_{je} + \cdots + \text{error},$$

where X_{jn} is the jth level of a service associated with the nth need, error is a random error term, and (of greatest interest) the b's and the c's are the coefficients indicating the relative impact of the associated service profile components on the overall ranking of the profiles by the individual. Each estimated b indicates the "direct effect" of associated service level on the overall profile score; each c indicates the "interaction effect" of two levels of two different services on the overall profile score.

Once the model is estimated, it is straightforward to calculate the expected Profile Score associated with any possible set of Xs (that is, any possible service profile), and then to select that service profile that maximizes the expected (predicted) value of Profile Score. That becomes the service profile recommended for the individual, subject, of course, to the assumptions of the model and also to resource constraints – that is, the "optimal" service profile must also be feasible. The latter issue either can be dealt with after the fact or in advance by including in the model, in the first place, only resource-feasible service profiles.

At this point, one might wonder why the multiple regression model is even necessary – why not just select the service profile that received the individual's highest rating? The answer is that this ignores the potential importance of service level trade-offs and other interaction effects[77] which cannot be readily addressed when service profile scores are considered one-at-a-time. To examine whether these interaction effects exist and to allow for their impact on the predicted Profile Score one is trying to maximize, a statistical model of the type above is required. (Note that while the model shows only two-way interaction terms, multi-way interactions can be considered.)

While attractive in principle, conjoint analysis can pose problems in practice. It can be a daunting task for an individual respondent to rate all feasible combinations of service profiles. For example, if five needs are considered and there are three service levels associated with each need, there are 243 possible profiles to rate. The resulting respondent burden[77] is not only a concern in its own right, but may lead to inaccurate and inconsistent service profile ratings, which would bias the estimated model and generate erroneous inferences. There are two general responses to this problem. First, one can use fractional factorial designs[78] to select from all possible profiles a modest-size sample of profiles, strategically chosen to permit one to estimate regression models that contain many important (but not all possible) interaction terms.

The second response is to adopt an entirely different modeling strategy. Specifically, one would estimate for each individual a relatively more simple model for deriving the (implied) rank order of all service profiles. Most critically, such an approach would not seek to estimate service level interaction effects and their implications for trade-offs (wherein arise the complications, and also the strengths, of the conjoint approach). Then one would periodically and selectively test whether the simplifications gained through the new model come at the cost of ignoring important interaction effects by constructing yet another model precisely to test for the importance of this "information leakage."

To be specific, the simple model noted above could take the form of what has become known as the "self-explicated utility model."[79] In this model, the individual is asked to rate the relative importance of all candidate needs (say, on a 0–1 scale) and then, in a separate operation, the relative importance (utility) of alternative ways of meeting each of these needs (so that each level of each service is rated, in turn, on a 0–1 scale, say). Then the overall score imputed to any service profile is the weighted average of the specified service levels, where the weight for each service level is the importance score for the need it addresses. For example, if controlling pain has an importance score of 0.8 (where 1.0 is "most important") and "taking narcotics" has a utility score of 0.1 (because the individual simply does not like the idea of being drugged), the corresponding score for the service profile is $0.8 \times 0.1 = 0.08$. Such computations are performed for each service level, and the results summed to get a self-explicated utility score.

Clearly, interaction effects cannot be accounted for under this approach. To determine whether that is an important issue, one can estimate what has been termed a "hybrid conjoint model"[80] by obtaining, from selected individuals, both their self-explicated utility scores *and* their conjoint model scores (based on their rating service profiles, as above). Then one specifies a new regression model of the following form: the dependent variable is now (Profile Score – Self-Explicated Utility Score), and the right-hand-side covariates are precisely those shown in the conjoint model above. If the conjoint model is adding very little systematic information to the self-explicated utility model, one would expect the estimated regression coefficients to be generally small and uninformative and the overall explanatory power of the model to be poor. This would be consistent with the conclusion that the interaction effects accounted for by the conjoint model are not relatively important. On the other hand, if such interaction effects are important, one would expect the hybrid conjoint model to indicate this – both overall, as reflected in the adjusted R^2 value, and via the signs and statistical significance of the estimated coefficients. Indeed, the signs and magnitudes of these estimated coefficients serve to indicate for which needs and service levels the interaction effects are most salient.

Recommendations

There is no gold standard for needs assessments. While many instruments have positive features, much needs to be done before one is developed that can be considered outstanding. Five recommendations are made below that, if followed, would produce such a product.

(1) The needs of patients with cancer and their families must be more thoroughly identified.

Approaches such as the critical incident technique and person-focused interviews (long used in market research) should be employed. Some studies may have used these methods in developing cancer needs assessments, but it is impossible to determine this from the limited descriptions found in the literature. Researchers should document in detail how needs were identified in research reports. Labels such as "semi-structured interviews" should be replaced by a description of the structure and process actually used.

(2) Research should determine how needs change over time, with consideration of key events across different types of cancer and at different stages across the disease continuum.

(3) Given the large number of needs that are likely to result from following the first two recommendations, research should examine the potential of modern measurement theory (e.g., IRT), coupled with computer-based needs assessment programs, to select needs to be presented to specific people in ways that reduce respondent burden and improve completion rates. More emphasis should be placed on ensuring that needs assessments have good test-retest reliability, are sensitive enough to detect differences, and focus on a set of needs that are mutually exclusive and exhaustive. More research is also required to understand relationships among needs, as well as the relationships between needs and outcomes such as satisfaction, HRQOL, and economic burden.

(4) Research should be directed at defining needs and ways of meeting needs more operationally. Tools such as hybrid conjoint analysis may provide more effective ways to estimate the relative importance of and trade-offs between needs. One of the side benefits of these tools is that they force needs assessment developers to identify alternative ways to meet those needs. Even if conjoint analysis is not pursued, research should move needs assessment beyond simply rating "extent of need" to identifying evidence-based ways to meet needs.

(5) We believe evaluations of needs assessments should place less emphasis on domains and more on item analysis. Artificial intelligence may provide a way to obtain mathematical operations that would explore individual needs, instead of pursuing the reductionist approach of creating and evaluating domains of needs. Specifically we are proposing that data mining be used to identify relationships among individual needs and between those individual needs and satisfaction and HRQOL. In particular we propose that this approach be used to better determine the relationship between interventions and specific individual needs.

Acknowledgments

I wish to acknowledge the fine work that has been done by Kuang Yi Wen, a graduate student who has been working with me on this project. She has helped with much of the literature review and analysis that is included in this paper.

A number of other people have reviewed the paper and provided very important insights. Primary among them are Neeraj Arora Ph.D. of the National Cancer Institute. He not only reviewed an early draft of the paper but also provided references and insights that really helped define many of the issues. Charles Darby of the Agency for Healthcare Research and Quality as well as Eric Boberg Ph.D., Roger Brown Ph.D., and Neeraj Arora Ph.D. (Yes, another one!) of the University of Wisconsin also provided valuable input.

REFERENCES

1 Maslow, A. (1943). A theory of human motivation. *Psychology Review* **50**:370–96.

2 Langley, G., Nolan, K., Nolan, T. *et al.* (1996). *The Improvement Guide.* San Francisco: Jossey-Bass.

3 Berwick, D. (1997). The total customer relationship in health care: broadening the bandwidth. *The Joint Commission Journal On Quality Improvement* **23**:245–50.

4 Ross, C., Steward, C., Sinacore, J. M. (1993). The importance of patient preferences in the measurement of health care satisfaction. *Medical Care* **31**:138–49.

5 Suchman, A. L., Markakis, K., Beckman, H. B. *et al.* (1997). A model of empathic communication in the medical interview. *Journal of the American Medical Association* **277**:678–82.

6 Guadagnoli, E., Ward, P. (1998). Patient participation in decision-making. *Social Science and Medicine* **47**:329–39.

7 Frosch, D. L., Kaplan, R. M. (1999). Shared decision making in clinical medicine: past research and future directions. *American Journal of Preventive Medicine* **17**:285–94.

8 Charles, C., Gafni, A., Whelan, T. (1999). Decision making in the physician-patient encounter: revisiting the shared treatment decision-making model. *Social Science and Medicine* **49**:651–61.

9 Maguire, P. (1999). Improving communication with cancer patients. *European Journal of Cancer* **35**:1415–22.

10 Cull, A., Stewart, M., Altman, D. (1995). Assessment of and intervention for psychosocial problems in routine oncology practice. *British Journal of Cancer* **72**:229–35.

11 Osoba, D. (1996). Rationale for the timing of health related HRQOL assessments in oncological palliative therapy. *Cancer Treatment Review* **22A**:69–73.

12 Ford, S., Fallowfield, L., Lewis, S. (1996). Doctor-patient interactions in oncology. *Social Science and Medicine* **42**:1511–19.

13 Holland, J. C., Almanza, J. (1999). Giving bad news: is there a kinder, gentler way? *Cancer* **86**:738–40.

14 Kim, M. K., Alvi, A. (1999). Breaking the bad news of cancer: the patient's perspective. *Laryngoscope* **109**:1064–7.

15 Sabo, D. (1990). Men, death anxiety and denial. In *Clinical Sociological Perspectives of Illness and Loss*, ed. D. Clark, J. Fritz, P. Rieder, pp. 71–84. Philadelphia, PA: Charles Press.

16 Peters-Golden, H. (1982). Varied perceptions of social support in the illness experience. *Social Science and Medicine* **16**:463–91.

17 Northouse, L., Peters-Golden, H. (1993). Cancer and the family: strategies to assist spouses. *Seminars in Oncology Nursing* **9**:74–82.

18 Cegala, D. J. (1997). A study of doctors' and patients' communication during a primary care consultation: implications for communication training. *Journal of Health Communication* **2**:169–94.

19 Northouse, L. (1988). Social support in patients and husbands adjustment to breast cancer. *Nursing Research* **37**:91–5.

20 Northouse, P., Northouse, L. (1987). Communication and cancer: Issues confronting patients, health professionals

and caregivers. *Journal of Psychosocial Oncology* **5**:17–46.

21 Vitaliano, P. (1997). Physiological and physical concomitants of caregiving; introduction to special issue. *Annals of Behavioral Medicine* **19**:75–7.

22 Schulz, R., Beach, S. (1999). Caregiving as a risk factor for mortality. *Journal of the American Medical Association* **282**:2215–19.

23 Morris, J., Sussa, S., Sherwood, S. *et al.* (1986). Last days: a study of the HRQOL of terminally ill cancer patients. *Journal of Chronic Disease* **39**:47–62.

24 Ward, S., Goldberg, N., Miller-McCauley, V. *et al.* (1993). Patient-related barriers to management of cancer pain. *Pain* **52**:319–24.

25 Bretsher, M., Rummons, R., Sloan J. *et al.* (1999). HRQOL in hospice patients. *Psychosomatics* **40**:309–13.

26 Silveira, M., De Piero, A., Gerrity, M. *et al.* (2000). Patients knowledge of options at the end of life. *Journal of the American Medical Association* **284**:2483–8.

27 Institute of Medicine (1997). *Approaching Death: Improving Care at the End of Life*, ed. M. Field, C. Cassel. Washington, DC: Institute of Medicine.

28 Lawton, M. (2000). *The End of Life: Scientific and Social Issues (Annual Review of Gerontology and Geriatrics)*. New York: Springer.

29 Mor, V., Masterson-Allen, S., Houts, P. *et al.* (1992). The changing needs of patients with cancer at home. *Cancer* **69**:829–38.

30 Northouse, L. (1988). A longitudinal study of the adjustment of patients and husbands to breast cancer. *Oncology Nurses Forum* **16**:511–16.

31 Ell, K., Nishimoto, R., Mantell, J. *et al.* (1988). Longitudinal analysis of psychological adaptation among family members of patients with cancer. *Journal of Psychosomatic Research* **32**:429–38.

32 Wilson, S., Morse, J. (1991). Living with a wife undergoing chemotherapy. *Image* **23**: 78–84.

33 Wilkerson, S. (1991). Factors which influence how nurses communicate with cancer patients. *Journal of Advanced Nursing* **16**:677–88.

34 Gustafson, D. (1991). Expanding on the role of patient as customer. *Quality Review Bulletin* **17**:324–5.

35 Ferrans, this volume, Chapter 2.

36 Marvel, M. K., Epstein, R. M., Flowers, K. *et al.* (1999). Soliciting the patient's agenda: have we improved? *Journal of the American Medical Association* **281**:283–7.

37 Grobe, M. E., Ahmann, D. L., Ilstrup, D. M. (1982). Needs assessment for advance cancer patients and their families. *Oncology Nursing Forum* **9**:26–30.

38 Longman, A. J., Atwood, J. R., Sherman, J. B. *et al.* (1992). Care needs of home-based cancer patients and their caregivers. *Cancer Nursing* **15**:182–90.

39 Thomas, S., Glynne Jones, R., Chait, I. (1997). Is it worth the wait? A survey of patients' satisfaction with an oncology outpatient clinic. *European Journal of Cancer Care in England* **6**:50–8.

40 Davis, S. W., Quinn, S., Fox, L. *et al.* (1988). Satisfaction among cancer outpatients. *Programs for Clinical Biological Research* **278**:227–32.

41 Darby, this volume, Chapter 14.

42 Schag, C. C., Heinrich, R. L., Ganz, P. A. (1983). Cancer Inventory of Problem Situations: an instrument for assessing cancer patients' rehabilitation needs. *Journal of Psychosocial Oncology* **1**:11–24.

43 Schag, C. C., Ganz, P. A., Heinrich, R. L. (1991). Cancer Rehabilitation Evaluation System-Short Form (CARES-SF). A cancer specific rehabilitation and quality of life instrument. *Cancer* **15**:1406–13.

44 Gates, M. F., Lackey, N. R., White, M. R. (1995). Needs of hospice and clinic patients with cancer. *Cancer Practice* **3**: 226–32.

45 Foot, G., Sanson-Fisher, R. (1995). Measuring the unmet needs of people living with cancer. *Cancer Forum* **19**: 131–5.

46 Bonevski, B., Sanson-Fisher, R., Girgis, A. *et al.* (2000). Evaluation of an instrument to assess the needs of patients with cancer. *Cancer* **88**:217–25.

47 McCusker, J. (1984). Development of scales to measure satisfaction and preferences regarding long-term and terminal care. *Medical Care* **22**:476–93.

48 Tamburini, M., Gangeri, L., Brunelli, C. *et al.* (2000). Assessment of hospitalized cancer patients' needs by the Needs Evaluation Questionnaire. *Annals of Oncology* **11**: 31–7.

49 Coyle, N., Goldstein, L., Passik, S. *et al.* (1996). Development and validation of a patient needs assessment tool (PNAT) for oncology clinicians. *Cancer Nursing* **19**:81–92.

50 Derdiarian, A. K. (1986). Informational needs of recently diagnosed cancer patients. *Nursing Research* **36**:276–81.

51 Mesters, I., Borne van den, B., Boer, M. D. *et al.* (2001). Measuring information needs among cancer patients. *Patient Education and Counseling* **43**:253–62.

52 Boberg, E., Gustafson, D., Hawkins, R. (2002). Assessing the unmet information, support and care delivery needs of men with prostate cancer. *Patient Education and Counseling* **49** (3):233–42.

53 Galloway, S., Graydon, J., Harrison, D. *et al.* (1997). Informational needs of women with a recent diagnosis of breast cancer: development and initial testing of a tool. *Journal of Advanced Nursing* **25**:1175–83.

54 McCarthy, M., Higginson, I. (1991). Clinical audit by a palliative care team. *Palliative Medicine* **5**:215–21.

55 Ellershaw, J. E., Peat, S. J., Boys, L. C. (1995). Assessing the effectiveness of a hospital palliative care team. *Palliative Medicine* **9**:145–52.

56 Emanuel, L. L., Alpert, H. R., Baldwin, D. C. *et al.* (2000). What terminally ill patients care about: toward a validated construct of patients' perspectives. *Journal of Palliative Medicine* **3**:419–31.

57 Kristjanson, L. J., Atwood, J., Degner, L. F. (1995). Validity and reliability of the Family Inventory of Needs (FIN): measuring the care needs of families of advanced cancer patients. *Journal of Nursing Measurement* **3**:109–26.

58 Kipatrick, M. G., Kristjanson, L. J., Tataryn, D. (1998). Measuring the information needs of husbands of women with breast cancer: validity and reliability of the Family Inventory of Needs-Husbands. *Oncology Nursing Forum* **25**: 1347–51.

59 Kristjanson, L. J. (1993). Validity and reliability testing of the FAMCARE scale: Measure Family Satisfaction with Advance Cancer Care. *Social Science and Medicine* **36**:693–701.

60 Chalmers, K. I., Luker, K. A., Leinster, S. J. *et al.* (2001). Information and support needs of women with primary relatives with breast cancer: development of the Information and Support Needs Questionnaire. *Journal of Advance Nursing* **35**:497–507.

61 Prigerson, H. G., Maciejewski, P. K., Reynolds, C. F. *et al.* (1995). Inventory of complicated grief: a scale to measure maladaptive symptoms of loss. *Psychiatry Research* **59**: 65–79.

62 Lev, E. L., Munro, B. H., McCorkle, R. (1993). A shortened version of an instrument measuring bereavement. *International Journal of Nursing Studies* **30**:213–26.

63 Gustafson, D. H., Arora, N. K., Nelson, E. C. *et al.* (2001). Increasing understanding of patient needs during and after hospitalization. *The Joint Commission Journal on Quality Improvement* **27**:81–92.

64 Reise, this volume, Chapter 21.

65 Miller, M. (1995). Coefficient alpha: a basic introduction from the perspectives of classical theory and structural equation modeling. *Structural Equation Modeling* **2**:255–73.

66 Novick, M., Lewis, C. (1967). Coefficient alpha and the reliability of composite measurements. *Psychometrika* **32**:1–13.

67 Siegel, K., Palamara, M., Karus, D. *et al.* (1992). Reducing the prevalence of unmet needs for concrete services of patients with cancer. *Cancer* **69**:1873–83.

68 Flanagan, J. (1954). The critical incident technique. *Psychology Bulletin* **51**:327–58.

69 Craig, T. J., Comstock, G. W., Geiser, P. B. (1974). Quality of survival in breast cancer care – control comparison. *Cancer* **33**:1451–7.

70 Fieldman, J. G., Gardner, B., Carter, A. C. *et al.* (1989). Relationship of race to functional status among breast cancer patients after surgery. *Journal of Surgical Oncology* **11**:333–9.

71 Lehmann, J. F., Delisa, J. A., Warren, C. G. *et al.* (1978). Cancer rehabilitation: assessment of need, development and evaluation of a model of care. *Archives of Physical Medicine and Rehabilitation* **58**:410–19.

72 Mor, V., Guadagnoli, E., Wool, M. (1987). An examination of the concrete service needs of advanced cancer patients. *Journal of Psychosocial Oncology* **5**:1–17.

73 Hilerman, J., Ackerman, N., Hassanein, R. (1992). Identifying the needs of home caregivers of patients with cancer. *Oncology Nursing Forum* **19**:771–7.

74 Leis, A., Kristjanson, L., Koop, P. *et al.* (1997). Family health and the palliative care trajectory: a cancer research agenda. *Prevention et Controle en Cancerologie* **1**:352–60.

75 Galloway, S. (1994). Meeting information needs of women with breast cancer (Abstract). *Canadian Oncology Nursing Journal* **14**:29.

76 Graf, M. A., Tanner, D. D., Swinyard, W. R. (1993). Optimizing the delivery of patient and physician satisfaction: a conjoint analysis approach. *Health Care Management Review* **18**:34–43.

77 Green, P. E., Srinivasan, V. (1978). Conjoint analysis in customer research: issues and outlook. *Journal of Customer Research* **5**:103–23.

78 Green, P. E. (1974). On the design of choice experiments involving multifactor alternatives. *Journal of Customer Research* **1**:61–8.

79 Huber, G. P. (1974). Multiattribute utility models: a review of field and field-like studies. *Management Science* **20**:1393–402.

80 Green, P. E. (1984). Hybrid conjoint analysis: an expository review. *Journal of Marketing Research* **21**:155–9.

16

Assessing the subjective impact of caregiving on informal caregivers of cancer patients

Claire Snyder, M.H.S.

National Cancer Institute, Bethesda, MD

Introduction

Cancer and its treatment affect not only the patients who have the disease but also their friends and family members who frequently play an important role in providing care. The impact on these "informal" caregivers is multidimensional, affecting many aspects of their everyday activities and emotional well-being. In many cases, caregivers who are also friends or relatives of patients provide emotional support, as well as assist with physical tasks and participate in the delivery of care. As a consequence, these informal caregivers may experience changes in their own social roles, may experience stress, anxiety and/or depression, or have physical effects. However, there are also positive aspects of providing care to a friend or family member, including satisfaction in caring for a loved one and in giving.

The impact on informal caregivers of caring for sick loved ones is of increasing importance as patients with cancer are living longer, policies are pushing care from the inpatient to the outpatient setting, and patients increasingly are preferring to receive care at home. Consequently, there are growing numbers of informal caregivers who are experiencing both the positive and negative impacts of caregiving. As informal caregivers continue to play an important part in the care of patients with cancer, the health care system needs to ensure that the patient is receiving quality care without undue strain on these individuals – strain that could compromise their ability to provide needed care to patients and which could also threaten their own health and well-being. While the degree of caregiver strain or burden is subjective, it can and should be assessed to ensure that caregivers are able to provide the care that patients need without putting themselves and the patient at risk. Thus, in addition to measuring the health-related quality-of-life effects of cancer and its treatment on patients, it is important to consider the impact of the disease and the caregiving role on patients' family members and friends.

The literature differentiates between objective and subjective caregiving impacts experienced by friends and family members of cancer patients.[1–5] For this chapter, the *objective impacts* are defined as those that describe the caregiver's activities but do not assess the caregiver's perception of the impact. Objective impacts include the number and types of caregiving tasks and the time spent on those tasks, including grocery shopping, assisting the patient with activities of daily living, and child care activities. *Subjective impacts* relate to the caregiver's feelings about the tasks s/he is performing for the patient and their psychosocial effects, including depression, anxiety, feelings of burden, and sense of satisfaction. For example, caring for a cancer patient may require financial outlays. The amount of these financial outlays is an objective effect; however, any stress experienced due to finances is considered a subjective impact. This chapter focuses on the various measures that have been developed to assess the subjective impact on informal caregivers of cancer patients.

Methods

Literature search

Two literature searches were conducted to identify articles relevant to subjective caregiver impact related to cancer. Both searches were conducted in MEDLINE through Internet Grateful Med. Searches covered the period 1966 through Spring 2001 and were limited to studies on human subjects that were reported in English. Searches were not limited by age, gender, or publication type.

The first search was for articles that had "caregiver" and "burden" or "impact" and "cancer" as subject headings. Seventy-nine abstracts were identified and reviewed for relevance. Articles were considered not relevant if they focused on caregivers of child patients (because the four cancers of interest here – lung, prostate, breast, and colorectal – affect adults); professional, paid caregivers (because this research is focused on unpaid informal caregivers), or if caregivers were used as proxies for patient responses (because our focus is on the impact on the caregivers themselves). From these 79 abstracts, 52 articles were selected for further review. While the Cancer Outcomes Measurement Working Group (COMWG) focuses primarily on breast, prostate, lung, and colorectal cancer, this review also included reports of other cancers.

The second search was for articles that had "caregiver" and "burden" or "impact" and "measure" as subject headings to identify instruments used to measure caregiver impact in other disease areas and to determine their applicability to cancer. Seventy-nine abstracts were identified and reviewed for relevance. From this search, articles were considered relevant only if they discussed a caregiver impact measurement model that used a structured questionnaire to assess impacts on the caregivers themselves; economic or financial impacts were not included. From these 79 abstracts, 31 articles were selected for further review. Articles that described

questionnaires developed specifically for use in non-cancer study populations were not generally abstracted.

Relevant articles were also identified from the reference lists of abstracted articles and the author's files. After further review, a total of 72 articles were deemed relevant and were abstracted.

Data abstraction

For each relevant article, the following data were abstracted: citation, definition of caregiver impact, intervention studied, study population, cancer type, part of the continuum of care, domains identified, and questionnaires used to assess the subjective caregiver impact. This information was used to develop a conceptual model of caregiver impact and to identify measures commonly used to assess the subjective impact of providing care to cancer patients.

Data related to the development and validation history of subjective caregiver impact questionnaires also were abstracted, including purpose for which the instrument was developed, length of questionnaire and item format, administration time, domains included, scoring methodology, validated modes of administration, validated translations/cultural adaptations, evidence of reliability (internal consistency, test-retest, other), evidence of validity (content, construct, criterion-related), evidence of responsiveness/sensitivity to change, interpretability (availability of normative data, clinically meaningful difference), and practical issues (respondent and administrative burden).

Analysis

The abstracted data were used to identify common themes in subjective caregiver impact and the most frequently used questionnaires that assess this outcome. First, a definition of subjective caregiver impact was developed. Then a conceptual model based on the concepts reported in the literature as being related to caregiver impact was constructed. The most commonly used questionnaires were compared and contrasted to identify their relative strengths and weaknesses based on attributes such as comprehensiveness, reliability, validity, responsiveness, interpretability, and practical matters.

Results

Definition

For this analysis, caregivers were considered to be the informal, unpaid care providers of patients with cancer. In the studies reviewed, caregivers were primarily spouses and adult children, but some informal caregivers were friends or neighbors. Most caregivers were women and frequently they were the wives or daughters of the cancer patient.

There were few definitions of caregiver "burden" or caregiver "impact" reported in the literature. In this review, the effect on the caregiver of caring for the patient with cancer is referred to as *subjective caregiver impact*. The word "impact" was selected over "burden" because the literature reports both positive and negative consequences of caregiving, and burden (with its negative connotation) is just one of many impacts of caregiving. Therefore, *subjective caregiver impact is defined here as the effect of the patient's disease and treatment on the informal caregiver's everyday life and overall well-being*. Objective measures, such as hours spent in caregiving activities or the economic cost of taking care of the patients, are not included in this definition, while the subjective evaluations of the impact of the hours spent caregiving or stress about finances are included.

Conceptual model

A conceptual model was constructed to further develop the concept of subjective caregiver impact (Figure 16.1). The model illustrates the content/definition of subjective caregiver impact. It is empirically based and not derived from a theoretical perspective.

The literature review identified four domains that are affected by caregiving, and these were used to construct the model. Each domain has the potential for positive and negative effects. The *emotional* domain relates to the impacts on the caregiver's feelings. The *social/role* domain addresses changes in how the caregiver relates to other people and the environment. The *physical* domain covers the physical demands of caregiving and the caregiver's own physical well-being. The *spiritual* domain focuses on caregivers' relationships to a higher spiritual power or to their general existential being. Each domain is described in more detail below.

Emotional

Many of the issues related to subjective caregiver impact fall into the emotional domain. Caring for a family member or friend can have a wide range of impacts on the caregiver's psychological and emotional well-being.[2,6–22] Depression[2,10,19,21–41] and anxiety[2,19,21–27,30,35,38,39,41–45] are the most commonly cited emotional impacts experienced by caregivers and stem from worry and concern about the patient's health and well-being.[11] Caregivers may experience uncertainty over the patient's health[44] and commonly feel helpless[19,21–24,26,30,42] and frustrated[12,15,24,30,42] as they try to care for the patient. They might be confused[19,21,22,25] over what to do and experience stress and strain related to their caregiving duties.[12,15,24,32,34,43,44,46]

In addition, caregivers may experience anger[15,19,21,22,24,25,28,42] and resentment.[13,24] These feelings might lead to conflict[32,34] and tension.[44,47] Caregivers might also feel guilty[32,34] and experience burn-out over time.[15]

Financial impact is another source of emotional distress for caregivers. They may worry about finances[24,48] and experience financial stress, strain, or burden.[13,14,17–22,25,28,33,40,49]

Fear is another common emotion experienced by caregivers.[50] The fear might be related to the cancer and its treatment[23,45] or death.[27] Ferrell and others identified the caregiver's fear that the patient will become addicted to painkillers,[26,30] which relates to

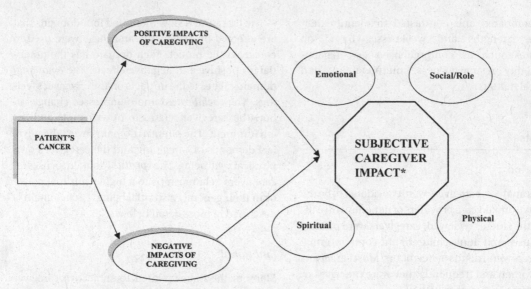

*One aspect of caregiver's health-related quality of life.

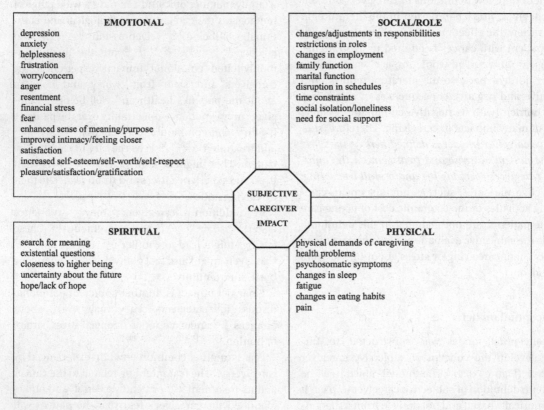

Figure 16.1. Conceptual model of subjective caregiver impact. Top section represents overall model and bottom section provides detail of the emotional, social/role, spiritual, and physical impacts.

the general concerns of caregivers about managing the patient's pain[51] and how they themselves are trying to deal with the patient's pain.[49]

Researchers have also cited many positive emotional impacts of caring for a friend or family member with cancer.[14,36] For example, caregivers may experience an enhanced sense of meaning or purpose.[40,48] The caregiving could also strengthen the emotional ties between the caregiver and patient leading to increased intimacy and feeling closer.[40] Caregivers might experience satisfaction[2,7,12,52] from their caregiving and have increased self-esteem, self-worth, and self-respect,[2,15,33,48,52,53] and they may also feel they are preventing the further deterioration of the patient.[48] These positive emotions lead to feelings of pleasure,[48] gratification,[2,52] and what some authors refer to as uplifts.[2,52] Caregiving may evoke positive emotions if caregivers feel they are filling a commitment/obligation successfully[15] or repaying earlier care received.[40] They may feel appreciated[48] and have a sense of attachment, responsibility, and pride.[13] Picot *et al.* summarized the rewards of caregiving as *external* ("verbal or nonverbal communication from God, health care professionals, and the carereceiver regarding the quality of the caregiver's caregiving") and *internal* ("the caregiver's personal feelings of achievement and growth") (p. 35).[54]

Social/Role

Caregivers may experience many and varied changes in their role responsibilities[7,13,17,18,20,23,27,28,31,37,40,44,45,47,55] and social[8,14,16,17–22,24,44,55,56] functioning.

Caregivers commonly experience changes and adjustments in role responsibilities,[10] related, in part, to taking on the patient's vacated roles and assuming the nursing care role.[6] Caregivers may experience restrictions in their roles[39,41] related to their ability to work,[57] and some caregivers may change employment.[58]

When a family member has cancer and other family members take up the caregiving roles, family function is affected.[7,18–22,25,40,49] These changes can lead to either enhancements or decrements in the

caregiver's relationship with the impaired person or other family members.[9,28,36,48] The families may experience changes in communication[43] and conflict.[42] Marital function is commonly affected,[19,21,22,24] leading sometimes to strain[39,41] or changes in marital cohesion.[55]

Caregivers also experience changes in their relationships with the world outside of their families. There is commonly an impact or disruption in their schedules.[19,21,22,25,32,33,38,40,46,49,50,52,53] Their activities and lives may be restricted and disrupted[39,41,43,46,59] because of caregiving demands. These demands can lead to time constraints,[45] leaving caregivers with little time for themselves[28] and their social lives and activities.[9,28] As a result, the caregiver may feel emotionally and socially isolated or lonely.[2,12,13,27,50]

A key aspect of the social/role domain is the need for social support.[20,35,40,45,46,56] The role of family and friend support, or abandonment, is key in how the caregiver perceives the impact of caregiving.[6,33,36,38,43,52,53] Some caregivers may perceive unmet needs for more help not only from family and friends but also need for professional support and information and services.[59]

Physical

Caring for a cancer patient may affect the caregiver's own physical well-being.[16] First, there are the actual physical demands of caregiving from assisting patients with their needs.[10,13,19,21,22,50] These caregiving tasks may impact the health of the caregiver[6,9,17–19,21,22,32,34,38–41,44,45,53] and lead to health problems[12,15,52] or psychosomatic symptoms.[19,21,22,39,41] The most commonly cited physical effects are changes in sleep,[8,23,47] fatigue,[2,8,12,17,24–27,30,34,35,40,45,60,61] and physical exhaustion.[34] Caregivers might also experience pain and changes in their appetite or eating habits.[23]

Spiritual

Being a caregiver may also affect the person's spirituality.[8] Caregivers may search for meaning and have existential questions related to their own health.[2] The caregiving experience might affect the caregiver's closeness to a higher spiritual being(s). Caregivers may also experience uncertainty about the future and feel hope or lack of hope. The spiritual domain is not well explored; more research is needed to improve our understanding of the role of this domain.

Overall description of measures

From the 72 articles reviewed, over 50 different instruments to measure subjective caregiver impact were identified. Few of these instruments were used in more than two different studies, but many studies used two or more instruments. In addition, there were studies that developed specific measures unique to their studies, and many studies used qualitative or semi-structured interviews or focus groups. Also, the names or titles used to identify the different questionnaires were not always used in a consistent manner, which made it difficult to determine whether the reference was to a previously used instrument or a different one. In some cases, the same name was used for an instrument in different studies, but the descriptions of the instruments indicated they were not the same. In other cases, slightly different names were used to identify the same instrument, and it was difficult to ascertain whether the reference was to the same or different instruments. Thus, there is little consistency in how subjective caregiver impact is assessed and reported, making it difficult to determine what questionnaires were used and how.

Some of the more commonly used instruments include the Center for Epidemiological Studies-Depression scale and the State-Trait Anxiety Inventory; other measures of depression, such as the Beck Depression Inventory and General Health Questionnaire, were also used but with less frequency. Other studies reported use of instruments that measured outcomes related to specific domains such as fatigue, family function, and social support. Several studies included a general health status measure, most commonly some form of the MOS SF-36.

Other studies focused specifically on caregiver issues related to managing the patient's pain, and these used questionnaires developed specifically for that purpose.

Many studies used some form of a multidimensional assessment of the subjective impact on caregivers. A wide range of such instruments was used; however, few were used more than three times. The Caregiver Reaction Assessment (or subscales thereof), the most commonly used measure, was used in over 10 studies. An instrument developed specifically for use in caregivers of cancer patients, the Caregiver Quality of Life Index-Cancer, was used three times.

The Caregiver Reaction Assessment and Caregiver Quality of Life Index-Cancer are described below and summarized in Table 16.1. In addition, brief summaries of less commonly used measures that have potential applicability in cancer follow.

Commonly used measures

Caregiver Reaction Assessment (CRA)

The Caregiver Reaction Assessment (sometimes referred to as the Caregiver Reaction Inventory) was developed by Given and others[53] in the USA to measure family members reactions to caring for older persons with physical impairments, Alzheimer's disease, and cancer.

To generate the items for the CRA, the researchers reviewed the literature and conducted in-depth interviews with caregivers to identify common themes. Once the themes were identified, the researchers generated 111 items, which after sorting was reduced to 101 items. The 101-item instrument was administered to a convenience sample of 99 caregivers to eliminate items that were unclear, had no variation, or did not correlate with other items. After elimination, 40 items remained, and during the exploratory and confirmatory factor analysis, the items were further reduced to produce the final 24-item instrument. This methodology should contribute to the instrument's content validity.

Table 16.1. Subjective Caregiver Impact Measures

	Caregiver Reaction Assessment	Caregiver Quality of Life Index-Cancer
Purpose for Which Developed	To measure family members reactions to caring for older persons with physical impairments, Alzheimer's disease, and cancer[53]	To assess health-related quality of life in caregivers of persons with cancer[19]
Length and Item Format	24 items with 5-point Likert scale from "Strongly Agree" to "Strongly Disagree"	35 items with 5-point Likert-type scale
Administration Time	In Dutch sample, 10 minutes on average for a trained research assistant to complete the CRA during a face-to-face interview[52]	10 minutes[19,21]
Domains Included	Impact on schedule (5 items); caregiver's esteem (7 items); lack of family support (5 items); impact on health (4 items); impact on finances (3 items)	No subscales
Scoring	Each subscale scored as average of item scores; range between 1.00 and 5.00 with higher score representing greater impact; no overall score[52]	Single total score
Practical Issues	97% completely filled out the CRA[52]	No missing data for the 263 caregivers who completed the packets;[19] no missing data for the 239 caregivers who completed the packets[21]
Validated Modes of Administration	Dutch version was both administered in face-to-face interviews and through self-report questionnaires[52]	Self-report questionnaires[21]
Validated Translations/Cultural Adaptations	Dutch[52]	None found
Evidence of Reliability (internal consistency, test-retest, other)	**Internal consistency:** alpha coefficient ranges from 0.80 for impact on health to 0.90 for caregiver's esteem in initial sample of 377 caregivers;[53] alpha coefficient ranges from 0.62 for lack of family support to 0.83 for financial problems in Dutch sample[52]	**Internal consistency:** Cronbach's alpha of 0.91 in a sample of 263 family caregivers;[19] Cronbach's alpha of 0.87 in a sample of 239 family caregivers of hospice patients[21] **Test-retest:** reliability of 0.95 in a sample of 263 family caregivers who completed two questionnaires 14 days apart[19]
Evidence of Validity (content, construct, criterion-related)	**Content:** items generated by project staff based on dimensions identified from a review of the literature and in-depth interviews with caregivers; all five project staff members had to agree on dimension to which items were related[53] **Construct:** exploratory factor analysis using a sample of 377 caregivers of elderly patients from lower Michigan yielded 5 subscales with a total of 24 items; confirmatory factor analysis, conducted in a sample of 276 caregivers of cancer patients and 101 caregivers of	**Content:** item pool generated through semi-structured interviews with patients, their caregivers, and healthcare professionals – 3 of the investigators analyzed the interviews to develop 120 phrases and after reduction for redundancy 91 items remained; item reduction through administration of initial pool of 91 items to 96 caregivers and 70 patients

(cont.)

Table 16.1. (*cont.*)

	Caregiver Reaction Assessment	Caregiver Quality of Life Index-Cancer
Evidence of Validity (cont'd)	Alzheimer's/dementia patients, demonstrated that factor loadings are the same for spouses vs. nonspouses and caregivers of Alzheimer's vs. caregivers of cancer patients; factors also demonstrated longitudinal stability;[53] correlations of the five subscales of the CRA with the number of patient dependencies in ADLs and caregivers' levels of depression provides additional support for construct validity;[53] 21 of 24 items loaded as hypothesized in the Dutch version and there was some indication that the health problems and disrupted schedule scales were not as independent as in other samples;[52] strong correlations were seen between scales specifically assessing burden and CRA subscales of disrupted schedule and health problems; there were high correlations between the impact on self-esteem and personal accomplishments, but the correlations indicate that impact of caregiving is not related to self-perceived pressure from caregiving, social activities changes, overall burden, and depression; personal accomplishment was either unrelated or had slight negative relationships to the four negative CRA subscales[52]	to obtain ranking of importance resulted in a final list of 35 items[19] **Construct:** in a sample of 263 family caregivers, convergent validity was supported by moderate correlations with overall mental health ($r = 0.64$), emotional distress ($r = -0.50$ to -0.52), burden ($r = -0.65$), and patient's performance status ($r = -0.47$), and divergent validity was supported by low correlations with overall physical health ($r = 0.13$), social support ($r = 0.22$), and social desirability ($r = 0.08$);[19] in a sample of 239 caregivers of hospice patients, construct validity was again supported by moderate correlations with overall mental health ($r = 0.68$) and low correlations with overall physical health ($r = 0.01$);[21] however, contrary to hypotheses, low correlations with patient's performance status ($r = 0.09$) rather than significant negative correlations were found[21]
Evidence of Responsiveness/ Sensitivity to Change	Evidence of longitudinal factor stability indicates suitability for measurement of change over time[53]	CQOLC was significantly negatively correlated with the patient's ECOG performance status and significantly negatively correlated to the number of treatment modalities the patient received in a cross-sectional sample;[19] contrary to hypotheses, low correlations with patient's performance status ($r = 0.09$) rather than significant negative correlations were found in a separate sample[21]
Interpretability (availability of normative data, clinically meaningful difference)	Not found	Not found

The instrument uses a 5-point Likert scale of responses from "Strongly Agree" to "Strongly Disagree." The 24 items are grouped into five domains, which are described by Given *et al.*[53] as follows. The *impact on schedule* subscale (5 items) assesses the degree to which caregiving interrupts usual activities, causes the elimination of some activities, and interferes with relaxation time. The *caregiver's esteem* subscale (7 items) addresses how caregiving affects the individual's self-esteem, including whether caregiving is enjoyable and rewarding or leads to resentment. The *lack of family support* subscale (5 items) measures how families support and work together with the caregiver and whether the caregiver perceives this support to be adequate. The *impact on health* subscale (4 items) assesses whether the caregiver is physically capable of and has the energy to provide care. Finally, the *impact on finances* subscale (3 items) addresses the impact of adequacy, difficulty, and strain of the financial situation on the caregiver and the family.

Each subscale is scored as the average of its item scores.[52] The scores range from 1.00 to 5.00, with higher scores representing a greater impact. There is no overall score. In a study conducted in the Netherlands of 181 partners of colorectal cancer patients, it took 10 minutes on average for a trained research assistant to complete the CRA in a face-to-face interview, and 97% of the sample completed it fully.[52] The Dutch version of the questionnaire was administered in both face-to-face interviews and as a self-report questionnaire,[52] and it is the only translation of the CRA instrument identified in the literature search.

In the initial validation sample of 377 caregivers in the US, Cronbach's alpha (used to measure the internal consistency reliability of each subscale) ranged from 0.80 for impact on health to 0.90 for caregiver's esteem.[53] However, in the Dutch study,[52] the reliability coefficients ranged from 0.62 for lack of family support to 0.83 for financial problems. Pasacreta *et al.*[13] used the CRA to assess a caregiver cancer education program; in this study, Cronbach's alpha ranged from 0.71 for impact on health to 0.85 for lack of support. Other studies[10,27,32,34,54,59,61,62]

used only subscales of the CRA, most commonly the impact on schedule and impact on health scales.

Given *et al.* also explored the construct validity of the questionnaire.[53] In an exploratory factor analysis using a sample of 377 caregivers of elderly patients from lower Michigan, 5 subscales with a total of 24 items were identified. Confirmatory factor analysis, conducted in a sample of 276 caregivers of cancer patients and 101 caregivers of Alzheimer's/dementia patients, demonstrated that the factor loadings are the same for spouses and nonspouses and for caregivers of Alzheimer's and cancer patients. The factors also demonstrated longitudinal stability (factorial invariance across comparison groups and measurement occasions).

In the translated Dutch version of the CRA, the factors were generally the same.[52] Specifically, 21 of 24 items loaded as hypothesized in the Dutch version, but there was some indication that the impact on health and impact on schedule scales were not as independent as in the other samples. The Dutch sample also provides further evidence of construct validity.[52] Strong correlations were seen between scales specifically assessing burden and CRA subscales of disrupted schedule and health problems. There were high correlations between the impact of caregiving on self-esteem and personal accomplishments, but the correlations indicate that impact of caregiving is not related to the self-perceived pressure from informal care, changes in social activities, overall burden, and depression. Personal accomplishment was either unrelated or had slight negative relationship to the four negative subscales of the CRA.

The only evidence of responsiveness (i.e., ability of an instrument to detect change) seen in the literature review was of longitudinal factor stability, indicating suitability for measurement of change over time.[53]

The literature review did not indicate the availability of normative data or consideration of what changes in the CRA scales should be regarded as clinically meaningful. However, to the extent that the CRA has been used more than other measures of multidimensional caregiver impact, there is relatively more knowledge of the characteristics and distributions of scores for various samples.

Caregiver Quality of Life Index-Cancer (CQOLC)

The Caregiver Quality of Life Index-Cancer was developed by Weitzner et al.[19,22] to assess health-related quality of life in caregivers of persons with cancer. The authors, following conceptual models developed by Ware and Cella, consider the quality of life of caregivers to be multidimensional, including areas of physical functioning, emotional functioning, family functioning, and social functioning.[22] The methodology used to develop the instrument contributes to its content validity.[19] Specifically, an item pool was generated through semi-structured interviews with patients, their caregivers, and health care professionals. Then, three of the researchers analyzed the interviews and developed 120 phrases. After reduction for redundancy, 91 items remained. The researchers then administered these 91 items to 96 caregivers and 70 patients to obtain a ranking of item importance. Items with a cumulative frequency of at least 60% for responses of "slightly important," "moderately important," or "extremely important" were retained.

The final questionnaire includes 35 items answered using a 5-point Likert-type scale. The CQOLC is not broken into subscales and thus only provides an overall score.[19] Administration time is approximately 10 minutes,[19,41] and there were no missing data for samples of 263 and 239 caregivers.[19,21] The only mode of administration found in the literature was self-report, and no validated language translations or cultural adaptations were found.

Several studies assessed the instrument's reliability. In a sample of 263 family caregivers of cancer patients, Cronbach's alpha was 0.91.[19] This study also assessed test-retest reliability over 14 days, which was 0.95.[19] In a separate study of 239 family caregivers of hospice patients, Cronbach's alpha was 0.87.[21]

The researchers also provide evidence of the instrument's construct validity. In the sample of 263 family caregivers,[19] convergent and divergent validity were assessed. Convergent validity was supported by moderate correlations with overall mental health, emotional distress, burden, and patient's performance status. Divergent validity was supported by low correlations with overall physical health, social support, and social desirability. In a separate study of 239 caregivers of hospice patients,[21] construct validity was again supported by moderate correlations with overall mental health and low correlations with overall physical health. However, contrary to the researchers' hypotheses, low correlations with patient's performance status rather than significant negative correlations were found. In a study comparing the quality of life among caregivers of cancer patients receiving curative treatments versus those receiving palliative care, CQOLC scores were lower for caregivers of patients receiving palliative care.[41]

The researchers provide some evidence of responsiveness. First, they hypothesized that the CQOLC would be statistically significantly negatively correlated with performance status, as they expect caregiver HRQOL to worsen as the patient's performance status worsens.[19,21] The hypothesis was sustained in one study but not the other. Specifically, in a cross-sectional sample, the CQOLC was significantly negatively correlated with the patient's ECOG performance status.[19] However, low correlations with patient's performance status (r = 0.09) rather than significant negative correlations were found in the hospice care study.[21] Also, as hypothesized in the cross-sectional sample, CQOLC scores were significantly negatively correlated with the number of treatment modalities the patient received.[19] Because some findings did not support the hypotheses, more study of the instrument's responsiveness is required.

There was no mention in the literature reviewed of the availability of normative data or definition of clinically meaningful difference. As the CQOLC is used more frequently, data on its performance and scoring may lead to improved interpretability.

Other caregiver impact measures

The CRA and CQOLC were the two most frequently used questionnaires found in the literature review;

however, the literature search also identified other instruments used in at least two studies. These questionnaires are briefly described below. Because this field is relatively young, there are many more questionnaires that may be of use but which were found in only one study. That they are not discussed here should not be taken as an indication that they are not appropriate and valid measures of subjective caregiver impact; rather, the evidence to date is insufficient to support an assessment.

Appraisal of Caregiving Scale (ACS)

Two versions of the Appraisal of Caregiving Scale were found in this literature review. The first, a study by Oberst and colleagues in 1989,[12] included 47 family members assisting patients receiving radiotherapy. This study used a 53-item version of the instrument, which was designed to assess "the meaning of the illness-caregiving situation in terms of the intensity of each of four appraisal dimensions: harm/loss (15 items), threat (15 items), challenge (15 items), and benign (eight items)" (p. 211). The items address various areas of stress response involved with caregiving, including caregiving tasks, relationships and interpersonal support, lifestyle, emotional and physical health, and overall personal impact. Each of the items is answered using a 5-point Likert-type format ranging from "very true" to "very untrue." Carey and colleagues,[7] used a 72-item version of the ACS in a study of 49 family caregivers of patients undergoing chemotherapy. In addition to the four appraisal dimensions used by Oberst *et al.* in the first study,[12] this version of the ACS included a benefit dimension. The stress response areas and format were also the same as reported in the first Oberst *et al.* study. Both studies reported internal consistency reliability coefficients above 0.70 for all domains.

Burden Scale

Schott-Baer and colleagues used the Burden Scale to assess caregiver burden in two studies that explored the relationship between dependent care, caregiver burden, self-care agency, and hardiness.[4,5] The instrument has a total of 14 items that use a 5-point Likert-scale, and includes objective and subjective subscales. Thus, only part of the questionnaire assesses subjective caregiver impact; the other part assesses objective caregiving events and activities. Cronbach's alpha coefficients in the two studies were above 0.70 except for the subjective subscale, which had an internal-consistency reliability of 0.69 in one of the studies.[4,5]

Caregiver Appraisal Scale

Lawton and colleagues have conducted research to develop this measure of subjective caregiving burden, caregiving satisfaction, caregiving impact, caregiving mastery, and traditional caregiving ideology in caregivers of demented and otherwise impaired patients.[63] However, confirmatory factor analyses in respite care and institutionalized samples raised some questions regarding the hypothesized factor structures. The studies did provide some support of the subjective burden, caregiving satisfaction, and caregiving impact factors. Cronbach's alpha for these three scales were 0.85, 0.67, and 0.70 in a respite sample and 0.87, 0.68, and 0.65 in an institutionalization sample, respectively. The investigators also assessed test-retest reliability over 16 weeks on average, which was 0.78 for subjective burden, 0.76 for caregiving satisfaction, and 0.75 for caregiving impact. Toseland and colleagues[39] used the Caregiving Mastery and Caregiving Satisfaction subscales in a study of a problem-solving intervention in caregivers of cancer patients but did not report their psychometric performance.

Caregiver Quality of Life Index (CQLI)

The CQLI was developed by McMillan and colleagues and tested on caregivers of cancer patients being managed in a hospice setting.[35] This questionnaire consists of four items that assess emotional, social, financial, and physical quality of life. The CQLI uses a 100 mm visual analogue scale anchored at "lowest quality" and "highest quality" and provides brief descriptions of the lowest and highest qualities. A single overall score is produced by summing and averaging the four items. The authors provide evidence of the validity and reliability of the CQLI. First, they support the content validity of the measure through discussion of its development. Also, they note that the CQLI distinguished between caregivers and a control group of non-caregiver adult volunteers. Internal consistency reliability at admission was 0.76. The CQLI was also used in a study by Weitzner et al.[21] to revalidate their own CQOLC in a home hospice setting. They found moderate correlations with the two instruments.

Zarit Burden Interview/Zarit Burden Inventory

Two studies[39,54] used a 22-item burden interview developed for caregivers of patients with dementia. The items query the impact of the patients' disability on the caregivers' lives and are answered using a 5-point scale ranging from "never" to "nearly always." In one study validating a new measure of perceived caregiver rewards, Cronbach's alpha for the Zarit Burden Interview was 0.91.[54]

Discussion

Informal caregivers are playing an increasing role in the care of friends or relatives who have cancer. Because cancer and its treatment affect not only the patient with the disease but also those caring for them, it is important to consider the impact on these caregivers. The impacts of caring for a cancer patient are wide-ranging, affecting the caregiver's emotional, social/role, physical, and spiritual well-being.

This review has focused on the two instruments that have been used three or more times to assess the subjective caregiver impact on the informal caregivers of cancer patients: the Caregiver Reaction Assessment and the Caregiver Quality of Life Index-Cancer. A comparison of their major characteristics follows.

The developers of the CRA and CQOLC used different conceptual bases for their instruments. The CRA was developed to assess the reactions of family members and the CQOLC was conceptualized as a health-related quality of life measure; this difference is evident in their item content (discussed below). Also, the CRA was developed to be applicable in multiple disease areas and has been developed and tested in caregivers of patients with physical impairments, Alzheimer's disease, and cancer, while the CQOLC was developed specifically for use in caregivers of cancer patients.

Due in part to their conceptual differences, the CRA and CQOLC include items that cover somewhat different content although there is quite a bit of overlap. The 24-item CRA is focused more specifically on the consequences of caregiving, including the impact on the caregiver's schedule, esteem, family support, health, and finances. Each domain includes multiple items that assess its particular outcomes. In contrast, the 35-item CQOLC covers a broader array of outcomes, including emotional aspects (e.g., sadness, guilt, frustration), changes in habits (e.g., sleep, sexual function), and spiritual issues. However, the CQOLC includes fewer items for certain issues covered in more depth by the CRA. In particular, the CRA provides much better coverage of the positive benefits of caregiving.

The scoring of the measures also differs. While the CRA produces subscale scores but no overall score, the CQOLC produces an overall score but no subscale scores. This difference may be important to researchers developing measurement strategies. For example, the CRA may be a more suitable instrument for studying the particular impacts of caregiving, but the CQOLC may be more appropriate for an overall assessment of impact. Further, the CRA is divided into subscales, so researchers may elect to use a few selected scales rather than the entire instrument. There were several examples of the use of selected scales in the literature.

Both questionnaires can be completed in a reasonable time (about 10 minutes), and studies have not reported problems with missing data on forms that have been completed. While the Dutch version of the CRA has been both self- and interviewer-administered, the CQOLC has only been evaluated as a self-administered instrument. More data on the relative performance of the different modes of administration is needed.

Use of these instruments in multinational studies may be challenging. No language translations were found in the literature for the CQOLC, and only a Dutch translation of the CRA was found. If the developers of these measures move forward with additional language translations, it will be important to consider the cultural validation of the instruments as well. Because cultures may vary in the familial caregiving role, adapting these measures for use in other countries and cultures will involve not only linguistic translations but also assessment of cultural validity. Exploration of cultural validity will be important even for continued use in the countries where they have been validated as these instruments have not been evaluated in culturally diverse samples to date.

Both the CRA and CQOLC produced adequate evidence of reliability. Cronbach's alpha for all domains of the CRA ranged from 0.80 to 0.90 in the initial validation study and remained high in most other published studies. However, the Dutch translation did not perform quite as well, with alpha coefficients for some measures falling below the 0.70 level. The CQOLC also had high internal consistency reliabilities (0.91 and 0.87) in its validation studies. In addition, test-retest reliability over 14 days for the CQOLC was 0.95.

The content validity of the CRA and CQOLC is supported by the methods used to develop them, which included interviews with caregivers to identify individual measurement items. In addition, there is evidence for construct validity for both of these measures. In general, the researchers found correlations in the hypothesized directions with similar measures. However, in one of the CQOLC studies, the score on the CQOLC did not correlate in the expected direction with ECOG performance status, suggesting the need to investigate the cause of this finding.

Evidence of responsiveness and information on interpreting the instruments were somewhat less well documented for the CRA and CQOLC. As these instruments are used in more studies, these issues should be studied in greater depth, in addition to continuing to assess their reliability and validity.

Future research

While increased attention has been paid to assessing caregiver impact in recent years, the field is still relatively young. Studies of caregiver impact tend to be non-randomized, cross-sectional assessments. Because many of the studies lack methodological rigor, their results can be difficult to interpret. Nevertheless, the science of assessing caregiver impact is improving over time as researchers begin to develop and use structured measures. And, as these measures begin to be used in longitudinal studies, our understanding of subjective caregiver impact will improve. Below are some suggestions for improving the state of the science.

While some authors provided definitions and conceptual models for assessing informal caregiver impact, this needs to be done more consistently. Models can assist in developing measurement strategies that would ensure the relevant concepts are covered and that the measurement instruments have been appropriately designed and validated.

In developing the conceptual model for this chapter, the literature suggested many and varied effects of caring for cancer patients. These impacts extend far beyond the concept of burden and include both positive benefits and negative consequences of caregiving. In assessing subjective caregiver impact, it is important to consider not only the commonly seen negative burden and strain measures but also to consider the positive effects. Further, because caregiver impact is multidimensional, researchers should consider instruments that include multiple domains. However, researchers who are interested in a particular outcome, e.g., depression, should consider instruments more specifically focused on that issue, perhaps used as a supplement to a more general caregiver impact instrument.

The four domains most commonly used to categorize the relevant concepts of caregiver impact are emotional, social/role, physical, and spiritual; of these, the concepts related to spiritual impact were relatively less well defined. While each of the four domains could benefit from further study and refinement, the spiritual domain, in particular, requires more research.

As the field grows, standardization in the way these measures are used and reported will be important. To minimize confusion in literature reviews, it would be helpful if the proper names of instruments were used consistently, and that newer questionnaires use names that can be clearly differentiated from other questionnaires. Perhaps more important to advancing the field would be a reduction in the number of instruments used to assess caregiver impact. In this review of 72 articles, over 50 different questionnaires were identified, but few of these questionnaires were used in more than two cancer studies even though many studies used multiple measures. More frequent use of a smaller number of instruments will lead to more comparability among studies and additional support for their reliability and validity. However, this suggestion is not to preclude using unique or less frequently used instruments to assess a more specific outcome (e.g., fatigue) with greater depth. There will always be a balancing act between improving comparability by using frequently used measures and improving sensitivity by using measures more specifically suited to the study. Also, as the field matures, some measures that had not been used frequently at the time of this review may be used more often.

It is also important to keep in mind the potential uses of caregiver impact information. For example, if measures can be used to identify "at risk" caregivers in need of support, steps may be taken to assist these informal caregivers so they can better care for their friend or family member with cancer. However, there are many factors that can contribute to a caregiver being "at risk." In addition to measures of subjective caregiver impact, demographics (e.g., age, sex, ethnicity, family status), clinical characteristics (e.g., comorbidities), individual difference variables (e.g., self-efficacy about ability to provide care, coping mechanisms), and objective burden variables (e.g., time spent caregiving, finances) may all affect caregivers' ability to assist their loved ones. In addition, patient variables (e.g., severity of disease, presence of comorbidities, self-efficacy) may also be key determinants of caregiver impact. Given the many and diverse patient and caregiver variables that can have an impact on caregivers lives, developing models to identify "at risk" caregivers remains an important challenge. Thus, assessing subjective caregiver impact and identifying factors that determine at-risk caregivers are important areas for further investigation.

Conclusions

Together the CRA and CQOLC form an excellent base for assessing subjective caregiver impact. The choice between the two should be determined by the specific research objectives of the planned study. It may also be necessary for these measures to be supplemented with more in-depth measures of particular outcomes of interest. In addition, these measures require further study to improve our understanding of their performance. As the field matures, other important measures of subjective caregiver impact may emerge.

But, is a measure of subjective caregiver impact necessary or could generic measures be used? The answer depends on the study's research question. Both the CRA and CQOLC specifically address impacts of caregiving that would not be included in a generic measure. For example, the CRA items are directly targeted at the impact of caregiving, including "stop work to care," "resent having to care," "difficult to get help," "healthy enough to care," and "difficult to pay." The CQOLC's items are also very specific to caregiving even though the instrument is conceptualized as a "quality of life" measure. Example items include "alteration in daily routine," "responsibility for patient's care," "family's interest in caregiving," and "management of patient's pain." Thus, if the research question were directed towards identifying the specific impact of caregiving, a caregiving-specific measure such as the CRA or CQOLC would be necessary. Alternatively, if the research question is more focused on assessing the overall health status of the caregiver, then a generic measure may be adequate. This strategy would allow for comparability with other studies and other populations. Finally, another option would be to use generic unidimensional measures that address impacts of caregiving such as fatigue and depression.

As the science of assessing subjective caregiver impact moves forward, the CRA and CQOLC and other measures may play a critical role. More importantly, researchers should seek to use measures more frequently and consistently to contribute to comparability across studies. These steps can help improve the state of the science of the increasingly important area of subjective caregiver impact. Such methodological improvements can lead to improved abilities to identify and assist at-risk caregivers in need of support so that caring for cancer patients does not lead to severe decrements in the caregivers' own health-related quality of life.

REFERENCES

1 Lim, Y. M., Luna, I., Caromwell, S. L. *et al.* (1996). Toward a cross-cultural understanding of family caregiving burden. *Western Journal of Nursing Research* **18**:252–66.

2 Nijboer, C., Tempelaar, R., Sanderman, R. *et al.* (1998). Cancer and caregiving: the impact on the caregiver's health. *Psycho-Oncology* **7**:3–13.

3 Ohaeri, J. U., Campbell, O. B., Ilesanmi, A. O. *et al.* (1999). The psychosocial burden of caring for some Nigerian women with breast cancer and cervical cancer. *Social Science and Medicine* **49**:1541–9.

4 Schott-Baer, D., Fisher, L., Gregory, C. (1995). Dependent care, caregiver burden, hardiness and self-care agency of caregivers. *Cancer Nursing* **18**:299–305.

5 Schott-Baer, D. (1993). Dependent care, caregiver burden, and self-care agency of spouse caregivers. *Cancer Nursing* **16**:230–6.

6 Buehler, J. A., Lee, H. J. (1992). Exploration of home care resources for rural families with cancer. *Cancer Nursing* **15**:299–308.

7 Carey, P. J., Oberst, M. T., McCubbin, M. A. *et al.* (1991). Appraisal and caregiving burden in family members caring for patients receiving chemotherapy. *Oncology Nursing Forum* **18**:1341–8.

8 Ferrell, B. R., Grant, M., Borneman, T. *et al.* (1999). Family caregiving in cancer pain management. *Journal of Palliative Medicine* **2**:185–95.

9 Gilbar, O. (1999). Gender as a predictor of burden and psychological distress of elderly husbands and wives of cancer patients. *Psycho-Oncology* **8**:287–94.

10 Given, C. W., Stommel, M., Given, B. *et al.* (1993). The influence of cancer patients' symptoms and functional states on patients' depression and family caregivers' reaction and depression. *Health Psychology* **12**:277–85.

11 Harrison, J., Haddad, P., Maguire, P. (1995). The impact of cancer on key relatives: a comparison of relative and patient concerns. *European Journal of Cancer* **31A**:1736–40.

12 Oberst, M. T., Thomas, S., Gass, K. *et al.* (1989). Caregiving demands and appraisal of stress among family caregivers. *Cancer Nursing* **12**:209–15.

13 Pasacreta, J. V., Barg, F., Nuamah, I. *et al.* (2000). Participant characteristics before and 4 months after attendance at a family caregiver cancer education program. *Cancer Nursing* **23**:295–303.

14 Rabins, P. V., Fitting, M. D., Eastham, J. *et al.* (1990). The emotional impact of caring for the chronically ill. *Psychosomatics* **31**:331–6.

15 Rusinak, R. L., Murphy, J. F. (1995). Elderly spousal caregivers: knowledge of cancer care, perceptions of preparedness, and coping strategies. *Journal of Gerontological Nursing* **21**: 33–41.

16 Siegel, K., Raveis, V. H., Houts, P. *et al.* (1991). Caregiver burden and unmet patient needs. *Cancer* **68**:1131–40.

17 Siegel, K., Raveis, V. H., Mor, V., Houts, P. (1991). The relationship of spousal caregiver burden to patient disease and treatment-related conditions. *Annals of Oncology* **2**:511–16.

18 Stommel, M., Given, C. W., Given, B. (1990). Depression as an overriding variable in explaining caregiver burdens. *Journal of Aging and Health* **2**:81–102.

19 Weitzner, M. A., Jacobsen, P. B., Wagner, H., Jr. *et al.* (1999). The caregiver quality of life index-cancer (CQOLC) scale: development and validation of an instrument to measure quality of life of the family caregiver of patients with cancer. *Quality of Life Research* **8**:55–63.

20 Weitzner, M. A., Knutzen, R. (1998). The impact of pituitary disease on the family caregiver and overall family functioning. *Psychotherapy and Psychosomatics* **67**:181–8.

21 Weitzner, M. A., McMillan, S. C. (1999). The caregiver quality of life index-cancer (CQOLC) scale: revalidation in a home hospice setting. *Journal of Palliative Care* **15**:13–20.

22 Weitzner, M. A., Meyers, C. A., Steinbruecker, S. *et al.* (1997). Developing a care giver quality-of-life instrument: preliminary steps. *Cancer Practice* **5**:25–31.

23 Blanchard, C. G., Albrecht, T. L., Ruckdeschel, J. C. (1997). The crisis of cancer: psychological impact on family caregivers. *Oncology* **11**:189–94.

24 Blood, G. W., Simpson, K. C., Dineen, M. *et al.* (1994). Spouses of individuals with laryngeal cancer: caregiver strain and burden. *Journal of Communication Disorders* **27**: 19–35.

25 Ferrell, B. R., Ferrell, B. A., Rhiner, M. *et al.* (1991). Family factors influencing cancer pain management. *Postgraduate Medical Journal* **67**(Suppl. 2):S64–9.

26 Ferrell, B. R., Grant, M., Chan, J. *et al.* (1995). The impact of cancer pain education on family caregivers of elderly patients. *Oncology Nursing Forum* **22**:1211–18.

27 Given, B. A., Given, C. W., Helms, E. *et al.* (1997). Determinants of family caregiver reaction: new and recurrent cancer. *Cancer Practice* **5**:17–24.

28 Given, B., Stommel, M., Collins, C. *et al.* (1990). Responses of elderly spouse caregivers. *Research in Nursing and Health* **13**:77–85.

29 Given, C. W., Given, B. A., Stommel, M. *et al.* (1999). The impact of new demands for assistance on caregiver depression: tests using an inception cohort. *The Gerontologist* **39**:76–85.

30 Juarez, G., Ferrell, B. R. (1996). Family and caregiver involvement in pain management. *Clinics in Geriatric Medicine* **12**:531–47.

31 Kozachik, S. L., Given, C. W., Given, B. A. *et al.* (2001). Improving depressive symptoms among caregivers of patients with cancer: results of a randomized clinical trial. *Oncology Nursing Forum* **28**:1149–57.

32 Kurtz, M. E., Given, B., Kurtz, J. C. *et al.* (1994). The interaction of age, symptoms, and survival status on physical and mental health of patients with cancer and their families. *Cancer* **74**:2071–8.

33 Kurtz, M. E., Kurtz, J. C., Given, C. W. *et al.* (1997). Predictors of postbereavement depressive symptomatology among family caregivers of cancer patients. *Support Care in Cancer* **5**: 53–60.

34 Kurtz, M. E., Kurtz, J. C., Given, C. W. *et al.* (1995). Relationship of caregiver reactions and depression to cancer patients' symptoms, functional states and depression – a longitudinal view. *Social Science and Medicine* **40**:837–46.

35 McMillan, S. C., Mahon, M. (1994). The impact of hospice services on the quality of life of primary caregivers. *Oncology Nursing Forum* **21**:1189–95.

36 Ohaeri, J. U., Campbell, O. B., Ilesanmi, A. *et al.* (1999). The opinion of caregivers of some women with breast and cervical cancer on aspects of the disease. *West African Journal of Medicine* **18**:6–12.

37 Raveis, V. H., Karus, D. G., Siegel, K. (1998). Correlates of depressive symptomatology among adult daughter caregivers of a parent with cancer. *Cancer* **83**:1652–63.

38 Summers, N., Dawe, U., Stewart, D. A. (2000). A comparison of inpatient and outpatient ASCT. *Bone Marrow Transplantation* **26**:389–95.

39 Toseland, R. W., Blanchard, C. G., McCallion, P. (1995). A problem solving intervention for caregivers of cancer patients. *Social Science and Medicine* **40**:517–28.

40 Weitzner, M. A., Haley, W. E., Chen, H. (2000). The family caregiver of the older cancer patient. *Hematology/Oncology Clinics of North America* **14**:269–81.

41 Weitzner, M. A., McMillan, S. C., Jacobsen, P. B. (1999). Family caregiver quality of life: differences between curative and palliative cancer treatment settings. *Journal of Pain and Symptom Management* **17**:418–28.

42 Holden, C. M. (1991). Anorexia in the terminally ill cancer patient: the emotional impact on the patient and the family. *The Hospice Journal* **7**:73–84.

43 Payne, S., Smith, P., Dean, S. (1999). Identifying the concerns of informal carers in palliative care. *Palliative Medicine* **13**:37–44.

44 Stetz, K. M. (1989). The relationship among background characteristics, purpose in life, and caregiving demands on perceived health of spouse caregivers. *Scholarly Inquiry for Nursing Practice* **3**:133–53.

45 Watt-Watson, J., Graydon, J. (1995). Impact of surgery on head and neck cancer patients and their caregivers. *Nursing Clinics of North America* **30**:659–71.

46 Pohl, J. M., Given, C. W., Collins, C. E. *et al.* (1994). Social vulnerability and reactions to caregiving in daughters and daughters-in-law caring for disabled aging parents. *Health Care for Women International* **15**:385–95.

47 Yates, P. (1999). Family coping: issues and challenges for cancer nursing. *Cancer Nursing* **22**:63–71.

48 Kramer, B. J. (1997). Gain in the caregiving experience: where are we? what next? *Gerontologist* **37**:218–32.

49 Ferrell, B. R., Rhiner, M., Cohen, M. Z. *et al.* (1991). Pain as a metaphor for illness. Part I: impact of cancer pain on family caregivers. *Oncology Nursing Forum* **18**:1303–9.

50 Smeenk, F. W. J. M., De Witte, L. P., Van Haastregt, J. C. M. *et al.* (1998). Transmural care of terminal cancer patients: effects on the quality of life of direct caregivers. *Nursing Research* **47**:129–36.

51 Ferrell, B. R., Cohen, M. Z., Rhiner, M. *et al.* (1991). Pain as a metaphor for illness. Part II: family caregivers' management of pain. *Oncology Nursing Forum* **18**:1315–21.

52 Nijboer, C., Triemstra, M., Tempelaar, R. *et al.* (1999). Measuring both negative and positive reactions to giving care to

cancer patients: psychometric qualities of the caregiver reaction assessment (CRA). *Social Science and Medicine* **48**:1259–69.

53 Given, C. W., Given, B., Stommel, M., Collins, C. *et al.* (1992). The caregiver reaction assessment (CRA) for caregivers to persons with chronic physical and mental impairments. *Research in Nursing and Health* **15**:271–83.

54 Picot, S. J. F., Youngblut, J., Zeller, R. (1997). Development and testing of a measure of perceived caregiver rewards in adults. *Journal of Nursing Measurement* **5**:33–52.

55 Given, B., Given, C. W. (1992). Patient and family caregiver reaction to new and recurrent breast cancer. *Journal of the American Medical Women's Association* **47**:201–6, 12.

56 Lyles, J., King, S., Given, B. A. *et al.* (1990). Social interaction, instrumental support, and family caregiver perception of support. *Behavior, Health, and Aging* **1**:105–20.

57 Curt, G. A. (2000). The impact of fatigue on patients with cancer: overview of FATIGUE 1 and 2. *The Oncologist* **5** (Suppl. 2):9–12.

58 Lang, D. A., Neil-Dwyer, G., Garfield, J. (1999). Outcome after complex neurosurgery: the caregiver's burden is forgotten. *Journal of Neurosurgery* **91**:359–63.

59 Fakhoury, W., McCarthy, M., Addington-Hall, J. (1996). Determinants of informal caregivers' satisfaction with services for dying cancer patients. *Social Science and Medicine* **42**:721–31.

60 Jensen, S., Given, B. (1993). Fatigue affecting family caregivers of cancer patients. *Supportive Care in Cancer* **1**:321–5.

61 Jensen, S., Given, B. A. (1991). Fatigue affecting family caregivers of cancer patients. *Cancer Nursing* **14**:181–7.

62 King, S., Collins, C., Given, B. *et al.* (1991). Institutionalization of an elderly family member: reactions of spouse and nonspouse caregivers. *Archives of Psychiatric Nursing* **5**:323–30.

63 Lawton, M. P., Kleban, M. H., Moss, M. *et al.* (1989). Measuring caregiver appraisal. *Journal of Gerontology* **44**:61–71.

17

Practical considerations in outcomes assessment for clinical trials

Diane L. Fairclough, Dr. P.H.

University of Colorado Health Sciences Center, Denver, CO

While clinical outcomes are often the primary method of evaluation in clinical trials, endpoints requiring patient-reported measures are essential. The scientific literature is full of reports where investigators make logical but unsubstantiated claims of quality-of-life benefits to patients based on the assumption that a change in treatment or a traditional biomedical outcome will improve the patient's quality of life. While in many cases this may be true, surprising results are sometimes obtained when the patient is asked directly. One classic example occurred with a study by Sugarbaker *et al.*[1] comparing two therapeutic approaches for soft-tissue sarcoma. The first was limb-sparing surgery followed by radiation therapy. The second treatment approach was full amputation of the affected limb. The investigator hypothesized that "Sparing a limb, as opposed to amputating it, offers a quality of life advantage." Rather than assuming this was true, the investigators tested their hypothesis. Subjects who received the limb-sparing procedures reported limitations in mobility and sexual functioning. These observations were confirmed with physical assessments of mobility and endocrine function. As a result of these studies, the original hypothesis was rejected, radiation therapy was modified, and physical rehabilitation was added to the limb-sparing therapeutic approach.[2]

There is a danger of adding patient-based outcomes to every clinical trial. If the majority of these studies either fail to answer clinically relevant questions or are methodologically weak, eventually a negative perception about patient-centered outcomes will grow in the research community. The purpose of this chapter is to address some of the practical considerations to incorporating patient-reported outcomes into oncology clinical trials and of implementing a successful trial. The scope of this discussion will be limited to patient-reported outcomes including symptom assessment, health-related quality of life (HRQOL), and satisfaction. Patient-reported data used in economic analyses (e.g., morbidity costs,[a] indirect costs of economic burden on the family and caregivers) will also be covered; however, patient-oriented outcomes that are obtained from hospital or insurance records are not included.

Measurement across stages of disease

There are important questions requiring patient-reported outcomes that can be answered across all stages of disease (prevention and screening, treatment, survivorship, and end of life). The characteristics of patient-oriented measures and the motivation for their measurement will differ with respect to the expected survival, age of the patients at diagnosis, and the specific morbidities associated with the disease and its treatment. At one extreme are cancers typically occurring in childhood where the majority will be long-term survivors. In these children, many of the side effects (alopecia, nausea, and vomiting), while distressing, are of short duration and reversible. These side effects are acceptable when there are long-term benefits such as increased survival. In these cases, the post-treatment and long-term survival periods as well as the long-term effects, such as diminished cognitive function and impaired reproductive capabilities that impact the patient's quality of life or create an economic burden, are the most relevant. At the other extreme, for cancers occurring in late adulthood that have no effective therapies, the expected survival is of a short duration and the quality of survival is what is important.

Assessment of patient-centered outcomes may not be necessary for all studies, and limited resources may not permit assessment in every clinical trial. More critically, without a well-defined research question, the study may never provide any meaningful information. Certain types of studies are more or less likely to influence clinical, regulatory, and payment decisions. For example, patient-centered outcomes are less likely to have much influence on clinical practice when the trial is examining an innovative breakthrough therapy for a diagnosis for which there is no effective alternative.[4,5] If the new therapy is successful in extending survival, it very likely will become the standard of care regardless of its economic cost or impact on quality of life. In contrast, patient-centered outcomes such as HRQOL are extremely important when the treatments are given with palliative intent.[5,6] Assessment of patient-centered outcomes are more likely to be useful when there are a number of competing therapies that have similar effectiveness in disease control and survival,[4,7,8] or when the therapy has a small benefit in increasing survival but is more toxic, leading to additional morbidity.[4,6,8] The latter might apply to diseases in which the median survival is expected to be long (e.g., early prostate cancer) or short (e.g., most metastatic cancers). When survival is expected to be long, the therapeutic options are often quite different, frequently employing different treatment modalities or watchful-waiting; the treatment (and no treatment) choices are likely to have differential HRQOL and economic impacts.[7] Adjuvant therapy for patients at risk of recurrence represents another setting where there may be considerable interest in the long-term impact of the therapies and the economic consequences.[7]

Even when patient-based outcomes are not part of the primary decision-making process about a therapeutic regimen, they may contribute in other ways.[8] For example, information about quality of life could guide the development of new regimens incorporating changes in schedule or supportive therapy to make the treatments more tolerable. Additionally, they may provide a basis for patient education about the timing and duration of certain side effects and anticipation of the need for additional supportive care or rehabilitation resources.

Hillner and Smith[9] raise similar issues in the context of economic analyses in their editorial "Does a Clinical Trial Warrant an Economic Analysis?" They suggest "the reader consider if there was a compelling case for doing an economic analysis, then scrutinize the technical performance and completeness of the assessments, and finally interpret the results and their transportability to one's own care setting." They also suggest the key maxim is that clinical economics are primarily driven by the clinical effectiveness of treatment. For example, an economic analysis for an innovative therapy that shows benefit for a condition for which there is currently no (other) effective treatment is unlikely to influence clinical practice. On the other hand, it may be of great interest for conditions where there are multiple effective therapies or for the management of non-life-threatening side effects of therapy. Considerations raised by Hillner and Smith[9] include: (1) Will the therapy be widely used in practice or is it limited to research institutions by technology? (2) Does the therapy change clinical practice? Will it replace, rather than supplement, other interventions? (3) Do the strategies differ substantially in cost, invasiveness, resource utilization, morbidity or mortality, or outcome (health status or preferences)? If a back-of-the-envelope calculation can answer the question, there is no need to perform a well-controlled economic analysis. An additional caution is the use of cost effectiveness when comparing treatment options that have very small differences in effectiveness.[b] These very small differences in effectiveness can translate into large differences in cost-effectiveness. In this setting, a cost-minimization analysis may be more appropriate, as our goal is to minimize the cost of providing the best care rather than making the choices between the treatment of different conditions. A number of other issues arise including questions such as whether costs should be collected only during the duration of treatment and what types of costs are relevant. These issues are discussed in more detail elsewhere in this book.[10,11]

Measurement across phases of drug development (Phase I, II, III, IV)

It is appropriate to start planning the collection of patient-centered outcomes measures during the early phases of drug development.[4,12] This planning is particularly important when appropriate well-validated instruments are not yet available for a particular disease or language. For example, it may be possible to identify toxicities/symptoms that are important to the patient in phase I/II trials before progressing to later phase studies. That said, patient-based outcomes should be employed cautiously in phase I and early phase II[c] trials. These trials enroll a very selective group of subjects who have failed treatment and rely on designs that minimize the number of patients exposed to previously untested treatments. It will not be possible to adequately validate instruments if the phase I/II patients have more advanced disease than larger phase III/IV studies. Answers to questions about feasibility may also not be valid as these trials are generally conducted solely in an inpatient setting in contrast to larger trials that rely on outpatient treatment to the greatest extent possible. Thus, neither instrument validation nor feasibility studies can be easily generalized to the more diverse populations that will participate in later trials under less intensive monitoring. Above all, it is important to be clear about what will be learned from these early trials.

Patient-centered outcomes are likely to be relevant and useful in most phase III studies, as well as randomized phase IV trials and large randomized phase II trials comparing different dose schedules. Confirmatory studies can be planned with focused objectives, adequate sample sizes, and validated assessment tools with careful attention to how the results will be used. Exploratory studies can be used to define hypotheses regarding the impact of disease and treatment on various dimensions of HRQOL and to explore the responsiveness of generic and disease-specific measures. When well-validated instruments do not exist or have not been validated for the population of interest, the early validation studies provide an opportunity to prepare for the later confirmatory studies. The usefulness of non-randomized phase IV trials should be evaluated carefully given the difficulty of interpretation of both between-group differences and within-group changes. Within-group changes are especially sensitive to bias in oncology patients who experience significant morbidity and mortality.[13]

Modes of data collection

The relative value of the different modes of data collection is primarily driven by their intended use. When patient-centered measures are used for screening in the clinic, rapid feedback is a priority. In contrast, when data are collected solely for research purposes, greater emphases on confidentiality, improved compliance (reduction of missing data), and reduced cost of data collection (personnel time) are often the primary considerations. The complexity of the measure (e.g., difficult skip logic within a questionnaire used to measure patient preferences or computer-adaptive testing) will also eliminate different modes of data collection from consideration.

Proxy measures from caregivers and family/significant others

There is a general consensus that it is preferable to obtain patient-oriented data (e.g., heath status and satisfaction measures) directly from the patient. The most compelling argument is the importance of the patient's assessment of health-related quality of life in the conceptual framework of clinical trial evaluation.[7] Secondary arguments rest on the levels of agreement between different observers. There are some exceptions to this rule. The first is when preference measures (utility measures) are to be obtained from a different perspective (e.g., general population), though it can be argued that these are no longer patient-centered measures. The second exception occurs when it is expected that a significant proportion of the patients are unable, or will become unable, to complete self-assessments due to significant levels of morbidity. In oncology, this issue applies to studies of patients with brain tumors, subjects in the terminal phases of care, and studies in young children.

Sprangers and Aaronson[14] performed a systematic review of research that included HRQOL assessments from both proxy raters and patients. While the results of the individual studies vary, certain themes emerge: (1) Agreement between patients and proxy respondents is in the moderate to good range (Correlation = 0.4–0.7), with stronger agreement occurring for measures of observable information (physical function) than for psychosocial function [14–17] or satisfaction.[18] (2) Health care providers and significant others tend to underestimate the patients' assessments.[14,15,17] (3) There is no clear trend indicating that health care providers are better raters than significant others (or vice versa). (4) Significant others' ratings tend to be more accurate when they live in close proximity to the patient,[18–21] but they are also influenced by the extent of caregiving function/burden. Groenvold et al.[21] examined the potential for different interpretation of questions by patients and researchers and noted that some patients reported only symptoms that they felt were relevant, specifically the symptoms related to their cancer diagnosis or treatment. Fitzsimmons et al.[22] observed that health professionals saw symptoms directly affecting the patient's HRQOL, but the patients' perception of HRQOL was mediated by the process of coping.

The critical question is whether bias (if any) increases as HRQOL gets poorer, as this is the setting where proxy measures are most likely to be used. The results are inconsistent. Sneeuw et al.[16] observed that the maximum levels of disagreement were found at intermediate levels of HRQOL, with smaller discrepancies noted for patients with good or poor HRQOL. Epstein et al.[18] observed that agreement between subject and proxy assessment of satisfaction was lower in those with worse overall health but found no differences for HRQOL scales. Not surprisingly, Novella et al.[17] observed that agreement decreased with increasing severity of dementia.

The issue of proxy assessment of patient preferences (utilities) is slightly different. The assessment of utilities using Time Trade-Off or Standard Gamble techniques requires a more time-consuming interview than is generally required for a health assessment questionnaire. This process may not be feasible for patients experiencing significant morbidity and may involve more stressful assessments by a patient realistically facing alternatives such as death. The use of multi-attribute assessment techniques with instruments such as the Health Utilities Index has partially addressed this issue.[23] There remains controversy as to whose preference scores should be used to determine the utilities for economic evaluations. The choice is between assessments by patients who have actually experienced the health state of interest versus respondents from a general population sample who have not experienced the health state. Some studies indicate no differences in the preferences,[24–26] while others observe that patients who have experienced the condition will give a higher value to the corresponding health state.[23,27] Some of the reasons suggested for this phenomenon are learned coping by patients,[24] avoidance of cognitive-dissonance resulting from a treatment choice, and exaggerated fear of disability and disease in healthy individuals.[24] When patients overvalue these health states the result is an undervaluing of prevention and treatment programs.

Self-administration versus interviewer administration (face-to-face or telephone)

Methods of administration that have been used successfully in clinical trials include pencil-and-paper self-report, in-clinic face-to-face assessments with trained interviewers, and centralized telephone administration with trained interviewers. Pencil-and-paper self-report is the most economical option but requires that patients be available on a regular basis. Interviewer administration is useful when the population has low literacy (children, immigrants), physical difficulty with pencil-and-paper forms (advanced neurological conditions, hospice patients), or the questionnaire involves complex skip patterns (Standard Gamble).

Schipper[28] cautions against using an instrument designed for self-administration by a third party, noting several issues. There is evidence that self-report data differs from interview-generated data in ways that cannot be predicted. This is particularly a problem when there is the potential for the influence of social desirability on the responses. Great care must be taken to ensure that patients do not feel the need to please the interviewer or clinical investigator. Similarly, patients may feel reluctant to answer honestly in the presence of family and friends. Administration at home may result in different responses than in a hospital environment,[29] although the findings on this are mixed. TeVelde et al.[30] did not observe any systematic differences when comparing administration of the CARES-SF by mail, in a telephone interview, or in the clinic. Interviews also require trained personnel to schedule and conduct the interview.

Regardless of mode of administration, it is preferable to use the same one throughout the study, unless it has been shown that responses are not affected by mode of administration. This advice is balanced by considerations of greater bias if this policy results in greater non-response among selected groups (e.g., those that are sicker). A compromise is required to balance feasibility and resources with ideal research conditions. The procedures selected should be carefully documented in the protocol and emphasized during training.

Face-to-face interview

Face-to-face interviews are the most susceptible to "social desirability" when topics include sexual habits or drug use,[31,32] although the results are mixed and some investigators have observed no differences.[33] In the context of HRQOL, assessment of spiritual well-being and sexual function may be susceptible to social desirability. Responses may be influenced by the extent to which the patient identifies the interviewer as part of the health care team. Weinberger et al.[34] observed that SF-36 scores gathered by personal interview were higher than through self-administration.

Telephone interview

Telephone interviews have the advantages of (a) controlling timing of administration, (b) reducing clinic and patient burden, (c) requiring fewer trained interviewers (in contrast to face-to-face interview), (d) being especially cost-effective when there are a large number of sites each studying a small number of patients,[35] (e) minimizing missing items (in contrast to self-administered), (f) not requiring a clinic visit, and (g) centralizing quality control.[35] Telephone interviews have the disadvantage of low response rates, largely due to problems with connecting to answering machines and changed numbers. There is a trend towards poorer response rates for younger subjects and for male subjects in both telephone and mail surveys.[36] One should also be concerned about a response bias if individuals who are experiencing more morbidity are easier to reach at home by telephone than healthy individuals. This concern is balanced by the possibility that individuals with more morbidity may find completion of a self-administered questionnaire tiring. The advantage of telephone or in-person interviews for those with poor literacy skills and visual disabilities may be balanced by those with auditory disabilities. Leidy et al.[37] suggest that there may be an advantage in studies with long follow-up or large, geographically diverse samples. Some studies show no or minimal differences in results when compared to self-administration,[37] but the results are typically mixed with both under-reporting and over-reporting of morbidity or health services utilization.[36]

Mailed self-assessment

The lowest cost approach is mailed self-assessment. Gasquet et al.[38] obtained a slightly higher return rate when satisfaction questionnaires were mailed to patients (45%) than when distributed at the time of discharge (40%), but both rates were low. Follow-up by two waves of mail reminders increased the rate to 67%, and an additional phone call increased rates to 80%. The disadvantage of mailed assessments is that there is little control over timing of assessment. TeVelde et al.[30] observed a higher proportion of missing items than occurred for telephone interviews or pencil-and-paper administration during a clinic visit. In the context of a general population survey, McHorney et al.[36] suggest that the cost savings of an initially mailed questionnaire could be used to support rigorous follow-up methods. This may be feasible in studies of prevention and of long-term survivors where there is little change in the patient-based outcomes over time, but not when assessing HRQOL during therapy.

Cost considerations

McHorney et al.[36] note that the total data collection costs for a telephone computer-assisted survey were almost double those for a mailed self-assessment ($48 vs. $27) in a national validation study. Cella[35] notes that centralized telephone data collection is more cost effective than in-clinic distribution of forms when there are a large number of sites or a small number of subjects per site because there are no on-site start-up costs. Overall, the cost of in-person interviews is highest, followed by telephone interviews, with mailed surveys having the lowest cost.

Medium for data collection

The different media for data collection are described below.

Standard pencil-and-paper

Self-assessment using paper forms is the most widely used mode of administration of patient-reported outcomes and the medium in which most questionnaires were developed and validated. It is also generally the most cost effective. Some of the disadvantages of paper forms are a higher rate of unintentionally skipped items and multiple responses to a particular question. Paper forms also require either manual scoring or data entry into computer databases.

Optical scanning

Paper forms are sometimes designed for optical scanning to process large amounts of data (large population-based surveys). With commercial programs, the time to set up the system is often very efficient. Velikova et al.[39] reported that it took 1 hour to set up optical scanning, but touch screens took 50 hours to program/debug. Some of the disadvantages of optical scanning are the requirement of special forms, which may be off-putting to patients. Further, while appropriate for healthy populations, the forms may require more hand-eye coordination than is appropriate for elderly or terminal patients. The major drawbacks are problems with changed answers and multiple answers that require personnel time to resolve. Velikova et al.[39] noted that only 12/158 (8%) optically-read questionnaires had no scanning, verification, or data base errors; each questionnaire averaged 5 minutes to process (1 minute scanning, 4 minutes problem resolution).

Computers

A potential advantage of computer administration is that forced completion of all questions can be built-in, though this feature may create an ethical problem. Velikova et al.[39] justified the use of a forced answer, as they felt adding an option to allow skipping a question would encourage patients to consider that a valid option. Kleinman and colleagues[40] describe a system where subjects are allowed to skip questions but, unfortunately, do not report the incidence of skipped items. Buxton et al.[41] observed that, even when skipped questions were allowed, all items of a 30-item questionnaire (QLQ-C30) were answered by the 178 patients when using a touch-sensitive video monitor. Other advantages include increased reliability because of perceived anonymity for sensitive questions (sexual function) and immediate scoring and printout of results. Yarnold et al.[42] tested multiple computer-based methods in the elderly and observed that touch screen had shorter training and completion times than speech recognition, trackball, or mouse entry. Crawley et al.[43] noted patients found the computer touch screen administration to be faster than pencil-and-paper. In terms of bias, there are varied results across studies. Velikova et al.[39] reported some small differences, whereas Burke et al.[44] and Yarnold et al.[42] reported no differences in SF-36 scores. It is unclear whether observed differences are systematic or the result of chance. Regarding disadvantages, Buxton and colleagues[41] noted that approximately 10% of a group of cancer patients were willing to participate but were unable to get to the touch-sensitive video monitor because of distance to the computer room and attachment to cumbersome medical equipment. High initial costs of computers may be overbalanced by personnel costs for handling optical scan forms.[39] Other practical issues with touch screens include the need to overcome the problem of build-up of static electricity with antistatic mats, and teaching appropriate sensitivity to the touch screen to balance problems of insensitivity of the screen with oversensitivity where trembling fingers cause skipping of questions.[39] Buxton et al.[41] noted problems with monitor responsiveness to touch that was later determined to be a technical problem requiring replacement of the computer.

Hand-held computers (personal data assistants, or PDAs)

Personal data assistants have the advantage of portability. Some of the disadvantages observed previously included small screens with poor contrast, batteries running low, and software design that prevented patients from changing responses.[39,45] These disadvantages have already been addressed through the fast pace of improved technology.

Audio (video)-CASI (computer-assisted self-interview)

Questions are delivered in both an audio (video) and computer display format, with answers recorded with numbered keys.[32] CASI allows complex branching, and it may facilitate responses by patients with a low literacy level.[31]

Cost considerations

Some authors note that an important difference between computer and pencil-and-paper is the initial outlay for equipment.[35,41,46] O'Connor et al.[46] added the need for locations where computer screens are shielded from general view. Buxton et al.[41] noted that the personnel time required to present the questionnaire and give initial instructions was similar for pencil-and-paper and computer administration. Replacement costs and the costs of having technical staff available to handle problems with computer devices are often ignored in these studies.

A note on study quality

The literature comparing different modes of data collection is quite diverse with heterogeneity of designs, small samples, and changing technology. In many feasibility studies, patients who were too ill or had cognitive disorders were excluded. In most reports, authors appear to have an a priori bias and have not established any criteria by which they would reject their hypotheses. In some studies, the authors declare an alternative mode of administration acceptable/equivalent even in the face of poorer psychometric properties. This general problem is in part due to the lack of established criteria for determining psychometric equivalence. What levels of discrepancy are acceptable and what are the appropriate statistics to measure the differences? Even published guidelines leave room for discretion: "Scores on conventional and computer administration may be considered equivalent when (a) the rank order of scores of individuals tested in alternative modes closely approximate each other, and (b) the means, dispersions, and shapes of the score distributions are approximately the same, or have been made approximately the same by rescaling the scores from the computer mode."[47]

Missing data

Hopwood et al.[48] surveyed 29 centers participating in one or more of three randomized trials for lung and head and neck cancer. They observed a very high proportion of preventable missing data. The three most commonly reported problems were staff that were not available, questionnaires that were not available, and staff that considered the patient to be too ill. Preplanning and budgeting have the potential to address the first two problems. Education is needed to address the third.

Data collection and management

It should be absolutely clear who is the key person at each clinical site responsible for administering the HRQOL assessment.[8,35,48] The responsibilities of this data coordinator include, in addition to the usual responsibilities associated with the clinical trial, knowing when the patient will arrive, making sure the patient receives the questionnaire prior to undergoing diagnostic or therapeutic procedures, having a quiet place for the patient to complete the assessment, and implementing follow-up procedures when the patient is not available as expected. At the time of the first assessment, this key person should emphasize the importance to the investigators of obtaining the patient's perspective, reviewing the instructions with the subjects, emphasizing that there are no correct or incorrect responses, encouraging subjects to provide the best answer they can to every question, and reminding them that repeat assessments will be sought at later dates (if applicable). This coordinator may have the responsibility of reviewing the forms for missing responses, but care must be taken to balance confidentiality with the need to minimize missing data. If the assessment

consists of an interview, sufficient trained personnel to schedule and conduct the interviews are required.

Another key to a successful study is a system that identifies when patients are due for assessments.[35] This may include preprinted orders in the patient's chart that identify which assessments should be administered at each clinic visit, or modifying data collection forms to remind data managers to gather data.[35] A central data management office where calendars and expectation notices are generated support this process. Stickers on patients' charts identifying them as part of a study, flow sheets, study calendars, and patient tracking cards[7] may all be helpful.

Avoiding missing data

While analytic strategies exist for dealing with missing data, they are less satisfactory than prevention. Some missing data, such as that due to death, is not preventable. In general, however, the best strategy is primary prevention: missing data should be minimized at the design and implementation stages of a study.[49,50] In most studies, a nurse or research coordinator is responsible for giving the HRQOL questionnaire to the patient. Various pressures and constraints facing these coordinators can lead to missing data, including lack of time and perceived physician support, inadequate protocols, lack of knowledge of the justification and rationale for collecting HRQOL data, lack of reminders, and lack of adequate sites for questionnaire completion.[50] Thus, having clearly specified procedures in the protocol for collecting HRQOL is the first step in minimizing missing data. This information should include the collection protocol if treatment schedule is disrupted, procedures for when the patient requires assistance, and a system for prompting nurses/research personnel that a HRQOL assessment is due.[8,35,49] It is also important to consider alternative methods to obtain follow-up data when patients do not complete questionnaires. Patients, research assistants, and primary investigators should be educated about the importance of collecting these assessments on all patients willing to complete them. Reluctance to approach all patients on all occasions will lead to selection bias. The timing and duration of assessments should also be reasonable. Practical considerations regarding frequency and duration of follow-up are important.

Secondary prevention of missing data consists of gathering information useful in the analysis and interpretation of the results, including collection of data on factors that contribute to missing assessments and data that are likely to predict the missing data. When constructing the set of possible reasons for missing data, the options should differentiate whether the non-response was likely to be related to the patient's HRQOL. For example, "Patient refusal" does not clarify this, but reasons such as "Patient refusal due to poor health" and "Patient refusal unrelated to health" are informative. Secondary prevention may include gathering concurrent data on toxicity, evaluations of health status by the clinical staff, or assessments from a caregiver.

Education

Education and training is an important part of minimizing missing data.[8,35] Training must begin at the investigator level and include research assistants (often nurses) as well as the patient. Vehicles for education include the protocol (with strong justifications for the assessments), symposia, videos, and written materials. Videos may be valuable as training vehicles both for research staff and patients. While there are often face-to-face training sessions at the initiation of a study, research personnel can change over time. Training tapes directed toward research personnel can deal with procedures in more detail than is possible in the protocol. Examples would include how to handle a patient who is unable to fill in the questionnaire and not letting family or friends assist. Training tapes are especially useful for providing positive ways of approaching the patient. For example, instead of referring to participation as burdensome, the assessment can be placed in a positive light.[51] Rather than "We have a lot of forms that you need to fill out," a better approach is, "We want to know more about the quality of life of people as they go through this treatment and the only way to know is

to ask you, so we're asking you to complete this brief questionnaire. It usually takes about 10 minutes."

Hopwood *et al.*[48] noted that, in three trials for lung and head and neck cancer, the most commonly cited factor affecting the distribution of questionnaires was the staff's judgment that the patient was too ill to complete a HRQOL assessment. Patient refusal was the least cited problem. It is understandable that study personnel are reluctant to approach patients when they appear to be feeling ill; but to minimize the bias from selecting out these patients, all subjects should be asked to complete the questionnaire. There are ways of encouraging ill patients, specifically by providing conditions that make it as easy as possible for them to complete the questionnaire. When a patient refuses, that refusal must be respected, of course.

Patient information sheets that explain the rationale behind the assessments will minimize missing data. These fact sheets can contain messages about the importance of the patient's perspective, that there are no "correct" answers, and reasons why it is important to respond to every question and to complete the follow-up questionnaires. In addition to the persuasive information, patients should be informed that they can refuse without affecting their treatment or relationship with their doctor.

Forms

The data collection forms should be attractive and professional in appearance, using fonts that are large enough to ensure readability (e.g., 12-point characters or greater). Two-sided forms should not be used as patients will often not look on the back of the page and, if forms are copied at the sites, there is a high probability that only the front side will be copied.[48]

Explicit procedures for follow-up

A practical schedule with assessments linked to planned treatment or follow-up visits can decrease the number of missing assessments. When possible, it is wise to link patient-reported outcomes with other clinical assessments. The availability of the patient increases the likelihood that the assessment will be completed. Staff may be more likely to remember when the assessment is scheduled if the timing is linked to clinical or laboratory follow-up. Finally, it is possible to link clinical events and laboratory values to the assessments. Less frequent assessment decreases patient burden slightly but may introduce confusion about the schedule and lead to missed assessments. If more frequent assessments are specified in the design, strategies for obtaining the additional assessments must be identified. If the duration of assessment continues after therapy is discontinued, this procedure should be clearly stated, and protocol flow charts for treatment and assessment schedules should clearly reflect the difference.

The protocol and training materials should include specific procedures to minimize missing data. These documents should clearly state the acceptable windows for each assessment[35] and whether follow-up by telephone or mail is allowed.[35] Documentation of the reasons for missing assessments can be combined with other questions about the conditions under which the HRQOL assessment was administered. For example, "What was the site and mode of administration?" and "Was any assistance given and, if so, by whom?"

Timing and administration

Frequency of evaluations

The frequency of assessments should correspond appropriately to the natural history of the disease and the likelihood of changes in the outcome within that period. Other considerations include having a practical follow-up schedule that includes the timing of therapeutic and diagnostic interventions. The assessments should be frequent enough to capture meaningful change, but not so frequent as to be burdensome to the patient or incongruent with the assessment tool. Assessments should not be more frequent than the period of recall defined for the instrument. Thus, if the instrument is based on recall over the previous month, assessments should not be

weekly or daily. Collection of patient-based measures used in economic analyses (e.g., sick days) should be frequent enough to ensure accuracy of the information with accurate recall rather than guessing, but not so frequent as to be overly burdensome.

Duration of HRQOL assessment

First, the HRQOL assessment should cover a time interval sufficient to observe changes in the outcome. Physiologic responses to a therapy may occur more rapidly than changes in HRQOL. This consideration is particularly relevant for chronic diseases that have associated physical or functional disabilities. For practical reasons, it is wise to define a specific limit to the duration of assessment, specifically avoiding statements such as "and every six months thereafter." This situation illustrates the need for a well-defined objective. For example, are the investigators interested in the HRQOL of subjects while on a therapy that is of limited duration, or is it especially important to understand the long-term impact of the treatment on HRQOL? If the former, the additional information that can be obtained from continued assessments may diminish after some point either because there is little or no change or because the number of subjects with assessments is too small to analyze. If none of the objectives of the study requires continued assessment, then follow-up beyond that point is unwarranted.

Assessment after discontinuation of therapy

A very clear policy needs to be developed for following patients who cannot follow the treatment protocol.[8] There are two major considerations. The first is scientific and depends on the research question. If the discontinuation of treatment limits any future therapy to more intensive and toxic treatments, or eliminates treatment options altogether as the disease progresses as is typical in cancer, the failure to continue patient-based assessment can lead to over-optimistic bias. A treatment arm with a high rate of dropout may appear artificially beneficial because only the healthiest of the patients are remaining on the treatment. On the other hand, discontinuation of assessment at the time treatment stops may make scientific sense in other settings such as prevention studies. The second consideration is practical. Off-treatment assessments are often difficult to obtain, especially if the patient no longer remains under the care of the same physician. If it is anticipated that patients are likely to change physicians, modes of administration such as telephone interviews or mailed assessments may be needed.

Timing of the initial HRQOL assessment

It is critical that the initial assessment occurs prior to randomization. Because the measurement of HRQOL is generally based on self-evaluation, there is a potential that the knowledge of treatment assignment will influence a subject's responses.[52] This concern is especially warranted when the patient is aware that one of the interventions is new, possibly more effective than standard therapy, and exciting to his or her physician. The possible exception occurs if the intervention is double-blinded and treatment starts within a reasonable period of time after randomization. In this case, it is allowable to obtain the initial assessment prior to the beginning of treatment but after randomization.

Timing of the follow-up HRQOL assessments

Similar attention should be paid to the timing of follow-up assessments. Assessments should be made consistently across treatment arms. Attention should be paid to the timing of diagnostic procedures. Especially with life-threatening diseases, the choices are not particularly easy. Prior to the testing, patients are likely to be experiencing stress in anticipation of the yet unknown results. After the test, the patients will either be experiencing great relief or anxiety.

Recall period is another important consideration. The period of accurate recall is between one and four weeks, with better recall of major events and more recent experiences. Schipper[28] notes that the side effects of chemotherapy in cancer patients may have a less adverse impact on a patient's HRQOL than similar side effects attributable to the disease. This observation may be true in other disease conditions as well. Testing immediately after toxicity occurs will emphasize that experience and de-emphasize the benefits of treatment and disease symptoms. It is important not to pick a particular timing that will automatically bias the results against one treatment arm. However, in studies where the timing and length of treatment differ across arms, this may be challenging if not impossible.

Timing of HRQOL assessments when therapy is cyclic

Treatment for cancer is generally cyclic, with administration of therapy only during the initial part of the cycle. Intense and toxic therapy is given often for one to two weeks, with a hiatus for another one or two weeks to allow for recovery from the toxic effects of the treatment. Thus, it may not be possible to identify a time when the HRQOL is "typical." For very practical reasons, HRQOL assessments have traditionally been scheduled to occur just prior to the beginning of the next cycle. Patients return to the clinic at this time for laboratory tests and other clinical evaluations; thus, they are consistently available for HRQOL assessment. As a result, there is potential for the measurement obtained just prior to the next cycle to overestimate the HRQOL over the entire cycle. More frequent assessment would solve this problem but must be weighed against the increased patient burden and the logistical issues of obtaining HRQOL assessments between patient visits.

Analysis

As most HRQOL studies consist of longitudinal assessments with measures that consist of multiple scales, the two most common analytic problems are missing data[53,54] and multiple endpoints.[55] Missing data are a concern because of the potential for biased estimates of HRQOL when the reasons for missing data are related to factors that affect the patient's HRQOL. The presence of multiple endpoints presents two potential problems: controlling Type I errors for multiple comparisons, and finding strategies for presenting HRQOL results in a manner that is clinically meaningful and easily interpretable.

Missing data are inevitable in any longitudinal study of free-living subjects where, over an extended period of time, patients may experience morbidity or mortality due to disease or its treatment. When missing data result from administrative problems, such as staff forgetting to give the forms to patients, they cause concern about the quality of the clinical trial. When the reasons are directly related to the patient's health-related quality of life, such as the patient being unable to complete the questionnaire because of severe toxicity or death, naive methods of analysis that ignore missing data or dropout may result in biased estimates. If patients who are experiencing a negative impact of the disease or therapy on their lives are less likely to complete the HRQOL assessments, simplistic analyses of available data may overestimate the HRQOL of the entire sample of subjects.

Two of the most commonly reported methods of analysis of HRQOL make the most restrictive assumptions about missing data: repeated univariate tests (t-tests, Wilcoxon rank sum tests) and multivariate analysis of variance (MANOVA) using only patients who have completed all of the scheduled assessments (Complete Cases). These approaches are based on the very strong assumption that data are missing completely at random (MCAR); if that assumption is violated, then the estimates of HRQOL may be seriously biased unless the proportion of subjects with any missing assessments is very small (<5% of the cases). On the other hand, an analysis of only complete cases could exclude more than half of the subjects and represent a very select subgroup of the entire sample. Repeated univariate tests also compare selected subgroups that change over time as more subjects drop out of the study. Another popular approach is to use the last observation (or value) carried forward (LOCF or LVCF), where the patient's last available assessment is substituted for each of the following missing assessments. This approach has limited utility[13,56] and should be employed with great caution. Unfortunately, it is often proposed as a standard analytic method without any thought as to whether it might result in an overly optimistic or overly pessimistic estimate of the true value.

Another popular method of addressing missing data is assigning a value of zero for those individuals who have died (or withdrawn). Gould[57] describes an approach where, if there is adequate documentation of the reasons for missing assessments, it may be possible to determine a reasonable ordering (or ranking) of HRQOL among the subjects. Heyting *et al.*[56] identifies some limitations, including reasons for dropout, that are not clearly ordered.

Likelihood-based methods[58–60] that use all the available data result in unbiased estimates when the missing data are ignorable or missing at random (MAR). Examples include maximum likelihood estimation of mixed effect models, growth curve models, and repeated measures models for incomplete data. Given that they are more efficient and have less restrictive assumptions about missing data, these likelihood based methods should be preferred over methods such as complete case MANOVA or repeated univariate methods.[53,61]

Non-ignorable missing data are the most likely type of missing data in trials where there is dropout due to toxicity, disease progression, or death. Studies with this type of missing data are also the most difficult to analyze. The primary reason is that there are numerous models for the missing data mechanism, and it is impossible to verify statistically the "correctness" of any particular model because the very data required to distinguish among models are missing. Little[60] describes two general classes of models: selection and mixture models. In the class of selection models, a statistical model is specified for the missing data mechanism. For example, dropout may be modeled as a function of patient characteristics, treatment outcomes, and measures of HRQOL. In addition to adjusting the HRQOL estimates for missing data, these models allow the investigator to make inferences about the relationship of HRQOL and other explanatory factors associated with missing observations. This might be particularly instructive, for example, if death or disease progression were the primary cause of dropout. Examples include a probit model,[62] a conditional linear model where the rate of change in an individual is modeled as a polynomial function of the time of dropout,[63] and empirical Bayesian estimation of the individual time gradients of HRQOL adjusted for informative right censoring.[64] Diggle and Kenward[65] describe a likelihood method with a marginal (and thus unconditional) model for the outcome and a conditional model for dropout given the observed measurements. When the change over time is not expected to be linear or the censoring times vary across patients, Schluchter[66] and DeGruttola and Tu[67] have proposed extensions of the random effects or two-stage mixed effects model. The time of censoring (or death) is incorporated into the second-stage model of the population parameters by allowing the time of censoring to be correlated with the random effects of the longitudinal model for HRQOL.[74]

In contrast to the selection models, the pattern mixture models do not require the specification of a particular model for the missing data mechanism. This strength is counter-balanced by the large number of potential patterns of missing data and the strong assumptions for the restriction required to estimate parameters in the (otherwise) under-identified models. The basic concept behind the pattern mixture models is described by Little.[60]

An alternative method of analysis uses the strategy of multiple imputation to estimate the missing data.[68–72] The motivations for this approach are that complete data methods such as MANOVA can be used to analyze the imputed data sets, and information about the reasons for missing data can be incorporated into the imputation scheme.[73]

Given the numerous potential methods of analysis for non-ignorable missing data, how do we choose among different strategies? In some cases, information such as the reason for missing assessments or a clearly defined objective will determine the "best" approach. But, in general, while certain approaches

may be eliminated from consideration, several possibilities will remain. A sensitivity analysis, in which the effect of the different methods of analysis is examined, is strongly recommended.[53,73,74]

Overall recommendations

Well-defined objectives established early in the design phase of the clinical trial

Providing sufficient background and a rationale to justify the resources required for an investigation of patient-reported outcomes will contribute to the success of the investigation. The rationale should address questions like "How exactly might the results affect the clinical management of patients?" and "How will the results be used when determining the effectiveness of the treatment arms?" The justification should include a motivation for the particular aspects of HRQOL or the economic assessments that will be measured in the trial (e.g., physical, functional, emotional) as they relate to the disease and its treatment.

The same demands for a rationale should be applied to all information collected in any clinical trial. However, investigators already have a habit of collecting laboratory and radiological tests so that minimal motivation is required to support this data collection. The same is not necessarily true for the collection of data that requires patient self-assessment, and greater motivation may be necessary. Writing a rationale for assessments also facilitates the development of well-defined research objectives.

Establishing specific procedures and resources for implementing the study

In many clinical trials, the decision to include HRQOL assessments is made at the end of the planning phase. Often, a questionnaire is added to the data collection with minimal appreciation for the amount of staff time required and with no allocation of additional resources. This generally results in overly ambitious assessment schedules and large amounts of missing data, which make analysis difficult and any results open to criticism. While this behavior has diminished over time, there are still too many trials in which the details of how the HRQOL assessments will be obtained are missing from the protocol and training materials. The specific procedures, and associated resources, for implementing any clinical trial should encompass all the components required for establishing efficacy and safety, including laboratory and radiological assessments, *and* for assessing those patient-reported outcomes incorporated in the trial design.

REFERENCES

1 Sugarbaker, P. H., Barofsky, I., Rosenberg, S. A., Gianola, F. J. (1986). Quality of life assessment of patients in extremity sarcoma clinical trials. *Surgery* **91**:17–23.

2 Hicks, J. E., Lampert, M. H., Gerber, L. H., Glastein, E., Danoff, J. (1985). Functional outcome update in patients with soft tissue sarcoma undergoing wide local excision and radiation. (Abstract). *Archives of Physical Medicine and Rehabilitation* **66**:542–3.

3 Brown, M. L., Lipscomb, J., Snyder, C. (2001). The burden of illness of cancer: economic cost and quality of life. *Annual Review of Public Health* **22**:91–113.

4 Revicki, D. A., Rothman, M., Luce, B. (1992). Health-related quality of life assessment and the pharmaceutical industry. *Pharmacoeconomics* **1**:294–408.

5 Slevin, M. L., Stubbs, L., Plant, H. J. *et al.* (1990). Attitude to chemotherapy: comparing views. *British Medical Journal* **300**:1458–60.

6 Brinkley, D. (1985). Quality of life in cancer trials. *British Medical Journal* **291**:685–6.

7 Moinpour, C., Feigl, P., Metch, B. *et al.* (1989). Quality of life endpoints in cancer clinical trials: review and recommendations. *Journal of the National Cancer Institute* **81**:485–95.

8 Gotay, C. C., Korn, E. L., McCabe, M. S., Moore, T. D., Cheson, B. D. (1992). Quality of life assessment in cancer treatment protocols: research issues in protocol development. *Journal of the National Cancer Institute* **84**:575–9.

9 Hillner, B. E., Smith, T. J. (1998). Does a clinical trial warrant an economic analysis? (Editorial). *Journal of the National Cancer Institute* **90**:724–5.

10 O'Brien, this volume, Chapter 25.

11 Hornbrook, this volume, Chapter 24.

12 Bungay, K. M., Boyer, J. G., Steinwald, A. B., Ware, J. E. (1996). Health-related quality of life: an overview. In *Principles of Pharmacoeconomics* (2nd Edition), ed. J. L. Bootman, R. J. Townsend, W. F. McGhan, pp. 128–48. Cincinnati, OH: Harvey Whitney Books Company.

13 Fairclough, D. L. (2002). *Design and Analysis of Quality of Life Studies in Clinical Trials*. Boca Raton, FL: Chapman and Hall/CRC.

14 Sprangers, M. A. G., Aaronson, N. K. (1992). The role of health care providers and significant others in evaluating the quality of life of patients with chronic diseases: a review. *Journal of Clinical Epidemiology* **45**:743–60.

15 Rothman, M. L., Hedrick, S. C., Bulcroft, K. A., Hickam, D. H., Rubinstein, L. Z. (1991). The validity of proxy-generated scores as measures of patient health status. *Medical Care* **29**:115–24.

16 Sneeuw, K. C. A., Aaronson, N. K., Sprangers, M. A. G., Detmar, S. B., Wever, L. D. V., Schornagel, J. H. (1998). Comparison of patient and proxy EORTC QLQ-C30 ratings in assessing the quality of life of cancer patients. *Journal of Clinical Epidemiology* **51**:617–31.

17 Novella, J. L., Jochum, C., Jolly, D., Morrone, I., Ankri, J., Bureau, F., Blanchard, F. (2001). Agreement between patient' and proxies' reports of quality of life in Alzheimer's disease. *Quality of Life Research* **10**:443–52.

18 Epstein, A. M., Hall, J. A., Togretti, J. *et al.* (1989). Using proxies to evaluate quality of life. *Medical Care* **27**(Suppl.): S91–8.

19 Nelson, L. M., Longstreth, W. T., Koepsel, T. D., van Belle, G. (1990). Proxy respondents in epidemiologic research. *Epidemiology Reviews* **12**:71–89.

20 Farrow, D. C., Samet, J. M. (1990). Comparability of information provided by elderly cancer patients regarding health and functional status, social network and life events. *Epidemiology* **1**:370–6.

21 Groenvold, M., Klee, M. C., Sprangers, M. A. G., Aaronson, N. K. (1997). Validation of the EORTC QLQ-C30 quality of life questionnaire through combined qualitative and quantitative assessment of patient-observer agreement. *Journal of Clinical Epidemiology* **50**:441–50.

22 Fitzsimmons, D., George, S., Payne, S., Johnson, C. D. (1990). Differences in perceptions of quality of life issues between health professionals and patient with pancreatic cancer. *Psycho-Oncology* **8**:135–43.

23 Gabriel, S. E., Kneeland, T. S., Melton, L. J., Moncur, M. M., Ettiger, B., Tosteson, A. N. A. (1999). Health-related quality of life in economic evaluations for osteoporosis: whose values should we use? *Medical Decision Making* **19**:141–8.

24 Llewellyn-Thomas, H., Sutherland, H. J., Tibshirani, R. *et al.* (1984). Describing health states. Methodologic issues in obtaining values for health states. *Medical Care* **22**: 543–52.

25 Patrick, D. L., Sittampalam, Y., Somerville, S. M. *et al.* (1985). A cross-cultural comparison of health status values. *American Journal of Public Health* **75**:1402–7.

26 Balaban, D. J., Sagi, P. C., Goldfarb, N. I., Mettler, S. (1986). Weights for scoring the quality of well-being instrument among rheumatoid arthritics. A comparison to general population weights. *Medical Care* **24**:973–80.

27 Sackett, D. L., Torrance, G. (1978). The utility of different health states as perceived by the general public. *Journal of Chronic Disease* **31**:697–704.

28 Schipper, H. (1990). Guidelines and caveats for quality of life measurement in clinical practice and research. *Oncology* **4**:51–7.

29 Wiklund, I., Dimenas, E., Wahl, M. (1990). Factors of importance when evaluating quality of life in clinical trials. *Controlled Clinical Trials* **11**:169–79.

30 TeVelde, A., Sprangers, M. A., Aaronson, N. K. (1996). Feasibility, psychometric performance and stability across modes of administration of the CARES-SF. *Annals of Oncology* **7**: 381–90.

31 Kissinger, P., Rice, J., Farley, T. *et al.* (1999). Application of computer-assisted interviews to sexual behavior research. *American Journal of Epidemiology* **149**:950–4.

32 Turner, C. F., Ku, L., Rogers, S. M. *et al.* (1998). Adolescent sexual behavior, drug use, and violence: increased reporting with computer survey technology. *Science* **280**: 867–73.

33 Skinner, H. A., Allen, B. A. (1983). Does the computer make a difference? Computerized versus face-to-face versus self-report assessment of alcohol, drug and tobacco use. *Journal of Consulting Clinical Psychology* **51**:267–75.

34 Weinberger, M., Oddone, E. Z., Samsa, G. P. *et al.* (1996). Are HRQOL measures affected by the mode of administration? *Journal of Clinical Epidemiology* **49**:135–40.

35 Cella, D. F. (1995). Methods and problems in measuring QOL. *Support Care in Cancer* **3**:11–22.

36 McHorney, D. A., Kosinski, M., Ware, J. E. (1994). Comparison of the cost and quality of norms for the SF-36 health survey collected by mail versus telephone interview: results from a national survey. *Medical Care* **32**:551–67.

37 Leidy, N. K., Elixhauser, A., Rentz, A. M. *et al.* (1999) Telephone validation of the QOL in epilepsy inventory-89 (QOLIE-89). *Epilepsia* **40**:97–106.

38 Gasquet, I., Falissard, B., Ravaud, P. (2001). Impact of reminders and methods of questionnaire distribution on patient response to mail-back satisfaction survey. *Journal of Clinical Epidemiology* **54**:1174–80.

39 Velikova, G., Wright, E. P., Smith, A. B. *et al.* (1999). Automated collection of quality of life data: a comparison of paper and computer-touchscreen questionnaires. *Journal of Clinical Oncology* **17**:998–1000.

40 Kleinman, L., Leidy, N. K., Crawley, J., Bonomi, A., Schoenfeld, P. (2001). A comparative trial of paper-and-pencil versus computer administration of the QOL in Reflux and Dyspepsia (QOLRAD) questionnaire. *Medical Care* **39**:181–9.

41 Buxton, J., White, M., Osoba, D. (1998). Patients' experiences using a computerized program with a touch-sensitive video monitor for the assessment of health-related quality of life. *Quality of Life Research* **7**:513–19.

42 Yarnold, P. R., Stewart, M. J., Stille, F. C. *et al.* (1996). Assessing functional status of elderly adults via microcomputer. *Perception and Motor Skills* **82**:689–90.

43 Crawley, J. A., Bleinman, L., Dominitz, J. (2000). User preferences for computer administration of quality of life instruments. *Drug Information Journal* **34**:137–44.

44 Burke, K. C., Baker, J. H., Hillis, A. (1995). Test-retest reliability in psychiatric patients of the SF-36 health survey. *International Journal of Methods in Psychological Research* **5**:189–94.

45 Drummond, H. E., Gosh, S., Ferguson, A. *et al.* (1995). Electronic quality of life questionnaires: a comparison of pen-based electronic questionnaires with conventional paper in a gastrointestinal study. *Quality of Life Research* **4**: 21–6.

46 O'Connor, K. P., Hallam, R. S., Hinchliffe, R. (1989). Evaluation of a computer interview system for use with neuro-otology patients. *Clinical Otolaryngology* **14**:3–9.

47 American Psychological Association (1986). *Guidelines of Computer Based Tests and Interpretation* (p. 18). American Psychological Association.

48 Hopwood, P., Harvey, A., Davies, J., Stephens, R. J. *et al.* (1997). Survey of the Administration of Quality of Life Questionnaires in three multicentre randomised trials in cancer. *European Journal of Cancer* **90**:49–57.

49 Fairclough, D. L., Cella, D. F. (1996). A Cooperative Group report on quality of life research: lessons learned. Eastern Cooperative Oncology Group (ECOG). *Journal of the National Cancer Institute* **40**:73–5.

50 Young, T., Maher, J. (1999). Collecting quality of life data in EORTC clinical trials – what happens in practice? *Psycho-Oncology* **8**, 260–3.

51 Cella, D. F., Skeel, R. T., Bonomi, A. E. (1993). *Policies and Procedures Manual*. Eastern Cooperative Oncology Group Quality of Life Subcommittee, Boston MA. (Unpublished).

52 Brooks, M. M., Jenkins, L. S., Schron, E. B., Steinberg, J. S., Cross, J. A., Paeth D. S. (1998). Quality of life at baseline: is assessment after randomization valid? *Medical Care* **36**:1515–19.

53 Fairclough, D. L. (1996). Quality of life in cancer clinical trials: now that we have the data, what do we do? *Journal of Applied Statistical Science* **4**:253–69.

54 Curren, D., Fayers, P., Molenberghs, G., Machin, D. (1998). Analysis of incomplete quality of life data in clinical trials. In *Quality of Life Assessment in Clinical Trials: Methods and Practice*, ed. M. Staquet, R. Hays, P. Fayers, pp. 249–80. Oxford: Oxford University Press.

55 Korn, E. L., O'Fallon, J. (1990). Statistical considerations. Statistics Working Group. In *Quality of Life Assessment in Cancer Clinical Trials*, Report on Workshop on Quality of Life Research in Cancer Clinical Trials, Division of Cancer Prevention and Control. Bethesda, MD: National Cancer Institute.

56 Heyting, A., Tolboom, J. T. B. M., Essers, J. G. A. (1992). Statistical handling of dropouts in longitudinal clinical trials. *Statistics in Medicine* **11**:2043–61.

57 Gould, A. L. (1980). A new approach to the analysis of clinical drug trials with withdrawals. *Biometrics* **36**:721–27.

58 Jennrich, R. I., Schluchter, M. D. (1986). Unbalanced repeated-measures models with structured covariance matrices. *Biometrics* **42**:805–20.

59 Laird, N. M. (1988). Missing data in longitudinal studies. *Statistics in Medicine* **7**:305–15.

60 Little, R. J. A. (1995). Modeling the dropout mechanism in repeated-measures studies. *Journal of the American Statistical Association* **90**:1112–21.

61 Zwinderman, A. H. (1992). Statistical analysis of longitudinal quality of life data with missing measurements. *Quality of Life Research* **1**:219–24.

62 Wu, M. C., Bailey, K. R. (1988). Analyzing changes in the presence of informative right censoring caused by death and withdrawal. *Statistics in Medicine* **7**:337–46.

63 Wu, M. C., Carroll, R. J. (1988). Estimation and comparison of changes in the presence of informative right censoring by modeling the censoring process. *Biometrics* **44**:175–88.

64 Mori, M., Woodworth, G. G., Woolson, R. F. (1992). Application of empirical Bayes inference to estimation of rate of change in the presence of informative right censoring. *Statistics in Medicine* **11**:621–31.

65 Diggle, P. J., Kenward, M. G. (1994). Informative dropout in longitudinal data analysis (with discussion). *Applied Statistics* **43**:49–93.

66 Schluchter, M. D. (1992). Methods for the analysis of informatively censored longitudinal data. *Statistics in Medicine* **11**:1861–70.

67 DeGruttola, V., Tu, X. M. (1994). Modeling progression of CD4-lymphocyte count and its relationship to survival time. *Biometrics* **50**:1003–14.

68 Rubin, D. B. (1987). *Multiple Imputation for Nonresponse in Surveys*. New York: John Wiley.

69 Rubin, D. B., Schenker, N. (1991). Multiple imputation in health-care data bases: an overview and some applications. *Statistics in Medicine* **10**:585–98.

70 Schafer, J. L. (1998). *Analysis of Incomplete Multivariate Data*. London: Chapman and Hall.

71 Crawford, S. L., Tennstedt, S. L., McKinlay, J. B. (1995). A comparison of analytic methods for non-random missingness of outcome data. *Journal of Clinical Epidemiology* **48**:209–19.

72 Lavori, P. W., Dawson, R., Shera, D. (1995). A multiple imputation strategy for clinical trials with truncation of patient data. *Statistics in Medicine* **14**:1913–25.

73 Fairclough, D. L. (2002). Multiple imputation for non-random missing data in longitudinal studies of health-related quality of life. In *Statistical Methods for Quality of Life Studies: Design, Measurement and Analysis*, ed. M. Mesbah, B. F. Cole, M.-L. T. Lee. Boston: Kluwer Academic Publishers, pp. 323–37.

74 Fairclough, D. L., Peterson, H., Cella, D., Bonomi, P. (1998). Comparison of model based methods dependent on the missing data mechanism in two clinical trials of cancer therapy. *Statistics in Medicine* **17**:781–96.

ENDNOTES

a. Morbidity cost is measured by lost income due to work disability and absenteeism associated with the disease.[3]

b. Estimates of cost-effectiveness will have very wide confidence intervals when small differences in effectiveness appear in the denominator.

c. In this discussion *Early Phase II* trial refers to a small non-randomized trial and *Late Phase II* trial refers to a large randomized trial with multiple dose levels and patients similar to those to be enrolled in later phase III and IV trials.

18

Statistical issues in the application of cancer outcome measures

Jeff A. Sloan, Ph.D.

Mayo Clinic, Rochester, MN

Introduction

Are there fundamental differences in the statistical analysis of patient-reported outcomes and other non-biomedical endpoints, on the one hand, and so-called "harder" endpoints such as survival, tumor response, or patient blood pressure on the other?

In this chapter we emphasize that, while the application and interpretation of statistical methods in the outcomes research literature to date has been highly variable, this is not a signal that standard statistical approaches are not up to the task. Rather, they need to be applied with intelligence, completeness, and due consideration to the unique aspects of outcomes research. To that end, this chapter will provide specific examples of how the standard statistical methods have been applied skillfully, while also indicating where the use of novel or modern methods can and should be explored. The idea is not to address all relevant statistical topics and approaches de novo, or to produce yet another primer on statistical methods; there are already texts for this. Our aim, rather, is to ask what is, and what should be, the interplay between each statistical topic and the construction and selection of a cancer outcome measure. If there were little linkage between the statistical topic, on the one hand, and the choice of endpoint measures on the other, then that topic would receive only modest attention. Where the interplay is significant, the spotlight rises accordingly.[1]

Two basic conclusions emerge in the chapter: (1) the standard scientific paradigm and existing statistical methods are all that is required to produce high quality, defensible, and credible outcomes research (though novel approaches may sometimes bring added value), and (2) outcomes research needs to be "demystified" and viewed as an achievable and integral part of clinical research. Only by accomplishing these two goals will cancer outcomes research make a convincing case for its existence. Otherwise, there is a danger it will eventually wither away as a passing fad in oncology research.

To tackle such a broad issue as statistical methods for cancer outcomes research, we organize the chapter's discussion into three general areas: (1) Study Design/Endpoint Selection, (2) Statistical Procedures/Analysis, and (3) Presentation / Interpretation of Results. While some statistical topics may fall into more than one general area, we will assign each topic to the area of primary importance. By taking this approach, the chapter asks what is, and what should be, the interplay between the outcome(s) under consideration, the construction and selection of appropriate outcome measures, the appropriate statistical analyses, and the methods of presentation.

The chapter is divided into four sections, each addressing issues using the trichotomization of topic areas noted above. The first section offers an overview of the "state of the science" by providing and commenting briefly on strategically chosen examples from the published literature, then identifying the most important challenges and barriers facing outcomes research in oncology. In response,

Table 18.1. Matching the outcomes research question to a common statistical approach: some representative examples

If your research question calls for . . .	then an appropriate method is . . . .
simple description of a population	means, medians, frequencies, percentages
quality monitoring of a system	outlier identification, z-scores
finding correlates of behavior (pairs of variables, both independent)	scatter plots, contingency tables, correlation coefficients
finding correlates of behavior (several variables, one or more dependent)	complex plotting, multiple regression, multicolinearity analysis
investigating how two or more variables interact to "produce" other variables	partial correlation, conditional analysis, complex graphical techniques, clustering
comparing how two separate groups of people score on a test	bar charts, t-tests or Wilcoxon tests, sign tests
comparing how more than two separate groups of people score on a test	bar charts, 1-way (ANOVA), Kruskal-Wallis, multiple comparisons procedures
comparing how two separate groups of people score on two tests	Hotelling's T^2, cluster analysis
comparing how more than two groups score on more than two tests	multivariate ANOVA or MANOVA
comparing how spouses differ	paired t-tests, difference scores
comparing how groups differ in the presence of other demographics	ANCOVA
examining how people perform over time	repeated measures ANOVA, profile analysis
assessing the reliability of a measurement tool, e.g., for health-related quality of life	Cronbach's alpha, Kendall's Tau, Cohen's Kappa, and related measures
examining the dimensionality of a measurement tool	factor analysis

the second section describes general aspects of a recommended model, or "gold standard," for statistical analysis in outcomes research. The third section discusses 12 elements of the recommended model and provides a number of examples specific to cancer outcomes research. The chapter concludes with suggestions for future research.

Throughout, the goal is to introduce the reader to the landscape of existing and possible future directions in cancer outcomes statistical methods. In the process, we summarize some of the mathematical and philosophical considerations surrounding this broad subject. We also supply concrete examples that demonstrate how outcomes research *can* be carried out with relative ease and simplicity. It can be made

very complex – but, in most cases, it does not need to be.

Examples of, and challenges in, the analysis of cancer outcomes data

That there is a wide body of existing statistical procedures for handling virtually any of the questions posed in cancer outcomes research is evident from Table 18.1. The emphasis there is on the linkage between the research question of interest and the appropriate approach(es) to statistical analysis.

Table 18.2 references a selection of well-known papers that well illustrate how to cope with the

Table 18.2. Selected readings on current methods in cancer outcomes research

Study design
1. Cleeland *et al.* (2000)[96]
2. Fairclough *et al.* (1999)[97]
3. Potosky *et al.* (2002)[98]
4. Stockler *et al.* (1999)[99]
5. Esper *et al.* (1997)[100]
6. Kemmler *et al.* (1999)[101]

The first paper describes the development of a new scale to measure patient symptoms, from item generation through to assessment of reliability and validity. The next two papers provide examples of how different aspects of HRQOL and clinical measures can be incorporated in a single study: Fairclough *et al.*, in the context of a randomized trial, and Potosky *et al.*, in the context of a large observational study. Stockler *et al.* and Esper *et al.* both describe the validation process for prostate cancer modules for two leading HRQOL measures, the EORTC QLQ-C30 and the FACT. The final paper exemplifies how to conduct a head-to-head comparison of instruments, in this case between the QLQ-C30 and the FACT.

Statistical analysis
1. Hakamies-Blomquist *et al.* (2000)[102]
2. Moinpour *et al.* (2000)[103]
3. McLachlan *et al.* (2001)[104]
4. Coates *et al.* (2000)[105]
5. Doyle *et al.* (2001)[106]
6. Zee (1998)[107]
7. Curran *et al.* (2000)[108]
8. Bernhard *et al.* (1998)[109]

The first paper is representative of a large scale, multi-site, cooperative group phase III clinical trial that is the gold standard for testing new cancer treatment modalities. The incorporation of and analysis of the HRQOL endpoints are simple and indicate that little special effort was required to carry out the necessary statistical analysis. The second paper exemplifies a comprehensive analysis of HRQOL data, again involving routine statistical methods, presented in accessible and understandable terms for the clinical audience. The third paper uses more complicated statistical methods i.e., multivariate modeling, because of the use of psychological measures. The fourth paper demonstrates how regression modeling of cancer outcomes measurement endpoints can be used to build prognostic models. The pitfalls, strengths, and weaknesses of each model are well described in this paper. Similarly the fifth paper demonstrates how simple regression modeling can be used to relate cost, outcomes, and HRQOL data using straightforward statistical methods. The sixth paper in this section demonstrates how complex models developed for survival analysis can be applied to research on cancer outcomes. This paper is a good example of how complex methodology can be applied to such work. It is also, unfortunately, an indication of how complex models can be both inaccessible and difficult in terms of interpretation of results. The seventh paper demonstrates how summary statistics can be used to circumvent the problem of longitudinal modeling and missing data. The methods are simple and straightforward and elegantly presented. The final methodological paper attempts to summarize the entire domain of statistical endeavors for outcomes research in cancer. Unfortunately it is also a typical example of the presentation of statistical challenges without an offering of complete solutions to the problems.

Presentation and interpretation of results
1. Madalinska *et al.* (2001)[110]
2. Bland, Altman (1996)[111]
3. Lee, Chi (2000)[112]
4. Chassany *et al.* (2002)[7]

The first paper is an example of standard reporting of results from a clinical trial using cancer outcome endpoints, with the use of simple analysis and straightforward reporting of average values in a tabular format with supporting p-values. The second paper shows how to present comparative data from competing measurement tools. The last two papers provide standards for reporting statistical results for HRQOL in clinical cancer trials. These recommendations could well be applied to any other endpoint in oncology research.

challenges that arise variously in study design, statistical analysis, and the presentation and interpretation of results. These papers underscore that the selection of well-validated and reliable measures is an integral part of outcomes analysis, and the analyst will sometimes want to conduct additional psychometric analysis to investigate the appropriateness of the measures selected. The papers in Table 18.2 also exemplify the types of studies and accompanying statistical analyses that may be required – from small observational studies to large clinical trials, and from simple summary statistics to complex modeling procedures. Also presented are examples of comprehensive approaches to presenting and interpreting the findings of outcomes research studies.

Beyond this brief summary, many chapters in this volume have provided concrete examples of both high quality and sometimes less-than-stellar analyses of outcomes data. In almost all applications, both strengths and shortcomings can be assessed through a careful examination of study design, choice of statistical procedures (given design), and presentation of findings.

In particular, did the design lead to: Designation of appropriate treatment arms or, more generally, study sub-groups (given the stated aims of the investigator)? Selection of appropriate endpoints and covariates, with special attention to patient-reported outcome measures such as health-related quality of life? Appropriate sample sizes, given the questions and the measures? And, more generally, the creation of a study structure that minimizes the need for complex and assumption-laden statistical procedures, in part, to compensate for design flaws? Next, were the statistical analyses appropriate, given the design? Finally, were the results presented clearly, accurately, and in an intuitively appealing way that spoke not only to the outcomes researcher but to the clinician, policy maker, provider, payer, patient, or other end users?

One needs to be reasonable and judicious in criticizing outcomes research studies, as it is all too easy to find flaws in virtually any research study or statistical method.[2] Much has been written about the frequent inadequacy of statistical analyses in medical research.[3,4] Fortunately, there are a number of important papers setting out detailed plans for how to carry out a complete statistical analysis of clinical trials data; as cases in point, see Fairclough (1997)[5] and Albert (1999)[6] for examples of how to deal with missing data and conduct longitudinal analysis.

Instead of cataloging how *not* to do cancer outcomes research, we instead list in Table 18.3 the main challenges that need to be surmounted. Most critical, of course, is avoiding the errors in study design that can lead to the "garbage in – garbage out" scenario. Among the various issues most often overlooked are simple power considerations (so that sample sizes are sufficient to permit detecting a meaningful difference in endpoints, if it exists), and the a priori specification of what results will be deemed a "success." The statistical analysis of patient-reported outcomes is complicated by missing data and concomitant confounding influences, but these problems can and do also arise when the focus is on traditional clinical endpoints, including survival. It is vital to explore the robustness of findings through the use of sensitivity analysis, so that any concerns over the "softness" of the endpoints can be dealt with directly and demonstrated (in most cases) to be unwarranted. Common problems in the presentation of findings include the absence of interpretation, or the misinterpretation, of p-values, and an inadequate explanation and reporting of complex analyses that were undertaken to supplement or replace traditional, more transparent approaches.

A paradigm, or "gold standard," for statistical analyses in cancer outcomes studies

This section will present what we consider to be a paradigm for carrying out statistical analyses within an outcomes research clinical study. There is no uniformly agreed upon approach to statistical analysis for outcomes research studies in oncology, which makes the delineation of a singular paradigm difficult. However, the goal of identifying guidelines for a uniform approach is achievable in general terms.[7]

Table 18.3. Challenges encountered in statistical analyses of outcomes research data

Study design

1. The outcomes are not well defined: Data are collected and analyzed without definition of endpoints, both primary and secondary. Such studies with both positive results and negative results leave the researcher with the problem of determining which of the results to believe.
2. Inappropriate choice of measurement tools: Measurement tools and items are not focused on the outcome(s) of interest.
3. Inadequate psychometric analysis: New measurement tools or selected items from existing tools are not examined for psychometric properties before use.
4. Measurement tools use different scales and approaches: Results are not interpretable or comparable to other studies or across measures without some form of data transformation.
5. Power analysis is missing or inappropriate: Results may be a function of sample size as much as a true indication of (non-)efficacy.
6. The study is not set up to interpret the clinical significance of results: The magnitude of effect observed cannot be interpreted in terms of its indication for changes in clinical practice.
7. Inadequate stratification to control for potential confounding variables: The primary endpoint is confounded with another variable so that it is difficult to attribute their relative impact on results.

Statistical analysis

8. Attrition: Missing data are present either in large quantities or in a nonrandom fashion, which complicates the application of standard statistical methods.
9. Heterogeneous sub-samples: Analyses fail to take into account imbalances between treatment groups.
10. Sensitivity analysis: Sensitivity analysis is either not performed or inadequate to state the threshold values which are likely to change the results of the analysis.
11. Too many variables per observations: Most multi-variable analytical procedures (e.g., regression) are not generalizable without 100+ observations and an observations to variables ratio of 20:1.

Presentation and interpretation of results

12. Results are presented only on "average patients": Study results often do not include distribution statistics, or the range of possible values of study results.
13. Results are presented as p-values without interpretation: Confidence intervals and interpretation of statistical significance are missing from presentation of results.
14. The clinical significance of results are not considered: The statistical significance of results (p-values) are reported without any consideration of clinical significance of study findings.
15. Results are presented only for complex models, without any presentation of results of basic statistical analyses: Results of basic statistical analyses are relegated to relative unimportance, with priority only given to results from more complex models.

In brief, outcome assessment should be held to the same standard – no more, no less – as any other form of scientific inquiry. Of primary importance is establishing a priori linkages among the research hypothesis, the tool selection, the study design, the statistical analysis, and the presentation of results; see Table 18.4. Because the resources for conducting an outcomes research study are limited, so must be the sample size; and sheer pragmatism typically dictates that a single primary endpoint be chosen and that a single statistical strategy or approach be linked to the analysis of that endpoint. Subsequent to this identification, the researcher is free to add as many secondary endpoints as are supportable scientifically. Rather than promoting any one strategy or approach to data analysis, we emphasize the need for multiple approaches to be considered via sensitivity analysis. This is particularly important in cancer outcomes research because results need to be demonstrable to a wide and sometimes skeptical audience. The basic paradigm proposed here might be characterized informally as "gonna get some data, what should our plans be?" as opposed to "got some data, what do we do with it now?"

Table 18.4. Elements of a general paradigm for designing, analyzing, and presenting cancer outcomes research

Study design

1. Create a priori linkage among research hypothesis, endpoints, measurement tools, study design, and statistical analysis.
2. Identify a single primary endpoint and related study design and statistical analysis.
3. Identify all secondary endpoints and related statistical tests.
4. Establish sample size and power specification for primary endpoint.
5. Specify the type of results that will be declared clinically significant.
6. Split significance levels appropriately to adjust for multiple endpoints, if necessary.
7. Stratify appropriately for potential confounding variables.

Statistical analyses

8. Separate primary analysis and supporting analyses.
9. Examine attrition patterns for missingness at random.
10. Carry out analyses verifying that underlying assumptions of statistical procedures are supported.
11. Analyze data using various approaches in a comprehensive sensitivity analysis so results are examined in the face of different assumptions. This should include intent-to-treat analysis.
12. Perform separate, complete analyses for differential effects on appropriately pre-specified subpopulations (e.g., minority or underserved patients).

Presentation and interpretation of results

13. Present descriptive statistics including range of values for important variables.
14. Present results for the "average" patient and "typical" individual patient profiles.
15. Use graphical displays to present data on each individual patient, including simultaneous examination of groups of patients to examine trends and differences.
16. Present results from basic models, before presentation of results from more complex modeling.
17. Present results from sensitivity analysis and threshold analysis.
18. Discuss results beyond p-values and confidence intervals, to include consideration of clinical significance.

Specific statistical issues in implementing the recommended paradigm

This section addresses issues in cancer outcomes research related to the recommendations summarized in Table 18.4. The first five issues deal with *study design and endpoints*.

Identifying and measuring endpoint(s)

Typically, an oncology research study begins by defining the primary and secondary endpoints. This is especially the case for randomized trials, established to test specific hypotheses subject to sample size and budget constraints that invariably require the investigator to prioritize objectives. Unambiguously defining the primary and secondary endpoints

upfront serves to focus the investigation and to clarify what it will mean for the study to have "significant" findings. In particular, it avoids the problem arising if there are several primary or co-equal main endpoints; unless care is taken to adjust the probability of a Type 1 error (α) for multiple testing appropriately, there is a misleadingly high probability that the study will yield at least one "significant" primary finding. As an initial step, it may be wise to carry out a pilot study or focus group to aid in identifying and selecting primary and secondary endpoints.

Outcomes research often has endpoints that are subjective, intangible, and multidimensional, e.g., health-related quality of life (HRQOL). The assumption underlying the use of such latent-variable constructs is that improvements in them will coincide with, or at least relate to, the corresponding measures based on respondent-reported data. There is a voluminous literature on this topic.[8]

The fact that the outcomes of interest may indeed be multidimensional makes the definition and choice of endpoints difficult, even in a seemingly simple situation. For example, post-mastectomy breast cancer patients often experience periods of augmented hot flash activity. In such studies we have used a bivariate endpoint reflecting both the frequency and intensity of hot flashes.[9]

Another example is that of patients with advanced cancer who often experience rapid weight loss (anorexia/cachexia). Studies have investigated ways that patients can maintain weight in the presence of an onerous tumor burden. The endpoints can be defined in several ways, i.e., weight gain, muscle mass and tone, enhanced appetite, nausea and vomiting, or a multidimensional HRQOL measure. Each of these presents measurement or data collection problems. Given the number of potential endpoints, we elect to choose one as primary and use the others to offer supportive evidence.[10]

Clinical response benefit

This refers to a composite endpoint as exemplified in a clinical trial of gemcitabine for pancreatic cancer.[11] In this trial, the patient's score on performance status, pain, and weight gain variables were classified in each case as either a positive, neutral, or negative indication. Overall response categories of "complete," "partial," or "non-response" in terms of clinical benefit were identified for all combinations of the three levels (positive, neutral, negative) of the three measured variables. This allowed each patient to be assigned a composite measure of clinical benefit.

The advantage of this approach is that all the standard methods used for tumor response data are applicable. Specifically, the proportion of patients who report a complete or partial clinical benefit response can be analyzed as a binomial variable. Standard approaches for analyzing response variable endpoints in phase II clinical trials apply.[3] Timed endpoints, such as time until the observance of a clinical benefit response, can be analyzed using standard survival analysis methods.[12]

Still, there are potential flaws to this novel and intuitively appealing approach. The response definition is ultimately arbitrary and leaves some wiggle room for interested parties to propose their own favored way to aggregate reported findings. The number of endpoints to be combined is arbitrary; an equally convincing case could have been made for more or fewer endpoints to be included in the definition of clinical response. Estimation of statistical power to detect a clinical benefit response is complicated by the fact that no a priori knowledge is generally available on how much these new composite endpoints are likely to change as a result of treatment. The fact that such an endpoint is a function of clinical variables that are influenced individually by tumor response does not mean the endpoint behaves statistically like tumor response. In the gemcitabine trial, differences were observed in only one of the three components of the clinical response benefit variable, raising the question of whether there was need for such a combined endpoint. Collectively, these concerns suggest that care must be taken in designing such composite clinical benefit endpoints. As experience with such endpoints accumulates and more is learned about their statistical properties and clinical interpretation, the approach may become more broadly acceptable.

Health-related quality of life assessment

The choice of HRQOL endpoints for outcomes research is challenging,[13–17] as discussed in a number of chapters in this volume. Specific dimensions of HRQOL likely to be affected by the treatment under consideration must be determined.[18–20] Typically, for the measures to be adequately responsive to the interventions under study, disease-specific instruments or items from existing generic tools relevant to dimensions under study should be chosen. Irrelevant constructs increase the likelihood that no impact will be observed since items with zero variance make the results less sensitive to change and bias the study towards an inflated Type II error rate (the latter being the probability of failing to identify a true difference in the interventions).[21,22] We recommend a "menu" approach to compiling appropriate HRQOL tools for clinical research studies. This involves detailing the specific constructs or dimensions that are likely to change and/or are of interest to the clinical investigation being considered. Then one compiles items for each HRQOL dimension from existing instruments that contain the prescribed construct, while ensuring the integrity of the psychometric properties of the original tool(s) from which the items were drawn. A unidimensional measure with a uniform response measurement scale should be employed when possible for consistency and ease of use. Custom-designed items for constructs not covered by existing instruments should be developed so that they belong along (or utilize) the same underlying measurement scale. We suggest measures that are simple, brief, and targeted at the HRQOL constructs that are likely to change as a result of the interventions of interest.

Item response theory (IRT), which has recently received considerable attention in the HRQOL literature, has the potential to reduce respondent burden while maintaining the same level of statistical confidence in the assigned scale score. Items intended to measure a construct can be analyzed as a hierarchy using IRT scoring procedures. Respondents need only complete those items that are most useful for the assessment of their own HRQOL level. Specifically, when used as the foundation for constructing "item banks" employed in computer adaptive assessment, IRT methods allow the respondent to be questioned in a strategic fashion, with each response guiding the choice of the next item. This economizes on the number of items – and the amount of time – required to assign the respondent a scale score with any given level of statistical precision.[23–27]

Stratification

A stratified study design is necessary in the presence of potentially confounding concomitant variables. For example, if we suspect there will be a gender difference in treatment response that varies by age, we would want to enroll (or sample) subjects so that for each treatment there is an adequate number of males and females in each specified age category (that is, level or stratum). A maximum feasible number of stratification levels per study has been proposed as being one half of the number of observations per treatment group (i.e., $n/2$),[28] where n is the group sample size. Suppose the study of interest involves 50 patients per treatment group. So, if we stratified by age (<50, $50+$), gender (male, female) tumor site (breast, colorectal, lung, other), we would have $2 \times 2 \times 4 = 16$ different levels of stratification variable, which is well below the recommended ceiling of ($50/2 =$) 25. Treatment assignment itself is often carried out by a method of randomly permuted incomplete blocks or by using a dynamic allocation procedure that balances the marginal distributions of the stratification factors (and thus their empirical weight) between the two treatment-sequence groups.[29] The aim of all such sample allocation procedures is to reduce or eliminate confounding.

Illness severity is an important stratification factor for outcomes studies involving cancer patients. We have demonstrated that a physician can provide reasonable estimates of expected remaining lifetime for patients in their care.[30] Figure 18.1 displays substantially different survival curves for a sample of advanced cancer patients stratified by physician estimate of expected survival, classified into an ordinal scale of "less than four months," "four months through six months," and "more than six months."

A recent development has been the GBU (or Good-Bad-Uncertain) Index, which extends the well-known indicator of physical well-being: the Eastern Cooperative Oncology Group (ECOG) performance status measure.[31] The ECOG measure classifies patients along a four point ordinal scale in terms of their ambulatory ability. As the acronym suggests, the GBU is a simple index for stratifying patients into those with good, bad, and uncertain prognosis. It includes four variables: the ECOG performance status, the physician's estimate of survival described earlier, as well as subjective measures of

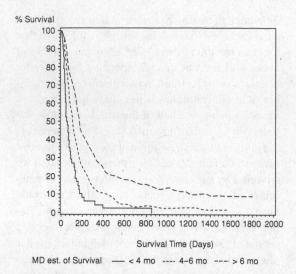

% Survival

Survival Time (Days)

MD est. of Survival —— < 4 mo ---- 4–6 mo ---- > 6 mo

Figure 18.1. Survival curves by physician estimate of survival.
Used with permission: Loprinzi, C. L., Kugler, J. W., Sloan, J. A.
et al. (1999). Randomized comparison of megestrol acetate
versus dexamethasone versus fluoxymesterone for the
treatment of cancer anorexia/cachexia. *Journal of Clinical
Oncology* **17**(10):3299–306.

the patient's appetite and physical status. The GBU
index thus improves the efficiency of the statistical
design.

Clinical significance

There are several ways of assessing clinical significance in the design phase, none of which have been
accepted as an optimal approach. A group of papers
published in the Mayo Clinic Proceedings in early
2002 analyzes the various aspects of assessing clinical significance.[32–37] We describe a simple framework, supplementary to the material presented elsewhere in this volume, that has evolved recently as
a facilitative tool for sample size determination in
outcomes research.[38,39]

This framework is based on a proposed unifying
theory that combines the effect sizes of Cohen[40] and
an empirical rule drawn from statistical theory. The
theory is unifying in the sense that it derives from
a striking universality in the use of one-half times
the standard deviation as a ballpark estimate for a

clinically significant effect. The determination of
clinical significance can be distilled into a trichotomy
of effect sizes distinguishing between small,
medium, and large impacts on patient well-being.[41]
A prior determination of sample size can then
be based upon judgments about whether a small,
moderate, or large effect size may be detectable.[42]
This approach has recently been validated using an
extensive search of the literature involving over 50
empirical studies.[43] The approach has also been
demonstrated to perform consistently whether one
is working with distribution-based or anchor-based
definitions for a clinically significant effect.

If reliable, empirically specific estimates of standard deviations for the particular study are available from the literature or pilot studies, the one-
half standard deviation approach can and should
supersede the use of the above general guideline
based on effect sizes. However, preliminary estimates of variance to determine power and sample
size are still subject to the test of whether they
are applicable to the proposed study. Andrew Vickers of the Memorial Sloan Kettering Institute for
Cancer Research (personal communication) has
demonstrated that standard deviation point estimates drawn from pilot studies have a 50% probability of resulting in an under-powered study. Gould[44]
has pointed out similar dangers, proposing interim
analyses to modify potentially inaccurate pilot data
estimates. Thus, while pilot data can be useful for
deriving a one-half standard deviation benchmark,
the accuracy of such estimates for power calculations
may not be any better than the effect size guidelines above. Whichever power analysis approach is
used for determining clinical significance, it is vital to
decide up front the benchmarks that will be considered as evidence that HRQOL has been significantly
altered.

The next five issues pertain to the *statistical analysis* of outcomes research data.

Multiple endpoints

It is useful to begin with an analysis of each endpoint
using univariate procedures, supplementing these

Table 18.5. O'Brien p-values for hot flash example

Endpoints Included	p-values
Hot flash frequency	
Hot flash severity	0.0071
Hot flash score	
	0.0005
Uniscale QOL	
	0.7528
Hot flash effect on QOL	
Toxicity incidence	

results by multivariate processes. A general method for analyzing multiple endpoints for clinical trials was proposed by O'Brien.[45] This allows for a single p-value to express the degree of difference in the relative rankings of treatment groups across an array of endpoints. An example of this technique can be found in a study of venlafaxine for hot flash activity in post-mastectomy patients.[46] Three primary measures of efficacy were included: hot flash frequency, severity, and a composite score. Data were also gathered on patient HRQOL and toxicity. Table 18.5 shows that a composite of the first three endpoints for hot flash activity was statistically significant in terms of the O'Brien p-value. But adding HRQOL to the composite reduced the p-value further. And the inclusion of myriad toxicity variables produced a non-significant p-value, indicating small differences in toxicity between the treatments that overwhelmed the impressively significant results for the other endpoints of the study.

In dealing with studies involving multiple endpoints, we need to decide whether to split the probability of a Type I error (α) (that is, the probability of rejecting the null hypothesis of no treatment effect when it is in fact true). A common approach involves dividing α by the number of hypothesis tests performed.[47] Hence, for three primary endpoints, one divides the overall experiment-wise (α) of 5% into three tests using a comparison-wise significance level of $5/3 = 1.67\%$. In theory, one would then ignore observed p-values between 0.05 and 0.0167. In reality, clinical investigators typically resist

ignoring a p-value of 2% or smaller, even if it is part of a trio of results, and instead commonly suggest that a "trend towards significance" has been observed. The discussion of results should turn to the context of the effect size observed and related clinical significance. If clinical significance has been addressed a priori, the splitting of the p-value becomes moot.

Several modeling procedures have direct application to the analysis of outcomes research studies involving multiple endpoints, with the aim of enhancing our understanding of the inter-relationships among endpoints. Causal relationships can be explored using structural equation modeling, factor analysis, and path models for the examination of latent variables.[48] Such approaches take into account multiple predictors of the variables of interest, as well as examining both direct and indirect causal relationships among variables.

Missing data and sample attrition

Missing data is a problem common to cancer outcomes research. The number of ways to handle this eventuality in the design and analysis phase of the trial is staggering.[5,49] We present a concrete example of how simple analytical methods can be applied.

In studies involving seriously ill patients, it is often reasonable to assume that missing data occur because patients are too ill to participate further in the trial due to random or systematic forces. One can choose to impute missing data in several ways. These include carrying forward the last score obtained or else assigning the minimum score observed before dropout, the maximum score observed, the average value, or a zero value (to reflect the fact that the patient is no longer living). Each approach has application in certain contexts. For example, it is often reasonable to assume that patients with missing data have, after dropout, an HRQOL no higher than their last provided observation or that HRQOL is close to zero. Imputing data using both assumptions provides a sensitivity analysis that reflects the best and worst case scenarios (Figure 18.2), with the true value of HRQOL likely lying in between.

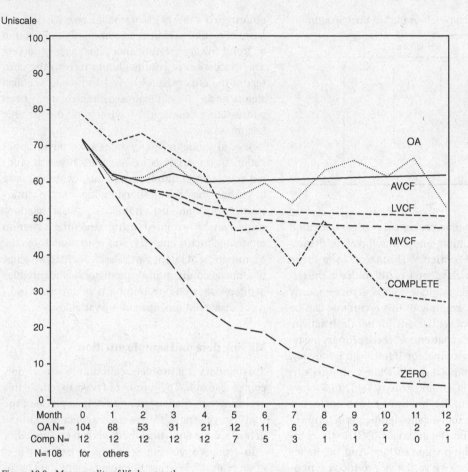

Figure 18.2. Mean quality of life by month.
Based on: Loprinzi, C. L., Kuross, S. A., O'Fallon, J. R. *et al.* (1994). Randomized, placebo-controlled evaluation of hydrazine sulfate in patients with advanced colorectal cancer. *Journal of Clinical Oncology* **12**:1121–5.

Figure 18.3 displays average HRQOL scores for patients with advanced cancer receiving hydrazine sulfate, causing attrition from 108 patients at baseline to two patients at twelve months.[50] The imputation methods used here provide markedly different HRQOL profiles over time. In particular the line marked (OA), representing the use of available data at each point, suggests high HRQOL. If we score missing data as zero, HRQOL for the baseline cohort of 108 patients drops sharply. The objective is to assess if the choice of imputation method alters the basic conclusions from the group comparison. Figure 18.3 indicates that irrespective of the use of the OA or the zero-carried-forward imputation method, the conclusion stands that HRQOL is the same for the placebo (PL) and hydrazine sulfate (HS) groups.

Intent-to-treat analysis

There have been many analyses of the advantages and disadvantages of applying the intent-to-treat

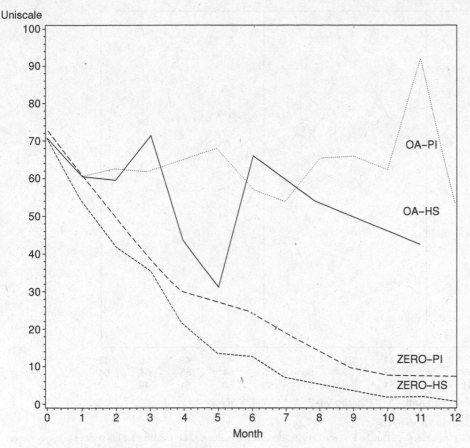

Figure 18.3. Mean quality of life by month and arm.
Based on: Loprinzi, C. L., Kuross, S. A., O'Fallon, J. R. *et al.* (1994). Randomized, placebo-controlled evaluation of hydrazine sulfate in patients with advanced colorectal cancer. *Journal of Clinical Oncology* **12**:1121–5.

(ITT) principle, and they will not be detailed here.[51] In brief, ITT characterizes results as a treatment failure if the patient is not reported to have a documented success. While this approach is somewhat conservative, it provides a rationale to address an unfortunate reality of clinical research. Patients may switch therapies after the initial, random assignment and for reasons that are often difficult to document and may reflect a purposive, or informative, response to the effectiveness of the therapy or its toxicities.[52]

An example of an ITT analysis can be found in the study of sucralfate for stomatitis in cancer patients.[53]

The trial involved 100 patients randomized to the treatment or placebo arm in a classic crossover design. Based solely on the data from patients who managed to complete the 10-week trial, sucralfate would have been found to be superior to the placebo for ameliorating chemotherapy-induced stomatitis. But an intent-to-treat analysis involving all 100 patients resulted in markedly different findings, indicating that sucralfate was inferior to placebo. The difference arises because only 3 of the 20 patients who failed to complete the trial were in the placebo arm, while the remaining 17 patients dropped out because of adverse effects of treatment. The ITT

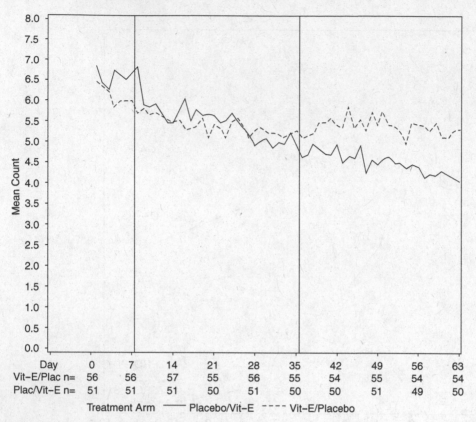

Figure 18.4. Mean total hot flashes by day.

Based on: Barton, D. L., Loprinzi, C. L., Quella, S. K. *et al.* (1998). Prospective evaluation of vitamin E for hot flushes in breast cancer survivors. *Journal of Clinical Oncology* **16**:495–500.

analysis thus appropriately concluded that sucralfate was not efficacious.

Longitudinal analysis

Longitudinal studies provide challenging problems for statistical analysis. As an example, consider Figure 18.4, which presents longitudinal HRQOL data for two patient groups. How does one make statistical comparisons between the two plotted profiles? The most direct and appropriate statistical analysis to analyze endpoints that include longitudinal profiles, as in this example, is the Area Under Curve (AUC) statistic. In Figure 18.4, the AUC statistic for each intervention corresponds to total number of hot flashes reported over the entire observation interval. Alternative statistical approaches include analyzing treatment group differences at each time point, calculating change from baseline scores to the end of the study, and using multiple regression (or analysis of covariance) models to account for the interrelationship among variables and among observations on the same variable, e.g., pattern-mixture models in recognition that repeated measures will be taken on each individual, some of whom will drop out over time. In fact, there have been entire texts dedicated to these issues without a consensus approach emerging.[54]

Fairclough[5] (among other authors) describes numerous methods for producing summary statistics for longitudinal profiles.

Selection bias

Observational studies are disadvantaged compared to randomized controlled trials in ensuring similarity between groups on all the important variables that could influence the outcomes of interest. For example, in cohort studies and case-control studies, the exposed and unexposed group and cases and controls nearly always differ in some important respect besides the exposure or treatment in question. The result will be a selection bias, which can take any of several forms: the Berkson bias (e.g., differential rates of hospital admissions for cases and controls), the Neyman bias (a type of incidence-prevalence bias that results in seeing more cases relative to controls because we are looking more often or more closely), unmasking (detection signals, wherein patients respond differently based on the knowledge of which cohort they are in), and non-response bias. Methods to compensate or correct for selection bias include the use of propensity scores and instrumental variable estimation. These techniques are designed to mitigate selectivity bias by removing the effects of (informative) imbalances across treatment groups in pre-treatment or pre-exposure characteristics that could influence the outcomes of interest. These methods have recently been used in outcomes research through application of two-stage least squares[55-60] or selectivity-corrected models.[61]

The final two issues deal with *interpretation and presentation of results* for a cancer outcomes research study.

Graphical presentation of results

Graphical methods are currently under-utilized in the presentation of outcomes research findings. Simple graphics of data on individual patients are often more informative than plots of group averages, particularly for studies with small sample sizes. We present two examples for summarizing and presenting clinical data.

The first example, the mirror image stream plot, is illustrated in Figure 18.5 using longitudinal data from one of the anorexia/cachexia studies described earlier.[10] The graph displays individual patient weights as a percentage of baseline weights over time for one of the treatment arms – megesterol acetate (left of vertical axis) versus the other treatment arm – fluoxetine (right of vertical axis). The horizontal reference line at the value 100 indicates stable weight. If the two treatment groups were equivalent, we should see a symmetric display on either side of the vertical reference line. Figure 18.5 shows that more patients on megesterol acetate achieve weight gain than do those receiving fluoxetine. The variability reflected in the picture also indicates that megesterol acetate is not uniformly successful in inducing weight gain for advanced cancer patients.

A second graphical presentation example, this time for meta-analysis, is Figure 18.6. Known as a Forrest plot, it presents the results of several studies on the differences in mouth soreness experienced by men and women undergoing standard chemotherapy treatment. One study by Sloan *et al.* revealed a statistically significant difference between men and women, with women reporting a greater amount of mouth soreness, contrary to four earlier studies on chemotherapy patients.[62] Further analysis, however, indicated that none of these studies had been powered to detect such differences. Figure 18.6 shows a consistent effect across studies with women reporting greater mouth soreness. This meta-analysis result has been replicated by a further study involving over 3000 patients.[63]

Role of complex statistical methods

One of the core messages of this chapter is the importance of considering the use of simple straightforward procedures, holding the more complicated analyses in abeyance until the basic questions have been answered or until clarity has been achieved about the gains and losses from the extra complexity. Basic statistical methods such as

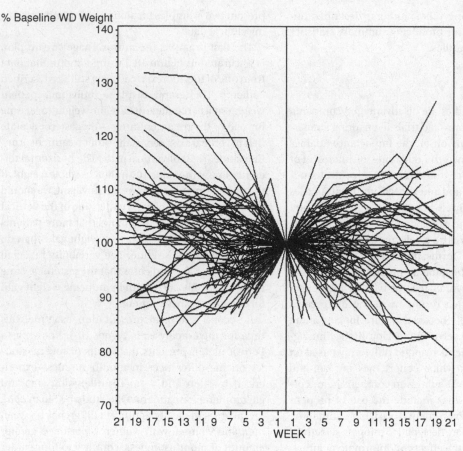

% Baseline WD Weight

Figure 18.5. Megesterol acetate (left) versus fluoxetine (right).

Used with permission: Loprinzi, C. L., Kugler, J. W., Sloan, J. A. *et al.* (1999). Randomized comparison of megestrol acetate versus dexamethasone versus fluoxymesterone for the treatment of cancer anorexia/cachexia. *Journal of Clinical Oncology* **17**:3299–306.

descriptive statistics to summarize distributions and simple hypothesis tests (see Table 18.1) are as fundamental to outcomes research as they are to any other scientific examination. Examples in this chapter and throughout the literature point to the usefulness of the simple t-test for comparing mean outcomes for different treatment groups, even when more complex statistical methodology is brought to bear.

Yet, there is a special role for complex statistical methodology in the interpretation of cancer outcomes research data. The complexity of the statistical methods should correspond to the complexity

of the study design. Specifically, the need for innovative and complex statistical methodology is in part a function of flaws or other more inherent difficulties in the basic research design, generating the potential for bias from several sources. This is frequently a characteristic of observational studies. In the absence of effective randomization, the analyst resorts to a variety of compensatory procedures.

Several complex models are becoming popular in cancer outcomes research. Rather than detailing any of these methods here, we suggest literature the interested reader can pursue for in-depth discussions. Examples of complex models

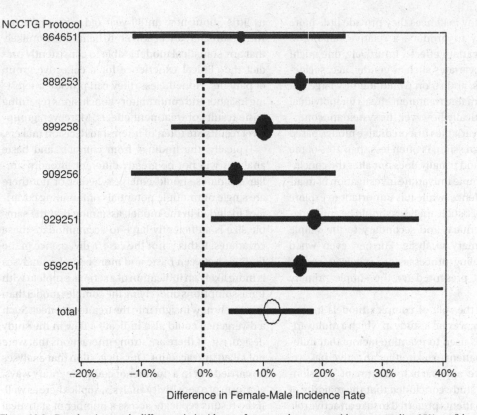

Figure 18.6. Female minus male difference in incidence of any mouth soreness with corresponding 95% confidence limits.

Note: In the individual studies the size of the circle is proportional to the sample size.

Used with permission: Sloan, J. A., Loprinzi, C. L., Novotny, P. J. *et al.* (2000). Sex differences in fluorouracil-induced stomatitis. *Journal of Clinical Oncology* **18**:412–20.

frequently used in outcomes research are structural equation modelling,[64–69] the Q-TWiST,[70–76] conjoint analysis,[77–79] instrumental variable estimation,[55–60] item response theory,[24–27,80–82] and Bayesian methods.[83–88]

Whenever one is working with a complex design or statistical analysis methodology, it is critically important to involve an experienced statistical consultant early in the development process. This allows difficult statistical issues to be addressed by the study design from the start. Considerations for flexibility of approach, validation of important assumptions underlying the requisite statistical theory, and the sensitivity of results relative to such assumptions can all be dealt with in advance rather than as an a posteriori rescue operation.

The complex nature of clinical practice can never be captured fully in a single statistical analysis. Further, the assumptions underlying most complex models are often not tenable when the models are adapted to the analysis of intangible constructs with inherent measurement error, non-normal distributions, and level of data measurement somewhere between ordinal and interval.

Thus while one can utilize complex models, it is a fallacy to expect they will necessarily guarantee a clearer vision of the clinical environment than basic techniques. At best, these models will allow for an investigation of the variability of the estimated treatment effect in the presence of, and while controlling for, the myriad of potentially confounding influences that are part of the reality of clinical practice. In many instances they provide little more than an ability to produce a relative ranking of the various covariate effects. Intuitively, one might assume that covariates such as gender, age, socioeconomic status, and so on would identify large differences in estimated treatment effects for individual patients. Statistically, however, the systematic contribution of such variables to a predictive model, based on multiple regression, is often less than 10% of the total variance and usually does not alter the conclusions from a simple univariate investigation of treatment effects. Hence, while it is important to explore complex models, such analyses should be confirmatory, supplementary, and secondary to the simple univariate primary analysis. Further, even when complex modeling processes are involved, results should be first presented for the simple primary analysis.

To illustrate the role of complex models in outcomes research, we cite a study in which a multivariable model was used to examine factors that influence a cancer patient to take either an active, passive, or collaborative approach to treatment decision-making.[89] The study concluded that the majority of breast cancer patients preferred to take an active role in treatment decision making whereas the majority of prostate cancer patients preferred to take a more passive role. Complex modeling was employed to examine the prognostic impact of selected covariates on the patient's role preference and revealed the significant effects of age, gender, and disease site. Collectively, however, the covariates accounted for only 11% of the total variability in role preference of the individual. This is not atypical of outcomes research in that a majority of the variance is left unexplained even after extensive modeling efforts to identify predictors.

Thus, while we can delineate a number of influences at the group level, there is an overriding individuality to treatment effects. In other words, patients are more than a simple aggregation of demographic and clinical variables. So while we can claim that, in general, older male patients and patients with less education and less income tend to be slightly more passive than other patients, these results tell

us little about how an 80-year-old male physician with colorectal cancer is likely to behave. It is unlikely that any statistical model is able to consistently predict the clinical experience for a collective group of patients. Nonetheless, they can provide interesting insights and confirmatory conclusions regarding basic results of treatment effects. Moreover, group-level results are often of interest to decision makers.

Typically, the findings from complex and basic analyses will not be greatly different. Broadly similar estimates should emerge whether or not there are single or multiple potential confounding covariates included in the model, assuming that the sample size is sufficiently large to accommodate these covariates. If this is not the case, a divergence in the findings between basic and more complex analyses is more likely an indication of a serious problem with the assumptions underlying the complex model than genuinely new insight into the treatment effect. Such a divergence could also indicate a flaw in the study design, e.g., if there are strong interactions that were not taken into account. Our suggestion that analyses be carried out in a number of complementary ways, as a form of a sensitivity analysis, applies here as well. If the results replicate across a number of statistical approaches, including basic and complex, one can have confidence that the findings are not driven simply by the assumptions underlying the statistical procedures and that the models have been adequately formulated.

The future

This section will delineate some research issues that need to be addressed. These involve issues of policy and communication of existing methods as well as new scientific endeavors.

1. *Methods to identify and compensate for "response shift."* A relatively new concept, response shift implies that patients adapt to their surroundings such that their HRQOL scores are significantly a function of a temporal alteration from homeostasis.[90,91] Simply put, as the patient

progresses through time, her perceptions about and evaluations of her actual and potential states of health may shift. She may now rate a given state of health either more, or less, desirable than she did or would have in the past, as her experiences with that state of health accumulate and are assimilated.

This makes it difficult for researchers to sort out, and perhaps even to define, the impact over time of a clinically efficacious treatment. How should one measure the amount of response shift present in a measured outcome? There is a need for new statistical models to deal with response shift and the determination of "treatment effects" in the face of substantial response shift.

2. *Methods for nonstandard use of standardized HRQOL instruments.* Standardized HRQOL instruments often are not relevant to a particular patient population or experimental setting. We need guidelines for deriving necessary information through a judicious choice of questions from standardized existing surveys. The trade-offs between the practical consideration of sensitivity of items to treatment with the comparability of outcomes across trials and patient groups must also be taken into account.

3. *Methods to establish the applicability of Item Response Theory to outcomes research.* IRT holds great promise for reducing respondent burden and increasing cross-study comparability of outcomes research. However, there needs to be more work comparing this methodology with classical test theory so that the value added of IRT can be demonstrated. The literature needs to provide an accessible approach for clinical researchers to understand and implement IRT in outcomes research.[92–94]

4. *Guidelines for constructing and validating new endpoints such as "clinical benefit response."* Dimension reduction by constructing composite endpoints is both exciting and disconcerting. Taking disparate endpoints, delineating all the possible combinations of responses, and then classifying each combination as evidence of a "clinical response" is an intuitively appealing approach in

that it mirrors tumor response assessment. The challenge is addressing the issues of when to combine, when not to combine, how to define the various categories of response, and how to assess relative robustness of such classification systems. All of these questions need further research.

A similar multivariate and correlated endpoint in nursing research, "symptom clusters," illustrates how to reflect the reality that multiple aspects of symptoms interrelate (such as fatigue, sleepiness, nausea, cognitive function, and mood). There has been little methodological work on how to assess these multivariate and correlated endpoints.

5. *Guidelines for assessing clinical significance.* The assessment of clinical significance has taken an important first step with the unified theory and approach recently proposed and discussed here earlier. The half standard deviation method needs to be further developed and verified as an acceptable practice, with guidelines for modification of the theory when needed. Ultimately what is needed is an approach that balances the need for psychometric validity with the pragmatic considerations of patient respondent burden and research resources.

6. *Improved training for statisticians in outcomes research.* Traditional training programs for statisticians, even biostatistics-oriented programs, include little exposure to outcomes research methodology. Additional opportunities should be created for statisticians interested in outcomes research to learn how existing and new methodologies can be applied. Perhaps additional post-doctoral programs offered through the National Cancer Institute, or the National Institutes of Health more generally, would produce a cadre of highly specialized statisticians with the skills necessary to tackle the specific problems set out in this section. Such training should strive to provide statisticians with the necessary communication skills to translate complex statistical theory into accessible language for clinical researchers.

7. *Role for Bayes methodology in outcomes research.* An approach fast gaining ground in outcomes

research is the application of the statistical paradigm known as Bayesian methodology.[83-88] This methodology is a logical, quantitative approach to organizing and synthesizing evidence based on observed data and prior beliefs. To date, virtually all randomized controlled trials in cancer (and other diseases as well) are designed and analyzed from the classical, or frequentist, statistical perspective, which (to simplify a bit) positions one to test the null hypothesis of "no treatment effect" and to reject that hypothesis if the study's p-value is sufficiently small. This is a critically important question. But by the same token, the frequentist approach does not justify one asking the often-asked question: What is the probability that Treatment A is better than Treatment B? But this is the kind of direct assessment that decision makers often seek in practice.

Bayes analyses permits such calculations based on observed data and past experience. To get a sense of how this works, consider this highly schematic Bayes analysis of whether treatment A or B is superior. The decision maker may have a *prior* (initial) probability that A is better than B. Then a randomized controlled trial (RCT) is performed and additional data emerge about A vs. B. Using the data combining rules of Bayesian statistics, the decision maker updates the prior probability with the *likelihood information* from the trial (that is, by the trial results) to obtain a *posterior probability* that A is better than B. The decision maker continues to collect information about A vs. B until the cost of doing so exceeds the value to the decision maker of increasing his confidence that A is in fact better than B. Note also that if there is no credible information about A vs. B prior to the RCT, the decision maker would adopt an "informationless" prior probability so that the posterior probability would be driven entirely by the trial data (and any subsequent data deemed to be relevant). Advocates of the Bayes approach point out that it not only uses all relevant information, but is grounded in what has become known as "statistical decision theory," wherein the decision maker collects and processes information coherently so as to maximize his utility function over feasible choices.

However, similar to item response theory, the Bayesian approach to data analysis has not yet made its way into the oncology clinical research environment, with a few exceptions. A recent oncology clinical trial was monitored by a Bayes method, which was demonstrated to have been a more efficient approach than the classical method.[95] The Bayes methods are complex, requiring intense numerical computations and considerable statistical expertise. The Bayesian paradigm is still not broadly understood in cancer outcomes research, and this alone may be one of the reasons for its slow acceptance.

Summary

We conclude by emphasizing several points. First, the application of statistical methods to cancer outcomes research need be no more complex than any other type of scientific inquiry. In this chapter we have discussed and shown by example the relative ease with which most statistical hurdles facing outcomes research studies can be overcome using standard methods with little need for adaptation. Second, it needs to be accepted that no single analytic approach will be *the* correct one, but some approaches will be more useful than others. It is expected that proposals will come forward with as varied a methodological underpinning as there are theoretical perspectives in statistical research. Consensus among methodologists will remain an ongoing challenge. However, the pursuit of different, competing approaches can provide a platform for testing the robustness of study findings through sensitivity analyses that use these alternative lenses to view the statistical issue at hand. Perhaps most critical is the need for dissemination of the importance of outcomes research and the demystifying of outcomes methodology to clinical researchers. The communication of this message remains a barrier to the general application of cancer outcomes research. It has been the aim of this chapter to contribute to that laudable goal.

REFERENCES

1 Sloan, J. A., Varricchio, C. (2001). Quality of life endpoints in prostate chemoprevention trials. *Urology* **57**:235–40.

2 Juni, P., Altman, D. G., Egger, M. (2001). Systematic reviews in health care: assessing the quality of controlled clinical trials. *British Medical Journal* **323**(7303):42–6.

3 Pocock, S. L. (1996). *Clinical Trials*. New York, NY: John Wiley & Sons.

4 Altman, D. G., Goodman, S. N., Schroter, S. (2002). How statistical expertise is used in medical research. *Journal of the American Medical Association* **287**(21):2817–20.

5 Fairclough, D. L. (1997). Summary measures and statistics for comparison of quality of life in a clinical trial of cancer therapy. *Statistics in Medicine* **16**:1197–209.

6 Albert, P. S. (1999). Longitudinal data analysis (repeated measures) in clinical trials. *Statistics in Medicine* **18**(13):1707–32.

7 Chassany, O., Sagnier, P., Marquis, P. *et al.* (2002). Patient reported outcomes: the example of health related quality of life – a European guidance for the improved integration of HRQOL assessment in the drug regulatory process. *Drug Information Journal* **36**:209–38.

8 Spilker, B. (ed.) (1996). *Quality of Life and Pharmacoeconomics in Clinical Trials*. New York, NY: Lippincott Raven.

9 Sloan, J. A., Loprinzi, C. L., Novotny, P. J. *et al.* (2001). Methodologic lessons learned from hot flash studies. *Journal of Clinical Oncology* **19**:4280–90.

10 Loprinzi, C. L., Sloan, J. A., Rowland, Jr., K. M. (2003). Methodologic issues regarding cancer anorexia/cachexia trials. In *Research and Palliative Care: Methodologies and Outcomes*, R. K. Portenoy, E. Bruera, eds. Oxford: Oxford University Press, pp. 25–40.

11 Burris, H. A., Moore, M. J., Andersen, J. *et al.* (1997). Improvements in survival and clinical benefit with gemcitabine as first-line therapy for patients with advanced pancreas cancer: a randomized trial. *Journal of Clinical Oncology* **15**(6):2403–13.

12 Marubini, E., Valsecchi, M. G. (1995). *Analyzing Survival Data from Clinical Trials and Observational Studies*. New York, NY: John Wiley & Sons.

13 Aaronson, N. K. (1991). Methodological issues in assessing the quality of life of cancer patients. *Cancer* **67**:844–50.

14 Cella, D. F. (1996). Quality of life outcomes: measurement and validation. *Oncology* **10**:233–46.

15 Cox, D. R., Fitzpatrick, R. (1992). Quality-of-life assessment: can we keep it simple? *Journal of Research Statistical Society* **155**:353–93.

16 Lara-Munoz, C., Feinstein, A. R. (1999). How should quality of life be measured? *Journal of Investigative Medicine* **47**(1):17–24.

17 Leplege, A., Hunt, S. (1997). The problem of quality of life in medicine. *Journal of the American Medical Association* **278**(1):47–50.

18 Fayers, P. M., Hopwood, P., Harvey, A. *et al.* (1997). Quality of life assessment in clinical trials – guidelines and a checklist for protocol writers: the U.K. Medical Research Council experience. *European Journal of Cancer* **33**:20–8.

19 Moinpour, C. M., Feigl, P., Metch, B. *et al.* (1991). Quality of life end points in cancer clinical trials: review and recommendations. *Journal of National Cancer Institute* **81**:485–95.

20 Sloan, J. A., Novotny, P. J., Loprinzi, C. L. (1998). Analyzing quality of life endpoints in clinical trials via the SAS system. *Proceedings of SAS Users Group International (SUGI)* **23**:1213–18.

21 Sloan, J. A., Loprinzi, C. L., Kuross, S. A. *et al.* (1998). Randomized comparison of four tools measuring overall quality of life in patients with advanced cancer. *Journal of Clinical Oncology* **16**:3662–73.

22 Sloan, J. A., O'Fallon, J. R., Suman, V. J. *et al.* (1998). Incorporating quality of life measurement in oncology clinical trials. *Proceedings of the American Statistical Association*: 282–7.

23 Hambleton, R. K. (2000). Emergence of item response modeling in instrument development and data analysis. *Medical Care* **38**(9 Suppl.):II60–5.

24 Cella, D., Chang, C. H. (2000). A discussion of item response theory and its applications in health status assessment. *Medical Care* **38**(9 Suppl.):II66–72.

25 McHorney, C. A., Cohen A. S. (2000). Equating health status measures with item response theory: illustrations with functional status items. *Medical Care* **38**(9 Suppl.): II43–59.

26 Jenkinson, C., Fitzpatrick, R., Garratt, A. *et al.* (2001). Can item response theory reduce patient burden when measuring health status in neurological disorders? Results from Rasch analysis of the SF-36 physical functioning scale (PF-10). *Journal of Neurology, Neurosurgery and Psychiatry* **71**(2):220–4.

27 Ware, J. E., Bjorner, J. B., Kosinski, M. (2000). Practical implications of item response theory and computerized

adaptive testing: a brief summary of ongoing studies of widely used headache impact scales. *Medical Care* **38**(9 Suppl.):II73–82.

28 Scott, N. W., McPherson, G. C., Ramsay, C. R. *et al.* (2002). The method of minimization for allocation to clinical trials: a review. *Controlled Clinical Trials* **23**(6):662–4.

29 Therneau, T. (1993). How many stratification factors is too many to use in a randomisation plan? *Controlled Clinical Trials* **14**:98–108.

30 Loprinzi, C. L., Kugler, J. W., Sloan, J. A. *et al.* (1999). Randomized comparison of megestrol acetate versus dexamethasone versus fluoxymesterone for the treatment of cancer anorexia/cachexia. *Journal of Clinical Oncology* **17**(10):3299–306.

31 Sloan, J. A., Loprinzi, C. L., Laurine, J. A. *et al.* (2001). A simple stratification factor for survival in advanced cancer patients: the Good/Bad/Uncertain index. *Journal of Clinical Oncology* **20**:1491–8.

32 Guyatt, G., Osoba, D., Wu, A. *et al.* (2002). Methods to explain the clinical significance of health status measures. *Mayo Clinic Proceedings* **77**:371–83.

33 Cella, D., Bullinger, M., Scott, C. *et al.* (2002). Group versus individual approaches to understanding the clinical significance of differences or changes in quality of life. *Mayo Clinic Proceedings* **77**:384–92.

34 Sloan, J., Aaronson, N., Cappelleri, J. *et al.* (2002). Assessing the clinical significance of single items relative to summated scores. *Mayo Clinic Proceedings* **77**:479–87.

35 Frost, M., Bonomi, A., Ferrans, C. *et al.* (2002). Patient, clinician and population perspectives on determining the clinical significance of quality of life scores. *Mayo Clinic Proceedings* **77**:488–94.

36 Sprangers, M., Moinpour, C., Moynihan, T. *et al.* (2002). Assessing meaningful change over time in quality of life: a users' guide for clinicians. *Mayo Clinic Proceedings* **77**:561–71.

37 Symonds, T., Berzon, R., Marquis, P. *et al.* (2002). The clinical significance of QOL results: practical considerations for specific audiences. *Mayo Clinic Proceedings* **77**:572–83.

38 Osoba, D., Rodrigues, G., Myles, J. *et al.* (1998). Interpreting the significance of changes in health-related quality of life scores. *Journal of Clinical Oncology* **16**:139–44.

39 Sloan, J. A., Vargas-Chanes, D., Kamath, C. C. *et al.* (2003). Detecting worms, ducks, and elephants: a simple approach for defining clinically relevant effects in quality-of-life measures. *Journal of Cancer and Integrative Medicine* **1**(1): 41–7.

40 Cohen, J. (1988). *Statistical Power Analysis for the Behavioral Sciences.* Hillsdale, NJ: Lawrence Erlbaum Associates.

41 Sloan, J. A., Dueck, A. (2004). Issues for statisticians in conducting analyses and translating results for quality of life end points in clinical trials. *Journal of Biopharmaceutical Statistics* **14**(1):73–96.

42 Sloan, J. A., Novotny, P. J., Loprinzi, C. L. *et al.* (1997). Graphical and analytical tools for the analysis of two-period crossover clinical trials. *Proceedings of SAS Users Group International (SUGI)* **22**:1312–17.

43 Norman, G. R., Sloan, J. A., Wyrwich, K. W. (2003). Interpretation of changes in health-related quality of life: the remarkable universality of half a standard deviation. *Medical Care* **41**(5): 582–92.

44 Gould, A. L. (2001). Sample size re-estimation: recent developments and practical considerations. *Statistics in Medicine* **20**(17–18):2625–43.

45 O'Brien, P. C. (1984). Procedures for comparing samples with multiple endpoints. *Biometrics* **40**:1079–87.

46 Loprinzi, C. L., Kugler, J. W., Sloan, J. A. *et al.* (2000). Venlafaxine in management of hot flashes in survivors of breast cancer: a randomized controlled trial. *Lancet* **356**:2059–63.

47 Benjamini, Y., Hochberg, Y. (1995). Controlling the false discovery rate: a practical and powerful approach to multiple testing. *Journal of the Royal Statistical Society, Series B, Methodological* **57**:289–300.

48 Loehlin, J. C. (1992). *Latent Variable Models.* Hillsdale, NJ: Lawrence Erlbaum and Associates.

49 Fairclough, this volume, Chapter 17.

50 McGinnis, W., Loprinzi, C. L., Buskirk, S. *et al.* (1997). Placebo-controlled trial of sucralfate for inhibiting radiation-induced esophagitis. *Journal of Clinical Oncology* **15**:1239–43.

51 Lachin, J. M. (2000). Statistical considerations in the intent-to-treat principle. *Controlled Clinical Trials* **21**(3):167–89.

52 Horne, A. D., Lachenbruch, P. A., Goldenthal, K. L. (2000). Intent-to-treat analysis and preventive vaccine efficacy. *Vaccine* **19**(2–3):319–26.

53 Martenson, J. A., Bollinger, J. W., Sloan, J. A. *et al.* (2000). Sucralfate in the prevention of treatment-induced diarrhea in patients receiving pelvic radiation therapy: A North Central Cancer Treatment Group Phase III double-blind placebo-controlled trial. *Journal of Clinical Oncology* **18**:1239–45.

54 Vickers, A. J., Altman, D. G. (2001). Analysing controlled trials with baseline and follow up measurements. *British Medical Journal* **323**:1123–4.

55 Cheung, Y. B. (2001). Adjustment for selection bias in cohort studies: an application of a probit model with selectivity to life course epidemiology. *Journal of Clinical Epidemiology* **54**(12):1238–43.

56 Gerstein, D. R., Johnson, R. A. (2000). Nonresponse and selection bias in treatment follow-up studies. *Substance Use and Misuse* **35**(6–8):971–1014.

57 Grasdal, A. (2001). The performance of sample selection estimators to control for attrition bias. *Health Economics* **10**(5):385–98.

58 Grimes, D. A., Schulz, K. F. (2002). Bias and causal associations in observational research. *Lancet* **359**(9302):248–52.

59 Oglesby, L., Rotko, T., Krutli, P. *et al.* (2000). Personal exposure assessment studies may suffer from exposure-relevant selection bias. *Journal of Exposure Analysis and Environmental Epidemiology* **10**(3):251–66.

60 Potosky, A. L., Legler, J., Albertsen, P. C. *et al.* (2000). Health outcomes after prostatectomy or radiotherapy for prostate cancer: results from the Prostate Cancer Outcomes Study. *Journal of the National Cancer Institute* **92**(19):1582–92.

61 Maddala, G. S. (1994). *Limited Dependent and Quantitative Variables in Econometrics.* Cambridge: Cambridge University Press.

62 Sloan, J. A., Loprinzi, C. L., Novotny, P. J. *et al.* (2000). Sex differences in fluorouracil-induced stomatitis. *Journal of Clinical Oncology* **18**:412–20.

63 Sloan, J. A., Goldberg, R. M., Sargent, D. J. *et al.* (2001). Women experience greater toxicity with fluorouracil-based chemotherapy for colorectal cancer. *Journal of Clinical Oncology* **19**:3539–46.

64 Bentler, P. M., Stein, J. A. (1992). Structural equation models in medical research. *Statistical Methods Medical Research* **1**(2):159–81.

65 Burgess, A. P., Carretero, M., Ellington, A. *et al.* (2000). The role of personality, coping style and social support in health-related quality of life in HIV infection. *Quality of Life Research* **9**(4):423–37.

66 de Boer, A., Spruijt, R. J., de Haes, J. C. (1998). Disease-specific quality of life: is it one construct? *Quality of Life Research* **7**(2):135–42.

67 Larsson, G., Larsson, B. W., Munck, I. M. (1998). Refinement of the questionnaire 'quality of care from the patient's perspective' using structural equation modeling. *Scandinavian Journal of the Caring Sciences* **12**(2):111–18.

68 Lehert, P. (2001). Quality-of-life assessment in comparative therapeutic trials and causal structure considerations in peripheral occlusive arterial disease. *Pharmacoeconomics* **19**(2):121–30.

69 Palta, M., Lin, C. Y. (1999). Latent variables, measurement error and methods for analysing longitudinal binary and ordinal data. *Statistics in Medicine* **18**(4):385–96.

70 Cole, B. F., Gelber, R. D., Kirkwood, J. M. *et al.* (1996). Quality-of-life-adjusted survival analysis of interferon alfa-2b adjuvant treatment of high-risk resected cutaneous melanoma: an Eastern Cooperative Oncology Group study. *Journal of Clinical Oncology* **14**(10):2666–73.

71 Cole, B. F., Solal-Celigny, P., Gelber, R. D. *et al.* (1996). Quality-of-life-adjusted survival analysis of interferon alfa-2b treatment for advanced follicular lymphoma: an aid to clinical decision making. *Journal of Clinical Oncology* **16**(7):2339–44.

72 Gelber, R. D., Goldhirsch, A., Cavalli, F. (1991). Quality-of-life-adjusted evaluation of adjuvant therapies for operable breast cancer. The International Breast Cancer Study Group. *Annals of Internal Medicine* **114**(8):621–8.

73 Gelber, R. D., Goldhirsch, A., Cole, B. F. (1993). Evaluation of effectiveness: Q-TWiST. The International Breast Cancer Study Group. *Cancer Treatment Reviews* **19**(Suppl. A):73–84.

74 Goldhirsch, A., Gelber, R. D., Simes, R. J. *et al.* (1989). Costs and benefits of adjuvant therapy in breast cancer: a quality-adjusted survival analysis. *Journal of Clinical Oncology* **7**(1):36–44.

75 Sloan, J. A., Sargent, D. J., Lindman, J. *et al.* (2002). A new graphic for quality adjusted life years (Q-TWiST) survival analysis: the Q-TWiST plot. *Quality of Life Research* **11**(1):37–45.

76 Sloan, J. A., Bonner, J. A., Hillman, S. L. *et al.* (2002). A quality-adjusted reanalysis of a Phase III trial comparing once-daily thoracic radiation vs. twice-daily thoracic radiation in patients with limited-stage small-cell lung cancer(1). *International Journal of Radiation Oncology, Biology, and Physics* **52**(2):371–81.

77 Moayyedi, P., Wardman, M., Toner, J. *et al.* (2002). Establishing patient preferences for gastroenterology clinic reorganization using conjoint analysis. *European Journal of Gastroenterology Hepatology* **14**(4):429–33.

78 Ryan, M., Shackley, P. (1995). Assessing the benefits of health care: how far should we go? *Quality Health Care* **4**(3):207–13.

79 Ryan, M., Farrar, S. (2000). Using conjoint analysis to elicit preferences for health care. *British Medical Journal* **320**(7248):1530–3.

80 Hays, R. D., Morales, L. S., Reise, S. P. (2000). Item response theory and health outcomes measurement in the 21st century. *Medical Care* **38**(9 Suppl.):II28–42.

81 Revicki, D. A., Cella, D. F. (1997). Health status assessment for the twenty-first century: item response theory, item banking and computer adaptive testing. *Quality of Life Research* **6**(6):595–600.

82 Teresi, J. A., Kleinman, M., Ocepek-Welikson, K. (2000). Modern psychometric methods for detection of differential item functioning: application to cognitive assessment measures. *Statistics in Medicine* **19**(11–12):1651–83.

83 Briggs, A. H. (1999). A Bayesian approach to stochastic cost-effectiveness analysis. *Health Economics* **8**(3):257–61.

84 Fryback, D. G., Chinnis, J. O., Ulvila, J. W. (2001). Bayesian cost-effectiveness analysis. An example using the GUSTO trial. *International Journal of Technology Assessment in Health Care* **17**(1):83–97.

85 Fryback, D. G., Stout, N. K., Rosenberg, M. A. (2001). An elementary introduction to Bayesian computing using WinBUGS. *International Journal of Technology Assessment in Health Care* **17**(1):98–113.

86 Hornberger, J. (2001). Introduction to Bayesian reasoning. *International Journal of Technology Assessment in Health Care* **17**(1):9–16.

87 Luce, B. R., Shih, Y. C., Claxton, K. (2001). Introduction. Bayesian approaches to technology assessment and decision making. *International Journal of Technology Assessment in Health Care* **17**(1):1–5.

88 Winkler, R. L. (2001). Why Bayesian analysis hasn't caught on in healthcare decision making. *International Journal of Technology Assessment in Health Care* **17**(1):56–66.

89 Degner, L., Sloan, J. A. (1995). Symptom distress in newly diagnosed ambulatory cancer patients and as a predictor of survival in lung cancer. *Journal of Pain and Symptom Management* **10**:1–8.

90 Schwartz, C. E., Sprangers, M. A. (1999). Methodological approaches for assessing response shift in longitudinal health-related quality-of-life research. *Social Science and Medicine* **48**:1531–48.

91 Sprangers, M. A., Van Dam, F. S., Broersen, J. *et al.* (1999). Revealing response shift in longitudinal research on fatigue – the use of the thentest approach. *Acta Oncologica* **38**:709–18.

92 Reise, this volume, Chapter 21.

93 Wilson, this volume, Chapter 23.

94 Hambleton, this volume, Chapter 22.

95 Vail, A., Hornbuckle, J., Spiegelhalter, D. J. *et al.* (2001). Prospective application of Bayesian monitoring and analysis in an "open" randomized clinical trial. *Statistics in Medicine* **20**:3777–87.

96 Cleeland, C. S., Mendoza, T. R., Wang, X. S. *et al.* (2000). Assessing symptom distress in cancer patients: the M. D. Anderson Symptom Inventory. *Cancer* **89**:1634–46.

97 Fairclough, D. L., Fetting, J. H., Cella, D. *et al.* (1999). Quality of life and quality-adjusted survival for breast cancer patients receiving adjuvant therapy. *Quality of Life Research* **8**:723–31.

98 Potosky, A. L., Reeve, B. B., Legler, J. L. *et al.* (2002). Quality of life following localized prostate cancer treatment initially with androgen deprivation therapy or no therapy. *Journal of the National Cancer Institute* **94**:430–9.

99 Stockler, M. R., Osoba, D., Corey, P. *et al.* (1999). Convergent, discriminative, and predictive validity of the PROSQOLI assessment and comparison with analogous scales from the EORTC QLQ-C30 and a trial-specific module. *Journal of Clinical Epidemiology* **52**:653–66.

100 Esper, P., Mo, F., Chodak, G. *et al.* (1997). Measuring quality of life in men with prostate cancer using the Functional Assessment of Cancer Therapy-Prostate Instrument. *Urology* **50**:920–8.

101 Kemmler, G., Holzner, B., Kopp, M. *et al.* (1999). Comparison of two quality-of-life instruments for cancer patients: the Functional Assessment of Cancer Therapy-General and the European Organization for Research and Treatment of Cancer Quality of Life Questionnaire-C30. *Journal of Clinical Oncology* **17**:2932–40.

102 Hakamies-Blomquist, L., Luoma, M., Sjostrom, J. *et al.* (2000). Quality of life for patients with metastatic breast cancer receiving either docetaxel or sequential methotrexate and 5-fluorouracil. A multi-center randomised phase III trial by the Scandinavian Breast Group. *European Journal of Cancer* **36**:1411–17.

103 Moinpour, C. M., Lovato, L. C., Thompson, I. M. *et al.* (2000). Profile of men randomized to the prostate cancer prevention trial: baseline health-related quality of life, urinary and sexual functioning, and health behaviors. *Journal of Clinical Oncology* **18**:1942–53.

104 McLachlan, S.-A., Allenby, A., Matthews, J. *et al.* (2001). Randomized trial of coordinated psychosocial interventions based on patient self-assessments versus standard care to improve the psychosocial functioning of patients with cancer. *Journal of Clinical Oncology* **19**:4117–25.

105 Coates, A. S., Hurny, C., Peterson, H. F. *et al.* (2000). Quality-of-life scores predict outcome in metastatic but not early breast cancer. *Journal of Clinical Oncology* **18**:3768–74.

106 Doyle, C., Crump, M., Pintilie, M. *et al.* (2001). Does palliative chemotherapy palliate? Evaluation of expectations, outcomes, and costs in women receiving chemotherapy for advanced ovarian cancer. *Journal of Clinical Oncology* **9**:1266–74.

107 Zee, B. C. (1998). Growth curve model analysis for quality of life data. *Statistics in Medicine* **17**:757–66.

108 Curran, D., Aaronson, N., Standaert, B. *et al*. (2000). Summary measures and statistics in the analysis of quality of life data: an example from an EORTC-NCIC-SAKK locally advanced breast cancer study. *European Journal of Cancer* **36**:834–44.

109 Bernhard, J., Cella, D. F., Coates, A. S. *et al*. (1998). Missing quality of life data in cancer clinical trials: serious problems and challenges. *Statistics in Medicine* **17**:517–32.

110 Madalinska, J. B. *et al*. (2001). Health-related quality-of-life effects of radical prostatectomy and primary radiotherapy for screen-detected or clinically diagnosed localized prostate cancer. *Journal of Clinical Oncology* **19**:1619–28.

111 Bland, J. M., Altman, D. G. (1995). Comparing two methods of clinical measurement: a personal history. *International Journal of Epidemiology* **24**(Suppl.):S7–14.

112 Lee, C. W., Chi, K. N. (2000). The standard of reporting of health-related quality of life in clinical cancer trials. *Journal of Clinical Epidemiology* **53**:451–8.

19

The clinical value and meaning of health-related quality-of-life outcomes in oncology

David Osoba, B.Sc., M.D., F.R.C.P.C.

QOL Consulting, West Vancouver, BC, Canada

The clinical value of measuring health-related quality of life

Common clinical outcomes

Before the modern era of objectivity in clinical oncology research, reports of the effects of therapy were often based on an individual clinician's experience (case reports and series). As awareness of the advantages of research objectivity increased, several clinical outcomes, including overall survival, median survival time, tumor-free survival, progression-free survival, time to progression, and frequency and duration of tumor response, were accepted and widely used. Of these, overall survival is considered as being the "hardest" endpoint, i.e., least likely to be subject to misinterpretation, and tumor response the "softest" endpoint.[1,2]

In addition, the concept of levels of evidence was introduced.[3–5] The highest level of evidence, Level I, consists of data from meta-analysis of several phase III randomized controlled clinical trials (RCTs) or a very large, phase III trial containing several hundred patients. The lowest level of evidence, Level IV, is data derived from small, uncontrolled case series or reports. Currently, institutions collaborate with each other to enroll the large number of patients needed to produce Level I evidence, and eligibility criteria for patient enrollment are increasingly stringent in order to control as many clinical variables as possible.

The interpretation of clinical trials has been aided by the collection of toxicity data. As with response and survival data, there has been an attempt to become more comprehensive by collecting very detailed information with uniform grading systems.[6] Some toxicity can be easily observed, e.g., oral mucositis or a skin rash, or can be given a numerical estimate, e.g., episodes of nausea/vomiting or diarrhea or changes in liver function tests or hemoglobin levels. However, other toxicity can only be inferred from subjective patient reporting, e.g., numbness of fingers and toes, pain, and fatigue. Toxicities elicited by questioning the patient are graded according to accepted scales and recorded by an observer, with a resulting potential for bias.

Assessment of function

In oncology, the concept of assessing the functional ability of a patient was introduced with the Karnofsky Performance Status Scale (KPS).[7] The KPS and its derivatives, such as the Zubrod (Eastern Cooperative Oncology Group) Performance Scale (ECOG),[8] are oriented primarily towards physical functioning. For example, items ask about whether the patient is able to dress him/herself and whether the patient spends less than or more than half his/her time in bed. Although the observer speaks to the patient and, ideally, also observes him/her, it is the observer who classifies the patient's performance status. Again, there is a potential for observer bias. Recently, there has been a move to use these scales as patient self-reported assessment tools.

Health-related quality of life (HRQOL) assessment

Social scientists, psychologists, educators, and others have a long history of developing tools for the assessment of psychological symptoms and status, and modern HRQOL measurement in clinical medicine has its roots in psychological research. Functional assessment, previously directed almost entirely to the physical functioning domain, now also includes psychological well-being, social interaction, cognitive functioning, as well as other domains and an assessment of symptoms.[9] Measurement of how this constellation of domains is affected by the health of an individual is known as HRQOL assessment (or measurement).

An important and distinguishing feature of HRQOL measurements is that they are all based on self-assessment by the subject, rather than by an observer. Indeed, important discrepancies have been reported between self-assessment and observer assessment.[10] Observers (proxies) are reasonably accurate in estimating physical functioning and most other domains as compared to patients' scores but, from the patient's perspective, tend to underestimate emotional functioning and overestimate symptoms like fatigue and insomnia.[11]

How does HRQOL assessment differ from symptom assessment?

With the emergence of a desire for greater objectivity in oncology, the use of symptoms as outcome measures in oncology was discouraged. Since observers have difficulty quantifying some symptoms, such as pain, fatigue, and insomnia, they were felt to be of little value in evaluating the effectiveness of therapy. However, an interest in adding symptom assessment to objective criteria, such as survival, has persisted.[12] Recently, there has been a greater interest in symptom assessment expressed, but cautions are still being sounded. For example, a standard definition of symptom palliation has been proposed which takes into account time of onset, degree and duration of symptoms, improvement, control, and prevention.[13]

The main differences between HRQOL assessment and symptom or toxicity assessment are that HRQOL assessment is:

(1) more comprehensive, and includes ability/level of functioning in several important domains of life (e.g., physical activity, social interaction, emotional well-being, and cognitive ability) as well as common or important symptoms such as pain and fatigue;

(2) always self-reported and, therefore, represents the patient's perspective rather than that of an observer;

(3) a patient-centered activity that emphasizes the patient's sense of well-being and functioning as the most important focus and goal of medical care;

(4) a more accurate appraisal of the effects of a disease and/or a medical intervention on the entire patient rather than only the manifestations of a disease or illness.

In most clinical trials, toxicity frequency and grade are still reported by observers and, thus, do not represent the patient's view of how the toxicity is affecting his/her functioning and well-being, i.e., HRQOL. As a result, the findings from the two methods do not necessarily provide identical responses.[14] When it is desirable to assess symptoms, it is preferable to use responses given directly by the patient.

A classification of uses of HRQOL assessment according to the purpose of assessment

When HRQOL outcomes were initially measured and their application to clinical medicine considered, only a few potential uses were envisioned.[15,16] These initial applications included aiding decision making in phase III randomized controlled trials when differences in survival were small, and describing HRQOL status in cancers (or other diseases) with a poor prognosis.

With the further development of HRQOL assessment and the increasing numbers of studies, it has become apparent that the potential uses are more extensive than originally envisaged. The reasons for

Table 19.1. Potential and demonstrated uses of HRQOL outcomes based on the purpose of the assessment

Screening
– identify cases for detailed study (case finding)
– assess needs for health services
– identify individuals who are eligible for entry into clinical trials

Profile Description
– conduct general population health studies, e.g. national census
– assess specific populations, e.g. cancers with a poor prognosis
– describe impact of disease or treatment (benefit or toxicity) on HRQOL
– provide prognostic and predictive information for response to treatment and survival
– assist in health resource allocation

Clinical Decision Making
– be the primary outcome in symptom control, palliative treatment, and supportive care
– use in clinical trials where survival differences are small
– decide which intervention is preferable in RCTs
– decide if an intervention improves baseline HRQOL
– determine effects of prevention trials
– monitor individual patients over time

Preference (Utility) Assessment
– combine HRQOL with survival (QALYs)
– assess health utility
– measure preference for certain HRQOL outcomes
– conduct economic evaluations

Facilitating Communication

obtaining HRQOL outcomes can be placed in a taxonomic framework based on the purpose of the assessment (Table 19.1).[17-19] These include screening, health profile description, clinical decision making, preference (utility) assessment, and facilitation of communication. Within each of these purposes, there are several applications.

Screening

The reason for screening groups of individuals for their HRQOL status is to identify individuals with a particular HRQOL attribute (e.g., depression) or need for health services (e.g., people with poor physical functioning) that would require more detailed assessment and, perhaps, intervention. Another possibility is to identify individuals who would fulfill

the eligibility criteria for participation in a particular clinical trial.[15,16] Up till the present, a person's performance status (e.g., KPS, ECOG) has often been used to determine eligibility. However, within a particular performance score, there may still be great HRQOL variability.[20,21] When HRQOL is an important outcome in a clinical trial, it would make sense to determine eligibility by stratification on HRQOL variables (e.g., emotional functioning, overall quality of life, or fatigue), rather than on performance status.

Profile description

There are many uses for describing the HRQOL profile of a sample of the population. The population may be as general as a cross-section of the citizenry of a country[22-25] or as specific as a group of patients with a particular cancer.[26] HRQOL profiles are descriptive and assist in improving our knowledge of the impact of a disease or condition, or of the impact of an intervention, on a group of individuals[27-35] (also see a review by Osoba[36]). Profiles of the general or specific population may assist in the allocation of health care resources.[37] Recently, it has been found that HRQOL status may be a better predictor of the likelihood of treatment benefit[38] and has been shown to be a better predictor of survival than the more commonly used performance status indicators.[39-48] This ability has been particularly apparent in patients with metastatic cancer[41] but may also apply to patients with localized disease.[47]

Clinical decision making

Clinical decision making, i.e., determining the appropriate choice of therapy, is dependent on having an accurate estimate of the benefit or harm accruing from a particular intervention. Such knowledge is required in day-to-day clinical practice when dealing with individuals. The treatment choices available to clinicians and patients should be evidence-based and tested by repeated experience. Today, the phase III trial is considered to be the most important source of evidence for evaluating the efficacy of therapy.[3-5] Although in oncology the traditional primary outcomes studied in phase III trials are overall survival, time to tumor progression, and toxicity, HRQOL outcomes are now being included. Differences in HRQOL outcomes are always important, but when differences in the traditional outcomes are small, a rational decision as to which treatment is preferable may still be made when HRQOL outcomes differ between the treatments.[30,32,49-51]

In phase III studies, a comparison of HRQOL scores should be made not only between treatment groups but, also, within treatment groups. A within-group assessment of change in HRQOL scores from baseline allows a calculation of the proportion of patients who have achieved a pre-set definition of improvement/deterioration in each treatment group. These proportions may then be compared between treatment groups and tested for statistical significance

(see below). Another reason for the within-group comparisons is that a beneficial treatment should result in an improvement of HRQOL scores as compared to before treatment. If there has been deterioration from baseline scores in both treatment groups and deterioration is greater in one group than another, a valid conclusion may still be that one treatment is preferable to the other, but an equally valid conclusion may be that neither treatment is of real benefit.

HRQOL data may be collected either as a primary or secondary outcome in clinical trials. When it is a *primary outcome*, HRQOL is the main outcome of interest, superseding all other outcomes, including survival. It is important as a primary outcome in palliation when the interventions are not expected to have a significant impact on survival. In addition, HRQOL may be a primary outcome when a particular treatment is expected to have less toxicity than another treatment in the absence of a difference in survival. An example of a clinical trial in which HRQOL was a primary outcome was the comparison of prednisone alone versus prednisone and mitoxantrone in men with hormone-refractory metastatic prostate cancer.[50,51] It was known beforehand that mitoxantrone would not affect survival, and the trial results bore out this expectation.[50] However, men who received mitoxantrone in addition to prednisone experienced better and longer pain relief[50] and reported improved global HRQOL and improvements in four functioning domains and nine symptoms.[51] Other similar situations are the use of erythropoietin for the treatment of anemia,[52] megestrol acetate for anorexia,[53-55] treatment of pain from bone metastases,[56] and a comparison of three cycles versus six cycles of chemotherapy for small-cell lung cancer.[49]

HRQOL outcomes have been used as *secondary outcomes* much more often than as primary outcomes in clinical oncology trials. The primary outcome in these trials has been survival. Although most investigators and regulatory agencies have placed greater emphasis on the survival data than on the HRQOL data, there have been instances in which HRQOL data have provided reasonable evidence for making a decision about which treatment is preferable. A few examples are α-interferon in metastatic colorectal cancer,[57] temozolomide in recurrent glioblastoma multiforme,[30] pegylated liposomal doxorubicin in AIDS-related Kaposi's sarcoma,[32] and continuous chemotherapy in advanced, metastatic breast cancer.[29]

Although it is clear that HRQOL outcomes may be helpful in phase III trials, they should also be included in phase II (non-randomized) studies[31] because treatments that do not result in improvement in HRQOL over the baseline status are of doubtful benefit even if they are associated with tumor responses. Additional reasons for conducting HRQOL assessments in phase II trials are to provide information about the required sample size in subsequent phase III studies and to validate further the reliability and validity of HRQOL instruments.

Recently, there has been a move to describe the HRQOL profile of patients enrolled in adjuvant therapy trials[58] and prevention trials.[59] The appropriate HRQOL outcome in these situations is the maintenance of HRQOL status until the recurrence/occurrence of disease. In prevention trials, HRQOL data can be used to ascertain whether the preventive intervention itself has a negative impact on HRQOL.

A practical use of HRQOL information would be the monitoring of individual patients over time in clinical practice. Although this application is appealing, it requires very precise assessment tools to be certain that the clinician is not misled into thinking that there has been a change in HRQOL when, in fact, the change is the result of measurement imprecision. Most HRQOL instruments in use today were developed for the purpose of group assessment. Although the internal consistency of the domains in these instruments meets commonly accepted standards (e.g., Cronbach's alpha coefficient of >0.7), they may not be sufficiently reliable to be dependable in individuals.[60,61] Nevertheless, current instruments may be useful for monitoring HRQOL in individuals if clinicians treat HRQOL assessments like a laboratory test, i.e., an adjunct to history-taking, physical examination, imaging procedures, and common

sense. An intelligent integration of the results of all of these procedures is required for good clinical practice.

Preference (utility) assessment

Utility assessment is often considered to be a form of HRQOL assessment, but the data are gathered with instruments that differ from the psychometrically-based instruments used to measure HRQOL.[62–65] Utility assessment is based on the desire to make rational decisions that take into account the preferences of individuals or groups for certain defined health states or outcomes. Utility scores (generally between 0 and 1) are combined with survival time (in years) to produce quality-adjusted life years.[63–65] This method and others like it are commonly used in cost-utility analyses. Additional details are provided in Chapter 4 by Feeny[66] and Chapter 25 by O'Brien[67] in this volume.

Facilitation of communication

The assessment of HRQOL can aid communication between health care professionals and the patient in several ways. First, the inclusion of questions about various aspects of health in HRQOL questionnaires encourages the patient to raise issues pertaining to these questions. Thus, they may be more likely to raise questions about aspects of their health that they may have thought their doctors and nurses were "too busy" to listen to. Second, discussion between patients and health care professionals is improved when the doctor (nurse) is aware of problems that the patient is experiencing in the domains included in questionnaires.[68] The presence of a set of questions covering several domains of health serves as an aid to the memory of patients and as a means of covering most of the important issues related to health. Third, information derived from HRQOL data can be used as a decision aid (e.g., decision boards) in determining preferences for treatment and future management of the patient's condition. Data from HRQOL results of clinical trials have been incorporated in decision boards to give patients information about the HRQOL consequences of particular treatments and aspects of their illness.[69,70]

In addition to aiding communication between health care professionals and patients, HRQOL data, collected and recorded in a systematic fashion, can also aid in communication between health care professionals. When the data are present in a patient's chart, they are available for use by doctors, nurses, social workers, and other professionals who have contact with the patient. Finally, HRQOL information can be used in communication between health care professionals and the public, third-party payers, and health care policy makers. Examples include national health surveys, health utility assessments, and economic evaluations.

Other taxonomies of the uses of HRQOL assessment are based on the type of assessment, i.e., whether it is evaluative or discriminative.[17,18] This classification may be combined with one based on uses, as described above, into a single taxonomy.[19]

A taxonomy of uses of HRQOL data based on the level of decision making

It is useful to classify HRQOL outcomes based on the levels of decision making in the health care system, i.e., at the micro, meso, and macro levels.[71]

At the *micro level*, decision making is centered on individual patients at the bedside (or in the office or clinic). In this setting, HRQOL instruments must possess high internal consistency and responsiveness to change[60,61] and provide individual-specific responses that have a minimum of error. The application of HRQOL measures to monitor the effects of disease and/or treatment in individual patients is being investigated.[72,73]

Meso level decision making is based on larger groups of patients at the level of health care institutions or clinical trials. The instruments must still have reasonably good internal consistency and responsiveness to change, but the high precision required at the individual level can be relaxed slightly because of the larger sample sizes.[60,61] In this setting, HRQOL measurement has been applied most frequently in samples of populations of patients with cancer as an evaluative tool in RCTs/phase III trials. It has also been used as a descriptive tool in phase II trials and in samples of patients who are not in trials. These studies have been carried out in a wide variety of clinical settings, ranging from prevention studies through therapeutic intervention to palliative care. Details of these studies can be found in other chapters in this volume and in previously published reviews.[36]

At the *macro level*, HRQOL measurement can be used, in addition to other measures, to describe and evaluate the health of the population for several reasons.[37,74,75] The HRQOL measures may range from subjective summary assessments through multidimensional measures of function and disability to preference-based utility measures. The combination of HRQOL measures with quality-adjusted life years (QALYs) and disability-adjusted life years (DALYs) attempts to integrate mortality and morbidity to produce summary health status scores. These summary scores are used, in turn, as the denominator in summary measures of health in cost-effectiveness studies comparing interventions[74,75] and to index the relative burden of cancer for various populations.[76-78] A detailed discussion of these uses and the issues surrounding them can be found in a review by Brown, Lipscomb, and Snyder[79] and in other chapters of this book.

Interpretation of the clinical meaning of HRQOL outcomes

HRQOL outcomes are most commonly reported as numerical data (scores) obtained from either psychometrically-based instruments or utility-based assessments.[80] The instruments are designed to give numerical values so that the data can be scored and analyzed statistically in ways that are not possible with descriptive terms.

While numerical data are appealing because of the ability to apply statistical analytic techniques, the use of numerical data can give rise to several difficulties. The main issue is that, unlike descriptive terms, the numbers are not themselves easily understood. Ideally, the numbers should be converted back to clinically relevant descriptive terms, but this translation is rarely done in reports of HRQOL data. Most commonly, the numbers are placed in the context of the range of possible scores for a given instrument. For example, a mean score of 40, in a range of 0 (lowest) to 100 (highest), implies that the function, or attribute, being scored is somewhat low within the possible range of scores for that attribute. A mean score of 40 may be statistically significantly lower than a score of 60 or 80, but the clinical meaning and relevance of the differences between these scores in terms of the attribute are unclear.

A second difficulty associated with numerical data is the interpretation of small differences in scores (over time within groups or between groups). A difference of 20 or 40 between two means seems large on a scale of 0–100 and would likely be statistically significant. Intuitively, it would seem to be clinically meaningful. However, a difference of 5 or 6 is more problematic. Such a difference between means, or between scores at different times for an individual, seems small. What meaning should be attributed to such a difference? The answer to this question is of vital importance as more and more investigators include HRQOL as an integral component of clinical studies, and as more and more decision makers are faced with the need to interpret and apply the results of these studies.

Thirdly, the heterogeneity of the users of HRQOL information will affect the interpretation of the meaningfulness of scores. Users range from individual patients and their home-based caregivers, to health care professionals involved in primary care (e.g., physicians, nurses), to hospital and clinic administrators, to policy makers at the macro level who are responsible for setting broad national policies for health care. Patients use HRQOL data to understand how their HRQOL may be affected by their cancer or treatment. Health care professionals are interested in knowing the magnitude of changes in HRQOL that would mandate a change in management of the disease, while at the meso and macro level, decision makers need to know how health service utilization may be affected. The significance or meaning of scores may be interpreted differently by these different groups in the context of their experience and how their decisions will be affected.[81]

The quality of the numerical data is strongly influenced by the degree, or proportion, of missing data.[82] Thus, minimizing the amount of missing data and applying appropriate techniques to deal with it, once it has occurred, are important.[83]

Aggregated versus disaggregated scores

Some HRQOL instruments have been designed to provide only aggregated, or summed, scores of the responses to the items in the instrument, while others emphasize the use of separate, or disaggregated, scores for each of the domains.[84] Intuitively, an aggregated score is appealing because of its simplicity and apparent ease of use, but disaggregated scores provide more detail.[16] Aggregated scores are made up of scores from more than one domain, some of which may have improved as a result of treatment and some of which may have deteriorated. Therefore, when aggregated, the summed scores may be the same between groups or over time within a group, and changes in domain scores may not be evident in the single score. Changes in domain scores may, therefore, be of importance in evaluating the impact of therapy on HRQOL, as for profile description or for clinical decision making. Both researchers and clinicians need detailed profiles of scores in individual domains to make informed decisions about the results of the assessment. Summed scores are of use in utility assessment and cost-utility calculations when a single number is required. They may also be useful in some screening procedures if there will be further assessment of the sample that has been identified as having the HRQOL attributes of interest.

Methods for interpreting HRQOL data

Distribution-based interpretations

Interpretation based on the statistical distribution of the results is the most commonly used method in clinical oncology.[80] Oncologists and policy makers are accustomed to looking for the statistical significance of between-groups differences in their studies of parameters such as overall survival and disease-free interval. The standard practice is to calculate probability (p) values of the observed difference having occurred by chance, based on the null hypothesis. The commonly accepted level of rejecting the null hypothesis is 0.05, i.e., a 1 in 20 probability that the result occurred by chance alone. The difficulty with this approach for interpreting differences in HRQOL scores is that small differences, e.g., 4 or 5 points or less on a 0–100 scale, may be statistically significant if the sample size is very large. Recent major clinical trials often have sample sizes of 300 or more patients, and, therefore, this situation is a real possibility. However, when decision makers are faced with interpreting small numerical differences, they are skeptical of their importance, regardless of the P-value. Conversely, large differences in HRQOL scores in a study with a relatively small number of patients may not reach statistical significance but may be meaningful. In this situation, and in general, effect sizes can provide important information.

The effect size is a distribution-based interpretation that is less dependent on sample size. It is an expression of the relative magnitude of change, is based on the variance of the data, and is expressed as the standard deviation (SD) of the mean.[85,86] The mean score at the baseline HRQOL assessment (for stable, untreated individuals) is subtracted from the mean score at a subsequent assessment and divided by the SD of the mean at baseline. Effect sizes up to 0.2 of one SD are considered unimportant, while those between 0.2 and 0.5 are important, but small. Those between 0.5 and 0.8 are moderate, and those greater than 0.8 are large. Since this interpretation is not as dependent on sample size as are tests of statistical significance, it is useful in studies involving small as well as large numbers of patients. However, it has not been used frequently in clinical oncology and is unfamiliar to many potential users of HRQOL information. An example from a recent study shows how the P-value was not statistically significant in subgroups of patients with small numbers, despite the magnitude of the change in HRQOL scores being the same as for the subgroups with larger numbers.

However, the effect sizes in these domains were similar regardless of whether the numbers of patients were large or small.[30]

King analyzed several clinical studies in a variety of cancers and found that effect sizes were in keeping with the magnitude of differences in QLQ-C30 scores between varying extents of disease.[87] Besides being unfamiliar, effect sizes have another difficulty. Little work has been done on relating them to the clinical meaning of changes in HRQOL scores in oncology, although there has recently been an effort in this direction (see below).[81,87] Thus, more investigation into their clinical relationships is still required.

Other distribution-based interpretations include the reliable change index, the proximity to the mean,[88] the unit of effectiveness, and estimates of the normative level of functioning.[89] Another method involves calculation of the standard error of measurement (SEM).[90–92] This value is the variability between the observed and the true scores and is calculated as the standard deviation of the baseline score multiplied by the square root of 1 minus the reliability (internal consistency) of the HRQOL instrument. It reflects within-person variability over time and is thought to be independent of sample size. One SEM appears to be equivalent to the minimum important difference in studies involving patients with heart and respiratory disease.

Anchor-based interpretations

Anchor-based interpretations[80] relate changes in scores from HRQOL instruments (target ratings) to other measures or ratings, or to other clinical or life events (anchor ratings). Examples of anchor ratings include global ratings of the minimum clinically important difference[93–94] or of subjective significance;[81] changes with therapy, with time, or with disease severity;[87] threshold effects; health care utilization; or changes with other life events, such as job loss, family illness, or divorce.[94] An additional approach would be to determine the predictive value of HRQOL scores (proportions of true and false positives as determined by receiver operating characteristic curves) and their correlations with events such as response to therapy and death.

Of the various anchors named above, very few have been used in the analysis of HRQOL data from oncology studies. The ones used most often have been global ratings, association with disease severity, and prediction of response to treatment or mortality.

Relationship of global ratings to magnitude of change in HRQOL scores

The use of global ratings as anchors requires a two-step process.[95,96] First, the degree of association of HRQOL scores with global ratings and disease severity is necessary in order to determine the degree of change required in a HRQOL score (on one or more domains), before it is perceived as a change on a global rating or an acknowledged change in disease severity. Second, if a particular HRQOL instrument and its domains have been "calibrated" in this way, then it must be shown repeatedly that a given change in the global rating should be associated with the same magnitude of change in HRQOL scores. If this relationship can be shown for various populations and forms of cancer, it may then be used to determine the proportions of individuals who experience this magnitude of change in clinical trials and clinical practice.

The most commonly used global rating, in diseases other than cancer, is the determination of the "minimum important difference" (MID).[93,94] This was originally defined as "the smallest difference in score in the domain of interest which patients perceive as beneficial and which would mandate, in the absence of troublesome side effects and excessive cost, a change in the patient's management." It is evident that this definition does not include a change for the worse, i.e., deterioration, but it could be taken as meaning that no deterioration is also a "benefit." It is also possible that a difference in HRQOL scores may not necessarily "mandate" a change in management in the light of other considerations, such as a long-term or ultimate benefit of continuing a treatment (e.g., when the deterioration is expected to be temporary or no other therapy is available). In studies of patients with asthma, the MID was calculated to be 0.5 on a 7-point scale (about 7% of the range of the scale).[93,94]

In oncology, a similar approach has been used but the difference in HRQOL scores is termed as being subjectively significant.[81] In essence, subjective significance is similar to the MID, but it includes the possibility of deterioration as well as benefit and does not suggest that the perception of subjective significance "mandates" a change in the patient's management. The amount of change in scores perceived to be of significance in the QLQ-C30 has been measured with the Subjective Significance Questionnaire (SSQ).[81] This assessment was designed to determine the numerical amount of change in four domains of the QLQ-C30 that corresponded to the perception of a change on items asking about the analogous domains in the SSQ. Thus, changes in the SSQ were used to calibrate a subjectively significant change in the QLQ-C30. Both the MID and SSQ are also known as global ratings and rely on the administration of the global rating (anchor) instrument together with the target instrument (a HRQOL questionnaire).

The SSQ asks patients to rate changes in their "physical condition," "emotional state," "enjoyment of social life," and "overall quality of life" since the last time they filled out the QLQ-C30. The response options are whether the change was "very much worse," "moderately worse," "a little worse," "about the same," "a little better," "moderately better," or "very much better."[81] In the initial studies, in patients with advanced metastatic breast cancer and extensive-stage small-cell lung cancer, each successive category of change in the SSQ items was associated with 5–10 points of change in the analogous QLQ-C30 domain scores (possible range 0–100). Subsequent studies in patients with stage I Hodgkin's disease and advanced ovarian cancer have confirmed this result (Osoba *et al.*, unpublished data). Thus, the smallest perceived change ("a little better" or "a little worse") on the SSQ was associated with changes in QLQ-C30 scores of between 5% and 10% of the possible range of scores.

Furthermore, when the SSQ ratings for the four domains that were assessed were associated with effect sizes, it was found that ratings of "a little worse" or "a little better" had effect sizes ranging from 0.34–0.51 to 0.09–0.51 (means of 0.40 and 0.33), respectively.[81] Ratings of "moderately worse" and "moderately better" had effect sizes ranging from 0.15–1.04 and 0.16–0.84 (means of 0.60 and 0.55), respectively. For ratings of "very much worse" and "very much better," they were 0.23–0.99 and 0.38–1.11 (means of 0.65 and 0.82), respectively. These ranges of effect sizes indicate approximately symmetrical effect sizes regardless of whether patients reported that their HRQOL was better or worse.

Recent work by Cella et al. dealt with changes in Functional Assessment of Cancer Therapy (FACT) scores as related to retrospective global ratings of change over two months.[97] The smallest change perceptible in FACT-G scores was about 5–7 points on a scale of 0–108. Effect sizes for the patients reporting "minimally worse" or "sizably worse" changes on the global ratings (these terms are those adopted by the authors after collapsing categories labeled "somewhat worse," "moderately worse," "a great deal worse," and a "very great deal worse") were generally in the same range as those reported by Osoba et al. for the patients reporting that they were "worse."[81] However, in the Cella et al. study, effect sizes for patients reporting that they were "better" were smaller than those in the Osoba et al. study. Thus, Cella et al. concluded that small improvements appear to be more meaningful than comparable declines.[97] Similar findings were also reported in a study of patients in a palliative care setting, with effect sizes being larger for patients reporting having "bad days" than for "good days,"[98] and in a study of patients receiving radiation therapy for laryngeal cancer who completed the FACT-Head and Neck questionnaire.[99]

The global rating approach used in the above studies was intended to determine how much change in the target instrument (e.g., the QLQ-C30 and FACT-G) scores is perceptible as a change by the subjects themselves. The use of this approach has some potential pitfalls. The instruments used to obtain global ratings are not themselves amenable to psychometric validation for internal consistency since, in each case, they consist of single items. Also, they have not been assessed for test-retest reproducibility. The wording of the items and the constructs they are intended to assess may not be the same as a patient's understanding of the wording of the analogous domains in the target instruments. When used to measure change in the QLQ-C30, it has been shown that scores at the ceiling have an effect on the strength of the correlations with the SSQ ratings[81,100] (Osoba et al., unpublished data). When only scores lying between 30–70 (0–100 point scale) were used, correlation coefficients were stronger than if the full range of scores from 0–100 were used (Osoba et al., unpublished data). Another consideration is the degree to which the target instrument responses and the anchor ratings are correlated. It has been suggested that recall bias[101] may be important in the retrospective assessment of change on health transition questionnaires. This may be true if the pre-test and post-test correlations are not mirror images of each other, and if the correlations with the target change scores are not stronger than with either pre-test or post-test scores.[102]

Some of these potential pitfalls have been investigated. Studies in several trials have shown reasonably strong correlations between either HRQOL change scores or on-trial HRQOL scores and global ratings, but correlations between global ratings and baseline HRQOL scores were weak or non-existent[103] (Osoba et al., unpublished data). Does this mean that recall bias is interfering with the patients' memories of their HRQOL status at baseline or that some other explanation is more likely? The length of the time intervals over which patients are asked to recall the pre-test state of their HRQOL may be a factor in the responses that are given on the global rating questionnaire (Osoba et al., unpublished data). They concluded that recall bias is not likely the best explanation. Other possibilities include the adaptation of patients to changing circumstances with resetting of their baseline HRQOL status ("response shift"),[104–106] and the use of thought processes in the ratings of global change that do not involve simple linear relationships. Nevertheless, whatever the explanation, it is clear that the discrepancy between the expectations based on theoretical grounds and the actual clinical results require further research.

It should be kept in mind that the use of global ratings, such as the SSQ in oncology, was intended as a tool to determine the magnitude of change in HRQOL scores that was perceptible as a change by patients. The SSQ and other health transition instruments composed of single items probably should not be used as stand-alone instruments to measure change in HRQOL.

Relationship to disease status, treatment toxicity, and response to treatment

HRQOL scores would be expected to change with and reflect the stage of disease, with better scores for patients with early-stage disease than advanced and metastatic disease.[87,107] Similarly, the severity of toxicity and responses (improvement or deterioration) to treatment should have effects on HRQOL. A summary of studies involving patients with breast cancer, head and neck cancer, melanoma, lung cancer, esophageal cancer, gynecological cancer as well as other sites,[87] and brain cancer,[107] showed differences in the QLQ-C30 scores reflective of disease stage and response to treatment. The analysis by King[87] included small sample sizes when patients were grouped by extent/severity of disease. In a reanalysis of the same data, studies with <100 patients were excluded (Osoba, unpublished data). This approach found that, as the stage of disease (tumor burden) increased from least extensive (no evidence of disease or localized with no weight loss) to moderately extensive (localized symptoms, locoregional disease or weight loss <10%) to most extensive (metastatic disease, weight loss >10%, systemic symptoms), mean HRQOL scores decreased from between 58–76 for least extensive, to 53–58 for moderately extensive, to 43–54 for most extensive disease. Scores for physical, role, and social functioning followed a similar pattern with very little overlap of the ranges of the scores. Fatigue scores increased with increasing disease burden, from 25–37 for least extensive to 39–63 for most extensive disease, again with little overlap in these ranges. Similar relationships were found between QLQ-C30 scores and

performance status. As the composition of patients with various performance status scores changed to include higher proportions with poorer performance status, QLQ-C30 scores worsened substantially. The changes associated with treatment were in the expected directions in that QLQ-C30 scores soon after treatment (7 days) showed decreases in the functioning scales scores (except for emotional functioning which tended to improve), while at later times and in those with improving performance status, HRQOL scores improved. King concluded that for the QLQ-C30 (range 0–100) "an improvement of 10 on the QOL scale may be considered clinically worthwhile." King also points out the importance of considering the clinical situation in each study since it may be important to take into account the deleterious effects of some side effects in relation to overall HRQOL scores before making a final decision about the clinical significance of the results.[87]

Ability to work and health care utilization

These measures have been used to assess functioning and health status; however, they have not yet been widely reported as anchors for HRQOL outcomes in patients with cancer.[108] It would be expected that as HRQOL status decreases, the ability to work (at a job or at home) would decrease while health care utilization would increase.

Mortality

Several studies in oncology have shown that patients with lower HRQOL status have shorter survival times than patients with higher scores.[39–47] Only one study, in esophageal cancer, has attempted to determine how much difference in HRQOL scores is associated with a finite difference in survival, i.e., 6 months, one year, etc.[46] In this study, a 10-point increase in the physical functioning score at baseline corresponded to a 12% reduction (95% confidence interval 4–18%) in the likelihood of death at any given time. It is unknown whether such a relationship would be constant for all cancer types or whether it would differ from one type of cancer to another.

Other considerations in the definition of clinically meaningful change

A recent workshop at the Mayo Clinic explored a large number of issues related to the interpretation of the results of HRQOL measurement and of meaningful change in HRQOL scores. In addition to a consideration of the distribution- and anchor-based methods[96] of interpretation, other issues were discussed. Most of these considerations remain unresolved and require further work. For example, are the results from group ratings applicable to individuals?[109] What is the place of single-item versus multiple-item measures?[110] It is clear that the perspectives of the users of HRQOL data will have an effect on what is considered to be an important (meaningful) change in scores, and these perspectives need to be explored in future work.[81,111,112]

How should clinicians interpret HRQOL data?

Clinicians should be aware of the following important issues: (1) Was a hypothesis stated about how HRQOL in general, or particular domains of HRQOL, would be affected by the intervention(s)? (2) Were well-validated instruments (questionnaires) used? (3) Was the sample size adequate? (4) Was the study design appropriate to the question being asked? (5) Were the appropriate statistical analyses used? (6) Were the results assessed for clinical significance as well as statistical significance? It is important that a definition of the threshold level (clinical significance) of change in HRQOL scores and its duration be given and justified. The most readily understood presentation of differences between groups is the calculation of the proportions of patients in each group that experienced a clinically significant threshold of change and the statistical significance of the differences in these proportions. This can be expressed as the proportions of patients whose HRQOL improved, remained stable, and deteriorated. The result is analogous to the well-known interpretation of the proportions of patients who achieved complete and partial responses, stable disease, and progression in tumor status. Similar guidelines have been suggested by others.[113–116]

Integration of HRQOL data with other clinical and laboratory data should be analogous to what is done presently with medical information collected on patients. HRQOL data should be viewed as another piece of information (analogous to the results of a laboratory test) that needs to be considered together with information from the patient's history, physical examination, and laboratory and imaging data when making decisions about the management and care of a particular patient. HRQOL data should not be used alone for decision making. The other clinical and investigative data also provide anchors for interpreting the HRQOL information. Finally, HRQOL data should also be used as a vehicle for improving communication between patients and health care professionals, between various health care professionals involved with the care of the patient, and between health care professionals and health care policy makers.

Some have suggested that the most valuable information for clinicians is data that can be translated into the number of patients needed to treat (NNT, the inverse of absolute risk reduction) to achieve a desired endpoint.[93,117] While this approach is attractive, it has not been used, as yet, by oncologists to any appreciable extent.

The interpretation of HRQOL data in day-to-day clinical practice is still problematic. The current HRQOL instruments were designed to collect data on groups of individuals and do not have the high degree of internal consistency that would be desirable in collecting data on an individual.[60,61,118] However, the emergence of questionnaires based on item response theory that are more individualized is likely to help in this regard.[119]

Interpretation of HRQOL data by regulatory agencies

Regulatory agencies are concerned primarily with the safety of new therapies and products, although efficacy or effectiveness must also be demonstrated. Both of these features determine the eventual labeling of the new therapy/product. Increasing numbers of clinical trials carried out by pharmaceutical companies have a HRQOL component. Regulatory agencies, therefore, should be familiar with the procedures and analyses involved in rigorous HRQOL assessment. Claims of HRQOL benefit from a new product or device must be scientifically substantiated, and guidelines to assist regulatory agencies and the pharmaceutical and medical devices industry have been developed.[120,121]

The guidelines for interpreting HRQOL data suggested above for clinicians also apply to regulatory agencies. Hypotheses must be stated a priori. It is important for pharmaceutical and medical device manufacturers not to seem to be on a "fishing expedition" when collecting HRQOL data. Well-validated instruments and appropriate analyses should be used, and the results should be interpreted in an unbiased manner. A potential difficulty arises with the conclusions drawn from multiple domain scores because some of the scores may be significantly improved with treatment while others may stay the same or worsen. If there is improvement in only one or two domains, claims for improved HRQOL should not be made, and only the domains showing improved scores should be claimed as showing improvement. If a majority of domains is improved, or if a domain asking about overall HRQOL/health is improved, then claims for improvement in HRQOL are justified. The magnitude of improvement should not only be statistically significant but also represent meaningful change by reaching a predetermined threshold level of change or by being correlated with independent anchor measures (see above). It is very important to show the proportions of patients who have achieved a predefined, meaningful change for better and for worse (e.g., a 10% change from baseline) and to determine whether the proportions are statistically significantly different in the treatment groups being evaluated in the study.

How should analysts conducting efficacy, effectiveness, or cost-effectiveness studies interpret HRQOL?

Efficacy studies are concerned with determining whether or not a particular intervention produces a more desirable outcome than another intervention in a predefined, selected sample of subjects meeting specific study entry criteria. Effectiveness studies are concerned with the same question, but in a broader sample of subjects who are representative of the population likely to receive the intervention in practice. In both instances, the interpretation of HRQOL data should follow the outline given above for clinicians and regulatory agencies.

In cost-effectiveness studies, a monetary value (e.g., dollars) is assigned to the cost required to achieve each unit of effectiveness. Therefore, HRQOL data are reduced to a single number and often combined with length of life. Each year of survival is multiplied by a number lying between 0 (death) and 1 (perfect health) to produce a QALY. Although this method is highly attractive because of its simplicity and because it yields a single number, there is a difficulty with this approach. The reduction of a complex, multidomain construct such as health or HRQOL to a single number may be too simple and omits much useful information. When scores from multiple domains are aggregated and averaged (with or without weighting), the likelihood that some domains improved while others worsened is ignored. Thus, an aggregate score, if measured repeatedly over time, may show no change, when there may have been major changes in domain scores. If QALYs are used to compare two groups of patients receiving different interventions in an RCT, a conclusion that the two groups do not differ may also be reached despite intergroup differences in some domain scores. In short, the importance of the information available in a multidomain assessment is not realized.

Recommendations

Clinical trials should be designed to use both distribution- and anchor-based approaches. The research question and the hypotheses about the expected outcomes should be clearly stated in protocols, and the HRQOL domains of interest should be specified. The magnitude of the change in scores that will be accepted as meaningful should be stated. Both improvement and deterioration in HRQOL scores should be shown and the proportions of patients with such changes calculated. Differences in proportions of patients should be tested for statistical significance, and the duration of HRQOL response should be shown for each treatment group.

Funding agencies should give well-designed HRQOL studies a high priority. The ultimate goal of such studies should be to provide a scientific basis for clinical interventions that enhance the HRQOL of patients and the general population. Intermediate goals include the development of more reliable and valid assessment methods (e.g., computer-adaptive testing based on item response theory), the interpretation of HRQOL outcomes in clinical terms, and improvement in communication between clinicians, policy makers, and patients. Attention needs to be given to the wide dissemination of results and the education of all parties concerned in the use of HRQOL outcomes in medical care. Education in the use of HRQOL outcomes needs to begin in the early phases of the training of health care professionals. These areas must be implemented on a broad front as soon as it is feasible.

At all stages of HRQOL research and clinical application, comprehensive consensus building and development is needed. This effort will help to define the major issues that require resolution and will provide a rational basis from which to continue research in this field.

Future needs

Some of the most pressing needs for future research in HRQOL include:

(1) The translation of HRQOL benefit into clinically meaningful and understandable terms:[122,123] For example, if a patient's physical functioning score improves by 20%, what does this mean in terms of what this patient can do now as compared to what s/he was able to do before the improvement?
(2) The tailoring of HRQOL assessment to individual circumstances: Computerized-adaptive testing is moving in this direction.

(3) A better understanding of how to deal with missing data in clinical trials: Although imputation of missing values is widely used, it has limitations because the imputed values cannot be proven to represent the true values. Other methods need to be explored further.
(4) Moving HRQOL assessment from the "lab" and clinical trials to the "bedside," i.e., everyday clinical practice: Ideally, all patients should be able to complete an HRQOL assessment at each visit to the clinic/doctor, and the results should be available for the consultation. These results then could be integrated with the findings from the history and physical examination and the results of laboratory tests and imaging studies to aid in clinical decision making.
(5) Teaching the basis and rationale for HRQOL assessment during medical and nursing undergraduate education: As yet, there is no coordinated effort by medical and nursing schools to adopt and develop a suitable curriculum for undergraduates.

Conclusions

The assessment of symptoms, whether originating from the disease or its treatment, is very important but, whether self-reported or not, is neither synonymous with, nor a substitute for, HRQOL assessment. The latter includes a self-reported assessment of functioning in at least three aspects of life (physical, emotional, and social domains) as well as of symptoms.

The interpretation of HRQOL results is a central issue in their measurement. Various approaches have been suggested to improve the interpretation of the data including distribution- and anchor-based approaches. Each approach has its advantages and disadvantages. Distribution-based approaches do not necessarily provide clinically meaningful interpretations of the results, while anchor-based approaches based on global ratings are difficult to validate psychometrically. To avoid the pitfalls of using only one approach, it is safer to use multiple approaches. A combination of distribution and anchor methods is desirable and, in addition, a combination of multiple anchors is probably better than one anchor alone. The use of global ratings in individuals allows a calibration of what constitutes a perceptible change in scores from a questionnaire. This information, in turn, provides a rational cut point for determining the proportions of patients achieving improvement or worsening of scores in HRQOL domains. In RCTs, the proportions of patients reporting an improvement in scores can be compared by tests for statistical significance to determine whether one treatment is preferable to another.

Clinical trials that show significant differences in the proportions of patients achieving HRQOL responses in pre-specified domains are important for clinical and regulatory decision making. Several studies indicate that a difference in HRQOL scores of 7–8% of the range of the scale is perceptible to patients and associated with clinically meaningful differences in disease severity and treatment effects. A slightly higher cut-off of 10% seems to be a reasonable lower limit to avoid the unnecessary inclusion of questionable or borderline improvements. Further research in this field will help to clarify the best approaches.

REFERENCES

1 Simon, R. (1993). Design and conduct of clinical trials. In *Cancer. Principles and Practice of Oncology,* (Fourth Edition), ed. V. T. DeVita Jr., S. Hellman, S. Rosenberg, pp. 416–40. Philadelphia, PA: JB Lippincott Co.

2 Warr, D., McKinney, S., Tannock, I. (1984). Influence of measurement error on assessment of response to anticancer chemotherapy: proposal for new criteria of tumor response. *Journal of Clinical Oncology* 2:1041–6.

3 Cook, D. J., Guyatt, G. H., Laupacis, A., Sackett, D. L. (1992). Rules of evidence and clinical recommendation on the use of antithrombotic agents. *Chest* 102 (Suppl. 4): 305S–11S.

4 Sackett, D. L. (1993). Rules of evidence and clinical recommendations for the management of patients. *Canadian Journal of Cardiology* 9:487–9.

5 Sackett, D. L., Cook, D. J. (1993). Can we learn anything from small trials? *Annals of the New York Academy of Sciences* 703:25–31.

6 Franklin, H. R., Simonetti, G. P., Dubbelman, A. C. *et al.* (1994). Toxicity grading systems. A comparison between the WHO scoring system and the Common Toxicity Criteria when used for nausea and vomiting. *Annals of Oncology* 5:113–17.

7 Karnofsky, D. A., Abelman, W. H., Craver, L. F., Burchenal, J. H. (1948). The use of nitrogen mustards in the palliative treatment of carcinoma. *Cancer* 1:634–56.

8 Zubrod, C. G., Schneiderman, M., Frei, E. III. *et al.* (1960). Appraisal of methods for the study of chemotherapy of cancer in man: comparative therapeutic trial of nitrogen mustard and triethylene thiophosphoramide. *Journal of Chronic Diseases* 11:7–33.

9 Ware, J. E., Jr. (1991). Measuring functioning, well-being, and other generic health concepts. In *Effect of Cancer on Quality of Life*, ed. D. Osoba, pp. 7–23. Boca Raton, FL: CRC Press.

10 Slevin, M. L., Plant, H., Lynch, D., Drinkwater, J., Gregory, W. M. (1988). Who should measure quality of life, the doctor or the patient? *British Journal of Cancer* 57: 109–12.

11 Sneeuw, K. C. A., Aaronson, N. K., Sprangers, M. A. G., Detmar, S. B., Wever, L. D. V., Schornagel, J. H. (1998). Comparison of patient and proxy EORTC QLQ-C30 ratings in assessing the quality of life of cancer patients. *Journal of Clinical Epidemiology* 51:617–31.

12 Osoba, D., Rusthoven, J. J., Turnbull, K. A., Evans, W. K., Shepherd, F. A. (1998). Combination chemotherapy with bleomycin, etoposide, and cisplatin in metastatic non-small-cell lung cancer. *Journal of Clinical Oncology* 3: 1478–85.

13 Stephens, R. J., Hopwood, P., Girling, D. J. (1999). Defining and analysing symptom palliation in cancer clinical trials: a deceptively difficult exercise. *British Journal of Cancer* 79:533–44.

14 Savage, C., Pater, J. L., Tu, D., Norris, B. (2002). He said/she said: how well do common toxicity criteria and quality of life agree on patient symptoms? *Proceedings of the American Society of Clinical Oncology* 21:382a (abstract 1540).

15 Osoba, D. (1991). Measuring the effect of cancer on quality of life. In *Effect of Cancer on Quality of Life*, ed. D. Osoba, pp. 25–40. Boca Raton, FL: CRC Press.

16 Osoba, D., Aaronson, N. K., Till, J. E. (1999) A practical guide for selecting quality-of-life measures in clinical trials and practice. In *Effect of Cancer on Quality of Life*, ed. D. Osoba, pp. 89–104. Boca Raton, FL: CRC Press.

17 Guyatt, G. H., Veldhuzen Van Zanten, S. J. O., Feeny, D. H., Patrick, D. L.. (1989). Measuring quality of life in clinical trials: a taxonomy and review. *Canadian Medical Association Journal* 140:1441–8.

18 Jaeschke, R., Guyatt, G. D., Cook, D. (1992). Quality of life instruments in the evaluation of new drugs. *Pharmacoeconomics* 1:84–94.

19 Osoba, D. (1995). Measuring the effect of cancer on health-related quality of life. *Pharmacoeconomics* 7:308–19.

20 Mackworth, N., Fobair, P., Prados, M. D. (1992). Quality of life self-reports from 100 brain tumor patients: comparisons with Karnofsky Performance Scores. *Journal of Neuro-Oncology* 14:243–53.

21 Schaafsma, J., Osoba, D. (1994). The Karnofsky performance status scale re-examined: a cross-validation with the EORTC-C30. *Quality of Life Research* 3:413–24.

22 Hjermstad, M. J., Fayers, P. M., Bjordal, K., Kaasa, S. (1998). Health related quality of life in the general Norwegian population assessed by the European Organization for Research and Treatment of Cancer Core Quality of Life Questionnaire: the QLQ-C30(+3). *Journal of Clinical Oncology* 16: 1188–96.

23 Klee, M., Roenvald, M., Machin, D. (1997). Quality of Life of Danish women: population-based norms for the EORTC QLQ-C30. *Quality of Life Research* 6:27–34.

24 Michelson, H., Bolund, C., Nilsson, B., Brandberg, Y. (2000). Health-related quality of life measured by the EORTC QLQ-C30 – reference values from a large sample of the Swedish population. *Acta Oncologica* 39:477–84.

25 Gandek, B., Ware, J. E., Aaronson, N. K. *et al.* (1998). Tests of data quality, scaling assumptions, and reliability of the SF-36 in eleven countries: results from the IQOLA project. *Journal of Clinical Epidemiology* 51:1149–58.

26 Fayers, P., Weeden, S., Curran, D. (1998). *EORTC QLQ-C30 Reference Values*. Brussels: EORTC Quality of Life Study Group, EORTC Data Centre.

27 Allen-Mersch, T. G., Earlam, S., Fordy, C., Abrams, K., Houghton, J. (1994). Quality of life and survival with continuous hepatic-artery floxuridine infusion for colorectal liver metastases. *Lancet* 344:1255–60.

28 Clavel, M., Soukop, M., Greenstreet, Y. C. A. (1993). Improved control of emesis and quality of life with ondansetron in breast cancer. *Oncology* 50:180–5.

29 Coates, A., Gebski, V., Bishop, J. F. *et al.* (1987). Improving the quality of life during chemotherapy for advanced breast cancer. A comparison of intermittent and continuous treatment strategies. *New England Journal of Medicine* 317:1490–5.

30 Osoba, D., Brada, M., Yung, W. K. A., Prados, M. (2000). Health-related quality of life in patients treated with temozolomide versus procarbazine for recurrent glioblastoma multiforme. *Journal of Clinical Oncology* 18:1481–91.

31 Osoba, D., Brada, M., Yung, W. K. A., Prados, M. (2000). Health-related quality of life in patients with anaplastic

astrocytoma during treatment with temozolomide. *European Journal of Cancer* 36:1788–95.

32 Osoba, D., Northfelt, D. W., Budd, D. W., Himmelberger, D. (2001). Effect of treatment on health-related quality of life in AIDS-related Kaposi's sarcoma; a randomized trial of pegylated liposomal doxorubicin versus doxorubicin, bleomycin and vincristine. *Cancer Investigation* 19:573–80.

33 Murray, N., Livingston, R. B., Shepherd, F. A. *et al.* (1999). Randomized study of CODE versus alternating CAV/EP for extensive-stage small-cell lung cancer: An intergroup study of the National Cancer Institute of Canada Clinical Trials Group and the Southwest Oncology Group. *Journal of Clinical Oncology* 17:2300–8.

34 Hürny, C., Bernhard, J., Coates, A. S. *et al.* (1996). Impact of adjuvant therapy on quality of life in women with node-positive operable breast cancer. International Breast Cancer Study Group. *Lancet* 347:1279–84.

35 Fairclough, D. L., Fetting, J. H., Cella, D., Wonson, W., Moinpour, C. M. (1999). Quality of life and quality adjusted survival for breast cancer patients receiving adjuvant chemotherapy. Eastern Cooperative Oncology Group (ECOG). *Quality of Life Research* 8:723–31.

36 Osoba, D. (1999). What has been learned from measuring health-related quality of life in clinical oncology. *European Journal of Cancer* 35:1565–70.

37 Cutler, D. M., Richardson, E. (1997). Measuring the health of the U.S. population. In *Brookings Papers on Economic Activity: Microeconomics*, ed. M. C. Bailey, P. C. Reiss, C. Winston, pp. 217–71. Washington, DC: Brookings Institute.

38 Osoba, D., Zee, B., Sadura, A., Pater, J., Quirt, I. (1993). Measurement of quality of life in an adjuvant trial of gamma interferon versus levamisole in malignant melanoma. In *Adjuvant Therapy of Cancer VII*, ed. S. E. Salmon, pp. 412–16. Philadelphia, PA: JB Lippincott Co.

39 Coates, A., Gebski, V., Signorini, D. *et al.* (1992). Prognostic value of quality-of-life scores during chemotherapy for advanced breast cancer. Australian New Zealand Breast Cancer Trials Group. *Journal of Clinical Oncology* 10:1833–8.

40 Coates, A., Porzsolt, F., Osoba, D. (1997). Quality of life in oncology practice: prognostic value of EORTC QLQ-C30 scores in patients with advanced malignancy. *European Journal of Cancer* 33:1025–30.

41 Coates, A. S., Hürny, C., Peterson, H. F. *et al.* (2000). Quality-of-life scores predict outcome in metastatic but not early breast cancer. *Journal of Clinical Oncology* 18: 3768–74.

42 Coates, A. S., Thomson, D., McLeod, G. R. M. *et al.* (1993). Prognostic value of quality of life scores in a trial of chemotherapy with or without interferon in patients with

metastatic malignant melanoma. *European Journal of Cancer* **29A**:1731–4.

43 Earlam, S., Glover, C., Fordy, C., Burke, D., Allen-Mersh, T. G. (1996). Relation between tumour size, quality of life, and survival in patients with colorectal liver metastases. *Journal of Clinical Oncology* **14**:171–5.

44 Kaasa, S., Mastekaasa, A., Lund, E. (1989). Prognostic factors for patients with inoperable non-small cell lung cancer, limited disease. *Radiotherapy Oncology* **15**:235–42.

45 Ganz, P. A., Lee, J. J., Siau, J. (1991). Quality of life assessment. An independent prognostic variable for survival in lung cancer. *Cancer* **67**:3131–5.

46 Blazeby, J. M., Brookes, S. T., Alderson, D. (2001). The prognostic value of quality of life scores during treatment for oesophageal cancer. *Gut* **49**:227–30.

47 Dancey, J., Zee, B., Osoba, D. *et al.* (1997). Quality of life scores: an independent prognostic variable in a general population of cancer patients receiving chemotherapy. *Quality of Life Research* **6**:151–8.

48 Herndon, J. E., Jr., Fleishman, S., Kornblith, A. B., Kosty, M., Green, M. R., Holland, J. (1999). Is quality of life predictive of the survival of patients with advanced non-small cell lung carcinoma? *Cancer* **85**:333–40.

49 Medical Research Council Working Party (1993). A randomized trial of three or six courses of etoposide, cyclophosphamide, methotrexate and vincristine or six courses of etoposide and ifosfamide in small cell lung cancer. (SCLC) II: quality of life. *British Journal of Cancer* **68**:1157–66.

50 Tannock, I. F., Osoba, D., Stockler, M. R. *et al.* (1996). Chemotherapy with mitoxantrone plus prednisone or prednisone alone for symptomatic hormone-resistant prostate cancer; a Canadian randomized trial with palliative end points. *Journal of Clinical Oncology* **14**:1756–64.

51 Osoba, D., Tannock, I. F., Ernst, S., Neville, J. (1999). Health-related quality of life in men with metastatic prostate cancer treated by prednisone alone or mitoxantrone and prednisone. *Journal of Clinical Oncology* **17**:1654–63.

52 Demetri, G. D., Kris, M., Wade, J., Degos, L., Cella, D. (1998). Quality-of-life benefit in chemotherapy patients treated with epoetin alfa is independent of disease response or tumor type: results from a prospective community oncology study. *Journal of Clinical Oncology* **16**:3412–25.

53 Rowland, K. M., Jr., Loprinzi, C. L., Shaw, E. G. *et al.* (1996). Randomized double-blind placebo-controlled trial of cisplatin and etoposide plus megestrol acetate in extensive-stage small-cell lung cancer: a North Central Cancer Treatment Group Study. *Journal of Clinical Oncology* **14**:135–41.

54 Simons, J. P., Aaronson, N. K., Vansteenkiste, J. F. *et al.* (1996). Effects of medroxyprogesterone acetate on appetite, weight, and quality of life in advanced-stage non-hormone-sensitive cancer: a placebo-controlled multicentre study. *Journal of Clinical Oncology* **14**:1077–84.

55 Bruera, E., Ernst, S., Hagen, N. *et al.* (1998). Effectiveness of megestrol acetate in patients with advanced cancer: a randomized, double-blind, crossover study. *Cancer Prevention and Control* **2**:74–8.

56 Porter, A. T., McEwan, A. J. B., Powe, J. E. *et al.* (1993). Results of a randomized phase III trial to evaluate the efficacy of strontium-89 adjuvant to local field external beam irradiation in the management of endocrine resistant metastatic prostate cancer. *International Journal of Radiation Oncology, Biology, and Physics* **25**:805–13.

57 Seymour, M. T., Slevin, M. L., Kerr, D. J. *et al.* (1996). Randomized trial assessing the addition of interferon α-2a to fluorouracil and leucovorin in advanced colorectal cancer. *Journal of Clinical Oncology* **14**:2282–8.

58 Ganz, P. A. (2001). Impact of tamoxifen adjuvant therapy on symptoms, functioning, and quality of life. *Journal of the National Cancer Institute Monograph* **30**:130–4.

59 Moinpour, C. M., Lovato, L. C., Thompson, I. M. *et al.* (2000). Profile of men randomized to the prostate cancer prevention trial: baseline health-related quality of life, urinary and sexual functioning, and health behaviors. *Journal of Clinical Oncology* **18**:1942–53.

60 Hays, R. D., Anderson, R., Revicki, D. (1993). Psychometric considerations in evaluating health-related quality of life measures. *Quality of Life Research* **2**:441–9.

61 Hays, R. D., Anderson, R. T., Revicki, D. (1998). Assessing reliability and validity of measurement in clinical trials. In *Quality of Life Assessment in Clinical Trials*, ed. M. J. Staquet, R. D. Hays, P. M. Fayers, pp. 169–23. Oxford: Oxford University Press.

62 Revicki, D. A., Kaplan, R. M. (1993). Relationship between psychometric and utility-based approaches to the measurement of health-related quality of life. *Quality of Life Research* **2**:477–87.

63 Torrance, G. W. (1986). Measurement of health state utilities for economic appraisal. *Journal of Health Economics* **5**:1–30.

64 Torrance, G. W., Feeny, D. (1989). Utilities in quality-adjusted life years. *International Journal of Technology Assessment in Health Care* **5**:559–75.

65 Kaplan, R. M., Feeny, D., Revicki, D. A. (1993). Methods for assessing relative importance in preference based outcome measures. *Quality of Life Research* **2**:467–75.

66 Feeny, this volume, Chapter 4.

67 O'Brien, this volume, Chapter 25.

68 Detmar, S., Muller, M. J., Schornagel, J. H., Wever, L. D., Aaronson, N. K. (2002). The role of health-related quality of life considerations in palliative chemotherapy treatment decisions. *Journal of Clinical Oncology* **20**: 1056–62.

69 Levine, M. N., Gafni, A., Markham, B., MacFarlane, D. (1992). A bedside decision instrument to elicit a patient's preference concerning adjuvant chemotherapy for breast cancer. *Annals of Internal Medicine* **117**:53–8.

70 Whelan, T. J., Levine, M. N., Gafni, A. *et al.* (1995). Breast irradiation postlumpectomy: development and evaluation of a decision instrument. *Journal of Clinical Oncology* **13**:847–53.

71 Osoba, D. (2002). A taxonomy of the uses of health-related quality of life (HRQOL) instruments in cancer care and the clinical meaningfulness of the results. *Medical Care* **40** (Suppl. 3):S31–8.

72 Detmar, S. B., Aaronson, N. K. (1998). Quality of life assessment in daily clinical oncology practice: a feasibility study. *European Journal of Cancer* **34**:1181–6.

73 Velikova, G., Brown, J. M., Smith, A. B., Selby, P. J. (2002). Computer-based quality of life questionnaires may contribute to doctor–patient interactions in oncology. *British Journal of Cancer* **86**:51–9.

74 Murray, C. J. L., Lopez, A. D. (1997). Global mortality, disability, and the contribution of risk factors: Global Burden of Disease Study. *Lancet* **349**:1436–42.

75 World Health Organization (2000). *The World Health Report 2000: Health Systems: Improving Performance.* Geneva: World Health Organization.

76 Goldie, A. J., Kuntz, K. M., Weinstein, M. C., Freedberg, K. A., Palefsky, J. M. (2000). Cost-effectiveness of screening for anal squamous intraepithelial lesions and anal cancer in human immunodeficiency virus-negative homosexual and bisexual men. *American Journal of Medicine* **108**:634–41.

77 Neilson, A. R., Whynes, D. K. (1995). Cost-effectiveness of screening for colorectal cancer: a simulation model. *IMA Journal of Mathematically Applied Medical Biology* **12**:355–67.

78 Norum, J. (2000). Adjuvant cyclophosphamide, methotrexate, fluorouracil (CMF) in breast cancer – is it cost-effective? *Acta Oncologica* **39**:33–9.

79 Brown, M. L, Lipscomb, J., Snyder, C. (2001). The burden of illness in cancer: economic cost and quality of life. *Annual Review of Public Health* **22**:91–113.

80 Lydick, E., Epstein, R. S. (1993). Interpretation of quality of life changes. *Quality of Life Research* **2**:221–6.

81 Osoba, D., Rodrigues, G., Myles, J., Zee, B., Pater, J. (1998). Interpreting the significance of changes in health-related quality-of-life scores. *Journal of Clinical Oncology* **16**: 139–44.

82 Bernhard, J., Gelber, R. D., ed. (1998). *Workshop on Missing Data in Quality of Life Research in Cancer Clinical Trials: Practical and Methodological Issues. Statistics of Medicine* **17**:511–796.

83 Fairclough, D. L. (2002). *Design and Analysis of Quality of Life Studies in Clinical Trials.* Boca Raton, FL: Chapman & Hall/CRC.

84 Sloan, this volume, Chapter 18, pp. 362–85.

85 Cohen, J. (1977). *Statistical Power Analysis for the Behavioural Sciences.* New York: Academic Press.

86 Kazis, L. E., Anderson, J. J., Meenan, R. F. (1989). Effect sizes for interpreting changes in health status. *Medical Care* **27** (Suppl. 3):S178–89.

87 King, M. T. (1996). The interpretation of scores from the EORTC Quality of Life Questionnaire QLQ-C30. *Quality of Life Research* **5**:555–67.

88 Jacobson, N. S., Roberts, L. J., Berns, S. B., McGlinchey, J. B. (1999). Methods for defining and determining the clinical significance of treatment effects: description, application and alternatives. *Journal of Consulting Clinical Psychology* **67**:300–7.

89 Salsburg, D. S., Turner, R. S. (1992). Defining clinically meaningful units of change for health outcome research. *Quality of Life Newsletter* **3**:1.

90 Wyrwich, K., Nienaber, N. A., Tierney, W., Wolinsky, F. (1999). Linking clinical relevance and statistical significance in evaluating intra-individual changes in health-related quality of life. *Medical Care* **37**:469–78.

91 Wyrwich, K., Tierney, W., Wolinsky, F. (1999). Further evidence supporting a SEM-based criterion for identifying meaningful intra-individual changes in health-related quality of life. *Journal of Clinical Epidemiology* **52**:861–73.

92 Wyrwich, K. W., Wolinsky, F. G. (2000). Identifying meaningful intra-individual change standards for health-related quality of life measures. *Journal of Evaluating Clinical Practice* **6**:39–45.

93 Jaeschke, R., Singer, J., Guyatt, G. H. (1989). Measurement of health status. Ascertaining the minimal clinically important difference. *Controlled Clinical Trials* **10**: 407–15.

94 Juniper, E. D., Guyatt, G. H., Willan, A., Griffith, L. E. (1994). Determining a minimal important change in a disease-specific quality of life questionnaire. *Journal of Clinical Epidemiology* **47**:81–7.

95 Ware, J. E., Keller, S. D. (1996). Interpreting general health measures. In *Quality of Life and Pharmacoeconomics in Clinical Trials*, ed. B. Spilker, pp. 445–60. Philadelphia, PA: Lippincott-Raven.

96 Guyatt, G., Osoba, D., Wu, A., Wyrwich, K., Norman, G. and the Clinical Significance Consensus Meeting Group (2002). Methods to explain the clinical significance of health status measures. *Mayo Clinic Proceedings* **77**:371–83.

97 Cella, D., Hahn, E., Dineen, K. (2002). Meaningful change in cancer-specific quality of life scores: differences between improvement and worsening. *Quality of Life Research* **11**:207–21.

98 Cohen, R. S., Mount, B. M. (2000). Living with cancer: "Good" days and "bad" days – what produces them? *Cancer* **89**:1854–65.

99 Ringash, G. J., Redelmeier, D. A., O'Sullivan, B., Bezjak, A. A. (1999). Asymmetry of good and bad minimal important differences in quality of life for laryngeal cancer patients. *Quality of Life Research* **8**:604 (abstract 214).

100 Rodrigues, G., Bezjak, A., Osoba, D. *et al.* (2000). Measuring patient perception of health-related quality-of-life changes using the Subjective Significance Questionnaire. *Quality of Life Research* **9**:256 (abstract 1404).

101 Ross, M. (1989). Relation of implicit theories to the construction of personal histories. *Psychological Reviews* **96**:341–7.

102 Norman, G. R., Stratford, P., Regehr, G. (1997). Methodological problems in the retrospective computation of responsiveness to change: the lesson of Cronbach. *Journal of Clinical Epidemiology* **50**:869–79.

103 Sneeuw, K., Muller, M., Aaronson, N. (2000). Interpreting the significance of changes in EORTC QLQ-C30 and COOP/WONCA scores. *Quality of Life Research* **9**:256 (abstract 1416).

104 Sprangers, M. A. G., Schwartz, C. E. (1999). Integrating response shift into health-related quality of life research: a theoretical model. *Social Science and Medicine* **48**:1507–15.

105 Sprangers, M. A. G., Schwartz, C. E. (1999). The challenge of the response shift for quality-of-life based clinical oncology research (Editorial). *Annals of Oncology* **10**:747–9.

106 Jansen, S. J. T., Stiggelbout, A. M., Nooij, E. M., Noordijk, E. M., Kievit, J. (2000). Response shift in quality of life measurement in early-stage breast cancer patients undergoing radiotherapy. *Quality of Life Research* **9**:603–15.

107 Osoba, D., Brada, M., Prados, M. D., Yung, W. K. A. (2000). Effect of disease burden on health-related quality of life in patients with malignant gliomas. *Neuro-Oncology* **2**:221–8.

108 Hornbrook, this volume, Chapter 24.

109 Cella, D., Bullinger, M., Scott, C., Gorkin, L., Barofsky, I., and the Clinical Significance Consensus Meeting Group. (2002). Group versus individual approaches to understanding the clinical significance of differences or changes in quality of life. *Mayo Clinic Proceedings* **77**:384–92.

110 Sloan, J. A., Aaronson, N., Cappelleri, J. C., Fairclough, D. L., Varricchio, C., and the Clinical Significance Consensus Meeting Group. (2002). Assessing the clinical significance of single items relative to summated scores. *Mayo Clinic Proceedings* **77**:479–87.

111 Frost, M. H., Bonomi, A. E., Ferrans, C. E., Wong, G. Y., Hays, R. D., and the Clinical Significance Consensus Meeting Group. (2002). Patient, clinician and population perspectives on determining the clinical significance of quality-of-life scores. *Mayo Clinic Proceedings* **77**:488–94.

112 Symonds, T., Berzon, R., Marquis, P., Rummans, T., and the Clinical Significance Consensus Meeting Group (2002). The clinical significance of quality-of-life results: practical considerations for specific audiences. *Mayo Clinic Proceedings* **77**:572–83.

113 Fayers, P., Machin, D. (2000). *Quality of Life: Assessment, Analysis and Interpretation*. Chichester: John Wiley & Sons.

114 Sprangers, M. A. G., Moinpour, C., Moynihan, T. J., Patrick, D. L., Revicki, D. A., and the Clinical Significance Consensus Meeting Group. (2002). Assessing meaningful change over time in quality of life: a users' guide for clinicians. *Mayo Clinic Proceedings* **77**:561–71.

115 Osoba, D. (1998). Guidelines for measuring health-related quality of life in clinical trials. In *Quality of Life Assessment in Clinical Trials*, ed. M. J. Staquet, R. D. Hays, P. M. Fayers, pp. 19–35. Oxford: Oxford University Press.

116 Staquet, M., Berzon, R., Osoba, D., Machin, D. (1996). Guidelines for reporting results of quality of life assessments in clinical trials. *Quality of Life Research* **5**:496–502.

117 Guyatt, G. H., Juniper, E. F., Walter, S. D., Griffith, L. E., Goldstein, R. S. (1998). Interpreting treatment effects in randomised trials. *British Medical Journal* **316**:690–3.

118 Nunnally, J. C., Bernstein, I. H. (1994). *Psychometric Theory* (3rd Edition), pp. 264–5. New York, NY: McGraw-Hill, Inc.

119 Revicki, D. A., Cella, D. F. (1997). Health status assessment for the twenty-first century: item response theory, item banking and computer adaptive testing. *Quality of Life Research* **6**:595–600.

120 Revicki, D. A., Osoba, D., Fairclough, D. *et al.* (2000). Recommendation on health-related quality of life research to

support labeling and promotional claims in the United States. *Quality of Life Research* **9**:887–900.

121 Leidy, N. K., Revicki, D. A., Geneste, B. (1999). Recommendations for evaluating the validity of quality of life claims for labeling and promotion. *Value in Health* **2**: 113–27.

122 Ganz, P. A. (1995). Impact of quality of life outcomes on clinical practice. *Oncology* **9** (Suppl. 11):61–5.

123 Osoba, D., Till, J. E., Pater, J. L., Young, J. R. (1995). Health-related quality of life: measurement and clinical application. A workshop report. *Canadian Journal of Oncology* **5**: 338–431.

20

Cross-cultural use of health-related quality of life assessments in clinical oncology

Neil K. Aaronson, Ph.D.

The Netherlands Cancer Institute, Amsterdam, the Netherlands

"Guests are advised to leave their values at the front desk."

(Notice posted in an Italian hotel lobby)

"Language is your most versatile scientific tool. Learn to use it with precision."

(Anonymous)

Introduction

Clinical research in oncology is increasingly characterized by multicenter efforts on an international scale. This has the advantage of improving the efficiency with which clinical trials can be conducted via rapid accrual of patients, and also facilitates the registration of new, effective therapies across national boundaries and health care systems. To carry out such international studies, it is essential that the outcomes of interest are standardized across participating countries. This presents few, if any, problems when focusing on biomedical outcomes such as tumor response or survival. However, when employing treatment outcomes of a more subjective nature, including patients' self-reported symptom experience, perceived health status, and quality of life, cross-cultural issues become of paramount importance. It is essential that the questions we ask and the responses we elicit from our patients maintain the same meaning when translated into different languages and applied in different cultural settings. Without such cross-cultural equivalence, the interpretation of patient-based data in multinational clinical investigations is at best problematic, and at worst impossible.

The past 15 years have witnessed major advances in the development of practical, reliable, and valid questionnaires for assessing the health-related quality of life (HRQOL) of patients with cancer. The most widely used HRQOL measures include the Functional Living Index – Cancer (FLIC),[1] the Cancer Rehabilitation Evaluation System (CARES and CARES-SF),[2,3] the Rotterdam Symptom Checklist (RSCL),[4] the European Organization for Research and Treatment of Cancer Core Quality of Life Questionnaire (QLQ-C30)[5], and the Functional Assessment of Cancer Therapy – General (FACT-G).[6] These questionnaires have proven their usefulness in documenting the symptom and functional health experience of patients with a range of cancer diagnoses and, perhaps more importantly, they have been applied successfully within the demanding settings of phase II and phase III clinical trials.

With the exception of the EORTC questionnaire, which was constructed in a multicultural (European) context, these questionnaires were developed and underwent initial psychometric testing in a single country and language (the FLIC, CARES, and FACT-G in the USA, among English-speaking patients; and the RSCL, in the Netherlands). For summary information on the development and testing of the original versions of these instruments, the reader is referred to Chapter 3 by Erickson in this volume.[7]

In this chapter, we review the published (English-language) literature pertaining to the translation, cultural adaptation, and psychometric evaluation of these five questionnaires for use in alternate languages and cultures. The psychometric evidence reviewed includes: (1) the adequacy of the measurement model as assessed empirically (e.g., with factor analysis or related correlational techniques); (2) internal consistency and test-retest reliability; (3) construct validity; and (4) responsiveness to change in health over time.

The Functional Living Index Cancer (FLIC)

Translation and cultural adaptation

Clinch reports that the FLIC has been translated into 19 languages, including most European languages, as well as Chinese (4 dialects), Japanese, Malay, and Thai.[8] Most of these translations were carried out using iterative, forward-backward translation procedures. However, the only languages for which some published information was found regarding the translation process were Chinese, Malay, and Japanese.[9,10]

The translation process presented a number of challenges that are instructive and illustrative for other cultural and language settings as well. First, the use of words that required a relatively high level of literacy and sophistication yielded better translations (i.e., more accurate and closer in meaning to the concepts being assessed), but were unlikely to be understood by the majority of patients, many of whom had low levels of education. Thus, the final choice of wording often represented a compromise between accuracy and practicality.

Second, because many elderly Chinese and Malay patients are illiterate, use was made of audiotaped versions of the questionnaire so that it could be administered in the form of a standardized interview. These oral language versions typically employed more colloquialisms than are available or necessary in the written language.

Third, among Malay patients, most of whom are Muslim, difficulties arose with the use of psychological terms such as "depression" and "feeling discouraged." The problem was not so much in generating appropriate translations, but rather that these patients considered it inappropriate to report such complaints or symptoms because doing so would suggest a lack of faith in Allah.

Finally, the use of the word "cancer" proved problematic because many of the older patients were not aware (i.e., informed) of their diagnosis. This is not uncommon in Asian cultures, and has been reported in studies conducted in other regions of the world as well, including some Western European countries.[11] In this case, the word "cancer" was replaced with the more general term "illness."

Psychometric performance of alternate language versions

King et al. investigated the measurement model and the psychometric characteristics of the FLIC based on a sample of 93 Australian patients with localized breast cancer and localized and advanced colorectal or ovarian cancer.[12] Factor analysis identified 7 factors, rather than 5 as in the original North American studies. Although 7 subscales were formed on the basis of these results, no further information was provided on the homogeneity (i.e., internal consistency reliability) of these subscales. Construct validity was examined by correlating the FLIC subscales with comparable scales of the EORTC QLQ-C30. The correlations were generally of a moderate magnitude, ranging from 0.35 to 0.74. The FLIC total score and 5 of the 7 subscale scores were also found to distinguish clearly between patient subgroups formed on the basis of clinical evidence of active disease and treatment status.

Mercier and colleagues carried out a cross-sectional study of the FLIC among 200 French-speaking patients undergoing outpatient treatment for breast or colorectal cancer.[13] Factor analysis yielded 5 factors very similar to those found in the original North American studies, with internal consistency reliability, as measured by Cronbach's coefficient alpha, ranging from 0.73 to 0.86. Evidence of the construct validity of 4 of the 5 FLIC subscales was supported by moderate correlations with comparable scales of the EORTC QLQ-C30 (ranging from 0.47 to 0.62). A much lower correlation (0.14) was observed between the FLIC and QLQ-C30 social functioning scales, despite the very similar content of these two scales. The overall FLIC score was found to vary significantly as a function of performance status, but was not related significantly to site of disease or disease status (primary versus recurrent). On average, patients required 11 minutes (standard deviation = 7 minutes) to complete the questionnaire.

Factor analysis of FLIC data, derived from a sample of 111 Chinese cancer patients with heterogeneous diagnoses, yielded a 5-factor solution very similar to that reported in the original North American studies.[9] The only additional psychometric data reported in this study related to the construct validity of the overall FLIC score. As hypothesized, mean scores on the FLIC varied significantly and in the expected direction as a function of stage of disease.

Finally, Forjaz and Guarnaccia compared FLIC total scores between a sample of Portuguese and American patients with hematological malignancies.[11] On average, the Portuguese patients reported significantly higher overall quality of life than their American counterparts. This difference remained significant when controlling statistically for differences in sociodemographic and clinical variables. Unfortunately, this study did not explore in any detail which HRQOL variables (i.e., FLIC items) accounted for the observed between-country differences in overall FLIC scores. It is also questionable whether adequate adjustments were made for case mix. Nevertheless, these findings suggest the need to exhibit caution when using the FLIC in cross-cultural investigations. To minimize the effect of unspecified cultural factors on self-reported HRQOL, patients should be stratified by country prior to randomization in phase III clinical trials.

The Cancer Rehabilitation Evaluation System (CARES) and CARES-Short Form (CARES-SF)

Translation and cultural adaptation

Only three published reports were identified that provided any information on the translation and/or cultural adaptation of the CARES or CARES-SF for use among non-English speaking patients.[14–16] Canales, Ganz, and Coscarelli employed iterative, forward-backward procedures to translate and pilot test a Spanish language version of the CARES for use among Hispanic-American patients.[14] In addition to completing the CARES, patients also underwent a qualitative interview. Several important issues arose during this pilot-testing phase. First, the questionnaire was written primarily in Castilian Spanish. This proved problematic for some questions, in which case the item wording was either changed to reflect more idiomatic use of the language or the idiomatic wording was added in parentheses.

Second, some patients had difficulty with the use of different verb tenses, probably reflecting low levels of formal education. This resulted in the decision to reword all items in the simple present tense.

Third, although Spanish grammar is sensitive to gender, for reasons of simplicity, most questions were phrased in the masculine form only. Exceptions included questions addressing sexuality, in which case both male and female forms were used.

Fourth, a number of problems were identified relating to the response choices and the layout of the questionnaire. Some difficulties were reported in equating numbers with words (e.g., "0" = "not at all"), and many patients also had difficulty in following the skip patterns built into the questionnaire. This may have reflected the patients' relatively low level of formal education rather than problems with the translation, per se. Some of these problems could be resolved by minor changes in the formatting of the questionnaire (e.g., by repeating instructions on every page as a memory cue).

Ultimately, although the translated version of the questionnaire was deemed technically adequate, attempts at conducting a larger validation study of the Spanish version of the CARES failed due to continued problems with its administration. Many patients were unable or reluctant to complete the questionnaire without assistance and, even with such assistance, there were substantial amounts of missing data (as high as 22%). Those patients who were able to complete the questionnaire required much more time than the English-speaking patients (mean of 56 minutes versus 20 minutes).

Rustoen et al.[16] and te Velde et al.[15] reported few problems in translating the CARES-SF into Norwegian and Dutch, respectively. Minor changes in item wording were introduced in the Dutch version with approval by the instrument's developers. The only important change was replacing the word "cancer" with "illness." This was done not because patients were unaware of their diagnosis (as was the case with the FLIC translation in Asia), but rather because it was deemed less confrontational to patients, particularly in longitudinal studies in which the questionnaire was to be administered serially.

Psychometric performance of alternate language versions

Te Velde and colleagues[15] examined the psychometric properties of the CARES-SF in a longitudinal study of 485 Dutch patients with varied diagnoses (primarily breast, lung, and colorectal cancer) and stage of disease receiving either outpatient chemotherapy or radiotherapy. All patients completed the CARES-SF at 3 points in time: prior to the start of treatment, 1 month, and 3 months later. A subset of patients completed the questionnaire on a fourth occasion for purposes of assessing test-retest reliability.

Both multitrait scaling and factor analysis confirmed the hypothesized scale structure of the questionnaire. Internal consistency reliability was above 0.80 for the physical functioning and psychosocial functioning scales, and above 0.90 for the global scale at all three assessment points. Lower values were obtained for the medical interaction (range = 0.61 to 0.74), marital interaction (range = 0.64 to 0.68), and sexual functioning (range = 0.49 to 0.56) scales. Test-retest reliability was good to excellent, ranging from 0.72 for the marital interaction scale to 0.91 for the physical functioning and global scales.

Known-groups comparisons, using either stage of disease or performance status ratings as grouping variables, supported the construct validity of 4 of the 5 summary scales (the exception being the marital interaction scale) and the global scale. The physical functioning and global scales were responsive to changes in patients' performance status over time.

The physical and sexual functioning scales and the global scale captured changes over time (i.e., deterioration) expected among patients with progressive disease.

Respondent burden was within acceptable limits, with patients requiring, on average, 11 minutes to complete the questionnaire. While the large majority of patients were able to complete the questionnaire without assistance, 82% reported difficulty with at least one item. Most often, this reflected difficulties in following the skip patterns and in understanding question-response combinations that contained double negations. Some patients reported that questions pertaining to sexuality were intrusive and chose not to complete them. Interestingly, some patients also reported being upset by items pertaining to future perspective (e.g., "I worry about whether my disease is progressing," "I worry about not being able to care for myself"), which they considered too confrontational.

Rustoen and coworkers carried out a cross-sectional, descriptive study of the HRQOL of Norwegian patients (N = 126) recently diagnosed with breast, gynecological, prostate, or colon cancer.[16] High internal consistency and test-retest reliability was observed for the global scale (0.89 and 0.83, respectively). Mean scores on the CARES-SF summary scales and global scale did not vary significantly as a function of age, gender, primary site of disease, time since diagnosis, or treatment status. Patients who were living with others reported significantly better physical, psychosocial, and sexual functioning, and better overall HRQOL than patients living alone. More highly educated patients reported significantly fewer problems in their interactions with medical personnel than those with lower levels of education.

The Rotterdam Symptom Checklist (RSCL)

Translation and cultural adaptation

No literature was found on the number of languages into which the RSCL has been translated, the availability of standardized procedures for carrying out such translations, or efforts undertaken to provide centralized quality control. While the RSCL has been used in several phase III multinational breast cancer clinical trials, including patients from ten primarily European countries,[17,18] in these trials it is simply stated that the questionnaire was translated into the requisite languages using forward-backward translation procedures.

The only published paper that provides a more detailed description of the translation process is a study of terminally ill cancer patients in Spain.[19] An iterative, forward-backward translation procedure was employed, involving dyads of bilingual translators. Additionally, independent teams provided quantitative ratings to identify items or response choices requiring further revision. Several pilot studies, involving groups of approximately 10 patients, were carried out to identify items that were unclear or difficult to answer, and the time required for completion of the questionnaire (on average, less than 10 minutes).

Psychometric performance of alternative language versions

Four publications were found that reported information relating to the psychometric characteristics of the RSCL in alternate languages. In the aforementioned phase III, multinational, adjuvant chemotherapy clinical trial in early breast cancer,[17] most of the psychometric analyses were carried out for the total study sample (N = 689, including patients from 13 countries, 10 of which were non-English speaking), and for 6 language/country clusters (English-speaking, Eastern European, Finnish, French, German, and "Latin" (Spanish, Portuguese, and Argentinean).

Factor analysis, based only on the total study sample, confirmed the two-factor structure (psychological and physical distress) of the symptom items of the RSCL. For the total sample, the internal consistency reliability for the psychological distress, physical distress, and activity scales was 0.88, 0.83, and 0.80, respectively. While the reliability estimates for the former two scales were highly consistent across language/country clusters, considerable variability was found for the activity scale (Cronbach's alpha ranging from 0.42 for the "Latin" cluster to 0.83 for the Eastern European cluster). Lower language/culture-specific scale reliability was attributed primarily to lack of score variability (i.e., ceiling effects).

No information was provided on the validity of the RSCL. However, statistically significant differences were observed between the language/country clusters in mean baseline scores for all three RSCL scales, with the Finnish sample consistently reporting the highest HRQOL and the French cluster the lowest. Mean change scores for the psychological and activity scales over a 3-month interval also varied as a function of language/country. It was hypothesized that these differences may have reflected, at least in part, a "regression to the mean" phenomenon. For example, the Finnish cluster, which reported the highest HRQOL at baseline, was the only one to report deterioration in HRQOL over time, while the German cluster, which reported the lowest HRQOL at baseline, exhibited the greatest improvement over time.

Ravaioli *et al.* reported on the use of the RSCL in a heterogeneous sample of Italian cancer patients with advanced disease receiving chemotherapy.[20] The internal consistency reliability of the psychological and physical distress scales was 0.76 and 0.85, respectively. Both scales were able to distinguish between patients receiving "high burden" versus "low burden" chemotherapy.

Paci administered the RSCL to a sample of 119 healthy Italian women attending a breast cancer screening program, and to 61 women treated previously for early breast cancer.[21] Most of the psychometric data pertain to the healthy sample only. Factor analysis results lent partial support to the hypothesized scale structure of the RSCL. Four factors were identified, the first of which paralleled the original psychological distress scale, with the latter three composed of subsets of items from the original physical distress scale. Nevertheless, when scored in accordance with the original two-factor scale structure, the internal consistency reliability estimates were high (0.91 and 0.87 for the psychological and physical distress scales, respectively).

The construct validity of the psychological symptom scale was examined by correlating it with the Spielberger State-Trait Anxiety Inventory (STAI). Although the authors did not highlight this finding, it is noteworthy that the RSCL scale correlated much more strongly with the trait version than with the state version of the STAI (r = 0.74 and 0.39, respectively). This raises some concern as to whether the RSCL scale is assessing current levels of psychological distress rather than a more stable personality characteristic, at least in this sample of healthy women. The mean scores on the RSCL scales were comparable between the healthy and breast cancer samples, and between women within the breast cancer sample who had undergone radical mastectomy versus breast-conserving therapy. Although these findings might be taken to suggest lack of (known groups) validity, it should be noted that the patient group was composed of women who were disease-free and in long-term follow-up, and that other studies have tended to find few if any significant differences in HRQOL between breast cancer patients treated with radical versus conservative surgery.[22-25]

Finally, Agra and Badía employed the RSCL in a cross-sectional study of 118 terminally ill cancer patients in Spain.[19] The internal consistency and test-retest reliability of the physical symptom, psychological symptom, and activity scales were uniformly high (alpha coefficients = 0.74, 0.79, and 0.87, respectively; test-retest correlations = 0.82, 0.78, and 0.87, respectively). The pattern of correlations observed between the RSCL scales and related scales of the Nottingham Health Profile supported the construct validity of the RSCL. The RSCL was also found to distinguish clearly between patient groups defined on the basis of Karnofsky performance status scores.

The European Organization for Research and Treatment of Cancer Core Quality of Life Questionnaire (EORTC QLQ-C30)

Translation and cultural adaptation

In contrast to other cancer-specific HRQOL questionnaires, the QLQ-C30 was developed and evaluated in an international, multicultural context. Thus, from the outset, issues of culture and language were incorporated into the choice of item content and wording. This is reflected in the relative simplicity and the absence of colloquial wording in the English-language version that has served as the parent instrument for all subsequent translations.

The EORTC has published standard guidelines and procedures for translating the QLQ-C30 into alternative languages.[26] These procedures are quite straightforward, involving iterative, forward and backward translations by teams of bilingual translators working independently of one another, and pilot-testing of the target language version among small groups (10–15) of patients. The pilot testing includes a structured interview and/or focus group exercises to identify items, response choices, or instructions that are difficult to understand or upsetting, and to elicit possible alternative wording. Procedures are also available for adapting existing translations of the questionnaire (e.g., French) for use in other settings (e.g., French-Canadian). The EORTC requires a written report documenting each step in the translation process, including copies of all forward and backward versions. Final review and approval of translations rests with the EORTC.

The QLQ-C30 is currently available in 37 languages, including all Western and most Eastern European languages, Arabic, (Taiwanese) Chinese, 4 Indian languages/dialects (Hindi, Gujarathi, Marathi, Telugu), Hebrew, Indonesian, Japanese, Korean, Malay, Persian, Thai, Turkish, and 3 African languages (Sotho, Xhosa, Zulu). Additionally, cultural adaptations are available for English (British versus American), Dutch (Afrikaans), French (Canadian), Portuguese (Brazilian), and Spanish (American, Argentinean, Mexican, Peruvian). Gender-specific versions of the questionnaire are available in those languages where this is grammatically appropriate.

Somewhat surprisingly, given the sustained effort that has gone into generating alternate language versions of the QLQ-C30, there are very few *published* reports describing problems encountered in the translation and cultural adaptation process. Whether this is because few problems or issues have been encountered that are worthy of reporting, or because investigators have simply chosen to focus on psychometric evaluation of the questionnaire is unclear.

Zhao and Kanda have described some of the changes that were necessary in adapting the Chinese version of the QLQ-C30 (developed in Hong Kong) for use in the People's Republic of China.[27] Most of these changes involved finding alternative wording more appropriate for "standard" Chinese as spoken on the mainland (e.g., "quality of life"). Kobayashi et al.[28] also reported difficulty in translating "quality of life" into Japanese.

Petersen et al. employed a more formal statistical method, Differential Item Function Analysis (DIF), to assess the equivalence of nine translated versions of the emotional functioning scale of the QLQ-C30.[29] DIF analysis aids in determining if a translated item functions in the same way as in the original, parent version. In this context, "function" refers to whether patients with the same level of the concept being measured (in this case, emotional distress) are equally likely to endorse an item, regardless of the translation used.[30,31] Based on these methods, several possible problems in translation were identified that had not been previously detected. For example, in the Swedish version of the QLQ-C30, the word "depressed" is translated as "feeling down." This latter, more colloquial term was purposively chosen because, in Swedish, the word "depressed" has a very serious, clinical connotation. The results of this DIF analysis illustrate how item wording can impact on threshold levels for endorsing an item, and consequently may affect the prevalence rates reported for certain symptoms or functional problems across languages and cultures.

Psychometric performance of alternate language versions

Ten studies, 8 of which employed non-English versions of the QLQ-C30, have examined empirically the measurement model of the QLQ-C30. Seven of these studies used multitrait scaling techniques as in the original international field study.[27,28,32–36] These studies have provided consistent support for the hypothesized scale structure of the questionnaire. In two studies, some evidence of scaling violations were observed for the role functioning scale (overlapping with the physical functioning scale),[36] and the cognitive functioning scale (overlapping with the emotional functioning scale).[27,36] Two studies employing factor analytic techniques and two studies using Mokken's latent non-parametric modelling yielded results very similar to those based on multitrait scaling.[36,37] Only one study[38] generated evidence of an alternative measurement model (a two-factor solution), but this was limited to the psychosocial items within the questionnaire.

Table 20.1 summarizes the results from 17 studies that evaluated the internal consistency reliability of the QLQ-C30 scales. With the exception of one Canadian study[35] and one study carried out among African-American patients,[39] all of these studies employed non-English versions of the questionnaire. Two studies used general population samples[40,41] and one involved patients with a range of chronic health conditions.[39]

With a few notable exceptions, the results of these studies lend strong support to the reliability of the QLQ-C30 scales for use at the level of group comparisons (i.e., alpha coefficient above 0.70).[42] In several studies[36,43] the role functioning scale exhibited relatively poor reliability (below 0.60), but these were all studies employing the original (1.0) version of the scale. The revised version of this scale has yielded consistently higher reliability coefficients (ranging from 0.68 to 0.91).[27,33,39–41,43,44]

The cognitive functioning scale has shown poor to moderate reliability (ranging from 0.37 to 0.77). This was already evident in the original international field study, and suggests that the two cognitive domains assessed by this scale (memory and concentration) are only modestly correlated with one another, at least at the relatively low levels of symptomatology typically observed in cancer patients.

The reliability of the emesis scale is highly variable across studies, with alpha coefficients ranging from 0.21 in a sample of Hawaiian patients of Japanese ancestry[42] to well above 0.80 in Japanese[28] and Chinese patients.[27] In the original field study, lower levels of reliability for this scale were observed

Table 20.1. Internal consistency reliability (Cronbach's alpha) of the QLQ-C30 Scales

Reference	Country	Sample (N)	Version	PF	RF	EF	CF	SF	QL	Pain	Fatigue	Emesis
Aaronson et al.[5]	Multiple	Lung (305)	1.0	0.68	0.54	0.73	0.56	0.68	0.86	0.82	0.80	0.65
Apolone et al.[32]	Italy	Breast (405)	1.0	0.64	0.85	0.87	0.77	0.83	0.90	0.82	0.85	0.58
		Colon (199)										
Arraras et al.[33]	Spain	Head and neck (201)	3.0	0.75[a]	0.91	0.69	0.57	0.77	0.92	0.76	0.81	0.63
				0.86	0.89	0.87	0.70	0.86	0.93	0.73	0.83	0.72
				0.72	0.90	0.70	0.65	0.75	0.91	0.76	0.79	0.60
Bjordal et al.[70]	Norway	Head and neck (204)	1.0	0.74	0.74	0.85	0.73	0.77	0.93	0.79	0.88	0.56
Bjordal et al.[71]	Multiple	Head and neck (1622)	3.0	0.84	–	–	–	–	–	–	–	–
Ford et al. [39]	USA	African-American	3.0	0.77	0.89	0.83	0.69	0.67	0.82	0.83	0.82	0.49
		Chronic dis (255)										
Gotay et al.[42]	(Ethnic)	Breast (126)	1.0	0.63	0.54	0.85	0.71	0.80	0.81	0.64	0.75	–
	Hawaiians,	Prostate (101)		0.59	–	0.83	0.63	0.60	0.68	0.68	0.79	0.37
	USA			0.50	0.56	0.77	0.37	0.80	0.80	0.61	0.79	0.21
				0.19	–	0.90	0.60	0.59	0.74	0.82	0.75	0.80
Hjermstad et al.[40]	Norway	General pop. (1965)	2.0	>0.70	>0.70	>0.70	>0.70	>0.70	>0.70	>0.85	>0.85	0.65
Kaasa et al.[34]	Norway	Palliative RT y (247)	1.0	0.77	0.68	0.80	0.62	0.78	0.88	0.89	0.87	0.81
				0.75	0.67	0.85	0.69	0.82	0.92	0.75	0.88	0.74
Kemmler et al.[46]	Germany	Breast (118)	1.0	0.77	0.86	0.79	0.66	0.75	0.94	–	–	–
Kobayashi et al.[28]	Japan	Lung (105)	1.0	0.83	0.74	0.90	0.63	0.72	0.88	0.87	0.90	0.86
Montazeri et al.[44]	Iran	Breast (168)	2.0	0.69	0.83	0.78	0.53	0.48	0.95	0.54	0.65	0.81
				0.71	0.77	0.83	0.51	0.52	0.98	0.67	0.83	0.81
Osoba et al.[35]	Canada	Breast (143)	1.0	0.71	0.66	0.85	0.63	0.82	0.89	0.83	0.87	0.60
		Ovarian (111)		0.75	0.53	0.84	0.58	0.83	0.94	0.83	0.90	0.78
		Lung (160)										
Osoba et al.[43]	Canada	Mixed (1181)	2.0	–	0.78	–	–	–	0.79	–	–	–
	Netherlands				0.88				0.92			
Ringdal et al.[36]	Norway	Mixed (177)	1.0	0.75	0.55	0.85	0.65	0.72	0.85	0.86	0.83	0.79
Schwarz et al.[41]	Germany	General pop. (2081)	3.0	0.81	0.89	0.90	0.68	0.86	0.89	0.84	0.80	0.65
Zhao et al.[27]	China	Gyn (191)	2.0	0.67	0.85	0.85	0.45	0.79	0.83	0.72	0.85	0.87

PF = physical function; RF = role function; EF = emotional function; CF = cognitive function; SF = social function; QL = overall quality of life
[a] Multiple alpha coefficients are due either to separate calculations per patient subgroup or to reliability estimates derived from different assessment points

in subsets of patients not receiving chemotherapy, suggesting that this may be an artifact of limited score variability.

Finally, in a study of Asian Pacific Islanders, the physical functioning scale performed very poorly in a subsample of Filipino-Hawaiians (alpha = 0.19).[42] The authors do not conjecture as to the reason for this rather perplexing finding, given the consistently higher reliability of this scale found across other languages and cultures.

One Norwegian study has evaluated the (4-day) test-retest reliability of the QLQ-C30 scales.[45] The reliability of the functioning and global HRQOL scales was consistently high, ranging from 0.82 for role and cognitive functioning to 0.91 for physical functioning. The reliability of the symptom scales – pain, fatigue and emesis – was 0.86, 0.83, and 0.63, respectively.

The validity of the questionnaire has been evaluated in three ways. Several studies have examined

Table 20.2. Known-groups validity of the EORTC QLQ-C30 scales

Reference	Grouping Variable	PF	RF	EF	CF	SF	QL	Pain	Fatigue	Emesis
Aaronson et al.[5]	Performance status	●	●	●	●	●	●	●	●	●
	Weight loss	●	●	○	○	○	●	○	●	○
	Treatment toxicity	○	●	●	●	●	●	●	●	●
Apolone et al.[32]	Gender	●	●	●	○	○	●	●	●	●
Arraras et al.[33]	Disease status	○	●	●	○	●	●	●	●	○
	Performance status	●	○	○	○	●	●	●	●	○
	Weight loss	●	●	○	○	●	●	●	●	○
Bjordal et al.[71]	Disease status	○	●	●	●	●	●	●	●	○
	Performance status	●	●	●	●	●	●	●	●	●
Kobayashi et al.[28]	Performance status	●	●	●	●	●	●	●	●	●
McLachlan et al.[72]	Performance status	–	●	○	○	●	●	–	–	–
	Chemotherapy (yes/no)	–	●	○	○	●	●	–	–	–
Montazeri et al.[44]	Disease stage	●	●	●	●	●	●	●	●	●
	Performance status	●	●	●	●	●	●	●	●	●
Osoba et al.[35]	Disease stage	●	●	○	○	●	●	●	●	○

PF = physical function; RF = role function; EF = emotional function; CF = cognitive function; SF = social function; QL = overall quality of life.

● = statistically significant (< 0.05) between-group difference in mean scores; ○ = no statistically significant difference in mean scores was observed.

the association between the QLQ-C30 scales and other instruments assessing similar constructs. Apolone and colleagues administered the QLQ-C30 and the SF-36 Health Survey to 588 Italian patients with either breast or colon cancer.[32] Correlations between corresponding scales of these two instruments ranged from 0.50 for the social functioning domain to 0.74 for the physical functioning domain.

In two German studies, correlations between related scales (at least in name) of the QLQ-C30 and the FACT-G were moderate for physical functioning and role functioning (r's ranging from 0.48 to 0.68), but lower for social and emotional functioning (r's ranging from 0.14 to 0.51).[46,47]

In a study of 247 Norwegian patients undergoing palliative radiotherapy, the correlation between the emotional functioning scale of the QLQ-C30 and the General Health Questionnaire (GHQ-20) was 0.62 and 0.71 at pre-treatment and post-treatment, respectively. Correlations between the QLQ-C30 pain scale and a visual analogue pain scale were 0.79 and 0.78.[34]

The known-groups validity of the QLQ-C30 has been investigated in eight studies, 6 of which were focused on non-English speaking patients. The results of these studies are summarized in Table 20.2. Grouping variables included stage of disease, disease status, performance status, weight loss, and treatment toxicity. Taken together, these studies provide strong and consistent evidence of the validity of the physical, role, and social functioning scales, the global HRQOL scale, the pain scale, and the fatigue scale (i.e., statistically significant group differences at the $p < 0.05$ level for 10/13, 14/15, 13/15, 15/15, 12/13, and 13/13 comparisons, respectively). The emotional and cognitive functioning scales yielded mixed results ($p < 0.05$ for 9/15 and 7/15 comparisons, respectively). This is not surprising in that the grouping variables used in these studies reflect differences in physical rather than psychosocial health. The emesis scale also exhibits moderate validity ($p < 0.05$ in 7/13 comparisons), again reflecting the limited score variability of this scale in settings where the prevalence of nausea and vomiting is low (e.g., at

Table 20.3. Responsiveness of the QLQ-C30 EORTC

Reference	PF	RF	EF	CF	SF	QL	Pain	Fatigue	Emesis
Aaronson et al.[5]	•	•	o	o	o	•	o	•	•
Apolone et al.[32]	•	•	o	•	•	•	•	•	
Arraras et al.[33]	•	•	o	•	•	•	o	•	•
Bjordal et al.[71]	•	•	o	o	•	•	•	•	•
Kaasa et al.[34]	•	•	o	o	o	o	o	•	•
Kobayashi et al.[28]	o	o	o	o	o	o	o	•	•
Osoba et al.[35]	•	•	•	•	•	•	o	•	•

PF = physical function; RF = role function; EF = emotional function; CF = cognitive function; SF = social function; QL = overall quality of life
• = statistically significant (< 0.05) change over time in mean scores; o = no statistically significant change over time in mean scores.

pre-treatment assessments, in studies not involving emesis-inducing chemotherapy).

Finally, Groenvold and colleagues[48] employed a mix of quantitative (i.e., comparison of patient versus proxy ratings) and qualitative (i.e., cognitive interviewing) methods to examine the validity of patients' responses to the QLQ-C30. The agreement between patients' and observers' ratings was high (median kappa = 0.85). Of particular interest, however, was the finding that some patients fail to report certain symptoms they are experiencing because they believe they are caused by health problems other than their cancer or its treatment (e.g., pain due to arthritis, depression due to other life events, etc.). Such unintended selective reporting may lead to systematic underreporting of symptoms, and may render some group comparisons problematic (e.g., comparison of patients' scores with general population norms, comparison of scores of patients receiving active treatment versus a control group). The authors suggest the use of explicit instructions (e.g., that the patient should report all symptoms without considering their cause) to reduce the risk of such selective reporting.

Responsiveness of the QLQ-C30 to changes in patients' health status over time has been investigated in seven studies, the results of which are summarized in Table 20.3. In some of these studies, the analysis simply compared mean baseline (typically pre-treatment) scores with mid-treatment or post-treatment scores for all patients. In other studies, more explicit hypotheses were tested by correlating changes in QLQ-C30 scores with changes observed on other indicators of health status (e.g., patients whose performance status had improved or deteriorated over time). The physical, role, and social functioning scales, the fatigue and emesis scales, and the global HRQOL scale appear to be most responsive, and the emotional functioning and pain scales least so. This latter finding may be due to the fact that pain control was seldom the treatment goal in the studies reviewed.

Lastly, several studies conducted in Scandinavia[40,49,50] and Germany[41] have generated general population normative data for the QLQ-C30. The EORTC has also published reference values for the QLQ-C30 for specific cancer patient populations (by stage of disease), using data obtained both from within the EORTC and from clinical trials and epidemiological studies conducted by the British Medical Research Council, the National Cancer Institute of Canada, and other collaborating organizations and individuals.[51] These data can be useful in interpreting QLQ-C30 scores by comparing them to background levels found in the general population or to score distributions found in groups of patients with similar clinical characteristics. They may also be useful in calculating sample sizes for studies in which HRQOL outcomes are of primary interest.

The Functional Assessment of Cancer Therapy – General (FACT-G) questionnaire

Translation and cultural adaptation

Translation and cultural adaptation of the FACT-G into alternate languages has been carried out in a systematic and standardized manner, with central coordination and quality control. The process includes: (1) forward translation from English to the target language by 2 bilingual speakers with the target language as their native tongue; (2) reconciliation of the forward translations; (3) backward translation of the reconciled version by one bilingual, native-English speaker; (4) independent review by 3 to 4 bilingual experts; (5) review by a centralized coordinating committee; (6) spelling and grammatical language verification; and (7) pilot testing with patients in the target language.[52,53]

An important feature of the FACT approach to translation is the use of a "decentering" technique. Essentially, this allows for modifications of the parent instrument (i.e., the original, English-language version of the FACT-G), based on difficulties encountered in generating equivalent or culturally appropriate translations. The developers of the FACT have also acknowledged that some items may be culturally inappropriate, and thus have allowed the option of administering the questionnaire without them. Examples include the item, "I worry about dying," which can be problematic in Japan and other countries where patients may not be aware they have cancer; and "I am satisfied with my sex life," which proved problematic in cultures where it is uncommon to inquire about sexuality, even in a medical setting (e.g., South Africa).[53]

The FACT-G is currently available in more than 40 languages, including all Western European and most Eastern European languages, as well as Afrikaans, Arabic, Chinese (simplified and traditional), Hebrew, Hindi, Indonesian, Japanese, Korean, Malay, Marathi, Pedi, Tagalog, Telugu, Thai, Tswana, and Zulu. Where deemed feasible, for languages for which variants are spoken in different countries (e.g., Spanish), a single, harmonized translation has been generated that can be used in a uniform manner worldwide.

Psychometric performance of alternate language versions

Nine published studies have explicitly evaluated the psychometric performance of alternate language versions or cultural adaptations of the FACT-G, including: (1) five studies of the Spanish version among Hispanics in the United States (including Puerto Rico),[54–57] and in Uruguay;[58] (2) a pilot study of the Dutch, French, German, Italian, Norwegian, and Swedish versions;[52] (3) one study of the Chinese version as used in Hong Kong;[59] (4) a study of the Pedi, Tswana, and Zulu versions in South Africa;[60] and (5) a study of the Malayalam version in India.[61] One additional study pertains to the use of the original (American) version of the FACT-G in the United Kingdom.[62] A number of these studies also report on other FACT scales (e.g., for breast or colorectal cancer),[55,56,59,61,62] but those data will not be reviewed here.

The measurement model underlying the FACT-G has been examined empirically (i.e., using factor analysis, multitrait scaling, or related techniques) only for the Chinese version of the questionnaire.[59] Using a forced, 5-factor solution, the pattern and strength of factor loadings were very similar to those reported in the original validation study.

Table 20.4 summarizes the results of nine studies that evaluated the internal consistency reliability of the FACT-G scales. The general pattern of results is very similar to that reported in the original, American study of the FACT-G (also presented in Table 5.4 for purposes of comparison). The scales with the highest levels of reliability across studies are physical and functional well-being, and the FACT-G total score, with coefficient alpha meeting or surpassing the 0.70 level recommended for group-level comparisons in 10/11, 11/11, and 11/11 tests, respectively. The

Table 20.4. Internal consistency reliability (Cronbach's alpha) of the FACT-G Scales

Reference	Country	Sample (N)	Version	PWB	SWB	RWD	EWB	FWB	FACT-G Total
Bonomi et al.[52]	Multiple European	Mixed (95)	3	0.84	0.63	0.83	0.75	0.86	0.89
Cella et al.[6]	USA	Mixed (466)	2	0.82	0.69	0.65	0.74	0.80	0.89
Cella et al.[54]	USA Hispanic Puerto Rico	Mixed (92)	2	0.82	0.74	0.75	0.66	0.83	0.89
Cella et al.[55]	USA Hispanic Puerto Rico	HIV (64)	2	0.90	0.65	0.85	0.72	0.86	0.91
Dapueto et al.[58]	Uruguay	Mixed (140)	2	0.79	0.65	0.66	0.60	0.72	0.83
Fallowfield et al.[62]	UK	Breast (268)	3	0.83	0.69	0.86	0.65	0.87	0.90
Mullin et al.[60]	South Africa	Breast (97)	3						
	Pedi	Other (53)		0.78	0.60	0.80	0.87	0.92	0.92
	Twsana			0.79	0.61	0.92	0.76	0.83	0.89
	Zulu			0.64	0.36	0.86	0.77	0.80	0.82
Pandey et al.[61]	India Malayalam	Breast (31)	4	0.75	0.63	–	0.84	0.84	0.90
Ward et al.[56]	USA Hispanic	Colon (93)	4	0.80	0.56	–	0.64	0.86	0.89
Yu et al.[59]	Hong Kong Chinese	Mixed (1,108)	3	0.75	0.53	0.37	0.65	0.75	0.85

PWB = Physical Well-Being; SWB = Social Well-Being; RWD = Relationship with Doctor; EWB = Emotional Well-Being; FWB = Functional Well-Being.

relationship with doctor scale has also exhibited satisfactory reliability (coefficient alpha > 0.70 in 7/9 tests). Lower and less consistent reliability estimates have been observed for the social and emotional well-being scales (coefficient alpha > 0.70 in 1/11 tests and 6/11 tests, respectively). None of these studies examined the test-retest reliability of the FACT-G scales.

Three studies have examined the validity of the FACT-G by comparing it with other instruments assessing similar HRQOL constructs. Cella and colleagues administered the FACT-G and the Profile of Mood States (POMS-SF) to a sample of 92 Spanish-speaking American and Puerto Rican cancer patients with varied diagnoses.[54] The pattern of correlations was consistent with expectations, and supportive of the validity of the FACT-G. For example, the FACT-G emotional and social well-being scales correlated most strongly with the POMS-SF depression scale ($r = -0.52$ and -0.73, respectively), while the FACT-G functional well-being scale correlated

highest with the POMS-SF vigor scale ($r = 0.71$). The overall POMS-SF score exhibited the highest correlation with the FACT-G emotional well-being scale ($r = 0.66$) and the total FACT-G score (0.54). Ward and colleagues found a similar pattern of associations between the FACT-G and the POMS-SF in a sample of Spanish-speaking patients with colorectal cancer.[56]

In a study of Chinese cancer patients residing in Hong Kong,[59] moderate correlations were observed between corresponding scales of the FACT-G and the abbreviated version of the World Health Organization Quality of Life Questionnaire (WHOQOL-BREF), ranging from 0.47 for the psychological health domain to 0.59 for the physical health domain. The correlation between the total FACT-G and WHOQOL-BREF scores was 0.72.

The known-groups validity of the FACT-G has been investigated in five studies of Spanish-speaking cancer patients in the USA[56,57] and Uruguay,[58] English breast cancer patients,[62] and Spanish-speaking

Table 20.5. Known-groups validity of the FACT-G

Reference	Grouping Variable	PWB	SWB	RWD	EWB	FWB	FACT-G Total
Cella et al.[55]	Disease stage	●	○	○	○	○	○
	Performance status	●	○	○	○	●	●
Dapueto et al.[58]	Performance status	●	●	○	●	●	●
Fallowfield et al.[62]	Disease stage	●	●	○	○	●	●
	Nature of treatment	●	●	○	○	○	○
Wan et al.[57]	Age	●	○	○	●	○	○
	Disease stage	●	○	○	○	○	●
	Performance status	●	○	○	●	●	●
	Spiritual belief	●	●	●	●	○	●
Ward et al.[56]	Disease stage	●	○	—	●	●	●
	Performance status	●	○	—	○	●	●

PWB = Physical Well-Being; SWB = Social Well-Being; RWD = Relationship with Doctor; EWB = Emotional Well-Being; FWB = Functional Well-Being.

● = statistically significant (< 0.05) between-group difference in mean scores; ○ = no statistically significant difference in mean scores.

patients in the USA with human immunodeficiency virus (HIV) infection[55] (Table 20.5). Grouping variables included age, disease stage, performance status, nature of treatment, and degree of spirituality. The strongest and most consistent evidence of validity was found for the physical well-being scale ($p < 0.05$ in 11/11 comparisons) and the total FACT-G ($p < 0.05$ in 8/11 comparisons). The social, emotional, and functional well-being scales yielded mixed results ($p < 0.05$ in 4/11, 5/11, and 6/11 comparisons, respectively). The relationship with doctor scale (which has subsequently been dropped from the FACT-G) performed worst, with statistically significant group differences noted in only 1 of 9 comparisons. A particularly interesting group contrast was noted by Wan and colleagues in their study of Hispanic patients.[57] Patients who reported strong spiritual beliefs had significantly higher scores on the physical, emotional, and functional well-being scales and the total FACT-G scale than those without such beliefs. The authors hypothesize that this may reflect an inverse relationship between spiritual beliefs and anxiety, a stronger sense of personal control (e.g., self-esteem and self-efficacy), and a smaller discrepancy between personal expectations and actual levels of functioning.

Only one study was found pertaining to the responsiveness of alternate language versions of the FACT-G to changes in patients' health condition over time. Among Spanish-speaking colorectal cancer patients in the USA, statistically significant changes, in the hypothesized direction, were observed for all of the functional scales and the total FACT-G scale for patients whose performance status had improved or deteriorated over time.[56] No published reports were identified that provide general population normative data or patient population reference data for alternate language versions of the FACT-G.

Summary and recommendations

One of the most striking findings to emerge from this review is the variability in the sheer volume of information available on the translation and cross-cultural validation of these five general cancer HRQOL questionnaires. Ideally, in carrying out such a review, formal criteria would be applied to evaluate both the process and the outcome of the efforts undertaken to establish the cross-cultural equivalence of these questionnaires. A number of taxonomies have been proposed for doing so, each of which employs somewhat different terminology, attributes, and criteria.[63–68] However, early on in the review process, it became apparent that the level of detail provided in the publications relating to these five HRQOL measures was insufficient to undertake such a detailed and formal analysis. Thus a somewhat less ambitious, more descriptive approach was taken.

For the FLIC, the CARES, the RSCL, and the QLQ-C30, three or fewer publications were identified that provided more than a cursory reference to the translation process. In contrast, many of the papers on the FACT-G provide relatively detailed information on the problems encountered in the translation process, and the approaches taken to resolving those problems. This should not be taken to mean that translation of the other instruments has been taken lightly or has been of an inferior quality. To the contrary, those reports that have been published suggest that careful attention has been paid to ensuring that the alternate language versions of all five questionnaires are conceptually and semantically equivalent to their parent versions.

Several important lessons can be distilled from these reports. First, generating high quality translations is a labor-intensive, time-consuming process. It requires input from multidisciplinary teams of linguists, health care professionals, patients, and methodologists over sustained periods of time. This needs to be taken into consideration when planning clinical investigations where it is known that additional translations will be needed. Although the time pressure involved in preparing trial protocols and opening studies to patient accrual is often severe, one cannot expect that new translations can be generated in a matter of weeks or even months.

Second, the availability of standardized translation guidelines and centralized review procedures can enhance enormously both the efficiency with which translations are produced and the quality of those translations. Both the EORTC and the FACT teams have such procedures and quality control mechanisms in place, which have allowed them to generate large numbers of translations in a relatively short period of time.

Third, despite the best efforts at producing high quality translations, it is essential to continue to monitor the use of questionnaires in cross-cultural settings, and to remain open to (and preferably solicit) feedback from local investigators regarding possible problems in item wording and questionnaire layout. Often, problems are reported only months or even years after a given translation has been in circulation.

Fourth, experience gained through the use of alternate language versions of a questionnaire can and should inform the further development and refinement of the original, parent instrument. The modifications introduced to the QLQ-C30 and the FACT-G have been based, in part, on such feedback.

Finally, it is important to maintain an optimal balance between the "art" and the "science" of questionnaire translation. Both qualitative and quantitative methods are useful and, in fact, necessary, to generate high quality translations in the first place, and to identify weaknesses in those translations once they have been put to use. As large-scale datasets become available on alternate language versions of a questionnaire, modern psychometric techniques, such as Differential Item Function Analysis (based on item response theory), offer sophisticated, quantitative methods for identifying questionnaire items that are not performing uniformly across languages and cultures, and that may require further refinement or possibly replacement.

Large differences were also found in the amount of information available on the psychometric characteristics of the five questionnaires. Relatively few reports were found for the FLIC, the CARES, and the RSCL, as compared to the QLQ-C30 and the FACT-G. In large part, this probably reflects the fact that both of the latter two instruments have a relatively stable group of investigators associated with them, facilitating a sustained and coordinated program of cross-cultural research.

In general, the cross-cultural studies of the psychometrics of these instruments have yielded few, if any, surprises. That is, findings with regard to the relative strengths and weaknesses of the alternate language versions of each questionnaire parallel closely those based on the validation studies of the original, parent versions of these instruments. For example, reports on alternate language versions of both the FLIC and the RSCL suggest that the measurement model (i.e., scale structure) underlying these questionnaires is somewhat unclear and unstable. This was already the case for the parent versions of these instruments. Importantly, the ambiguous scale structure of these questionnaires, combined with the absence of explicit scoring procedures for the parent versions, has resulted in inconsistent and somewhat idiosyncratic reporting of results in the literature. In some cases, only total scale scores are reported. In other instances, subscales are employed that contain different sets of items or results are reported at the individual item level only. This obviously hampers the possibility of comparing results across studies. It should be noted that the evidence pertaining to the other psychometric attributes of alternate language versions of these two instruments are much more consistent and, in general, quite positive.

Findings pertaining to alternate language versions of the CARES, the QLQ-C30, and the FACT-G are quite consistent and, in general, provide strong support for their scale structure, reliability, construct validity, and responsiveness. While some of the scales of these questionnaires exhibit lower or less stable reliability estimates than others (e.g., the medical interaction, marital interaction, and sexual functioning scales of the CARES; the cognitive functioning and emesis scales of the QLQ-C30; the social and emotional well-being scales of the FACT-G), this was already known from the original psychometric reports on the parent instruments.

There are notable differences in the geographical regions that have been the focus of methodological research on the five questionnaires. For example, most research on the FLIC has been carried out in the Asian-Pacific Region, on the FACT-G in ethnic minority groups in the USA (specifically, Spanish-speaking populations), and on the RSCL and the QLQ-C30 in Western Europe. This reflects, in large part, the home base of the principal investigators and the network of collaborators associated with these measures. Little attention has been paid to evaluating alternate

language versions of any of these measures for use in Eastern Europe or among the major ethnic minority groups in Western Europe (e.g., Turkish, Moroccan, South Asian, African, and Caribbean immigrants). Well-validated HRQOL instruments for use among these populations are needed for several reasons: (1) following the opening of the political and geographic boundaries in Europe, there has been an influx of Eastern European participants in multinational cancer clinical trials; and (2) the first generation of ethnic minority immigrants are now reaching the age at which steep increases in the incidence of cancer can be expected. In a similar vein, future efforts should be directed toward evaluating the performance of these measures as a function of age (particularly among the elderly) and socioeconomic status.

Overall, the large majority of the empirical evidence supports the psychometric robustness of the alternate language versions of the five questionnaires reviewed. There are few, if any, empirical grounds for preferring or recommending the use of one instrument above the others. Yet, particularly for the two questionnaires that are currently most widely used (and for which the largest amount of psychometric information has been reported) – the QLQ-C30 and the FACT-G – there appear to be fairly distinct "spheres of influence." The large majority of US-based HRQOL studies in oncology have employed the FACT-G, while for Europe and Canada the QLQ-C30 has typically been the instrument of choice.

While perhaps understandable from a sociological perspective (i.e., a preference for "home-grown" products), one can question whether this is a desirable situation in scientific terms. Ultimately, the choice of HRQOL measures to be used in any given study should be based on methodological and/or substantive considerations rather than on geography or politics. Given the few differences in the psychometric characteristics of these questionnaires, content-related issues become paramount. Although the QLQ-C30 and the FACT-G appear to address similar HRQOL domains, they are somewhat different in their focus and in their specific item content. In general, the QLQ-C30 places greater emphasis on physical health issues (e.g., symptoms and functional health problems), while the FACT-G tends to be more psychosocially oriented. This holds true even for scales that, at first glance, appear to address the same HRQOL issues. For example, while the QLQ-C30 social functioning scale addresses the effect of physical health on social role functioning, the FACT-G social well-being scale focuses on issues of social support and emotional closeness. This may, in large part, explain the low correlation observed between these two scales ($r = 0.14$).[46,47] There are also differences between these two measures in the range of topics addressed (e.g., the QLQ-C30 includes items on cognitive functioning, while the FACT-G addresses sexuality and future perspective). Thus, only by examining the specific content and wording of the questionnaires can one decide which is most suitable and appropriate. While this holds true regardless of the language or country in which a study is to be conducted, it may be of even greater importance in the light of cultural norms, traditions, and values.

The relatively high level of psychometric robustness observed for these five questionnaires across languages and cultures should not be taken to suggest that HRQOL is culturally invariable. Clearly, there are differences in the prevalence of self-reported functional health problems and symptoms across countries and cultures. In part, this may be a function of cultural differences in symptom perception and in the tendency to report problems when they are present. While such differences may not affect the assessment of HRQOL in the context of multinational, randomized clinical trials, they can influence significantly the results of epidemiological studies whose aim is to compare the health status and HRQOL of patient populations across geographic and cultural boundaries. In this regard, future efforts should be directed at generating country- and culture-specific normative or reference data (preferably stratified by age, gender, and socioeconomic status) for these questionnaires that can serve as benchmarks against which the results of any specific HRQOL study can be interpreted.

Currently, innovative projects are being conducted that employ statistical techniques based on item response theory to understand better the relationship between, and the relative positioning on a health continuum of items drawn from different HRQOL questionnaires.[69] This is the first step in developing computer-adaptive assessment procedures whereby, rather than having all patients complete the same series of questions (i.e., fixed length questionnaires), the choice and sequencing of questions for any given patient depends on that patient's responses to previously posed questions.[30,31] If these projects prove successful, the next generation of HRQOL measures may minimize, if not entirely transcend, the challenges associated with deciding which questionnaire to use in a given study. However, until such time these newer measurement systems become available, those interested in assessing the HRQOL of patients with cancer, whether they be American, French, or Chinese, will need to choose between currently available questionnaires. Hopefully, this review will aid in making a rational choice by, if nothing else, providing reassurance that the current generation of measures will be relatively robust, regardless of the language or culture in which the research is to be conducted.

REFERENCES

1 Schipper, H., Clinch, J., McMurray, A. *et al.* (1984). Measuring the quality of life of cancer patients: the Functional Living Index-Cancer: development and validation. *Journal of Clinical Oncology* **2**:472–83.

2 Ganz, P. A., Schag, C. A., Lee, J. J. *et al.* (1992). The CARES: a generic measure of health-related quality of life for patients with cancer. *Quality of Life Research* **1**:19–29.

3 Schag, C. A., Ganz, P. A., Heinrich, R. L. (1991). Cancer Rehabilitation Evaluation System–short form (CARES-SF). A cancer specific rehabilitation and quality of life instrument. *Cancer* **68**:1406–13.

4 de Haes, J. C., van Knippenberg, F. C., Neijt, J. P. (1990). Measuring psychological and physical distress in cancer patients: structure and application of the Rotterdam Symptom Checklist. *British Journal of Cancer* **62**:1034–8.

5 Aaronson, N. K., Ahmedzai, S., Bergman, B. *et al.* (1993). The European Organization for Research and Treatment

of Cancer QLQ-C30: a quality-of-life instrument for use in international clinical trials in oncology. *Journal of the National Cancer Institute* **85**:365–76.

6 Cella, D. F., Tulsky, D. S., Gray, G. *et al.* (1993). The Functional Assessment of Cancer Therapy scale: development and validation of the general measure. *Journal of Clinical Oncology* **11**:570–9.

7 Erickson, this volume, Chapter 3.

8 Clinch, J. (1996). The Functional Living Index-Cancer: ten years later. In *Quality of Life and Pharmacoeconomics in Clinical Trials* (2nd Edition), ed. B. Spilker, pp. 215–25. New York: Lippincott-Raven.

9 Goh, C. R., Lee, K. S., Tan, T. C. *et al.* (1996). Measuring quality of life in different cultures: translation of the Functional Living Index for Cancer (FLIC) into Chinese and Malay in Singapore. *Annals of the Academy of Medicine of Singapore* **25**:323–34.

10 Eguchi, K., Fukutani, M., Kanazawa, M. *et al.* (1992). Feasibility study on quality-of-life questionnaires for patients with advanced lung cancer. *Japanese Journal of Clinical Oncology* **22**:185–93.

11 Forjaz, M. J., Guarnaccia, C. A. (2001). A comparison of Portuguese and American patients with hematological malignancies: a cross-cultural survey of health-related quality of life. *Psycho-Oncology* **10**:251–8.

12 King, M. T., Dobson, A. J., Harnett, P. R. (1996). A comparison of two quality-of-life questionnaires for cancer clinical trials: the functional living index–cancer (FLIC) and the quality of life questionnaire core module (QLQ-C30). *Journal of Clinical Epidemiology* **49**:21–9.

13 Mercier, M., Bonneterre, J., Schraub, S. *et al.* (1998). The development of a French version of a questionnaire on the quality of life in cancerology (Functional Living Index-Cancer: FLIC). *Bulletin du Cancer* **85**:180–6.

14 Canales, S., Ganz, P. A., Coscarelli, C. A. (1995). Translation and validation of a quality of life instrument for Hispanic American cancer patients: methodological considerations. *Quality of Life Research* **4**:3–11.

15 te Velde, A., Sprangers, M. A., Aaronson, N. K. (1996). Feasibility, psychometric performance, and stability across modes of administration of the CARES-SF. *Annals of Oncology* **7**:381–90.

16 Rustoen, T., Moum, T., Wiklund, I. *et al.* (1999). Quality of life in newly diagnosed cancer patients. *Journal of Advanced Nursing* **29**:490–8.

17 de Haes, J. C., Olschewski, M. (1998). Quality of life assessment in a cross-cultural context: use of the Rotterdam Symptom Checklist in a multinational randomised trial comparing CMF and Zoladex (Goserlin) treatment in early breast cancer. *Annals of Oncology* **9**:745–50.

18 Kramer, J. A., Curran, D., Piccart, M. *et al.* (2000). Randomised trial of paclitaxel versus doxorubicin as first-line chemotherapy for advanced breast cancer: quality of life evaluation using the EORTC QLQ-C30 and the Rotterdam symptom checklist. *European Journal of Cancer* **36**:1488–97.

19 Agra, Y., Badia, X. (1998). Spanish version of the Rotterdam Symptom Check List: cross-cultural adaptation and preliminary validity in a sample of terminal cancer patients. *Psycho-Oncology* **7**:229–39.

20 Ravaioli, A., Buda, P., Fava, C. *et al.* (1996). Assessment of the RSCL quality of life instrument during chemotherapy in an Italian setting. *Quality of Life Research* **5**:491–5.

21 Paci, E. (1992). Assessment of validity and clinical application of an Italian version of the Rotterdam Symptom Checklist. *Quality of Life Research* **1**:129–34.

22 Fallowfield, L. J. (1995). Assessment of quality of life in breast cancer. *Acta Oncologica* **34**:689–94.

23 Ganz, P. A., Desmond, K. A., Leedham, B. *et al.* (2002). Quality of life in long-term, disease-free survivors of breast cancer; a follow-up study. *Journal of the National Cancer Institute* **94**:39–49.

24 Ganz, P. A., Schag, A. C., Lee, J. J. *et al.* (1992). Breast conservation versus mastectomy. Is there a difference in psychological adjustment or quality of life in the year after surgery? *Cancer* **69**:1729–38.

25 Kiebert, G. M., de Haes, J. C., van de Velde, C. J. (1991). The impact of breast-conserving treatment and mastectomy on the quality of life of early-stage breast cancer patients: a review. *Journal of Clinical Oncology* **9**:1059–70.

26 Cull, A., Sprangers, M., Bjordal, K. *et al.* (2002). *EORTC Quality of Life Group Translation Procedures.* Brussels: European Organization for Research and Treatment of Cancer.

27 Zhao, H., Kanda, K. (2000). Translation and validation of the standard Chinese version of the EORTC QLQ-C30. *Quality of Life Research* **9**:129–37.

28 Kobayashi, K., Takeda, F., Teramukai, S. *et al.* (1998). A cross-validation of the European Organization for Research and Treatment of Cancer QLQ-C30 (EORTC QLQ-C30) for Japanese with lung cancer. *European Journal of Cancer* **34**:810–5.

29 Petersen, M. A., Groenvold, M., Bjorner, J. *et al.* (2003). Use of differential item functioning analysis to assess the equivalence of translations of a questionnaire. *Quality of Life Research* **12**(4):373–85.

30 Reise, this volume, Chapter 21.

31 Hambleton, this volume, Chapter 22.

32 Apolone, G., Filiberti, A., Cifani, S. *et al.* (1998). Evaluation of the EORTC QLQ-C30 questionnaire: a comparison with SF-36 Health Survey in a cohort of Italian long-survival cancer patients. *Annals of Oncology* **9**:549–57.

33 Arraras, J. I., Arias, F., Tejedor, M. *et al.* (2002). The EORTC QLQ-C30 (version 3.0) quality of life questionnaire: validation study for Spain with head and neck cancer patients. *Psycho-Oncology* **11**:249–56.

34 Kaasa, S., Bjordal, K., Aaronson, N. *et al.* (1995). The EORTC core quality of life questionnaire (QLQ-C30): validity and reliability when analysed with patients treated with palliative radiotherapy. *European Journal of Cancer* **31A**:2260–3.

35 Osoba, D., Zee, B., Pater, J. *et al.* (1994). Psychometric properties and responsiveness of the EORTC Quality of Life Questionnaire (QLQ-C30) in patients with breast, ovarian and lung cancer. *Quality of Life Research* **3**:353–64.

36 Ringdal, G. I., Ringdal, K. (1993). Testing the EORTC Quality of Life Questionnaire on cancer patients with heterogeneous diagnoses. *Quality of Life Research* **2**:129–40.

37 Ringdal, K., Ringdal, G. I., Kaasa, S. *et al.* (1999). Assessing the consistency of psychometric properties of the HRQoL scales within the EORTC QLQ-C30 across populations by means of the Mokken Scaling Model. *Quality of Life Research* **8**:25–43.

38 McLachlan, S. A., Devins, G. M., Goodwin, P. J. (1999). Factor analysis of the psychosocial items of the EORTC QLQ-C30 in metastatic breast cancer patients participating in a psychosocial intervention study. *Quality of Life Research* **8**: 311–17.

39 Ford, E. M., Havstad, S. L., Kart, C. S. (2002). Assessing the reliability of the EORTC QLQ-C30 in a sample of older African American and Caucasian adults. *Quality of Life Research* **10**:533–41.

40 Hjermstad, M. J., Fayers, P. M., Bjordal, K. *et al.* (1998). Health-related quality of life in the general Norwegian population assessed by the European Organization for Research and Treatment of Cancer Core Quality-of-Life Questionnaire: the QLQ = C30 (+3). *Journal of Clinical Oncology* **16**:1188–96.

41 Schwarz, R., Hinz, A. (2001). Reference data for the quality of life questionnaire EORTC QLQ-C30 in the general German population. *European Journal of Cancer* **37**:1345–51.

42 Gotay, C. C., Holup, J. L., Pagano, I. (2002). Ethnic differences in quality of life among early breast and prostate cancer survivors. *Psycho-Oncology* **11**:103–13.

43 Osoba, D., Aaronson, N., Zee, B. *et al.* (1997). Modification of the EORTC QLQ-C30 (version 2.0) based on content validity and reliability testing in large samples of patients with cancer. The Study Group on Quality of Life of the EORTC and the Symptom Control and Quality of Life Committees of the NCI of Canada Clinical Trials Group. *Quality of Life Research* **6**:103–8.

44 Montazeri, A., Harirchi, I., Vahdani, M. *et al.* (1999). The European Organization for Research and Treatment of Cancer Quality of Life Questionnaire (EORTC QLQ-C30): translation and validation study of the Iranian version. *Supportive Care in Cancer* **7**:400–6.

45 Hjermstad, M. J., Fossa, S. D., Bjordal, K. *et al.* (1995). Test/retest study of the European Organization for Research and Treatment of Cancer Core Quality-of-Life Questionnaire. *Journal of Clinical Oncology* **13**:1249–54.

46 Kemmler, G., Holzner, B., Kopp, M. *et al.* (1999). Comparison of two quality-of-life instruments for cancer patients: the functional assessment of cancer therapy-general and the European Organization for Research and Treatment of Cancer Quality of Life Questionnaire-C30. *Journal of Clinical Oncology* **17**:2932–40.

47 Kopp, M., Schweigkofler, H., Holzner, B. *et al.* (2000). EORTC QLQ-C30 and FACT-BMT for the measurement of quality of life in bone marrow transplant recipients: a comparison. *European Journal of Haematology* **65**:97–103.

48 Groenvold, M., Klee, M. C., Sprangers, M. A. *et al.* (1997). Validation of the EORTC QLQ-C30 quality of life questionnaire through combined qualitative and quantitative assessment of patient-observer agreement. *Journal of Clinical Epidemiology* **50**:441–50.

49 Klee, M., Groenvold, M., Machin, D. (1997). Quality of life of Danish women: population-based norms of the EORTC QLQ-C30. *Quality of Life Research* **6**:27–34.

50 Michelson, H., Bolund, C., Nilsson, B. *et al.* (2000). Health-related quality of life measured by the EORTC QLQ-C30–reference values from a large sample of Swedish population. *Acta Oncologica* **39**:477–84.

51 Fayers, P., Weeden, S., Curran, D. (1998). *EORTC QLQ-C30 Reference Values*. Brussels: European Organization for Research and Treatment of Cancer.

52 Bonomi, A. E., Cella, D. F., Hahn, E. A. *et al.* (1996). Multilingual translation of the Functional Assessment of Cancer Therapy (FACT) quality of life measurement system. *Quality of Life Research* **5**:309–20.

53 Lent, L., Hahn, E., Eremenco, S. *et al.* (1999). Using cross-cultural input to adapt the Functional Assessment of Chronic Illness Therapy (FACIT) scales. *Acta Oncologica* **38**:695–702.

54 Cella, D., Hernandez, L., Bonomi, A. E. *et al.* (1998). Spanish language translation and initial validation of the functional assessment of cancer therapy quality-of-life instrument. *Medical Care* **36**:1407–18.

55 Cella, D. F., McCain, N. L., Peterman, A. H. *et al.* (1996). Development and validation of the Functional Assessment of Human Immunodeficiency Virus Infection (FAHI) quality of life instrument. *Quality of Life Research* **5**:450–63.

56 Ward, W. L., Hahn, E. A., Mo, F. *et al.* (1999). Reliability and validity of the Functional Assessment of Cancer Therapy-Colorectal (FACT-C) quality of life instrument. *Quality of Life Research* **8**:181–95.

57 Wan, G. J., Counte, M. A., Cella, D. F. *et al.* (1999). The impact of socio-cultural and clinical factors on health-related quality of life reports among Hispanic and African-American cancer patients. *Journal of Outcome Measurement* **3**:200–15.

58 Dapueto, J. J., Francolino, C., Gotta, I. *et al.* (2001). Evaluation of the Functional Assessment of Cancer Therapy-General Questionnaire (FACT-G) in a South American Spanish speaking population. *Psycho-Oncology* **10**:88–92.

59 Yu, C. L., Fielding, R., Chan, C. L. *et al.* (2000). Measuring quality of life of Chinese cancer patients: a validation of the Chinese version of the Functional Assessment of Cancer Therapy-General (FACT-G) scale. *Cancer* **88**:1715–27.

60 Mullin, V., Cella, D., Chang, C. H. *et al.* (2000). Development of three African language translations of the FACT-G. *Quality of Life Research* **9**:139–49.

61 Pandey, M., Thomas, B. C., Ramdas, K. *et al.* (2002). Quality of life in breast cancer patients: validation of a FACT-B Malayalam version. *Quality of Life Research* **11**:87–90.

62 Fallowfield, L. J., Leaity, S. K., Howell, A. *et al.* (1999). Assessment of quality of life in women undergoing hormonal therapy for breast cancer: validation of an endocrine symptom subscale for the FACT-B. *Breast Cancer Research and Treatment* **55**:189–99.

63 Flaherty, J. A., Gaviria, F. M., Pathak, D. *et al.* (1988). Developing instruments for cross-cultural psychiatric research. *Journal of Nervous and Mental Disease* **176**:257–63.

64 Guillemin, F., Bombardier, C., Beaton, D. (1993). Cross-cultural adaptation of health-related quality of life measures: literature review and proposed guidelines. *Journal of Clinical Epidemiology* **46**:1417–32.

65 Hays, R. D., Anderson, R., Revicki, D. (1993). Psychometric considerations in evaluating health-related quality of life measures. *Quality of Life Research* **2**:441–9.

66 Herdman, M., Fox-Rushby, J., Badia, X. (1998). A model of equivalence in the cultural adaptation of HRQoL instruments: the universalist approach. *Quality of Life Research* **7**:323–35.

67 Hui, C., Triandis, H. C. (1985). Measurement in cross-cultural psychology: a review and comparison of strategies. *Cross Cultural Psychology* **16**:131–52.

68 Stewart, A. L., Napoles-Springer, A. (2000). Health-related quality-of-life assessments in diverse population groups in the United States. *Medical Care* **38**:II102–24.

69 Cella, D., Chang, C. H., Lai, J. S. *et al.* (2002). Advances in quality of life measurements in oncology patients. *Seminars in Oncology* **29**:60–8.

70 Bjordal, K., Kaasa, S., Mastekaasa, A. (1994). Quality of life in patients treated for head and neck cancer: a follow-up study 7 to 11 years after radiotherapy. *International Journal of Radiation Oncology, Biology, and Physics* **28**:847–56.

71 Bjordal, K., de Graeff, A., Fayers, P. M. *et al.* (2000). A 12 country field study of the EORTC QLQ-C30 (version 3.0) and the head and neck cancer specific module (EORTC QLQ-H&N35) in head and neck patients. EORTC Quality of Life Group. *European Journal of Cancer* **36**:1796–807.

72 McLachlan, S. A., Devins, G. M., Goodwin, P. J. (1998). Validation of the European Organization for Research and Treatment of Cancer Quality of Life Questionnaire (QLQ-C30) as a measure of psychosocial function in breast cancer patients. *European Journal of Cancer* **34**:510–17.

21

Item response theory and its applications for cancer outcomes measurement

Steven P. Reise, Ph.D.

University of California at Los Angeles, Los Angeles, CA

Introduction

Each year new health-related quality of life (HRQOL) questionnaires are developed or revised from previous measures in the hope of obtaining instruments that are more reliable, valid within the study population, and sensitive to a patient's change in health status. Also, it is important that the measures provide interpretable scores that accurately characterize a patient's HRQOL. While several quality instruments have emerged in cancer outcomes research, we presently lack the ability to crosswalk scores from one instrument to another so that researchers are able to combine or compare results from multiple studies when different instruments are used. Developing these psychometrically strong measures requires analytical methods that will allow researchers to choose the best set of informative questions to match study objectives and to crosswalk scores from one assessment to another, despite use of different sets of questions.

There has been growing interest in learning how applications of item response theory (IRT) modeling can be used to respond to these analytical needs of the cancer outcomes measurement field. This interest is generated by the ability of IRT models to analyze item and scale performance within a study population; to detect biased items that may occur when translating an instrument from one language to another, or when respondents from two different groups hold culturally different meanings for the item content; to link two or more instruments on a common metric and thus facilitate crosswalking of scores; and to create item banks that serve as a foundation for computerized adaptive assessment.[1,2]

In the past, HRQOL instruments were developed under the principles of classical test theory (CTT), which required long questionnaires to meet the minimal criteria for reliability. Often this practice resulted in surveys that included redundant questions that differed only in phrasing. For example, the SF-36[3] Vitality subscale asks respondents, "How much of the time during the past 4 weeks . . . (1) Did you feel full of pep; (2) Did you have a lot of energy; (3) Did you feel worn out; and (4) Did you feel tired?" Not surprisingly, internal consistency measures (coefficient alpha) will find these four highly correlated items to have very high reliability. While long questionnaires may work well in educational testing, the cancer population cannot tolerate this burden. A better alternative would be to select the minimal set of reliable and valid questions that target the study population. However, this approach may pose another obstacle. If different instruments are created that are tailored to a specific population, then we lack the ability to compare patient scores across survey forms. For example, a physical functioning scale may look very different if created for a young population than for an elderly population. Because CTT statistics, such as item-total score correlation or the proportion of items endorsed, are dependent on the sample of respondents in which they are calculated, crosswalking scores from one instrument to another is impossible unless both instruments were created with the same number of questions that share similar statistical properties.

IRT makes full use of the information provided by individuals' responses to each question in a scale, and simultaneously estimates both the properties of the items and persons to develop a probabilistic model that places individuals' scores and item properties on the same metric. This is different from the CTT approach, which typically uses the sum score to determine a person's score without taking into account the relative difficulty of the set of items they endorsed.

IRT models characterize each question in a scale with a set of properties that describe an item's relationship with a measured construct, such as depression or fatigue, as well as how the item functions within the study population. If the IRT model assumptions are met, item properties are invariant with respect to the sample of respondents, and respondent scores are invariant with respect to the set of questions used in the scale. After using IRT to assign the item properties (i.e., calibrate the items), researchers can choose the most salient items that target a patient's level of function with the fewest number of questions. This method will result in different groups receiving a different set of items; however, items calibrated by the best fitting IRT model will lead to results that are comparable on a similar metric, e.g., the metric for the construct HRQOL.

Despite this potential, there are a number of obstacles that prevent greater use of IRT methods in cancer outcomes assessment. An advanced knowledge of measurement theory is required to understand the mathematical complexities of the IRT models; to evaluate if the assumptions of the IRT models are met; and to choose the best model within a family of over a hundred IRT models.[4] In addition, the supporting software and literature is not well adapted for the field of health outcomes measurement. Also, real-world research within this field that demonstrates the strengths of IRT modeling over traditional procedures is lacking.

This chapter is the first of a set of chapters discussing the applications of IRT modeling to health outcomes measurement. The focus here is on the principles of IRT modeling, and a number of basic questions will be addressed: (1) what are IRT models;

(2) what assumptions do they make about the data; (3) how are these assumptions evaluated; (4) how are IRT item properties and person scores estimated; (5) how is IRT model-fit assessed; (6) how does IRT differ from CTT; and (7) what advantages do IRT models have over traditional methods. The chapter will attempt to define this methodology in the context of health outcomes measurement, providing examples of how IRT can be used to improve questionnaires for HRQOL assessment. Table 21.1 provides basic definitions for many of the IRT concepts discussed in this text and in the IRT literature. Readers are encouraged to refer to this table whenever a term is unclear.

Hambleton (Chapter 22, this volume)[5] continues this discussion in the next chapter by illustrating how IRT can be used to build instruments based on a study's objective, link instruments that measure similar domains on the same metric, create item banks, and develop computerized adaptive tests. These computer-adaptive tests combine the features of IRT modeling with advances in computer technology to accurately measure a cancer patient's HRQOL with a minimal set of questions. Following Hambleton's chapter, Wilson (Chapter 23, this volume)[6] presents a methodological approach to validate the structure of a scale with results from an IRT analysis, discusses the strengths and limitations for using a single summary score verses reporting sub-domain scores, and illustrates how multidimensional IRT models may be used to improve individual domain scores. Finally, in Invited Chapter B, McHorney and Cook[7] provide a unique perspective of the role of psychometrics in health outcomes measurement, examining further the implications of IRT for item banking and computerized adaptive assessment.

To illustrate this complex methodology, response data from the SF-36 Mental Health subscale will be used to discuss the IRT models. These data are drawn from 6151 participants who responded to the full SF-36,[1,8–10] which contains 36 items designed to assess a patient's health status. Demographic details, response rates, and data collection procedures are provided elsewhere,[11] but they are not relevant to the present didactic discussion. This chapter is not a psychometric report of the SF-36 instrument; rather,

Table 21.1. Commonly used terms seen in IRT literature

Term	Also Known As . . .	Definition
Latent variable (θ, theta)	Trait. Construct. Ability	The unobservable construct being measured by the questionnaire (e.g., depression level, fatigue)
Item threshold (b, β)	Item location. Item difficulty. Item intensity	Locates an item along the θ continuum indicating the level of the underlying variable (e.g., depression) needed to endorse the question (e.g., suicidal thoughts?) with a specified probability typically set at 0.50.
Item discrimination (a, α)	Item slope	Describes the strength of an item's ability to discriminate among people with trait θ levels below and above the item thresholds b. The a parameter may also be interpreted as describing how an item may be related to the trait measured by the scale.
Item response curve (IRC) Category response curves (CRC)	Item characteristic curve. Item trace lines. Item response function	The IRC or CRC models the relationship between a person's probability for endorsing an item category and the level on the construct θ measured by the scale.
Information function – for item (IIF) – for scale (SIF)	Test information. Information curve	An index, typically displayed in a graph, indicating the range of trait level θ over which an item or scale is most useful for distinguishing among individuals. For any item, the IIF or SIF characterizes the precision of measurement for persons at different levels of θ, with higher information denoting better precision (lower standard error).

the five items from the Mental Health (MH) sub-scale serve to facilitate the discussion of IRT modeling. The item content for the MH subscale is shown in Table 21.2 and descriptive statistics are given in Table 21.3. Note that all items are scored on a 6-point graded scale with higher scores representing better mental health. As a measure of internal consistency, the Cronbach's alpha reliability coefficient for the five items is 0.85.

Item response theory basics

IRT measurement models are a class of statistical procedures used to develop measurement scales with desirable psychometric properties. The chief analytic objective of IRT modeling is to calibrate an item response curve (IRC; also referred to in the literature as a category response curve, item characteristic curve, or item trace line) for each item in a scale. An IRC models the (assumed-to-be) non-linear

Table 21.2. Items included in the SF-36 Mental Health (MH) Subscale*

Question (over the past four weeks . . .)[a]	Short Description
Have you been a very nervous person?	nervous person
Have you felt so down in the dumps that nothing could cheer you up?	down in the dumps
Have you felt calm and peaceful? (reverse scored)	calm and peaceful
Have you felt downhearted and blue?	downhearted & blue
Have you been a happy person? (reverse scored)	happy person

* The 36-Item Health Survey was developed at RAND as part of the Medical Outcomes Study. Items reprinted with permission.
[a] Responses to these items are "All of the time," "Most of the time," "A good bit of the time," "Some of the time," "A little of the time," and "None of the time."

relationship between a latent variable (e.g., mental health, fatigue, pain, or other dimension of HRQOL) and the expected item score (i.e., the expected item

Table 21.3. Item and scale descriptives of the MH scale

Item	Mean	S.E.[a]	Variance	Skew	S.E.[a]	Kurtosis	S.E.[a]	Alpha[b]
Nervous person	4.873	0.015	1.362	−1.156	0.031	1.038	0.062	
Down in the dumps	5.350	0.013	0.994	−1.790	0.031	3.197	0.062	
Calm and peaceful	4.013	0.016	1.488	−0.571	0.031	−0.501	0.062	
Downhearted and blue	5.015	0.013	1.043	−1.177	0.031	1.490	0.062	
Happy person	4.437	0.014	1.170	−0.910	0.031	0.406	0.062	
Scale	23.681	0.056	19.054	−1.102	0.031	1.109	0.062	0.8526

[a] Standard error of the previous statistic.

[b] Cronbach's alpha reliability for scale of five items.

response). For the SF-36 MH subscale, the IRC models the association between individuals' responses to an item such as "have you been a happy person" and their mental health status. People with good mental health will be expected to endorse *most of the time* they are happy.

The latent variable in IRT models represents the individual-differences construct the researcher is attempting to assess and is often referred to as the latent "trait" in some literature. Typically, the researcher wants to estimate the individual's most likely position, via a scale score, along this latent trait continuum. The simplest forms of the IRT models are those that model data with two response options per question, such as True or False, Agree or Disagree, or Yes or No. Therefore, we will introduce the basic concepts of IRT models for dichotomous data, and then move to the more commonly occurring case of more than two response categories (polytomous response data) per question.

IRT modeling was originally developed in educational measurement, and it has a rich history (over 75 years) in advancing the theory of modern measurement and the application of these concepts to different fields of measurement. For a good review of the history of IRT modeling, see Bock,[12] Lord,[13] and Wright.[14]

Unidimensional IRT model for dichotomous response data

IRT models for dichotomous response items differ in the number of item parameters needed to describe the relationship between a person's level on the measured construct and his or her response to an item. The most common IRT model applied to dichotomous response data in health outcomes research is the 2-parameter logistic model (2PLM). Most of the models discussed in this chapter build off the 2PLM model, so it will provide a good basis to discuss the differences among IRT models. Equation 21.1 provides the formula for the IRC in the 2PLM.

$$P(X_i = 1|\theta, a_i, b_i) = \frac{1}{1 + e^{-a_i(\theta - b_i)}} \quad (21.1)$$

In Equation 21.1, the person parameter, θ (theta), represents the latent variable or construct (e.g., mental health) the scale is measuring. People vary in their level on this construct from one extreme to another, so estimates of theta will be on a continuous scale. Further, IRT assumes this construct is the only systematic variable that gives rise to a person's response to an item. Any other covariance among item responses not accounted for by this single construct is viewed as random noise. In IRT modeling, it is customary to fix the θ scale to have a mean of zero and a variance of 1.0 in the population. Thus, the metric by which individual differences are represented in IRT (i.e., the θ metric) can be thought of as like a Z-score metric. The item parameters in Equation 21.1 are defined as: 1) b is an item threshold (called item "difficulty" in educational testing), and 2) a is an item discrimination (or slope) parameter. Thus, $P(X_i = 1|\theta, a_i, b_i)$ represents the probability, P, that persons endorse (e.g., say "true" to) an item i conditional on their level on the underlying

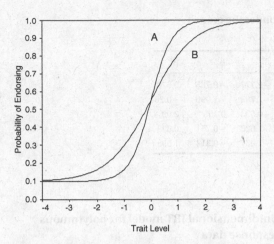

Figure 21.1.   Two item response curves that vary in discrimination.

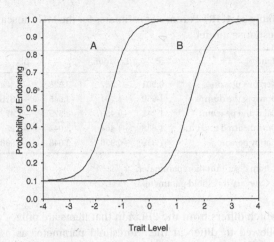

Figure 21.2.   Two item response curves that vary in difficulty.

construct, θ, as well as the difficulty b and the discrimination ability a of the question. This relationship, described in Equation 21.1, is modeled by a logistic function, which approximates an ogive function, but requires less mathematical computational burden.

In the 2PLM, items are allowed to vary on two characteristics. First, items vary in their ability to discriminate among individuals. This is indexed by the a parameter, which typically ranges between 0.5 and 1.5 in value. The larger the a parameter, the steeper the IRC at its inflection point (i.e., the point where the slope changes over from continuously increasing to continuously decreasing). In turn, steeper slopes indicate that the IRC increases relatively rapidly such that small changes on the latent variable (e.g., small changes in mental health status) lead to large changes in item endorsement probabilities. The a parameter also may be interpreted as describing how an item is related to the latent variable measured by the scale, and it can be thought of as a measure of the correlation between the item score and the overall scale score. Figure 21.1 displays the IRCs for two (hypothetical) items that differ in discrimination. The item parameters for item A are: $a = 1.5$ and $b = 0.0$, and the item parameters for item B are: $a = 0.75$ and $b = 0.0$. In Figure 21.1, item A has more discrimination power (thus, more related to the latent variable) than item B.

Second, in the 2PLM, items are allowed to vary in their threshold. The item-threshold parameter (b) is on the same scale as the latent variable (θ), and threshold values typically range from −2.5 to 2.5. In IRT terminology, the item threshold in the 2PLM refers to the level of the latent variable an individual needs in order to endorse the item with 50% probability. If endorsing an item reflects better mental health, then items like "I am happy throughout the day" will have high threshold values (large positive b values) as only people with good mental health, θ, will endorse true to this question. Questions like "I have suicidal thoughts" will have a low threshold value (large negative b value) because many people will respond false to this question. Figure 21.2 displays the IRCs for two items that differ in threshold (but not in discrimination ability). The parameters for item A are: $a = 1.5$ and $b = −1.5$, and the parameters for item B are: $a = 1.5$, and $b = 1.5$. The item threshold can also be thought of as a measure of difficulty (in educational research) or intensity,[7] in that for any given probability of endorsing, it takes a higher level of the latent construct to endorse item B than item A. Similarly, at any level of the latent construct, the probability of endorsing A is at least as great as endorsing B.

Another commonly used IRT model for dichotomous response data in health outcomes measurement is the 1-parameter logistic model (1PLM),

Table 21.4. IRT Parameter estimates for the MH subscale under the graded response model

Item	α^a	Location	β_1^b	β_2^b	β_3^b	β_4^b	β_5^b
Nervous person	0.901	−1.587	−3.528	−2.424	−1.777	−0.785	0.578
Down in the dumps	1.959	−1.701	−3.045	−2.316	−1.783	−1.096	−0.264
Calm and peaceful	1.241	−0.459	−2.529	−1.477	−0.533	0.155	2.09
Downhearted and blue	1.838	−1.461	−3.043	−2.257	−1.628	−0.751	0.373
Happy person	1.329	−0.958	−3.048	−1.988	−1.037	−0.314	1.598

[a] Item discrimination parameter.
[b] Category threshold parameter.

which differs from the 2PLM in that items are only allowed to differ in their threshold parameter as shown in Equation 21.2:

$$P(X_i = 1|\theta, a, b_i) = \frac{1}{1 + e^{-a(\theta - b_i)}}, \qquad (21.2)$$

where the discrimination parameter a for the 1PLM is constrained to be equal to one across all items and thus drops out of the model.

This simplest form of the IRT model is also called the Rasch[15] model, which carries with it several unique properties comprising what has been termed *specific objectivity*. This means that comparison of any two items' threshold parameters are assumed to be independent of the group of subjects being surveyed, and the comparison of any two subjects' trait levels (i.e., scores) does not depend on any subset of items being administered.[16] Because only one overall discrimination parameter (and not one for each item) is being estimated, Rasch models will require smaller sample sizes than 2PLMs to achieve any given level of precision in the estimates of person and item properties. However, these ideal properties hold only when the data adequately fit the model, and critics argue that the constraint that all items are equally related to the underlying variable in health outcomes measures is rarely observed. Nevertheless, there is a whole Rasch family of models for both dichotomous and polytomous response data that are built on this principle, and those researchers who believe specific objectivity is essential for valid measurement are dedicated to using only such Rasch models.

Unidimensional IRT model for polytomous response data

Most questionnaires used in health outcomes research contain items that are responded to on a multi-point scale (e.g., on a 5-point graded scale ranging from very dissatisfied to very satisfied). One popular IRT model appropriate for such an ordered Likert-type response format is the graded response model (GRM).[17] Note that there are many alternative polytomous IRT models in the literature, including the partial credit[18,19] and the rating scale model,[20] which belong to the Rasch family of models.

The GRM model is a simple generalization of the 2PLM (Equation 21.1). In the GRM, each item is described by one discrimination parameter a and threshold parameters (or category difficulties) equal in number to one minus the number of response categories ($m = k − 1$). For example, an item with six response categories will have five threshold parameters located along the latent variable θ continuum describing where each of the six response categories map on the latent construct. The a parameter in the GRM model reflects an item's discrimination, with higher values indicating better items, that is, items that provide better differentiation among respondents who are high or low on the latent variable.

To illustrate application and interpretation of the GRM, item parameters for the SF-36 MH subscale were estimated using the software program PARSCALE™.[21] The resulting item parameter estimates are shown in Table 21.4. All item

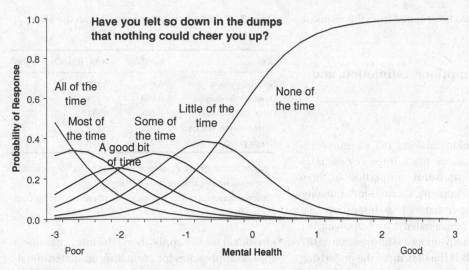

Figure 21.3. IRT GRM category response curves for the polytomous response question, "Have you felt so down in the dumps that nothing could cheer you up?".

discrimination parameter estimates are fairly large, indicating that all items provide reasonably good differentiation among individuals and that all items are highly related to the latent variable, mental health. The item *nervous person* has the lowest discrimination parameter ($a = .90$), indicating it is less related to the mental health dimension than the other four items. Likewise, the item *down in the dumps* has the highest discrimination value ($a = 1.96$), indicating it is a very good measure of mental health.

With Likert-type response items, it is important to explore the spread of the threshold parameters within an item. In the MH subscale, it appears that most of the threshold parameters are negative. This reflects the relative "easiness" of the response categories. In other words, most people in our sample responded in the higher categories (indicating positive mental health). Furthermore, there are several items with threshold parameters that are tightly clustered together, which indicates that the item may have too many response options. Threshold parameters that go lower than –3.0 or higher than 3.0 indicate that the response categories are too easy or too difficult. This may be evidence that the item content is too extreme, causing either ceiling or floor response effects. (Note that the Location statistic for

each item in Table 21.4 is simply the algebraic mean of the estimated threshold parameters, providing a summary indicator of the item's positioning along the construct.)

To illustrate the GRM, Figure 21.3 shows the category response curves (CRCs) for the *down in the dumps* question. CRCs are nothing more than the polytomous extension of the IRC described previously for dichotomous IRT models. CRCs graph the probability of responding in a specific category (from *all of the time* to *none of the time*) conditional on the latent variable, mental health. This item is particularly interesting because all the threshold parameters are negative, indicating that only people with very poor mental health (i.e., very depressed) are likely to endorse *most of the time* or *all of the time* they are so "down in the dumps that nothing could cheer them up." Most respondents across the mental health continuum, starting about one standard deviation below the population mean (set at 0), are likely to say *little of the time* or *none of the time* they could not be cheered up. Also, the GRM shows that the response category *a good bit of the time* is rarely endorsed, and that it would be better to have five category responses for the question. Examination of the GRM for the other four items in the MH scale also indicates that *a good bit of the time* should be dropped from the response options.

IRT model assumptions, estimation, and evaluation of fit

Assumptions

The parametric, unidimensional IRT measurement models described above make three key assumptions about the statistical properties of item responses: (1) monotonicity, (2) unidimensionality, and (3) local independence. It is important that these assumptions be evaluated *prior* to applying IRT models because the advantages of implementing IRT can be realized only if the data meet the underlying assumptions. It should be noted, however, that IRT models are fairly robust to minor violations (e.g., of the unidimensionality assumption) and that no real data ever meet the assumptions perfectly.[22-24]

In general terms, the *monotonicity* assumption means that as levels of the latent variable increase (e.g., mental health increases from poor to good), individuals have a higher probability of endorsing item response categories indicating better mental health. This assumption is logical; it would be impossible to use the models described above – which define monotonically increasing IRCs – if the response propensities do not increase systematically with increases on the latent variable. For dichotomous or polytomous items, respectively, the most direct way to evaluate the monotonicity assumption is through inspection of graphs of summed scale scores versus item endorsement rates or versus item means.

The second assumption is *unidimensionality*. A scale is considered unidimensional when the common variance among the items can be accounted for by a single latent variable. In other words, no other variable, except the respondents' level on mental health, accounts for the variation in responses to the five items on the MH subscale. Although numerous indices for assessing dimensionality have been proposed,[25] there is no single gold-standard test for deciding whether a data set is sufficiently unidi-

Table 21.5. Dimensionality statistics on the MH subscale

Item	Loading[a]	Item/Total Correlation[b]
Nervous person	0.650	0.729
Down in the dumps	0.869	0.819
Calm and peaceful	0.766	0.811
Downhearted and blue	0.852	0.828
Happy person	0.765	0.798

[a] Factor loading after extracting one factor from a polychoric correlation matrix among these five items.
[b] Pearson correlation between each individual item and the composite total.

mensional for IRT application. The most commonly applied approaches for evaluating unidimensionality are: (1) conduct a factor analysis of polychoric or tetrachoric correlations,[26] or (2) conduct a full-information item factor analysis.[27] In either case, what the researcher is looking for is: (1) a large ratio of the 1st to 2nd eigenvalues (e.g., 3 to 1), which in turn indicates a strong common dimension running through the items; (2) all items load highly on (i.e., correlate highly with) a single common factor (e.g., loading greater than 0.40); and (3) residuals after extracting one factor are small, indicating that the first dimension accounts for a high percentage of item covariance. By implication, the above analyses are an evaluation of between-item (common) variance and not an indicator that all the reliable variance within each item is due to only one systematic factor.

The dimensionality of the MH subscale was investigated by conducting an exploratory factor analysis on a smoothed matrix of polychoric correlations using MicroFACT.[28] The results of these analysis are shown in Table 21.5. Factor loadings were all very high, ranging from 0.65 to 0.87, indicating that all items belong on this scale. Moreover, additional calculations (not shown) indicate that the ratio of the first to second eigenvalue was 5.9, the goodness-of-fit index (GFI) was 0.996, and all residuals were very small (i.e., mean residual = 0.001, SD = 0.054). Combined, these results indicate that the MH subscale is appropriate for IRT modeling. It is interesting to note from Table 21.5 that the item *nervous person* has the lowest factor loading and lowest item-total score correlation, which is consistent with GRM finding that the item has the lowest discrimination ability of the five-item set.

The third assumption is *local independence*, which means that once one common factor has been extracted from an item covariance matrix, the residuals are zero. In other words, local independence means that, after accounting for the latent variable, item responses are independent (of one another). Unidimensionality and local independence might appear to be the same concept, but they are not.[29] A highly unidimensional test can still display violations of local independence (called local dependence). Violations of local independence occur when item responses are linked for reasons beyond a common latent variable. For example, when two items have highly similar item content, responses can be influenced by a specific factor having little to do with the common latent variable. Local dependence must be guarded against because its occurrence will lead to a false impression of a scale's psychometric properties. Specifically, local dependence causes a measure to look better than it really is (e.g., spuriously high internal consistency reliability).

Extended discussion of local independence is beyond the present scope. However, several researchers have described procedures for detecting violations of local independence for dichotomous items.[30,31] Rather than perform statistical tests of local independence, IRT researchers often attempt to limit its occurrence by writing items whose responses depend only on individuals' positions on the latent variable and not on their responses to previous items.

Estimating IRT model item and person parameters

In most IRT applications, both item parameters and person (trait) parameters are unknown and must be estimated, using a maximum-likelihood (ML) method, from the same data. Estimating item parameters with unknown trait θ levels is analogous to performing a logistic regression with unknown predictor values. Joint maximum likelihood, marginal maximum likelihood, and conditional maximum likelihood are three popular methods for estimation with unknown trait levels; in the estimation of IRT model parameters, these three ML approaches differ only in how the probability of the observed response patterns is conceptualized. If item responses are locally independent, we can write out the likelihood of any item response pattern (X) as Equation 21.3.

$$L(X \mid \theta) = \Pi_{j=1}^{J}(P_j|\theta)^{x_j}(1 - P_j \mid \theta)^{(1-x_j)} \tag{21.3}$$

This fundamental equation states that the likelihood of any response pattern (X) can be defined as the serial product of the individual item response probabilities (assume $x_j = 1$ indicates an item endorsement and $x_j = 0$ indicates a non-endorsement for dichotomous response data). Finding the maximum of this equation plays a central role in using a respondent's item response pattern to estimate his or her location on the latent variable. For a fuller discussion of the methods for item and person parameter estimation, see Embretson and Reise[32] or Baker.[33]

In HRQOL assessment, deriving the individual's estimated position along the latent trait (the person score) is clearly of central interest, and IRT and CTT approach this in quite different ways. In CTT, individual item scores are often summed together to form a person's raw or transformed score. This procedure assumes that equal ratings on each scale item (e.g., a *some of the time* response) represent equal levels of the underlying construct. IRT, on the other hand, estimates an individual's score on a latent construct based on *all* the information in the person's response pattern. That is, IRT takes into consideration each response to an item, and utilizes the difficulty and discrimination parameters of the category response curve associated with that response to determine a person's score. As indicated above, to estimate a person's level on a latent variable (the score), one finds the maximum of a likelihood function created from the product of the IRCs associated with a person's item response pattern. Specifically, the estimated trait level for a person maximizes the likelihood function (as in Equation 21.3) of his or her response pattern, given the item properties. Thus, to find the appropriate trait level estimate, one must a) represent the likelihood of a response pattern under various trait levels and b) conduct a search process that yields the trait level that gives the highest likelihood.[32]

While scoring a respondent in IRT is more complex, it has a major advantage over CTT. In CTT, the summed scale score is dependent on the difficulty of the items used in the selected scale and, therefore, is not an accurate measure of a person's level on a latent variable. In IRT, respondent scores are invariant to the set of items given to them. Thus, individuals who endorse 4 out of 10 items will have the same summed raw score but may have different IRT estimated scores if they have different response patterns. For example, one person may answer more of the highly discriminating and difficult items and receive a higher latent score than one who answered the same number of items with low discrimination or difficulty. The advantages of IRT scores over CTT scores are highlighted later in this chapter.

Evaluating IRT model-fit

After testing model assumptions and estimating a model, the fit of the estimated item parameters has to be considered. IRT differs in a number of ways from other data modeling methods, such as structural equation modeling, in how it evaluates model-fit. In IRT, there is no standard set of fit indices recognized as useful across a wide variety of research settings. Second, IRT researchers are generally not concerned about global fit, but rather are concerned with the fit of a model on an item-by-item, or person-by-person, basis. Third, the goal of IRT modeling is to estimate a set of item and person parameters that reproduce observed item responses. Thus, IRT models are considered to have a good fit to the data to the degree that they can be used to predict item responses.

There are both graphical[34] and empirical[35] approaches for evaluating item-fit. In graphical approaches, a researcher attempts to compare an estimated IRC (or CRC) with the actual observed

item responses. Discrepancies between the IRC and the observed data (i.e., large residuals) indicate poor item-fit. However, interpreting fit plots is inevitably a subjective process. Partly for this reason, numerous statistical approaches for evaluating item-fit have emerged.[36–38] The majority of these statistics are based on evaluation of the residuals between an IRC and the observed data. The most commonly used software packages such as PARSCLALE[TM,21] and BILOG[TM,39] provide a chi-square item-fit index. IRT item-fit assessment is an evolving topic and much research is needed, especially in identifying the practical consequences of misfit.

Although most IRT fit research is concerned with item-fit, some researchers have focused on the complementary topic of person-fit.[40–42] Person-fit statistics evaluate the degree of consistency between individuals' estimated trait levels and their observed item response pattern. For example, if an individual responds she cannot walk 10 steps on one item (an easy item), but then on another item responds she can run a mile (a difficult item), that is an inconsistency. This is not the forum to review the computational details of the many statistical indices to detect either item-fit or person-fit. Nevertheless, it is important to note person-fit assessment in this context because it nicely illustrates an advantage of IRT over CTT. Specifically, IRT is a formal measurement model of item response behavior that simultaneously considers item and person characteristics. Thus, IRT modeling allows for the development of statistical tests of the consistency of an individual's data with the proposed measurement model. CTT does not provide an easy mechanism for studying or evaluating person-fit. Such IRT-generated indices may be of particular value to HRQOL researchers in identifying bogus or invalid response protocols.

Key IRT model features and comparison to CTT approach

Traditional psychometric procedures based on CTT are relatively simple to implement and have served measurement researchers well for many years. IRT modeling, on the other hand, is technically complex, makes strong assumptions, requires special software to estimate models, and is not generally well understood among social science and medical researchers. Given these impediments, it is fair to ask why health outcomes researchers should consider applying IRT models to evaluate and revise their instruments. To address this question, the following section reviews two key properties of IRT models: invariance and information. Then, four IRT applications for health outcomes research are briefly described and, in each case, the advantages of IRT modeling over traditional procedures are discussed.[43]

Property of item and person parameter invariance

Many psychometricians have proposed that the property of *invariance* is the most critical advantage of IRT modeling over CTT psychometrics. If all assumptions are met and the data fit an IRT model, then IRT models contain the properties of person and item parameter invariance. Item parameter invariance means that the psychometric properties of items (item discrimination and difficulty) do not change as a function of the sample. Person invariance means that an individual's standing on the latent variable continuum does not depend on what particular items they respond to. IRT models have the invariance property because they simultaneously include both item and person characteristics into the measurement model (i.e., the IRC or CRC). Before elaborating more on these properties, we first consider invariance (or the lack thereof) in CTT.

In CTT, item and person indices are sample dependent. Item difficulty is defined as the mean item response (or proportion correct); easy items have high mean scores and difficult items have low mean scores. However, an item's difficulty depends on the mean ability or trait level of the respondent sample. An IQ test administered to an intelligent sample will look easy, but will look challenging if given to a not-so-intelligent sample. In turn, item discrimination is defined by an item score-scale score correlation; highly discriminating items have high

item-scale correlations and poorly discriminating items have low correlations with the total scale score. However, an item-scale correlation is highly dependent on the variability of the sample. In particular, item-scale correlations are lower the more homogeneous the sample since there is less variability in the construct for any item, even a very discriminating one, to capture.

In CTT, comparison of respondents who took different mental health measures rests on the assumption that people have been administered "parallel forms" of the scales (i.e., instruments whose item sets are of very similar difficulty and discrimination ability). Moreover, comparison of individuals on a construct depends on the particular scale form being administered. Obviously, if one person receives items from the SF-36 MH subscale and a second person receives another researcher's favorite "mental health" scale, the resulting raw scores are not comparable, even though the items may all measure the same construct. In CTT, individuals' raw scale scores (e.g., sum of item raw scores) are an estimate of their "true" scores – but, in turn, true scores are scale dependent. Relatedly, in CTT an individual's raw scale score depends on the difficulty of the items administered. A person may score high if given a set of easy items, and low if given a set of difficult items.

For non-psychometricians, the concept of invariance in IRT is often very confusing. One reason is that IRT item and person parameters are both, in one specific sense, sample dependent much like CTT. However, although the values of the estimated item parameters may change when estimated for different samples, IRT item and person parameters are invariant under a linear transformation. That is, assuming model-fit, item and person parameters can always be transformed to be on a common scale and can be compared across samples of persons and items, respectively. This requires some explanation.

IRT parameters are sample dependent in the following sense. In order to estimate item parameters, a calibration sample is needed. Further, the scale of the item parameters is undefined until the scale of the latent variable is defined. It is customary to solve the identification problem by standardizing scores in the calibration sample to have a mean of 0 and a variance set to 1.0. Because of this metric-fixing standardization, values of the estimated item parameters are influenced by the characteristics (level and dispersion) of the calibration sample in much the same way they are in CTT. So, particular IRT item parameter values may change depending on the qualities of the calibration sample. In turn, by the same logic, the value of a person's score in IRT (i.e., his or her estimated position on the latent variable) also depends on characteristics of the original calibration sample.

Despite this calibration sample dependence, IRT item and person parameters are still considered invariant – specifically, they are invariant over a linear transformation. (This means that if X is an IRT item or person parameter and m and n are real numbers with m non-zero, then X' = mX + n is an equally valid expression of the parameter.) This may not sound like much of a difference, but the implications are rather dramatic. Specifically, item parameters calibrated on the basis of different samples are linearly transformable to be on the same scale and are comparable (assuming model-fit, of course). That is, two researchers can administer the MH scale to distinctively different samples, estimate IRT parameters, and then directly compare the results. Moreover, individuals can be administered completely different MH measures, or sets of items within a scale, and their scores can be compared on the same latent trait scale. Using IRT, a researcher may administer one respondent one set of three items on the MH subscale and another respondent a different set of three MH items, and their "scores" would still be perfectly comparable. The subsequent sections elaborate more on the consequences of the item and person parameter invariance property. However, before addressing this further, we discuss a second important IRT feature, the concept of information.

Judging the precision of the estimate: Information and standard error

In CTT, the most common method of judging scale score precision is through a measure of internal consistency such as coefficient alpha,[44] defined as follows:

$$r_{ii'} = \alpha = \frac{K}{K-1}\left(1 - \frac{\sum_{k=1}^{K}\sigma_k^2}{\sigma^2}\right), \tag{21.4}$$

where K refers to the items (k = 1 . . . K), σ_k^2 is the (within-item) variance for item k, and σ^2 is the total variance (both within and between items). It is also standard practice to judge the error surrounding an individual's observed test score by the standard error of measurement (SEM):

$$SEM = \rho\sqrt{1 - r_{ii'}}. \tag{21.5}$$

Clearly, indices of internal consistency reliability are sample dependent because their value depends on the item variances and covariances and on the total test score variance in a particular sample. Consequently, measurement error, which is assumed constant for all individuals regardless of their raw score, also depends on sample characteristics (e.g., mean and variability).

In IRT, the concepts of reliability and standard error of measurement are replaced with the concepts of information and conditional standard errors. In this regard, the concepts of item and scale information functions are critical in IRT modeling. Information functions can be computed for items and scales in both dichotomous and polytomous IRT models. At the item level, the estimated parameters of the IRCs or CRCs can be converted into an item information function (IIF). An IIF indicates an item's ability to discriminate among contiguous scores at various locations along the latent variable continuum. Not surprisingly, information is related to reliability in that items with high information provide greater precision in measuring respondents' levels on the latent variable, for levels located around the item thresholds. Therefore, the information function describes the level of measurement precision across the entire trait continuum.

In dichotomous IRT models, items with large discrimination values provide more information than items with small discrimination values. In turn, item

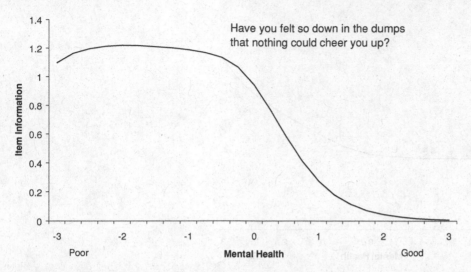

Figure 21.4. Item information function for the question, "Have you felt so down in the dumps that nothing could cheer you up?".

information is maximized around the item's threshold parameter value and then tapers off in ranges away from the item's threshold. This makes logical sense. Consider an item such as "I can easily run a marathon." Such an item would be psychometrically useful (i.e., informative) in differentiating among a group of good athletes. On the other hand, the item is worthless for differentiating among poor athletes because they would all fail to endorse it. So, the maximum of the information curve would appear in the high regions of physical functioning and would taper off in regions measuring respondents low on physical functioning.

In polytomous IRT models, such as the GRM, information functions follow the same basic principles as with dichotomous items. Specifically, information is maximized around the threshold parameters, and items with high discrimination parameters tend to provide more information than items with low discrimination parameters. However, because a multipoint item has several thresholds, information is not peaked around a single value, but rather is more evenly spread out over the entire latent variable range.[45] The IIF for the question *down in the dumps* is presented in Figure 21.4. The IIF is high across low levels of the underlying construct, indicating the item is reliable for measuring respondents with poor

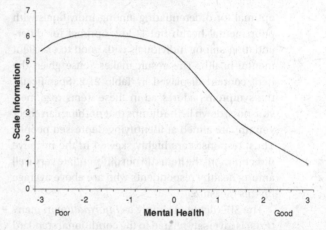

Figure 21.5. Scale information function for the SF-36 Mental Health subscale.

mental health; and the IIF tapers off at the high end of the continuum, indicating the item is not useful for discriminating among people with good mental health.

Because of the property of local independence among item responses, IIFs can be summed across items to form the scale information function (SIF). The SIF in Figure 21.5 shows that the MH subscale provides a lot of information in the low range, but much less in the high range. In short, this scale is

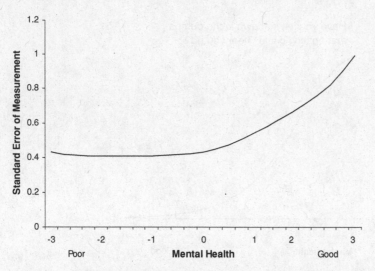

Figure 21.6.   Standard error of measurement function for the SF-36 Mental Health subscale.

optimal for differentiating among individuals with poor mental health but is less optimal for differentiating among individuals with good to excellent mental health. This result makes sense given the item content displayed in Table 21.2. Specifically, the symptoms addressed in these items (e.g., nervousness, down in the dumps that nothing can cheer you up) are aimed at identifying depressed people. Thus, responses are highly skewed in the negative direction, and the items do not differentiate very well among healthy respondents who are above average on this measure.

The SIF (denoted simply as *Information* in many texts) is inversely related to the conditional standard error of measurement (SEM):

$$SEM(\theta) = \frac{1}{\sqrt{Info(\theta)}}. \qquad (21.6)$$

The SEM function for the MH subscale is shown in Figure 21.6, which provides a visual depiction of where along the latent variable MH continuum the item set is most discriminating (informative). In contrast to CTT, where test reliability and standard error are assumed to be constant for all raw scale scores, the SIF (Figure 21.5) shows that the precision of measurement differs along various ranges of the latent variable. In turn, Figure 21.6 shows precisely

how the standard error of measurement changes as a function of differential precision of scores at different ranges of the latent variable.

Four applications of invariance and information

The concepts of invariance and information, two distinguishing characteristics of IRT measurement models, have important applications for all phases of assessment ranging from scale development and item analysis to scale scoring. The following sections describe four major ways in which an IRT approach to psychometrics may differ from a CTT approach. The discussion is necessarily brief, but references are provided where appropriate.

Scale development and analysis

Traditional scale development practice focuses on the creation of a specific fixed-length paper-and-pencil scale that can reliably tap into an individual difference construct. Questions for such a scale may be selected using quantitative methods such as factor analysis, perhaps followed by item analysis looking at item means and item-scale correlations.

A measure of internal consistency, such as coefficient alpha, will likely be calculated as well. Regardless, once the scale is created, it is fixed in stone; in CTT, change the measure and one has changed what is being measured because one has changed the true score distribution. If one or two items from the MH subscale are eliminated, new research results would not be comparable to old results. Moreover, traditional scale construction practice often leads to scales that are most precise for people near the mean on the construct – the group that researchers often care least about.

IRT psychometrics, in particular the concept of information, leads researchers away from the creation of fixed-length measures and toward the creation of item banks.[46] Item banks are sets of scale items, all of which are intended to measure the same construct and have been fit to an IRT model. The psychometric properties of each item, as well as the bank as a whole, are judged by information functions as presented previously. Item banks serve not only as a foundation for computerized adaptive testing (CAT; see Hambleton, Chapter 22, this volume),[5] but also as a basis for constructing fixed-length scales for specific purposes. That is, because IRT recognizes that scale items perform differentially for people with different trait levels, subsets of items can be selected from a bank to tailor scale properties to the particular needs of the measurement situation. For example, from an item bank, a fixed-length mental health scale might be constructed that maximizes measurement precision for people with poor mental health.

Beyond the construction of new measures based on item banks, IRT also has advantages in terms of the psychometric analysis of existing measures. For example, instead of comparing two competing measures in terms of reliability, measures can be compared in terms of their information. It is possible that two equally reliable measures provide different amounts of information in different ranges along the latent variable continuum. Furthermore, in contrast to CTT, under an IRT framework individuals who have taken different scales can be compared with each other.[47] Of course, this assumes that both scales

have been fit with an IRT model and that the metrics have been linked in some way.[2,48]

Computerized adaptive testing

In aptitude testing, computerized adaptive testing is perhaps the most important and the most successful application of IRT to date. In fact, over one million computerized adaptive Scholastic Aptitude Tests have been administered.[49] CAT is not possible under a CTT framework because comparing individuals on the same scale depends on the administration of parallel forms (as defined earlier). In IRT, because of the person invariance property, an individual's standing on a latent trait continuum can be estimated using their responses to any subset of items that have been calibrated under an IRT model.

IRT modeling is the foundation of CAT because IRT psychometrics incorporates both item and person characteristics into the same model. Moreover, IRT models recognize that different items provide different amounts of information in different trait ranges. In turn, this allows individuals to be administered sets of items that are tailored to their specific trait level. The end result is that compared to traditional paper-and-pencil tests, CAT allows respondents to receive 50% fewer items with little loss of measurement precision.[50–53]

Differential item functioning

In any applied measurement context, it is important to understand whether a scale is invariant across different populations. In order for scale scores to be comparable across different groups, the items must measure the same construct in the same way across different groups. In CTT, this principle is reflected in, and is a direct consequence of, the parallel forms assumption – that any two scales have item sets of comparable difficulty and discrimination ability. This fundamental measurement tenet is well recognized among health measurement specialists. For example, the health-related quality of life literature is replete with studies that examine the psychometric properties of scales across clinical versus non-clinical populations, men versus women, and across culturally or ethnically diverse populations.[54,55]

Unfortunately, it is extremely difficult to assess item or scale invariance with CTT methods because CTT item statistics are sample dependent. Consider the following example. An item has a mean of 2.3 and item-scale correlation of 0.55 in a sample of men, and a mean of 3.2 and item-scale correlation of 0.45 in a sample of women. Does this item function differently for men and women or are these observed differences in item statistics due to real and valid gender differences in mean level and variability on the latent trait? Moreover, if this item truly does work differently for men and women, what is the impact of the bias on their scale scores?

These questions are difficult to address using traditional CTT-based procedures, but become much easier with IRT methods because of their invariance property.[56] In IRT terminology, an item is considered invariant when it has the same relationship with a latent variable across two or more groups. This will occur when the item has the same IRC across two or more groups. Differential item functioning (DIF) is said to occur when the IRCs (for the same item) are not equivalent across groups. Because of the invariance property of IRT item parameters, it is relatively easy to compare IRCs computed within different groups (after the item parameters have been linked), even if the groups differ in mean and variance on the trait.

In fact, a popular IRT program called BILOG-MG[TM,57] is specifically designed to facilitate the linking of scales across diverse samples and the identification of DIF. In addition to this program, the IRT literature offers several procedures for detecting DIF and assessing the consequences of DIF for trait score estimation.[58-60] Many empirical examples of DIF detection can be found in the quality-of-life domain[55] as well as in the personality domain.[61,62] A thorough treatment of this important topic is presented in Holland and Wainer.[63]

Optimal scaling/scale score interpretation

In CTT, an individual's absolute standing on a trait continuum is usually indexed by the simple raw score (i.e., the sum of all item scores). As noted, the raw score is an estimate of an individual's (CTT-defined) true score, which in turn is scale dependent. In CTT, individuals can be compared only if they have been administered parallel scales. To make a raw score meaningful, it is usually compared to relevant population norms (e.g., clinical norms, healthy population norms, ethnic group norms). This type of comparison mandates the calculation of a standardized score (Z-score, T-score) that requires that the mean and standard deviation on the scale be known in some population. Thus, an individual's relative standing on a construct is sample (i.e., norm-group) dependent. The same raw scale score can look quite different, in terms of relative standing, depending on what norms it is compared to. For this reason, it is often said that CTT allows for normed-based measurement.

The raw score scale has certain well-known deficiencies in terms of scaling properties.[64,65] For example, one cannot assume that equal differences in levels on the latent variable correspond to equal differences in raw scores.[22,66] Furthermore, the summed raw scale score and the relative scaling of individuals on the raw score continuum are dependent on the difficulty of the items used in the scale. Also, raw scores do not take into account differences in item response patterns.[67] Finally, using the raw score metric may lead to erroneous identification or misidentification of interaction effects.[68]

In contrast to CTT, because person parameters (i.e., latent variable scores) and item parameters are imbedded in the same measurement model, IRT modeling facilitates a content-based interpretation of a person's score on a latent variable. Consider the IRCs shown in Figure 21.1. Observe that if we know an individual's estimated position on the latent variable, we can evaluate these IRCs and know exactly what type of item content the person is likely to endorse or not endorse. For example, if those items represent two health-related behaviors or symptoms, we could interpret any theta estimate in terms of the probability of engaging in those behaviors or of having those symptoms. Of course, with IRT we are still free to develop norms for specific groups based on the latent trait metric.

In IRT, an individual's item response patterns are used to estimate her position on a latent trait continuum. Because item properties are explicitly accounted for in the IRT model, a person's location on the latent variable scale can be estimated using any subset of items with known item parameters. Thus, scores from different tests – even tests that are not parallel – can be compared on the same metric. Estimates of a respondent's position on the latent variable are not scale dependent like true scores are in CTT. A person's position on a latent variable metric does not depend on a particular set of items being administered. Finally, the IRT scaling of individual differences is maximally efficient;[9] no weighting of item responses can be more precise than IRT scoring. In turn, this potentially leads to better (more accurate) group comparisons.

Summary: the future role of IRT in cancer outcomes assessment

Key IRT model features and several advantages of IRT over CTT have been discussed in terms of scale development, scale analysis, and scale administration. In terms of a psychometric framework, IRT and CTT have major differences. In CTT, weak but unrealistic assumptions are made (e.g., error constant across the true score range), item and person indices are sample dependent, and comparison of individuals depends on parallel instruments. In IRT, strong but realistic assumptions are made (e.g., monotonicity), item and person indices are incorporated into the same model, item and person indices have the property of invariance, and comparison of people is possible with any subset of items calibrated to the same scale.

Earlier we discussed a need in the cancer outcomes measurement field for an analytic tool to facilitate development of instruments that are more reliable, sensitive, and valid, as well as tools that would allow us to link instruments together. IRT has the potential to answer that call. With the use of the IRT information functions, developers can choose the most reliable items that match the study population. This approach increases precision in measurement, increases the sensitivity of the instrument to measure change in health status in the study population, and reduces the burden to respondents by not asking them questions that do not add any information in estimating their scores. The invariance property of IRT models allows researchers to link instruments on the same metric, but also provides a tool in DIF to detect cultural differences in questionnaire responses. Finally, cancer outcomes experts can capitalize on IRT's ability to sort out the contribution of each question to measuring the underlying construct(s) of interest in order to better understand and improve the content validity of HRQOL instruments.

However, it is important to point out that none of these advantages of IRT has been convincingly empirically demonstrated, as of yet, in health outcomes research. There is not a large body of literature demonstrating that when IRT methods are used, better (i.e., more valid, efficient) results occur or that substantive conclusions change. In addition, with IRT methods, there is the veritable Devil in the technical details. Empirical issues – such as how to construct a calibration sample, what type of estimation algorithm works best, when and what type of prior distributions should be used, how should scales be linked, and how should latent variable scores be estimated – are extremely complex topics. Researchers will inevitably need to find a balance between the added complexity of IRT and the benefit of using such models.

Finally, IRT is certainly not the solution to all measurement problems, and this may be especially true in health outcomes research. IRT modeling and its associated applications (e.g., item banking, adaptive testing) are likely not worth the effort if a researcher is working with very short scales (e.g., 1, 2, or 3 items). Also, some constructs relevant to outcomes assessment are very specific (e.g., nausea and vomiting) or narrow in their conceptual bandwidth; it is likely that very few items are valid indicators of such narrow constructs, and IRT application may not be called for.

Most importantly, IRT is a latent variable measurement model: it is assumed that there is a *latent* variable that "causes" item responses. In all social and medical fields, some important constructs are not latent variables (e.g., attractiveness, social class). For such "emergent" constructs that are defined by their indicators (e.g., owning a house defines high social class, but high social class does not cause house owning), IRT modeling is not appropriate. In the end, the nature and context of the measurement problem must guide the choice of measurement model.

Acknowledgments

I would like to thank Ron Hays and Leo Morales for providing access to the SF-36 data used in this study. The data were originally collected with support from a grant from the Medical Quality Commission to RAND (R. Hays, Principal Investigator). Thanks to Matt Henson for help with tables, figures, and analyses.

REFERENCES

1 McHorney, C. A., Cohen, A. S. (2000). Equating health status measures with item response theory: illustrations with functional status items. *Medical Care* **38**:43–59.

2 Ware, J. E., Bjorner, J. B., Kosinski, M. (2000). Practical implications of item response theory and computerized adaptive testing: a brief summary of ongoing studies of widely used headache impact scales. *Medical Care* **38**:73–83.

3 Medical Outcomes Trust (1991). *Medical Outcomes Trust: Improving Medical Outcomes from the Patient's Point of View*. Boston, MA: Medical Outcomes Trust.

4 van der Linden, W. J., Hambleton, R. K. (ed.) (1997). *Handbook of Modern Item Response Theory*. New York: Springer.

5 Hambleton, this volume, Chapter 22.

6 Wilson, this volume, Chapter 23.

7 McHorney, Cook, this volume, Invited Paper B.

8 Hays, R. D., Morales, L. S. (2001). The RAND-36 measure of health-related quality of life. *Annals of Medicine* **33**:350–7.

9 Hays, R. D., Sherbourne, C. D., Mazel, R. M. (1993). The RAND 36-item Health Survey 1.0. *Health Economics* **2**:217–27.

10 Ware, J. E., Sherbourne, C. D. (1992). The MOS 36-item short-form health survey (SF-36), conceptual framework and item selection. *Medical Care* **30**:473–83.

11 Morales, L. S., Cunningham, W. E., Brown, J. A. *et al.* (1999). Are Latinos less satisfied with communication by health care providers? *Journal of General Internal Medicine* **14**: 409–17.

12 Bock, R. D. (1997). A brief history of item response theory. *Educational Measurement: Issues and Practice* **16**:21–33.

13 Lord, F. M. (1980). *Applications of Item Response Theory to Practical Testing Problems*. Hillsdale, NJ: Lawrence Erlbaum Associates.

14 Wright, B. D. (1997). A history of social science measurement. *Educational Measurement: Issues and Practice* **16**:33–45.

15 Rasch, G. (1960). *Probabilistic Models for Some Intelligence and Attainment Tests*. Copenhagen: Denmarks Paedagogiske Institute.

16 Mellenbergh, G. J. (1994). A unidimensional latent trait model for continuous item responses. *Multivariate Behavioral Research* **29**:223–36.

17 Samejima, F. (1969). Estimation of latent ability using a response pattern of graded scores. *Psychometric Monograph*, No. 17.

18 Masters, G. N. (1982). A Rasch model for partial credit scoring. *Psychometrika* **47**:149–74.

19 Masters, G. N., Wright, B. D. (1996). The partial credit model. In *Handbook of Modern Item Response Theory*, ed. W. J. van der Linden, R. K. Hambleton. New York: Springer.

20 Andrich, D. (1978). Application of a psychometric model to ordered categories which are scored with successive integers. *Applied Psychological Measurement* **2**:581–94.

21 Muraki, E., Bock, R. D. (1997). *PARSCALE: IRT Based Test Scoring and Item Analysis for Graded Open-ended Exercises and Performance Tasks*. Chicago: Scientific Software.

22 Cooke, D. J., Michie, C. (1997). An item response theory analysis of the Hare psychopathy checklist – revised. *Psychological Assessment* **9**:3–14.

23 Drasgow, F., Parsons, C. (1983). Applications of unidimensional item response theory models to multidimensional data. *Applied Psychological Measurement* **7**: 189–99.

24 Reckase, M. D. (1979). Unifactor latent trait models applied to multifactor tests: results and implications. *Journal of Educational Statistics* **4**:207–30.

25 Hattie, J. (1985). Methodology review: assessing unidimensionality of tests and items. *Applied Psychological Measurement* **9**:139–64.

26 Reise, S. P., Waller, N. G. (2001). Dichotomous IRT models. In *Advances in Measurement and Data Analysis,* ed. F. Drasgow, Schmitt, pp. 88–122. Williamsburg, VA: Jossey-Bass.

27 McLeod, L. D., Swygert, K. A., Thissen, D. (2001). Factor analysis for items scored in two categories. In *Test Scoring,* ed. D. Thissen, H. Wainer, pp. 141–86. Mahwah, NJ: Lawrence Erlbaum Associates.

28 Waller, N. G. (2000). *MicroFACT 2.0 User's Manual.* St. Paul, MN: Assessment Systems Corporation.

29 McDonald, R. P. (1981). The dimensionality of tests and items. *British Journal of Mathematical and Statistical Psychology* **34**:100–17.

30 Chen, W., Thissen, D. (1997). Local dependence indexes for item pairs using item response theory. *Journal of Educational and Behavioral Statistics* **22**:265–89.

31 Yen, W. M. (1984). Effects of local item dependence on the fit and equating performance of the three-parameter logistic model. *Applied Psychological Measurement* **8**: 125–45.

32 Embretson, S. E., Reise, S. P. (2000). *Item Response Theory for Psychologists.* Mahwah, NJ: Lawrence Erlbaum Associates.

33 Baker, F. B. (1992). *Item Response Theory Parameter Estimation Techniques.* New York: Marcel Dekker, Inc.

34 Kingston, N., Dorans, N. (1985). The analysis of item-ability regressions: an exploratory IRT model-fit tool. *Applied Psychological Measurement* **9**:281–8.

35 McKinley, R., Mills, C. (1985). A comparison of several goodness-of-fit statistics. *Applied Psychological Measurement* **9**:49–57.

36 Hambleton, R. K., Robin, F., Xing, D. (2000). Item response models for the analysis of educational and psychological test data. In H. E. A. Tinsley, S. D. Brown (ed.), *Handbook of Applied Multivariate Statistics and Mathematical Modeling,* pp. 553–85. San Diego, CA: Academic Press.

37 Orlando, M., Thissen, D. (2000). Likelihood-based item-fit indices for dichotomous item response theory models. *Applied Psychological Measurement* **24**:50–64.

38 Rogers, H., Hattie, J. (1987). A Monte Carlo investigation of several person and item-fit statistics for item response models. *Applied Psychological Measurement* **11**:47–57.

39 Mislevy, R. J., Bock, R. D. (1989). *BILOG 3: Item Analysis and Test Scoring with Binary Logistic Models.* Mooresville, IN: Scientific Software.

40 Meijer, R. R., Sijtsma, K. (1995). Detection of aberrant item score patterns: a review of recent developments. *Applied Measurement in Education* **8**:261–72.

41 Reise, S. P., Waller, N. G. (1993). Traitedness and the assessment of response pattern scalability. *Journal of Personality and Social Psychology* **65**:143–51.

42 Zickar, M. J., Drasgow, F. (1996). Detecting faking on a personality instrument using appropriateness measurement. *Applied Psychological Measurement* **20**:71–88.

43 Embretson, S. E. (1996). The new rules of measurement. *Psychological Assessment* **8**:341–9.

44 Cronbach, L. J. (1951). Coefficient alpha and the internal structure of tests. *Psychometrika* **16**:297–334.

45 Dodd, B. G., DeAyala, R. J. (1994). Item information as a function of threshold values in the rating scale model. In *Objective Measurement: Theory and Practice,* ed. M. Wilson, Vol. 2, pp. 201–317. Norwood, NJ: Ablex.

46 Flaugher, R. (2000). Item pools. In *Computerized Adaptive Testing: A Primer* (2nd Edition), ed. H. Wainer, N. J. Dorans, D. Eignor *et al.,* pp. 37–60. Mahwah, NJ: Lawrence Erlbaum Associates.

47 Orlando, M., Sherbourne, C. D., Thissen, D. (2000). Summed-score linking using item response theory: application to depression measurement. *Psychological Assessment* **12**: 354–9.

48 Vale, D. C. (1986). Linking item parameters onto a common scale. *Applied Psychological Measurement* **10**:133–44.

49 Wainer, H., Eignor, D. (2000). Caveats, pitfalls, and unexpected consequences of implementing large-scale computerized testing. In *Computerized Adaptive Testing: A Primer* (2nd Edition), H. Wainer, N. J. Dorans, D. Eignor *et al.,* pp. 37–60. Mahwah, NJ: Lawrence Erlbaum Associates.

50 Weiss, D. J. (1985). Adaptive testing by computer. *Journal of Consulting and Clinical Psychology* **53**:774–89.

51 Drasgow, F., Olson-Buchanan, J. B. (1999). *Innovations in Computerized Assessment.* Mahwah, NJ. Lawrence Erlbaum Associates.

52 Wainer, H., Dorans, N. J., Eignor, D. *et al.* (2000). *Computerized Adaptive Testing: A Primer* (2nd Edition). Mahwah, NJ: Lawrence Erlbaum Associates.

53 van der Linden, W. J., Glas, C. A. W. (2000). *Computerized Aadaptive Testing: Theory and Practice.* London: Kluwer Academic Publishers.

54 Bjorner, J. B., Kreiner, S., Ware, J. E. *et al.* (1998). Differential item functioning in the Danish translation of the SF-36. *Journal of Clinical Epidemiology* **51**:1189–202.

55 Gandek, B., Ware Jr., J. E., Neil, K. A. *et al.* (1998). Tests of data quality, scaling assumptions, and reliability of the SF-36 in eleven countries: results from the IQOLA project. *Journal of Clinical Epidemiology* **51**:1149–58.

56 Millsap, R. E., Everson, H. T. (1993). Methodology review: statistical approaches for assessing measurement bias. *Applied Psychological Measurement* **17**:297–334.

57 Zimowski, M. F., Muraki, E., Mislevy, R. J. *et al.* (1996). *BILOG-MG: Multiple-group IRT Analysis and Test Maintenance for Binary Items*. Chicago: Scientific Software.

58 Kim, S., Cohen, A. (1998). Detection of differential item functioning under the graded response model with the likelihood ratio test. *Applied Psychological Measurement* **22**: 345–55.

59 Raju, N. S. (1988). The area between two item characteristic curves. *Psychometrika* **53**:495–502.

60 Reise, S. P., Smith, L., Furr, R. M. (2001). Invariance on the NEO PI-R Neuroticism Scale. *Multivariate Behavioral Research* **36**:83–110.

61 Thissen, D., Steinberg, L., Gerrard, M. (1986). Beyond group-mean differences: the concept of item bias. *Psychological Bulletin* **99**:118–28.

62 Reise, S. P., Widaman, K. F., Pugh, R. H. (1993). Confirmatory factor analysis and item response theory: two approaches for exploring measurement invariance. *Psychological Bulletin* **114**:352–66.

63 Holland, P. W., Wainer, H. (1993). *Differential Item Functioning*. Hillsdale, NJ: Lawrence Erlbaum Associates.

64 Yen, W. M. (1986). The choice of scale for educational measurement: an IRT perspective. *Journal of Educational Measurement* **23**:299–325.

65 Thissen, D., Orlando, M. (2001). Item response theory for items scored in two categories. In *Test Scoring*, ed. D. Thissen, H. Wainer, pp. 73–140. Mahwah, NJ: Lawrence Erlbaum Associates.

66 Cella, D., Chang, C. (2000). A discussion of item response theory and its applications in health status assessment. *Medical Care* **9**:66–72.

67 Santor, D. A., Ramsay, J. O. (1998). Progress in the technology of measurement: applications of item response models. *Psychological Assessment* **10**:345–59.

68 Embretson, S. E. (1996). Item response theory models and spurious interaction effects in factorial ANOVA designs. *Applied Psychological Measurement* **20**:201–12.

22

Applications of item response theory to improve health outcomes assessment: developing item banks, linking instruments, and computer-adaptive testing

Ronald K. Hambleton, Ph.D.

University of Massachusetts at Amherst, Amherst, MA

Introduction

For the field of health outcomes assessment to move forward, researchers must integrate advances in measurement theory with improvements in computer technology. We need health outcomes researchers and patient advocates to guide the development of tailored health-related quality-of-life (HRQOL) instruments that meet the criteria for validity, reliability, and sensitivity to change in health status while minimizing the burden of questions for the cancer patient. Also, to accurately characterize a patient's HRQOL after disease onset or treatment (a call for more specific than generic measures), we need the ability to crosswalk scores from one instrument to another despite groups of patients receiving different sets of questions.

In Chapter 21, this volume, Reise[1] discusses the shortcomings of traditional (i.e., classical test theory, CTT) methods that have been used to direct the development and analysis of HRQOL instruments. CTT item statistics are dependent on the particular sample of respondents, while patient scores are dependent on the particular choice of items. Such dependencies hinder the ability of researchers to combine results from studies using different HRQOL measures or to create tailored instruments by choosing specific questions from other instruments. Reise[1] also explains how item response theory (IRT), with the properties of item parameter invariance (over samples of respondents) and respondent parameter invariance (over samples of items or questions), provides a flexible tool for instrument developers to link sets of questions measuring the same domain on a common metric and to create computerized adaptive assessments.

The current chapter builds on Reise's introduction to the basic concepts, assumptions, popular models, and important features of IRT and discusses the applications of IRT modeling to health outcomes assessment. In particular, we highlight the critical role of IRT modeling in: developing an instrument to match a study's population; linking two or more instruments measuring similar constructs on a common metric; and creating item banks that provide the foundation for tailored short-form instruments or for computerized adaptive assessments.

An *item bank* combines high quality items from multiple instruments (i.e., captures the best items from many different questionnaires) into a single data resource. Response data on these items are collected from a representative sample, and item properties are assigned to each question using IRT modeling methods. Once the items have been IRT-calibrated, researchers may pick a set of informative items from the item bank that target their study population, or a computer can select the best set of items based on an individual's responses to earlier questions. Scores from any set of items collected from the item bank are comparable because of the IRT property of invariance.

Both tailored instruments and computerized adaptive assessments will result in shorter questionnaires and lower measurement error than traditional HRQOL instruments. The advantage of a computerized adaptive assessment is its ability to cover multiple health domains in a short amount of time and provide instant, accurate reports of a patient's health status to a care provider or researcher. For a range of clinical and observational settings, these instruments can exist on multiple platforms, including laptop computers, handheld devices, the Internet, telephone interviews, or interactive voice recognition technology.

This chapter will serve as a didactic and will use actual data to illustrate the applications of IRT models for health outcomes assessment. Readers will be shown how to select the best IRT model based on the characteristics of the data; how to identify the strengths and limits of a data set to match a study population; how to link two sets of items together on a common metric; and how to create item banks. Because suitable data are not available on multiple instruments, the data at hand will be manipulated to illustrate the tools of IRT.

This didactic will consider: the investigative process for evaluating IRT model assumptions; choosing and interpreting the IRT model; evaluating model fit; evaluating item and scale performance; developing an item bank; adding items to a bank; linking instruments on a common metric; crosswalking or "equating" scores from one instrument to another; and detecting item bias. Every attempt is made to keep the terminology consistent with the preceding chapter by Reise.[1] Readers are encouraged to keep Table 21.1 in Reise as a reference for the common IRT terms and definitions.

Data in the examples are from responses to the Patient Satisfaction with Medical Care Questionnaire (PSQ-III), a 50-item revised version of the Patient Satisfaction Questionnaire[2,3] developed for use in the Medical Outcomes Study.[4] In that survey, participants were asked to indicate how they feel about the medical care they receive in general, with no reference to a specific time frame or visit.[5] Table 22.1 lists the 50 questions from the PSQ-III that are used in the analyses for this chapter. Response options are on a Likert-type five-point scale: *strongly agree, agree, uncertain, disagree, strongly disagree.* All items (i.e., questions) were scored such that a higher score reflects a higher state of satisfaction with medical care. Respondents (N = 2914) were patients who had a physician's diagnosis of one of four chronic medical conditions: diabetes, hypertension, depression, and heart disease. Roughly 40% were male and 58% percent were married. The average age of respondents was 54.8 years, with a standard deviation of 15.5.

Assessing IRT model assumptions, fitting the model, and evaluating the fit

Before any interpretation of IRT results can begin, one must confirm that the assumptions of the IRT models are satisfied. As reviewed in Reise,[1] IRT models are based on strong assumptions about the data. The assumption of unidimensionality means that the items in the scale are measuring a single dominant trait. In practice, most instruments are measuring more than a single trait, but good model fit will require only a reasonably good approximation to the unidimensionality assumption. A previous review[5] of the structure of the PSQ-III found the 50 items loaded onto six dimensions of medical care that influence patients' assessments of their satisfaction (time, technical, interpersonal, communication, financial, access), and the six factors load on a higher order factor of *general satisfaction* with medical care. To support this earlier finding, we performed a principal components analysis (PCA) on the data. PCA is a multivariate statistical procedure for evaluating the dimensionality of a scale based on the correlation among items and variability observed in the scale.

Figure 22.1 shows the scree plot for the largest 25 eigenvalues from a PCA of the 50-item instrument. Eigenvalues provide a measure of the amount of variance accounted for by each orthogonal factor within a scale. Note that while a large first factor exists (accounting for over 35% of the variability), the second factor is relatively large also (8% of the variability). This result was not surprising, as the survey was specifically designed to reflect different aspects of health care satisfaction. By conventional standards, however, the first factor is dominant; it accounts for more than 20% of the variability, and the first

Table 22.1. Questions (some abbreviated) in the Patient Satisfaction with Medical Care Questionnaire *

Item	Question
1	If I need hospital care, I can get admitted without any trouble.
2	Doctors need to be more thorough in treating and examining me.
3	I am very satisfied with the medical care I receive.
4	I worry sometimes about having to pay large medical bills.
5	It is easy for me to get medical care in an emergency.
6	Doctors are good about explaining the reason for medical tests.
7	I am usually kept waiting for a long time when at the doctor's office.
8	My doctor's office has everything to provide complete medical care.
9	The doctors who treat me should give me more respect.
10	Sometimes it is a problem to cover my cost for a medical care visit.
11	The medical care I have been receiving is just about perfect.
12	Sometimes doctors make me wonder if their diagnosis is correct.
13	During my visits, I am allowed to say everything I think is important.
14	I feel confident that I can get the medical care I need without being set back financially.
15	They are careful to check everything when treating and examining me.
16	It's hard for me to get medical care on short notice.
17	The doctors who treat me have a genuine interest in me as a person.
18	Sometimes doctors use medical terms without explaining what they mean.
19	Sometimes I go without medical care I need because it is expensive.
20	The office hours when I can get medical care are convenient for me.
21	There are things about the medical system I receive my care from that need to be improved.
22	The office where I get medical care should be open for more hours.
23	The medical staff that treats me knows the latest medical developments.
24	I have to pay for more of my medical care than I can afford.
25	I have easy access to the medical specialists I need.
26	Sometimes doctors make me feel foolish.
27	Regardless of the health problems I have now or will experience later, I feel protected from financial hardship.
28	Where I get care, people wait too long for emergency treatment.
29	Doctors act too businesslike and impersonal toward me.
30	There is a crisis in health care in the United States today.
31	Doctors never expose me to unnecessary risk.
32	The amount I pay to cover my medical care needs is reasonable.
33	There are things about the medical care I receive that could be better.
34	My doctors treat me in a very friendly and courteous manner.
35	Those who provide my medical care sometimes hurry too much.
36	Some of the doctors I have seen lack experience with my condition.
37	Places where I can get medical care are very conveniently located.
38	Doctors sometimes ignore what I tell them.
39	When receiving medical care, they should pay more attention to my privacy.
40	If I have a medical question, I can reach a doctor without any problem.
41	Doctors rarely give me advice about ways to stay healthy.
42	All things considered, the medical care I receive is excellent.
43	Doctors listen carefully to what I have to say.
44	I feel insured and protected financially against all possible medical problems.
45	I have some doubts about the ability of the doctors who treat me.
46	Doctors usually spend plenty of time with me.
47	Doctors always do their best to keep me from worrying.
48	I find it hard to get an appointment for medical care right away.
49	I am dissatisfied with some things about the medical care I receive.
50	My doctors are very competent and well-trained.

* The PSQ was developed at RAND as part of the Medical Outcomes Study. Items reprinted with permission.

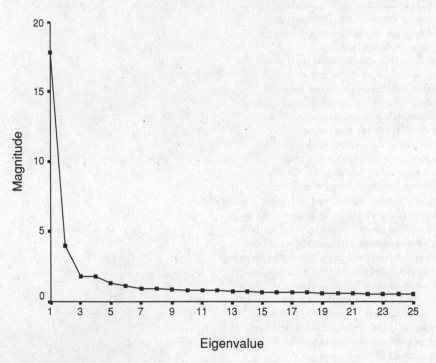

Figure 22.1. Plot of the largest 25 eigenvalues from a principal components analysis of the Satisfaction with Medical Care Survey (Number of items = 50).

eigenvalue is four or five times larger than the second factor (with our data, the ratio exceeds 4). At the same time, the second, although the less significant factor, is not of trivial size. Still, based on relevant experience and recognizing that other analyses of model fit will follow, it is definitely reasonable to regard the unidimensionality assumption as essentially met.

Another critical assumption is that the chosen IRT model adequately fits the data. To the extent that the basic IRT assumptions, such as local independence, monotonicity, and unidimensionality, are violated, the IRT model will show poorer fit to the data. Because of the Likert-type (polytomous) response format of the data, Samejima's[6] graded response model (GRM) is an excellent choice from among the family of IRT models that provides a relatively straightforward interpretation of item response behaviors. Evaluating IRT model fit requires first fitting the GRM model to the data, which involves estimation of item and ability parameters and item-level fit statistics.

Using the IRT software program, PARSCALE™,[7], GRM item parameters were estimated for each of the 50 questions of the PSQ-III, and each item's parameter estimates and fit statistics are reported in Table 22.2. To illustrate the GRM, Figures 22.2 and 22.3 present the category response curves (CRC) for the two questions "I am very satisfied with the medical care I receive" (#3) and "Sometimes doctors use medical terms without explaining what they mean" (#18), respectively. The CRC displays the probabilities for responding to each of the five response categories as a function of patients' level of satisfaction with their medical care. The first question (#3) functions well, since each response category maps to a different segment of the θ continuum of patient satisfaction. Patients very dissatisfied with their medical care are likely to answer *strongly disagree* with the

Table 22.2. Summary of graded response model item and fit statistics for the Satisfaction with Medical Care Survey

Item	a_i	b_{i1}	b_{i2}	b_{i3}	b_{i4}	Fit Chi^2	df
1	0.63	−4.04	−3.32	−1.86	0.14	34.11	25
2	0.75	−2.23	−0.81	−0.11	1.82	173.83	30
3	1.42	−2.58	−1.78	−1.13	0.39	51.22	19
4	0.23	−4.54	−1.23	−0.13	3.14	86.67	39
5	0.60	−4.05	−3.21	−1.72	0.62	75.31	27
6	1.10	−2.65	−1.54	−1.1	0.76	41.78	24
7	0.59	−3.14	−1.52	−1.05	1.91	102.88	32
8	0.75	−3.36	−2.41	−1.19	0.91	129.43	27
9	0.73	−3.02	−1.83	−1.27	0.98	127.75	28
10	0.33	−5.26	−2.8	−2.11	1.31	106.96	33
11	1.30	−2.38	−1.34	−0.59	1.05	95.44	21
12	0.86	−2.56	−0.63	0	1.88	128.60	26
13	1.23	−2.91	−1.93	−1.64	0.34	51.56	19
14	0.59	−3.2	−2.17	−0.99	1.26	119.25	30
15	1.41	−2.42	−1.3	−0.67	0.91	60.37	20
16	0.78	−2.93	−1.7	−1.07	1.17	58.90	28
17	1.32	−2.55	−1.73	−0.87	0.65	32.46	20
18	0.75	−3.09	−1.12	−0.77	1.61	109.63	27
19	0.56	−3.51	−2.33	−1.93	0.41	87.32	27
20	0.83	−3.3	−2.15	−1.89	0.86	57.83	25
21	0.92	−2.1	−0.65	0.31	2.04	150.07	27
22	0.65	−3.19	−1.74	−0.49	2.27	114.61	30
23	0.87	−3.43	−2.79	−0.71	1.28	74.52	24
24	0.42	−4.56	−2.71	−1.8	1.55	94.51	31
25	0.95	−2.76	−1.91	−1.01	1.06	83.17	25
26	1.01	−2.79	−1.44	−1.1	0.94	61.81	24
27	0.41	−3.43	−1.97	−0.09	2.71	150.10	34
28	0.78	−2.91	−1.76	−0.35	1.63	85.41	28
29	1.18	−2.55	−1.54	−1.13	1.02	61.63	22
30	0.72	−3.49	−2.32	−0.56	1.69	104.91	28
31	0.42	−4.39	−2.32	−1.13	2.76	104.42	32
32	0.89	−2.3	−0.33	0.7	2.52	170.17	28
33	1.25	−3.01	−2.38	−1.97	0.28	62.35	17
34	1.24	−2.14	−0.92	−0.6	1.37	61.57	22
35	0.85	−2.57	−1.37	−0.59	1.67	157.20	27
36	0.62	−3.91	−2.43	−2.1	1.34	114.48	26
37	1.24	−2.33	−1.13	−0.56	1.28	75.31	22
38	0.55	−3.76	−1.93	−0.93	2.26	195.25	31
39	1.07	−2.49	−1.39	−0.8	1.1	49.94	25
40	0.71	−2.81	−1.3	−0.88	1.77	118.69	27
41	2.01	−2.59	−1.63	−1.09	0.49	21.46	13
42	1.88	−2.59	−1.51	−0.95	0.7	21.07	15
43	0.53	−3.13	−1.78	−0.17	2.13	160.45	33
44	1.15	−2.5	−1.56	−1.01	0.95	100.02	23
45	1.23	−2.38	−1.17	−0.77	1.3	63.94	21
46	1.13	−2.85	−1.51	−0.75	1.38	61.09	22
47	0.87	−2.57	−1.3	−0.96	1.37	81.53	26
48	1.33	−2.17	−0.83	−0.47	1.27	71.19	21
49	1.32	−2.83	−2.37	−1.34	0.54	101.43	17
50	1.13	−2.73	−1.76	−1.2	0.8	75.16	23

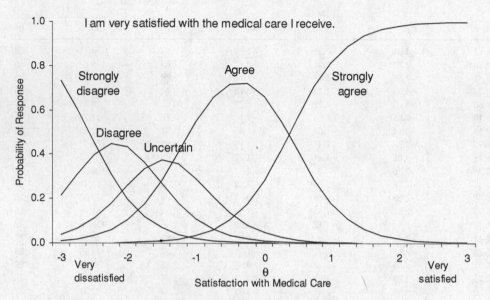

Figure 22.2.   IRT GRM category response curves for the item, "I am very satisfied with the medical care I receive."

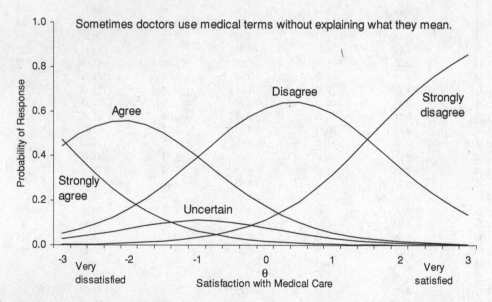

Figure 22.3.   IRT GRM category response curves for the item, "Sometimes doctors use medical terms without explaining what they mean."

statement "I am very satisfied with the medical care I receive." As one moves across the latent variable continuum (i.e., along the horizontal axis), it is evident that as satisfaction increases, individuals are more likely to agree with this statement and thus endorse the appropriate response category. To contrast the differences among the GRM item properties, the next item in Figure 22.3 has lower discrimination ability (i.e., lower item-scale correlation) than the item in Figure 22.2 ($a = 0.75$ and $a = 1.42$, respectively); this is reflected graphically by the steepness of their curves. This makes sense when reading the item content; the first question, "I am very satisfied with the medical care I receive," is more related (i.e., has higher discrimination) to the underlying construct, *satisfaction with medical care*, than the second item "Sometimes doctors use medical terms without explaining what they mean." The first question focuses directly on what we are trying to measure, while the second is more of an indirect measure of patient satisfaction.

Another key difference clearly evident from the two-item CRC plots is that each of the five response categories in Figure 22.3 does not solely represent a section of the construct continuum as they do in Figure 22.2. We see that patients who are dissatisfied with their medical care ($\theta < -1$) will likely *agree* that, "Sometimes doctors use medical terms without explaining what they mean." Patients with average levels of satisfaction in the population ($-1 < \theta < 1.6$) typically *disagree* with this statement, and very satisfied patients ($\theta > 1.6$) *strongly disagree* with this statement saying their doctors explain complicated medical terms. This CRC graph shows that the response categories *strongly agree* and *uncertain* were little endorsed, and test developers may want to consider dropping the number of response categories from five to three in revised questionnaires.

One strong impression from a review of the item statistics in Table 22.2 is that the discriminating powers of the 50 items vary substantially (from 0.23 to 2.01), reflecting that some items measure a patient's satisfaction more directly than others, and more weight is given to those items when estimating a person's level of satisfaction. This suggests that choosing an IRT model that allows the item discrimination parameter to vary is quite important for achieving model fit. Thus, the partial credit model, a Rasch model, which constrains the discrimination power of each item to be equivalent, may not be suitable for these data. For instrument developers wishing to reduce the number of items in the PSQ-III, plots of CRCs can be used to identify the more informative items, i.e., those having high discrimination and spread of response categories that contribute the greatest to the estimation of trait scores, and to eliminate the less informative items that contribute the least to these estimates. Consequently, the more informative CRCs become the building blocks for instruments.

With the item parameter estimates in hand (see Table 22.2 for a summary), the assumption of model fit can be checked by computing standardized residuals and examining their size and pattern.[7,8] The IRT score of an individual's placement along the construct continuum can be usefully divided into 12 intervals. In each interval the actual performance of respondents can be compared to the predicted performance by the best fitting IRT item statistics. For example, consider Figure 22.2 and respondents with trait scores around $\theta = -2.0$. Here, we would predict that about 20% of the respondents would choose *strongly disagree*, 43% would choose *disagree*, 26% would choose *uncertain*, 11% would choose *agree*, and 0% would choose *strongly agree*. Each of these expectations could be compared to the frequency distribution of choices for respondents near −2.0 on the trait scale (the difference between the actual performance and the expected performance, assuming the model to be true, is called the "raw residual") and converted to standardized residuals (SRs) by dividing the raw residual by the standard error. The computations would be repeated for other intervals along the trait score scale and then repeated for each item. Such computations can be tedious, but computer programs do exist for such analyses. For example, POLYFIT[9] was designed specifically to assess goodness-of-fit for polytomous IRT models. The program provides SRs across

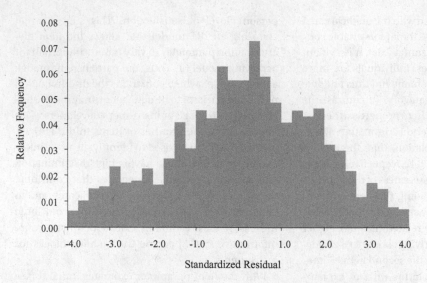

Figure 22.4. Distribution of standardized residuals obtained after fitting the graded response model to the Satisfaction with Medical Care Survey.

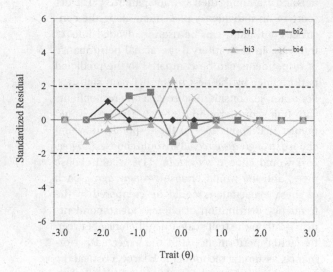

Figure 22.5. Standardized residual plot for item 1 that shows excellent fit (Item: "If I need hospital care, I can get admitted without any trouble").

12 trait-level intervals, in addition to chi-square fit statistics (see Table 22.2) at the item and scale levels and a distribution of the standardized residuals. This distribution can prove useful for assessing fit because the SRs from a good fitting model will be approxi-

mately normally distributed. Standardized residuals can also be pictured using output from the POLYFIT[9] program.

Figure 22.4 shows the distribution of SRs for all items and score categories. Their distribution is not very different from a normal distribution, and it is therefore reasonable to assume a good model fit. But as noted earlier, we would want to explore model fit using different approaches before drawing a final conclusion, and possibly consider dropping several of the seriously misfitting items.

Analysis of SRs at the item level can also help gauge how a particular item and set of score categories are functioning. Figures 22.5 and 22.6 display the standardized residuals for two items from the PSQ-III: "If I need hospital care, I can get admitted without any trouble" and "Doctors need to be more thorough in treating and examining me," respectively.

The standardized residuals are reported for each of the 12 trait-score categories and organized to highlight the SRs associated with each score category. (The "strongly disagree" score category was deleted from the analyses because it was selected by very few respondents.) In Figure 22.5, the fit is excellent. Of nearly 48 SRs, only one exceeds a value of 2.0. In Figure 22.6, the model fit appears poor. About 30% of the SRs exceed an absolute value of 2.0. Given that the standardized residuals should be normally distributed if there is good model fit, one might expect about 5% of the SRs to exceed an absolute value of 2.0. Clearly, in this case, model fit is not adequate and further diagnostic work is in order.

The overall conclusion from our estimation of model parameters and goodness of fit work is that the graded response model fits the PSQ-III data quite well, despite the presence of a second trait influencing scores. There also appears to be some substantial variation in the item statistics. This feature opens up some possibilities in any redesign of the instrument, including deleting some items (if deletion does not distort the construct in a meaningful way).

Building and evaluating instruments

To this point it has been assumed that the PSQ-III measures an essentially unidimensional construct of *general patient satisfaction with their medical care*, and the focus has been on determining if the IRT GRM fits the data. With the item parameters estimated, IRT can also play an important part in instrument development and/or redesign. For example, we might want an instrument that is highly reliable for measuring respondents' view of their medical care, from very dissatisfied to very satisfied, across the entire trait continuum. On the other hand, we might be interested in creating an instrument focused on only one area of the trait continuum, e.g., people who are dissatisfied with their medical care. Such an instrument would lead to precise estimates of patient satisfaction at the lower end of the trait continuum and substantially less precision in trait estimation at the upper end of the scale.

Reise[1] introduced the IRT concept of item and scale information functions that indicate the contribution a specific question, or set of questions, makes to assessment across the trait θ continuum. In a general sense, an item's "information" could be regarded as the proportional contribution it makes to

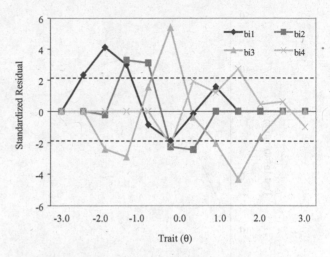

Figure 22.6. Standardized residual plot for item 2 that shows problematic model fit (Item: "Doctors need to be more thorough in treating and examining me").

an overall instrument score, conditional on the item's location along the trait continuum. In practice, desired instrument information (i.e., the amount of precision desired along the trait continuum) is specified at each trait score of interest. This is often called the "target information function." Then, the instrument development task is to select items that meet the content and statistical specifications and any constraints (e.g., number of items, sub-domain coverage) that are imposed.

Figure 22.7 displays the scale information function for the 50-item Satisfaction with Medical Care Questionnaire. Normally, information in the region of about 20 is quite sufficient (the corresponding measurement error associated with trait estimation is about 0.23, or less than one-fourth of the standard deviation of trait scores on the survey). This corresponds to a classical parallel reliability estimate (Cronbach's alpha) in excess of 0.90. In Figure 22.7, the information function is very high, suggesting excellent measurement of trait scores across the full continuum of patient satisfaction.

The scale information function is obtained by summing the information functions for each of the 50 items. The implications of adding or subtracting

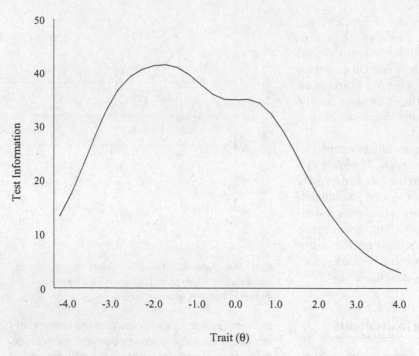

Figure 22.7.   Scale information function for the 50-item Satisfaction With Medical Care Survey.

items from the instrument would then be easy to see. For example, if 10 items were deleted, the information could be recalculated easily. The exact implications of redesigning the instrument by deleting items would be known immediately. In a similar way, the implications of adding items or substituting one set of items for another could be determined (assuming, of course, that the new items had been IRT-calibrated on the same trait score scale). Design and redesign of instruments is done by looking at the test information function resulting from particular selections of items.[1,10-12] Of course, item deletions or additions should be carried out under the guidance of a content expert to make sure the multifaceted nature of the measured construct is reflected in the pool of items.

Taking this a step further, assume that an instrument is needed to identify respondents who are *dissatisfied* with their health care. Presuming that the underlying trait being measured is health care

satisfaction, the information function shown in Figure 22.7 would be acceptable. The PSQ-III is doing its best measuring for respondents with low scores (i.e., scores of generally dissatisfied respondents). However, if we wished to focus on respondents responding as *highly satisfied* with their health care (those with the highest trait levels), the instrument could be revised by adding items that provide information at the higher end of the trait continuum. These items can be spotted as those with high levels of item discrimination a and with item thresholds b in the region of 1.0 to 4.0.

Scale information is inversely linked to the precision with which trait scores are estimated:[1]

$$SE(\theta) = \frac{1}{\sqrt{I(\theta)}}$$

The more information provided by an instrument at a trait score, the smaller the error in trait score estimation. Again, in most practical work, the goal

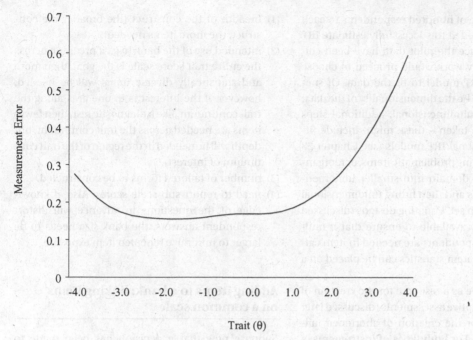

Figure 22.8. Measurement error at each trait score for the Satisfaction With Medical Care Survey.

is to get scale information into the region of 10 to 20. This level of information corresponds, roughly, to classical reliability estimates in the region of 0.90 and higher.

Figure 22.8 provides the standard errors of trait score estimation corresponding to the instrument information function displayed in Figure 22.7. Here it can be seen that the instrument is providing excellent precision across nearly the full trait scale. Standard errors below .30 are highly satisfactory for nearly all uses of individual trait scores. With trait scores scaled to a mean of zero and a standard deviation of one (as they are in the example), standard errors of 0.20 are quite small, suggesting that, at least from the perspective of trait score estimation, the instrument could be considerably shortened. Of course, if item level data are also being used for, say, diagnostic work, or subscale reporting is being done,[13] shortening the instrument may be inconsistent with other goals for the instrument and should not be done.

Developing item banks

An item bank is a collection of questions, taken from existing instruments or developed by an expert panel, which measures a particular content/behavior domain. Normally, these items have been calibrated (i.e., classical and IRT statistics have been estimated) and the content of each item has been stored in the bank, so that, at the time of instrument development, items can be selected to meet any desired set of content and statistical specifications. Software is readily available for storing items and their associated statistics. It is not uncommon to have 20 to 30 pieces of information stored on each item, e.g., classical and IRT statistics, detailed content information, date of last use, number of words in the item, reading difficulty, information about scoring, and average response time.

Development of the item bank is a multi-stage process. After questions have been written, reviewed, and edited, a pilot study is conducted to obtain item statistics. A couple of hundred respondents to each item would be needed to successfully estimate IRT item statistics. Once the pilot data have been collected, preliminary work would proceed to choose an appropriate IRT model to fit the data. Of special interest would be the dimensionality of the data. If the data are multidimensional, additional steps would need to be taken – these might include fitting multidimensional IRT models (see Chapter 23 by Wilson[14]), deleting problematic items, or reorganizing the content domain into smaller unidimensional sets of items and then fitting unidimensional IRT models to each set. Equating designs (discussed below) are readily available to ensure that if multiple groups of respondents are needed in item calibration, all of the item statistics can be placed on a common scale.

Item banks serve as a resource for the creation of computerized adaptive assessments (discussed later in this chapter) or the creation of shortened tailored instruments. For both types of instruments, a subset of informative questions are selected to provide the greatest amount of precision for measuring a study population. Because the set of items comes from the same item bank, scores on any set of items are comparable on a similar measurement scale. For example, with a *patient satisfaction with medical care* item bank, one researcher may select ten items designed to accurately measure people who are dissatisfied with their medical care, while another researcher may select ten items that measure satisfaction across the whole trait continuum. Scores from the two different instruments can be compared because they are standardized to the same metric. Standard errors of measurement will differ between these cases because the first set of items covers a more narrow range (dissatisfaction) than the other ten items (covering full range of satisfaction).

Whether the application is computerized adaptive testing or tailoring short-form assessments, the item bank must contain a statistically diverse set of items to permit good estimation of trait scores along the entire trait score continuum. The desired size of an item bank depends on several factors:

(1) breadth of the construct (the broader the construct, the more items needed).
(2) intended use of the bank (e.g., if precision across the entire trait score scale is the goal, then more and statistically diverse items will be needed; however, if the interest is in one area along the trait continuum, like a diagnostic test, then fewer items are needed across the trait continuum, but depth will be needed in the region of the trait continuum of interest).
(3) number of tailored forms to be constructed.
(4) need to report sub-scale scores. Also, if knowledge of the questions in advance will distort respondent answers, the bank size needs to be larger to minimize repeated item exposure.

Adding items to a bank: linking items on a common scale

Suppose now that a decision has been made to expand the newly created *patient satisfaction with medical care* (PSMC) item bank from the current 50 items to 90 items. Perhaps the goal is to add 40 items that might be helpful in assessing respondents who have high satisfaction with their medical care (i.e., the goal is to improve measurement of respondents at the high end of the trait continuum).

One technical problem immediately arises when new items are being added to an existing bank: respondents answering the new items may not be equivalent on the patient satisfaction trait to those respondents who were used to calibrate items in the original 50-item PSQ-III instrument. Thus, to maintain comparability of item statistics, they must be "equated." This means that an adjustment in the new item statistics, obtained with the new respondent sample, must be made in order to control for any difference in the trait scores of respondents taking the two forms of the instrument. In other words, the distribution of satisfaction scores will likely be different between the original calibration sample and the sample responding to the new set of patient satisfaction questions, so we need some way to equate the metric from the new respondent sample to the

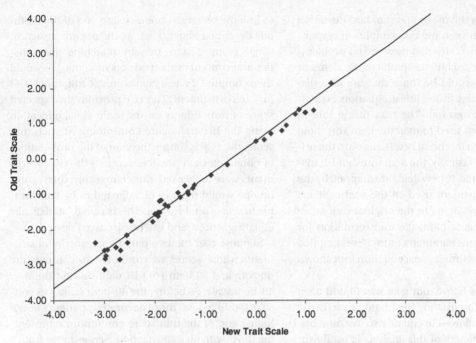

Figure 22.9. Plot of 40 thresholds from 10 common items used in linking the old (50-item) scale to the new (40-item) scale.

original sample. This adjustment would be estimated by including a common set of questions from the original PSQ-III, called the "anchor set of items," in the administration of the set of questions that also contains the 40 new items.

Because anchor items are drawn from the bank (in this example, the original 50 PSQ-III questions make up the PSMC bank), their item statistics (e.g., item discrimination, item thresholds) are already known. These anchor item statistics will be linearly related to the item statistics estimated from any other sample of respondents because of the IRT item invariance property. Once the linear transformation from the new to the original item statistics has been obtained for the anchor items, statistics for new items (the non-anchor items) obtained from the second sample can be transformed to statistics that would have been obtained had the 40 new questions been administered to the original (calibration) sample of respondents. Thus, comparing the performance of the original sample and the new sample of respondents on the anchor items is the key to deciding if a linear

mathematical adjustment is needed to equate the 40 new items on the same scale with the 50 original PSQ-III items. Normally, anchor items are selected to be broadly representative of the item bank (or the original instrument). Ten to fifteen anchor items are usually sufficient to accomplish the task. Other linking (equating) designs are possible (e.g., single group, randomly equivalent groups, and multiple variations), but will not be considered further here.[10,12]

To carry forward our example of adding 40 new items to the original 50-item PSMC bank, we will pretend that ten anchor items were selected from the original bank based on their statistical quality, their coverage across the trait continuum, and their item content representation. These anchor items and the 40 new items were then administered to a new sample of respondents. Figure 22.9 shows the plot of IRT item thresholds (four per item) for the ten anchor items in the original and new respondent samples. The item statistics should be the same except for sampling error and a linear adjustment for differences in the mean and standard deviation of trait scores between the two samples of respondents. The plot indicates that there are no problematic items in the anchor set (problematic items or item thresholds would be those that are at a distance from the best fitting linear equation exceeding two standard errors). The best fitting line in Figure 22.9 is then used to map the item threshold statistics obtained for the 40 new items onto the original trait scale. Basically, the item threshold statistics obtained for the 40 new items are mapped by the same linear adjustment used on the anchor items to equate the new items to the original trait score scale. In a similar fashion, the transformation for the discrimination a parameter estimates is handled with a related best fitting linear equation (not shown here).

In the example above, our goal was to add a set of new items to an existing item bank. Exactly the same steps are followed to equate two instruments; however, the difficulty of this analysis is establishing that the two instruments are sufficiently similar in content that equating makes sense (for example, does it make sense to treat scores from the two instruments interchangeably?) and then finding a link that can be used to carry out the equating. Sometimes an anchor set of items from one of the instruments could be administered along with the second instrument. Other designs might include a single group of respondents taking both instruments (i.e., single group design), or a large group of respondents randomly assigned to take one of the two instruments (i.e., randomly equivalent groups designs). These points will be developed further in the next section.

Crosswalking scores between instruments

Suppose the instrument developer has two scales, both of which measure a patient's satisfaction with medical care, and would like to crosswalk scores from one instrument to the other either for comparing respondents or for combining study results from using the different scales. First, we would need to link the two instruments using one of the methods described above, such as the anchor design or single group design, thereby matching the statistics and content of the two sets of items. We would then compute the test characteristic function (TCF) for each instrument. The TCF provides the expected score of respondents on the scale at each location along the IRT trait score continuum. At each trait score, the TCF is simply the sum of the probabilities of obtaining each possible score. If the two instruments were to be used interchangeably, then scores on one would need to be adjusted to be comparable to scores on the other. This is called "statistically equating scores" and will be discussed next.

Suppose that the two patient satisfaction instruments whose scores we would like to compare are our original 50-item PSQ-III data set and the new 40-item scale. As before, the 40-item scale was constructed to assess, more accurately, patients at the higher end of the trait score continuum representing those with high satisfaction. Scores range from 0 to 4 on each item (each question has five response categories), and so maximum scores on the original and new instruments are 200 and 160, respectively. Figure 22.10 shows the TCFs for the original and new instruments. Scores on each instrument corresponding to the same trait θ score are considered to be statistically equivalent – for example, a respondent with a trait score of $\theta = 0.10$ would have an expected score of 148 on the original 50-item instrument and an expected score of 78 on the new 40-item instrument. Though the two instruments vary in both length and difficulty, these two expected scores are considered statistically equivalent. Table 22.3 provides the complete conversion table for linking scores from the original instrument to the new one.

Any number of tailored instruments constructed from questions in an item bank can have scores statistically linked in exactly the same way. Of course, it is even easier to link scores from two instruments from the same item bank, since trait scores from any collection of items are reported on a common scale and therefore are directly comparable. Here, the instrument developer is capitalizing on the property of "ability parameter invariance." It is important,

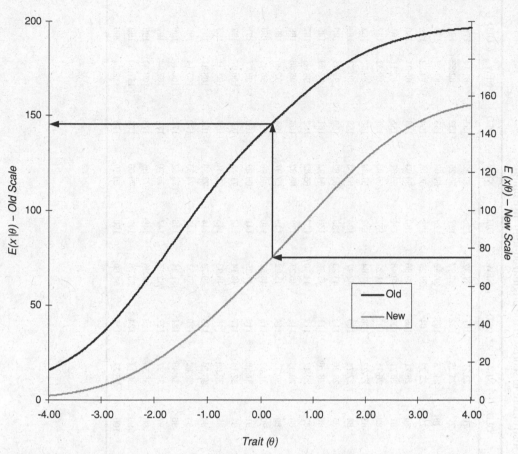

Figure 22.10   TCFs for obtaining a conversion of scores between the two instruments.

though, to keep in mind the standard error of each trait score in making any comparisons.

When we discuss the notion of "crosswalking scores" or "linking instruments together on a common metric," we are talking about linking two sets of items which measure the same construct (such as patient satisfaction). If the assumption of unidimensionality does not hold within both item sets, this IRT linking procedure cannot be carried out successfully. This method contrasts with other attempts by researchers to derive scores from one multidimensional instrument to predict scores on another multidimensional instrument. For example, Nichol *et al.*[13] use linear regression techniques to estimate a Health Utility Index score from scores from the SF-36. To use the IRT technique illustrated above, we would need to link scores from the two instruments on a domain-by-domain basis, i.e., link the depression items from Instrument A to depression items from Instrument B, link physical functioning items from Instrument A to physical functioning items from Instrument B, and so on.

Computerized adaptive assessment

The concept of computerized adaptive assessment (typically referred to as computer-adaptive testing, CAT, to denote its development in the field of educational measurement) is an extension of the idea expressed above. Respondents may be administered,

Table 22.3. Conversion table linking scores on the new instrument to scores on the original 50-item instrument

OLD	NEW	OLD	NEW	OLD	NEW	OLD	NEW	OLD	NEW	OLD	NEW	OLD	NEW	OLD	NEW
1	0.01	26	4.84	51	13.02	76	23.77	101	37.32	126	55.42	151	81.14	176	114.00
2	0.04	27	5.14	52	13.42	77	24.25	102	37.92	127	56.25	152	82.33	177	115.55
3	0.10	28	5.43	53	13.75	78	24.73	103	38.52	128	57.08	153	83.52	178	117.22
4	0.18	29	5.73	54	14.09	79	25.22	104	39.25	129	58.06	154	84.72	179	118.86
5	0.28	30	6.04	55	14.51	80	25.71	105	39.86	130	59.03	155	85.91	180	120.61
6	0.39	31	6.33	56	14.93	81	26.21	106	40.48	131	59.87	156	87.11	181	122.33
7	0.52	32	6.63	57	15.36	82	26.71	107	41.22	132	60.85	157	88.32	182	124.01
8	0.67	33	6.94	58	15.73	83	27.22	108	41.84	133	61.84	158	89.52	183	125.91
9	0.83	34	7.23	59	16.10	84	27.74	109	42.47	134	62.83	159	90.73	184	127.88
10	1.00	35	7.52	60	16.56	85	28.26	110	43.23	135	63.82	160	91.93	185	129.78
11	1.17	36	7.87	61	16.94	86	28.78	111	43.86	136	64.82	161	93.29	186	131.74
12	1.38	37	8.18	62	17.33	87	29.42	112	44.50	137	65.82	162	94.65	187	133.73
13	1.57	38	8.51	63	17.81	88	29.95	113	45.27	138	66.82	163	95.86	188	135.84
14	1.80	39	8.84	64	18.21	89	30.49	114	45.92	139	67.97	164	97.06	189	138.04
15	2.02	40	9.13	65	18.62	90	31.03	115	46.57	140	68.98	165	98.42	190	140.20
16	2.27	41	9.49	66	19.12	91	31.58	116	47.35	141	69.99	166	99.77	191	142.45
17	2.47	42	9.85	67	19.54	92	32.14	117	48.14	142	71.15	167	100.97	192	144.75
18	2.73	43	10.17	68	19.97	93	32.69	118	48.93	143	72.31	168	102.32	193	147.07
19	2.96	44	10.50	69	20.49	94	33.26	119	49.73	144	73.33	169	103.81	194	149.45
20	3.22	45	10.84	70	20.92	95	33.82	120	50.53	145	74.35	170	105.14	195	151.82
21	3.49	46	11.18	71	21.37	96	34.40	121	51.34	146	75.52	171	106.47	196	154.17
22	3.74	47	11.53	72	21.82	97	34.97	122	52.15	147	76.70	172	107.94	197	155.39
23	4.00	48	11.89	73	22.27	98	35.55	123	52.96	148	77.88	173	109.40	198	158.21
24	4.29	49	12.26	74	22.83	99	36.14	124	53.78	149	79.06	174	111.00	199	159.58
25	4.56	50	12.64	75	23.30	100	36.73	125	54.60	150	80.10	175	112.58	200	159.99

in principle, any set of items from the bank of items measuring the construct of interest, such as *satisfaction with medical care*. Trait scores estimated for respondents are comparable because the properties of the items (IRT item threshold and discrimination parameters) administered to separate respondents are taken into account in the trait estimation process. All trait scores are reported on the trait score scale and are comparable to each other or to benchmark (or cutoff) scores that may be placed on the trait score scale. One benchmark might be a point on the scale that represents "good health" as defined by a panel of experts. If respondents do not have to rate the same items in order to be compared, or even rate sets of items matched on difficulty, then they do not need to rate even the same number of items.

With computer-adaptive assessment, respondents are administered items that maximize the precision of trait estimation (high scoring respondents would generally see "harder" items and lower scoring respondents would generally see "easier" items). The corresponding information function for the items administered to each respondent is used to obtain a standard error, so that the respondent's scores can be compared to other respondent scores and to benchmarks. In addition, trait score distributions can be produced for the total group of respondents or any sub-groups of interest. Only enough items need be administered to a respondent to achieve some desired level of precision (for example, a standard error of about 0.33 is common). In principle then, the number of items administered to respondents in a CAT will be highly variable. Normally, respondents receive middle-difficulty items to start, and then they are branched to harder or easier items based upon their responses. If prior information were available about the respondent sample or even individual respondents, the information could be used to determine the best starting point for the computerized instrument administration. In practice, instrument length can usually be cut at least 50% with a CAT administration.

In summary, it is straightforward to link new items to the scale created by the original set of items (the original instrument), and it is straightforward to equate statistically various forms of instruments or even non-equivalent samples of items that may be constructed from the bank of calibrated items. And, with CAT, respondents may see unique sets of non-equivalent items and still be confidently compared with each other; alternatively, the trait scores could be combined for research studies. The key is to keep the standard error associated with each trait score low.

Detecting potentially biased test items

It is common for instrument developers to worry about item-level bias in their instruments. Item bias occurs when an item functions differently in two populations even though the differences between the populations on the measured construct have been determined or taken into account in the calculation of scores. Item bias is a source of invalidity in the instruments and should be removed. Such bias may be due to gender, race, age, culture, method of instrument administration (e.g., mail or telephone), educational background, use of language, or other factors. To the extent that bias is present, systematic errors are present in the instrument trait scores. IRT offers a convenient way to spot items that may be biased. Note the operative words here are "may be biased," because items identified as potentially biased may still be quite acceptable as measures of the construct of interest. Other times, problems are identified that highlight unfairness in the instrument. For example, some of the vocabulary or concepts may be unfamiliar to respondents for whom the instrument language is not their native (or first) language.

Figure 22.11 shows the plot of item difficulty parameter estimates (averaging across the four thresholds for each item) for males and females for the 50 items in the PSQ-III. What is expected is what is seen – a tight scatterplot about a straight line. The scatter, indicating departures from linearity, reflects sampling error. But there does appear to be one item, a b-value of −1.0 for females and −1.5 for males, which is somewhat off the best fitting line. This is

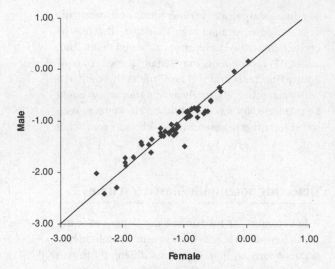

Figure 22.11.   Comparison of *b*-parameter estimates (50 items, reported on the Male scale).

the item, "I have easy access to the medical specialists I need." The expected score function is shown in Figure 22.12, and it suggests that the item is more favorable to males than to females. (The curve for females is the lower curve in the figure.) It appears that for males and females matched on trait scores (i.e., same levels of satisfaction), males are more likely to agree with this item than females. All things considered, it is more likely that the finding is correct and informative rather than representing some source of bias in the item. But the point must be checked prior to assuming that there is nothing about the item that places females at a disadvantage. Detection of biased items (or differential item functioning, DIF, in the IRT literature) must be carried out with the guidance of a content expert who can provide insight into the behaviors behind responses to the items.

Summary

In this chapter, we have discussed and illustrated several types of IRT analyses. We began by investigating the extent to which data from the Patient Satisfaction

with Medical Care Questionnaire (PSQ-III) meet the assumption of instrument unidimensionality when fitted by the two-parameter IRT graded response model (GRM) for polytomous response data. The assumption seems to be met by the data. We proceeded next to fit the GRM to the 50-item questionnaire and investigated the properties of the items and scale using the category response curves and the information functions. Possibilities for redesign were considered. Next, we demonstrated how 40 new items can be added to the original 50 items to create a *general satisfaction with medical care* item bank that serves as the foundation for the creation of short-form tailored instruments or computer-adaptive assessments. The issue of linking new items to the bank and the original trait scale was addressed using an anchor test design (in our example, including 10 items from the original instrument). A similar approach would be used to link different health-related instruments to a common scale. With the equating methods described above, we discussed how we can crosswalk scores from one instrument to another with use of the test characteristic function. Taking advantage of the invariance properties of the IRT models and the improvements in computer technology, we discussed the premise of computer-adaptive testing and how it can be incorporated in health outcomes assessment. Finally, an investigation of the PSQ-III instrument for potentially gender-biased items illustrated how IRT models can detect biased or differentially functioning items.

Item response theory is not a magic wand to wave over a vague definition of the construct of interest and a poorly written set of items to produce a reliable and valid instrument. But in the hands of serious instrument developers, IRT models such as the GRM for handling polytomous response data can provide many advantages for developing tests, equating forms, identifying bias, reporting scores, and making it feasible to implement innovative test designs such as computer-adaptive assessments. Hopefully, the examples in this chapter will prove to be useful to health-related instrument developers in their work. Readers are encouraged to study McHorney and Cook's review[15] (Invited Paper B in this volume)

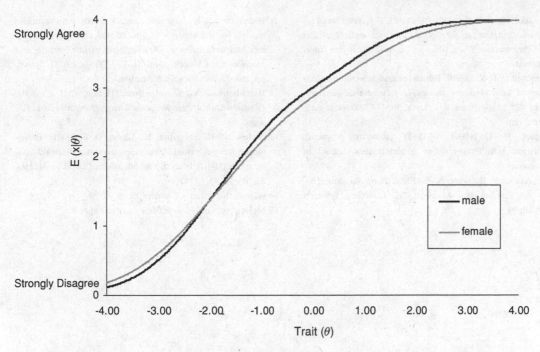

Figure 22.12. Comparison of male and female expected score functions for item 49 ("I have easy access to the medical specialists I need").

of the application of these IRT methods in health outcomes research. IRT would appear to be the measurement framework for the next generation of instruments.

Acknowledgment

The author wishes to acknowledge the important role of Tim O'Neil from the University of Massachusetts at Amherst in the preparation of this chapter. He was responsible for conducting many of the analyses, preparing the tables and figures, and assisting in the interpretation of results.

REFERENCES

1 Reise, this volume, Chapter 21.

2 Ware, J. E., Snyder, M. K., Wright, W. R. (1976). *Development and Validation of Scales to Measure Patient Satisfaction with Medical Care Services: Volume I, Part A. Review of Literature, Overview of Methods, and Results Regarding Construction of Scales.* NTIS Publication No. PB 288-329. Springfield, VA: National Technical Information Service.

3 Ware, J. E., Snyder, M. K., Wright, W. R. (1976). *Development and Validation of Scales to Measure Patient Satisfaction with Medical Care Services: Vol. I, part B. Results Regarding the Construction of the Patient Satisfaction Questionnaire and Measures of Other Health Care Perceptions.* NTIS Publication No. PB 288–330. Springfield, VA: National Technical Information Service.

4 Tarlov, A. R., Ware, J. E., Greenfield, S. *et al.* (1989). Medical outcomes study: an application of methods for evaluating the results of medical care. *Journal of the American Medical Association* 262:907–13.

5 Marshall, G. N., Hays, R. D., Sherbourne, C. D. *et al.* (1993). The structure of patient satisfaction with outpatient medical care. *Psychological Assessment* 5(4):477–83.

6 Samejima, F. (1969). Estimation of latent ability using a response pattern of graded scores. *Psychometrika Monograph* 17, Richmond, VA: William Byrd Press.

7 Muraki, E., Bock, R. D. (1993). *PARSCALE: IRT-based Test Scoring and Item Analysis for Graded and Open-ended Exercises and Performance Tasks*. Chicago: Scientific Software International.

8 Hambleton, R. K. (1989). Principles and selected applications of item response theory. In *Educational Measurement*, (3rd Edition), ed. R. L. Linn, pp. 147–200. New York: Macmillan.

9 Rogers, H. J. (1996). POLYFIT [software program]. Amherst, MA: University of Massachusetts School of Education.

10 Embretson, S. E., Reise, S. P. (2000). *Item Response Theory for Psychologists*. Mahwah, NJ: Lawrence Erlbaum Publishers.

11 Hambleton, R. K., Robin, F., Xing, D. (2000). Item response models for the analysis of educational and psychological test data. In *Handbook of Applied Multivariate Statistics and Mathematical Modeling*, ed. H. E. A. Tinsley, S. D. Brown, pp. 553–85. San Diego, CA: Academic Press.

12 Hambleton, R. K., Swaminathan, H., Rogers, H. J. (1991). *Fundamentals of Item Response Theory*. Newbury Park, CA: Sage.

13 Nichol, M. B., Sengupta, N., Globe, D. R. (2001). Evaluating quality-adjusted life years: estimation of the health utility index (HUI2) from the SF-36. *Medical Decision Making* **21**:105–12.

14 Wilson, this volume, Chapter 23.

15 McHorney, Cook, this volume, Invited Paper B.

23

Subscales and summary scales: issues in health-related outcomes

Mark Wilson, Ph.D.

University of California at Berkeley, Berkeley, CA

Introduction

Many regard health as a multidimensional construct. Correspondingly, a number of health-related quality-of-life (HRQOL) instruments are built around a framework of subscales,[1-3] with each subscale intended to capture a particular dimension (e.g., physical, social, emotional) of the overall construct (HRQOL). The validity of the total instrument is based on the strength of the validity of the underlying subscales. Not infrequently, the instrument's scoring algorithm will also allow the derivation of summary scores. That is, the items used to construct the instrument's N subscales are further aggregated to yield M (<N) summary scales; when M = 1, the instrument yields an overall summary score.[2]

A fundamental assumption in both Classical Test Theory (CTT) and Item Response Theory (IRT) is the unidimensionality of the latent trait. In the case at hand, this means the unidimensionality of each of the HRQOL instrument's subscales and, for that matter, the unidimensionality of any summary scales. If the analyst insists that health is a multidimensional construct, at least two important questions arise.

First, must we therefore derive and apply each subscale using information collected only from the items on *that* subscale, so that each subscale in the multidimensional construct essentially "floats on its own bottom"? Or, alternatively, is there some way to strengthen each subscale by drawing strength from the ensemble of information available across all related subscales? The central purpose of this chapter is to discuss and then demonstrate how multidimensional item response modeling (MIRM), an emerging subfield of modern measurement, may be applied to strengthen each subscale by capitalizing on relevant information possibly lurking in other subscales (or, strictly speaking, the items comprising those subscales).

One implication of this inquiry is that a traditionally derived (say, via unidimensional IRT) subscale with r items could be replaced by constructing a corresponding MIRM-derived subscale containing r' (< r) items, with no loss in reliability or construct validity. This could be especially important where time and resource constraints, including concerns about respondent burden, serve to limit the number of items that can be included on any one subscale. But, as will be seen, these advantages are obtained at the cost of greater computational complexity. Thus, the user ultimately has to weigh the benefits and costs of a MIRM strategy compared with today's dominant approach, which is to derive each subscale independently, or "consecutively," using only the items selected for that subscale.

The second question pertains to the derivation of summary scale and aggregate scale scores when one insists, at the same time, that health is a multidimensional construct comprising N fundamental subscales. Specifically, what are the available and defensible options for deriving summary and aggregate scores? We will necessarily touch on this question in the course of analyzing the first (and main) question, then discuss it briefly near the end.

Our illustrative analyses to compare subscale construction and performance under a MIRM approach versus the consecutive approach will be carried out with data from a recent application of the well-known SF-36 Health Survey. The SF-36 is a CTT-derived multidimensional instrument in which 35 out of its 36 items are used to create the following eight subscales (under the consecutive approach, of course): physical functioning (PF), role-physical (RP), bodily pain (BP), general health (GH), vitality (VT), social functioning (SF), role-emotional (RE), and mental health (MH). In addition, factor-analytical methods were applied to the 35 items to derive two summary scales: the physical health scale (PHS) and the mental health scale (MHS).[3] As Ware and Gandek note, the SF-36 has proven useful in comparing general and specific populations, estimating the relative burden of different diseases, differentiating the health benefits produced under a wide range of treatments, and screening individual patients.[3] A detailed assessment of the psychometric performance and characteristics of the SF-36 is reported in McHorney et al.[4]

We note at the outset that the analyses pursued in this chapter will be IRT (not CTT) based, and we will find it useful to derive eight subscales, two summary scales, and an aggregate health status scale, using raw data on the SF-36 items. This is all for the purpose of comparing the MIRM and unidimensional (consecutive) IRT-based approaches to scale development. While it might be of some interest, a further analysis comparing these findings with what would emerge from the current (CTT-based) SF-36 would entail a lengthy detour and, if done adequately, would not advance our central objective of examining the potential of multidimensional modeling to strengthen subscale construction.

The logic of subscale construction points to several issues that will be explored in the sections that follow.

First, establishing the validity of the entire instrument must entail the establishment of the validity of each of the subscales. Unfortunately, this basic step is often not closely attended to in instrument construction. The validity of the subscales is sometimes seen as self-evident, or is not brought into question. In the next section, we describe a framework, called the "four building blocks,"[5] that is designed to address the issue of the validity of each subscale in turn. (This framework could, and arguably should, be applied to the construction of any scale, not just the subscales in a multidimensional instrument.)

Second, whatever the intent of the instrument developer, users may want to utilize information from both the summary scales and the individual subscales. This leads to an important question: Which is better, the summary measure or the subscale measures (or can we find a way to have the advantages of both)? The third point is that the subscale measures may yield a description of the respondent, as a profile of subscale scores, that is more complex and hence potentially more useful than summary measure(s). Yet, the subscales themselves may each be less reliable than the summary measure(s), which reduces the confidence one places in that more complex portrait. To address this issue, a multidimensional item response model is introduced and applied in the section that follows. This MIRM is used to compare the summary scale and subscale perspectives, pointing the way to a compromise between the two perspectives. The chapter concludes with a brief discussion of the computational resources required to implement the MIRM approach.

The four building blocks

The perspective embraced in this chapter is that any instrument intended to measure a latent trait ought to embody a set of attributes that are detailed below in "The Four Building Blocks" of measurement: the construct map, items design, outcomes space, and the measurement model. While a consideration of these might appear, at first pass, to be a digression into elementary modern measurement, these building blocks in fact constitute important desiderata to the analysis of scales and subscales from a unidimensional or multidimensional item response perspective. Taken together, the building blocks define a conceptual framework for carrying out a MIRM analysis and for comparing the findings with subscales or scales derived via the traditional, consecutive approach. These building blocks will now be discussed in turn.

Construct map

An instrument always results from something more basic: first there is always an idea or a concept that is the theoretical object of our interest – this will be called the "construct" – and the instrument is designed on that basis. A construct could be part of a theoretical model of attitudes, say, towards well-being; or it could pertain to cognition about something, such as understanding of evolution; or it could relate to some other outcome variable, such as "need for achievement;" or a personality variable, such as a bipolar tendency. The construct could be from the domain of educational achievement, or it could be health related such as "quality of life," or a sociological construct such as stratification or migrant assimilation. The type of construct described in this chapter is one that is particularly suitable for a visual representation in what we call a *construct map*.

The most important features of a construct map[6] are that:

(1) there is a coherent and substantive definition for the content of the construct;

(2) there is an idea that the construct is composed of an underlying continuum; in other words, the respondents, in principle, can be ordered from more to less (or less to more) of the construct, so that one can make a comparison among pairs of respondents in terms of having more, the same, or less of the construct; and

(3) this continuum can be "mapped out" in terms of the responses to the items (either of individual items or groups of items).

In this conception (which, as we will see later, is consistent with the requirements of the Rasch item response theory model), the ordering of the respondents implies simultaneously an ordering of the items, and vice versa. The content of a construct is usually delimited by the intended use of the instrument. A construct can be most readily mapped where it has a single underlying continuum, implying that, for the intended use of the instrument, the measurer wants to array the respondents from high to low, or from one extreme to the other in some context. Note this does not imply that this ordering of the

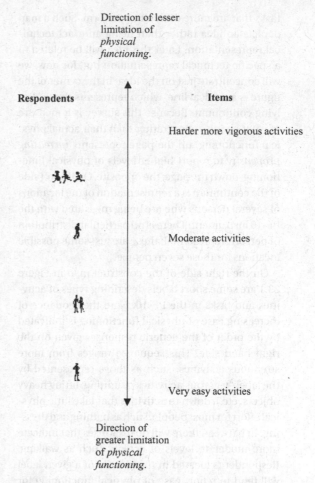

Figure 23.1. A construct map for a "physical functioning" instrument.

respondents is their only relevant feature. As mentioned above, where a construct has multiple underlying continua, the four building blocks approach can be applied to each in turn (which is, of course, the strategy to be deployed in this chapter).

One example of a construct that may be mapped in this way is the Physical Functioning subscale (PF-10) of the SF-36 health survey.[3,7] A sketch of the construct map for the PF-10 is shown in Figure 23.1. People who have less physical functioning would be placed below people who have more physical functioning. Likewise, activities or tasks that are easier to perform physically are located below activities or tasks that are more difficult to perform. Such a map depicts an idea rather than being an exact technical representation. Later this idea will be related to a specific technical representation but, for now, we will concentrate just on the idea. In the center of the figure is a vertical line, which represents the underlying continuum. Because this survey is a measure of what people report rather than their actual physical functioning, up the page represents *increasing propensity* to report higher levels of physical functioning; down the page, the opposite. On the left side of the continuum is a representation of the locations of several persons who are being measured with the PF-10 instrument. There is no particular distribution of persons represented; these are just some possible locations for these seven people.

On the right side of the construct map in Figure 23.1 are some short labels describing types of activities and tasks in the PF-10. Note the sequence of increasing ease of physical functioning is indicated by the order of the generic responses given on the right hand side. This sequence ranges from more strenuous activities, such as those represented by the label "vigorous activities" (running, lifting heavy objects, etc.), down to activities that take little physical effort for most people, such as bathing and dressing. In between there will be responses that indicate more moderate levels of activity such as walking. Respondents located in the vicinity of a given label will tend to report ease of physical functioning for those tasks implied by the label. Respondents located above that label will tend to report greater ease of physical functioning on those tasks, and respondents below that label will tend to report less ease of physical functioning on those same tasks.

Thus, the three people at the top of Figure 23.1, who are hence highest on the PF construct, would tend to respond positively to questions that ask about vigorous activities and all the activities below vigorous activities. But for the person lowest on Figure 23.1, just about the opposite would be true, that is, the person would tend to respond positively only to questions about activities requiring a very low level of physical functioning. People between the highest and lowest positions would tend to give answers that were somewhat in between these two extremes. The whole structure is a construct based on the idea of a continuum, and the representation is a construct map.

In the following sections, the remaining building blocks are described. These can guide the creation of an instrument on the basis of this construct map and, eventually, when data have been collected, they can facilitate a comparison of the empirical results with the original construct map. When the two are found to be consistent, this provides evidence supporting the *construct validity* of the instrument.

Items design

The measurer next must think of some way that this theoretical construct could be manifested in a real-world situation. At first, this will be not much more than a hunch, but later this hunch will become more crystallized and settle into a certain pattern. For example, the PF-10 items probably began as informal questions that a health researcher asked a patient. Typically, there will be more than one real-world manifestation used in the instrument; these parts of the instrument are generically called "items," and the way they are organized will be called the *items design*.

An item can take on many forms, but the most common in the HRQOL arena is probably the Likert-type item (i.e., with the possible responses ranging from "Strongly Agree" to "Strongly Disagree"). This is an example of a forced-choice item, where the respondent is given only a limited range of possible responses. There are many variants of this, ranging from questions about which activities a respondent prefers to a respondent's ranking of activities. The items design for the PF-10 is illustrated in Figure 23.2.

Outcome space

The next task is to make an inference from the persons' responses on questions to locate them on the construct map. The first step in the inference is a decision about which aspects of the response to the

The following items are about activities you might do during a typical day. Does your health now limit you in these activities? If so, how much?

1. Vigorous activities, such as running, lifting heavy objects, participating in strenuous sports (*Vigorous Activities*)
2. Moderate activities, such as moving a table, pushing a vacuum cleaner, bowling, or playing golf (*Moderate Activities*)
3. Lifting or carrying groceries (*Lift/Carry*)
4. Climbing several flights of stairs (*Several Stairs*)
5. Climbing one flight of stairs (*One Flight Stairs*)
6. Bending, kneeling, or stooping (*Bend/Kneel/Stoop*)
7. Walking more than a mile (*Walk More Mile*)
8. Walking several blocks (*Walk Several Blocks*)
9. Walking one block (*Walk One Block*)
10. Bathing or dressing yourself (*Bathing/Dressing*)

Figure 23.2. Items designed for the "physical functioning" subscale (PF-10) of the SF-36.[*]

[*] The 36-Item Health Survey was developed at RAND as part of the Medical Outcomes Study. Items reprinted with permission.

item will be used as the basis for the inference and how those aspects of the response will be categorized and then scored. This defines the *outcome space*.[8] Examples of outcome spaces include responses of "strongly disagree" to "strongly agree" in a Likert-type instrument; the question and prompt protocols in a standardized open-ended interview[9] and the subsequent categorization of the responses; and the translation of a physical performance into ordered levels using a "scoring guide."

Sometimes the categories themselves are the final product of the outcome space, and sometimes the categories are scored in such a way that they can (a) serve as convenient labels for the outcome categories, and (b) be manipulated in various ways. To emphasize this distinction, the latter case may be called a "scored" outcome space. The original (fixed-choice) outcome space for the PF-10 construct has three categories: "Yes, limited a lot," "Yes, limited a little," and "No, not limited at all." But to simplify the analysis, one may choose to re-score these three into dichotomous categories: Both the "Yes" options are scored 0, and the "No" response is scored 1. (While

such a dichotomization is not required, of course, we adopt it here for the empirical analyses below.)

Measurement model

The final building block in the design of the instrument is the measurement model. Its purpose is to provide a principled way to use the information about respondents and responses, as coded in the outcome space, to locate *both* the respondents *and* the item responses on the construct map. This requires that the measurement model be based on item response theory rather than classical test theory, as Reise discusses elsewhere in this volume.[10] In CTT, the respondent locations on the underlying continuum of interest are reflected by their "true scores" (T), estimated on the basis of their raw scores (X) with allowance for measurement error (E); specifically, the relationship is expressed as $X = T + E$. Unfortunately, this framework provides no straightforward way to locate the item responses on the same metric as the respondents, which means the items themselves (or, more precisely, their scale "locations") can play no formal role in assessing the construct validity of the scale once estimated.

Any measurement model that does allow respondents and items to be located on the same metric (in line with the fourth building block) must enable one, *ipso facto*, to

(1) interpret the distance between respondent and item response options on the construct map, and
(2) interpret the distance between different item responses on the construct map (and also the difference between different respondents).

To make sense of these requirements, we must explain what "distance" means. On a geographical map, distance and direction have meaning with respect to the surface of the earth. For example, 1 mile north might equal 1 inch "up" the map. On the construct maps in this chapter, distance between respondents and responses will indicate, and be gauged by, the *probability* of making that response. To express this mathematically, assume that person n's position on the construct map is represented by

θ_n and the location of item i is represented by δ_i. Then the probability that person n will choose the positive response to the item, Prob(positive response), will be given by some function, f, of the "difference" between the person and the item:

$$\text{Prob(positive response)} = f(\theta_n - \delta_i). \qquad (23.1)$$

This can be interpreted as follows:

(1) a zero distance between a person and an item would mean that person is likely to choose the positive response with a certain pre-specified probability (conventionally set at 0.50);
(2) a person located *above* a response on the construct map would indicate a greater (than 0.50) probability of choosing the positive response;
(3) a person located *below* a response on the construct map would indicate a lesser (than 0.50) probability of choosing the positive response.

If the logistic function is then chosen as the function f in Equation 23.1, the resulting model is known as the Rasch[11] model, which can be used as a foundation for more complex models. Denote person n's response to item i as X_{ni}, with 1 indicating a positive response and 0, a negative response. Then, under the Rasch model, the probability of a positive response is

$$\text{Prob}(X_{ni} = 1 | \theta_n, \delta_i) = \frac{e^{(\theta_n - \delta_i)}}{1 + e^{(\theta_n - \delta_i)}} \qquad (23.2)$$

The logistic function is a natural choice for f, since it allows one to map discrete choice (for example, yes-no) responses onto the 0–1 continuum, as probability theory requires. It can readily be shown that the logistic model implies that the difference, $\theta_n - \delta_i$, can be expressed as $\ln[\text{Prob}(X_{ni} = 1) / \text{Prob}(X_{ni} = 0)] = \theta_n - \delta_i$. That is, the distance between respondent and item (or between any two respondents, or between any two items) can be expressed as the log odds ratio, so that the logit becomes the fundamental unit of measurement on the scale. Moreover, there is a direct, albeit nonlinear, correspondence between the logit and the probability that person n will endorse item i: the greater the positive (negative) distance between the person and the item, the higher (lower) the probability the person will endorse the item. Table 23.1 provides a summary of convenient benchmarks for this translation.

Table 23.1. Logit differences and probabilities for the Rasch model

$\theta - \delta$	Probability
−4.0	0.02
−3.0	0.05
−2.0	0.12
−1.0	0.27
0.0	0.50
1.0	0.73
2.0	0.88
3.0	0.95
4.0	0.98

Equation 23.2 can be readily expanded to include the possibility of polytomous items (e.g., the partial credit, rating scale, and graded response models[12–14]), and the incorporation of other item characteristics such as the "slope" parameter (which indicates that some items may have a more intense relationship with the underlying latent variable than others[15]). Note that this extension, including such an item-by-item varying slope parameter, is not compatible with the fundamental idea of the construct map as discussed here.[5] In particular, it would lead to a violation of the requirements for using the construct map, as given in (1)–(3) on p. 470. (This is because the slope parameter of non-Rasch models – which, in general, varies item-by-item – interacts with, and therefore does not leave invariant, the "true" distance between a person and an item, as defined in Equation 23.1.) Some specific varieties of item response models, including ones that include slope parameters, are introduced in two other chapters in this volume.[10,16]

The PF-10 scale has already been described above, and we discussed how the three response categories recognized in its outcome space can be collapsed into two; this means recoding the responses "Limited a lot" and "Limited a little" to "0," and recoding "Not limited at all" to "1." Using a large data set of patients' responses to these PF-10 items,[4] we have generated

```
          Respondents              Item  Responses
 Logit    Score

          (less limited)                 Vigorous Activities
  4.0                            |
                                 |
          9  XXXXXXXXXXXXXXXXXXXX |
  3.0                            |
                                 |
                                 |
          8  XXXXXXXXXXXXXXX     |
  2.0                            |
                                 |
                                 |  Several Stairs
          7  XXXXXXXXXXXXXX      |
                                 |  Walk More Mile
  1.0                            |
          6  XXXXXXXXXXXX        |  Bend/Kneel/Stoop
                                 |  Moderate Activities
   .0     5  XXXXXXXXXXX         |
                                 |  Lift/Carry
                                 |  Walk Several Blocks
          4  XXXXXXXXXX          |
 -1.0                            |  One Flight Stairs
                                 |
          3  XXXXXXX             |
 -2.0                            |
                                 |
          2  XXXXXXX             |  Walk One Block
 -3.0                            |
                                 |
          1  XXXXXXXXXX          |
 -4.0                            |
          (more limited)         |  Bathing/Dressing
```

Figure 23.3. A Wright map for the dichotomized PF-10 instrument (each X represents approximately 18 respondents).

and displayed in Figure 23.3 an empirical version of a construct map, called a "Wright map" (in honor of Benjamin D. Wright of the University of Chicago Department of Education).

The Wright map allows one to check for evidence of construct validity by investigating how well the instrument designer's intentions, as represented in the construct map, are reflected by empirical results and, specifically, by the item locations on the Wright map. Comparing this Wright map in Figure 23.3 to

the construct map in Figure 23.1, we can notice several ways in which they differ. First, the Wright map is not just a sketch of the idea of the construct, but rather an empirical map based on respondents' self-reports. A histogram of the respondents is shown on the left-hand side of the map. It is vertically oriented, which is unusual for a histogram, to make it match the orientation of the construct map. What is even more unusual is that the bars of this histogram are not evenly arrayed. That is because the locations of the bars are the *estimated* locations of the respondents, which can take on real number values; they need not be located at integer values as are raw scores. Each bar corresponds to a particular score. Thus the location of the respondents who had a raw score of 5 is 0.04 (which is indistinguishable from 0.0 in Figure 23.3). And the difference between the locations for those respondents who scored 5 and those who scored 6 is less than that between the locations for those who scored 6 and 7. The units for that continuous scale are shown on the far left-hand side, in the column headed "logit," which are units of the difference $(\theta_n - \delta_i)$ in Equations 23.1 and 23.2, as discussed above. Each location (i.e., each histogram bar) corresponds to a raw score on the instrument, ranging from 1 to 9. Thus a respondent with a score of 1 is estimated to be located at -3.65 logits, and a respondent with a score of 6 is located at 0.65 logits.

Most researchers find it useful to translate the logits back into probabilities. To do this using Table 23.1, just find the difference between the respondent location and the item location, then look up the probability. (If a probability table is not readily accessible, one can always resort to a calculator to compute the probability from Equation 23.2.) These logits can also be re-scaled by any linear transformation to values that typical users of the information might find more comfortable (e.g., eliminating negative numbers) while retaining the same mathematical relationship with the probabilities.

The right hand side of the map in Figure 23.3 shows the *calibrated* item locations; these correspond to the δ's in Equation 2. Notice, for instance, that the respondents with a score of 6 are at the same point on the map as the "Bend/Kneel/Stoop" item. This means that they have approximately a 50% probability of responding "Not limited at all" to that item. Noting that the item "Several Stairs" is about 1 logit above this location, we can see from Table 23.1 that the probability these same respondents would render the response "Not limited at all" to this particular item is approximately 0.27. And noting that "Walk Several Blocks" is about 1 logit below this location, we can say that the probability of respondents with a raw score of 6 giving this same response

("Not limited at all") to that item is approximately 0.73. Using the benchmarks in Table 23.1, the reader can practice translating the logit differences implicit in Figure 23.3 into probability statements about expectations for respondents giving a "Not limited at all" response.

There are many issues and possibilities that one could pursue with the results illustrated in Figure 23.3 in hand. For example, an investigation of fit is a very important step in any such analysis, but the central issue at the moment is whether the intent of the construct map has been realized, so we will dispense with that otherwise essential element. That is, how well has the empirical Wright map replicated the intended 3-level construct map? In this case, if one judges the "Vigorous Activities" question in the PF-10 to belong to the highest level in Figure 23.1, the "Walk One Block" and the "Bathing/Dressing" questions as belonging to the lowest level, and the remaining questions as all belonging in the middle category, then the rank correlation between the Wright map and the construct map is 0.83. The two rankings are very close, even though the construct map is divided into only three levels, and for all practical purposes we can conclude they are essentially the same. (The rank correlation is typically the appropriate measure here: an expectation like that shown in Figure 23.1 will be a qualitative one based on theory, and there will be, at most, a ranking of the expected locations.) The high correlation found here should not be surprising: the expectations shown in the construct map (Figure 23.1) were based on the accumulation of experiences from many years, many researchers, and many studies.[3] From the CTT perspective, the PF-10 subscale has long demonstrated strong construct validity.[17]

Multidimensional models and the "balance of error"

Having examined how to look at the construct of a subscale of a HRQOL instrument (using an IRT-derived version of the PF-10 as the example), we shift back to the larger perspective of the

Table 23.2. Two fictitious respondents to the SF-36.

Summary Scale	Sub Scales	Sid	Nancy
Physical health (PHS)		60	38
	physical functioning	65	30
	role-physical	60	28
	bodily pain	80	40
	general health	30	50
Mental health (MHS)		20	42
	vitality	30	40
	social functioning	5	45
	role emotional	25	35
	mental health	15	38

Table 23.3. Reliability coefficients for the SF-36 models.[a]

		Approach	
Scale	# Items	Consecutive	Multidimensional
Subscales			
General Health (GH)	5	0.80	0.86
Physical Functioning (PF)	10	0.94	0.94
Role-Physical (RP)	4	0.76	0.94
Role-Emotional (RE)	3	0.68	0.89
Social Functioning (SF)	2	0.74	0.92
Bodily Pain (BP)	2	0.72	0.93
Vitality (VT)	4	0.89	0.96
Mental Health (MH)	5	0.91	0.93
Summary scales			
Physical Health Scale (PHS)	21	0.98	0.91
Mental Health Scale (MHS)	14	0.99	0.97

[a] Note: Reliability for the Omnibus Summary Scale was 0.92.

multidimensional (multi-construct) instrument. If each of the eight (SF-36 item-based) subscales we derive independently passed muster as an instrument – according to the Four Building Blocks paradigm – the whole instrument can be seen as measuring an 8-dimensional construct; call this the *subscales perspective*. At the same time, it is possible that summary scales, including a physical health scale (PHS) and a mental health scale (MHS), both derived anew here from the SF-36 items *via* IRT, will likewise pass muster. If so, the whole instrument can be seen as measuring a 2-dimensional construct; call this the *summary scale perspective*. (Of course, the limiting case of the latter is when a single aggregate scale is derived.) If the eight subscales do not individually pass muster but the summary scales do, then the summary scale perspective is the appropriate one.

Consider a pair of fictitious respondents, Sid and Nancy, to illustrate this issue. Assume for simplicity that each of the summary scales (including a total scale) and the subscales have been re-scaled to have a range of 0 to 100, with lower scores representing a poorer quality of life. Suppose that both Sid and Nancy have total (overall) scores of 40 and that their patterns of subscale and summary scale (PHS and MHS) scores are as shown in Table 23.2. While Sid and Nancy have the same total score, the interpret-

ation of what the total "means" would appear to differ markedly: Sid is much more variable than Nancy at the PHS/MHS summary scale level, and the same is reflected at the level of the eight subscales.

For an overall evaluation of a program's effectiveness, a policy maker may not be concerned by this underlying variability: the overall summary may be satisfactory, or the PHS/MHS level of summary may suffice in level of detail. However, a clinician or a policy analyst concerned about how an intervention affects various aspects of HRQOL will likely regard as important the more detailed information available at the 8-subscale level, and would be keenly interested in (if not disturbed by) the variability hidden in the higher levels of summary.

So the crucial question is: can one have both perspectives without losing too much of the instrument's good measurement characteristics? An initial answer to that question is found in the column labeled "Consecutive" in Table 23.3. This shows the subscale and summary scale reliabilities, with each scale having been derived "consecutively" using information from only the items assumed to comprise the scale itself. The reliabilities in this column suggest that the answer is "sometimes yes, sometimes no." A strong determining factor is the number of items in the subscale. The PF-10 is doing as well (in terms of reliability) as the Omnibus Summary Scale (the total score scale) and almost as well as the PHS summary scale. The VT and MH subscales, even though they have only 4 and 5 items, respectively, are doing just about as well as the PF. (Note that both the VT and MH items have six response categories, which similarly enhances reliability.) But most of the smaller subscales (RP, RE, SF, BP) are not doing very well, as indicated by reliabilities that are considerably lower. In contrast, the PHS and MHS summary scales are doing very well.

Although one can almost invariably increase reliability to acceptable levels just by increasing the number of items in each subscale, this is not possible in many practical situations, particularly where respondent burden will mean that answers are either missing or not trustworthy. Thus, one is forced into an unwanted trade-off situation where the need for more detailed information must be balanced against the need to keep the instrument short – one might call this the "balance of error." This conflict between response burden and measurement error is reflected in the HRQOL context as a conflict between the need for detailed information (subscale perspective) and the need to summarize a patient's health status in an aggregate way to make policy decisions (summary scale perspective). One must seek further options in order to break out of this impasse.

This is where multidimensional item response models come into the picture. MIRMs open up the possibility of bringing the full information from all of the items into the estimation of each individual subscale. In MIRMs, observations may be related to multiple constructs.[18,19] For instance, responses to questions about a person's general health might be attributable to the respondent's perception of their general well-being, as well as their perceptions of specific aspects of their health. The multiple subscales of an instrument (the SF-36, for example) can thus be considered multiple dimensions of health.

There are both technical and practical reasons for using a multidimensional model of this sort to describe a subscale context. In technical terms, if one is interested, for example, in finding the pairwise correlations between the respondents' perceptions of (overall) physical health and their perceptions of specific aspects of physical health, a multidimensional model allows one to make an unbiased estimate of this correlation. This contrasts with the consecutive approach, which produces correlations that tend to be reduced (biased in a downward direction) due to unreliability in the subscales.[20,21] In practical terms, as pointed out above, there are often situations where one is constrained to obtain responses on fewer items per subscale than would be optimal. This can be both planned, such as when one can afford to gather information on only a small number of items for each subscale, and unplanned, such as when there is a lot of missing data in a long survey form or in a longitudinal measurement design. In such situations, multidimensional models can effectively compensate for data sparseness by using the available information from one subscale to improve estimation on another.

The relationship of the Four Building Blocks approach to assessing the construct validity of such a multidimensional measurement model is straightforward: the construct validity of each of the subscales is established and investigated, in turn, using the principles incorporated in the building blocks. The multidimensional model is *confirmatory*; hence, its usefulness is dependent on the (demonstrated) validity of the subscales. This is in contrast to the situation in classical (exploratory) factor analysis, where the usefulness of the subscales is dependent on the validity of the measurement model. Once the data are gathered, the multidimensional model makes maximum use of the information to generate unbiased estimates of the pairwise correlations between subscales. These cross-scale correlations are the vehicles for bringing full-sample information to bear on the estimation of each subscale. The larger (in absolute value) these correlations, the stronger the cross-scale effects; on the other hand, were the correlations (essentially) zero, the subscale estimates from the multidimensional approach would be essentially the same as under the consecutive approach.

We now implement the MIRM approach with a particular measurement model that can be viewed as a direct extension of the model in Equation 2. Dubbed the multidimensional random coefficients multinomial logit model (MRCML model) by its authors,[20,21] it permits the subscales to be calibrated simultaneously so that the estimated pairwise relationships between the subscales are not biased by measurement error (as can be the case under an alternative, "concurrent" approach to estimation[22]).

There is also allowance both for items that are on only one subscale and items that are on more than one subscale. The former is often called a "between-item" situation, and the latter, a "within-item" situation.[20,21] Consider a very simple example with two dimensions (and thus subscales) and three dichotomous items, wherein the first item is on the first subscale, the second is on the second subscale, and the third is on both subscales. The equivalent MRCML model would be:

$$\text{Probability}(X_{n1} = 1 | \theta_{1n}, \delta_1) = \frac{e^{(\theta_{1n} - \delta_1)}}{1 + e^{(\theta_{1n} - \delta_1)}}$$

$$\text{Probability}(X_{n2} = 1 | \theta_{2n}, \delta_2) = \frac{e^{(\theta_{2n} - \delta_2)}}{1 + e^{(\theta_{2n} - \delta_2)}} \qquad (23.3)$$

$$\text{Probability}(X_{n3} = 1 | \theta_{1n}, \theta_{2n}, \delta_3) = \frac{e^{(\theta_{1n} + \theta_{2n} - \delta_3)}}{1 + e^{(\theta_{1n} + \theta_{2n} - \delta_3)}}$$

where now θ_{dn} is the measure of person n on dimension d, and the other symbols are as defined earlier. Thus the two dimensions are "between items" for items 1 and 2, and "within items" for item 3. This model can be described in a quite general setting,[20,21] and examples of its use in diverse contexts can be found in the literature.[20,21,23-28] Just as the inclusion of a slope parameter is incompatible with the use of a construct map in the unidimensional case,[5] as noted when Equation 23.2 was discussed, the same is true in the multidimensional case.

To estimate the full MRCML model for all eight subscales and also two summary scales, we applied the ConQuest software[28] to the complete set of SF-36 item responses. The computational algorithm is based on an iterative maximum likelihood procedure that yields, in the end, estimates of each respondent along each subscale or summary scale, estimates of each item along each applicable scale (depending on whether the situation is between-item or within-item), and estimates of all pairwise correlations between scales. (For each subscale, one can envision the final product as portrayed symbolically in Figure 23.3.)

Also emerging from these computations are the subscale and summary scale reliabilities, and these are shown in Table 23.3 under the heading "Multidimensional." It is immediately evident that the reliabilities for the subscales that were low under the Consecutive approach are now considerably higher; and, arguably, *all* of the subscale reliabilities are now high enough to be used for the measurement of individuals (though some may raise doubts about GH). Thus, we illustrate how we can break free from the unwanted "balance of error" between number of items and number of subscales by drawing on the total information in the response vector to support the measurement in each subscale.

Of course, the gain is not without cost. The advantages of using all of the respondent's information in the estimation of each subscale might also be seen as generating some less-than-desirable byproducts or implications. The estimated θ for a person on any given subscale will now be sensitive to (a) the responses that person made on the subscale, and (b) the locations of that person on the other subscales. The effects of these other subscales will be influenced by the correlation of the various subscales, and this will mean that two respondents with the same response pattern within a given subscale may not have the same estimated θ when the rest of the response string is used. Essentially, the responses on all the other subscales will tend to act as a "damper" on the estimates within that subscale.

As in the "simple" unidimensional case, the Four Building Blocks are of central relevance to the assessment of the subscales and summary scales obtained under this multidimensional approach; in particular, the construct map and the Wright map retain their interpretability. In a MIRM approach, the construct validity of each subscale is built up (individually) guided by the principles embodied in the Four Building Blocks. Parenthetically, it is interesting to note that, in contrast, the summary scale reliabilities are higher for the consecutive approach than for the multidimensional approach, although only one is substantially higher. This might be a fluke, or it might indicate a limit to the advantage of the multidimensional approach. Further research will be necessary to determine which is the case.

Deriving an aggregate score for a multidimensional instrument

For certain types of studies, e.g., the evaluation of interventions or the tracking of population trends in HRQOL, the analyst may want an overall summary measure of the multidimensional construct. As far as we can see, there are two broad options, each of which entail assumptions that some may find objectionable.

(1) *Item aggregation.* Submit all, or a selected subset, of the items from which the N subscales are constructed to a standard unidimensional IRT (or, if one is so inclined, CTT) analysis to derive one overall scale for something called "health-related quality of life." From an IRT perspective, the model would be in the spirit of Equation 23.2. This is precisely how we derived, using the SF-36 items, the Omnibus Summary Scale whose reliability is reported in Table 23.3.

There might be the concern, however, that the same items being employed judiciously to estimate N purportedly unidimensional subscales are, at the same time, fully capable of estimating one unidimensional summary scale. Thus there is the risk of an ill-defined summary construct. While unidimensionality is an ideal that is never perfectly realized, this approach does suggest there is some unresolved "tension" between assuming and confirming that valid subscales exist, and then proceeding, for practical reasons, to produce a global summary scale using (some subset of) the very same items. If one estimates both the unidimensional (summary) model and the multidimensional model, care must

be taken not to confuse the two sets of estimated parameters and scales. Ways have been proposed to set up the analysis so that the two sets of results share a similar metric,[29] but there is no established tradition for how this is to be done. Finally, one must be aware that when multiple subscales are contributing items to the summary scale, the greater the number of items on a given subscale, the greater its potential influence *ipso facto* in the estimated summary scale.

(2) *Subscale aggregation.* Derive an aggregate score for HRQOL by adding up the subscale scores, on a weighted or unweighted basis. This option further divides into two pathways: (1) aggregations that use only information internal to the scale estimation process, and (2) aggregations that employ also external information, e.g., preference weights supplied by the decision maker, to achieve the subscale aggregation.

There are numerous examples of (1), especially in CTT-based subscales where the total scale score is simply the straight sum of item scores; for example, see the Brady *et al.* analysis of the well-known FACT-G instrument.[30] (We note that the FACT-G now also offers the option of computing an IRT-based "standardized" score derived via the single-scale approach described in the first bullet; personal communication with David Cella.) To pursue scale-score aggregations in a CTT-based framework is to assume that these scores can be defensibly melded into a conceptually interpretable total score. In an IRT framework, it is not clear what the theoretical requirements or justifications are for direct subscale score summation.

Under pathway (2), the analyst would derive a summary score as a weighted average of subscale scores, where the weight for each subscale would reflect a judgment about its relative importance in forming the total picture. One possibility is that the weights would be derived from preferences scores, indicating the relative importance of the subscale dimension in the overall calculus of HRQOL. See Chapter 4 by Feeny in this volume for a detailed discussion of the derivation and use of preference weights to compute quality-adjusted life-year measures.[31] To our knowledge, psychometrically derived subscales, either by CTT or IRT, have not yet been aggregated via preference weighting, but this remains one possible option for coming up with an aggregate measure of HRQOL, and would be consistent with the MRCML approach.

Discussion

This chapter has provided a framework for relating the qualitative, conceptual foundations of instrument development to the quantitative, empirical results obtained when one actually measures a person's HRQOL. This framework, called the Four Building Blocks, consists of the Construct Map, Items Design, Outcome Space, and Measurement Model. The items in the PF-10 subscale of the SF-36 Health Survey were used to illustrate the steps through the building blocks, culminating in the Wright Map in Figure 23.3. When the empirical results in the Wright map match the qualitative intentions in the construct map, the instrument can be said to show evidence of construct validity. In an instrument composed of multiple constructs, where one wants to estimate a person's standing on each construct (the subscale perspective), this process should be repeated for each subscale.

Of course, there are other measurement issues besides construct validity that need to be considered, and reliability is one that is very prominent. Reliability becomes critical when one is contrasting the summary scale perspective (where the focus is on measuring overall summary measures) with the subscales perspective (where the focus is on measuring each subscale). This is because practical issues of respondent burden work to minimize the number of questions that can be asked, and hence can severely limit the number of items within each subscale. In our Rasch-based illustrative analysis of the SF-36 items, this meant that four of the eight subscales we estimated had low reliabilities. Multidimensional measurement models offer one way to break out of this dilemma, because they allow the estimation to take advantage of *all* the information in a person's responses to the entire set of questions. When

applied to the SF-36 raw data here, multidimensional measurement resulted in greatly improved reliabilities for those subscales that had low reliabilities when scaled on their own. Although this is an important advantage, there are some trade-offs in embracing the MIRM approach, and these were discussed.

This introductory discussion of the relationships between subscales and summary scales has been primarily focused at a conceptual, rather than technical level. In addition, there is a rich historical debate about many of these issues, and that has not been reviewed. The aim here has been to illustrate some of the major ideas and issues so that the interested reader can begin to explore the techniques, their backgrounds, and applications themselves.

Practical considerations: learning more about these methods

What are the software options for the outcomes researcher who wants to use multidimensional modeling? The *ConQuest* package[28] was successfully used to carry out the analyses in this chapter. While it is possible to extract results out of this program without much literacy in item response modeling, interpreting those results appropriately requires a basic familiarity with IRT and applied statistics (or consultants who can bring this knowledge and experience to bear). Another recent software program that is available is Muthen's *M-Plus*.[32] While this program starts from a different perspective than ConQuest, it can be used in a similarly wide range of situations, including multidimensional applications.[33] The SAS procedure NLMIXED can also be used to calibrate multidimensional item response models.[34]

Recommendation for further research and applications

We need to better understand how to communicate the results of multidimensional analyses and make them more interpretable to researchers and other users of information from multidimensional scales. (Of course, the same perhaps holds true for all of item response theory.) In particular, new ways to display the relationships among the potentially many dimensions are needed – ways that encompass the complexity of multidimensional covariation.

As well, we need standard approaches for presenting the results of such multidimensional analyses within the HRQOL context, for use with contemporary instruments such as the FACT-G and the EORTC QLQ-C30. Most likely, this would be best done in a computerized format, since the multiplicity of the inter-relationships makes it difficult to convey patterns in a static paper format.

Beyond that, there are many interesting and important issues that arise in the application of measurement models to HRQOL. By analogy to the situation in the psychometric modeling of cognition, there are a host of measurement approaches that can be applied to modeling the potential complexities of HRQOL constructs[35] and to incorporating substantive data analyses to enhance the overall quality of measurement.[36]

Acknowledgments

I would like to thank Derek Briggs and Diane Allen of UC Berkeley Graduate School of Education for providing analyses, reflections, and advice for this paper. I would also like to thank Bryce Reeve for arranging for me to have access to the data used and for very helpful comments and perspectives.

REFERENCES

1 Aaronson, N. K., Ahmedzai, S., Bergman, B. *et al.* (1993). The European Organization for Research and Treatment of Cancer QLQ-C30: a quality-of-life instrument for use in international clinical trials in oncology. *Journal of the National Cancer Institute* 85:365–76.

2 Cella, D. F., Tulsky, D. S., Gray, G. *et al.* (1993). The Functional Assessment of Cancer Therapy scale: development and validation of the general measure. *Journal of Clinical Oncology* 11:570–9.

3 Ware, J. E., Gandek, B. (1998). Overview of the SF-36 Health Survey and the International Quality of Life Assessment (IQOLA) Project. *Journal of Clinical Epidemiology* 51: 903–12.

4 McHorney, C. A., Ware, J. E., Lu, J. F. R. *et al.* (1994). The MOS 36-Item Short-Form Health Survey (SF-36): III. Tests of data quality, scaling assumptions and reliability across diverse patient groups. *Medical Care* 32(4):40–66.

5 Wilson, M. (2001). On choosing a model for measuring. Paper presented at the *International Conference on Objective Measurement 3*, Chicago, IL.

6 Masters, G. N., Adams, R. A., Wilson, M. (1990). Charting student progress. In *International Encyclopedia of Education: Research and Studies. Supplementary Volume 2*, ed. T. Husen, T. N. Postlethwaite, pp. 628–34. Oxford: Pergamon Press.

7 Raczek, A. E., Ware, J. E., Bjorner, J. B. *et al.* (1998). Comparison of Rasch and summated rating scales constructed from the SF-36 Physical Functioning items in seven countries: Results from the IQOLA Project. *Journal of Clinical Epidemiology* 51:1203–11.

8 Masters, G. N., Wilson, M. (1997). Developmental Assessment. *Berkeley Evaluation and Assessment Research Center Research Report.* University of California, Berkeley. (see http://bear.soe.berkeley.edu/)

9 Patton, M. Q. (1980). *Qualitative Evaluation Methods.* Beverly Hills, CA: Sage.

10 Reise, this volume, Chapter 21.

11 Rasch, G. (1960). *Probabilistic Models for Some Intelligence and Attainment Tests.* Copenhagen: Danmarks Paedogogiske Institut. [also, 1980 University of Chicago Press, Chicago]

12 Andrich, D. (1978). A rating formulation for ordered response categories. *Psychometrika* 43:561–73.

13 Masters, G. N. (1981). A Rasch model for partial credit scoring. *Psychometrika* 47:149–74.

14 Samejima, F. (1969). *Estimation of Latent Ability Using a Response Pattern of Graded Scores.* Psychometrika Monograph Supplement No. 17.

15 Hambleton, R. K., Swaminathan, H., Rogers, H. J. (1991). *Fundamentals of Item Response Theory.* Newbury Park: Sage.

16 Hambleton, this volume, Chapter 22.

17 American Educational Research Association, American Psychological Association, National Council for Measurement in Education. (1999). *Standards for Educational and Psychological Testing.* Washington, DC: American Educational Research Association.

18 Reckase, M. D. (1972). *Development and Application of a Multivariate Logistic Latent Trait Model.* Unpublished doctoral dissertation, Syracuse University, Syracuse, NY.

19 Sympson, J. B. (1978). A model for testing with multi-dimensional items. In *Proceedings of the 1977 Computerized Adaptive Testing Conference*, ed. D. J. Weiss, pp. 82–98. Minneapolis: University of Minnesota, Dept. of Psychology, Psychometric Methods Program.

20 Adams, R. J., Wilson, M. (1995). Formulating the Rasch model as a mixed coefficients multinomial logit. In *Objective Measurement: Theory into Practice. Volume III*, ed. G. Engelhard & M. Wilson, pp. 143–66. Norwood, NJ: Ablex.

21 Adams, R., Wilson, M., Wang, W. (1997). The multidimensional random coefficient multinomial logit model. *Applied Psychological Measurement* **21**(1):1–23.

22 Davey, T., Hirsch, T. M. (1991). Concurrent and consecutive estimates of examinee ability profiles. Paper presented at the Annual Meeting of the Psychometric Society, New Brunswick, NJ.

23 Briggs, D. C., Wilson, M. (2003). An introduction to multidimensional measurement using Rasch models. *Journal of Applied Measurement* **4**(1):87–100.

24 Wang, W. (2000). Direct estimation of correlations among latent traits within IRT Framework. MPR-online **4**(1) 47–70. (http://www.mpr-online.de/)

25 Wang, W., Wilson, M. (1996). Comparing open-ended items and performance-based items using item response modeling. In *Objective Measurement: Theory into Practice, Volume III*, ed. G. Engelhard, M. Wilson pp. 167–94. Norwood, NJ: Ablex.

26 Wang, W., Wilson, M., Adams, R. J. (1997). Rasch models for multidimensionality between and within items. In *Objective Measurement: Theory into Practice, Volume IV*, ed. M. Wilson, G. Engelhard, K. Draney, pp. 139–56. Norwood, NJ: Ablex.

27 Wang, W., Wilson, M., Adams, R. J. (1998). Measuring individual differences in change with Rasch models. *Journal of Outcome Measurement* **2**(3):240–65.

28 Wu, M., Adams, R. J., Wilson, M. (1998). *ACERConQuest*. Hawthorn, Australia: ACER Press.

29 Paek, I., Peres, D., Wilson, M. (2002). Constructing one scale to describe two statewide exams. Paper presented at the International Objective Measurement Workshop, New Orleans, LA.

30 Brady, M. J., Cella, D. F., Mo, F. *et al.* Reliability and validity of the Functional Assessment of Cancer Therapy – Breast Quality of Life Instrument. *Journal of Clinical Oncology* **15**:974–86.

31 Feeny, this volume, Chapter 4.

32 Muthén, L. K., Muthén, B. O. (1998). *M-Plus User's Guide*. Los Angeles: Muthén & Muthén.

33 Muthén, B. O., Khoo, S. T. (1998). Longitudinal studies of achievement growth using latent variable modeling. *Learning and Individual Differences, Special issue: Latent growth curve analysis* **10**:73–101.

34 SAS Institute Inc. (1999). *SAS OnlineDoc (Version 8)* [software manual on CD-ROM]. Cary, NC: SAS Institute Inc.

35 Pellegrino, J., Glaser, R., Chudowsky, N. (ed.) (2001). *Knowing What Students Know: The Science and Design of Educational Assessment*. Washington, DC: National Academy Press.

36 De Boeck, P., Wilson, M. (2004). *Explanatory Item Response Models*. New York: Springer-Verlag.

24

On the definition and measurement of the economic burden of cancer

Mark C. Hornbrook, Ph.D.

Center for Health Research Northwest/Hawai'i, Kaiser Permanente Northwest Region, Portland, OR

Introduction

Economic analysis should play an essential role in controlling cancer, including defining priorities for research, treatment, screening, and prevention because society's resources are limited.[1-6] Competing demands for resources can give rise to decisions with myriad unforeseeable effects on costs, outcomes, and benefit distribution. Patients, families, physicians, and other providers face difficult trade-offs among alternative cancer prevention, screening, treatment, and palliation regimens with differing costs, probabilities of successful outcomes, side effects during treatment, and levels of uncertainties associated with estimates of these parameters. Even seeking additional information to reduce uncertainty about regimen options is costly, and the information gained will be of little value if it is wrong or irrelevant.

The concept of economic burden of disease is central to considerations of how to achieve an optimal resource allocation to and within health care.[7-11] Diseases that place the highest economic burdens on society, for example, should receive greater priority in medical and health services research compared to other diseases. Moreover, cancer treatments and prevention services that provide greater reductions in cancer's overall economic burden should receive greater priority in making coverage decisions, developing clinical practice guidelines, and making clinical decisions. Models that forecast cancer's economic burden are needed to understand the relative ranking among the sources of burden; to identify potential disease management opportunities so that appropriate practice guidelines can be developed, tested, and implemented; and to decompose total burden imposed by all comorbidities into cancer-related and cancer-unrelated.[12]

The term "burden" appears often in the cancer literature and denotes many concepts derived from both private and societal perspectives, including mortality,[13] years of life lost,[13] incidence and prevalence,[14-18] treatment side effects,[19-20] comorbidities,[21] stress and related emotional effects of cancer on patients,[20] effects of cancer on caregivers,[22] medical care utilization,[13] self-care demands,[23] cost of illness,[1-4] and disability-adjusted life-years lost.[13] The multiplicity of meanings of the term and the resulting absence of a consistent, comprehensive definition causes difficulties in estimating the actual burden of cancer.

We assign a specific meaning to the concept of economic burden of disease that recognizes both efficiency and equity effects. From an efficiency perspective, burden is defined to include the value of all market and non-market resources diverted to the prevention, diagnosis, and treatment of cancer and its sequelae.[1-4,24] Economic burden incorporates not only the cost of formal medical and long-term care, but also informal caregiving. It includes the value of lost market productivity attributable to cancer and, in principle, the value of forgone non-market productivity, including "leisure" time. A full accounting of burden must also include the intangible psychosocial costs – pain, suffering, self-esteem loss, and overall reduction in health-related quality of life – that accompany a serious disease.[5-6]

In assessing the economic burden of cancer in a given instance, the *perspective* of the analysis must be specified, e.g., the patient, the payer or provider, or society at large. Most recent economic evaluations in health care implicitly or explicitly assume some form of the societal perspective, incorporating and valuing all costs and benefits at their social opportunity cost, regardless of who incurs the costs or who obtains the benefits.[5] For example, say the economic cost (the value of the resources required) to produce a chemotherapy outpatient visit is $300, and the patient with insurance pays 10% of this out of pocket and the third-party payer covers the remaining costs. Thus, the "economic burden" induced by this visit is $30 from the patient's perspective and $270 from the insurer's perspective, totaling $300 from the societal perspective. But, suppose the patient cannot afford the 10% copayment for an expensive medication and does not pick up the prescription. Then the burden becomes the value of the incremental disease severity, reduced functioning, and years of life lost as the disease progresses.

From an equity perspective, cancer's economic burden also includes the societal value of the reduction in well-being for cancer patients who cannot afford care or who make relatively small productivity contributions to the economy (e.g., disabled, unemployed, and retired persons). These persons incur the burden of cancer as solely reductions in health and welfare because they are unable to demonstrate their willingness-to-pay to avoid cancer through the marketplace. Ubel *et al.*[25,26] define the term "societal value" as the overall value that society assigns to health care programs based on how they affect people's health, including valuing whose health is affected by how much.

This chapter is thus organized around the major categories of cancer's economic burden: (1) *Formal Medical Care Costs Induced by Cancer*; (2) *Formal Long-term Care Costs Induced by Cancer*; (3) *Lost Productivity and Household Costs Induced by Cancer*; (4) *Other Societal Costs Induced by Cancer*; and (5) *Total Societal Value Lost from Cancer*.[1-6] Burden is most often valued in monetary units so that the multiple components can be summed for research and policy applications. However, some applications focus on the health status and psychosocial impacts of disease, and the corresponding metric is some variant of the quality-adjusted life year (QALY).[11]

As a guide to the sections that follow, we will define three methodological approaches to estimating burden and then three areas of application. The methodological approaches may be termed *macrocosting*, *microcosting*, and *modeling*.[5-6] In macrocosting, we combine aggregated data from a variety of sources to estimate burden for the populations or groups of interest. For example, in projecting the direct cost burden of cancer, estimates of disease incidence might come from data set A, the intensity of resource consumption for those with cancer from data set B, and the unit costs of the resources consumed from data set C. While macrocosting allows one to make judicious use of a variety of information sources, there is the ever-present threat to validity: the various pieces and parts of the cost equation may not yield the correct total picture of burden for the population of interest. (More formally, macrocosting generally assumes linear separability and direct additivity across all the cost elements, a generally untested and usually unstated assumption.)

By contrast, microcosting methods involve collection and analysis of data on the same individuals, which avoids this confounding of interactive relationships among the components of burden. On the other hand, the scope and depth of the burden assessment is limited by the quantity and quality of the burden-related data collected on *those* individuals.

To compensate for the limitations of microcosting data, and also to strengthen macrocosting applications, analysts frequently adopt modeling methods. These include statistical and decision analytic approaches to cope with a variety of challenges related to "missingness" in the data, including extrapolating beyond the range of observed values, interpolating synthetic estimates of missing values for specific individuals, and modeling censored and non-normal distributions (primarily costs and utilization rates).

Macrocosting, microcosting, and modeling methods have three types of applications. The first is estimating the population-level burden of cancer, using surveillance data and other (macro-, micro-, and modeling-derived) information to chart the burden of cancer on society and the progress being achieved in reducing this burden over time. The unit of analysis may be an entire nation or group of nations, or it may be a state or some other geopolitically defined entity. Frequently, the policy maker is interested in the prevalence cost of cancer – that is, the aggregate cost burden associated with existing cancer cases (new and ongoing) over some fixed time interval, usually a year, e.g., the total cancer-related direct medical costs in the USA in 2002.

The second type of application is at the individual patient level, where the focus is on understanding the burden of cancer for particular types or categories of individuals. For example, what is the cost impact of intervention A vs. B in a clinical trial comparing the two? What is the total economic burden of lung cancer in an observational study of patients diagnosed at different stages, with different levels of insurance coverage, varying amounts of social support, and undergoing different treatment regimens? What is the net economic impact of a new colorectal cancer prevention program? Most such analyses will employ both microcosting and modeling approaches, with the former typically playing the major role when the key data are being collected expressly for the study itself. In contrast to population-level studies, the emphasis in most patient-level studies is on the incidence cost of cancer – that is, the lifetime (or multi-period) cost of new cancer cases arising within some fixed time period, usually a year.

The third type of application requiring burden estimates is economic evaluations – cost-effectiveness analyses (CEA), cost-benefit analyses (CBA), and decision analyses. Economic evaluations typically involve a combination of microcosting and modeling approaches, but often with a heavy emphasis on modeling. Modeling addresses the common need

to draw conclusions beyond the timeframe encompassed by any available patient-level data set and the desire to incorporate the effects of uncertainty and the concomitant value of information into the analyses.

In all three areas of application, our interest is frequently on the burden associated with or attributable to cancer, rather than simply the total burden (cancer plus other diseases) on patients and their families with cancer. As will be seen, estimating the attributable cost of cancer is a recurring challenge.

The aim of this chapter is not to provide a comprehensive review of the literature on measuring the burden of cancer, but rather to draw selectively from that literature to illustrate approaches and to suggest where further work is needed. We address the opportunities and challenges of measuring total societal burden in a way that might account or adjust for equity as well as efficiency effects, and we point to approaches for improving and standardizing data collection instruments to enhance the comparability of cancer burden estimates over time. At the moment, there is general agreement among health economists about "cost concepts" – but there are virtually no widely used, standardized data collection instruments (in sharp contrast to the HRQOL field).

Formal medical care costs induced by cancer

Formal medical care services are provided to prevent, screen, diagnose, and treat cancer and the side effects of treatments; to monitor for tumor progression and recurrence; and to provide palliative and end-of-life care for cancer patients and their families. Figure 24.1 summarizes cost elements by type of provider, type of technology, and purpose of the service. These services correspond to data elements contained in medical records, insurance claims, and encounter data systems.

Before embarking on a selective review of efforts to measure medical care costs in cancer, we note

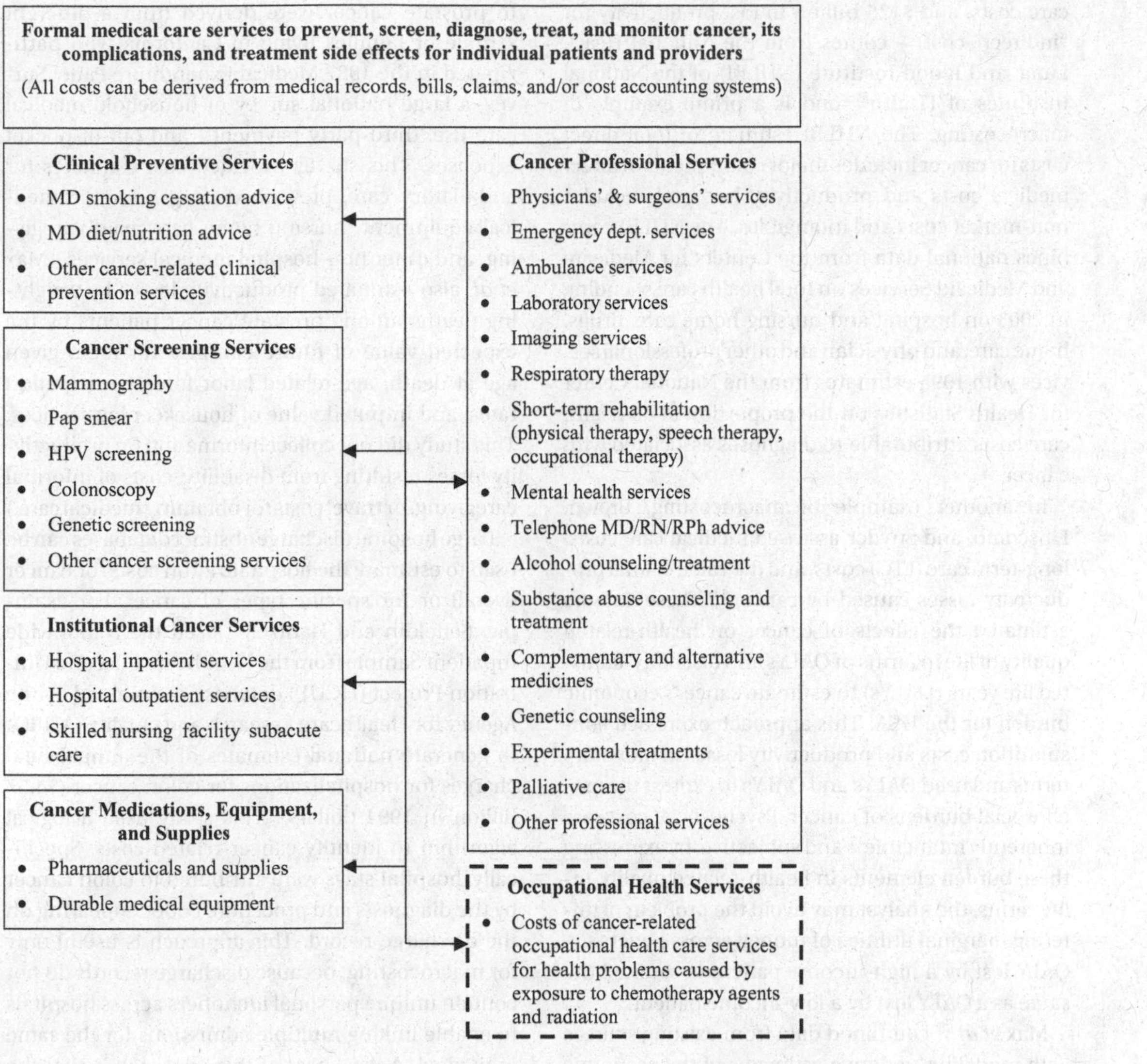

Formal medical care services to prevent, screen, diagnose, treat, and monitor cancer, its complications, and treatment side effects for individual patients and providers

(All costs can be derived from medical records, bills, claims, and/or cost accounting systems)

Clinical Preventive Services

- MD smoking cessation advice
- MD diet/nutrition advice
- Other cancer-related clinical prevention services

Cancer Screening Services

- Mammography
- Pap smear
- HPV screening
- Colonoscopy
- Genetic screening
- Other cancer screening services

Institutional Cancer Services

- Hospital inpatient services
- Hospital outpatient services
- Skilled nursing facility subacute care

Cancer Medications, Equipment, and Supplies

- Pharmaceuticals and supplies
- Durable medical equipment

Cancer Professional Services

- Physicians' & surgeons' services
- Emergency dept. services
- Ambulance services
- Laboratory services
- Imaging services
- Respiratory therapy
- Short-term rehabilitation (physical therapy, speech therapy, occupational therapy)
- Mental health services
- Telephone MD/RN/RPh advice
- Alcohol counseling/treatment
- Substance abuse counseling and treatment
- Complementary and alternative medicines
- Genetic counseling
- Experimental treatments
- Palliative care
- Other professional services

Occupational Health Services

- Costs of cancer-related occupational health care services for health problems caused by exposure to chemotherapy agents and radiation

Figure 24.1. Formal medical care costs induced by cancer.

two significant challenges facing all such studies. First, one must identify what portion of the services consumed is attributable to cancer (and not to competing disease risks). Second, one must attach measures of economic value to those services in a way that accurately indexes the burden cancer has imposed (from the perspective selected for analysis). We will discuss approaches to dealing with

both challenges after surveying some representative applications.

Population-level burden of cancer

The most recently published estimate of the aggregate economic burden of cancer in the USA – $190 billion total, representing $64.2 billion in direct health care costs, and $125 billion in lost productivity (or "indirect" cost) – comes from the National Heart, Lung, and Blood Institute (NHLBI) of the National Institutes of Health[27] and is a prime example of macrocosting. The NHLBI estimate of total direct costs for cancer includes major components of direct medical costs and productivity loss and excludes non-market costs and intangibles. The NHLBI combines national data from the Centers for Medicare and Medicaid Services on total health care spending in 2003 on hospital and nursing home care, drugs, home care, and physician and other professional services with 1995 estimates from the National Center for Health Statistics on the proportion of all health care costs attributable to diagnoses associated with cancer.

In another example of macrocosting, Brown, Lipscomb, and Snyder assessed medical care costs, long-term care (LTC) costs, and the value of total productivity losses caused by cancer.[11] These authors estimated the effects of cancer on health-related quality of life in terms of QALYs and disability-adjusted life years (DALYs) to estimate cancer's economic burden for the USA. This approach expressed consumption costs and productivity losses in monetary terms and used DALYs and QALYs to express the psychosocial burdens of cancer. Psychosocial costs are inherently intangible[11] and subjective; by expressing these burden elements in health-related quality-of-life terms, the analyst may avoid the problem of differing marginal utilities of money across patients. A QALY lost by a high-income patient is counted the same as a QALY lost by a low-income patient.

Max et al.[28] combined data from existing sources with modeling to derive estimates of the economic burden of prostate cancer in California for 1998. Hospitalization costs for prostate cancer were separately derived from a statewide hospital discharge abstract database. Eligible cases were selected on the basis of any mention of prostate cancer among principal and secondary diagnoses. Total charges were converted to estimates of economic resource costs using hospital-specific overall ratio of costs-to-charges (RCC) and imputed costs for HMO hospitalizations. Other direct medical care costs related

to prostate cancer were derived from a different sample of families living in California who participated in the 1987 Medical Expenditure Panel Survey, a large national survey of household medical care use, third-party payments, and out-of-pocket expenses. This survey provided cost estimates for ambulatory care, prescribed drugs, durable medical equipment, nursing home care, paid caregiving, and other non-hospital medical services. (Max et al. also estimated productivity losses by weighting deaths among prostate cancer patients by the expected value of future earnings for men, given age at death, age-related labor force participation rates, and imputed value of housekeeping services. This study did not collect information on productivity losses resulting from disability, costs of informal caregiving, or travel costs for obtaining medical care.)

Large hospital discharge abstract databases can be used to estimate the hospitalization costs for cancer overall or for specific types of cancer. For example, Seifeldin and Hantsch[29] used the Nationwide Inpatient Sample from the Healthcare Cost and Utilization Project (HCUP) database maintained by the Agency for Healthcare Research and Quality (AHRQ) to generate national estimates of the annual total charges for hospitalizations for colon cancer ($4.57 billion in 1994 dollars). This study used a logical algorithm to identify cancer-related costs. Specifically, hospital stays were attributed to colon cancer by the diagnosis and procedure codes appearing on the discharge record. This approach is useful only for macrocosting, because discharge records do not contain unique personal identifiers across hospitals to enable linking multiple admissions for the same individual. A weakness of this approach is that the entire hospital stay is assigned to the cancer, regardless of whether comorbidities were also treated during the same stay, because it is not possible to assign inpatient days and services to separate diseases in these data.

A frequent shortcoming of many macroeconomic cancer burden estimates is that the data are derived from different time periods, because it is unlikely that estimates of all medical care costs of cancer are available for the same year. In the Max et al.

study,[28] for example, the hospitalization data were for 1998 and the household expenses were for 1987. This approach assumes that changes in the technology of prostate cancer treatment had no effect on the relative ratio of hospital to household expenses over this 11-year period.

Patient-level burden of cancer

The prime arenas for microcosting burden analyses are clinical trials and observational studies; cost-effectiveness analyses also have been conducted alongside trials examining therapeutic strategies for a specific cancer.[30-32] Trials typically focus on medical care costs for only a limited follow-up period, so modeling approaches must address right-censoring of the cost burden estimates.

In an observational study, Du et al.[33] estimated the costs of treating pancreatic cancer at a single tertiary cancer center in Detroit, Michigan. Such facility-based expenses can be helpful in measuring medical care costs of cancer to the extent that patients receive all their care at the facility for the cancer disease episode. Since the median survival among the patient sample was only seven months, patients had less time to seek alternative sources of care. Such a facility-based approach omitted costs incurred prior to the referral to the cancer center and, hence, represents only a minimum threshold estimate of economic burden for pancreatic cancer.

An observational study using the Surveillance, Epidemiology, and End Results (SEER) cancer registries linked to Medicare claims for 1990 through 1998 is an excellent example of the macrocosting approach applied to patient-level burden analysis. Nationally representative estimates of treatment costs for elderly women with early-stage breast cancer were generated to compare the per-patient cost of modified radical mastectomy versus breast-conserving surgery and radiation therapy.[34] Brown et al.[35] used SEER-Medicare data to estimate the life-cycle medical care costs of colorectal cancer. Five years of Medicare claims data were extracted to estimate cancer costs by phase of care: "initial" (the first 12 months of care), "terminal" (the final 12 months

before death), and "continuing" (the period between initial and terminal).

Fireman et al.[36] used the Northern California SEER registry to identify Kaiser Permanente enrollees diagnosed with one of seven cancer sites. The investigators reviewed medical records to extract data on cancer-specific utilization (which involved specification of a cancer care episode algorithm). Estimates of average HMO production costs were applied to each service unit, multiplied by the volume of each service consumed by each patient, and summed to the total cost of cancer care for each patient. Taplin et al.[37] estimated the average and incremental medical care costs of three cancers – colon, prostate, and breast – in a single HMO. The average cost data were extracted from the HMO's financial information system, which provides encounter-specific average cost data. The incremental cost analysis was the difference in average annual costs of patients with the selected cancers and the annual costs of all other members of the HMO without the cancer of interest matched by sex and age group. The Fireman and Taplin HMO-based studies have methodological significance because they are not based on billed charges or paid claims (as were the other studies cited above), but rather on HMO production costs – a distinction discussed in more detail below.

Measuring attributable costs

At least three broad approaches can be used to estimate the direct costs of care that arise from, and thus may be attributable to, a given disease of interest (in our case, cancer).

The "top-down" strategy partitions total health care costs for the population of interest algorithmically into a mutually exclusive and exhaustive set of disease-specific categories. This approach was illustrated by Hodgson and Cohen[38] for circulatory diseases and has been adopted by NHLBI[27] for their disease-specific estimates. It has the advantage of ensuring that total costs across all diseases will not exceed aggregate estimated costs. On the other hand, the algorithms that allocate costs to diseases, particularly for population-level analyses where the strategy is most commonly seen, are often arbitrary. For example, 100% of the cost of a given hospitalization might be attributed to the first-listed diagnosis on the claims form. This approach is not well suited to estimating changes in the burden of cancer, because it assumes that cancer is independent of all other diseases.

The *comparison sample strategy* first derives total costs for the identified sample of patients with cancer, with no effort to separate out cancer from noncancer. Then a comparison sample of patients is matched to the cancer patient sample in all measurable respects, except the absence of a cancer diagnosis. For example, the cancer and comparison samples might be closely matched by age, gender, race/ethnicity, and possibly other exogenous covariates predictive of cost. Then the attributable cost of cancer in the patient sample is the difference between mean total cost in that sample and mean total cost in the comparison sample. Such computations can be carried out by patient subgroup, as well as for the total sample.

In cancer costing, the comparison sample strategy has been employed by Etzioni *et al.*,[39–40] Warren *et al.*, [34] Brown *et al.*,[35] and Taplin *et al.*[37] Each of these studies estimates direct cost at the patient level; Brown *et al.*[11] report estimates of population-level attributable direct cost of cancer for selected years.

Because the incident cases of cancer – unlike any other chronic disease – are recorded in good-to-high quality registries in most regions of the USA now, we can assume that individuals found in linked registry-claims data bases are "true positive" cancer cases, and that disease site(s) will be correctly identified. But this does not address the problem of attributing services to diseases among the great majority of cancer patients who have comorbidities. Careful study of pre- and post-diagnosis encounters is required to identify services specifically related to cancer.

The *microcosting strategy* defines the cancer care episode as a series of temporally contiguous health care services provided to treat specified cancer-related health problems.[41,42] Care episodes are typically differentiated by the patient's reasons for seeking care and by the clinician's goals in ordering services. Services should also be organized according to their technical relationships to metaplastic and neoplastic disease processes. A heuristic classification of various types of cancer care episodes can serve as a roadmap in decomposing total cancer-related health care utilization in a defined population (see Figure 24.2). The utility of the care episode concept for analysis of health care delivery has been demonstrated in several studies.[43–47]

In one of the few comparative analyses of the attributable cost approaches discussed so far, Ward *et al.*[48] evaluated three alternative algorithms. These were (a) attributing 100% of the cost of hospitalization to the first-listed diagnosis; (b) attributing a portion of the cost of hospitalization to the disease of interest, depending on its position in the list of diagnoses and the clinical relevance of any comorbidities; and (c) analyzing incremental cost based upon the hospitalization experiences of an age- and gender-matched cohort using regression analysis – a variant of the comparison sample approach. Algorithm (a) yielded the lowest cost estimate, and (b) yielded the highest.

Defining the various types and components of cancer care episodes listed in Figure 24.2 requires strong clinical knowledge of cancer and its epidemiology, prevention, diagnosis, and treatment. A cancer diagnosis may appear in reports from pathologists, radiologists, and surgeons, as well as in the notes of attending physicians. Information on cancer diagnoses will also appear in electronic information systems, including insurance claims, inpatient utilization files, ambulatory care utilization files, pathology data systems, dispensing data systems, computerized patient record systems, and so on. Three approaches, one prospective and two retrospective, are available for defining cancer care episodes, as described below.

(1) *Concurrent episode coding*: On-line, real-time coding by treating clinicians is the gold standard for defining cancer care episodes. Treating clinicians know their reasons for ordering each service and can assign the relevant ICD-9-CM or ICD-10 codes to each service during the order-entry process. The

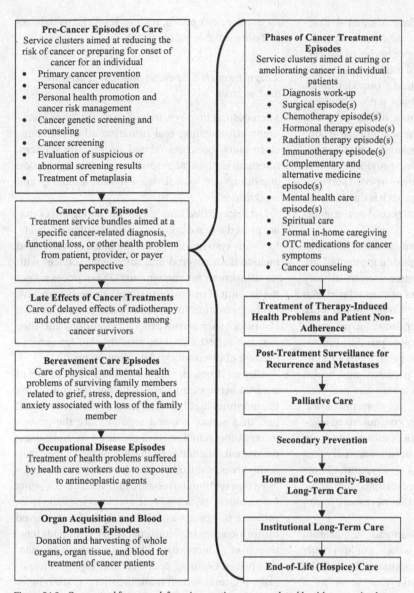

Figure 24.2. Conceptual framework for microcosting cancer-related health care episodes.

problem-oriented medical record (POMR)[49–53] is one approach to structured documentation that supports episode measurement. The POMR approach, if followed rigorously, reduces the difficulty of abstracting utilization by episode. All orders are linked to a specific health problem, and the status of each problem – continuing or resolved – is documented at each contact. Automated medical record systems (such as http://www.epiccare.com/) are available in a growing number of settings[54,55] but have not been used in published studies of cancer burden. The major question regarding the validity of this approach is the extent to which ordering clinicians follow appropriate episode coding principles.

(2) *Retrospective episode coding*: Manual abstraction of hard copy or electronic medical records is the traditional method of defining episodes of cancer-related services. Medical record technicians analyze all elements of the patient's chart – provider notes, laboratory test results, consultant reports, surgical reports, hospital discharge notes, imaging reports, and so on – and reconstruct the sequence and content of care processes.[41,42] Unrelated comorbid conditions are identified, and services provided for these diseases are separated from cancer-related services. The major weakness of this approach is that it is only as good as the quality of medical record documentation.

(3) *Retrospective computerized episode algorithms*: Software products, termed "episode groupers," are applied to claims and encounter data to identify temporally contiguous clusters of care related to a specific medical condition.[44,46] While much work remains to standardize the terminology, measurement, and process of health care episodes, proprietary companies began in the early 1990s to market episode software grouper products, and health plans have begun to use them to measure and evaluate health care delivery.[44,46] All currently available products use retrospective computerized algorithms to group clusters of services into discrete care episodes, which then are output into summary files with the episode as the unit of observation. Claims and encounter data (in standard formats such as the UB-92) supply all the information necessary to run episode groupers.

Standardization and widespread application of such microcosting approaches could greatly improve the quality and comparability of the cancer-specific utilization data that serve as a basis for direct cost estimation. However, there are some important limitations. Since most health insurance policies do not cover complementary and alternative medicine (CAM) treatments, household surveys are required to capture patients' use of acupuncture, naturopathy, and other types of CAM therapies.[56] Another constraint is that for Medicare beneficiaries participating in the program's managed care option (as opposed to the traditional fee-for-service option), patient-level claims data are still not available for cost analysis.

Assigning costs to specific medical procedures and services

Microcosting involves, in addition to episode measurement, assigning real (inflation-adjusted) monetary units to cancer-related health care services. Alternative physical resource-to-dollar conversion algorithms are available, each with strengths and weaknesses.

List Prices/Billed Charges are the asking prices that are posted when a good or service is offered for sale. In claims systems, list prices are billed amounts and include both covered and uncovered services with no adjustment for copayments. These prices reflect the amount of revenue the supplier wishes to receive as compensation for providing the good or service. List prices vary across providers/vendors, and they may not reflect amounts actually paid for services because of discounts and disallowments.[57]

Allowed Amounts represent discounted prices of covered services and are the basis for computing the amounts that both the insurer and insured will pay. In a sense, allowed amounts are the payer's internal fee schedule and are used in computing the patient's liabilities from the payer's perspective – deductibles, coinsurance, and uncovered services – as well as withholds, rebates, and volume discounts for providers. Withholds are amounts withheld from provider payments as a hedge against unexpected future increases in volume of claims. Withholds have the effect of increasing uncertainty about transaction prices. Contract providers and suppliers (especially pharmaceutical manufacturers) grant rebates and volume discounts to insurers and HMOs as an inducement to increase consumption of their services and products. Since these discounting schemes are usually based on annual volume, the billed price will be the list price, but the transaction price will not be known until the amount of the discount or rebate is computed sometime after the end of the year. Using Allowed Amounts to measure medical care cost burden removes some of the variation in list prices but may understate opportunity costs if providers are allowed to bill patients for the difference between the billed amount and the allowed amount (balance billing; see below).

Paid Amounts are the dollars paid by third-party insurers for medical care services, that is, partial transaction prices, from hospital accounts receivable records or insurer benefit payment records. Paid amounts omit payments by patients for deductibles, coinsurance, and balance billing. Furthermore, paid amounts omit any provider withholds, rebates, and discounts. In their patient-level analysis of direct costs attributable to breast cancer and colorectal cancer, respectively, Warren *et al.*[34] and Brown *et al.*[35] defined costs as the amount Medicare paid providers, plus the estimated deductibles and copayments that patients paid. Under Medicare, there are no withholds, rebates, or discounts to complicate or distort these estimates, although this generally will not be the case in the private sector.

Balance Billing is the difference between allowed amount and billed amount that is collected from the patient if the patient's insurance company permits balance billing (Medicare, Medicaid, and many HMOs do not permit this practice).[58] The amount of consumer out-of-pocket expenses represented by balance billing can be substantial. Methods for capturing balance billing include household expenditure diaries, interviews,[59–61] and provider accounts receivable data. Tracking household expenditures is costly and requires considerable effort from patients (keeping receipts and recording all cash and credit payments for medical care).

Private sector claims processing systems have different methods for adjustments to deal with disallowed claims, risk-sharing contracts, and allowable expenses, which heightens the challenge the analyst faces in "rolling up" all claims related to the same occasion of service and computing the final adjudicated amount paid.

Revenues received by health care providers represent the most accurate approach to capturing balance billing, since consumer surveys are subject to recall losses, and respondent compliance with expenditure diaries is not perfect. However, providers view their accounts receivable data as highly proprietary and resist releasing these data to outside researchers.

Production Costs are the resource-related expenses incurred by providers to produce a particular medical care service, device, or supply item. Using production costs avoids many of the difficulties associated with computing transaction prices for medical care services.

Well-known sources of production cost estimates are the Medicare Cost Reports (MCRs) for hospitals and HMO cost management information systems (CMISs). However, with either the MCRs or the CMISs, distortions caused by differences in overhead allocation practices across providers and health plans must be identified and removed. While MCRs appear to apply a standard method for converting departmental overhead allocations to a consistent scheme, Medicare regulations permit hospitals and health plans some latitude, so they may be tempted to report costs in ways that maximize their Medicare payments. If so, MCRs may be a better reflection of "price" than "cost." Nevertheless, researchers have used the MCRs to develop both facility-level and department-level ratios of costs-to-charges (RCC), which are then used (via simple multiplication and addition) to convert service charges to an approximation of production costs.[62] Distinct from the RCC approach, analysts can attempt to assign fixed and variable costs to each service by detailed analysis of internal accounting systems for hospitals, medical groups, and HMOs. Because of the time intensity of understanding complex financial data systems, this approach is usually adopted in studies with only one or two provider organizations.

Capitation and other forms of risk-sharing contracts between HMOs and providers create special challenges to estimating production costs. Managed care systems will usually create pseudo-claim records for services covered through capitation contracts so they can track utilization events, but these claims do not show the true costs of services. The average cost per service must be estimated after the close of the fiscal year so that the total costs of the contract can be spread over the realized utilization.

Production costs will naturally incorporate geographic variation in costs of inputs, such as building rents, wage rates, and energy prices. In most applications, cost estimates should be standardized across geographic regions, and there are well-known indices for doing this.[24]

Costing Algorithms are required to measure medical care production costs in the absence of detailed, patient-level cost accounting systems by converting recorded resource use into dollar values. Relatively standardized costing systems have been developed for hospital care, nursing home care, medications, and ambulatory care. The important steps are to define a set of basic utilization elements for which average production costs can be derived from the general ledger, incorporate adjustments for resource intensity wherever possible, and watch for dead-ended costs and services that do not show up in patient-related cost accounts. A commonly applied approach is to apply Medicare Prospective Payment System payment rates for Diagnosis Related Groups (DRGs) to compute an overall average payment rate for each hospital stay.[34] A method that preserves more of the variation in resource use is to assign average DRG-weighted costs per day to each day of the stay. Yet more variation in resource use can be preserved by weighting each day of the stay by the average cost of the particular nursing unit, and each minute of operating room time and recovery room time by the average cost per minute.

Ambulatory care costing algorithms employ the CPT-4 procedure coding system and then apply the Resource-Based Relative Value Scale (RBRVS) to estimate the relative resource intensity of various procedures. An RBRVS-to-dollar conversion coefficient is applied to enable aggregation to total costs. The Medicare Fee Schedule, which is an RBRVS-based system, could be used as a standard national fee schedule, although it is limited to services used primarily by older patients. All-payer RBRVS systems that cover all services are now available.[63–66]

Skilled nursing facilities (SNF) have a Medicare-mandated prospective reimbursement system, called Resource Utilization Groups (RUG), that can be used to estimate production costs.[67–70] Non-SNF nursing home care is not generally covered by Medicare, and there is no nationally standardized prospective reimbursement system. Non-SNF nursing home costs can be estimated as an average cost per day by level of care – heavy, medium, and light – using data from selected Medicaid programs or private sector sources.

To measure the cost of outpatient prescription drugs, one can estimate the acquisition costs for the product and add a dispensing fee to cover pharmacy overhead and pharmacist labor expense. Alternatively, drug costs can be estimated by applying a suitable discount to the average retail ("Red Book")[57] price or the average wholesale price, which can be obtained from pharmaceutical benefits management companies or consulting firms specializing in drug costs.

Economic evaluations

Simulation modeling usually combines micro-costing and macrocosting techniques. The study population may be derived from primary data collection or created randomly by Monte Carlo or multi-sampling techniques. The parameters for forecasting cancer incidence, treatment options, late effects, and outcomes may be derived from a clinical trial, published aggregate estimates, and expert opinion. For instance, Loeve *et al.*[71] developed a simulation model to predict costs and savings for colorectal cancer under various screening scenarios. Tsao *et al.*[72] developed a simulation model to estimate the treatment costs of cutaneous melanoma using published and unpublished data from two teaching hospitals. Grover and colleagues[73] used a Markov state-transition simulation model to forecast prostate cancer incidence, progression, and direct medical costs, based on patient age, tumor stage and grade, and treatment modalities for Canadian men.

Elsewhere in this volume (Chapter 25), O'Brien[74] provides an excellent discussion of how decision

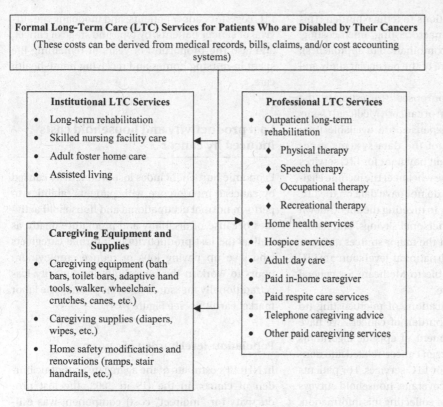

Figure 24.3. Formal long-term care costs induced by cancer.

analytic methods can be used to combine economic burden data from a variety of sources to investigate the cost-effectiveness of cancer interventions. He illustrates how the macrocosting approach can be applied in a patient-level analysis by drawing costs and QALY data from multiple relevant microcosting sources. O'Brien also discusses how to represent uncertainty about the model's parameter estimates using probability distributions, and to derive overall uncertainty about the cost-effectiveness recommendation through either Bayesian statistical approaches or probabilistic sensitivity analysis (usually carried out from a Classical perspective). Fairclough (Chapter 17 in this volume)[75] provides a complementary discussion of how to correct for missing data and other empirical shortcomings that can arise in the microcosting analyses.

Formal long-term care costs induced by cancer

Many types of cancer are survivable, but patients may incur functional impairments (e.g., amputations, nerve damage) from the cancer or its treatment that may require rehabilitation and continuing care. This care may involve patient placement in institutions such as nursing homes, foster care homes, or assisted living facilities. Rehabilitation services, formal caregiving, and caregiving equipment and supplies may be required, as well as special adaptive equipment related to mobility, hearing, vision, or other tasks. Figure 24.3 summarizes the key elements of such long-term (that is, non-medical care) costs – which, like medical care costs, should be considered for inclusion in population-level and patient-level studies of cancer burden, and in economic evaluations of interventions to reduce burden. This will, likewise, require macrocosting, microcosting, or modeling (or some combination of approaches), depending on the nature of the particular study and the available data.

For macrocosting purposes (to estimate the population-level burden of cancer), Medicaid claims data on formal LTC expenses are available from states, but the quality of the data systems varies widely. Because Medicaid payment for LTC services is available only for those who meet the income eligibility requirements, we do not have data on the LTC expenses incurred prior to meeting the spend-down thresholds. Medicaid, personal savings, and family contributions represent the major sources of financing of LTC expenses. No national-level source of LTC expense data comparable to Medicare for general medical care is available.

With regard to applications of microcosting (to estimate patient-level burden of cancer), we have yet to see the development of episode algorithms for discriminating between cancer-related and non-cancer-related claims for LTC services. For patients who do not have LTC coverage, household surveys are the major method for collecting this information. Cross-sectional surveys reduce respondent burden, compared to weekly or monthly expense diaries, but diaries provide higher quality data. Expense diaries combined with telephone or personal interviews provide cued recall.[76] Because many cancer patients requiring long-term care are among the frail elderly, who typically have multiple health problems, there are particular challenges in estimating the attributable cost of cancer. Note also that family out-of-pocket expenses on end-of-life care may be substantial.[77,78]

Because of the high proportion of LTC costs paid out-of-pocket and the expense and burden of primary data collection for such data, modeling approaches are needed to cope with missing data and related problems. Such approaches might include: assigning estimated nursing home and home health costs from age- and gender-matched cohorts of patients for whom data are available; extrapolating from pre-existing estimates of formal LTC costs for cancer patients; and modeling the survival of cancer patients, by type and stage of cancer, and also the proportion of years of remaining life spent in nursing homes and receiving home health care.

Lost productivity and household costs induced by cancer

Economic burden includes lost productivity caused by cancer's interference with patients' abilities to perform normal occupational and household activities because of disability and premature death, as well as the lost productivity of informal caregivers who give up paying jobs or reduce employment hours to work in the household. Productivity loss is traditionally measured in terms of foregone labor market earnings (see Figure 24.4).

Population-level burden of cancer

In NHLBI's estimate of the aggregate economic burden of cancer in the US in 2003, the lost productivity (or "indirect" cost) component was estimated to be $125 billion – or about two-thirds of the $190 billion total.[27] These indirect costs were partitioned into morbidity costs, about $16 billion, and mortality costs, $109 billion. In this traditional cost-of-illness typology, morbidity costs are measured by the income lost because of work disability and absenteeism attributable to cancer, while the mortality costs associated with a given year are typically measured as the total lifetime productivity lost due to cancer-attributable deaths in *that* year.[11]

The typical method for estimating productivity loss is to assume that the average cancer patient would have continued to work for as long as the average age- and gender-matched worker who did not have cancer, at the average wage stream for their remaining productive years. As with any application of the attributable-cost methodology, this approach assumes that cancer patients are sufficiently similar to the average worker of the same age and gender that

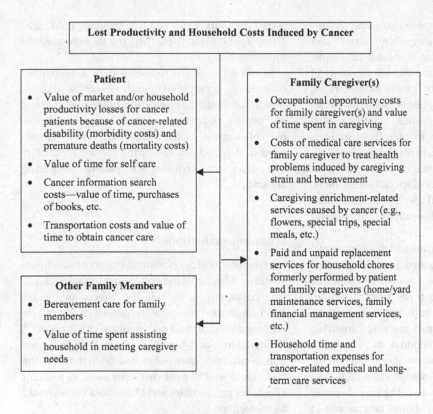

Figure 24.4. Lost productivity and household costs induced by cancer.

productivity differences are cancer-associated. This approach is imminently practical, requiring only macro data on wages, employment patterns, and average age at diagnosis; average age at retirement because of cancer; and average age of cancer-related death for cancer patients.[1,5–6]

Across all health problems, the total value of informal caregiving in the United States has been estimated at $196 billion for 1997.[79] In valuing informal caregiving specifically for cancer, Hayman et al.[80] used data from the first wave (1993) of the Asset and Health Dynamics (AHEAD) Study, a nationally representative longitudinal survey of persons aged 70 or older, to estimate the incremental costs of informal caregiving. They used regression modeling to estimate the attributable cost of caregiving for cancer patients in comparison with patients of similar age, gender, functional status, and social support.

Cancer treatment was associated with an incremental increase of 3.1 hours of informal caregiving per week, which translates into an additional average yearly cost of $1200 per patient and just over $1 billion nationally.[80]

Patient-level burden of cancer

Within the context of clinical trials and prospective observational studies, household surveys and employer sick leave records can be used to estimate the productivity and time loss effects of cancer. Economic burden also includes self-care and family care, i.e., caregiving tasks performed by family members for the cancer patient. Such informal caregiving time should be valued and added to the total burden, because patients would have to hire someone to perform these activities if family members did not.[81]

Family members who provide caregiving to cancer patients often experience high stress and role strain, which may lead to health problems. Ideally, cancer burden should include the costs of health care consumption by cancer caregivers for caregiving-induced health needs, such as stress, depression, anxiety, and injuries. Economic burden also includes changes in household budgets caused by accommodations to special needs of cancer patients and performance of care enrichment activities, such as purchases of special meals, diets, furniture, and clothing, and also (it can be argued) the extra spiritual care often required of patients and families.

The value of the patient's time and that of patients' escorts, when present, required to consume cancer care services should be counted in economic burden. Also included are travel costs to obtain health care service, e.g., auto mileage, parking, and bus/taxi fare. Cancer patients with caregiving responsibilities for young children, ill persons, or frail/disabled persons will make other arrangements to discharge these responsibilities when their cancer interferes with role activities. The cost of respite care for the cancer patient should be counted in economic burden. Similarly, the costs of hiring out household services that used to be performed by the cancer patient or family caregiver should be assessed.

When individuals retire from paid employment, their productivity consists of contributions to the effective and efficient functioning of their household, as well as contributions to the community through volunteer work and to their extended families by childcare, assistance with home maintenance, and household chores. A comprehensive approach would model functional health status trajectories and include the threshold when one is no longer able to perform regular household chores. The economic burden of cancer for the retired individual would be the difference between his/her productivity contributions to the household in the absence of cancer and the contributions now expected, given cancer. To index the economic value of a retiree's household contributions, the typical approach is to assign the market cost of a housekeeper, paid caregiver, or others who could carry out these household functions.[27]

To obtain such microcosting data may require household surveys or family expense diaries, which for budgetary and administrative reasons are usually restricted to small samples. A number of survey instruments have been developed and tested for measuring formal and informal caregiving activities for patients requiring assistance.[77–81]

Economic evaluations

In assessments of the economic impact of new interventions, whether at the population or patient level, it is customary to include the effects on market and non-market productivity, as well as the effects on direct medical and non-medical (LTC) costs.[1–3] Similarly, in a cost–benefit analysis of an intervention conducted from what has been termed the "human capital" (or net cost) approach, all relevant effects on productivity and household costs should be recognized.[6]

However, in cost-effectiveness analysis, the commonly recommended practice is to exclude both morbidity costs and mortality costs from the numerator of the cost-effectiveness (C-E) ratio, while including in the numerator only the *patient and caregiver time costs* associated with receiving the interventions, plus the so-called *"friction" costs* incurred by employers when attempting to replace the labor productivity lost due to illness.[5] The rationale is that the great bulk of the market and non-market productivity impacts of the interventions will be captured, instead, in the C-E ratio's denominator – assuming that a suitably comprehensive measure of quality-adjusted life years is selected to gauge intervention effectiveness. When the analyst believes that the impact of the intervention at issue on morbidity and/or mortality costs will in fact be significant, it is prudent to carry out cost-of-illness or cost-benefit analyses in addition to a QALY-based cost-effectiveness analysis.[5]

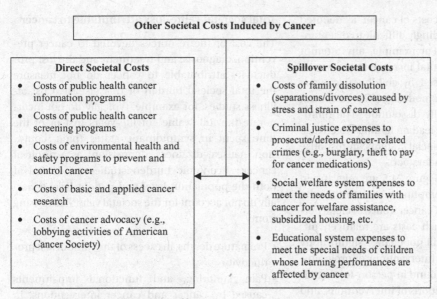

Figure 24.5. Other societal costs induced by cancer.

Other societal costs of cancer

There are certain additional costs attributable to cancer that are typically borne not by individual patients or families, but rather by public and private institutions in society. Such costs arise either directly from public health and private advocacy efforts to prevent or treat cancer, or indirectly as "spillover" costs imposed on societal institutions, such as the education or criminal justice system; see Figure 24.5.

Societal costs incurred directly in response to the cancer burden include the value of resources devoted to public health initiatives for cancer prevention and screening, basic and applied cancer research, environmental and food safety regulations related to cancer prevention, and cancer-related advocacy activities (Figure 24.5). Such activities represent (or nearly so) the economist's concept of "public goods." For example, consumption of a cancer prevention education program by one person does not diminish the quantity of information available for another person to consume. The costs incurred by individuals who undertake specific actions to reduce their cancer risks will be counted by various methods outlined earlier in this chapter, but this will not capture the costs of producing and distributing a televised tobacco smoke avoidance program, for example. The same goes for the costs of enforcing environmental health and safety regulations and for producing new medical research knowledge to find new cancer treatments.

The methods for measuring such costs are specific to each element. For example, cancer research and advocacy costs can be obtained from budget documents of public and private research funding agencies. Venture capital investment in cancer research is more difficult to measure accurately because of the proprietary nature of these efforts. Media tracking services can provide information on media buys for public service messages related to cancer. The Cost of Cancer Treatment Study is attempting to produce generalizable estimates of the total incremental costs of government-sponsored cancer clinical trials.[82] For this study, costs will be measured using microcosting methods from a combination of billing records, medical records, and personal interviews for a sample of 1500 cancer patients. There is a well-developed methodology in the field of environmental economics for measuring the costs of regulatory enforcement.[83-88]

The spillover societal costs of cancer, as denoted in Figure 24.5, are exceedingly difficult to disentangle from other causes. For example, any attempt to estimate the incremental increase in the separation/divorce rates caused by childhood cancers would require a complex modeling effort to control for other causes of family dissolution. The multifaceted causal pathways leading families to engage with public and private social systems, in response to cancer, are not well understood.

The cost elements in Figure 24.5 are relevant, in principle, to studies attempting to account for the total economic burden of cancer from a societal perspective. But because such costs are relatively difficult to measure, and will not change significantly in response to individual interventions or programs, they are virtually never found in person-level studies and economic evaluations of interventions, and only rarely seen in population-level reports of disease burden.

Extensions

There are two significant challenges in measuring the economic burden of cancer comprehensively and fairly. The first is that even the most exhaustive efforts to measure the economic opportunity costs of the resources consumed and the lost productivity incurred because of cancer will fail to account for all important aspects of burden. We discuss what is being missed in Figures 24.1–24.5, and approaches to measuring it. The second challenge is that current measures of economic burden are substantially influenced by the prevailing distributions of income, wealth, labor market opportunities, and access to health care. Because the poor, the young, the elderly, the unemployed, and others in economically disadvantaged positions may not generate as much market-measured costs or productivity losses in response to their cancers as the economically advantaged, the burdens they bear may be undercounted or uncounted. This raises fundamental equity concerns, and the challenge is how to address them analytically.

Total societal value-loss attributable to cancer

The cost of the resources devoted to cancer prevention, diagnosis, and treatment and the lost productivity attributable to cancer do not measure the total societal burden of this disease. Cost-of-illness studies, for example, typically do not incorporate the full "value" of life-years lost or of the time spent in symptomatic states (pain, confusion, nausea, dizziness, depression) as a result of cancer.[1] Economic burden studies conducted at both the population level and patient level generally do not account for the societal value-loss arising from:

- Premature deaths, in excess of the value of lost productivity
- Pain, suffering, and functional impairments caused by cancer and cancer interventions, in excess of the associated resource costs and the value of lost productivity
- Caregiver strain and health status effects, in excess of the resource costs and the value of lost productivity
- Family and friends' suffering in response to the cancer patient's pain, suffering, and impairments
- Family and friends' bereavement from the cancer patient's death
- Fear, anxiety, and phobias arising from the fear of cancer among both high-risk and average-risk individuals

There are, in principle, two general pathways available for measuring economic burden to account for some or all of the elements above, while at the same time accounting for some or all of the cost elements displayed in Figures 24.1–24.5.

First, preference-based measures of health status that take the form of the QALY[5] or the DALY[11] are aimed at reflecting the full impact of disease and disability on life and limb. Specifically, within each of the major QALY measurement systems commonly used today (the Health Utilities Index (HUI), the Quality of Well-Being (QWB) Index, and the EuroQol EQ-5D), the preference weight for each health state is intended to capture the total utility (or more likely, disutility) associated with being in that state.[89] Such preference weights therefore incorporate, in principle, both the market and non-market implications of being in these health states. Death may have less disutility than some poor health states for some people.

As Feeny (Chapter 4)[89] and O'Brien (Chapter 25)[74] in this volume indicate, QALYs have been widely used in the cost-utility variant of cost-effectiveness analysis, with a number of prominent applications to cancer. Whether the "costs" measured in the numerator of the cost-effectiveness ratio in conjunction with the "utility effects" captured via the QALY in the denominator together encompass the *total* impact of the interventions being compared on burden (and without double-counting) is a subject of ongoing debate among CEA experts.[5-6] Feeny cites a number of patient-level applications of burden measurement using QALYs, and Brown *et al.*[11] show how QALYs and DALYs can be used in population-level assessments of cancer burden.

It must be noted, however, that among the societal value-loss elements listed above, today's QALY' is largely geared to capturing the total effects (not just the "pure health" effects) of the first two items – premature mortality and morbidity for the cancer patient.

Yet, from the perspective of many economists, a significant shortcoming of the QALY for burden measurement is not that it fails to encompass effects beyond premature mortality and morbidity, but that it actually fails to provide a valid measure of the full societal value-loss for *any* burden element. Rather, to accurately determine this total value-loss, one would ideally wish to know the maximum amount the relevant decision maker would be willing to pay to avoid the cancer, that is, the decision maker's willingness-to-pay (WTP) to avoid the aggregate burdens generated by the disease.[5-6, 74]

WTP calculations of the value of life without cancer can, in principle, be derived in one of two ways. Either we can ask individuals how much they would be willing to pay to achieve (modest, realistic) improvements in the probability of avoiding cancer, after presenting them with accurate data on the conse-quences, including death, of getting cancer. Or, we can attempt to observe how much they are willing to pay to reduce the probability of cancer. Either way, we can use the WTP data to calculate the value of avoiding cancer in the following (highly stylized) way. Suppose the population average WTP for reducing the lifetime risk of cancer from 0.10 to 0.05 is $50 000. Then the implied value of avoiding the cancer (and thus, the value-loss generated by cancer for the average individual) can be calculated as $50 000/(0.10 − 0.05) = $1 million.

However, neither approach to obtaining WTP estimates is without problems. The stated-preference approach is at risk of eliciting unrealistic answers to what is a hypothetical question. The revealed-preference approach is grounded in observational reality, but inferences about willingness to pay are complicated by the fact that the "price" of cancer care the individual faces is heavily influenced by insurance coverage; that the individual may not be adequately informed about costs, risks, and benefits; and that many medical decisions are made jointly by the individual and provider.

Such difficulties notwithstanding, it is well-known from microeconomic theory that the "value" a society places on achieving any given outcome can be measured as the direct algebraic sum of the willingness to pay that each and every member of society has for achieving the outcome. Ideally, this aggregate value would encompass all the elements in Figures 24.1–24.5, plus those in the bullet list above.

While there have been virtually no published studies applying the WTP approach in patient-level analyses in cancer or in economic evaluations of cancer interventions, there is at least one notable effort to do so at the population level. In a much-discussed recent investigation of the total economic value of medical research in the USA, Murphy and Topel[90] used data from a variety of sources to estimate the parameters of a microeconomic model of consumer utility maximization, from which they derive a rather astounding conclusion. Finding a cure for cancer, so that cancer-attributable deaths are eliminated forever, would generate about $48 trillion in economic value.

A major driver in these calculations is the assumption that economic burden attributable to a cancer death is not the sum simply of the resource cost of treatment and lost productivity. Rather, it is the WTP-based value of the life lost, assumed in the Murphy-Topel analyses to be $1.5 million on average. The fact that neither society as a whole, nor most of its members individually, could practically afford to spend dollar amounts on cancer equivalent to the corresponding WTP values assumed here is worthy of some discussion. Nonetheless, through the willingness-to-pay approach, which is grounded in basic microeconomics, we do have a means for valuing any and all aspects of disease burden. Note also that QALY estimates can be converted into WTP estimates once the decision maker designates the marginal willingness to pay per QALY gained (this is the λ parameter discussed by O'Brien in Chapter 25).[74]

A variation on the theme for value/burden measurement is the "willingness to accept" (WTA) approach. In the case at hand, the relevant question would be: How much would you have to be paid in order to be willing to increase your risk of cancer by some specified amount? For reasons both economic and cognitive, a WTA question and a WTP question about the same amount of risk change may not yield the same response.

Equity concerns in measuring the economic burden of cancer

Resources consumed and productivity lost due to cancer are confounded by variations in income, wealth, human capital endowments, and other factors affecting both financial and physical access to health care and the calculated value of one's economic contributions to society. How might the policy analyst respond to this challenge? Could either or both of the two approaches just discussed for improving the comprehensiveness of cancer burden estimates provide ways to assess the equity implications of current burden estimates or perhaps even correct, or compensate for, equity effects?

First, the preference weights used in the major QALY measurement systems (the HUI, QWB, EQ-5D) already address important aspects of the equity issue. That is, the mean preference weight attached to each health state is derived typically from population-representative, community-based samples.[89] It is not clear why any respondent's ratings for states of health would be constrained or circumscribed by such factors as income or access to care. Thus, the portion of the cancer burden measured (or purported to be measured) by QALYs would seem not to raise equity concerns, at least not in the same way as health care expenditures and lost productivity measures, which are conditional on economic position and opportunity. In fact, the US Panel on Cost-Effectiveness in Health and Medicine recommended measuring the health effects in economic evaluations using QALYs that employ community preferences.[5] Recently, however, Nord [91,92] and Ubel [25,26] have taken to task the traditional QALY approach: weighting states by community-average preferences serves to foreclose societal options to value differently the QALYs received by different individuals. In response, Nord and Ubel have advocated and illustrated the Person Trade-off (PTO) technique for collecting population-based information on the relative value of health gains for different members of society. For example, the PTO might ask how many patients age 65 and over with stage 3 colon cancer, who each would receive one extra year of life from cancer treatment, would be equivalent to 10 000 healthy female patients age 40–60 who each received an expected 0.10 extra years of life (a little more than a month) from mammography. Such questions are cognitively challenging but allow the decision maker to acquire a new form of information about the perceived equity of alternative distributions of health (and health gains) across important societal groups.

Finally, while the willingness-to-pay approach to burden measurement arguably offers the most comprehensive assessment, it would also appear to be at direct risk to income and wealth effects. We would expect WTP to be directly influenced by ability to pay, and evidence to date suggests this is generally the case.[5,6,74] There has been virtually no treatment of this topic in the disease burden literature, but a potential solution is suggested in the cost-benefit analysis models first proposed by Harberger[93] and expanded upon by others.[94] In computing the costs incurred or the benefits to be gained from a proposed project, calculations could be adjusted using "equity weights" that transform the raw cost and benefit projected for each population group into fairness-adjusted estimates. Determining such equity weights is extraordinarily controversial, and as a first pass, Harberger has suggested they be inversely proportional to income or wealth.

In the end, the decision maker will surely be asked to explain and defend any such equity adjustments. And when that day comes, it should well be noted that *not* adjusting burden estimates for variations in economic status and opportunity requires its own defense.

Acknowledgments

Martha Swain provided substantial technical editing assistance. Daphne Plaut performed on-line bibliographic searches and reference retrieval. Christina Gullion, Richard Meenan, and Dawn Provenzale provided comments on earlier versions of this manuscript.

REFERENCES

1 Hodgson, T. A., Meiners, M. R. (1982). Cost of illness methodology: a guide to current practices and procedures. *Milbank Memorial Fund Quarterly/Health and Society* **60**(3):429–62.

2 Hodgson, T. A. (1983). The state of the art of cost-of-illness estimates. *Advances in Health Economics and Health Service Research* **4**:129–64.

3 Rice, D. P., Hodgson, T. A., Kopstein, A. N. (1985). The economic costs of illness: a replication and update. *Health Care Financing Review* **7**(1):61–80.

4 Hodgson, T. A. (1994). Costs of illness in cost-effectiveness analysis. A review of the methodology. *Pharmacoeconomics* **6**:536–52.

5 Gold, M. R., Siegel, J. E., Russell, L. B. *et al.* (1996). *Cost-Effectiveness in Health and Medicine.* New York: Oxford University Press.

6 Drummond, M. F., O'Brien, B., Stoddart, G. L. *et al.* (1997). *Methods for the Economic Evaluation of Health Care Programmes,* (2nd Edition). Oxford: Oxford University Press.

7 Rice, D. P., Hodgson, T. A. (1981). Social and economic implications of cancer in the United States. *Vital and Health Statistics, Series 3* **20**:1–43.

8 Brown, M. L. (1990). The national economic burden of cancer: an update. *Journal of the National Cancer Institute* **82**(23):1811–14.

9 Evans, W. K., Will, B. P., Berthelot, J. M. *et al.* (1995). The cost of managing lung cancer in Canada. *Oncology (Huntington)* **9**(11 Suppl):147–53.

10 Schuette, H. L., Tucker, T. C., Brown, M. L. *et al.* (1995). The costs of cancer care in the United States: implications for action. *Oncology* (Huntington) **9**(11 Suppl):19–22.

11 Brown, M. L., Lipscomb, J., Snyder, C. (2001). The burden of illness of cancer: economic cost and quality of life. *Annual Review of Public Health* **22**:91–113.

12 Koopmanschap, M. A., van Roijen, L., Bonneux, L. *et al.* (1994). Current and future costs of cancer. *European Journal of Cancer* **30A**(1):60–5.

13 Gross, C. P., Anderson, G. F., Powe, N. R. (1999). The relation between funding by the National Institutes of Health and the burden of disease. *New England Journal of Medicine* 17;**340**(24):1881–7.

14 Forbes, J. F. (1997). The incidence of breast cancer: the global burden, public health considerations. *Seminars in Oncology* **24**(1 Suppl. 1):S20–35.

15 Young, T. K., Kliewer, E., Blanchard, J. *et al.* (2000). Monitoring disease burden and preventive behavior with data linkage: cervical cancer among aboriginal people in Manitoba, Canada. *American Journal of Public Health* **90**(9):1466–8.

16 Wunsch-Filho, V., de Camargo, E. A. (2001). The burden of mouth cancer in Latin America and the Caribbean: epidemiologic issues. *Seminars in Oncology* **28**(2):158–68.

17 Merrill, R. M., Weed, D. L. (2001). Measuring the public health burden of cancer in the United States through lifetime and age-conditional risk estimates. *Annals of Epidemiology* **8**:547–53.

18 Satcher, D. (2001). The unequal burden of cancer. *Cancer* **91**(1 Suppl.):205–7.

19 Longman, A. J., Braden, C. J., Mishel, M. H. (1996). Side effects burden in women with breast cancer. *Cancer Practice* **4**(5):274–80.

20 Longman, A. J., Braden, C. J., Mishel, M. H. (1999). Side-effects burden, psychological adjustment, and life quality in women with breast cancer: pattern of association over time. *Oncology Nursing Forum* **26**(5):909–15.

21 Mandelblatt, J. S., Bierman, A. S., Gold, K. *et al.* (2001). Constructs of burden of illness in older patients with breast cancer: a comparison of measurement methods. *Health Services Research* **36**(6 Pt 1):1085–107.

22 Nijboer, C., Tempelaar, R., Sanderman, R. *et al.* (1998). Cancer and caregiving: the impact on the caregiver's health. *Psycho-Oncology* **7**(1):3–13.

23 Munkres, A., Oberst, M. T., Hughes, S. H. (1992). Appraisal of illness, symptom distress, self-care burden, and mood states in patients receiving chemotherapy for initial and recurrent cancer. *Oncology Nursing Forum* **19**(8):1201–9.

24 Luce, B. R., Manning, W. G., Siegel, J. E. *et al.* (1996). Estimating costs in cost-effectiveness analysis. In *Cost Effectiveness in Health and Medicine*, ed. M. Gold, J. E. Siegel, L. B. Russell, M. C. Weinstein, pp. 176–213. New York: Cambridge University Press.

25 Ubel, P. A. (2000). *Pricing Life*. Cambridge, MA: MIT Press.

26 Ubel, P. A., Richardson, J., Menzel, P. (2000). Societal value, the person trade-off, and the dilemma of whose values to measure for cost-effectiveness analysis. *Health Economics* **9**:127–36.

27 National Heart, Lung, and Blood Institute. *Fact Book for Fiscal Year 2002*. Bethesda, MD, 2002. Available at: http://www.nhlbi.nih.gov/about/02factbk.pdf. Last accessed on September 12, 2004.

28 Max, W., Rice, D. P., Sung, H. Y. *et al.* (2002). The economic burden of prostate cancer, California, 1998. *Cancer* **94**(11):2906–13.

29 Seifeldin, R., Hantsch, J. J. (1999). The economic burden associated with colon cancer in the United States. *Clinical Therapeutics* **21**(8):1370–9.

30 Evans, W. K. (1998). Cost-effectiveness of vinorelbine alone or vinorelbine plus cisplatin for stage IV NSCLC. *Oncology (Huntington)* **12**(3, Suppl. 4):18–25.

31 Wirt, D. P., Giles, F. J., Oken, M. M. *et al.* (2001). Cost-effectiveness of interferon alfa-2b added to chemotherapy for high-tumor follicular non-Hodgkin's lymphoma. *Leukemia and Lymphoma* **40**(5–6):565–79.

32 Ramsey, S. D., Moinpour, C. M., Lovato, L. C. *et al.* (2002). Economic analysis of vinorelbine plus cisplatin versus paclitaxel plus carboplatin for advanced non-small-cell lung cancer. *Journal of the National Cancer Institute* **94**(4): 291–7.

33 Du, W., Touchette, D., Vaitkevicius, V. K. *et al.* (2000). Cost analysis of pancreatic carcinoma treatment. *Cancer* **89**(9):1917–24.

34 Warren, J. L., Brown, M. L., Fay, M. P. *et al.* (2002). Costs of treatment for elderly women with early-stage breast cancer in fee-for-service settings. *Journal of Clinical Oncology* **20**(1):307–16.

35 Brown, M. L., Riley, G. F., Potosky, A. L. *et al.* (1999). Obtaining long-term disease specific costs of care: application to Medicare enrollees diagnosed with rectal cancer. *Medical Care* **37**(12):1249–59.

36 Fireman, B. H., Quesenberry, C. P., Somkin, C. P. *et al.* (1997). Cost of care for cancer in a health maintenance organization. *Health Care Financing Review* **18**(4):51–76.

37 Taplin, S. H., Barlow, W., Urban, N. *et al.* (1995). Stage, age, comorbidity, and direct costs of colon, prostate, and breast cancer care. *Journal of the National Cancer Institute* **87**(6):417–26.

38 Hodgson, T. A., Cohen, A. J. (1999). Medical care expenditures for selected circulatory diseases: opportunities for reducing national health expenditures. *Medical Care* **37** (11):994–1012.

39 Etzioni, R., Urban, N., Baker, M. (1996). Estimating the costs attributable to a disease with application to ovarian cancer. *Journal of Clinical Epidemiology* **49**:95–103.

40 Etzioni, R., Ramsey, S. D., Berry, K. *et al.* (2001). The impact of including medical care costs when estimating the costs attributable to a disease: a colorectal cancer case study. *Health Economics* **10**:245–56.

41 Hornbrook, M. C., Hurtado, A. V., Johnson, R. E. (1985). Health care episodes: definition, measurement and use. *Medical Care Review* **42**:163–218.

42 Hornbrook, M. C. (1995). Definition and measurement of episodes of care in clinical and economic studies. In *Cost Analysis Methodology for Clinical Practice Guidelines Conference Proceedings*, ed. M. L. Grady, K. A. Weis, AHCPR Publication No. 95–0001, pp. 15–40. Rockville, MD: US Department of Health and Human Services, Public Health Service, Agency for Health Care Policy and Research.

43 Steinwachs, D. M. (1992). Episode of care framework: utility for medical effectiveness research. *Medical Effectiveness Research Data Methods*, M. Grady, ed. AHCPR Publication No. 92–0056. Rockville, MD: US Department of Health and Human Services, Public Health Service, Agency for Health Care Policy and Research.

44 Rosen, A. K., Mayer-Oakes, A. (1998). Developing a tool for analyzing medical care utilization of adult asthma patients on indemnity and managed care plans: can an episode of care framework be used? *American Journal of Medical Quality* **13**(4):203–12.

45 Rosen, A. K., Houchens, R. L., Gibson, T. B. *et al.* (1998). Developing episodes of care for adult asthma patients: a cautionary tale. *American Journal of Medical Quality* **13**(1):25–35.

46 Rosen, A. K., Mayer-Oakes, A. (1999). Episodes of care: theoretical frameworks versus current operational realities. *Joint Commission Journal of Quality Improvement* **25**(3):111–28.

47 Ettner, S. L., Hermann, R., Tang, H. (1999). Differences between generalists and mental health specialists in the psychiatric treatment of Medicare beneficiaries. *Health Services Research* **34**:737–60.

48 Ward, M. M., Javitz, H. S., Smith, W. M. *et al.* (2000). A comparison of three approaches for attributing hospitalizations to specific diseases in cost analyses. *International Journal of Technology Assessment in Health Care* **16**(1):125–36.

49 Weed, L. J. (1968). Medical records that guide and teach. *New England Journal of Medicine* **278**(11):593–600.

50 Weed, L. J. (1971). The problem oriented record as a basic tool in medical education, patient care and clinical research. *Annals of Clinical Research* **3**(3):131–4.

51 Reinstein, L. (1977). Problem-oriented medical record: experience in 238 rehabilitation institutions. *Archives of Physical Medicine and Rehabilitation* **58**(9):398–401.

52 Fernow, L. A., Mackie, C., McColl, I. *et al.* (1978). The effect of problem-oriented medical records on clinical management controlled for patient risks. *Medical Care* **16**(6):476–87.

53 Lloyd, S. C. (1984). Computer-generated progress notes in an automated POMR. *Journal of Medical Systems* **8**(102):35–42.

54 Hornbrook, M. C., Goodman, M. J., Fishman, P. A. *et al.* (1998). Health-based payment and computerized patient record systems. *Effective Clinical Practice* **1**(2):66–72.

55 Hornbrook, M. C., Goodman, M. J., Fishman, P.A. *et al.* (1998). Building health plan databases to risk-adjust outcomes and payments. *International Journal for Quality in Health Care* **10**(6):531–8.

56 DiGianni, L. M., Garber, J. E., Winer, E. P. (2002). Complementary and alternative medicine use among women with breast cancer. *Journal of Clinical Oncology* **20**(18 Suppl.):34S–8S.

57 Medical Economics Staff (2002). *200 Red Book*. Montvale, NJ: Thomsen Medical Economics. Inc. See http://www.medec.com/html/products/productdetail/redbook.html, last accessed March 21, 2003.

58 Physician Payment Review Commission (1990). *Annual Report to Congress 1990*. Washington, DC: US Government Printing Office.

59 Birenbaum, L. K., Clarke-Steffen, L. (1992). Terminal care costs in childhood cancer. *Pediatric Nursing* **18**(3):285–8.

60 Moore, K. (1998). Out-of-pocket expenditures of outpatients receiving chemotherapy. *Oncology Nursing Forum* **25**(9):1615–20.

61 Agency for Healthcare Research & Quality. *Medical Expenditure Panel Survey*. Available at http://www.ahrq.gov/data/mepsix.htm. Last accessed on September 12, 2004.

62 Friedman, B., De La Mare, J., Andrews, R. *et al.* (2002). Practical options for estimating cost of hospital inpatient stays. *Journal of Health Care Finance* **29**:1–13.

63 Hsiao, W. C., Braun, P., Dunn, D. L. *et al.* (1992). An overview of the development and refinement of the Resource-Based Relative Value Scale. The foundation for reform of U.S. physician payment. *Medical Care* **30**(11 Suppl.):NS1–12.

64 Berlin, M. F., Faber, B. P., Berlin, L. M. *et al.* (1997). RVU costing applications. *Healthcare Financial Management* **51**(11):73–4, 76.

65 Grimaldi, P. L. (2002). Medicare fees for physician services are resource-based. *Journal of Health Care Finance* **28**(3):88–104.

66 Bronstein, J. M., Adams, E. K. (2002). Rural-urban differences in health risks, resource use and expenditures within three state Medicaid programs: implications for Medicaid managed care. *Journal of Rural Health* **18**(1):38–48.

67 Fries, B. E., Schneider, D. P., Foley, W. J. *et al.* (1989). Case-mix classification of Medicare residents in skilled nursing facilities: resource utilization groups (RUG-T18). *Medical Care* **27**(9):843–58.

68 Fries, B. E. (1990). Comparing case-mix systems for nursing home payment. *Health Care Financing Review* **11**(4):103–19.

69 Fries, B. E., Schneider, D. P., Foley, W. J. *et al.* (1994). Refining a case-mix measure for nursing homes: resource utilization groups (RUG-III). *Medical Care* **32**(7):668–85.

70 Carpenter, G. I., Main, A., Turner, G. F. (1995). Casemix for the elderly inpatient: resource utilization groups (RUGs) validation project. Casemix for the Elderly Inpatient Working Group. *Age and Ageing* **24**(1):5–13.

71 Loeve, F., Brown, M. L., Boer, R. *et al.* (2000). Endoscopic colorectal cancer screening: a cost-saving analysis. *Journal of the National Cancer Institute* **92**(7):557–63.

72 Tsao, H., Rogers, G. S., Sober, A. J. (1998). An estimate of the annual direct cost of treating cutaneous melanoma. *Journal of the American Academy of Dermatology* **38**(5 Pt 1):669–80.

73 Grover, S. A., Coupal, L., Zowall, H. *et al.* (2000). The clinical burden of prostate cancer in Canada: forecasts from the Montreal Prostate Cancer Model. *Canadian Medical Association Journal* **162**(7):977–83.

74 O'Brien, this volume, Chapter 25.

75 Fairclough, this volume, Chapter 17.

76 Miller, L. L., Hornbrook, M. C., Archbold, P. G. *et al.* (1996). Development of use and cost measures in a nursing intervention for family caregivers and frail elderly patients. *Research in Nursing and Health* **19**(4):273–85.

77 Chochinov, H. M., Kristjanson, L. (1998). Dying to pay: the cost of end-of-life care. *Journal of Palliative Care* **14**(4):5–15.

78 Emanuel, E. J., Fairclough, D. L., Slutsman, J. *et al.* (2000). Understanding economic and other burdens of terminal illness: the experience of patients and their caregivers. *Annals of Internal Medicine* **132**(6):451–9.

79 Arno, P. S., Levine, C., Memmott, M. M. (1999). The economic value of informal caregiving. *Health Affairs (Millwood)* **18**(2):182–8.

80 Hayman, J. A., Langa, K. M., Kabeto, M. U. *et al.* (2001). Estimating the cost of informal caregiving for elderly patients with cancer. *Journal of Clinical Oncology* **19**(13):3219–25.

81 Harrow, B. S., Tennstedt, S. L., McKinlay, J. B. (1995). How costly is it to care for disabled elders in a community setting? *Gerontologist* **35**(6):803–13.

82 Goldman, D. P., Schoenbaum, M. L., Potosky, A. L. *et al.* (2001). Measuring the incremental cost of clinical cancer research. *Journal of Clinical Oncology* **19**(1):105–10.

83 Hahn, R. W. (ed.). *Risks, Costs, and Lives Saved: Getting Better Results from Regulation.* New York: Oxford University Press.

84 McGarity, T. O., Ruttenberg, R. (1997). Counting the cost of health, safety, and environmental regulation. *Texas Law Review* **80**:1997–2058.

85 Harrington, W., Morgenstern, R. D. (2000). On the accuracy of regulatory cost estimates. *Journal of Policy Analysis and Management* **19**:297–318.

86 Morganstern, R. D., Pizer, W. A., Shih, J. S. (2001). The cost of environmental protection. *The Review of Economics and Statistics* **83**:732–8.

87 Joshi, S., Krishnan, R., Lave, L. (2001). Estimating the hidden costs of environmental regulation. *The Accounting Review* **76**:171–98.

88 Freeman, A. M. (2002). Environmental policy since earth day I: what do we know about the benefits and costs? *Agricultural and Resource Economics Review* **31**:1–14.

89 Feeny, this volume, Chapter 4.

90 Murphy, K. M., Topel, R. H. (2003). The Economic Value of Medical Research. In *Exceptional Returns: the Economic Value of America's Investment in Medical Research*, ed. R. H. Topel, K. M. Murphy. Chicago, IL: University of Chicago Press.

91 Nord, E. (1999). *Cost-value Analysis in Health Care.* Cambridge: Cambridge University Press.

92 Nord, E., Pinto, J. L., Richardson, J. *et al.* (1999). Incorporating societal concerns for fairness in numerical valuations of health programmes. *Health Economics* **8**:25–39.

93 Harberger, A. C. (1978). On the use of distributional weights in social cost–benefit analysis. *Journal of Political Economy* **86**(2), Part 2, S87–S120.

94 Boardman, A. E., Greenberg, D. H., Vining, A. R. *et al.* (1996). *Cost–Benefit Analysis: Concepts and Practice*, pp. 37–47. Prentice Hall, Upper Saddle River, NJ.

25

Cost-effectiveness analysis in cancer: toward an iterative framework for integration of evidence from trials and models

Bernie J. O'Brien, Ph.D.

McMaster University and Centre for Evaluation of Medicines, St Joseph's Hospital, Hamilton, ON, Canada

Introduction

Cost-effectiveness analysis is now an integral part of technology assessment and addresses the question of whether a new treatment or diagnostic intervention offers good value for money. Economic evaluation has been most prominent and formalized in the context of public-payer reimbursement of new medicines. For example, the national Pharmaceutical Benefits Scheme in Australia and the Ontario Drug Benefit Plan in Canada both require economic evidence from manufacturers in support of new submissions for formulary listing.[1,2] In the UK, the National Institute of Clinical Excellence (NICE) uses economic evidence in setting guidance for the use of new technologies in the National Health Service.[3] In the USA, the Public Health Service has issued influential guidelines in how health care cost-effectiveness studies should be conducted.[4]

Cancer is a leading cause of death and disability, and advances in diagnosis and treatment often come at a high price that generates economic scrutiny and policy debate. For example, in their recent initial evaluation of a group of drugs known as taxanes (e.g., paclitaxel and docetaxel) for the British National Health Service, NICE raised doubts about their cost effectiveness,[5] which led to appeals from manufacturers, lobbying from patient groups, and intense media coverage. Many other examples exist, covering the range from cancer screening (e.g., mammography for women between 40 and 50 years), cancer diagnosis (PET scanning for staging of lung cancer), and cancer treatment (e.g., Herceptin® for metastatic breast cancer or surgery for prostate cancer). All of the major academic cancer journals regularly publish economic evaluations.

In this chapter we have two goals. The first is to offer an overview and assessment of economic evaluation in cancer care, illustrating both decision-analytic modeling approaches and prospective cost-effectiveness trials. The second goal is to make an argument about the relation between modeling and trial-based data collection. Specifically, we contend that the primary role of data gathering in clinical trials and elsewhere should be to update a pre-existing model of cost effectiveness and to give more precise estimates of model parameters. Using the Bayesian reasoning of observed data being used to update prior information, new evidence should be used to reduce both structural (related to the model structure itself) and parameter (related to the estimated values of the parameters in the model) uncertainty in a cost-effectiveness model. We characterize this process as an iterative loop, where the value of new information in reducing decision uncertainty plays a key role in the decision to conduct further data collection. We conclude that the iterative loop for evidence synthesis provides a logical framework for adaptive cost-effectiveness analysis and efficient data collection.

Economic evaluation: rationale and basic techniques

The rationale for economic evaluation derives from the concept of economic efficiency. The fundamental scarcity of resources, coupled with the multitude of health care programs that are competing for funding and priority, forces the need to make choices. For the economist, an important principle guiding choice is the notion of efficiency; stated simply, this is an attempt to achieve the mix of programs and services that maximize the health benefit from the available resources for the population being served. The logic of efficiency can be applied at different "levels" in health care delivery, whether it is allocating a local cancer care budget between competing programs or allocating resources more broadly between competing health care priorities in different disease areas. Operationally, the quest for efficiency requires us to identify, measure, and value both the costs and outcomes of alternative programs so that comparisons can be made.

There are four basic types of economic evaluation,[6-8] and they differ based on how the outcomes of interest are measured.

Cost-minimization analysis (CMA)

Traditional guidance suggests that CMA can be used when it has been established that the health outcomes of two alternatives are not different, because it then makes sense to choose the less costly option. But assuming or establishing the equivalence of outcomes is fraught with conceptual and empirical problems,[9] and this technique should be used with caution. We strongly discourage the use of this method.

An example of CMA in cancer treatment is the comparison between an oral versus intravenous etoposide in the treatment of small cell lung cancer. The results from a randomized multi-center clinical trial indicated no difference in efficacy between groups in terms of overall response rates and toxicities. Consequently, the authors only compared resource use for the oral and intravenous treatment approaches and estimated the difference in total cost per course of therapy was US$349 less for the oral therapy.[10]

Cost-effectiveness analysis (CEA)

CEA measures program benefits in terms of program-specific outcome units such as "cases detected" for a screening program or "life-years gained" for a treatment program. CEA is most appropriate for comparisons of alternative therapies to treat the same condition because it addresses the conditional question: *given* that we want to achieve some specific outcome, what is the least-cost way of achieving it? An example would be the comparison of different chemotherapy regimens in small cell lung cancer in which the results of cost-effectiveness analysis might be reported in terms of the cost per relapse.

An example of a CEA is a retrospective economic evaluation of a randomized clinical trial performed by the Canadian National Cancer Institute on chemotherapy for lung cancer.[11] The study compared two chemotherapeutic regimens (vindecine + cisplatin (VP) and cyclophosphamide + doxorubicin + cisplatin (CAP)) with best supportive care (BSC). A detailed costing study of hospital-based services from the viewpoint of the public health care plan was performed based on the resource utilization in two centers, which were claimed to be representative of oncology centres in Canada. The mean survival and mean costs were 24 weeks and CDN$8600 for BSC, 37 weeks and CDN$12 200 for VP, and 32 weeks and CDN$7600 for CAP. Therefore, using survival as the outcome measure, CAP was cost saving compared to BSC at CDN$6200 per year of life gained and VP cost CDN$49 700 per life-year gained compared to CAP.

Cost-utility analysis (CUA)

CUA is an extension of CEA and permits the comparison of programs in circumstances where there is no single unidimensional measure of outcome. So, not only are the number of years of life counted, but consideration is given for the quality (or utility) associated with health states experienced during those years of life. In cancer treatment this is clearly a common situation. The outcome measure in CUA is typically survival time weighted for reductions in quality of life by estimated utility weights; the composite metric of outcome is known as quality-adjusted life-years (QALYs). Feeny discusses these utility weights in detail in Chapter 4 in this volume.[12] In addition to permitting the multidimensionality of outcomes to be captured, having estimates of cost per QALY permits a broader comparison across treatment programs; for example, for the same resources, does a new treatment in prostate cancer produce more or less QALYs than a program to increase the frequency of cervical cancer screening?

In passing, a minor issue of nomenclature should be noted: some analysts (including, for example, the US Panel on Cost-Effectiveness in Health and Medicine[4]) do not make a distinction between CEA and CUA, but consider QALYs as a permissible outcome measure for CEA. In the majority of this chapter we will use the term "cost-effectiveness analysis" in this more general sense of including CUA.

An example of CUA is the study by Hayman et al.[13] comparing conservative surgery for breast cancer with and without radiation therapy. The estimates for the quality-of-life weightings (utilities) for non-metastatic health states were collected from 97 breast cancer patients who had been treated with lumpectomy and radiation therapy using the standard gamble technique. In addition, the utilities of 20 medical oncology nurses were also collected for the same outcomes and used in the sensitivity analysis. Expert judgment was used to estimate utilities for metastatic health states. Baseline results showed no gain in survival with the addition of radiation, with both strategies having a life expectancy of 7.81 years. However, there was an increase in *quality-adjusted* life-years with the addition of radiation therapy, with an additional cost per patient of US$9800. This implied that when quality of life is included, the strategy of adjunctive radiation therapy had a CE ratio of US$28 000 per QALY, well within the range of what is generally considered good value for money.

Weeks[14] has argued that approaches to economic evaluation, such as CUA, that incorporate evidence on preference-based quality of life are important in cancer evaluations to capture trade-offs between quantity and quality of health outcomes. However, readers should be cautious in using these results uncritically. In their comprehensive review of cost-utility assessments in oncology from 1975 through 1997, Earle et al.[15] raised concerns about the quality of the preference-based methods adopted in some studies.

Cost-benefit analysis (CBA)

CBA is a technique for broad program comparisons, within and between sectors of the economy (e.g., health, education, defense), to inform resource allocations. With direct links back to market-based welfare economic theory, the operational challenge of CBA is that both costs and outcomes need to be converted into monetary units to permit an assessment of net benefit. Although CBA is widely used in environmental and transport program evaluation, where benefits – including health – are monetized using consumer willingness-to-pay, the use of CBA in health care evaluation has been limited.[6,16,17]

Ortega et al. made an attempt at cost-benefit analysis and estimated willingness-to-pay for the benefit of prophylactic epoetin alfa to reduce anemia by face-to-face interviews of cancer patients undergoing chemotherapy. When balanced against the total cost of the drug, the net incremental cost of US$2943 suggests that these patients were not willing to pay a sufficient amount to cover the cost of epoetin alfa to avoid anemia.[18] The main problem with this study, as argued by O'Brien and Gafni,[16] is that the relevant question for willingness-to-pay is not what patients are willing to pay at the point of service, but is an insurance-based question for all persons at risk of using a program or service in the future. An example of such an insurance-based willingness-to-pay approach in oncology is found in the study by O'Brien et al.,[19] which estimated how much additional insurance enrollees in a managed care organization would pay for coverage of colony

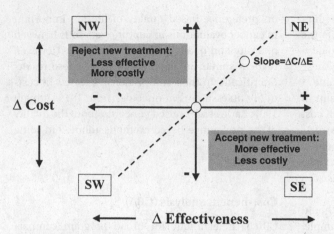

Figure 25.1. The cost-effectiveness plane. The origin is the comparator therapy from which is plotted the coordinates for the new therapy; its incremental effectiveness (ΔE) and incremental cost (ΔC). The slope of the dashed line from the origin bisecting this point (ΔE, ΔC) is the incremental cost-effectiveness ratio (ICER = ΔC/ΔE).

stimulating growth factor, which is used for prophylaxis of chemotherapy-induced neutropenia.

Making decisions: the cost-effectiveness plane

One useful diagram that helps orient new readers to the methods of economic evaluation and its relation to decision making is the cost-effectiveness plane shown in Figure 25.1. The plane defines an x-y coordinate space where the results of an incremental cost-effectiveness analysis can be plotted. The x-axis is the difference (new treatment minus comparator) per patient in the mean effect (ΔE), and the y-axis is the difference in mean cost (ΔC). For ease of reference, the points of the compass are used to refer to the four quadrants defined. For the moment, assume the x-y coordinate for the new treatment (ΔE, ΔC) is known with certainty, and this point is plotted on the plane. Clearly, any programs falling in either the northwest or southeast quadrants are eliminated by the logic of dominance; programs that increase costs and lower effects should never be adopted, and programs that lower costs and increase effectiveness should always be adopted.

Most programs fall into the northeast quadrant and offer additional effectiveness at added cost. In this circumstance, it is useful to extend a straight line from the origin (the comparator therapy) that

bisects the (ΔE, ΔC) coordinate; the slope of this line (dashed line in Figure 25.1) is the ratio ΔC/ΔE and is known as the incremental cost-effectiveness ratio (ICER). Whether a program in the northeast quadrant is economically attractive will depend upon the relation between the observed ICER and some predefined ceiling ratio (λ), which can be thought of as Society's willingness-to-pay for an additional unit of health outcome. If the ICER $\leq \lambda$, the program's cost-effectiveness is acceptable.

It will be immediately evident to most readers that an important omission from our discussion of the cost-effectiveness plane is any consideration of uncertainty. The location of (ΔE, ΔC) will not be known precisely but estimated and subject to sampling error and other forms of measurement error. In the extreme, it may not be known whether the joint distribution of (ΔE, ΔC) lies in one or more quadrants.

Our brief overview of economic evaluation methods highlights two key points, which are developed further below: (1) With the exception of CBA, which is seldom used in health care, the vast majority of economic evaluations generate *estimates* of incremental cost-effectiveness or cost-utility (e.g., a new cancer treatment, compared to usual care, has a cost-effectiveness of $30 000 per life-year gained). Cost-effectiveness data, therefore, tell us the price of achieving a specified outcome, and whether this is good value for money is a value judgment based on what Society is willing to pay (i.e., sacrifice elsewhere) for improved health. Every time a decision is made using cost-effectiveness data, an implicit monetary valuation of health outcomes is made implicitly or explicitly. (2) All estimates of cost-effectiveness are subject to uncertainty because the true values of parameters in the analysis are not known. As we will show, careful analysis and presentation of uncertainty is an important feature of contemporary economic evaluation that can provide key insights into the value of collecting new data to reduce parameter imprecision and decision error.

Decision analytic cost-effectiveness models

There are two stylized ways to proceed in the construction of an economic analysis of the type described above; the first is to construct a decision-analytic model, and the second is to conduct a pragmatic trial where cost and effect data are collected as part of a randomized controlled trial of two or more therapies. We describe each of these in turn and then argue that the combination of both approaches is the best way forward.

A typical cost-effectiveness model uses tools of decision analysis to construct a mathematical model of a treatment comparison. Such a model relates multiple inputs of cost and effect parameters, derived from multiple sources, to make predictions about outputs that are of relevance to decision makers, such as expected program costs and expected QALYs. Components of modeling can be structured into four broad activities: model structure design, data incorporation, data modeling, and model validation.

Model structure

The starting point in the design of a decision model is a decision tree, which is a systematic and quantitative method for representing, in schematic form, all the important outcomes of a decision

and explicitly estimates the expected value of each alternative.[20,21] To illustrate, the decision tree from the study by Marshall et al.[22] on the potential cost-effectiveness of screening for lung cancer with helical CT scanning in a high-risk cohort is shown in Figures 25.2 and 25.3. Figure 25.2 illustrates the decision tree at a summary level, distinguishing between a strategy of screening for lung cancer and no screening for lung cancer. In this study, survival was stratified by gender, age group, stage of cancer, and tumor size using data from the Surveillance, Epidemiology and End Results (SEER) registry database; this detail of stratification for individuals with lung cancer is illustrated in Figure 25.3. The time horizon of the model was 5 years and, therefore, manageable within a decision tree framework.

Decision trees are appropriate for modeling interventions where events occur over a relatively short time period and the required structure is not too complex; the disadvantage of using trees to model longer duration or more complex structures is that they become too "bushy" and difficult to manage.[23–25] A common approach to the design of models over longer periods of time, and where complex disease history must be characterized, is the use of stochastic compartment models such as Markov State-Transition models. In a typical Markov model, the analyst defines a finite number of "states" that a patient can be in over time. Each state might have QALY weights and costs associated with a sojourn time, and the model proceeds by taking the expectation of these outcomes conditional upon the specified probabilities for transitions between states. The most common analytic procedure is the Markov Cohort simulation method described by Sonnenberg and Beck[26] and further discussed in Briggs and Sculpher.[27]

One of the early applications of the Markov model approach in cancer is the study by Hillner and Smith[28] on the efficacy and cost-effectiveness of adjuvant chemotherapy in women with node-negative breast cancer. Adaptations of this model have subsequently been used by other groups to evaluate other treatments in breast cancer.[13] Nine health states were used in the model using annual intervals for movements between states. All women

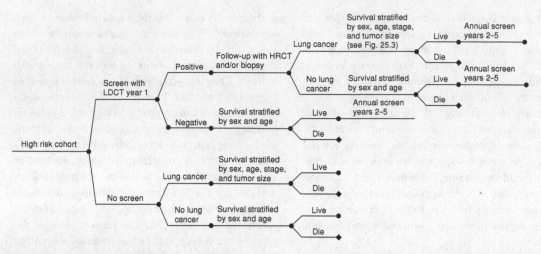

Figure 25.2. A decision tree of screening a high-risk cohort for lung cancer with low dose computed tomography (LDCT) compared to no screening. Patients with a positive result are followed up with high resolution CT (HRCT) and/or biopsy. Survival is stratified by gender, age, stage of cancer, and tumor size as illustrated in Figure 25.3. Present figure used with permission: Marshall, D. A., Simpson, K. N., Earle, C. C. *et al.* (2001). Economic decision analysis model of screening for lung cancer. *European Journal of Cancer* **37**:1759–67.

started in the well state without metastatic disease and moved through the states based on assigned probabilities until all women in the cohort died or reached the age of 90. In the first year, the cohort that received chemotherapy could experience minor (nausea and vomiting without hospitalization) or major toxicity (complications sufficient to require hospitalization) or death. If there was no recurrence of breast cancer, the patient returned to being well in the next year of the model. In each subsequent year, a woman could remain free of recurrence (well) or have her first recurrence of breast cancer. If a first recurrence occurred, the patient might respond to salvage therapy (post-first-recurrence state) or die. Once a patient had a first recurrence, it was not possible to return to the well state. A maximum of three recurrences were considered. The structure and possible transitions for the Markov model are illustrated in Figure 25.4.

Data incorporation

The philosophy guiding the incorporation of data into models is that of "the best available data." Models synthesize evidence from many different sources of empirical data, including clinical trials, observational studies, and public health statistics, into a logical framework to answer clinical and policy questions.[29–32] It may be logical to incorporate parameters such as a treatment efficacy from a meta-analysis of randomized trials, but other parameters are difficult or impossible to observe in most randomized trials; for example, long-term safety of a new therapy or patient compliance with medication in real-world settings. We return to the issue of trial-based data and modeling below.

Data modeling

The ISPOR (International Society for Pharmacoeconomics and Outcomes Research) Task Force on modeling includes a discussion of data modeling, which is defined as the mathematical steps that are taken to transform empirical observations into a form that is useful for decision modeling.[29] Virtually every economic evaluation includes some form of data modeling to generate the results. This includes transforming interval probabilities into an appropriate format and time

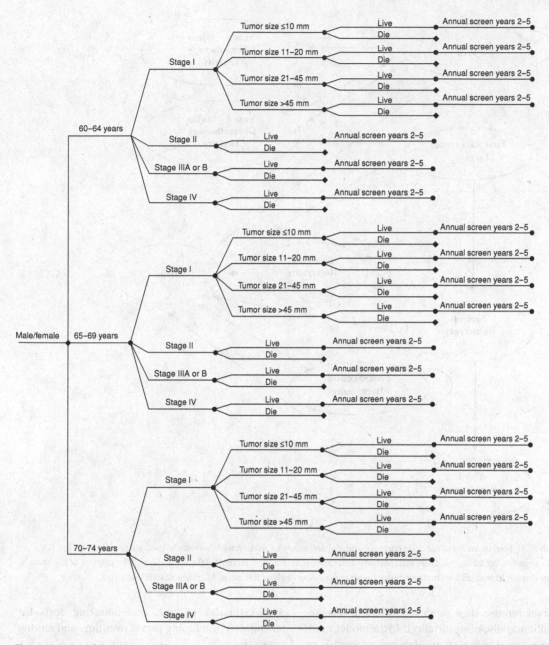

Figure 25.3. Partial decision tree of lung cancer screening showing survival stratification based on Surveillance, Epidemiology and End Results (SEER) data. Survival is assigned by gender, age, stage of cancer, and tumor size over 5 years. Used with permission: Marshall, D. A., Simpson, K. N., Earle, C. C. *et al.* (2001). Economic decision analysis model of screening for lung cancer. *European Journal of Cancer* **37**:1759–67.

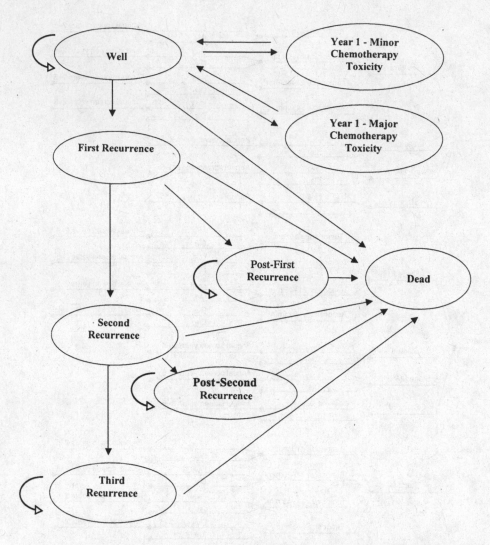

Figure 25.4. Markov model of cancer recurrence and chemotherapy for women who have undergone surgery for Stage I or IIA (node-negative) breast cancer. Used with permission: Hillner, B. E., Smith, T. J. (1991). Efficacy and cost-effectiveness of adjuvant chemotherapy in women with node-negative breast cancer. *New England Journal of Medicine* **324**:160–68.

interval for use in a model, combining disease-specific and all-cause mortality into the model, modeling survival using an underlying parametric or non-parametric distribution function, modeling the effect of risk factors on baseline probabilities or rates of disease incidence or mortality, estimating multi-attribute utilities from domain-specific utilities, transforming available price and charge information into estimates of cost, and adjusting costs for changes in purchasing power over time and among countries.

Model validation

Model validation refers to tests to confirm the internal and external consistency of the model with known facts and includes both debugging and calibration.[33] Validation may include (a) ensuring the face validity of the model, (b) corroboration or convergent validity to compare the results of the model that were developed independently, and (c) predictive validity to determine whether a model produces results that actually occur. McCabe and Dixon[34] provide a good overview of the literature describing the steps and approaches to model validation. They then go on to present a framework for assessing the validity of cost-effectiveness models that includes evaluating the structure, inputs, and results from the model and assessing the value of the model to the decision maker.

An example of a model that underwent extensive verification and calibration is the Montreal Prostate Cancer Model.[35] This is a Markov state-transition model that was used to estimate the direct medical costs associated with each treatment modality to forecast the total lifetime clinical and economic burden of prostate cancer among a cohort of Canadian men aged 40–80 years in 1997. The model was validated specific to tumor stage and grade using: (1) national population cancer statistics from the National Cancer Institute of Canada (NCIC); (2) long-term survival data from a population-based study of nearly 60 000 men with clinically localized prostate cancer: and (3) observed survival rates from the Connecticut Tumor Registry.

Randomized cost-effectiveness trials

The second approach to conducting cost-effectiveness analysis is to collect data on use of resources and costs prospectively for each patient as part of a randomized trial.[36–38] One of the attractions of this approach is that patient-level data on both costs and effects are available for analysis. However, as discussed later, this kind of data can introduce biases related to both patient inclusion criteria and protocol effects. This approach has been adopted in a number of cancer treatment trials, and the National Cancer Institute (NCI) and the

American Society of Clinical Oncology (ASCO) jointly produced an economics workbook that aimed to identify and elucidate important characteristics of economic evaluations in cancer clinical trials.[8] The intention was that it should be a practical reference outlining considerations in the planning and implementation of an economic analysis alongside a cancer clinical trial, including the types of costs specific to cancer that should be collected, the design of data collection forms, and details about statistical issues in the analysis of economic data from clinical trials.

Examples of prospective economic evaluations alongside clinical cancer trials include studies by Schulman et al.[39] and Drummond.[36] Schulman et al.[39] undertook an economic study accompanying a multi-center, randomized, controlled clinical trial of sequential interleukin-3 followed by GM-CSF (colony stimulating factor) compared to CSF alone. Over the 13-month study period, they showed that there was no significant effect on the costs of care for patients undergoing bone marrow transplantation (GM-CSF alone = US$79 892 and GM-CSF plus IL-3=US$89 651). This study demonstrated the feasibility of prospective economic evaluation of medical therapy in cancer trials.

There are several limitations to trial-based cost-effectiveness analysis, and these arise largely because, in most cases, the economic analysis is a so-called "piggyback" analysis into an existing trial designed to test an efficacy hypothesis. Elsewhere we have discussed several reasons why some form of modeling is needed to adapt, modify, or extend trial-based observations,[40] and others have concluded that modeling is "an inevitable fact of life" in economic evaluation.[41] Consider now four groups of issues that limit the usefulness of trial-based evaluation.

Wrong comparator therapy

Comparators, such as placebo, that may be required for efficacy decisions, such as licensing of new pharmaceuticals, may have limited relevance for reimbursement decisions if a new therapy will replace an existing therapy. For example, in evaluating the cost-effectiveness of trastuzumab (Herceptin®) for treatment of metastatic breast cancer, the most relevant treatment alternative is standard chemotherapy. In the pivotal randomized controlled trial of trastuzumab, women who had not previously received adjuvant therapy with anthracycline were treated with doxorubicin or epirubicin; those who had previously received adjuvant anthracycline were treated with paclitaxel.[42]

If head-to-head trials of active therapies are not available, some form of statistical modeling based on indirect meta-analysis is required. This is feasible provided that the two therapies to be compared have both been studied in a trial with a common third comparator. For example, an inference about A versus B can be made provided that both A and B have been compared to C in similar patient populations. Bucher *et al.* have demonstrated this methodology using data on prophylactic treatments for pneumocystis carinni in HIV-infected patients.[43]

Protocol effects

Some aspects of cost or outcome that are observed in a clinical trial would not be part of usual care outside the research setting. There are numerous examples of protocol effects, including the effects of blinding, where resources may be consumed to protect knowledge of treatment assignment. For example, regular blood tests for toxicity for an investigational drug are required, but the tests would also have to be undertaken for an existing drug with a known toxicity profile. Freemantle and Drummond[44] argue that cost-effectiveness trials should not be blinded.

Efficacy versus effectiveness endpoints

Outcomes such as change in tumor size are intermediate markers of therapeutic success (efficacy) and may not be the most relevant *effectiveness* endpoints for economic evaluation where, as noted above, the focus is on final health outcomes such as improvements in survival and/or quality of life. If a trial provides only an intermediate marker as a primary endpoint, it may be necessary either to analyze (potentially underpowered) secondary endpoints such as survival, or undertake statistical modeling using, for example, extra-trial observational data relating changes in the intermediate outcome to endpoints such as survival. Another modeling approach would be a Markov model of disease progression that relates intermediate and final outcomes. Similarly, where the objective of the CEA is to include some measure of health-related quality of life (HRQOL), and the clinical trial does not include outcome measures that are preference based, some kind of mapping is needed to translate the results into CEA metrics.

For example, evidence from randomized controlled trials for screening for colorectal cancer exists only for fecal occult blood testing. However, various models of cost-effectiveness have been developed to demonstrate the potential cost-effectiveness (in terms of costs per life-year or quality-adjusted life-year saved) of using colonoscopy for colorectal cancer screening by combining data relating intermediate outcomes to survival. The model by Ness *et al.*[45] uses a discrete event simulation to combine data on colonoscopy testing parameters to detect colorectal cancer (including small, intermediate, and large polyps) with a detailed model of the natural history of colorectal neoplasia and disease progression. The model predicts the number of colonoscopies performed, the number of cases of colorectal cancer, the number of colorectal cancer deaths, as well as the costs and quality-adjusted life-years per person. The authors conclude that one time colonoscopy screening between 50 and 54 years of age is cost-effective (US$3625 per quality adjusted life-year) compared to no screening and screening at older ages in both men and women.

Truncated follow-up time

Randomized trials of cancer therapies have finite periods of follow-up and vary among days, weeks, or years. A challenge for conducting cost-effectiveness analysis is that important and attributable costs and outcomes may be sufficiently "downstream" that they are not observed during the trial. Particularly for chronic diseases such as cancer, adopting sufficiently long time horizons for analysis is of key importance for unbiased estimates of cost-effectiveness. The US Public Health Service Panel[4] took a strong view on this issue and recommended that studies adopt the time horizon of a patient's lifetime. Although some have taken the view that it "is inappropriate to model economic benefits after stopping long-term treatment and policy decisions should not be based on such models,"[46] we believe that some form of extrapolation beyond clinical trial observation is necessary for most cost-effectiveness studies, and particularly so for chronic diseases such as cancer.

Integration of evidence from trials and models

In summary, there is no simple dichotomy between modeling and trial-based cost-effectiveness studies; the former attempt to integrate trial and other evidence into a model, and the latter require modeling to adapt, adjust, or extend observations made in an experiment to be relevant to a reimbursement policy decision. To some extent this can be seen as a trade-off between internal and external validity; trials provide unbiased estimates of efficacy in selected populations but may not provide generalizable estimates of effectiveness.

Approaches to the integration of evidence from experimental and observational sources include the General Accounting Office's report on Cross-Design Synthesis,[30] and the work of Eddy *et al.*[47] on the Confidence Profile Method for meta-analysis. In what follows, we apply such an approach to general integrative reasoning to cost-effectiveness evidence from trials and models. We first explain how new advances in the analysis of uncertainty in cost-effectiveness data provide a framework for estimating the value of collecting new data. We then use this Bayesian reasoning to propose an adaptive process for model building and new data collection.

The new analytics of uncertainty in cost-effectiveness analysis

Several related topics are receiving increased attention and, together, are enhancing our ability to define, estimate, cope with, and, in some cases, reduce the uncertainty accompanying estimates of cost-effectiveness.

Sensitivity analysis

For many years the conventional approach to assessing parameter uncertainty in a cost-effectiveness analysis has been by one-way or multi-way sensitivity analyses.[48,49] In a one-way sensitivity analysis, the analyst identifies the key model parameters to which the model results are anticipated to be sensitive. In an exploration of "what if," each of these parameters is then changed one at a time to determine the effect on the results. Specifically, the focus is on the range of values of the parameter for which the CE ratio falls below the designated threshold value for determining whether the intervention is "cost-effective." A multi-way sensitivity analysis proceeds in a similar way, but the analyst varies more than one parameter at the same time.

More recently, probabilistic approaches to evaluating uncertainty have been advocated so that the results of a sensitivity analysis convey information about both the range of possible results and the probability of each result.[50,51] Probabilistic sensitivity analysis makes it possible to assign ranges and distributions to uncertain variables in a model. The parameters to consider might include estimates related to (a) the probabilities of a pathway in a decision tree or transition probabilities in a Markov model, (b) estimates of resource use and health outcomes, and (c) estimates of the values associated with the resource use (costs) and health outcomes (utility weights). By assigning a distribution to each such parameter, a probabilistic sensitivity analysis can be undertaken by sampling from these parameter distributions simultaneously in a (second-order) Monte Carlo simulation.[48] Such an approach provides the simulated joint density between costs and effects and permits the analyst to compute, for the cost-effectiveness ratio, analogues of conventional measures of precision for parameters, such as 95% confidence intervals. A detailed illustration of how probabilistic sensitivity analysis can be applied to a model of alternative treatments for reflux disease can be found in the paper by Briggs *et al*.[52]

There have also been advances in methods for statistical analysis of data on observed costs and effects from trial-based cost-effectiveness studies. Non-parametric re-sampling methods such as bootstrapping are increasingly being used for estimating standard errors and confidence intervals for cost and effect means.[53] Parametric methods such as Fieller's Theorem, where cost and effect differences are assumed to follow a bivariate normal distribution, have also been shown to have good coverage properties in computing confidence intervals for the cost-effectiveness ratio.[54,55] A comprehensive review of statistical methods in cost-effectiveness methods can be found in the paper by Briggs *et al*.[51]

New directions in uncertainty: net benefit analysis

While the computation of 95% confidence intervals for cost-effectiveness ratios has an intuitive appeal, there are some problems to this approach that limit its usefulness. A key problem identified by Stinnett and Mullahy[56] is that of negative cost-effectiveness ratios, which can occur in two different ways: ΔC negative and ΔE positive (southeast quadrant in Figure 25.1); ΔC positive and ΔE negative (northwest quadrant in Figure 25.1). The first case has the interpretation of dominance to accept the new treatment; the second case has the complete opposite interpretation. The issue is that a statistical distribution of the incremental cost-effectiveness ratio, for example, by bootstrapping, will simply order replicates of the ratio from low to high and will not distinguish between these negative ratios, which will all be placed in the left tail of the distribution. A confidence interval based on such a distribution will be incorrect for purposes of coherent decision making within the cost-effectiveness framework. A further

problem with presenting uncertainty for the cost-effectiveness ratio is that the mean of the ratio is not the same as the ratio of the means; it is the latter which is the relevant parameter.[57]

These problems led Stinnett and Mullahy to suggest a simple transformation of the cost-effectiveness ratio into a conditional net benefit statistic,[56] where net benefit can either be computed in terms of health units or monetary units.[58] To illustrate, consider the computation of the Net Monetary Benefit (NMB) of an intervention. From our earlier discussion, define:

ΔE = difference in mean effect (treatment − control)

ΔC = difference in mean cost (treatment − control)

λ = what Society is willing to pay for one more unit of health effects

As indicated earlier, the usual decision rule for cost-effectiveness is whether the incremental ratio lies below the threshold willingness-to-pay:

$$\Delta C/\Delta E < \lambda$$

Although λ may be (indeed, typically now is) an unknown parameter to the analyst setting up the CEA, its value must be determined by the decision maker when a decision is made. Put another way, when a choice is made between the two alternatives, it is *as if* the decision maker has arrived at some determination about the value of λ. Therefore, one can multiply through by λ and transform the decision rule into Net Monetary Benefit that is conditional on λ

$$NMB(\lambda) = \lambda \Delta E - \Delta C$$

All units of measurement are now commensurate (for example, in dollars or Euros), and the decision rule is whether NMB is greater or less than zero. The net benefit estimator is normally distributed for sufficiently large sample sizes (under the central limit theorem), regardless of whether the individual cost and effect distributions are normal or not. This greatly simplifies the calculation of confidence intervals for the estimate of net benefit. The estimate of the variance of NMB is simply the sum of the squared variances for effect and for cost, minus twice the covariance.[51]

New Bayesian cost-effectiveness insights: the value of information

So far, we have implicitly assumed that the desire to characterize uncertainty in cost-effectiveness derives from the goal of hypothesis testing and inference in the classical statistical sense. Clearly such an approach is possible with NMB, where one can test the hypothesis that NMB = 0, assuming it is distributed normally, and accept or reject the hypothesis conditional upon the data and the assumed acceptable Type 1 error, which is usually set to 5%.

An alternative paradigm to classical frequentist statistical inference is offered by Bayesian methods. A comprehensive introduction to Bayesian methods and reasoning in health care research is beyond the scope of this chapter and readers are referred to other sources.[59–61] The key elements of Bayesian reasoning stem from the principles of statistical decision theory: an analyst specifies a prior probability distribution for a decision parameter, such as NMB above, and then updates this decision parameter as new data are collected. The three key elements are: (1) *prior probability* distribution for the decision parameter, which can be "flat" (uninformative), or based on previous data (empirical Bayes), or simply a subjective probability statement; (2) *data likelihood*, which reflects the probability (or likelihood) of having observed the new data collected from a trial or other source, given alternative assumptions about the true value of the decision parameter; and (3) *posterior probability* distribution, which is derived by updating the prior distribution with the data likelihood information. Relatively simple analytic methods exist for computing the posterior distribution of a decision parameter based on the prior distribution and the likelihood data when the functional forms for the latter two are selected so as to be "conjugate" to each other. To take a specific example, suppose that prior to a trial, our uncer-

tainty about the 1-year survival probability for a patient with advanced stage lung cancer is modeled as a beta probability distribution (whose mean is our best guess about the survival probability). If the data on survival from a subsequent trial is assumed to arise from a binomial (event, no event) distribution, it is straightforward to combine this new (likelihood) information with the prior distribution to derive the corresponding posterior distribution on 1-year survival; the latter will also be beta in form, and the beta and binomial are said to be conjugate distributions. When conjugates do not naturally exist for the problem at hand, there are new methods of numerical integration such as Markov Chain Monte Carlo (MCMC) achieved by a technique known as Gibbs Sampling.[61]

Returning to our question of cost-effectiveness, Claxton[62] has argued strongly that the "classical" frequentist approach to inference and hypothesis testing is "irrelevant" if one adopts the Bayesian posture, because the optimal decision rule is to adopt the strategy with the highest expected value for the decision parameter, i.e., NMB. Expressed in terms of frequentist logic, decision makers who seek to maximize expected utility should always use an alpha (type 1 error) of 0.5 (not 0.05) – sometimes referred to as "playing the winner" – where the focus of decision making is exclusively on the first moment (statistically speaking) of the outcome distribution, which is the mean or expected value. The normative premise that a societal decision maker should consider only the expected value can be contested on a descriptive basis for (most) health care decisions conducted at a sub-societal level. For example, some authors have suggested incorporating risk aversion into cost-effectiveness,[63] and others have described how portfolio theory from financial economics might be applicable to resource allocation decisions among risky health investment projects.[64]

However, if we accept Claxton's line of argument that a cost-effectiveness decision rule should be based on expected value, what role is there for analyzing and presenting uncertainty? The answer lies in the relation between the acquisition of new information for specific parameters of the problem and the use of this new information to increase precision and reduce decision error.

Expected value of information

In the spirit of sensitivity analysis, an emerging approach in cost-effectiveness analysis is to calculate the Expected Value of Perfect Information (EVPI).[65,66] In simple terms, EVPI proceeds by assuming perfect information for one or more parameters in the decision problem. Given that the decision variable (NMB) is in monetary units here, this permits a computation of the expected cost of uncertainty for any specified value of λ, which is the value of a unit of health outcome. By applying EVPI analysis, one can get a sense of the "importance" of uncertainty in a parameter to the decision problem. It is not at all the case that "perfect information" about a given parameter will lead to a "perfect" decision, but rather a different and possibly better decision than the one made given the *current* level of uncertainty about the parameter. For example, if perfect information for a parameter has very low value (i.e., it would not change the decision), it may not be worthwhile to collect further data on that parameter. This form of analysis can be extended naturally to the computation of the Expected Value of Sample Information (EVSI), where the costs of sampling are also included.

EVPI has been proposed as a new measure to evaluate the sensitivity of models that can incorporate both the probability of a decision change and the marginal benefit of such a change into a single measure. As an example, Claxton *et al.*[67] demonstrated how the EVPI can be estimated for the decision to adopt a new pharmaceutical for the population of patients with Alzheimer's disease in the USA based on a probabilistic analysis of a published decision analysis model. The EVPI was estimated as $339 million at a time horizon of 210 weeks, and under the assumption that a decision maker would be willing to pay $50 000 per quality-adjusted life-year. This represents the maximum value of acquiring additional information. Providing that the actual cost of the research is less than $339 million, then obtaining the

information would be potentially cost-effective. This kind of analysis can direct the focus of future research towards the specific variables for which better estimates would be most valuable. Figure 25.5 shows the EVPI associated with the Alzheimer's disease model inputs at 210 weeks under the assumption that a decision maker would be willing to pay $50 000 per quality-adjusted life-year. The results showed that the model parameter for which EVPI is greatest ($270 million) was the efficacy duration. Based on this, undertaking research with an increased follow-up time for treatment with the new medication seems worthwhile because it potentially contributes the most information to the model (Figure 25.5). Obtaining better estimates of other parameters, such as the estimate of the relative risk ratio (RRR) beyond 24 weeks and the estimate of direct costs, may not be as helpful.

EVPI is a useful tool because it provides a bridge between the imprecision of the evidence we have for the current decision (e.g., to reimburse this treatment or not) and how much we should be willing to pay to increase that precision, based upon our forecast of how we will reduce "incorrect" decisions with the new information. No decision can ever be without risk of being incorrect, and gathering new evidence always costs money. What EVPI related to net benefit offers is a formal framework for quantifying how much decision makers should be willing to pay to reduce such uncertainty, conditional upon the data and the declared monetary value of health outcomes (λ).

An iterative framework for integrating trials and models

Our contention is that there is no dichotomy between trials and models for cost-effectiveness analysis, and that a conceptual framework that permits the adaptive integration of the two, in the context of uncertain information, would be helpful. The framework is outlined in Figure 25.6.

The point of entry into the framework for a given decision problem is the prior knowledge – with its

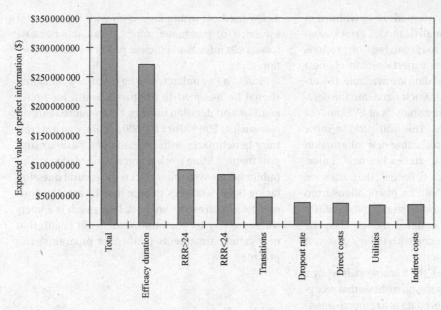

Figure 25.5. Expected value of perfect information for various model inputs evaluated over a time horizon of 210 weeks under the assumption that a decision maker would be willing to pay $50 000 per quality-adjusted life-year. RRR > 24 = relative risk ratio beyond 24 weeks of follow-up. Used with permission: Claxton, K., Neumann, P. J., Araki, S. *et al.* (2001). Bayesian value-of-information analysis. An application to a policy model of Alzheimer's disease. *International Journal of Technology Assessment in Health Care* **17**(1):38–55.

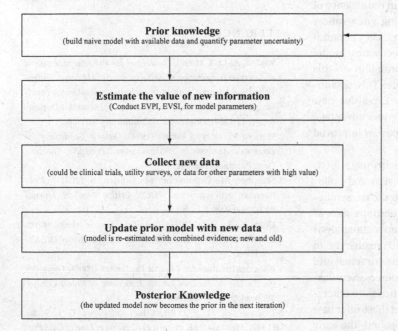

Figure 25.6. An iterative-adaptive loop for cost-effectiveness evidence synthesis.

attendant uncertainty – systematically quantified in a probabilistic decision analytic model. Prior knowledge may be based on meta-analysis of previous studies, but also includes expert opinion of "best guess" where no observed data are available. Uncertainty can similarly be parameterized into the decision model to permit some analysis of EVPI and/or EVSI as discussed above. This will provide some insight into the value of collecting new information for specific parameters in studies like new clinical trials. Once new data are collected, they are used to update the prior probability distributions from the model to generate the posterior probabilities for parameters and the updated model. Then the iterative process begins again with today's posterior becoming tomorrow's prior.

At its most general level, the framework is really a way of thinking about research synthesis that recognizes that collection of new data is a resource intensive exercise. The key to understanding the framework is to recognize that new cost-effectiveness information has value only if it is predicted to have a high probability of changing the decision (e.g., reimbursement) from what it would be in the absence of the new data. For example, launching a new cancer clinical trial to further estimate an efficacy parameter may be inefficient if the cost-effectiveness model indicates that having perfect information on this parameter has zero expected value. This circumstance can easily arise for a very expensive new medicine with very small effectiveness advantage and where societal willingness-to-pay for improved health is low.

The proposed framework also helps us to focus on some key elements of the research and policy agenda that require urgent attention. First, synthesis of evidence to inform policy questions such as cost-effectiveness requires more than meta-analysis of randomized trials; it requires the creative use of statistical tools to bring together experimental and observational data from multiple sources. New flexible frameworks for evidence synthesis are emerging using Bayesian principles,[60] and these offer new insights and exciting challenges. Second, the early use of cost-effectiveness modeling in the life cycle of

a new medical technology, even with limited prior evidence for parameter values, is valuable because it can help inform an efficient policy for data collection.

Finally, a key unknown is the monetary value that should be assigned to improved health for policy analysis and decision making. Often quoted thresholds such as $50 000 or $100 000 per life-year are arbitrary benchmarks with no evidential basis to support them.[68] More work is urgently needed to solicit public values systematically on the central question facing those who seek to base health care decisions on cost-effectiveness analysis: how much is Society willing to pay for the improvements in health that new cancer treatments (and other programs) can provide?

Acknowledgments

I am indebted to Deborah Marshall for her help in developing this chapter.

REFERENCES

1 Woden, A. C. T. (1990). *Guidelines for the pharmaceutical industry on preparation of submissions to the Pharmaceutical Benefits Advisory Committee: including submissions involving economic analysis.* Commonwealth of Australia: Department of Health, Housing and Community Services.

2 Ontario Ministry of Health (1994). *Ontario Guidelines for Economic Analysis of Pharmaceutical Products.* Toronto: Drug Programs Branch.

3 Sculpher, M., Drummond, M., O'Brien, B. (2001). Effectiveness, efficiency and NICE. *British Medical Journal* **322**(7292):943–4.

4 Gold, M. R., Siegel, J. E., Russell, L. B. *et al.* (1996). *Cost-effectiveness in Health and Medicine.* Oxford: Oxford University Press.

5 National Institute for Clinical Excellence (2000). *Guidance on the Use of Taxanes for the Treatment of Breast Cancer.* Technology Appraisal No. 6.

6 Drummond, M. F., O'Brien, B. J., Stoddart, G. L. *et al.* (1997). *Methods for Economic Evaluation of Health Care Programmes* (2nd Edition). Oxford: Oxford University Press.

7 Schulman, K., Glick, H., Yabroff, R. *et al.* (1995). Introduction to clinical economics: assessment of cancer therapies. *Journal of the National Cancer Institute Monographs* **19**:1–9.

8 National Cancer Institute and American Society of Clinical Oncology (1998). Integrating economic analysis into cancer clinical trials: The National Cancer Institute – American Society of Clinical Oncology economics workbook. *Journal of the National Cancer Institute Monographs* **24**:1–28.

9 Briggs, A. H., O'Brien, B. J. (2001). The death of cost-minimisation analysis? *Health Economics* **10**:179–84.

10 Pashko, S., Johnson, D. H. (1992). Potential cost savings of oral versus intravenous etoposide in the treatment of small cell lung cancer. *Pharmacoeconomics* **1**:293–7.

11 Jaakkimainen, L., Goodwin, P., Pater, J. *et al.* (1990). Counting the costs of chemotherapy in a National Cancer Institute of Canada randomized trial in non-small cell lung cancer. *Journal of Clinical Oncology* **8**(8):1301–9.

12 Feeny, this volume, Chapter 4.

13 Hayman, J. A., Hillner, B. E., Harris, J. *et al.* (1998). Cost-effectiveness of routine radiation therapy following conservative surgery for early-stage breast cancer. *Journal of Clinical Oncology* **16**(3):1022–9.

14 Weeks, J. (1996). Taking quality of life into account in health economic analyses. *Journal of the National Cancer Institute Monographs* **20**:23–7.

15 Earle, C. C., Chapman, R. H., Baker, C. S. *et al.* (2000). Systematic overview of cost-utility assessments in oncology. *Journal of Clinical Oncology* **18**(18):3302–17.

16 O'Brien, B., Gafni, A. (1996). When do the "dollars" make sense? Toward a conceptual framework for contingent valuation studies in health care. *Medical Decision Making* **16**:288–9.

17 Diener, A., O'Brien, B., Gafni, A. (1998). Health care contingent valuation studies: a review and classification of the literature. *Health Economics* **7**:313–26.

18 Ortega, A., Dranitsaris, G., Puodziunas, A. L. (1998). What are cancer patients willing to pay for prophylactic epoetin alfa? *Cancer* **83**:2588–96.

19 O'Brien, B., Goeree, R., Gafni, A. *et al.* (1998). Assessing the value of a new pharmaceutical: a feasibility study of contingent valuation in managed care. *Medical Care* **36**(370):384.

20 Petitti, D. B. (1994). *Meta-Analysis, Decision Analysis, and Cost-Effectiveness Analysis: Methods for Quantitative Synthesis in Medicine*. New York: Oxford University Press.

21 Weinstein, M. C., Fineberg, H. V., Elstein, A. S. *et al.* (1980). *Clinical Decision Analysis*. Philadelphia: W.B. Saunders Company.

22 Marshall, D. A., Simpson, K. N., Earle, C. C. *et al.* (2001). Economic decision analysis model of screening for lung cancer. *European Journal of Cancer* **37**:1759–67.

23 Detsky, A. S. (1989). Are clinical trials a cost-effective investment. *Journal of the American Medical Association* **262**:1795–800.

24 Naglie, G., Krahn, M. D., Naimark, D. *et al.* (1997). Primer on medical decision analysis: Part 2 – Estimating probabilities and utilities. *Medical Decision Making* **17**:136–41.

25 Naimark, D., Krahn, M. D., Naglie, G. *et al.* (1997). Primer on medical decision analysis: Part 5 – Working with Markov processes. *Medical Decision Making* **17**:152–9.

26 Sonnenberg, F. A., Beck, J. R. (1993). Markov models in medical decision making: a practical guide. *Medical Decision Making* **13**:322–38.

27 Briggs, A. H., Sculpher, M. J. (1998). An introduction to Markov modelling for economic evaluation. *Pharmacoeconomics* **13**(4):397–409.

28 Hillner, B. E., Smith, T. J. (1991). Efficacy and cost-effectiveness of adjuvant chemotherapy in women with node-negative breast cancer. *New England Journal of Medicine* **324**:160–8.

29 Weinstein, M. C., O'Brien, B., Hornberger, J. *et al.* for the ISPOR Task Force on Good Research Practices – Modeling Studies (2003). Principles of good practice for decision analytic modeling in health-care evaluation. *Value in Health* **6**(1):9–17.

30 United States General Accounting Office (1992). *Cross Design Synthesis: A New Strategy for Medical Effectiveness Research*, pp. 1–121, Washington, DC: General Accounting Office/PEMD-92-18.

31 Sculpher, M., Fenwick, E., Claxton, K. (2000). Assessing quality in decision analytic cost-effectiveness models. *Pharmacoeconomics* **17**:461–77.

32 Brennan, A., Akehurst, R. (2000). Modeling in health economic evaluation. What is its place? What is its value? *Pharmacoeconomics* **17**(5):445–9.

33 Weinstein, M., Toy, E. L., Sandberg, E. A. *et al.* (2001). Modeling for health care and other policy decisions: uses, roles, and validity. *Value in Health* **4**(5):348–61.

34 McCabe, C., Dixon, S. (2000). Testing the validity of cost-effectiveness models. *Pharmacoeconomics* **17**(5):501–13.

35 Grover, S. A., Coupal, L., Zowall, H. *et al.* (2000). The economic burden of prostate cancer in Canada: forecasts from the Montreal Prostate Cancer Model. *Canadian Medical Association Journal* **162**(7):987–92.

36 Drummond, M. (1995). Economic analysis alongside clinical trials: practical considerations. *Journal of Rheumatology* **22**:1418–19.

37 Bennett, C. L., Golub, R., Waters, T. M. *et al.* (1997). Economic analyses of Phase II Cooperative Cancer Group clinical trials: are they feasible? *Cancer Investigation* **15**(3):227–36.

38 Bennett, C. L., Waters, T. M. (1997). Economic analyses in clinical trials for cooperative groups: operational considerations. *Cancer Investigation* **15**(5):448–53.

39 Schulman, K., Dorsainvil, D., Yabroff, K. R. *et al.* (1998). Prospective economic evaluation accompanying a trial of GM-CSF/IL-3 in patients undergoing autologous bone marrow transplantation for Hodgkin's and non-Hodgkin's lymphoma. IL-3 BMT Study Team. *Bone Marrow Transplantation* **21**(6):607–14.

40 O'Brien, B. (1996). Economic evaluation of pharmaceuticals: Frankenstein's monster or vampire of trials? *Medical Care* **34**(12):DS99–DS108.

41 Buxton, M. J., Drummond, M. F., van Hout, B. A. *et al.* (1996). Modelling in economic evaluation: an unavoidable fact of life. *Health Economics* **6**:217–27.

42 Slamon, D. J., Leyland, J., Shak, S. *et al.* (2001). Use of chemotherapy plus a monoclonal antibody against HER2 for metastatic breast cancer that overexpresses HER2. *New England Journal of Medicine* **344**(11):783–92.

43 Bucher, H. C., Guyatt, G. H., Griffith, L. E. *et al.* (1997). The results of direct and indirect treatment comparisons in meta-analysis of randomized controlled trials. *Journal of Clinical Epidemiology* **50**(6):683–91.

44 Freemantle, N., Drummond, M. (1997). Should clinical trials with concurrent economic analyses be blinded? *Journal of the American Medical Association* **277**(21):1677.

45 Ness, R. M., Holmes, A. M., Klein, R. *et al.* (2000). Cost-utility of one-time colonoscopic screening for colorectal cancer at various ages. *American Journal of Gastroenterology* **95**(7):1800–11.

46 Pharoah, P., Freemantle, N., Mason, J. (1998). Economic benefit analysis of primary prevention with pravastatin. Modelling economic benefits after such long term treatment is inappropriate. *British Medical Journal* **316**(7139): 1241–2.

47 Eddy, D. M., Hasselblad, V., Shachter, R. (1990). An introduction to a Bayesian method for meta-analysis – the confidence profile method. *Medical Decision Making* **10**:15–23.

48 Briggs, A. H. (2000). Handling uncertainty in cost-effectiveness models. *Pharmacoeconomics* **17**(5):479–500.

49 Briggs, A., Sculpher, M., Buxton, M. (1994). Uncertainty in the economic evaluation of health care technologies: the role of sensitivity analysis. *Health Economics* **3**(2):95–104.

50 Doubilet, P., Begg, C. B., Weinstein, M. C. *et al.* (1985). Probabilistic sensitivity analysis using Monte Carlo simulation. A practical approach. *Medical Decision Making* **5**(2): 157–77.

51 Briggs, A. H., O'Brien, B. J., Blackhouse, G. (2002). Thinking outside the box: recent advances in the analysis and presentation of uncertainty in cost-effectiveness studies. *Annual Review of Public Health* **23**:377–401.

52 Briggs, A. H., Goeree, R., Blackhouse, G. *et al.* (2002). Probabilistic analysis of cost-effectiveness models: choosing between treatment strategies for gastroesophageal reflux disease. *Medical Decision Making* **22**(4):290–308.

53 Briggs, A. H., Wonderling, D. E., Mooney, C. Z. (1997). Pulling cost-effectiveness analysis up by its bootstraps: a non-parametric approach to confidence interval estimation. *Health Economics* **6**(4):327–40.

54 Willan, A., O'Brien, B. J. (1996). Confidence intervals for cost-effectiveness ratios in clinical trials: A new method using Fieller's Theorem. *Health Economics* **5**:297–305.

55 Willan, A. R., O'Brien, B. J. (1999). Sample size and power issues in estimating incremental cost-effectiveness ratios from clinical trials data. *Health Economics* **8**(3):203–11.

56 Stinnett, A. A., Mullahy, J. (1998). Net health benefits: a new framework for the analysis of uncertainty in cost-effectiveness analysis. *Medical Decision Making* **18**(Suppl.):S65–80.

57 Stinnett, A. A., Paltiel, A. D. (1997). Estimating CE ratios under second-order uncertainty: the mean ratio versus the ratio of means. *Medical Decision Making* **17**(4):483–9.

58 Tambour, M., Zethraus, N., Johannesson, M. (1998). A note on confidence intervals in cost-effectiveness analysis. *International Journal of Technology Assessment in Health Care* **14**:467–71.

59 Hornberger, J. (2001). Introduction to Bayesian reasoning. *International Journal of Technology Assessment in Health Care* **17**(1):9–16.

60 Spiegelhalter, D. J., Myles, J. P., Jones, D. R. *et al.* (2000). Bayesian methods in health technology assessment: a review. *Health Technology Assessment* **4**(38):1–129.

61 Gelman, A., Carlin, J. B., Stern, H. S. *et al.* (1995). *Bayesian Data Analysis*. London: Chapman & Hall.

62 Claxton, K. (1999). The irrelevance of inference: a decision-making approach to the stochastic evaluation of health care technologies. *Journal of Health Economics* **18**(3):341–64.

63 Zivin, J. G. (2001). Cost-effectiveness analysis with risk aversion. *Health Economics* **10**(6):499–508.

64 O'Brien, B. J. (2000). Building uncertainty into cost-effectiveness rankings: portfolio risk-return tradeoffs and implications for decision rules. *Medical Care* **38**(5):460–8.

65 Felli, J. C., Hazen, G. B. (1998). Sensitivity analysis and the expected value of perfect information. *Medical Decision Making* **18**(1):95–109.

66 Claxton, K., Neumann, P. J., Araki, S. *et al.* (2000). Bayesian value-of-information analysis. An application to a policy model of Alzheimer's disease. *International Journal of Technology Assessment in Health Care* **17**(1):38–55.

67 Claxton, K., Neumann, P. J., Araki, S. *et al.* (2001). Bayesian value-of-information analysis. An application to a policy model of Alzheimer's disease. *International Journal of Technology Assessment in Health Care* **17**(1):38–55.

68 Hirth, R. A., Chernew, M. E., Miller, E. *et al.* (2000). Willingness-to-pay for Quality-Adjusted Life Year: In search of a standard. *Medical Decision Making* **20**:332–42.

26

Data for cancer outcomes research: identifying and strengthening the empirical base

Carolyn C. Gotay, Ph.D.[1] and Joseph Lipscomb, Ph.D.[2]

[1]Cancer Research Center of Hawai'i, Honolulu, HI
[2]National Cancer Institute, Bethesda, MD

Introduction

It is clear from earlier chapters that data for measuring, interpreting, explaining, and predicting cancer outcomes are currently available from a variety of sources. Cancer registries, medical records, administrative claims data, and patient and provider surveys yield, individually or in concert, information about a range of outcomes that matter to decision makers. These outcomes include not only survival, disease-free survival, tumor progression, and a host of other biomedical endpoints, but important patient-reported outcomes that are the focus of this book – health-related quality of life (HRQOL), patient perceptions of and satisfaction with care, and the economic burden of cancer and its treatment. Moreover, these same data sources also yield, with varying degrees of completeness, information on a variety of factors associated with variations in cancer outcomes. These include socioeconomic and other demographic descriptors, comorbidities and other clinical determinants, and provider and health system variables.

At the moment, no single database or system provides sufficiently comprehensive information on the full range of variables required for cancer outcomes research. Rather, what we have is a substantial number of public agencies and private organizations doing an increasingly good job at collecting important pieces, components, and parts of the data required for the cancer outcomes research agenda of today and tomorrow.

In the immediate future and beyond, new prevention, diagnostic, treatment, and palliative modalities will continue to emerge. Public and private payment systems will continue to evolve, as pressures for both cost containment *and* quality assurance grow. Patients, families, and institutional purchasers will have heightened incentives to seek "value for money" in cancer care, and providers will become increasingly accountable for the quality and cost of the care they deliver. As a result of these forces, decision makers across the board will demand more and better cancer outcomes research. The statistical modeling and analytical tools to meet these challenges are rapidly developing.[1-3] The central issue addressed in this chapter is whether the currently available data are adequate to the task and, if not, what needs to be done. Consequently, the chapter will critically review existing sources of data to support outcomes research, and will identify current and emerging mechanisms for enriching the empirical base. This will lead us to examine the need for, routes to, and challenges in creating a "national cancer data system" for monitoring trends in cancer outcomes and supporting research to improve outcomes. While data for tracking cancer risk factors and behaviors and prevention activities will be briefly considered, the primary focus is on individuals diagnosed with cancer.

Methods

This chapter drew on the published literature (through MEDLINE searches whose key words included "outcomes," "quality of life," and the names of relevant organizations or data mechanisms), websites maintained by sponsors of data sources or mechanisms, and reports issued by public agencies and private organizations. Of particular importance were two reports issued by the Institute of Medicine's (IOM's) National Cancer Policy Board, which both identified current cancer outcomes data sources and mechanisms and discussed the framework for a national cancer data system.[4,5] We also benefited significantly from a video conference focus group (conducted in July 2001) consisting of key individuals from a number of organizations that support cancer outcomes data collection and analysis. Focus group participants were asked about strengths and weaknesses of their data source or mechanism for cancer outcomes research, challenges in linking data bases, and the characteristics of an ideal infrastructure for assessing cancer outcomes. (See the Appendix 26.A for focus group participants.)

Identifying data sources and mechanisms

We will distinguish four general sources of data and then identify major public and private mechanisms in the USA for collecting and, in some instances, combining these data to supply the empirical base for cancer outcomes research. The four sources discussed here are cancer registries, medical records, administrative data (especially insurance claims yielding information on patterns of care and resource use and cost), and surveys (of patients, providers, and others including the at-risk population). Within each source, there are a number of distinct variations on the theme.

Data mechanisms are defined here as the organizational means or structures by which data are collected, processed, combined or linked, and then made available for outcomes research. A mechanism may be a single entity (e.g., the Department of Veterans Affairs collecting and analyzing its own outcomes data), or a collaborative or consortium arrangement (e.g., the HMO Cancer Research Network, as discussed below). Such data mechanisms may be provided by, or supported through, a broad range of public agencies and private organizations involved variously in delivering, producing, or paying for cancer interventions; regulating, monitoring, or setting standards for cancer care; or conducting or sponsoring data collection and outcomes research. The distinction between a data source and mechanism will not always be sharply defined; in particular, a cancer registry can be viewed as both a source of data and the mechanism (organizational vehicle) through which data are collected and made available for outcomes research.

While this chapter's inventory of sources and mechanisms is not exhaustive, we have tried to include those that are important individually and that, taken together, could contribute significantly to the development of a coordinated data system to support cancer outcomes research in the USA.

Data sources

With some notable exceptions, the sources of data relevant to cancer outcomes research were generally not designed for *that* purpose but rather to support other disease monitoring, care delivery, or administrative activities. For that reason alone, it will not be surprising that no one source can supply the information needed for the breadth of outcomes research questions discussed in this volume. Nonetheless, each source brings significant value to the enterprise.

Cancer registries

The three major national cancer registry programs in the USA are described in Table 26.1.

The National Cancer Institute's (NCI) Surveillance, Epidemiology, and End Results (SEER) Program is the oldest (dating from 1973) and best established registry system, with rigorous quality-control procedures long in place and nearly complete case identification (estimated at over 95%) for the populations covered.[6] In addition, because SEER registries are required to track the vital status of each patient, the SEER data base remains the most authoritative source of information on cancer survival in the

Table 26.1. National cancer registries

Registry	Sponsor(s)	Coverage	# Annual Cases	Outcomes Research Data
Surveillance, Epidemiology, and End Results (SEER) Program	National Cancer Institute	26% of US population, including 9 states (California, Connecticut, Hawaii, Iowa, Kentucky, Louisiana, New Jersey, New Mexico, Utah), 3 metropolitan areas (Atlanta, Detroit, and Seattle-Puget Sound), and 3 supplementary sites (rural counties in Georgia, Native Americans in Arizona, and Alaskan Natives residing in Alaska)	170 000	Incidence by primary tumor site, stage at diagnosis, first course of treatment, mortality, demographics (age, sex, race/ethnicity)
National Program of Cancer Registries (NPCR)	Centers for Disease Control and Prevention	45 states, the District of Columbia, and 3 territories	1 million	Incidence by primary tumor site, stage at diagnosis, first course of treatment, mortality, demographics
National Cancer Data Base (NCDB)	Commission on Cancer of the American College of Surgeons and the American Cancer Society	Inpatient cancer admissions at over 1500 hospitals in 50 states and the District of Columbia	800 000+	First course of treatment (surgical and other details), recurrence, mortality, and demographics

USA. Given the recent addition of three new states (Kentucky, Louisiana, and New Jersey) and the portions of California not previously covered, SEER now includes 26% of the US population, with African-Americans, Hispanics, and Native Americans now represented roughly in proportion to their numbers in the entire US population. All of the SEER registries are certified by the North American Association of Central Cancer Registries (NAACCR), meaning that at least 90% of new cases are identified within two years of diagnosis and other data quality standards are met.[7]

Established in 1994 at the Centers for Disease Control and Prevention (CDC), the Congressionally mandated National Program of Cancer Registries (NPCR) now covers about 96% of the US population (inclusive of SEER-covered areas). By 2003, 32 of the 45 NPCR states had NAACCR-certified registries, and there are ongoing efforts to continue the progress

being achieved in data quality control and completeness, including obtaining follow-up information on patient survival status.

Created in 1992 as a joint project of the Commission on Cancer of the American College of Surgeons and the American Cancer Society, the National Cancer Data Base (NCDB) now includes an estimated 60% of the nation's annual incidence of 1.3 million cancer cases. In a given year, roughly 1500 hospitals and other facilities across the 50 states report patient-level data to the Commission on Cancer as one requirement for their affiliation with and approval by the Commission.[8] The NCDB offers a comparatively detailed look at aspects of the inpatient care of cancer patients treated at these facilities; but, by the same token, there is no requirement, yet, to obtain follow-up survival status on all patients nor to track care received in other settings.

All three registry systems collect information directly relevant to outcomes research: tumor type, date of diagnosis, stage at diagnosis, first course of treatment (to the extent this information can be obtained from the institutions reporting cases), demographics (age, sex, race/ethnicity), and follow-up vital status (i.e., date of death). In addition, the NCDB includes details about cancer surgeries, reconstructive procedures, and other interventions occurring during the index hospitalization.

Strengths and limitations

For supporting outcomes research, all three registry systems have certain common strengths and limitations, but there are also important differences. Both SEER and NPCR are population based, which facilitates statistically sound analyses of incidence, therapy choices (at least for the first course of treatment), and survival, by tumor type and stage at diagnosis. Incidence data from the NCDB are not representative of well-defined populations, since cancers diagnosed in non-hospital settings will generally not be reported to NCDB and therefore case ascertainment will be incomplete. That said, this registry system's relatively extensive inpatient treatment data provide good support for certain types of patterns-of-care studies. Moreover, the NCDB can provide a sampling frame for selecting cases for a variety of outcomes studies. Because SEER now offers up to 30 years of historical incidence data, it is an ideal vehicle for studies of long-term cancer survivors. Because NPCR is virtually nationwide, it can potentially support investigations of regional differences in cancer outcomes and other studies nationwide in scope.

But these registry systems share common limitations, as the National Cancer Policy Board noted in reporting an analysis by Weeks.[5] Treatment data are limited to first course and even then, information is frequently missing about chemotherapy drugs and regimens and other therapies delivered in physician offices. There is generally no information on diagnostic procedures or co-morbid conditions at the time of diagnosis. Most significantly, data on outcomes are limited to survival (so, for example, tumor recurrence status is not available). There is no information on the types of patient-reported outcomes discussed throughout this volume.

To address these limitations, both the SEER Program and the NCDB have been supporting targeted studies in which registry data are augmented by additional information – from medical records, patient interviews, or insurance claims – to provide a more complete longitudinal picture of the cancer patient's diagnosis, course of therapy, and outcomes. Since 1990, the NCDB has published about 100 such patient care evaluation studies examining patterns of care across a range of tumor sites.[8] Since 1988, the NCI has sponsored about 65 SEER patterns-of-care/quality-of-care studies [9] (most augmented by medical chart abstraction to learn about cancer care in the community post-initial therapy) and over 100 SEER "special studies," in which investigators linked registry data with medical records and/or patient surveys.[10] A prime example of the latter is NCI's Prostate Cancer Outcomes Study (PCOS), which is tracking over 3500 men prospectively following their diagnosis with prostate cancer.[11] In addition, NCI has created, and a number of investigators are now using, the SEER-Medicare Linked Database, which combines high-quality registry data with Medicare claims data to generate detailed information on patterns of care for patients age 65 and over.[12] Through 2003, there have been over 100 published papers using SEER-Medicare to examine patterns of care, adherence to quality-of-care standards, and the economic cost of cancer and cancer treatment.

Enhancements to support outcomes research

It follows that for registry data to play an increasingly important role in cancer outcomes research, several developments (already underway) should be accelerated where possible.

First, efforts should continue to create and implement a uniform set of data items which, once collected by hospital and other registrars, would jointly satisfy the three different cancer staging systems currently employed by SEER, NPCR, and NCDB; a "Stage Task Force" has recommended such an efficient (labor-saving) approach.[13]

Second, opportunities for comparing outcomes research studies across registry systems, including formal meta-analyses, would be greatly enhanced if SEER, NPCR, and NCDB moved, to the extent feasible, toward common reporting requirements in general. (For an excellent summary of how the three systems differ, see Appendix E of the 2000 National Cancer Policy Board Report.[5])

Third, for all three registry systems there is still a notable time lag, often 1–2 years, between the date of diagnosis and when the patient's data enter the registry. Such lags not only serve to delay the analysis and publication of findings about incident cases occurring in any given year, but also pose more subtle difficulties for certain linked data analyses. For example, investigators wishing to obtain patients' assessment of their health-related quality of life near the time of their diagnosis and treatment may be stymied if the patients cannot be identified in the registry until a year or more after diagnosis. In response, there needs to be greater emphasis on "rapid case ascertainment," with the aim of entering patients in the registry nearer the time of diagnosis (e.g., within 6 months). The feasibility of this has been well demonstrated by PCOS, and future advances in medical informatics (discussed below) should hasten progress.

Fourth, each registry system should continue to strive for complete case ascertainment, within the constraints and limitations imposed by the system's purpose and purview. Cases with missing treatment or outcomes data may be systematically "different" than fully reported cases, which threatens the generalizability of analyses. But even if each system flawlessly collected all the data it targeted, the treatment and outcomes profile of the cancer patient, from diagnosis to death, would be far from complete. This leads now to the final point.

Fifth, there should be a heightened focus on linking registry data with information from the other major data sources – administrative data, medical records, and surveys – to produce a comprehensive, longitudinal picture of the cancer patient's status at diagnosis, treatment patterns, and outcomes (vital, biomedical, and patient-reported). An

excellent illustration of how high-quality registry data can be combined with hospital discharge, physician specialty, and US Census data to assess the quality of colorectal cancer care in California is reported by Ayanian et al.[14] Hillner et al.[15] show how state registry data can be linked with private insurance claims data to study lung cancer patterns of care in both the non-elderly and elderly populations.

Finally, if one takes a broadened view of cancer outcomes research to include investigating the linkages between genetic risk factors, environmental exposures, incidence, screening, diagnosis, treatment, and outcomes – as explicitly underscored in 1999 by NCI's Surveillance Implementation Group (SIG)[16] – then cancer family registries and disease screening become important, as well. Prime examples include NCI's family registries for breast and ovarian cancers[17] and for colon cancer[18] and the privately supported Gilda Radner Familial Ovarian Cancer Registry.[19] Likewise, mammography registries play an important role in the linked data sets created by NCI's Breast Cancer Surveillance Consortium.[20]

Administrative data and medical records

As indicated above, information collected routinely in the process of delivering, documenting, and paying for medical care can be used effectively to support cancer outcomes research. Central to such applications are administrative data documenting the time trail and other details about claims for services rendered, and patient medical records and charts. These data sources, used separately or (even better) in concert, can provide the clinical and significant aspects of the non-clinical information for studies gauging the burden of disease and the impacts of interventions on health-related and economic outcomes.

Administrative data

The potential contributions of insurance claims information to cancer outcomes research have been most decisively demonstrated by the marriage of Medicare administrative files (which cover

Americans 65 years of age and older) with SEER registry data. But there are also a number of recently completed or ongoing efforts to use other types of claims data – both public and private, and with or without a registry linkage – to conduct cancer outcomes studies. The examples that follow will suggest both the strengths and limitations inherent in administrative data and lay the groundwork for considering how these might be managed.

The potential for Medicare data (certainly when combined with SEER) to inform the cancer care policy debate was emphasized by the National Cancer Policy Board[4,5] and is well illustrated in the study by Bach et al.[21] of black-white treatment and survival differences for early-stage non-small-cell lung cancer. Combining SEER data with Medicare-derived information on coexisting illnesses, type of Medicare (insurance) coverage, survival status, and (confirmatory observations on) initial course of therapy and patient demographics for nearly 11 000 patients over the 1985–93 period, the authors derived their influential findings. Both surgery rates and 5-year survival were significantly lower for blacks than whites; but among all patients undergoing surgery, there was no race difference in survival, and likewise for patients not undergoing surgery. While the Bach et al. study focused on initial treatment, the power of Medicare data to provide longitudinal information on medical care utilization is illustrated by Schrag et al.[22] and a number of the other publications cited at http://healthservices.cancer.gov/seer-medicare. Moreover, these data have been shown to be useful in identifying cancer incidence[23] and patient's stage of disease.[24]

While Medicare claims files are nationally uniform, well-documented, and generally well understood by many outcomes researchers, Medicaid claims files have constituted a comparatively heterogeneous, variably documented, and not well explored "national set" of data bases that vary, state by state, in content and accessibility. This stems from the fact that the Medicaid program, although designed to provide care for individuals with low income and resources, is interpreted and administered on a state-by-state basis, with the consequence that many aspects of the program, including eligibility criteria, vary significantly across states. Thus, unlike SEER-Medicare, Medicaid claims do not constitute true population-based data, even for the economically disadvantaged parts of the population generally served by the program. Yet, these data do have the potential to inform important analyses of disparities in utilization and outcomes, since they focus almost entirely on the poor and under-insured, and cover all age ranges – not just the 65 and over population found in Medicare. The potential for registry-linked Medicaid data to support cancer outcomes research is well illustrated in Bradley et al.,[25] where about 600 of the 5700 women with documented breast cancer in the Metropolitan Detroit SEER registry were currently Medicaid enrolled. The authors found that low socioeconomic status was significantly associated with late-stage breast cancer diagnosis, type of treatment received, and mortality, and that race was not a significant independent predictor of these unfavorable outcomes. To further examine the potential of fruitful SEER-Medicaid linkages, NCI has initiated an exploratory analysis to determine the number of persons in the California Cancer Registry who are MediCal eligible, and the availability and quality of their enrollment and claims data (personal communication, Joan Warren, Ph.D., NCI, May 15, 2003).

The large number of private insurance databases in the USA represents a significant, and still largely untapped opportunity to support claims-based cancer outcomes research in large-population samples, focusing particularly on the non-poor non-elderly. Exemplary applications include both Hillner et al.[15] and the study by McKee et al.,[26] in which the claims for a large carrier (covering 25% of all privately insured persons in Western New York state) were linked with medical records and registry data to investigate whether high-volume medical practices delivered more guideline-compliant breast cancer care. They found that practice volume was positively correlated with the use of breast-conserving surgery, but, on the other hand, not related to the rate of positive biopsy. In a test of the feasibility and accuracy of linking SEER data with the claims from one large private insurer in Iowa, Doebbeling et al.[27] reported that about 96% of matched incident cases (from the state SEER registry in 1994) had identifiable claims data. Finally, contract research organizations, under contract to pharmaceutical or other firms, are exploiting a number of commercially available (and generally proprietary) claims-based data systems to conduct client-focused outcomes research (personal communication, Clark Paramore, MSPH, MEDTAP International, May 14, 2003). Examples of data systems intended to provide fully integrated claims (inpatient, outpatient, drugs, and more) include MEDSTAT MarketScan[TM] (http://www.medstat.com), Ingenix LabRx (http://www.ingenix.com), and Lifemetrix (http://www.lifemetrix.com).

Medical records

Generally regarded as the authoritative source of data on patient diagnoses, treatments rendered and prescribed, and biomedical outcomes (including signs, symptoms, side effects, functional status, and survival), the medical record continues to play an important role in cancer outcomes research. These data are of central import to a number of investigations, including patterns-of-care/quality-of-care studies such as those using SEER registries or the National Cancer Data Base as the sampling frame for patients. Apart from some notable exceptions (including, for example, PCOS), large-sample, multisite investigations – like the SEER-Medicare study by Bach et al.[21] – have generally not found it feasible to use medical records to augment patient profiles. There have been at least two inhibiting factors. First, while 17–30% of US physicians surveyed nationally now report using electronic medical records in their practices,[28] most medical records and charts in most medical centers, of all sizes, remain non-automated. (A noteworthy exception is the US Department of Veterans Affairs, where medical records in many medical centers are now fully automated, with computerized records and clinical reminders.)[29] Extracting patient data accurately remains an expensive,

labor-intensive process in most settings and prohibitively costly for many large studies. Second, approval by Institutional Review Boards (IRBs) and patient consent are required for access to and use of medical records for research purposes, again imposing significant costs to broad-scale applications (for more on the potential impact of privacy regulations, see the final section below).

Strengths and limitations

Administrative data files provide automated, low-cost access to information of critical importance to many studies of cancer treatment, follow-up care, and outcomes: patient diagnoses, demographics, the nature and pattern of services received over time, and vital status (over the period for which the patient is enrolled in the insurance plan). Consequently, such data contribute substantially to studies about the pattern and quality of cancer care and economic burden – including calculation of the attributable (net) cost of cancer. Regarding the latter, Etzioni et al.[30] demonstrate how (registry-linked) claims data can be applied to estimate the difference over time between the total (observable) cost incurred by cancer patients and a demographically matched, but non-cancer, sample; this difference is interpreted as the attributable cost of cancer.

The major limitations of administrative data lie in what is *not* found there. Any given claims file includes only those individuals covered; and, for each individual, only those services included in the plan. Thus, the Medicare files generally exclude the non-elderly, and omit data on such uncovered services as outpatient prescription drugs and most nursing home care. Moreover, for the covered patient there is limited clinical detail (beyond what can be inferred from diagnostic and procedure codes) and no patient-reported outcomes of the type emphasized in this volume. Because public and private payer insurance systems presently operate in "silos" administratively, there is no natural mechanism to follow enrollees who change plans. Some (difficult-to-estimate) portion of this disenrollment will come from enrollees who change plans *because* they now have cancer and seek a different coverage option. From a statistical perspective, this constitutes "informative right-censoring," which can lead to biased inferences. One of the major analytical advantages of Medicare's coverage-to-death policy is that it effectively avoids such patient selectivity threats to validity.

Compared with claims, medical records provide greater, more authoritative clinical detail and arguably *some* information on patient-reported outcomes (PROs), if one accords PRO-status to recorded indications of disease symptoms and treatment side effects. But with rare exception, patient-reported measures of health-related quality of life or satisfaction with care are still not routinely incorporated into medical records (automated or not).[31] The labor intensity of data abstraction (which is exacerbated if records for a given patient must be accessed from multiple sites, as often the case in panel studies), can be mitigated through greater automation. But informed consent hurdles in using medical records for outcomes research will likely impose significant administrative costs for the foreseeable future.

Enhancements to support outcomes research

To improve the utility of administrative and medical records data for cancer outcomes research, it is important to accelerate current efforts to link, to automate, and to augment.

Specifically, with SEER-Medicare as the model, public and private research support should focus on linking high-quality registry data with state Medicaid files *and* with private insurance claims data. This would significantly enhance the opportunity for large-sample studies of health and cost outcomes across all age categories and socioeconomic strata. For Medicaid data, such linkages will not be easy because of changing rules about eligibility and coverage. Another challenge lies with successfully linking (or otherwise pooling) the claims data from multiple payers within a given geopolitical area. Beyond the information-technology difficulties that arise in linking data for the individual covered by multiple

payers (e.g. because of disenrollments/re-enrollments), the area's competing health plans may be reluctant to share (even de-identified) patient data or other proprietary information that either reflects upon or might influence market performance and profitability.

The National Cancer Policy Board of the IOM has urged federal agencies to support public-private partnerships to spur the adoption of "computer-based patient records systems" as one cornerstone of a national cancer data system.[5] In fact, the trend toward automation of medical records (and provider-patient interchanges of all types) is steadily accelerating, with more than 70 electronic medical record vendors in the USA by mid-2003[32] and with several of these (e.g., EpicCare, ChartWare, Health Probe) receiving top ratings in a recent provider survey conducted by the American Academy of Family Physicians.[32] Meanwhile, clinical data collection design systems, like MedQuest,[33] are emerging that allow investigators to more efficiently enter, merge, sort, and analyze clinical data obtained from either traditional medical charts or electronic records. (This system has been adopted by NCI's Cancer Care Outcomes Research and Surveillance (CanCORS) Consortium.)[34]

Finally, there is the issue of whether and how administrative data or medical records could be augmented, on a routine basis, to include a parsimonious set of patient-reported outcomes that convey information beyond that provided by biomedical indicators. If so, the array of endpoints available for analysis in registry-claims-records linked analyses would be enriched accordingly. Because this clearly would involve substantial administrative costs, it should be weighed against an alternative strategy, noted by the National Cancer Policy Board[5] and illustrated in PCOS. That strategy is to supplement routine data collection with surveys of patients and survivors to generate linked data sets augmented with patient-reported outcomes. Ideally, this would yield data sufficiently broad and rich to support studies across the major tumor sites, phases of care, geographic regions, and population subgroups.

Surveys

Certain data of central importance to cancer outcomes research cannot efficiently, or even feasibly, be obtained through registries, administrative files, or medical records (in their present forms). In this section we provide an overview of how surveys are presently being used, and could be further enhanced, to fill these information gaps. The critical point throughout is that surveys constitute the primary source of information on patient-reported outcomes – HRQOL, perceptions and evaluations of cancer care, and important aspects of the economic impact of cancer and its interventions.

Because the scope of outcomes research encompasses the full cancer continuum (from prevention to end of life), there is a correspondingly wide array of potentially relevant surveys. In Tables 26.2 and 26.3 and the discussion below, we offer a simple typology for characterizing the surveys of interest here, and highlight well-known or otherwise representative examples (from a large universe of ongoing efforts).

Health knowledge, practices, and outcomes

In Table 26.2, the first four entries under "Population Surveys" constitute major sources of data for tracking and analyzing prevention activities, screening, risk factors, health behaviors, and other variables directly relevant to studies along that range of the cancer continuum. The potential of the National Health Interview Survey[36] to support cancer prevention research is well illustrated by Freedman et al.,[37] who used data from the 2000 NHIS' Cancer Control Module to estimate that more than 2 million women who would be eligible for tamoxifen chemoprevention for breast cancer according to FDA criteria were not receiving it. The California Health Interview Survey[38] (CHIS) likewise now contains an (NCI-supported) Cancer Control Module; and while obviously not national in scope, CHIS does yield a demographically diverse sample including large numbers of Hispanics and African Americans. The CDC's Behavioral Risk Factor Surveillance System[39] provides state-level estimates

of not only the propensity to engage in a wide range of unhealthy (and some healthy) behaviors, including tobacco use and weight control, but also asks about the elapsed time since the most recent colorectal cancer screening test. The National Health and Nutrition Examination Survey[40] permits population-based analyses of the interaction among risk factors, behaviors, biomedical outcomes, and health status. Another important effort in this vein is the Tobacco Use Supplement to the US Census Bureau's Current Population Survey, a large (N = 240 000), nationally representative survey that supports both US-wide and state-level studies to monitor tobacco use and evaluate control programs.[41]

The final two Population Surveys noted in Table 26.2 (HOS and CAHPS®) demonstrate how a large health care payer (in this case, Medicare) can use well-known survey tools to monitor and evaluate an "intervention" (Medicare Managed Care) on a national scale. The utility of the Medicare Health Outcomes Survey[42] for assessing HRQOL among cancer survivors is illustrated in Baker et al.,[43] who found that they scored significantly poorer on all 8 subscales of the SF-36 than a matched sample of patients without cancer. The Centers for Medicare & Medicaid Services (CMS) is using the Consumer Assessment of Health Plans (CAHPS®) instrument to track and analyze enrollees perceptions and evaluations of their managed care plan;[44] see Chapter 14 by Darby[45] in this volume for a discussion of the CAHPS® and competing instruments for assessing patient satisfaction and other aspects of the care experience.

Virtually the only way to measure and understand the *perceived* impact of disease and its treatments on the health-related quality of life of the cancer patient, survivor, or caregiver is to inquire directly, through surveys that may be administered in person, by mail, over the phone, or electronically over the web. A substantial portion of the large HRQOL literature in cancer has been analyzed elsewhere in this volume: within treatment trials for breast, colorectal, lung, and prostate cancer,[46–49] for survivorship[50] and end-of-life care,[51] for caregivers,[52] and across a range of applications using

Table 26.2. Selected population, patient, and provider surveys on health knowledge, practices, and outcomes

Survey/Instrument(s)	Sponsor(s)	Coverage	Sample size	Data for outcomes research
Population Surveys				
National Health Interview Survey (NHIS)	National Center for Health Statistics-CDC	Civilian non-institutionalized US population	40 000 households and over 100 000 individuals annually, oversampling Blacks and Hispanics and using computer-assisted personal interviewing	Single-item health status; functional limitations; activities of daily living (ADLs), and instrumental ADLs; disability; disease conditions; demographics; health care and utilization and health insurance; for 1987, 1992, and 2000, an NCI-supported Cancer Control Supplement (Topical Module) on risk factors including family history, screening, health behaviors, and selected service utilization (e.g., genetic testing, smoking, hormone use, diet, colorectal and prostate cancer screening).
California Health Interview Survey (CHIS)	California Dept. of Health Services, UCLA Center for Health Services Research, and the Public Health Institute	Civilian non-institutionalized CA population	55 000 households and over 120 000 individuals in all 58 CA counties, fielded initially in 2000–2001; telephone based	Broadly similar to NHIS: physical and mental health status of CA adults and children; prevalence and management of chronic diseases; diet and exercise; health insurance coverage; access and barriers to preventive and other health services; NCI-supported Cancer Control Module on risk factors, screening, behaviors, and selected service utilization.
Behavioral Risk Factor Surveillance System (BRFSS)	National Center for Chronic Disease Prevention and Health Promotion-CDC	Civilian non-institutionalized US population age 18 and over	State-based sampling frame targeting 150 000 annually across all 50 states; telephone based	Behavioral risk factors (e.g., smoking, alcohol abuse, obesity); disease screening, including for colorectal cancer; HRQOL; health status; demographics.
National Health and Nutrition Examination Survey (NHANES)	National Center for Health Statistics-CDC	Civilian non-institutionalized US population	5000 persons annually, oversampling Blacks, Hispanics, and adolescents; personal interview, physical examination, lab tests	Detailed assessment of disease prevalence, clinical measures, risk factors, and health behaviors; physical activity and functioning; demographics.

(cont.)

Table 26.2. (*cont.*)

Survey/Instrument(s)	Sponsor(s)	Coverage	Sample size	Data for outcomes research
Medicare Health Outcomes Survey (HOS)	Centers for Medicare and Medicaid Services (CMS), in cooperation with National Committee for Quality Assurance (NCQA)	Enrollees nationwide in Medicare managed care plans (Medicare+Choice)	For each plan, 1000 enrollees randomly sampled to complete self-administered mailed questionnaire, then followed up 2 years later. First cohort in 1998 comprised national sample of 280 000, with 167 000 respondents	Health status (SF-36 and single-item question); self-reported co-morbidities (for risk adjustment); demographics.
Medicare Managed Care Consumer Assessment of Health Plans (CAHPS®)	CMS, with instrument developed by research consortium (Research Triangle Institute, Rand, and Harvard) through a cooperative agreement with Agency for Healthcare Research and Quality (AHRQ)	Enrollees nationwide in Medicare + Choice managed care plans	For each plan, 600 enrollees (in plan for at least 6 months) randomly sampled annually to complete self-administered mailed questionnaire; mail and telephone follow up as needed. First cohort in 1998; by 1999, national sample of 202 000 from 367 plans, with 166 000 responding	Includes rating of personal doctor, specialist (if used), overall health care, and health care plan, with this instrument also asking about ease of obtaining medical equipment; speech, and occupational therapy; home health services; and prescription drugs. Asks about advice on quitting smoking, getting vaccinations, personal doctor's knowledge for medical decision making, and health plan handling of complaints.

Patient and Survivorship Surveys

Study of Cancer Survivors –II (SCS-II)	American Cancer Society	Adults with one of 6 major tumor sites (breast, colorectal, prostate, urinary bladder, skin melanoma, uterine) surviving for at least 2 years post diagnosis	Cross-sectional samples of survivors at 2, 5, and 10 years after diagnosis, drawn from NPCR registries, with anticipated sample of 25 000 persons yielding 15 000 completed interviews over time	HRQOL (via SF-36); pain and other symptom reports; social support resources; needs assessment; medical care use; perceptions about cancer survivorship; demographics.
Health, Eating, Activity, and Lifestyle (HEAL) Study	NCI, with patient recruitment through 3 SEER registries (Seattle, WA; New Mexico; and Los Angeles, CA)	Women diagnosed with early-stage breast cancer	SEER population-based sample of 1065 women physically examined and interviewed at baseline, again at 24 months, and (for more limited information) at 60 months	Diet, weight and body composition, and physical activity; a battery of clinical measures; breast cancer recurrence and survival; HRQOL (including SF-36 and Piper Fatigue Scale) and social support; sources of and need for information; demographics.

Table 26.2. (*cont.*)

Survey/Instrument(s)	Sponsor(s)	Coverage	Sample size	Data for outcomes research
Assessment of Patients' Experience of Cancer Care (APECC) Study	NCI, in collaboration with Northern California Cancer Center	Adults diagnosed with and surviving at least 12 months with either bladder cancer, colorectal cancer, or leukemia	SEER-population-based sample of 600 patients completing computer-assisted telephone interview between 12 and 24 months after cancer diagnosis	Health history; perceptions of cancer care over past 12 months (with items from Consumer Assessment of Health Plans (CAHPS) and Picker Survey as points of departure); use of complementary and alternative therapies; decision making preferences regarding follow-up tests, side-effects management, and treatment for recurrent cancers; information seeking needs and behaviors; HRQOL (SF-36 and single-item question); self-appraisal of current health; demographics.
Provider Surveys				
Physician Survey on Cancer Susceptibility Testing	NCI (with data collected by private contractor)	US physicians in primary care (general internists, family and general practitioners, ob/gyn) and specialty care (oncologists, gastroenterologists, urologists, and general surgeons)	National probability sample of 1250 from American Medical Association's Physician Masterfile in 2000, with multiple modes of administration (mail, phone) of questionnaire	Use of, knowledge about, and attitudes toward genetic testing for cancer susceptibility; medical practice arrangements; personal and family history of cancer; patterns-of-care factors; race/ ethnicity.
Survey of Colorectal Cancer Screening Practices	NCI (with data collected by private contractor)	US physicians in primary care (general internists, family and general practitioners, ob/gyn) and specialty care (gastroenterologists, general surgeons, diagnostic radiologists), and health plan medical directors	National probability sample of 2225 physicians from AMA Physician Masterfile in 2000; 180 health plan respondents from SMG Marketing Groups' data base	Use of, knowledge about, and attitudes toward colorectal cancer screening, including perceptions of barriers to achieving high screening rates; health plan guidelines, policies, and practices about colorectal cancer screening.

generic preference-based[53] or non-preferenced-based[54] measures. Moreover, approaches to measuring and addressing patient perceptions, concerns, and needs have been discussed by Darby[45] and Gustafson.[55]

While all of these PRO applications require *ipso facto* that patients or others be surveyed, most have yielded outcomes data that are study specific – that is, aimed at testing particular hypotheses or addressing targeted questions. It has not been the business

Table 26.3. Selected resource use and cost surveys

Survey/Instrument(s)	Sponsor(s)	Coverage	Sample size	Data for outcomes research
National Hospital Discharge Survey (NHDS)	National Center for Health Statistics (NCHS)	US non-institutional hospitals (excluding federal, military, and VA) located in all 50 states and the District of Columbia	About 275 000 discharges annually from a random sample of about 470 hospitals	For each inpatient discharge, information on length of stay, expected sources of payment, diagnoses, surgical procedures, demographics (including age, race, sex, ethnicity, and marital status), hospital bed size, and geographic location.
Healthcare Cost and Utilization Project (HCUP)	Federal-state-industry partnership organized by the Agency for Healthcare Research and Quality (AHRQ)	All non-federal hospital discharges in 29 states (with additional sampled information on inpatient admissions and ambulatory surgery within these states)	*State Inpatient Databases (SID):* the universe of non-federal hospital discharge abstracts in 29 states; contains 26 million discharges annually (80% of US total); available 1995–2000 *Nationwide Inpatient Sample (NIS):* stratified random sample of SID, yielding representative 20% sample of US community hospitals; 7 million discharges annually from 28 states; available 1988–2000 *State Ambulatory Surgery Databases:* hospital-based same-day surgeries in 15 states; available 1997–2000	For each admission, over 100 variables including diagnoses, procedures, admission and discharge status, demographics (including age, sex, median income for ZIP code, and for some states, race), expected payment source(s), total charges, length of stay, hospital characteristics (including ownership, bed size, and teaching status), and hospital and county identifiers that permit linkage to other data bases.
National Ambulatory Medical Care Survey (NAMCS)	NCHS	Civilian non-institutionalized US population	3-stage sampling plan (primary sampling unit, then physician practices, then patient visits) to get representative data; about 3000 practices surveyed, with each providing data on 30 visits in a selected week; annually since 1989	For each encounter, information includes reason for visit, type of physician seen, diagnosis, expected source(s) of payment, diagnostic and screening services ordered or provided during the visit, ambulatory surgical procedures, medication therapy, disposition of case, duration of visit.
Medical Expenditure Panel Survey (MEPS)	AHRQ	Civilian, non-institutionalized US population	About 25% of NHIS households randomly sampled, with 2 panels followed at any point in time and each panel followed for 2 years. In 2000, about 10 000 households and 26 000 persons interviewed. Uses both computer-assisted personal interviews (CAPI) and self-administered questionnaires. Began in 1997	*Household component:* self-report medical conditions and utilization; adults complete EQ-5D (including visual analog scale), SF-12, instrumental activities of daily living (IADLs), and sensory limitations form.

Table 26.3. (*cont.*)

Survey/Instrument(s)	Sponsor(s)	Coverage	Sample size	Data for outcomes research
				Provider component: surveys physicians, hospital, and home health providers to supplement Household component. *Insurance component*: surveys employers and union leaders on insurance benefits available to Household component respondents. *Nursing Home component*: survey of nursing homes and residents (to capture NH experience of those in Household component sample). Demographics collected on all household members.
Medicare Current Beneficiary Survey (MCBS)	Centers for Medicare and Medicaid Services (CMS)	Medicare population (including institutionalized)	Rotating (replenished) stratified random sample of 12 000 enrollees, each (since 1994) interviewed 12 times over a 4–year period to yield a total of 3 years of cost and service use data	Longitudinal observations on health service use, sources and amounts of payment (public and private, including out of pocket), health status and functioning, and behavioral and demographic information (including income, assets, living arrangements, family supports, and access to medical care). For institutionalized, facility questionnaire includes health status, residence history, insurance coverage, and use and costs of health care services. MCBS files link to Medicare claims and other administrative data to enhance analytic capabilities.
Study of Assets and Health Dynamics among the Oldest Old (AHEAD)	National Institute on Aging, via contract with Institute for Social Research, University of Michigan	National panel survey of non-institutionalized persons age 70+	About 7400 persons interviewed biennially in person, by phone, or by proxy since 1993, with sample replenished as needed and with over-sampling of Blacks, Hispanics, and Florida	Cognitive performance; physical and functional health; economic status (assets and income), dissaving, and Medicaid eligibility; family structure, caregiving, and financial transfers; housing; health care use and expenditures; demographics.

of these studies to develop large-scale, population-representative, ongoing PRO databases comparable to the prevention and screening information sets currently available, for example, from the NHIS. However, the Patient and Survivorship Surveys noted in Table 26.2, as well as the Breast Cancer Surveillance Consortium, the Prostate Cancer Outcomes Study, and new work emerging from the CanCORS Consortium (see below), point the way to the development of such PRO databases.

NCI's ongoing Health, Eating, Activity, and Lifestyle (HEAL) Study[56] (see Table 26.2) demonstrates how breast cancer patients can be identified by high-quality registries, then followed over time via personal interviews and clinical assessments to generate a profile of information on risk factors, health behaviors, disease recurrence and survival, various biomedical indicators, and HRQOL (using the SF-36 and the Piper Fatigue Scale). The American Cancer Society's Study of Cancer Survivors-II,[57] launched in 2003, calls for identifying from registry rolls three large, cross-sectional samples of survivors at 2, 5, and 10 years after diagnosis with any of six common cancers. Survivors' HRQOL (indexed by the SF-36) can be analyzed in relation to measures of coping skills, social support, resource use, and a number of other (self-reported) variables – at three different time points beyond the initial diagnosis. NCI's Assessment of Patients' Experience of Cancer Care (APECC) Study,[58] also begun in 2003, is gathering extensive descriptive and evaluative information from survivors identified by a SEER registry with any of three cancers (bladder, colorectal, or leukemia). Data will include perceptions about and evaluations of cancer care, the nature and quality of the medical decision-making process, and HRQOL as measured by the SF-36 and the one-item, Excellent-Very Good-Good-Fair-Poor scale.

In addition, there are several other federally sponsored ongoing, national-level data collection efforts, which do identify cancer patients either by clinical records or respondent self-report and which may potentially provide information useful to survivorship or end-of-life studies. A prime example is the National Long-Term Care Survey,[59] an ongoing cross-sectional effort to study changes in physical and mental health, insurance coverage and financial status, and family support systems for persons 65 and over.

Provider surveys can likewise provide valuable information not otherwise available from standard administrative and clinical records. The two entries in Table 26.2 demonstrate the potential to acquire data shedding light on decision making about the use of screening modalities, new technologies, and other factors influencing patient outcomes. NCI's Physician Survey of Cancer Susceptibility Testing[60] examines factors bearing on the propensity of both primary care providers and specialists to offer or recommend genetic testing for inherited mutations associated with increased cancer risk. The National Survey of Colorectal Cancer Screening Practices[61] asks national-level health plans about coverage of CRC screening, barriers to successful screening, and programs to promote and monitor screening. Note that both surveys use as the sampling frame the American Medical Association's "AMA Physician Masterfile" (http://ama-assn.org/ama/pub/category/2673.html), thus illustrating the frequently employed strategy of using provider organization membership roles to identify survey candidates. As another example, analyses of survey data on physician-radiologists from NCI's Breast Cancer Surveillance Consortium have demonstrated that provider attributes are associated with variations in care.[62] Finally, provider surveys relevant to cancer outcomes research can also focus on institutions (e.g., nursing homes) or facilities. An important example of the latter is the National Survey of Mammography Facilities, an NCI-sponsored survey of over 1000 provider organizations in 1992 that collected data on facility characteristics and personnel, procedures performed, procedure volume and charges, and other institutional features.[63]

Resource use and cost

Table 26.3 includes six national-level surveys of individuals or institutions that provide data on aspects of the economic burden of cancer, and the utilization and cost of interventions. None of these surveys is designed expressly for cancer (or for any other disease); rather, cancer patients, overall and by tumor type, are sampled roughly in proportion to their presence in the overall sampling frame.

Potentially excellent sources of data for patterns-of-care and economic cost studies focusing expressly on the inpatient admission for cancer care are the National Center for Health Statistics's (NCHS) National Hospital Discharge Survey (NHDS)[64] and AHRQ's Healthcare Cost and Utilization Project (HCUP).[65] In particular, HCUP includes for each admission over 100 variables covering not only all of the information normally available from administrative claims data but also hospital-level descriptors (ownership, size, teaching status) and identifiers allowing linkage to other data sets pertaining either to the hospital or the patient's county of residence. With such a county linkage, it is possible to assign proxy values to patient-level variables otherwise missing from administrative files using the Area Resource File (ARF).[66] The ARF is a federally supported, county-specific health resources information system containing over 7000 variables on such relevant topics as health facilities and physicians, economic status, and socioeconomic characteristics of the population for every county in the USA. Consequently, the researcher lacking direct observations from the NHDS (or, for that matter, from many other standard data sources) on the individual patient's income, education, and other socioeconomic variables can link to the ARF and assign to the patient the mean values of these variables for the patient's county or zip code. (This was the approach taken, for example, by Bradley et al.[25] in their SEER-Medicaid analysis.)

Population-based encounter-level data on outpatient visits are available from NCHS's National Ambulatory Medical Care Survey (NAMCS),[67] the nation's foremost ongoing data collection project on outpatient care. The NAMCS has a multi-stage sampling scheme yielding U.S. representative data on visits by diagnosis and including information on procedures and services performed, sources of payment, and case disposition in random samples of encounters in more than 3000 medical practices nationwide each year.

Two large-scale, ongoing, and potentially very useful population-based surveys of individuals' medical care use and expenditures, health status, and indicators of HRQOL are the AHRQ's Medical Expenditure Panel Survey (MEPS)[68] and CMS's Medicare Current Beneficiary Survey (MCBS).[69] Constructed from a 25% random sample of NHIS households, the MEPS currently includes at any moment about 10 000 US households and 26 000 individuals. Each household is interviewed a targeted three times over a two-year period for information on health service use, cost, and payment sources including private insurance coverage; self-reported medical conditions and HRQOL as measured by the EQ-5D, SF-12, and instrumental activities of daily living (IADLs); and a number of demographic variables. Using MEPS data, Thorpe and Howard[70] found that 11% of all cancer patients under age 65 are uninsured, a figure that rises to 15% for African Americans and 20% for Hispanics. Uninsured cancer patients receive significantly less health care than the insured – but controlling for insurance status, utilization did not differ significantly by race.

The MCBS is an ambitious effort to measure health care use and expenditures comprehensively and longitudinally in a large nationally representative sample of Medicare enrollees age 65 and over. Each individual in this annually replenished, stratified random sample of about 12 000 is followed for four years to collect a targeted three years worth of data on a host of variables: health care utilization (including prescription drugs), income status, health status, family and social support, and demographic information. Many self-reported variables are verified or amplified by reference to Medicare's administrative claims files. These include not only short-term inpatient and various provider files (from Medicare Part B), but also the Minimum Data Set (MDS),[71] which contains detailed clinical and health status data on each enrollee's routine nursing home care, and the Outcomes and Assessment Information

Set (OASIS),[72] which includes health and functional status, socio-demographic, environmental, and social support information on all adult enrollees using home health care.

Detailed information on physical and cognitive functioning, economic status and decision making, housing, family structure, caregiving, and health care expenditures for a nationally representative sample of the elderly is available from the Study of Assets and Health Dynamics in the Oldest Old (AHEAD) study.[73-74] About 7400 persons (or their proxies) are interviewed biennially in AHEAD, an ongoing project based at the University of Michigan and supported by the US National Institute on Aging. Hayman et al.[75] used these data to estimate that the annual economic opportunity cost of informal caregiving for elderly patients with cancer in the USA is about $1200 per patient, or $1 billion nationally (1998 dollars).

Strengths and limitations

The principal value of surveys for cancer outcomes research is their ability to provide important information not otherwise available in health system data files and records. Surveys provide the opportunity to obtain from cancer patients, and also family members and caregivers, assessments of HRQOL, the quality and effectiveness of the care delivery process, resources devoted to otherwise undocumented care (e.g., prescription drugs, complementary and alternative medicines), and certain demographic data not otherwise collected. Virtually by definition, the only way to elicit a "patient-reported outcome" is from the patient (or, on occasion, a designated surrogate).

Similarly, surveys of physicians, institutions, and other health care providers can yield valuable information regarding knowledge of, attitudes about, and approaches to using – or not using – particular cancer interventions (e.g., genetic testing or colorectal cancer screening). Sometimes one survey in a study can provide information that strengthens data collection efforts elsewhere in the study. For example, in the CanCORS Consortium project now underway,[34] patients identified via rapid case ascertainment

from registry files are being asked to identify all of their care providers, who will then be surveyed about their approaches to cancer therapy and decision making styles.

The principal limitations of surveys closely mirror the major challenges facing the successful measurement of patient-reported outcomes in any environment (including clinical trials): validity, reliability, responsiveness, comparability (across studies), and feasibility (administrative and financial). Particular concerns may include the credibility of respondent self-reports (especially for resource use and expenditure questions), respondent burden, and non-response biases. The surveys in Tables 26.2 and 26.3 that include HRQOL components all use generic measures, with four (MHOS, SCS-II, HEAL, and APECC) adopting the SF-36 and one (MEPS) using the closely related SF-12. Not surprisingly, none of these large-scale, population-based surveys include a general cancer or cancer site-specific HRQOL measure. Consequently, and in contrast to the HRQOL instrumentation found in most cancer treatment trials, these surveys understandably lean in the direction of facilitating comparisons across multiple disease types and population subgroups, and this necessarily comes at the expense of sensitivity to respondent differences *within* a disease type (e.g., cancer). Finally, there is general concordance among the surveys in Table 26.3 about the major components of health care utilization and expenditures, but not an evident consensus about the precise battery of questions to pose. An implication of Hornbrook's analyses[76] is that such broadly concordant yet somewhat disparate approaches to cost data collection reduce comparability across surveys.

Finally, surveys of the kind reviewed here represent costly *new* investments (typically ranging from six to seven figures annually) in information for research and policy development. This contrasts with the outcomes research-relevant data emerging from registries, administrative files, and medical records, which (while also very expensive in absolute terms) are already being collected for health system purposes.

Enhancements to support outcomes research

Several potential modifications to the surveys noted in Tables 26.2 and 26.3 should be carefully evaluated. On either an ongoing or periodic basis, comprehensive national-level surveys such as the MEPS and MCBS could include a "cancer patient module" to collect general cancer or cancer site-specific information on HRQOL, patient perceptions of care, and economic burden. To complement this, cancer patients could be over-sampled, either overall or by tumor type. The inclusion of additional cancer-related items should be preceded by appropriate cognitive testing of the expanded survey(s),[77] and the performance of these new items should be analyzed by modern psychometric approaches guided by item response theory.[3] At the same time, efforts should be undertaken to standardize survey items capturing resource use and cost.

While such survey expansions would be administratively ambitious and costly, they would enhance opportunities to track cancer outcomes on a population basis, and to conduct cancer outcomes research routinely for a much broader patient base than presently possible.

Data mechanisms

We now briefly discuss the alternative organizational means, or vehicles, currently or potentially available for collecting, preparing, linking, or using data to support cancer outcomes research. Such mechanisms may be private, public, or mixed (public-private). They may involve either a single organization (e.g., an HMO), a consortium formed to collect and analyze data for specific projects or other objectives, or a network of pre-existing (e.g., registries) and new (e.g., surveys) data sources that support multiple outcomes research studies over time and across populations.

Single organizations

There are several private-sector health care delivery organizations in the USA with a sufficiently large patient population and demonstrated commitment to studying evidence-based medicine that each alone is presently a viable platform for cancer outcomes research. Prominent cases in point include non-profit, staff model HMOs, like Kaiser Permanente[78] and Group Health Cooperative of Puget Sound,[79] that have created the research infrastructure to collect and analyze data from our four major sources – registries, medical records, administrative files, and surveys – on their enrolled populations. A striking example of how a research-oriented provider organization can investigate the outcomes of cancer care from the patient's perspective is the Mayo Clinic's evaluation of prophylactic mastectomy in a large case series of surgeries spanning a third of a century.[80]

The largest Federal health care delivery systems in the USA are continuing to enhance their data systems in ways that can serve to support cancer outcomes research. The US Department of Veterans Affairs (VA) has created the VA Information Resource Center (VIReC) to facilitate access to and provide expert consultation about the agency's most prominent outcomes research databases, which encompass inpatient and outpatient care, extended and long-term care, and services rendered outside the VA system.[29] The Indian Health Service is strengthening patient- and provider-oriented data collection within its Resource and Patient Management System, including development of an electronic health record that builds upon the VA's successfully implemented system.[81] The Department of Defense (DoD)'s Military Cancer Institute (based at Walter Reed Army Medical Hospital) is accelerating efforts to link DoD tumor registry data with medical records, administrative files, and pathology data to create an integrated patient information data set (dubbed ACTEURS) to improve care management and support outcomes research (personal communications with John Potter and John Powers, DoD, April 2003).

It is noteworthy that the agency above that has arguably advanced the furthest in building information systems to support cancer outcomes research – the VA – is continuing to invest in new data collection and linkage in recognition of gaps that persist.

For example, the VA's Colorectal Cancer Quality Enhancement Research Initiative (CRC QUERI) project, co-supported by NCI, is building a CRC screening assessment and surveillance data system to track the follow-up care of positive screens.[82] The CRC QUERI is also developing an outcomes research and quality surveillance data system (in conjunction with its participation in NCI's CanCORS project[34]) that will link registry and medical records information with patient and provider survey interviews. This underscores again that no matter how advanced the evolving information technology within a health care delivery system (public or private), the incorporation of patient-reported outcomes into analytical databases will continue to require special efforts – until the day comes when they are collected routinely to inform patient-provider decision making.

Consortia and networks

Public and private health care providers, research organizations, and funders can, and do, create collaborative mechanisms for outcomes data generation and analysis. The resulting consortia and networks are intended to draw strength from the ensemble of partnering organizations, affording, for example, larger and more diverse sample sizes than any one organization alone could bring to bear. We turn first to some prime examples, focusing on major consortia established to conduct specific cancer research studies or to monitor the quality, cost, and accessibility of cancer care over time in defined populations. Then we discuss how cancer outcomes research could be enhanced by harnessing the potential of existing cancer delivery and research organizations and also general practice provider networks already formed to conduct population-based outcomes research (though not necessarily oriented to cancer).

Collaboratives in progress

We start with consortia formed to carry out pre-specified research projects, then move on to confederations that conduct multiple, perhaps evolving outcomes research and monitoring activities over time.

Cancer Care Outcomes Research and Surveillance Consortium (CanCORS)

In 2001, NCI launched a 5-year, $35 million project to conduct large, prospective cohort studies on newly identified lung and colorectal cancer patients.[34] Carried out through a cooperative agreement with 7 multidisciplinary research teams from around the country and a statistical coordinating center, CanCORS is investigating the impact of targeted interventions on patient-centered outcomes, examining dissemination of state-of-the-art therapies, studying modifiable risk factors, and analyzing population disparities in cancer care utilization and outcomes. To accomplish this, investigators are linking registry data with medical record information, administrative data, and patient and provider survey information to build a comprehensive, longitudinal picture of each sample patient (for colorectal, N = 5500; for lung, N = 4500). To minimize the time gap between cancer diagnosis and the collection of patient-reported outcomes – which is especially important for obtaining accurate evaluations related to the initial course of treatment – participating SEER and NPCR registries are using "rapid case ascertainment." Because CanCORS is investigating the administrative feasibility, resource cost, and research payoff of collecting and linking all major sources of cancer outcomes data, it should significantly inform discussions about the architecture and engineering of a national cancer data system for the USA.

National Initiative on Cancer Care Quality (NICCQ) of the American Society of Clinical Oncology (ASCO)

Launched in 2000, this privately supported initiative is investigating patterns of care, and clinical and patient-reported outcomes for over 1000 breast cancer and 1000 colorectal cancer patients sampled from hospitals contributing to the National Cancer Data Base in five US cities.[83] Research teams based at Harvard School of Public Health and RAND are linking patient medical records with telephone interview data to examine whether cancer care following diagnosis was consistent with national norms (as defined by NICCQ expert panels) and also the patient's recalled perceptions of and satisfaction with that care. A major long-term objective of this 5-year, $5 million project is to test the feasibility of a national system for cancer quality evaluation.

Breast Cancer Surveillance Consortium

Established in 1994 by NCI in response to the Mammography Quality Standards Act of 1992, this consortium of seven geographically dispersed research teams has enhanced understanding of US breast cancer screening practices by assessing the accuracy, cost, and quality of screening programs through a coordinated strategy of data collection, analysis, and publication.[20,84] To investigate the impact of screening on cancer outcomes, data on screening practices are linked with information from population-based cancer registries; likewise, data on tumor pathology and biologic characteristics, as well as patient demographics and risk factor information, can be linked to registries. This permits study of staging and survival for breast cancers detected by mammography compared with those detected in other ways. The consortium's database includes information on more than 4 million screening mammographies for close to 2 million women, over 30 000 of whom have subsequently developed breast cancer.

HMO Cancer Research Network (CRN)

This consortium of 10 large non-profit health plans, covering more than 9 million lives across the USA, conducts a program of health services and outcomes research to increase the effectiveness, and cost-effectiveness, of preventive, curative, and supportive cancer interventions.[85] Launched in 1999 with financial support from NCI, the HMO CRN's multidisciplinary research teams use a variety of linked information sources – automated clinical and financial databases, chart reviews, and surveys of patients, providers, and health plan managers. Seven of the 10 plans have their own tumor registries, and the other three identify incident cancer

cases using diagnostic codes; seven plans have rapid case ascertainment systems in place. Current projects utilizing these linked data resources examine tobacco control in managed care, late-stage diagnoses suggesting screening failure, and the risks and benefits of early screening and prophylactic mastectomy in women at high risk of breast cancer.

National Comprehensive Cancer Network (NCCN)

One major aim of this confederation of 19 large US cancer centers is to enhance the effectiveness and efficiency of cancer care delivery through the collection, synthesis, and analysis of outcomes data.[86] The NCCN Oncology Outcomes Database, created in 1997 and focusing initially on breast cancer, is designed to link detailed clinical, administrative, and economic information on the patient's cancer care and outcomes, both biomedical and patient-reported. Early applications have included examining the adherence of NCCN clinicians and institutions to the NCCN guidelines for breast cancer diagnosis and treatment at 5 member institutions treating over 7000 new cases a year. The NCCN intends to expand participation in the outcomes database to additional member institutions and to add new tumor sites, starting with non-Hodgkin's lymphoma.

NCI's Clinical Trials Cooperative Group and Community Clinical Oncology Programs (CCOPs)

Begun in the 1950s, the Cooperative Group program currently comprises 9 groups of investigators conducting at any one time about 150 Phase III and 200 Phase II treatment trials and enrolling approximately 30 000 new patients annually.[87] Some groups focus on specific cancers (e.g., gynecologic), others on specific treatment modalities (e.g., radiation therapy), one on the common clinical expertise of group members (i.e., pediatrics), and several are multimodal, studying various cancers and approaches to therapy. The 50 CCOP organizations and 10 additional Minority Based CCOPs (drawing from catchment areas with a high proportion of minority residents) were created to increase enrollment in Cooperative Group trials[88] and now contribute about one-third of all newly enrolled patients.

While the Cooperative Group program began with an exclusive focus on treatment, and patient survival remains the primary endpoint in the majority of trials, health-related quality-of-life measures are being increasingly included. A 2003 review of all NCI-sponsored treatment trials either active, approved, in review, or temporarily closed to accrual found that 31% (59/189) of Phase III trials had one or more HRQOL endpoints, as did 4% (34/810) of Phase I, II, or I/II trials (personal communication, Mason Schoenfeldt, EMMES Corp., under contract to NCI, July 2003). In addition, with increasing knowledge about cancer prevention and control, the Groups are now conducting large-scale prevention trials – one of the largest of which examined whether tamoxifen could prevent breast cancer in healthy, high-risk women. In this study, HRQOL measures played a particularly important role in capturing the intervention's full impact on the participants.[89]

Realizing the potential of existing mechanisms – and envisioning new ones

The quantity and quality of information for cancer outcomes research can be enhanced by taking better advantage of existing infrastructures for data collection and analysis, and possibly developing new mechanisms. We examine several options, starting with existing vehicles.

NCI's Cooperative Groups and CCOPs

That the current clinical trials infrastructure is possibly well poised to carry out cancer outcomes research inside, alongside, or outside of randomized treatment or prevention trials has been well illustrated.[89–92] But many conclusions from a recent paper examining the strengths and weaknesses of Cooperative Groups for conducting behavioral research[93] apply here, as well. Groups have access to a large and varied population that encompasses virtually all areas of the country. Consequently, studies can be tailored to specific populations (e.g., specific tumor sites, therapies, or demographics), institutions, or organizations. Recent cancer prevention research has demonstrated that Groups can provide access to populations other than cancer patients. In addition, Groups have developed rigorous systems of data collection and analysis, with multidisciplinary participation in study design and execution.

Nonetheless, outcomes research – with a focus on patient-reported endpoints and possibly conducted in community settings, and not just randomized trials – is still a relatively new enterprise for Cooperative Groups, whose members remain substantially engaged in clinical care and typically focused on biomedical endpoints. While protocols for collecting traditional treatment-related data have become routinized, obtaining patient-reported outcomes poses new challenges. Such data must be gathered in "real time," often under challenging circumstances (rather than retrieved retrospectively from patient charts). Because only 2–4% of adult cancer patients are presently enrolled in treatment trials, and these individuals must meet eligibility criteria, study populations may differ in important ways from the general population of cancer patients. The frequent observation that the elderly are underrepresented in treatment trials was recently documented in an analysis of studies undertaken by the Southwest Oncology Group.[94] The same may be true for non-English speaking patients, those with significant comorbidities, and other subgroups. In response, NCI and other organizations that support cancer trials should accelerate efforts to increase enrollment in trials, so that studies are better powered to detect not only overall effects by treatment arm but also subgroup differences.

To enhance the contributions of the clinical trial Group mechanism to cancer outcomes research, trial sponsors and end users of the data – including the Food and Drug Administration (FDA) and purchasers – should clearly signal to the Cooperative Groups (and other trialists) what is expected in terms of study designs, choice of outcome measures (including HRQOL), and key questions for analysis.

Comprehensive Cancer Centers (CCC)

An NCI-designated Comprehensive Cancer Center must show reasonable depth and breadth in each of three research areas: basic, clinical, and prevention/control/behavioral/population-based; moreover, the center must demonstrate a strong body of interactive research that bridges these three areas.[95] The third research area is defined to encompass not only preclinical and clinical outcomes, but also psychosocial, including HRQOL, and health-services-related, including patterns of care and cost-effectiveness analysis. All the while, many of NCI's 39 CCCs have individual investigators or research teams contributing significantly to cancer outcomes research. For example, the majority of lead and co-investigators in the CanCORS consortium are affiliated with CCCs, as are a majority of the Cancer Outcomes Measurement Working Group participants whose research interests lie predominantly in cancer. The 19 institutional members of the National Comprehensive Cancer Network *are* NCI CCCs.

But despite these and many other linkages, the potential contributions of comprehensive cancer centers to outcomes research have yet to be realized. As amply demonstrated in the projects noted above, the CCCs can contribute importantly to outcomes measure development and testing, to population-based (as well as center-based) patterns-of-care and quality-of-care studies, and to translation of evidence-supported guidelines into oncology practice. For all this to occur, however, cancer centers may require strong, new signals that in progressing successfully along the "discovery-development-delivery" continuum of cancer research,[96] there should be greater focus on applied research that accelerates the journey from the development and evaluation of new interventions to their use by those in need.

Primary Care Practice-Based Research Networks (PBRNs) and the Integrated Delivery System Research Network (IDSRN)

Created by the Agency for Healthcare Research and Quality (AHRQ), these two networks – each linking health services and outcomes research with community-based health care delivery – have considerable untapped potential for supporting cancer-oriented studies and demonstration projects.

Each of the 19 PBRNs receiving planning grants from AHRQ in 2000 is a group of ambulatory care practices affiliated with each other and typically with an academic or professional organization to investigate a variety of health care delivery questions.[97] To take just one example, the Case Western Reserve University has organized the Research Association of Practicing Physicians (RAPP), a network of 116 practices in northeast Ohio, to investigate structure-process-outcome linkages in primary care. The PBRNs together provide research access to over 5000 primary care providers and 7 million patients in 49 states.

The IDSRN is presently a confederation of nine organizations, each consisting of a health services and outcomes research unit working with one or more health care delivery systems "collaborators" for the purpose of conducting cutting-edge measurement, evaluation, and dissemination research.[98] For example, Weill Medical College of Cornell University in New York City serves as the IDSRN research unit (or "partner") collaborating with a number of NYC institutions including NY Presbyterian Healthcare System, the Mailman School of Public Health at Columbia University, and Memorial Sloan-Kettering Cancer Center. To qualify, each IDSRN partner must collect and maintain administrative, claims, medical encounter, and other data on a clinically and demographically diverse population. The nine organizations together provide health care services to an estimated 55 million Americans annually.

The NCI-supported HMO Cancer Research Network is demonstrating the outcomes research payoff from harnessing the collective expertise and data collection potential of research-oriented care delivery organizations. Fully exploiting the potential of the PBRNs and the IDSRN for cancer outcomes research will likely require new partnerships between AHRQ and organizations, both public and private, committed to improving cancer care in the community.

Industry-supported mechanisms

Could a cooperative cancer outcomes data system be created? Each of the pharmaceutical and medical device companies conducting Phase II and Phase III trials and post-marketing surveillance (including "Phase IV" trials) for its cancer-related products collects, analyzes, and maintains an enormous amount of biomedical, administrative, and sometimes patient-reported data to support FDA labeling claims and subsequent marketing activity. It is not evident from the published literature that any company pools data from its own trials over time in order to carry out large-scale (meta-analytic) investigations of intervention-outcome linkages in a given disease area (like cancer). It is clear, and not surprising, that the outcomes research community has not had general access to these proprietary trial data, even after the data's commercial value has ended. Nor does it appear that firms working in the same disease area have found motive or opportunity to pool their trials' data (post the period of commercial utility) to support studies that might yield deeper insights into structure-process-outcome linkages. While clinical trial samples in cancer are generally not population-based, they are frequently diverse in many important ways. The merger of several such trial samples could well yield a quite diverse sample overall, while being sufficiently large to permit subgroup analyses with adequate power. In-depth analyses with such data could well improve each firm's ability to interpret the findings from subsequent trials. Finally, the pooling of industry trial data with similar data from the NCI Cooperative Groups could potentially yield similar benefits.

To create and successfully maintain such a cooperative outcomes data system (focusing largely or exclusively on clinical trials, at least initially) is a hugely complex undertaking. Challenges loom in working out a data sharing agreement that adequately protects each participating firm's perceived commercial interests, surmounts patient confidentiality and other legal issues, and emerges as affordable and administratively manageable. One option would be a public–private arrangement, in which the public partner(s) provides administrative and some financial support and serves as the "honest broker" to encourage each firm to perceive much more reward than risk from collaborating.

Towards a national cancer data system

Based on the National Cancer Policy Board's recommendations on enhancing data systems for monitoring and improving the quality of cancer care[5]; observations from a focus group of data experts convened to inform the COMWG (see the Appendix 26.A); and related points noted across this chapter, several major conclusions emerge. These are taken up successively in the paragraphs that follow.

A high-quality system of cancer registries across the USA should be the firm foundation of a national cancer data system that supports population-based surveillance and outcomes research to identify and understand structure-process-outcome relationships, variations in patterns and quality of care, and disparities in utilization and outcomes. There should be a heightened and sustained focus on rapid case ascertainment, standardizing the data to establish cancer stage and comorbidities, and inclusion of information on chemotherapy and other treatment rendered in outpatient settings. The major national registry systems – SEER, NPCR, and NCDB – should seek to learn from such registry-based projects as NCI's CanCORS and ASCO's NICCQ whether certain additional data elements are so central to cancer outcomes research they should be collected routinely on every incident case.

Most quality, cost, and access issues can best be analyzed with data providing adequate detail on episodes (complete histories) of cancer care – charting the patient's medical care utilization and outcomes from diagnosis through treatment, the survivorship period, and end of life. This requires linking information from some or all of the major data sources discussed in this chapter: registries, medical records, administrative data including insurance files, and surveys (of patients, but possibly also of their health care providers and caregivers). It is not feasible, or necessary, to build such linked data sets on every new cancer case. Rather, this should be done selectively so as to support a strategically planned portfolio of outcomes research studies that, taken together, would address the major issues across tumor types, population groups, and geographic regions.

To ensure that the emerging national data system encompasses the cancer continuum, there should be additional emphasis on surveys of prevention, screening, and health-related behaviors in at-risk populations. In addition, direct capture of use of services, such as for screening and tobacco cessation programs, is being done already in data systems like those established by the Breast Cancer Surveillance Consortium and the HMO Cancer Research Network (discussed above). Increased automation, particularly through electronic health records, should both improve the accuracy and lower the cost of data capture.

Trends well underway to implement more effective and efficient data collection technologies – including electronic medical records, web-based applications, hand-held devices, and item-response-theory-based approaches to survey administration – should be accelerated.

For private health care provider organizations and the pharmaceutical and device industry to voluntarily participate fully in a national cancer data system, positive incentives should be created and disincentives addressed. When such entities contribute important data and allow it to be linked to other sources, there should be clear public recognition of the contributions to cancer outcomes research. At the same time, there should be adequate protections against disclosure of sensitive commercial information (e.g., pricing strategies, market share, product line planning) or patient data not conforming to confidentiality rules (see below).

A national data system should incorporate evidence-based core measures, or indices, of cancer care quality. This would facilitate the monitoring of trends, cross-sectionally and over time, in who gets (and does not get) cancer care regarded generally as high quality.

The data privacy regulations following implementation of the Health Insurance Portability and Accountability Act (HIPAA) of 1996 are already increasing the administrative and resource costs of high-quality health services and outcomes research. HIPAA's "privacy rule," which went into effect April 18, 2003, pertains to "protected health information" that is under control of a "covered entity" and which may be transmitted electronically by the latter to a range of users, including researchers.[99] By implication, the privacy rule applies to a wide range of health care delivery and research entities engaged in collecting and transmitting data useful to cancer outcomes research. But in the end, these new regulations may not pose a significant roadblock. This is because the Privacy Rule provides for a number of ways that covered entities (e.g., health plans) can use and disclose protected health information beyond simply getting the individual's written authorization. Alternative pathways include de-identifying the individual's data, producing data sets with limited individual identifiability and then establishing "data use agreements" between all organizations involved in the transmission and use of the information, and obtaining Institutional Review Board (IRB) waiver of additional authorization requirements.[100]

Federal agencies, professional organizations, and institutions engaged in medical education should collaborate to create and support new training opportunities in outcomes, health services, and surveillance research. There is a particular need for well-prepared analysts and well-informed policy makers at the state level. These individuals would support registry-based data collection and analysis that contribute not only to the national agenda in outcomes and health services research, but to the development and implementation of state-level plans for cancer prevention and control.

The leadership for a national cancer data system in the USA may not reside, finally, with one single entity, either currently existing or new. Rather, it is more likely to be provided through a "coordinated confederation" of public and private organizations significantly involved in cancer data collection, analysis, and policy application. Federal financial and organizational support will likely remain critically important, since not all private partners will have either the incentive or resources to invest heavily in a data system. But the support and active participation of cancer advocacy, education, provider organizations, and the business community is important, not only to supplement public dollars but to inform and energize the public at large. Few things in cancer outcomes research are less exciting on the surface, but more important over the long term, than a high-quality, population-based data system to chart progress, identify failures, and point the way to improvement.

REFERENCES

1 Sloan, this volume, Chapter 18.

2 O'Brien, this volume, Chapter 25.

3 Reise, this volume, Chapter 21.

4 National Cancer Policy Board, Institute of Medicine (1999). *Ensuring Quality Cancer Care*, ed. M. Hewitt, J. V. Simone. Washington, DC: National Academy Press.

5 National Cancer Policy Board, Institute of Medicine (2000). *Enhancing Data Systems to Improve the Quality of Cancer Care*, ed. M. Hewitt, J. V. Simone. Washington, DC: National Academy Press.

6 National Cancer Institute. "Surveillance, Epidemiology, and End Results (SEER) Program." Available at http://seer.cancer.gov. Last accessed September 9, 2004.

7 Centers for Disease Control and Prevention. "National Program of Cancer Registries." Available at http://www.cdc.gov/cancer/npcr/. Last accessed September 9, 2004.

8 Commission on Cancer, American College of Surgeons. "National Cancer Data Base (NCDB)." Available at http://www.facs.org/dept/cancer/ncdb/. Last accessed September 9, 2004.

9 National Cancer Institute. "SEER Pattern of Care/Quality of Care Studies." Available at http://www.healthservices.cancer.gov/surveys/poc. Last accessed September 9, 2004.

10 National Cancer Institute. "Rapid Response Surveillance Studies." Available at http://outcomes.cancer.gov/methods/quality/seer-rrss.html. Last accessed September 9, 2004.

11 Potosky, A. L., Harlan, L. C., Stanford, J. L. *et al.* (1999). Prostate cancer practice patterns and quality of life: the Prostate Cancer Outcomes Study. *Journal of the National Cancer Institute* 91(20):1719–24.

12 National Cancer Institute. "SEER-Medicare Linked Data Base." Available at http://healthservices.cancer.gov/seer-medicare/. Last accessed September 9, 2004.

13 Edge, S. B., Fritz, A., Clutter, G. G. *et al.* (1999). A unified cancer stage collection system: preliminary report from the Collaborative Stage Task Force/American Joint Committee on Cancer. *Journal of Registry Management* 26(2): 57–61.

14 Ayanian, J. Z., Zaslavsky, A. M., Fuchs, C. F. *et al.* (2003). Use of adjuvant chemotherapy and radiation therapy for colorectal cancer in a population-based cohort. *Journal of Clinical Oncology* 21:1293–300.

15 Hillner, B., McDonald, K., Desch, C. *et al.* (1998). A comparison of patterns of care of nonsmall cell lung carcinoma patients in a younger and Medigap commercially insured cohort. *Cancer* 83(9):1930–7.

16 Surveillance Implementation Group (1999). *Cancer Surveillance Research Implementation Plan*. National Cancer Institute, National Institutes of Health. Available at http://dccps.nci.nih.gov/DCCPS/SIG. Last accessed September 9, 2004.

17 National Cancer Institute. "Breast and Ovarian Cancer Family Registries." Available at http://epi.grants.cancer.gov/BCFR/index.html. Last accessed on April 26, 2003.

18 National Cancer Institute. "Colon Cancer Family Registries." Available at http://epi.grants.cancer.gov/CCFR/index.html. Last accessed on April 26, 2003.

19 Gilda Radner Familial Ovarian Cancer Registry (located at Roswell Park Cancer Institute, Buffalo, NY). Available at http://www.ovariancancer.com/. Last accessed on April 26, 2003.

20 Ballard-Barbash, R., Taplin, S. H., Yankaskas, B. C. *et al.* (1997). Breast Cancer Surveillance Consortium: a national mammography screening and outcomes database. *American Journal of Radiology* 169:1001–8.

21 Bach, P. B., Cramer, L. D., Warren, J. L. *et al.* (1999). Racial differences in the treatment of early-stage lung cancer. *New England Journal of Medicine* 341(16): 1198–205.

22 Schrag, D., Cramer, L. D., Bach, P. B. *et al.* (2001). Age and adjuvant chemotherapy use after surgery for stage II colon cancer. *Journal of the National Cancer Institute* 93(11): 850–7.

23 Warren, J. L., Feuer, E., Potosky, A. L. *et al.* (1999). Use of Medicare hospital and physician data to assess breast cancer incidence. *Medical Care* 37(5):445–56.

24 Cooper, G. S., Yuan, Z., Stange, K. C. *et al.* (1999). The utility of Medicare claims data for measuring cancer stage. *Medical Care* **37**(7):706–11.

25 Bradley, C. J., Given, C. W., Robert, C. (2002). Race, socioeconomic status, and breast cancer treatment and survival. *Journal of the National Cancer Institute* **94**(7): 490–6.

26 McKee, M. D., Cropp, M. D., Hyland, A. *et al.* (2002). Provider case volume and outcome in the evaluation and treatment of patients with mammogram-detected breast carcinoma. *Cancer* **95**:704–12.

27 Doebbeling, B. N., Wyant, D. K., McCoy, K. D. *et al.* (1999). Linked insurance-tumor registry database for health services research. *Medical Care* **37**(11):1105–15.

28 CyberAtlas Staff. "U.S. doctors behind in adoption of electronic records." *Harris Interactive*. Available at http://cyberatlas.internet.com/markets/healthcare/article /0,,10110_897031,00.html. Last accessed September 9, 2004.

29 U.S. Department of Veterans Affairs. "Information about VIReC (VA Information Resource Center)." Available at http://www1.va.gov/hsrd/fr/loi/virec.htm. Last accessed September 9, 2004.

30 Etzioni, R., Urban, N., Baker, M. (1996). Estimating the costs attributable to a disease with application to ovarian cancer. *Journal of Clinical Epidemiology* **49**(1):95–103.

31 Donaldson, M. S. (2004). Taking stock of health-related quality-of-life measurement in oncology practice in the United States. *Journal of the National Cancer Institute Monograph* **33**:155–67.

32 Rehm, S., Kraft, S. (2001). Electronic medical records: the FPM vendor survey. *Family Practice Management* **8**:45–54.

33 Centers for Medicare & Medicaid Services (DHHS). "MedQuest." Available at http://cms.hhs.gov/medquest. Last accessed September 9, 2004.

34 Ayanian, J. Z., Chrischilles, E. A., Wallace, R. B. *et al.* (2004). Understanding cancer treatment and outcomes: the Cancer Care Outcomes Research and Surveillance Consortium. *Journal of Clinical Oncology* **22**:2992–6.

35 Board on Health Care Services, Institute of Medicine (2003). *Key Capabilities of an Electronic Health Record System*, Board on Health Care Services. Washington, DC: National Academy Press.

36 National Cancer Institute. "What is the Health Interview Survey?". Available at http://appliedresearch.cancer.gov/ surveys/nhis/ Last accessed on September 4, 2004.

37 Freedman, A. N., Graubard, B. I., Rao, S. R. *et al.* (2003). Estimates of the number of U.S. women who could benefit from Tamoxifen for breast cancer chemoprevention. *Journal of the National Cancer Institute* **95**:526–32.

38 National Cancer Institute. "What is the California Health Interview Survey?" Available at http://appliedresearch.cancer.gov/surveys/chis/. Last accessed September 9, 2004.

39 Centers for Disease Control and Prevention. "Behavioral Risk Factor Surveillance System." Available at http://www.cdc.gov/brfss/. Last accessed on September 27, 2004.

40 National Center for Health Statistics. "National Health and Nutrition Examination." Available at http://www. cdc.gov/nchs/nhanes/htm. Last accessed September 9, 2004.

41 National Cancer Institute. "What Is the TUS-CPS?" Available at http://riskfactor.cancer.gov/studies/tus-cps/. Last accessed on September 9, 2004.

42 Centers for Medicare & Medicaid Services. "Medicare Health Outcomes Survey." Available at http://cms.hhs.gov /surveys/hos/. Last accessed September 9, 2004.

43 Baker, F., Haffer, S. C., Denniston, M. (2003). Health-related quality of life of cancer and noncancer patients in Medicare managed care. *Cancer* **97**:674–81.

44 Goldstein, E., Cleary, P. D., Langwell, K. M. *et al.* (2001). Medicare managed care CAHPS®: a tool for performance improvement. *Health Care Financing Review* **22**(3):101–7.

45 Darby, this volume, Chapter 14.

46 Ganz, Goodwin, this volume, Chapter 5.

47 Moinpour, Provenzale, this volume, Chapter 8.

48 Earle, Weeks, this volume, Chapter 7.

49 Litwin, Talcott, this volume, Chapter 6.

50 Zebrack, Cella, this volume, Chapter 11.

51 Ferrell, this volume, Chapter 12.

52 Snyder, this volume, Chapter 16.

53 Feeny, this volume, Chapter 4.

54 Erickson, this volume, Chapter 3.

55 Gustafson, this volume, Chapter 15.

56 National Cancer Institute. "What is the Health, Eating, Activity, and Lifestyle (HEAL) Study?" Available at http:// appliedresearch.cancer.gov/surveys/heal. Last accessed on September 9, 2004.

57 American Cancer Society. Research Program and Funding – Behavioral Research Center. Available at http://www.cancer.org/docroot/RES/RES_0.asp. Last accessed on September 27, 2004.

58 National Cancer Institute. A pilot evaluation of the Consumer Assessment of Health Plans instrument in a cancer population. Available at http://outcomes.cancer.gov/ methods/quality/seer_rrss.html. Last accessed on September 13, 2004.

59 Center for Demographic Studies (Duke University). "The National Long Term Care Survey (NLTCS)." Available at http://www.nltcs.eds.duke.edu/index.htm. Last accessed September 9, 2004.

60 National Cancer Institute. "What is the Physician Survey on Cancer Susceptibility Testing?" Available at http://riskfactor.cancer.gov/studies/physician/. Last accessed September 9, 2004.

61 National Cancer Institute. "National Survey of Colorectal Cancer Screening Practices." Available at http://healthservices.cancer.gov/surveys/colorectal/. Last accessed September 9, 2004.

62 Sickles, E. A., Wolverton, D. E., Dee, K. E. (2002). Performance parameters for screening and diagnostic mammography: specialist and general radiologists. *Radiology* **224**:861–9.

63 Brown, M. L., Fintor, L. (1995). The use of mobile units to deliver screening mammography services in the United States: results from the National Survey of Mammography Facilities. *Radiology* **195**:529–32.

64 National Center for Health Statistics. "National Hospital Discharge Survey Description." Available at http://www.cdc.gov/nchs/about/major/hdasd/nhdsdes.htm. Last accessed September 9, 2004.

65 Agency for Healthcare Research and Quality. "Healthcare Cost and Utilization Project (HCUP): 1988–2000: a Federal-State Industry Partnership in Health Data." Available at http://www.ahrq.gov/data/hcup/. Last accessed September 9, 2004.

66 Quality Resource Systems, Inc. "The Area Resource File System" (maintained under contract from the Bureau of Health Professions, U.S. Health Resources and Services Administration). Available at http://www.arfsys.com/. Last accessed September 9, 2004.

67 National Center for Health Statistics. "What is the National Ambulatory Medical Care Survey?" Available at http://www.cdc.gov/namcs/. Last accessed September 9, 2004.

68 Agency for Healthcare Research and Quality. "Medical Expenditure Panel Survey (MEPS)." Available at http://www.meps.ahrq.gov. Last accessed September 9, 2004.

69 Centers for Medicare & Medicaid Services. "Medicare Current Beneficiary Survey: Overview." Available at http://www.cms.hhs.gov/MCBS/default.asp. Last accessed September 9, 2004.

70 Thorpe, K. E., Howard, D. (2003). Health insurance and spending among cancer patients. *Health Affairs*. Available at http://www.healthaffairs.org/WebExclusives.php and also summarized in volume 22, number 3 (May/June): 12.

71 Centers for Medicare & Medicaid Services. "The Minimum Data Set 2.0." Information Site. Available at http://www.cms.hhs.gov/medicaid/mds20/. Last accessed September 9, 2004.

72 Centers for Medicare & Medicaid Services. "OASIS Overview." Available at http://www.cms.hhs.gov/oasis/hho.view.asp. Last accessed on September 9, 2004.

73 Institute for Social Research, University of Michigan. "Study of Assets and Health Dynamics Among the Oldest Old (AHEAD). Available at http://hrsonline.isr.umich.edu/. Last accessed September 9, 2004.

74 Soldo, B. J., Hurd, M. D., Rodgers, W. L. *et al.* (1997). Asset and Health Dynamics among the oldest old: an overview of the AHEAD Study. *Journal of Gerontology B: Psychological Science and Social Science* **52B**:1–20.

75 Hayman, J. A., Langa, K. M., Kabeto, M. U. *et al.* (2001). Estimating the cost of informal caregiving for elderly patients with cancer. *Journal of Clinical Oncology* **19**:3219–25.

76 Hornbrook, this volume, Chapter 24.

77 Willis, Reeve, Barofsky, this volume, Invited Paper C.

78 Selby, J. V. (1997). Linking automated databases for research in managed care settings. *Annals of Internal Medicine* **127**:719–24.

79 Wagner, E. H., Thompson, R. S. (1988). Cancer prevention and HMOs. *Cancer Investigation* **6**(4):453–9.

80 Hartmann, L. C., Schaid, D. J., Woods, J. E. *et al.* (1999). Efficacy of bilateral prophylactic mastectomy in women with a family history of breast cancer. *New England Journal of Medicine* **340**(2):77–84.

81 U.S. Indian Health Service. "EHR Overview, Site Planning and Schedule." Available at http://www.ihs.gov/generalweb/webapps/ehr/save/index.asp. Last accessed September 9, 2004.

82 U.S. Department of Veterans Affairs. "Quality Enhancement Research Initiative," available at http://www1.va.hsrd/research/queri/ and "Colorectal Cancer Quality Enhancement Research Initiative," http://www.hsrd.minneapolis.med.va.gov/CRC/CRCHome.asp. Last accessed on July 5, 2003.

83 Schneider, E. C., Epstein, A. M., Malin, J. L. *et al.* (2004). Developing a system to assess the quality of cancer care: ASCO's National Initiative on Cancer Care Quality. *Journal of Clinical Oncology* **22**:2985–91.

84 National Cancer Institute. "Breast Cancer Surveillance Consortium." Available at http://breastscreening.cancer.gov. Last accessed on September 9, 2004.

85 National Cancer Institute. "HMO Cancer Research Network." Available at http://crn.cancer.gov. Last accessed September 9, 2004.

86 National Comprehensive Cancer Network. "Oncology Outcomes Database." Available at http://www.nccn.org/professionals/outcomes_database.asp. Last accessed September 9, 2004.

87 National Cancer Institute. "Cancer Therapy Evaluation Program." Available at http://CTEP.cancer.gov. Last accessed September 9, 2004.

88 National Cancer Institute. "Community Clinical Oncology Program." Available at http://www3.cancer.gov/prevention/ccop/. Last accessed September 9, 2004.

89 Day, R., Ganz, P. A., Costantino, J. P. *et al.* (1999). Health-related quality of life and tamoxifen in breast cancer prevention: a report from the National Surgical Adjuvant Breast and Bowel Project P-1 Study. *Journal of Clinical Oncology* **17**(9):2659–69.

90 Schink, J. C., Weller, E., Harris, L. S. *et al.* (2001). Outpatient taxol and carboplatin chemotherapy for sub-optimally debulked epithelial carcinoma of the ovary results in improved quality of life: an Eastern Cooperative Group phase II study (E2E93). *Cancer Journal* **7**(2): 155–64.

91 Cella, D., Eton, D. T., Fairclough, D. L. *et al.* (2002). What is clinically meaningful change (CMC) on the Functional Assessment of Cancer Therapy – Lung (FACT-L) questionnaire? An analysis of data from ECOG 5592. *Journal of Clinical Epidemiology* **55**:286–95.

92 Wenzel, L. B., Donnelly, J. P., Fowler, J. M. *et al.* (2002). Resilience, reflection, and residual stress in ovarian cancer survivorship: a Gynecologic Oncology Group study. *Psycho-Oncology* **11**:142–53.

93 Gotay, C. C., Moinpour, C. M., Moody-Thomas, S. *et al.* (2000). Behavioral science research in the cooperative group setting: the Southwest Oncology Group experience. *Journal of the National Cancer Institute* **92**:1381–7.

94 Hutchins, L. F., Unger, J. M., Crowley, J. J. *et al.* (1999). Underrepresentation of patients 65 years of age or older in cancer-treatment trials. *New England Journal of Medicine* **341**(27):2061–7.

95 National Cancer Institute. "Policies and Guidelines Relating to the Cancer-Center Support Grant." Available at http://www3.cancer.gov/cancercenters/ccsg.comp_pt1_1to2.html. Last accessed September 9, 2004.

96 National Cancer Institute. "The Nation's Investment in Cancer Research: A Plan and Budget Proposal for Fiscal Year 2005." Available at http://plan.cancer.gov. Last accessed on September 13, 2004.

97 Agency for Healthcare Research and Quality. "Primary Care Practice-Based Research Networks: Fact Sheet." Available at http://www.ahrq.gov/research/pbrnfact.htm. Last accessed on September 9, 2004.

98 Agency for Healthcare Research and Quality. "Integrated Delivery System Research Network (IDSRN): Field Partnerships to Conduct and Use Research." Available at http://www.ahrq.gov/research/idsrn.htm. Last accessed September 9, 2004.

99 U.S. Office of Civil Rights. "Office for Civil Rights – HIPAA. Medical Privacy – National Standards to Protect the Privacy of Personal Health Information." Available at http://www.hhs.gov/ocr/hipaa. Last accessed on September 9, 2004.

100 National Institutes of Health. "Protecting Personal Health Information in Research: Understanding the HIPAA Privacy Rule." Available at http://privacyruleandresearch.nih.gov. Last accessed on September 9, 2004.

APPENDIX 26.A

Participants in Videoconference Focus Group on Cancer Outcomes Data Infrastructure, Conducted July 6, 2001

Phyllis Wingo, Centers for Disease Control and Prevention

Susan Desharnais, Monica Morrow, and Joanne Sylvester, American College of Surgeons

Denise Hynes, Department of Veterans Affairs

Mark Hornbrook, Kaiser-Permanente Center for Health Research, Portland, OR

Janet Mitchell, Health Economics Research, Inc.

Carolyn C. Gotay, Cancer Research Center of Hawai'i, University of Hawai'i

Brenda Edwards, Joseph Lipscomb, and Joan Warren, National Cancer Institute

Facilitator: Ellen Tobin, Cancer Care Strategies, Inc.

27

Use of health-related quality-of-life measures by industry and regulatory agencies in evaluating oncology therapies

Dennis A. Revicki, Ph.D.

MEDTAP International, Bethesda, MD

Introduction

More than 50 years ago, clinical researchers in oncology recognized that the outcomes of chemotherapy extended beyond survival and other clinical endpoints.[1] The earliest effort to systematically measure the impact of cancer therapy on patient functional status was by Karnofsky et al.[2] During the past 30 years, significant advances have been made in understanding the impact of cancer and oncology treatments on patient health-related quality of life (HRQOL) and other patient-reported outcomes.[3–8] HRQOL measures extend patient outcomes assessment beyond survival, toxicity, and clinical efficacy and reflect the patient's perspective on the impact of disease and its treatment on functioning and well-being. Frequently, an important objective for evaluating HRQOL outcomes is demonstrating the value of new oncology treatments relative to other competing treatments. The pharmaceutical industry's intent in funding clinical trials with HRQOL measures is to achieve labeling and/or promotional claims for marketing to physicians, pharmacists, health care decision makers, and patients.[9,10]

Although HRQOL outcomes have been used in evaluating oncology treatments, the use of these endpoints in drug development and the regulatory approval process is a relatively new phenomenon. In the past, the Food and Drug Administration (FDA) has encouraged the measurement of survival, symptom, and HRQOL endpoints in evaluating oncology treatments.[11] During the past 17 years, no new cancer chemotherapy has been approved based primarily on HRQOL endpoints.[12,13] More recent statements by FDA officials continue to express skepticism about the value of HRQOL in evaluating oncology treatments.[13] For many oncology researchers, HRQOL is viewed as the ultimate outcome of health care interventions; however, no single outcome, such as survival, tumor response, symptoms, or HRQOL, adequately describes the comprehensive effects of disease and treatment.[14–16]

The primary objective of this chapter is to describe the application and use of HRQOL and other patient-reported outcomes in the evaluation and approval of new oncology treatments. The intent is to summarize the regulatory agency and pharmaceutical industry perspectives on the use of HRQOL endpoints in the drug development, approval, and marketing process. The report will provide recommendations for improving the application, use, and interpretation of HRQOL data associated with new cancer therapies and will outline methodological and statistical challenges related to HRQOL endpoints in oncology clinical trials. It will examine how HRQOL assessments add value, beyond safety and efficacy data, in understanding the impact of treatment on patients with cancer. In addition, the chapter will review how these data inform the drug evaluation and approval process and product labeling and marketing.

HRQOL outcomes in the drug development and approval process

Summary of drug development phases

After pre-clinical evaluation, there are four phases in the new drug development and approval process. The initial three phases are conducted during the pre-approval phases to study a specific indication for a new drug or a new indication for an existing drug. Phase IV studies are conducted after regulatory approval and after the drug enters the market, and they are usually focused on establishing safety in a more generalizable patient population.

In oncology, phase I studies are conducted with small groups of metastatic cancer patients to evaluate toxicity, pharmacokinetic, and pharmacodynamic outcomes. Phase I studies concentrate on safety endpoints, with no or only limited focus on clinical efficacy. During phase IIa and IIb, randomized clinical trials are conducted to broaden the preliminary safety assessments and to determine the most effective dosage of the experimental treatment. Phase IIa and IIb oncology clinical trials attempt to balance toxicity with potential clinical efficacy, but these studies are usually not powered to evaluate clinical efficacy.

For some oncology chemotherapies (e.g., palliative care), there is a growing acceptance in the pharmaceutical industry and in regulatory agencies that HRQOL data can add valuable information to understanding the risks and benefits of a new drug. HRQOL measures are often included in phase IIb and IIIa studies to evaluate safety, efficacy, and HRQOL endpoints. During phase III clinical trials, the experimental cancer treatments are frequently compared to chemotherapy regimens with established clinical effects, depending on the cancer indication. Phase III clinical trials are often conducted in patients with advanced metastatic cancer, and, because of expected disease progression and survival rates, these patients present challenges to the evaluation of treatment differences. Phase IIIa and IIIb clinical trials are designed to provide evidence for the safety and efficacy of the experimental therapy

sufficient to convince regulatory review agencies that the new product is approvable. Fast-track applications for new pharmaceutical therapies[17] often combine phase II and III clinical trials to determine toxicity and clinical efficacy where the disease indication is life threatening and where there are few effective treatment options. In this case, phase IV post-approval studies may be conducted to further evaluate the safety and efficacy of the new treatment. Other post-approval phase IV studies may evaluate outcomes, such as HRQOL, treatment satisfaction, and cost-effectiveness, in more heterogeneous patient populations. Phase IV studies cannot now be used to establish new indications for a drug's use beyond what is on the approved label.

HRQOL in oncology clinical trials

HRQOL and other patient-reported outcome measures are most often incorporated into phase II, III, or IV clinical trials, depending on whether there is some evidence that these data may accelerate regulatory approval or contribute to marketing the new product after approval for safety and efficacy. HRQOL outcomes are included in phase IIa and IIb studies to pilot test the instruments and to obtain descriptive statistics and variance estimates necessary for powering subsequent phase III clinical trials. Some researchers advocate the application of HRQOL instruments in phases I through IV clinical trials (I. Barofsky, personal communication, November 1999). Many industry-sponsored clinical trials include HRQOL measures in phase II studies.

There is evidence from recent reviews[4–8] that HRQOL instruments are frequently included in cancer clinical trials. Clinical trials sponsored by government agencies (e.g., the National Cancer Institute) and the pharmaceutical industry that are designed to compare chemotherapy regimens often include measures of patient-reported symptoms and HRQOL. The National Cancer Institute does not have an official policy requiring inclusion of HRQOL measures in clinical trials; however, if these outcomes are included, the selected instruments must be reliable, valid, and appropriate for addressing the research question, and should also be an integral part of the clinical trial protocol. The development of psychometrically sound cancer-specific HRQOL instruments, such as the EORTC Quality of Life Questionnaire,[18] Functional Assessment of Cancer Therapy (FACT),[19] Functional Living Index-Cancer,[20] Quality of Life-Cancer Scale,[21] and other cancer- or treatment-specific scales,[22,23] has further encouraged their addition to cancer clinical trial protocols. Currently, there are numerous examples of clinical studies in which HRQOL endpoints provided additional insight into the combined effects of clinical response and toxicity.[8,22]

Regulatory perspective on HRQOL endpoints

In the United States, the FDA has made several statements encouraging the use of patient-reported symptom, HRQOL outcome, and clinical effectiveness data in evaluating oncology products.[11,12,24,25] More recently, Richard Pazdur, Director of the Oncology Division within the FDA, indicated that HRQOL should not be considered in drug approvals, although patient-reported cancer-related symptoms might be helpful in evaluating new therapies.[13] It is also clear that some persons within the FDA make no distinction between symptom scales and measures of HRQOL and quality of life.[12] During the Oncology Division Advisory Committee (ODAC) Quality of Life Subcommittee meeting held in June 2000, several ODAC members suggested that disease-related symptoms were equivalent to HRQOL. This viewpoint about HRQOL and health outcome terminology may have resulted from the numerous alternative definitions of HRQOL,[26–33] some including symptom domains, and also from the many frequently used cancer-specific HRQOL instruments that include symptom items.[18,19,23] Measures of disease-related symptoms and functional status are conceptually closer to clinical endpoints and, thus, may be viewed as more clearly linked to clinical effectiveness measures. HRQOL research methodology workshops held within the FDA over the past three years have educated FDA staff in health outcomes terminology, HRQOL measures and methods,

and other related research issues. To further assist FDA staff, efforts are underway to clarify definitions and terminology of patient-reported outcomes and HRQOL.[34]

The FDA is responsible for ensuring that approved drugs are safe and effective. Labeling claims must be approved by the FDA. Promotional claims are reviewed by the FDA, and a response is issued if it is thought that the claim is not supported by scientific research. The FDA has responsibility for ensuring that any claims related to clinical efficacy, safety, or HRQOL are based on adequate research designs, statistical methods, and measurements. A key issue for the FDA is the review and decision making for any HRQOL claims associated with products under accelerated review. In this case, FDA reviewers usually have only 30 days to review and comment on the HRQOL results, but review periods are often sufficient for this purpose. However, approved labeling on HRQOL benefits can appear in various sections of the product package information, and often there is not sufficient time for the FDA to carefully consider these data.

Recent changes in FDA legislation have placed more focus on HRQOL, patient-reported outcomes, and health economics.[35] The FDA, in general, views HRQOL outcomes as one of a number of clinical effectiveness endpoints. The importance placed on HRQOL endpoints in the study protocol influences the amount of attention paid to them; HRQOL is not of primary importance in all clinical trials. Although the FDA has considerable expertise in reviewing and evaluating clinical efficacy and toxicity data, it has significantly less experience with HRQOL methods and outcomes. There has been some inconsistency within the FDA over the past 10 years, resulting in some confusion among HRQOL researchers, industry personnel, and clinicians regarding the standards used for evaluating promotional or labeling claims of HRQOL effects. HRQOL measures are most helpful when a therapy is designed to improve patient functioning and well-being; the study is an equivalence trial with HRQOL benefits; treatment has a small impact on survival; there are no objective markers of disease activity; or evaluation of treatment is based primarily on patient perceptions.[36] HRQOL data may be most useful in differentiating products with comparable biomedical clinical outcomes.

From the perspective of the FDA, the incorporation of HRQOL and other patient-reported outcomes in pivotal clinical trials and new drug applications may add to the understanding of the effectiveness of experimental oncology treatments. Within the FDA, there is often uncertainty about different HRQOL and patient-reported outcomes terminology and concern about multi-domain instruments and outcomes. FDA personnel are most comfortable when the clinical efficacy and HRQOL outcomes show trends in the same direction for an oncology treatment. Explicatory information needs to be provided in new drug applications to increase the confidence of FDA reviewers in accepting HRQOL endpoints, i.e, the endpoints are not an afterthought and the instruments and methods conform to the state of the art in HRQOL research. FDA staff has expressed concern about lowering the standards too far in negotiations for promotional and labeling claims.

The FDA perspective focuses on ensuring that any statements about HRQOL and other patient-reported outcomes are conveyed in a fair and accurate manner based on the best scientific methods and measures available. This focus is not confined just to HRQOL outcomes. For example, the FDA recently issued a guidance stating that subjective and vague terminology describing side effects, such as describing adverse effects as "well tolerated," is viewed as misleading.[37] In general, the FDA has objected to vague and overly broad claims of HRQOL or quality-of-life benefits. Statements of HRQOL improvement must be supported by well-controlled clinical trials, psychometrically sound instruments, and adequate statistical methods.[9,10] The communication of patient health outcomes must be clear, unambiguous, and based on adequate scientific methods. The FDA Division of Drug Marketing, Advertising, and Communication (DDMAC) has the responsibility for reviewing the promotion of claims on a product's clinical and HRQOL effects, and it is concerned that HRQOL findings are communicated in clear and unambiguous terms.

A recent policy analysis by Morris and Miller[38] noted an inconsistency between the FDA's policies for substantiation of HRQOL claims in labeling and its substantiation of HRQOL claims in advertising. Apparently, it is more difficult to obtain approval of an advertising claim if data supporting the advertising are not included in the product label. However, the Morris and Miller review does not consider the past application of varied evaluation criteria across FDA sections and changes over time in FDA attention to HRQOL data. In the past, it was easier to insert information on HRQOL outcomes in the clinical studies section (i.e., the standards were lower than for promotional claims) because the FDA was focusing most of its attention on other parts of the product package insert (i.e., toxicity) and was not fully aware of HRQOL measurement methods and scientific rigor. Currently, more consistent standards are used in reviewing both labeling and promotional claims for HRQOL benefits. Burke[39] states that the same level of substantiation is required for HRQOL and other patient-reported outcomes claims as for clinical efficacy claims. Clearly, consistency is necessary for effective regulation. Morris and Miller[38] recommend basing HRQOL advertising claims, in the absence of a labeling claim, on the Federal Trade Commission's (FTC) competent and reliable scientific evidence standard.[40] The FTC standard may not be workable, given that the FDA views HRQOL as an additional clinical benefit measure.

HRQOL labeling and promotional claims assist in the translation of clinical effects of a new treatment into patient functioning and well-being. HRQOL information plays an important role in communicating the real value of oncology treatments to physicians and patients. The FDA and DDMAC have been very open about seeking assistance from scientific experts, outcomes research organizations (i.e., the International Society for Quality of Life Research and the International Society for Pharmacoeconomics and Outcomes Research), and industry researchers in developing standards for evaluating the adequacy of HRQOL claims. The Patient Reported Outcomes

Harmonization effort, which includes representatives from industry and the outcomes research field, is one example of current activities toward increasing consistency in standards for HRQOL research evidence.[34]

Industry perspective on HRQOL endpoints

The pharmaceutical industry is interested in demonstrating the clinical value of its products. To the extent that HRQOL and other patient-reported outcomes data help in demonstrating this health value from the perspective of the treating physician and the patient, these endpoints will be included in clinical trials. There is some variation among industry researchers as to where the bar should be set in terms of scientific methods and instrumentation for HRQOL outcomes. Some in industry think these standards should be kept flexible and simple; however, the majority of industry researchers believe that the standards for research and evidence in HRQOL should conform to the state of the art in methods and instrumentation. These differences make it difficult for the pharmaceutical industry to hold, and communicate, one perspective related to HRQOL research, although the Pharmaceutical Research and Manufacturers of America (PhRMA)[41] has recently made statements about regulatory issues and HRQOL assessment.

In the pharmaceutical industry, HRQOL outcomes are used most often to support patient-based effectiveness outcomes, with primary emphasis placed on documenting safety and clinical efficacy. There are regulatory, marketing, and treatment reasons for planning and conducting HRQOL outcomes studies.[42] Increasingly, clinical studies are designed and conducted with the specific purpose of securing a HRQOL labeling or promotional claim. Symptom scales and HRQOL measures can be useful in documenting treatment effects when survival and clinical response endpoints are equivocal.

Obtaining a HRQOL labeling or promotional claim provides excellent opportunities for marketing new products. Several oncology products have achieved approval of HRQOL or related claims, and there is continued research focus by industry in evaluating HRQOL outcomes in cancer clinical trials. Even if a FDA-approved claim is not obtained, there may be important marketing and sales advantages associated with positive HRQOL results in published articles. In disease indications where there are many competing products, HRQOL data may provide a competitive advantage.[42] HRQOL data are used by industry to differentiate products and to demonstrate patient outcomes benefits, or the absence of ill effects, for oncologists and patients.

Physicians working in oncology are sensitized to the trade-offs between survival, clinical response, and toxicity; and HRQOL outcomes provide integrated data on the impact of these factors on patient functioning and well-being.[8] HRQOL studies are designed to provide clinicians and patients with comprehensive information on the effects of cancer chemotherapy. It is recognized in oncology that survival for some cancers comes at some cost in terms of functioning and well-being[14,43] and that HRQOL assessments help quantify these effects in meaningful ways.

Finally, given the increase in consumer and patient involvement in medical decision making, industry increasingly uses the results of HRQOL studies in direct-to-consumer marketing. HRQOL data have the potential for assisting pharmaceutical companies in describing their products on dimensions that have meaningful relevance to patients and their families.[42,44]

For industry, HRQOL outcomes have the potential for translating clinical outcomes into functioning and well-being effects that may hold value for physicians and patients.[44] Positive HRQOL findings may result in increased market share and sales, but note that a strong marketplace performance depends on both the successful dissemination of findings and the marketing activities of competitors. Few studies, because of analytic complexity, attribution issues, and the number of alternative factors influencing sales, have focused on estimating the potential increases in pharmaceutical sales. Jack[45] has demonstrated that marketing and sales of a pharmaceutical product can increase following the publication of a HRQOL outcomes study. It is difficult to quantify the incremental value of HRQOL outcomes studies in sales of pharmaceuticals. Future research needs to attempt to estimate the incremental marketing and sales value of positive HRQOL findings.

Currently, industry continues to support the inclusion of HRQOL and related patient outcomes in cancer clinical trials. From the industry's perspective, a clear and consistently applied FDA guidance for substantiating claims for HRQOL benefits for labeling or advertising would be beneficial. The inconsistency in FDA reviews and decision making[38] makes it difficult to plan effectively to support HRQOL claims. There is a concern among industry researchers that the scientific burden for substantiating claims of HRQOL effects may be greater than for clinical effectiveness. Standards for documenting HRQOL effects should be consistent with the standards for documenting clinical effects.

Documenting evidence for HRQOL labeling and promotional claims

Past and current guidance and standards

Although the FDA encouraged the application of cancer-related symptom and HRQOL outcomes in evaluating the effectiveness of new oncology agents,[24] no published guidance or standards for designing and conducting HRQOL research have been published by the FDA. For the past three years, a task force on HRQOL and patient-reported outcome assessment has been meeting within the FDA, and a draft guidance document has been developed. It is uncertain when this guidance will be issued, but there is optimism that it will be soon. There is an evolving consensus within the FDA regarding some standards for HRQOL clinical trials. Based on presentations by FDA officials, information necessary for substantiating a claim of HRQOL benefit includes specification of research objectives and hypotheses, rationale for measuring HRQOL domains and for the selection of instruments, evidence of instrument reliability and validity, an a priori data analysis plan, fair and complete reporting of results, and guidelines on interpretation of clinical significance. A patient-reported outcomes harmonization effort has been underway for the past year to provide assistance to the FDA in developing scientific and methodological standards for HRQOL research as part of drug development and evaluation.[34]

There are FDA-approved HRQOL claims for more than 20 products and about 25% are for oncology indications.[46] Using information provided by the FDA[46] and a recent review (B. Crawford, personal communication, August 2001), we identified seven oncology products with approved labeling or promotional claims for HRQOL benefits. These examples may prove informative in understanding the methods and instruments used to support HRQOL claims in the past. However, statements made by Laurie Burke, FDA DDMAC, suggest that past decisions and experience may not always be informative about future FDA reviews and decision making.[39,46] FDA experience with reviewing HRQOL data is increasing, and it is anticipated that more consistent standards of evidence will be used in judging future HRQOL claims.

Table 27.1 summarizes the seven oncology agents by indication, company, HRQOL instrumentation, domains evaluated, and the approved claim. Most often, information about a product's HRQOL effects is located in the "Clinical Studies" or related section of the product label. There is substantial variation in the amount of detail provided in the product label. In particular, the study designs and statistical methods and results are not consistently described across labels, and information is provided on the domains of HRQOL measured and those domains that differ between treatments. A variety of symptom-based and HRQOL instruments are used to assess patient health outcomes in these clinical trials.

Added value of HRQOL data

HRQOL measures are frequently included in phase II and III clinical trials comparing oncology

Table 27.1. Selected FDA approved HRQOL claims for oncology products

Indication	Product	Sponsor	HRQOL Instrument	Domains	Label Claim	References
Metastatic colorectal cancer	Camptosar® injection (irinotecan hydrochloride).	Pharmacia and Upjohn	EORTC QLQ-C30.	Global health status (functional (i.e., cognitive, emotional, social, physical, role), and symptom(i.e., fatigue, appetite loss, pain assessment, insomnia, constipation, dyspnea, nausea/vomiting, financial impact, diarrhea) subscales.	In study 1, patients receiving irinotecan reported significantly better results for global health status on two of five functional subscales and on four of nine symptom subscales. In study 2, the multivariate analysis on all 15 subscales did not indicate a statistically significant difference between irinotecan and infusional 5-FU.[47]	Cunningham et al.[48] Rougier et al.[49]
	Casodex® (bicalutamide).	Astra Zeneca	ECOG Performance Status, assessments of pain, QOL questionnaire (33 multiple choice questions).	QOL questionnaire: social functioning, emotional well-being, vitality, activity limitation, bed disability, overall health, physical capacity, general symptoms, treatment-related symptoms.	Assessment of the QOL questionnaires did not indicate consistent significant differences between the two treatment groups.[50]	Schellhammer et al.[51] Schellhammer et al.[52]
Non-small-cell lung cancer	Gemzar Injection® (gemcitabine hydrochloride).	Eli Lilly	FACT-L, EORTC QLQ-C30, QLQ-LC13.	FACT-L Domains: physical, social, emotional, and functional well-being, lung cancer symptoms EORTC Domains: physical and psychological functioning, symptoms related to lung cancer and its treatment.	In both studies, no significant differences were observed in QOL between the Gemzar plus cisplatin and the comparator arm.[53]	Cardenal et al.[54] Sandler et al.[55]
	Navelbine® Injection (vinorelbine tartrate).	Glaxo Wellcome	Modified SWOG QOL questionnaire.	SWOG Domains: role functioning, physical functioning, symptom distress, global QOL.	Quality of life was not adversely affected by Navelbine when compared to control.[56]	Le Chevalier et al.[57] Wozniak et al.[58] Crawford et al.[59]
	Taxol® (paclitaxel).	Bristol- Myers Squibb	FACT-L, EORTC QLQ-C30, QLQ-LC13.	FACT-L Domains: physical well-being, functional well-being, lung cancer symptoms, social well-being, emotional well-being, relationship with doctor.	The Lung Cancer Symptoms subscale showed a lesser rate of deterioration for the treatment arm of Taxol 135 mg/m/ 24 hours plus cisplatin compared to the cisplatin/etoposide arm.[60]	Bonomi et al.[61] Giaccone et al.[62]

Cancer type	Product	Company	Instrument	Measures	Results	Reference
Thyroid cancer	Thyrogen® (thyrotropin alfa)	Genzyme	SF-36, Profile of Mood States (POMS).	SF-36 domains: physical functioning, physical role, bodily pain, emotional role, general health, vitality, social functioning, and mental health; POMS domains: fatigue-inertia, depression-dejection, vigor-activity, confusion-bewilderment, tension-anxiety, anger-hostility.	Following Thyrogen, no change was observed in any of the 8 domains of the SF-36. Following thyroid hormone withdrawal, statistically significant negative changes were observed in 4 of the 8 SF-36 domains. These 4 domains were physical functioning, physical role, bodily pain, and emotional role. No change was observed in the following scales: general health, vitality, social functioning, and mental health.[63]	Haugen et al.[64] Ladenson et al.[65]
Metastatic breast cancer	Aredia® (pamidronate disodium)	Novartis	Spitzer QOL Index, ECOG Performance Status, pain scores severity v frequency.	QOL, pain relief.	Decreases in pain scores from baseline occurred at the last measurement for those Aredia patients with pain at baseline (p=0.026) but not in the placebo group. At the last measurement, a worsening from baseline was observed in the placebo group for the Spitzer quality of life score (p<0.001) and ECOG performance status (p<0.001) while there was no significant deterioration from baseline in these parameters observed in Aredia-treated patients.[66]	Theriault et al.[67] Hortobagyi et al.[68]

treatments. Despite this frequency of application, skeptics counter that HRQOL endpoints add little new information not captured by traditional safety and efficacy data. Therefore, there is little actual need for HRQOL data, and these data are of only limited use for regulatory or clinical decision making. However, the American Society of Clinical Oncology[14] notes that no single endpoint, including survival, adequately represents the results of cancer treatment. There is evidence that HRQOL outcomes have added value in understanding the effectiveness of oncology and other medical treatments.[8,16,34] HRQOL outcomes can provide additional data on effectiveness not captured by clinical efficacy outcomes, differentiate treatments with comparable clinical efficacy or survival, provide more meaningful endpoints to clinicians and patients, perhaps best measure treatment effectiveness for chronic diseases without objective clinical endpoints, and have prognostic value in oncology and other diseases.[16] In sections that follow, research will be summarized which illustrates the relationship between HRQOL and clinical status, the value of HRQOL endpoints in cancer studies, and the prognostic value of HRQOL endpoints.

Relationship between HRQOL and clinical status

HRQOL is a quantitative indicator of the impact of disease and treatment that is related to but not perfectly correlated with biologic, physiologic, and clinical markers of disease activity.[34] HRQOL endpoints are not the same as measures of symptoms or toxicity, although HRQOL measures the effects of the underlying disease and treatment-related benefits and side effects. Clearly, HRQOL outcomes are expected to change with and reflect changing disease stage, frequency and severity of treatment-related toxicity, and treatment response.[8]

Cancer disease stage is consistently associated with HRQOL scores. For example, King[69] examined 14 studies using the EORTC QLQ-C30 in different cancers (e.g., colorectal, breast, lung) and found relationships between QLQ-C30 scores and disease stage and treatment response. In general, cancer patients

with advanced or metastatic disease reported lower (worse) HRQOL scores compared to those patients with early stage disease. Treatment-related toxicity and response to treatment were related to HRQOL scores. Osoba[8] re-evaluated the largest of these studies and determined a strong consistent relationship exists between disease stage and EORTC QLQ-C30 global quality of life scores and for social, physical, and role functioning scores. HRQOL scores varied in expected directions based in part on treatment response and changing performance status ratings. HRQOL increased for those patients with improving performance status scores.[8,69]

Treatment differences and HRQOL

HRQOL outcomes have been included as primary or secondary endpoints in many oncology clinical trials.[3-8] HRQOL provides an integrated assessment, from the patient's perspective, of the effects of clinical response and toxicity on functioning and well-being. HRQOL data are useful for interpreting clinical outcomes and in clinical decision making. For example, HRQOL was the primary outcome in a clinical trial comparing prednisone versus combined prednisone and mitoxantrone in men with hormone-refractory metastatic prostate cancer.[70,71] No survival differences were expected or observed in this study. Patients in the combined prednisone-mitoxantrone treatment group reported decreased pain and improved global quality of life, physical function, and emotional function.[71] Other clinical trials have demonstrated HRQOL effects associated with treatment of anemia in cancer patients,[72] anorexia treatment,[73-75] and different cycles for chemotherapy for small cell lung cancer.[76] Most often, HRQOL outcomes are considered secondary endpoints in cancer clinical trials, with the primary endpoint being survival or tumor response. Although the major emphasis has traditionally been on the clinical efficacy endpoints, HRQOL outcomes have proven valuable in differentiating treatments with comparable survival or clinical outcomes. Examples of these clinical trials include temozolamide treatment for recurrent glioblastoma multiforme[77] and anaplastic astrocytoma,[78] alpha-interferon in metastatic colorectal cancer,[79] pegylated liposomal doxorubicin in AIDS-related Kaposi's sarcoma,[80] and chemotherapy in advanced metastatic breast cancer.[81,82]

HRQOL endpoint data can provide additional insight into the effects of chemotherapy. For example, Fairclough et al.[83] compared HRQOL in a clinical trial of breast cancer patients receiving either increased dose intensity for 16 weeks or standard cyclophosphamide, doxorubicin, and 5-fluorouracil (CAF) therapy. HRQOL was assessed using the Breast Chemotherapy Questionnaire (BCQ).[84] BCQ scores decreased more (worsened) in the 16-week intense chemotherapy group compared to the CAF group during treatment. No differences were observed between the two treatment groups four months after treatment ended. A slightly increased 4-year survival advantage was observed for the 16-week intensive chemotherapy group, and a Q-TWiST analysis suggested that this treatment group was associated with a 2 to 2.4 month increase in quality-of-life adjusted survival.[83] In addition, the BCQ detected a clinically meaningful treatment difference in fatigue which was not captured by the toxicity measures.

Industry-sponsored oncology clinical trials have included HRQOL outcomes as secondary endpoints to evaluate the effectiveness of therapies from the patient's perspective. HRQOL labeling and promotional claims have been supported by HRQOL assessments in clinical trials comparing treatments for colorectal cancer,[48,49] non-small-cell lung cancer,[54,55,57–59,61,62] thyroid cancer,[64,65] metastatic breast cancer,[67,68] and metastatic prostate cancer.[51,52,70,71] HRQOL data from these clinical trials have shown to be useful in demonstrating the clinical value of new cancer treatments and can assist oncologists and their patients in making decisions about the best treatment for individuals and groups of patients.[8]

Prognostic value of HRQOL measures

A number of studies have demonstrated that HRQOL measures predict survival in cancer and other diseases, even after controlling for sociodemographic, performance status, and clinical status variables.[8,16,22] Several studies in oncology patient samples have shown that patients with better HRQOL have longer survival times than those patients with lower HRQOL scores.[85–93] For example, Dancey et al.,[90] in a study of 474 patients with various cancers, demonstrated that global quality-of-life and psychological well-being scores were independent predictors of survival, after controlling for cancer type and severity and performance status. Blazeby et al.,[93] in a study of esophageal cancer patients, showed that a 10-point increase in physical function scores at baseline was associated with a 12% decrease in the likelihood of death. The relation between impaired HRQOL and mortality across different cancers and other diseases provides strong support for the construct validity and importance of HRQOL. Despite this research evidence, many physicians do not know that baseline HRQOL is an independent prognostic factor in survival among cancer patients.[94] Additional translational research is needed to provide physicians with guidance as to how to interpret and use HRQOL data in clinical practice.

Use of HRQOL data and future directions

Standards for documenting HRQOL labeling or promotional claims

Evidence requirements for a HRQOL claim should be based on accepted scientific standards of HRQOL research. The evidence for documenting claims of the HRQOL benefits of therapy must be consistent with the existing regulatory standards for claims of clinical efficacy.[9,10] The evidentiary requirements for labeling and promotional claims should also be consistent. The changes in evidentiary requirements for clinical effectiveness as part of the FDA Modernization Act of 1997[35] apply to HRQOL and other patient-reported outcomes.

Recent articles[9,10,41,95] and meetings of the PRO Harmonization Group[34] provide insight into evolving standards for documenting HRQOL claims. First, the evidence supporting a HRQOL claim requires two well-designed randomized clinical trials with unequivocal findings. The results from multiple studies are necessary when HRQOL outcomes are secondary endpoints or when results across clinical trials are equivocal. It may be possible to achieve an approved claim based on one well-designed and well-implemented clinical trial. However, this clinical trial needs to include comprehensive assessment of HRQOL outcomes, representative patient populations, few missing data, and acceptable statistical power. The study needs to yield unequivocal HRQOL results which are supported by additional confirmatory evidence. In addition, to provide sufficient evidence for HRQOL benefits, there must be consistency in the results from the clinical efficacy and HRQOL data analyses and in any subgroup analyses performed on the HRQOL data for a single clinical trial.

To justify a labeling or promotional claim, the HRQOL component to the clinical trial must also explicitly document the rationale for measuring HRQOL, provide the rationale for the specific HRQOL domains assessed and for selecting the HRQOL instrumentation, document the psychometric characteristics (i.e., reliability, validity, responsiveness) of the HRQOL instruments, describe procedures for ensuring quality data collection, and provide an a priori statistical analysis plan. The statistical analysis plan should be filed before subject recruitment and follow-up is completed and before any treatment blinding is broken. The data analysis plan should provide details on methods for handling missing item-level and form-level data, multiplicity in endpoints, longitudinal data structure, and statistical analyses for comparing treatment groups.

The key to a successful promotional or labeling claim rests in using HRQOL measures with documented psychometric qualities.[9,10,95] Standards for evaluating the reliability and validity of psychological and HRQOL instruments have been published.[10,95-98] Basically, evidence of the reliability, validity, and responsiveness of the instrument(s)

and information for clinical interpretation need to be documented for the HRQOL and other patient-reported outcomes included in the clinical study. This evidence must include data on the instrument's internal consistency and test-retest reliability, content and construct validity, and responsiveness to clinical or other relevant changes.[10] Acceptable psychometric qualities must be demonstrated in the target patient population participating in the clinical trial, ideally from an independent study.

Methods and statistical analysis advances

Three main research method and data analysis advances may assist investigators, industry, and regulatory agencies in dealing with problems in HRQOL studies in oncology: (1) research and methods focused on evaluating responsiveness and clinical interpretation of HRQOL measures; (2) item response theory models and computer-adaptive testing; and (3) methods for statistically analyzing HRQOL when there are missing data.

Although data on responsiveness and clinical significance have been inconsistently provided for many cancer-specific HRQOL instruments, research is focusing on assessing the responsiveness of HRQOL instruments and on providing guidelines for interpretation. Responsiveness to changes in patient clinical status is important for comparing treatment differences in clinical trials. Research attention is continuing to focus on providing insight into the interpretation of changes or differences in HRQOL scores. Further research and clinical trial experience is needed on the main cancer-specific HRQOL instruments, such as the FACT and the EORTC QLQ measures; and with experience, guidelines will evolve for recognizing important differences. The series of articles produced by the Clinical Significance Consensus Meeting Group should provide the beginning of consensus on evaluating responsiveness and clinical interpretation issues for HRQOL measurement.[99-102] More research is needed, but there is evidence from psychometric evaluation studies and clinical trials on practically significant changes in cancer-specific HRQOL instruments. For further discussion on defining clinical significance, see Chapter 19 by Osoba in this volume.[8]

Item response theory (IRT) methods and analyses for evaluating the measurement characteristics of tests have been available for more than 40 years but only recently have been applied to health status and HRQOL data.[103–107] IRT models are mathematical equations summarizing the relationship between the respondent's underlying level on a latent construct (e.g., HRQOL) and the probability of a specific item response using a nonlinear monotonic function.[103, 104] The chapters by Reise,[105] Hambleton,[106] and Wilson[107] in this volume provide an introduction to IRT models and their applications for measuring HRQOL in oncology.

Several potential advantages of IRT measurement approaches have been identified for HRQOL assessment, including more comprehensive and accurate evaluation of item characteristics, evaluating group differences in item and scale functioning, evaluating scales with items with different response formats, improvement of existing health status measures, computer-adaptive testing, and modeling longitudinal change in HRQOL.[108] Item banking and computer-adaptive testing have implications for more precise, efficient, and less burdensome measurement of HRQOL endpoints.[106] In computer-adaptive testing, subsets of items measuring a domain of interest are administered to patients according to item characteristics and are targeted to the person's level on the domain. Different patients are administered different subsets of items that best place them on the underlying HRQOL domain continuum. Clearly, the IRT model techniques can be used effectively to measure changes in health outcomes over time using combinations of items that best measure the person's domain level at any point in time. Additional applications of IRT models in HRQOL measurement are needed, but research is continuing. Combined with the use of computer-administered instruments, it is likely that, in the future, patient outcomes assessment in oncology clinical trials will become more efficient and less burdensome to patients. There are a number of technical and conceptual challenges that must be addressed

before IRT-based instruments in HRQOL studies are widely used.[106, 108]

In addition, issues of multiplicity of endpoints, informative missing data, and longitudinal data structure complicate the statistical analysis of HRQOL outcomes in oncology clinical trials.[10, 101, 109–112] In many cancer clinical trials, missing data are unavoidable due to toxicity, disease progression, or mortality. Most missing HRQOL endpoint data in oncology studies are non-ignorable, which complicates the statistical analyses. Fortunately, there has been considerable research on statistical methods for handling missing HRQOL outcomes data in clinical trials[111–114] and in various imputation methods.[110, 113, 115] Repeated measures mixed models are increasingly used in clinical trials to compare treatment effects on HRQOL over time.[111, 112]

Analyzing data from studies with non-ignorable missing data is difficult; there are a number of potential models, but it is not possible to determine the statistically best model without access to the missing data.[109, 112] Selection models and pattern mixture models can be used to analyze HRQOL studies with non-ignorable missing data.[111, 112] For a more complete discussion of techniques to address missing data, refer to the book by Fairclough.[112]

Finally, although there have been few (if any) attempts to use Bayesian techniques to analyze HRQOL data, the application of Bayesian methods[116] to HRQOL data from cancer clinical trials should be explored. Proponents argue this would provide a more comprehensive and coherent way to incorporate uncertainty into data analyses. These methods have been used in economic studies and in several studies for analyzing clinical endpoints.

Summary and conclusions

The evaluation of HRQOL and other patient-reported outcomes endpoints continues to increase and provide useful information on the effects of cancer chemotherapy. There is interest from physicians, patients, and health care decision makers in understanding the impact of treatment on patient functioning and well-being. Any labeling or promotional claims of HRQOL effects should be based on sound scientific evidence. Clearly, HRQOL claims, as for any health outcome claim, require a well-documented rationale for measuring HRQOL and, if relevant, selected domains of HRQOL, and for selecting generic or disease-specific instruments to assess these domains. Instruments should have sufficient evidence of reliability, construct validity, and responsiveness in the patient population participating in the planned cancer clinical trial. The trial planners need to address data collection procedures, training for clinical center research staff in the collection of HRQOL data, methods for minimizing missing item and form data, and a data analysis plan. Before study recruitment ends and before database closure and lock, a statistical analysis plan needs to be filed that summarizes the methods used to handle missing form data, multiplicity in endpoints, and longitudinal data structure, and that also specifies how statistically significant results will be interpreted for practical significance.

The challenge for academic researchers, industry representatives, and regulatory agency reviewers is to reach consensus on the standards for scientific evidence to support HRQOL and patient-reported outcomes claims for labeling and advertising. Consistency in the application of scientific standards for evaluating labeling and advertising claims is developing within the FDA and other regulatory agencies. These standards must be based on consensus among the HRQOL scientific community as to state-of-the-art research methods, instrumentation, and assessment procedures. There are a number of initiatives underway involving international outcomes research organizations, academic researchers, the FDA, and industry researchers.

The findings from HRQOL studies provide patients, physicians, and health care decision makers with more comprehensive data about the effect of treatment on physical, social, and psychological functioning and well-being. These HRQOL data also assist the pharmaceutical industry in documenting and communicating the value of its oncology products to physicians and patients. A HRQOL claim for labeling or promotion must be based on consistent evidentiary standards. These evidentiary requirements must be based on accepted scientific standards of HRQOL research and should be consistent with the evidence needed for efficacy claims. The focus of these studies should be on evidence-based medical practice, where treatment decision making is based on the available scientific research. Any treatment intended to improve or maintain HRQOL should provide evidence from well-controlled clinical trials using sound measurement. HRQOL data add to other available health outcome data, such as toxicity and efficacy outcomes, and allow patients and their physicians to select the best treatment based on the research evidence. HRQOL scientists, industry researchers, and regulatory agency staff must work together to ensure that HRQOL promotional and labeling claims are based on sound science, and that the results of the studies are communicated accurately and unambiguously to consumers.

REFERENCES

1 Barofsky, I., Sugarbaker, P. (1990). Cancer. In *Quality of Life Assessments in Clinical Trials*, ed. B. Spilker, pp. 419–40. New York: Raven.

2 Karnofsky, D., Abelman, W., Craver, L. *et al.* (1948). The use of the nitrogen mustards in the palliative treatment of carcinoma. *Cancer* 1:634–56.

3 Kiebert, G., Curran, D., Aaronson, N. (1998). Quality of life as an endpoint in EORTC clinical trials. *Statistics in Medicine* 17:561–9.

4 Litwin, Talcott, this volume, Chapter 6.

5 Ganz, Goodwin, this volume, Chapter 5.

6 Moinpour, Provenzale, this volume, Chapter 8.

7 Earle, Weeks, this volume, Chapter 7.

8 Osoba, this volume, Chapter 19.

9 Leidy, N., Revicki, D., Geneste, B. (1999). Recommendations for evaluating the validity of quality of life claims for labeling and promotion. *Value in Health* 2:113–27.

10 Revicki, D., Osoba, D., Fairclough, D. *et al.* (2000). Recommendations on health-related quality of life research to support labeling and promotional claims in the United States. *Quality of Life Research* 9:887–900.

11 Johnson, J. R., Temple, R. (1985). Food and Drug Administration requirements for approval of new anticancer drugs. *Cancer Treatment Reports* **69**:1155–7.

12 Beitz, J. (1999). Quality-of-life end points in oncology drug trials. *Oncology* **13**:1439–42.

13 F-D-C Reports. (2002). Oncologic NDA approval standards: FDA asks "what stands behind" response rate. *Pink Sheet* **64**:34–5.

14 American Society for Clinical Oncology (1996). Outcomes of cancer treatment for technology assessment and cancer treatment guidelines. *Journal of Clinical Oncology* **14**: 671–9.

15 Berzon, R. (1998). Understanding and using health-related quality of life instruments within clinical research studies. In *Quality of Life Assessment in Clinical Trials: Methods and Practice*, ed. M. Staquet, R. Hays, P. Fayers, pp. 3–18. New York: Oxford University Press.

16 Revicki, D. A. (2000). The added value of health-related quality of life evidence: is safety and efficacy enough? Presented at the annual meeting of the International Society for Quality of Life Research, Vancouver, British Columbia, Canada.

17 Food and Drug Administration (1998). Guidance for Industry: Fast Track Drug Development Programs – Designation, Development and Application Review. Available at: http://www.fda.gov/cder/guidance. Accessed September 9, 2004.

18 Aaronson, N., Cull, A., Kaasa, S. *et al.* (1996). The European Organization for Research and Treatment of Cancer (EORTC) modular approach to quality of life assessments in oncology: an update. In *Quality of Life and Pharmacoeconomics in Clinical Trials* (2nd Edition), ed. B. Spilker, pp. 179–90. Philadelphia, PA: Lippincott-Raven.

19 Cella, D., Bonomi, A. (1996). The Functional Assessment of Cancer Therapy (FACT) and Functional Assessment of HIV Infection (FAHI) quality of life measurement system. In *Quality of Life and Pharmacoeconomics in Clinical Trials*, (2nd Edition), ed. B. Spilker, pp. 203–14. Philadelphia, PA: Lippincott-Raven.

20 Clinch, J. J. (1996). The Functional Living Index-Cancer: ten years later. In *Quality of Life and Pharmacoeconomics in Clinical Trials*, (2nd Edition), ed. B. Spilker, pp. 215–25. Philadelphia, PA: Lippincott-Raven.

21 Padilla, G., Grant, M., Ferrell, B., Presant, C. (1996). Quality of Life-Cancer. In *Quality of Life and Pharmacoeconomics in Clinical Trials*, (2nd Edition), ed. B. Spilker, pp. 301–8. Philadelphia, PA: Lippincott-Raven.

22 Osoba, D. (1999). What has been learned from measuring health-related quality of life in clinical oncology? *European Journal of Cancer* **35**:1565–70.

23 Osoba, D. (1999). Quality of life instruments in oncology. *European Journal of Cancer* **35**:1571–80.

24 McCabe, M. S., Shoemaker, D., Temple, R. J. *et al.* (1996). Regulatory perspectives on quality of life issues. In *Quality of Life and Pharmacoeconomics in Clinical Trials*, (2nd Edition), ed. B. Spilker, pp. 569–74. Philadelphia, PA: Lippincott-Raven.

25 Beitz, J., Gnecco, C., Justice, R. (1996). Quality of life endpoints in cancer clinical trials. *Journal of the National Cancer Institute Monographs* **20**:7–9.

26 Bergner, M. (1989). Quality of life, health status, and clinical research. *Medical Care* **27**(Suppl.):S148–56.

27 Ferrans, this volume, Chapter 2.

28 Patrick, D. L., Erickson, P. (1993). *Health Status and Health Policy*. New York: Oxford University Press.

29 Schipper, H., Clinch, J. J., Olweny, C. L. (1996). Quality of life studies: definitions and conceptual issues. In *Quality of Life and Pharmacoeconomics in Clinical Trials*, (2nd Edition), ed. B. Spilker, pp. 11–24. Philadelphia, PA: Lippincott-Raven.

30 World Health Organization (1958). *The First Ten Years of the World Health Organization*. Geneva: World Health Organization.

31 Cella, D., Tulsky, D. (1990). Measuring quality of life today: methodological aspects. *Oncology* **5**:29–38.

32 Gill, T. M., Feinstein, A. R. (1994). A critical appraisal of the quality of quality-of-life measurements. *Journal of the American Medical Association* **272**:619–26.

33 Leplege, A., Hunt, S. (1997). The problem of quality of life in medicine. *Journal of the American Medical Association* **278**:47–50.

34 Acquadro, C., Berzon, R., Leidy, N. K. *et al.* for the PRO Harmonization Group (2004). Incorporating the patient's perspective into drug development and communication: an ad hoc task force report of the Patient-Reported Outcomes (PRO) Harmonization Group meeting at the Food and Drug Administration, February 16, 2001. *Value in Health* **6**(5):522–31.

35 Food and Drug Administration Modernization Act, 1997. Available at: http://www.fda.gov/cder/guidance. Accessed September 9, 2004.

36 Smith, N. D. (1993). Quality of life studies from the perspective of an FDA reviewing statistician. *Drug Information Journal* **27**:617–23.

37 Food and Drug Administration. (2000). Guidance to Industry: Content and Format of the Adverse Reactions Section of Labeling for Human Prescription Drugs and Biologics. Available at: http://www.fda.gov/cder/guidance. Accessed September 9, 2004.

38 Morris, L. A., Miller, D. (2002). The regulation of patient reported outcome claims: need for a flexible standard. *Value in Health* **5**:372–81.

39 Burke, L. B. (2000). Acceptable evidence for pharmaceutical advertising and labeling. Presented at Drug Information Association Workshop on Pharmacoeconomic and Quality of Life Labeling and Marketing Claims. New Orleans, Louisiana.

40 Federal Trade Commission. (1984). Policy statement regarding Advertising Substantiation Program. *Federal Register* **49**(50):30999–1001.

41 Santanello, N. C., Baker, D., Cappelleri, J. C. *et al.* (2002). Regulatory issues for health-related quality of life – PhRMA Health Outcomes Committee Workshop, 1999. *Value in Health* **5**:14–25.

42 Revicki, D. A., Rothman, M., Luce, B. (1992). Health-related quality of life assessment and the pharmaceutical industry. *Pharmacoeconomics* **1**:394–408.

43 National Institutes of Health Consensus Development Panel. (2001). National Institutes of Health Consensus Development Conference Statement: Adjuvant therapy for breast cancer, November 1–3. *Journal of the National Cancer Institute* **93**:979–89.

44 Morris, L. A., Beckett, T., Lechter, K. (1996). A marketing perspective: theoretical underpinnings. In *Quality of Life and Pharmacoeconomics in Clinical Trials*, (2nd Edition), ed. B. Spilker, pp. 541–8. Philadelphia, PA: Lippincott-Raven.

45 Jack, W. (1991). Pharmaceutical differentiation through quality of life measurement: a case study. *Journal of Pharmaceutical Marketing Management* **10**:33–53.

46 Burke, L. B. (2000). Regulatory issues in the use of patient reported outcomes in drug labeling and advertising. Presented at the Health-Related Quality of Life Workshop. Rockville, MD: Center for Drug Evaluation and Research, Food and Drug Administration.

47 Camptosar (Irinotecan hydrochloride) Injection Package Insert. Kalamazoo, MI: Pharmacia & Upjohn Company, 2000.

48 Cunningham, D. C., Pyrhonen, S., James, R. D. *et al.* (1998). Randomised trial of irinotecan plus supportive care versus supportive care alone after fluorouracil failure for patients with metastatic colorectal cancer. *Lancet* **352**:1413–18.

49 Rougier, P., Van Cutsem, E., Bajetta, E. *et al.* (1998). Randomised trial of irinotecan versus fluorouracil by continuous infusion after fluorouracil failure in patients with metastatic colorectal cancer. *Lancet* **352**:1407–12.

50 Casodex® (Bicalutamide tablets) Package Insert. Wilmington, DE: AstraZeneca Pharmaceuticals, 2000.

51 Schellhammer, P., Sharifi, R., Block, N. *et al.* (1996). Maximal androgen blockade for patients with metastatic prostate cancer: outcome of a controlled trial of bicalutamide versus flutamide, each in combination with luteinizing hormone-releasing hormone analogue therapy. Casodex Combination Study Group. *Urology* **47**(1A Suppl):54–60.

52 Schellhammer, P., Sharifi, R., Block, N. *et al.* (1995). A controlled trial of bicalutamide versus flutamide, each in combination with luteinizing hormone-releasing hormone analogue therapy, in patients with advanced prostate cancer. Casodex Combination Study Group. *Urology* **45**: 745–52.

53 Gemzar (Gemcitabine HCl) for Injection Package Insert. Indianapolis, IN: Eli Lilly and Company, 1998.

54 Cardenal, F., Lopez-Cabrerizo, M. P., Anton, A. *et al.* (1999). Randomized phase III study of gemcitabine-cisplatin versus etoposide-cisplatin in the treatment of locally advanced or metastatic non-small-cell lung cancer. *Journal of Clinical Oncology* **17**:12–18.

55 Sandler, A. B., Nemunaitis, J., Denham, C. *et al.* (2000). Phase III trial of gemcitabine plus cisplatin versus cisplatin alone in patients with locally advanced or metastatic non-small-cell lung cancer. *Journal of Clinical Oncology* **18**: 122–30.

56 Navelbine (vinorelbine tartrate) Injection Package Insert. Research Triangle Park, NC: GlaxoWellcome Inc., 2000.

57 LeChavalier, T., Brisgand, D., Douillard, J. Y. *et al.* (1994). Randomized study of vinorelbine and cisplatin versus vindesine and cisplatin versus vinorelbine alone in advanced non-small-cell lung cancer: results of a European multicenter trial including 612 patients. *Journal of Clinical Oncology* **12**:360–7.

58 Wozniak, A. J., Crowley, J. L., Balcerzak, S. P. *et al.* (1998). Randomized trial comparing cisplatin with cisplatin plus vinorelbine in the treatment of advanced non-small-cell lung cancer: a Southwest Oncology Group Study. *Journal of Clinical Oncology* **16**:2459–65.

59 Crawford, J., O'Rourke, M., Schiller, J. H. *et al.* (1996). Randomized trial of vinorelbine compared with flourouracil plus leucovorin in patients with stage IV non-small-cell lung cancer. *Journal of Clinical Oncology* **14**:2774–84.

60 Taxol® (paclitaxel) Injection Package Insert. Princeton, NJ: Bristol-Myers Squibb Co., 2000.

61 Bonomi, P., Kim, K. M., Fairclough, D. *et al.* (2000). Comparison of survival and quality of life in advanced non-small-cell lung cancer patients treated with two dose levels of paclitaxel combined with cisplatin versus etoposide with cisplatin: results of an Eastern Cooperative Oncology Group trial. *Journal of Clinical Oncology* **18**:623–31.

62 Giaccone, G., Splinter, T. A. W., Debruyne, C. *et al.* (1998). Randomized study of paclitaxel-cisplatin versus cisplatin-teniposide in patients with advanced non-small-cell lung cancer. *Journal of Clinical Oncology* **16**:2133–41.

63 Thyrogen (thyrotropin alfa) for Injection Package Insert. Cambridge, MA: Genzyme Corporation, 1999.

64 Haugen, B. R., Pacini, F., Reiners, C. *et al.* (1999). A comparison of recombinant human thyrotropin and thyroid hormone withdrawal for the detection of thyroid remnant or cancer. *Journal of Clinical Epidemiology and Metabolism* **81**:3877–85.

65 Ladenson, P. W., Braverman, L. E., Mazzaferri, E. L. *et al.* (1997). Comparison of administration of recombinant human thyrotropin with withdrawal of thyroid hormone for radioactive iodine scanning in patients with thyroid carcinoma. *New England Journal of Medicine* **337**: 888–95.

66 Aredia (pamidronate disodium) for Injection Package Insert. East Hanover, NJ: Novartis Pharmaceutical Co., 1999.

67 Theriault, R. L., Lipton, A., Hortobagyi, G. N. *et al.* (1999). Pamidronate reduces skeletal morbidity in women with advanced breast cancer and lytic bone lesions: a randomized, placebo-controlled trial. *Journal of Clinical Oncology* **17**:846–54.

68 Hortobagyi, G. N., Theriault, R. L., Lipton, A. *et al.* (1998). Long-term prevention of skeletal complications of metastatic breast cancer with pamidronate. *Journal of Clinical Oncology* **16**:2038–44.

69 King, M. T. (1996). The interpretation of scores from the EORTC Quality of Life Questionnaire QLQ-C30. *Quality of Life Research* **5**:555–67.

70 Tannock, I. F., Osoba, D., Stockler, M. R. *et al.* (1996). Chemotherapy with mitoxantrone plus prednisone or prednisone alone for symptomatic hormone-resistant prostate cancer: a Canadian randomized trial with palliative end points. *Journal of Clinical Oncology* **14**:1756–64.

71 Osoba, D., Tannock, I. F., Ernst, S. *et al.* (1999). Health-related quality of life in men with metastatic prostate cancer treated by prednisone alone or mitoxantrone and prednisone. *Journal of Clinical Oncology* **17**:1654–63.

72 Demetri, G. D., Kris, M., Wade, J. *et al.* (1998). Quality-of-life benefit in chemotherapy patients treated with epoetin alpha is independent of disease response or tumor type: results from a prospective community oncology study. *Journal of Clinical Oncology* **16**:3412–25.

73 Rowland, K. M., Loprinzi, C. L., Shaw, E. G. *et al.* (1996). Randomized double-blind placebo-controlled trial of cisplatin and etoposide plus megestrol acetate in extensive-stage small-cell lung cancer: a North Central Cancer Treatment Group study. *Journal of Clinical Oncology* **14**:135–41.

74 Simons, J. P. F., Aaronson, N. K., Vansteenkiste, J. F. *et al.* (1996). Effects of medroxyprogesterone acetate on appetite, weight, and quality of life in advanced-stage non-hormone-sensitive cancer: a placebo-controlled multicentre study. *Journal of Clinical Oncology* **14**:1077–84.

75 Bruera, E., Ernst, S., Hagen, N. *et al.* (1998). Effectiveness of megestrol acetate in patients with advanced cancer: a randomized, double-blind, crossover study. *Cancer Prevention and Control* **2**:74–8.

76 Medical Research Council Working Party (1993). A randomized trial of three or six courses of etoposide, cyclophosphamide, methotrexate and vincristine or six courses of etoposide and ifosfamide in small cell lung cancer. II: quality of life. *British Journal of Cancer* **68**:1157–66.

77 Osoba, D., Brada, M., Yung, W. K. *et al.* (2000). Health-related quality of life in patients treated with temozolomide versus procarbazine for recurrent glioblastoma multiforme. *Journal of Clinical Oncology* **18**:1481–91.

78 Osoba, D., Brada, M., Yung, W. K. *et al.* (2000). Health-related quality of life in patients with anaplastic astrocytoma during treatment with temozolomide. *European Journal of Cancer* **36**:1788–95.

79 Seymour, M. T., Slevin, M. L., Kerr, D. J. *et al.* (1996). Randomized trial assessing the addition of interferon alpa-2a to flourouracil and leucovorin in advanced colorectal cancer. *Journal of Clinical Oncology* **14**:2282–8.

80 Osoba, D., Northfelt, D. W., Budd, D. W. *et al.* (2001). Effect of treatment on health-related quality of life in AIDS-related Kaposi's sarcoma: a randomized trial of pegylated liposomal doxorubicin versus doxorubicin, bleomycin and vincristine. *Cancer Investigation* **19**:573–80.

81 Coates, A., Gebski, V., Bishop, J. F. *et al.* (1987). Improving the quality of life during chemotherapy for advanced breast cancer: a comparison of intermittent and continuous treatment strategies. *New England Journal of Medicine* **317**:1490–5.

82 Tannock, I. F., Boyd, N. F., DeBoer, G. *et al.* (1988). A randomized trial of two dose levels of cyclophosphamide, methotrexate, and fluorouracil chemotherapy for patients with metastatic breast cancer. *Journal of Clinical Oncology* **6**:1377–87.

83 Fairclough, D. L., Fetting, J. H., Cella, D. *et al.* (1999). Quality of life and quality adjusted survival for breast cancer patients receiving adjuvant therapy. *Quality of Life Research* **8**:723–31.

84 Levine, M., Guyatt, G., Gent, M. *et al.* (1988). Quality of life in stage II breast cancer: an instrument for clinical trials. *Journal of Clinical Oncology* **6**:1798–810.

85 Kaasa, S., Mastekaasea, A., Lund, E. (1989). Prognostic factors for patients with inoperable non-small cell lung cancer, limited disease. *Radiotherapy Oncology* **15**:235–42.

86 Ganz, P., Lee, J., Siau, J. (1991). Quality of life assessment: an independent prognostic variable for survival in lung cancer. *Cancer* **67**:3131–5.

87 Coates, A., Grebski, V., Signorini, D. *et al.* (1992). Prognostic value of quality-of-life scores during chemotherapy for advanced breast cancer. Australian New Zealand Breast Cancer Trials Group. *Journal of Clinical Oncology* **10**:1833–8.

88 Earlam, S., Glover, C., Fordy, C. *et al.* (1996). Relation between tumor size, quality of life, and survival in patients with colorectal liver metastases. *Journal of Clinical Oncology* **14**:171–5.

89 Coates, A., Porzsolt, F., Osoba, D. (1997). Quality of life in oncology practice: prognostic value of EORTC QLQ-C30 scores in patients with advanced malignancy. *European Journal of Cancer* **33**:1025–30.

90 Dancey, J., Zee, B., Osoba, D. *et al.* (1997). Quality of life scores: an independent prognostic variable in a general population of cancer patients receiving chemotherapy. *Quality of Life Research* **6**:151–8.

91 Coates, A., Hurny, C., Peterson, H. *et al.* (2000). Quality-of-life scores predict outcome in metastatic but not early breast cancer. *Journal of Clinical Oncology* **18**:3768–74.

92 Langendijk, J. A., Aaronson, N. K., ten Velde, G. P. *et al.* (2000). Pretreatment quality of life of inoperable non-small cell lung cancer patients referred for primary radiotherapy. *Acta Oncology* **39**:949–58.

93 Blazeby, J. M., Brookes, S. T., Alderson, D. (2001). The prognostic value of quality of life scores during treatment for oesophageal cancer. *Gut* **49**:227–30.

94 Bezjak, A., Ng, P., Skeel, R. *et al.* (2001). Oncologists' use of quality of life information: results from a survey of Eastern Cooperative Oncology Group physicians. *Quality of Life Research* **10**:1–13.

95 Chassany, O., Sagnier, P., Marquis, P. *et al.* for the European Regulatory Issues on Quality of Life Assessment Group (2002). Patient-reported outcomes: the example of health-related quality of life – a European guidance document for the improved integration of health-related quality of life assessment in the drug regulatory process. *Drug Information Journal* **36**:209–18.

96 Scientific Advisory Committee of the Medical Outcomes Trust (2002). Assessing health status and quality-of-life instruments: attributes and review criteria. *Quality of Life Research* **11**:193–205.

97 Hays, R. D., Anderson, R. T., Revicki, D. A. (1998). Assessing reliability and validity of measurements in clinical trials. In *Quality of Life Assessment in Clinical Trials: Methods and Practice*, eds. M. Staquet, R. Hays, P. Fayers, pp. 169–82. New York, NY: Oxford University Press.

98 Guyatt, G. H., Kirshner, B., Jaeschke, R. (1992). Measuring health status: what are the necessary measurement properties? *Journal of Clinical Epidemiology* **45**:1341–5.

99 Guyatt, G., Osoba, D., Wu, A., Wyrwich, K., Norman, G. and the Clinical Significance Consensus Meeting Group (2002). Methods to explain the clinical significance of health status measures. *Mayo Clinic Proceedings* **77**:371–83.

100 Cella, D., Bullinger, M., Scott, C. *et al.* and the Clinical Significance Consensus Meeting Group (2002). Group versus individual approaches to understanding the clinical significance of differences or changes in quality of life. *Mayo Clinic Proceedings* **77**:384–92.

101 Sprangers, M., Moinpour, C., Moynihan, T. *et al.* and the Clinical Significance Consensus Meeting Group (2002). Assessing meaningful change over time in quality of life: a users' guide for clinicians. *Mayo Clinic Proceedings* **77**:561–71.

102 Sloan, J., Aaronson, N., Cappelleri, J. *et al.* and the Clinical Significance Consensus Meeting Group (2002). Assessing the clinical significance of single items relative to summated scores. *Mayo Clinic Proceedings* **77**:479–87.

103 Hambleton, R., Robin, F., Xing, D. (2000). Item response models for the analysis of educational and psychological test data. In *Handbook of Applied Multivariate Statistics and Mathematical Modeling*, eds. H. Tinsley, S. Brown. San Diego: Academic Press.

104 Embretson, S., Reise, S. (2001). *Item Response Theory for Psychologists*. Mahwah, NJ: Lawrence Erlbaum Associates.

105 Reise, this volume, Chapter 21.

106 Hambleton, this volume, Chapter 22.

107 Wilson, this volume, Chapter 23.

108 Hays, R., Morales, L., Reise, S. (2000). Item response theory and health outcomes measurement in the 21st century. *Medical Care* **38**(Suppl. II):II-28–42.

109 Fairclough, D. (1998). Methods of analysis for longitudinal studies of health-related quality of life. In *Quality of Life Assessment in Clinical Trials: Methods and Practice*, ed. M. Staquet, R. Hays, P. Fayers, pp. 227–45. New York, NY: Oxford University Press.

110 Curran, D., Fayers, P., Molenberghs, G. *et al.* (1998). Analysis of incomplete quality of life data in clinical trials. In *Quality of Life Assessment in Clinical Trials: Methods and Practice*,

ed. M. Staquet, R. Hays, P. Fayers, pp. 249–80. New York, NY: Oxford University Press.

111 Fayers, P., Machin, D. (2000). *Quality of Life: Assessment, Analysis and Interpretation*. New York: John Wiley & Sons.

112 Fairclough, D. (2002). *Design and Analysis of Quality of Life Studies in Clinical Trials*. Boca Raton, FL: Chapman Hall/CRC Press.

113 Mesbah, M., Cole, B. (ed.) (2002). *Statistical Methods for Quality of Life Studies: Design, Measurement, and Analysis*. Amsterdam: Kluwer Academic Publishers.

114 Hedeker, D., Gibbons, R. (1997). Applications of random-effects pattern mixture models for missing data in longitudinal studies. *Psychological Methods* **2**:64–78.

115 Revicki, D., Gold, K., Buckman, D. *et al.* (2001). Imputing physical function scores missing owing to mortality: results of a simulation comparing multiple techniques. *Medical Care* **39**:61–71.

116 Luce, B., Shih, Y. C. T., Claxton, A. (2001). Special Section: Bayesian approaches to technology assessment and decision making. *International Journal of Technology Assessment in Health Care* **17**(1):1–125.

28

Reflections on COMWG findings and moving to the next phase

Carolyn C. Gotay, Ph.D.[1], Joseph Lipscomb, Ph.D.[2] and Claire Snyder, M.H.S.[2]

[1] Cancer Research Center of Hawai'i, Honolulu, HI
[2] National Cancer Institute, Bethesda, MD

Introduction

The perspectives of individuals who receive cancer-related interventions provide important information about diagnosis, treatment, and continuing care. These patient-centered data also have implications for the effectiveness of interventions and the quality of cancer care and can thus be an important resource for decision makers who deliver, pay for, regulate, and evaluate cancer care. At the same time, measuring such outcomes poses challenges different from those of biomedical outcomes. In particular, certain patient-centered outcomes (e.g., health-related quality of life) are subjective, by design, and not directly verifiable by physiological or other objective indicators, while others (e.g., economic outcomes) are not generally part of standard clinical information systems. Because of the growing importance of outcomes data, the National Cancer Institute (NCI) convened the Cancer Outcomes Measurement Working Group (COMWG) to assess the current state of the science and to provide recommendations for future research to improve the field. This book reports on findings from the COMWG effort.

The COMWG focused on three primary outcomes – health-related quality of life (HRQOL), patient needs and satisfaction, and economic burden – in the four cancers that affect the largest numbers of individuals in the USA: breast, colorectal, lung, and prostate. The group also considered outcomes measurement across the entire spectrum of cancer prevention, treatment, survivorship, and end-of-life care. COMWG members provided critical review and discussion of current literature in specified topics, as well as identification of areas where more work is needed.

Because the COMWG was not a Federal advisory committee or consensus panel, its findings reflect only the individual judgments and perspectives of its members, and the chapters vary accordingly in emphasis and conclusions. In this summary chapter, we will highlight several cross-cutting issues and themes that emerged across the individual chapters, as well as in other relevant literature. We should note from the outset that the majority of our discussion focuses on HRQOL, since this area has received much more attention in the research literature than the other outcomes. The following working definition was provided to promote effective communication and consistency across analyses: HRQOL includes patient-reported symptoms, functional status, and global well-being (see Chapter 1 by Lipscomb *et al.* in this volume for additional detail).[1] In addition to HRQOL, we include discussion of patient perceptions of care (including satisfaction), needs assessment, and economic burden.

While we draw on, and cite, work of the COMWG authors, this chapter does not necessarily represent the views of those individuals or the group as a whole. Our aim is to provide a selective overview of what we regard as some of the most important issues in cancer outcomes measurement at the present time.

In particular, we discuss the research on the quality of the tools currently available to measure HRQOL, the relationship among different cancer outcomes, new directions in cancer outcomes measurement, and how the study purpose affects choice of assessment tools. We conclude by describing research priorities for moving the field forward.

What is the quality of current tools used to measure cancer-related outcomes?

For the outcome measures that are the primary focus of this book – HRQOL, perceptions of and satisfaction with care, and economic impact – we wanted a broad, internally consistent framework for evaluating instrument quality and value to decision makers. This would then allow us to use clearly articulated principles to evaluate the quality of existing instruments, identify the need for improvements, and address conceptual and interpretative issues. To accomplish this goal, we adopted the well-known typology of instrument attributes and review criteria recommended by the non-profit Medical Outcomes Trust (MOT)[2] (see Chapter 1 by Lipscomb *et al.* in this volume).[1] The performance of any given outcome measure could then be assessed by the degree to which its instrumentation "measures up" to the criteria defined for each attribute: i.e., conceptual and measurement model, reliability, validity, responsiveness, interpretability, respondent and administrative burden, alternative forms (i.e., modes of administration), and cultural and language adaptations (including instrument translation). In fact, the MOT paradigm proved useful for establishing a common terminology and evaluation framework for the COMWG chapter tables comparing HRQOL instrument performance within the four major cancer sites (breast,[3] colorectal,[4] lung,[5] and prostate[6]); in end-of-life care[7] and caregiver impact[8] applications; and of cross-cutting generic measures.[9] The chapters on patient perspectives on care, needs assessment, and survivorship (Darby,[10] Gustafson,[11] Zebrack and Cella[12]) also used a similar framework.

Positive accomplishments of cancer outcome measures to date

By applying this framework, we can draw a number of conclusions about the research contributions of cancer outcome measures to date:

(1) In contrast to perceptions by some skeptics, assessing HRQOL in a research context is feasible. Patients do not resent being asked about personal aspects of their lives, nor do they object to using numerical, somewhat abstract scales to indicate their responses. HRQOL assessment can be incorporated in clinical protocols without posing undue burdens to either patients or clinicians. HRQOL assessment can be accomplished in the context of clinical trials, the application where the largest amount of research has focused to date; in observational studies of treatment outcomes;[13] and in descriptive studies of the impact of cancer in selected populations.[14]

(2) The quantity and quality of such research has increased markedly in the past 15 years (witness the dates of the citations throughout this book and see also the historical perspective provided by Spilker in Invited Paper A in this volume),[15] and some of the methodological improvements are only now being observed in the scientific literature. For example, Fairclough (Chapter 17, this volume)[16] discusses a number of techniques to avoid or minimize missing data, such as designating responsible staff to manage the enterprise, training data collectors and study respondents, and budgeting adequate resources for monitoring and patient follow-up as well as considering the adoption of multiple modes of survey administration, e.g., paper-and-pencil self-assessments, in-person interviews, telephone surveys, or electronic (including web-based) approaches. Some of these technologies are just becoming available in the clinical setting.

Sloan[17] argues that the statistical analysis of HRQOL and other patient-reported outcomes poses no greater problem, fundamentally, than encountered with more traditional biomedical measures. He concludes it is vital to have a clear statistical modeling plan specified in advance; to pursue complex statistical modeling approaches only after careful, basic analyses have been completed; to conduct sensitivity analyses to examine robustness of study findings as a routine matter; and to present findings clearly and transparently, emphasizing not only summary statistics but graphical displays and other approaches to reveal important variations within the sample.

(3) There are numerous HRQOL questionnaires currently available that have been developed with careful consideration of most of the MOT criteria.[2] Some of the most common approaches include (a) generic measures, designed to be used in any disease group or a general population, (b) general cancer measures, developed for use across cancer types, (c) cancer-specific measures, designed to be used in specific cancers, (d) general cancer core questionnaires supplemented with cancer-specific modules, which combine the general cancer and cancer-specific approaches, and (e) targeted, unidimensional measures, which focus in depth on specific aspects of HRQOL (including symptoms like pain, nausea, and fatigue) and can be used alone or in combination. Global measures and preference-based measures were also reported, although less frequently. Many of these questionnaires post impressive data supporting their reliability and validity, and recent attention has also focused particularly on responsiveness, interpretability, and cultural and language adaptations (see Chapter 20 by Aaronson).[18] In contrast, the areas of patient perceptions of care (including satisfaction) and needs assessment are less mature than HRQOL assessment; and Darby[10] and Gustafson[11] both report there have been few studies assessing these measures' validity, reliability, and responsiveness (with the interesting exception of Hambleton's analysis[19] here of the Patient Satisfaction with Medical Care Questionnaire (PSQ-III)).

(4) Outcomes measurement can be applied across the continuum of cancer prevention and care. Mandelblatt and Selby[20] discuss how individual assessments can be used in cancer prevention and screening, where the emphasis is on not harming healthy individuals (as opposed to treating patients with cancer). Zebrack and Cella[12] point out that outcomes assessment is equally applicable in cancer survivorship, since the impact of cancer and its treatment does not cease when treatment ends, and the long-term effects of cancer have important consequences on functioning and well-being. Finally, as Ferrell[7] notes, when patients are terminally ill, comfort and well-being should be the focus. The importance of understanding the psychological, social, and behavioral factors influencing HRQOL outcomes across the cancer continuum has recently been underscored by Holland.[21]

(5) The primary areas where outcomes assessments, and most often HRQOL measurement, have been used to date are clinical trials and observational studies of cancer treatment. The most frequent research questions have been determining the preferable intervention in randomized clinical trials and identifying short- and long-term effects of cancer therapy.

(6) The contributions and findings of the HRQOL outcomes data and generalizations that could be drawn for particular cancers reflect both the prevalence of research and the current state of diagnosis and cancer therapy. However, interesting and useful findings that demonstrate the sensitivity and responsiveness of the HRQOL measures used have emerged in all disease sites.

In breast cancer, many studies have been reported, partially due to the relatively high prevalence of breast cancer and the fact that it is not rapidly fatal in most cases. Based on the patterns they observed in the data, Ganz and Goodwin[3] are able to draw generalizations about HRQOL in breast cancer. For example, younger patients and those with more advanced disease report more distress; survivors generally have good HRQOL compared to control groups; HRQOL improves in the year post-diagnosis and worsens with recurrence; and psychological interventions confer significant benefits for breast cancer patients. These authors are also able to conclude that, surprisingly, HRQOL in adjuvant chemotherapy in breast cancer has been studied only infrequently, and that HRQOL data have not contributed to the interpretation of most of the biomedical breast cancer treatment studies reported to date.

The analyses for each of the other three cancer sites yielded somewhat different conclusions. There was considerably less literature available for review in lung and colorectal cancer, partly because both of these cancers are generally diagnosed at an advanced stage when there is less life expectancy and opportunity to measure HRQOL. In both of these sites, studies of both primary and adjuvant treatments were common. Earle and Weeks[5] note that, in lung cancer, health care professionals underestimate HRQOL compared to patient ratings. In prostate cancer, a disease where the current therapeutic modalities for early stage disease have long-term consequences on sexual and bladder function, measures of impotence, incontinence, and other symptoms were frequently reported. Litwin and Talcott[6] also remark that HRQOL data have shown that patient impairments in these areas are much more common than clinicians realized.

Challenges regarding cancer outcome measures

The preceding discussion has identified a number of real accomplishments in cancer outcomes measurement; current questionnaires have satisfied many of the MOT criteria[2] and made contributions to understanding the effects of cancer on the individual and groups of individuals (the reader is referred to other chapters in the book for detailed discussion). However, there are several significant areas where more instrument development is warranted.

(1) Perhaps the most pressing need is in the area of conceptual and measurement models. As Ferrans[22] describes in detail, HRQOL has yet to be consistently defined and, as such, different and sometimes competing definitions may be used. Darby[10] points out that the same is true for patient satisfaction. Erickson[9] observes that even when two measures purport to assess the same domains, they may use very different items to measure what is theoretically the same concept. As HRQOL questionnaires vary widely in their domains and items, much confusion remains as to what HRQOL really is.

However, there seem to be a few points of agreement on defining and conceptualizing HRQOL, and the same points generally hold for patient perceptions of care and the assessment of patient needs. It is widely (though not universally) agreed that HRQOL (as defined here) is an unobservable, or "latent," construct that can acquire operational meaning only through an appropriately specified and estimated *psychometric* measurement model. Second, a key aspect of HRQOL, patient reports and evaluations on care experiences, and patient needs assessments is that they reflect the patient's perspective. Third, there is general agreement that HRQOL, patient perceptions of care, and patient needs should be regarded as multidimensional constructs. HRQOL nearly always includes physical and mental/emotional health, with less consensus about additional domains such as social functioning, spiritual well-being, symptoms, role functioning, and domains that may be particularly relevant in certain contexts (e.g., sexual functioning in prostate cancer, fertility concerns in survivorship). Measures of patient satisfaction or care experiences frequently include domains such as provider communication and access. The domains of patient needs tend to be much less clearly specified, and assessment of individual needs (as opposed to domains) is the more common measurement strategy.

While these points of agreement are useful for capturing important areas and generating topics for questionnaires, they are less helpful in understanding *what* about these domains needs to be measured. Ferrans[22] distinguishes between different kinds of HRQOL questions that patients may be asked: objective conditions (e.g., did you go for a long walk today?), perceived status (e.g., could you go for a long walk today?), and evaluation (e.g., how satisfied are you with your physical functioning today?). Litwin and Talcott[6] and Darby[10] make similar distinctions regarding symptoms and patient care experiences, respectively. It is not obvious that these are the same questions, and that they would yield the same answers. In fact, it is likely that they would not. In particular, the evaluation approach may be more subject to influence by factors such as patient expectations, previous experience, and predispositions, which may be good or bad depending on the intent of the analysis. The interrelationships among these different ways of asking the HRQOL question have not been examined in depth and deserve consideration.

With respect to measurement models, the need for additional attention is at least as pressing. For HRQOL (and also patient perceptions of care and needs assessment), conceptual models are required that include a theory that specifies which dimensions are to be included in the HRQOL measurement model, how the various domains relate to one another, their relative importance, and a causal pathway that clearly distinguishes causal and indicator variables (in the terminology of Fayers and Machin)[23] and specifies the relationships between them.

Structural equation modeling (SEM) may offer a useful platform for exploring a number of these conceptual model / measurement model issues. SEM facilitates building causal models that depict relationships among sets of survey items, on the one hand, and the scale and subscales posited to represent a complex construct such as "health-related quality of life."[2,23] While each subscale must adhere to an assumption of unidimensionality, one can allow for interactive relationships among subscales and also between subscales and other patient-reported (e.g., symptoms) and biomedical (e.g., toxicity) outcomes, as well as with exogenous factors like respondent age, race, sex, and education. To date, there have been comparatively few applications of SEM to HRQOL, as Fayers and Machin[23] note, and we await further evidence about whether this approach's potential to clarify causal relationships can be realized in practice.

A note about economic outcomes: in contrast to HRQOL and patient needs, there are usually no latent, or implicitly defined, constructs used in gauging the economic impact of cancer. Rather, one is trying to determine the economic opportunity cost of cancer-induced resource use (e.g., a hospital stay) from the perspective of the relevant decision maker. To be sure, opportunity cost might be difficult to observe when there are no market prices to indicate

cost incurred or saved; but then the task reverts to finding surrogate measures ("shadow prices") of resource use, e.g., the foregone market earnings of the family caregiver.[25] It might be pointed out that the relationship between economic analyses and patient-perceived economic problems (measured on a number of HRQOL questionnaires) has yet to be explored.

(2) A number of COMWG chapters called for enhancing the content-related validity of the instrument(s) for measuring the outcome of interest – that is, improving the extent to which the instrument (with its particular item content) is appropriate for the intended application. For example, Moinpour and Provenzale[4] conclude that social functioning is inadequately assessed in HRQOL measures applied to colorectal cancer patients undergoing treatment. Zebrack and Cella[12] find that current multidimensional HRQOL measures may not capture elements important to cancer survivors, such as fear of recurrence or chronic physical compromise. Williams,[26] a prostate cancer survivor, believes that current HRQOL instruments fail to capture the depth of suffering faced by patients and their families.

In response, we propose that, on a selected basis, HRQOL scales undergo a multi-step examination, using both qualitative and quantitative analysis, to identify omitted or misspecified items and pave the way for creation of items (or whole scales) with greater content validity. For any given category of instruments (e.g., for long-term survivorship), such an examination might entail: item response theory (IRT) analyses to check for gaps in the measurement continuum (if relevant survey data already exist); focus groups to evaluate item content and presentation; and creation of new items, or scales, that would then be subject to cognitive testing and IRT analysis of item performance. Such an interactive approach to content assessment and improvement is recommended by Willis et al.[27]

There are a variety of ways newly created or modified items might be put into practice: as new entries on an existing scale, as items comprising an entirely new and different scale, as items comprising a module attached to an existing general cancer instrument (as both Erickson[9] and Barry and Dancey[28] suggest), or as elements in an item bank.

(3) While many available instruments have demonstrated construct validity, construct validation is a continuing process, with ongoing gathering and evaluation of evidence that an instrument measures the construct (e.g., HRQOL) it is intended to measure. The important task for the research agenda is identifying the most salient threats to construct validity in the measurement of patient-reported outcomes. Particular attention should perhaps be accorded to IRT-based models, which have a shorter history of application to behavioral and evaluative constructs compared with classical test theory (CTT) models, to test whether these IRT models add value and facilitate use and interpretation of HRQOL assessment.[24]

(4) The reliability of many HRQOL questionnaires has been examined and found acceptable. However, one potential threat to reliability (and hence, to the validity of conclusions that can be drawn) that has received considerable attention is "response shift." As analyzed by Schwartz and Sprangers,[29,30] this phenomenon is defined by the degree to which the very meaning of the patient's self-evaluation of a construct like HRQOL changes over time as a result of a change in (1) internal standards of measurement of the construct (literally, an intra-personal scale recalibration), (2) the values placed on the domains comprising the construct, or (3) the patient's own definition (or concept) of the construct itself. As Ferrans[22] emphasizes, a deeper understanding of whether response shift influences HRQOL assessments in oncology could open the way to conceptual models that better account for the complex relationship between changes in "objective" biomedical outcomes and comparatively malleable measures of HRQOL. The importance of this issue in interpreting the meaning of HRQOL change for those with chronic disease has been underscored in empirical analyses, e.g., see Patrick et al.[31]

(5) Finally, interpretation of HRQOL data is critical to the appropriate use of such information. Osoba[32] discusses this issue in detail, and Sloan[17] provides additional suggestions for analysis. A recent

series of meetings sponsored by the Mayo Clinic has also yielded insights into the issue of clinical interpretability.[33] Considerable progress has been made in terms of knowing how big a difference in scores on HRQOL questionnaires is seen as meaningful by patients, and the extent to which such scores are associated with differences that make sense to clinicians. Osoba's evidence-based conclusion that a "small perceptible meaningful" change in an HRQOL score appears to be about 7% of the full scale breadth (perhaps bracketed by 5% and 10%) is a genuinely surprising if not felicitous finding – yet one bearing ongoing investigation by anchor-based approaches, as he rightly emphasizes.[32] Among such anchors, we would suggest, should be those having what might be called "decision significance": the relationship between observed changes in HRQOL scores and choices, real or hypothetical, made by patients or other decision makers.[34] Specifically, how large must the change in HRQOL be before a patient not only perceives a change, but a change "significant enough" to influence selection of therapy, evaluation of the therapy chosen, or other behavioral-based anchors? This question is critical in determining whether HRQOL provides added value. Future research is warranted to answer this question.

What is the relationship among different cancer outcomes?

The COMWG efforts focused on three "non-traditional" outcomes (HRQOL, needs and patient perceptions, and economic burden). These outcomes, of course, need to be interpreted in the context of other outcomes important for cancer patient well-being, such as response, toxicity, survival, and disease-free survival. The relationships among the three COMWG outcomes were discussed by some writers. Gustafson[11] suggests that patient needs, and how well they are met, may be causal variables that affect HRQOL. In a recent conference presentation, Wasson noted that assessment of patient needs and problems provides a link between HRQOL research and clinical practice, as satisfaction assessment provides information about concrete areas of care that can be improved and lead to improvements in HRQOL.[35] The earlier discussion about the need for models of HRQOL and satisfaction as individual variables certainly applies to any efforts to integrate findings from these three kinds of outcomes.

However, to date, a more frequent research question has been whether HRQOL data provide additional information beyond that which is learned from standard biomedical variables. One of the most pressing questions asked by all parties, including the funders of HRQOL research is, "Do such data actually add anything beyond standard outcomes? Do they contribute to the interpretation of clinical trials of cancer treatment?" The authors of chapters in this book were asked to examine these questions, which were referred to as the "value added" issue, in their reviews. Specifically, the authors were asked to consider if HRQOL data reveal information beyond that available from traditional biomedical outcomes in ways that (1) influence the overall interpretation of a study and therefore (2) may appropriately inform decision making.

While many of the chapters include discussion of this issue, the authors of the disease-specific papers (those on breast,[3] colorectal,[4] lung,[5] and prostate[6] cancers) were asked to examine the patterns of outcomes in studies that included both biomedical and HRQOL or other patient-reported outcomes. The tables in the respective chapters provide detailed information about the specific measures that were used in the studies they examined. While there were some exceptions, an overriding conclusion across all chapters was that there was no consistent pattern of covariation between HRQOL and biomedical outcomes; in particular, if survival improved, HRQOL did not also consistently improve. In fact, findings reflected almost all logical possibilities: e.g., better survival and better HRQOL, better survival but no difference in HRQOL, no difference in survival and differences in HRQOL, better survival and worse HRQOL, and better survival and differences on some HRQOL measures and not others. This is consistent with other reviews that have examined this issue.[36,37]

What are the implications of concordance: that is, when biomedical outcomes and HRQOL are consistent with prior hypotheses about their covariation? There are at least two potential interpretations: (a) that HRQOL is redundant and does not add any new information, or (b) in the case of, for example, improved survival and improved HRQOL, that data may indicate that the advantages of the therapy in terms of increased survival are important enough to be reflected in patients feeling better and having higher functioning. With respect to (a), given the significance of increasing survival for both clinicians and patients,[38,39] HRQOL data may have a limited impact on study interpretation when survival differences are found. In the words of some of the COMWG members, "Survival trumps all." On the other hand, possibility (b) also may be persuasive, particularly when a therapy results in increased survival times of only a few months (not uncommon in trials of advanced disease). Such information could be useful to clinicians to support the value of the therapy from the patient's perspective.

What about the situation when biomedical outcomes and HRQOL data are inconsistent, and thus contrary to expectations? This was a more common finding in these reviews. In particular, there were a number of studies when a difference in biomedical outcomes was found, but there was no difference in HRQOL. There are, again, several possible interpretations of such findings (see discussions by Barry & Dancey[28] and Moinpour & Provenzale[4]): (a) the HRQOL measurement tool was not sensitive enough to detect real differences in patient well-being, (b) the HRQOL measurement tool did not focus on the right aspects of HRQOL, (c) the timing of the HRQOL assessment was not appropriate to when patients perceived such effects, (d) the trial had methodological flaws that affected the HRQOL data, such as small sample size or large amounts of missing data, or (e) the (statistically significant) difference in biomedical outcomes did not in fact correspond to a clinical benefit (or harm) that was both perceptible and important to the patient – consistent with the observation that there was no clinically meaningful change in HRQOL. This final possibility (in contrast to the others) points to a plausible scenario in which HRQOL data provide unique information that the apparent clinical impact of therapy does not translate into patient-perceived benefits.

There are many other potential scenarios as well, such as significant changes in biomedical outcomes and HRQOL, but in opposite directions, and HRQOL findings that are broadly divergent (e.g., improvement on one dimension and deterioration on another). These scenarios convey the complexity of trying to interpret outcomes that do not necessarily covary as predicted. Given the multiple possible explanations for any set of findings, in our opinion, it is premature to conclude that HRQOL data do or do not contribute to treatment decision making based on clinical trials. Careful attention needs to be given to selection of HRQOL measures for a clinical trial and to understanding the inter-relationships between and among the various outcome measures. It may be advisable to follow up clinical trials with in-depth examination of such questions in selected patients, perhaps using methods such as cognitive interviewing, as described by Willis and colleagues.[27] For example, a patient who had experienced disease remission but who reported low HRQOL could be asked questions such as, "What was it like participating in this clinical trial? What are the reasons that you answered this question the way you did? How did the treatment affect your daily life? What does HRQOL mean to you?"

What are new directions in cancer outcomes measurement and analysis?

One of the purposes of the COMWG was to explore new methodological and analytic approaches that could move the field forward. One frequent observation of HRQOL questionnaires is that there are a lot of them, yet there are few head-to-head comparisons. In addition, there is the question of how to measure "cancer-related HRQOL" in patient groups as diverse as, for example, newly diagnosed, symptomatic lung cancer patients, and long-term survivors of breast cancer, who may have quite different levels of concerns. The COMWG membership included three psychometricians (Reise,[24] Hambleton,[19] and Wilson[40]) who are experts in item response theory (IRT) modeling, an analytic technique that offers the potential to address concerns like those listed above. IRT is long-established in educational testing research, but it is only recently being applied in the HRQOL area. The technique has considerable promise in cancer outcomes measurement, as we discuss below.

An important, recurring question is whether classical test theory (CTT) or item response theory (IRT) provides the better basis for assessing and evaluating HRQOL and other patient-reported outcomes that involve latent-variable constructs. A CTT approach to estimating an individual's HRQOL level is based on the sum (possibly weighted) of survey item responses, while an IRT approach makes use of the *pattern* of item responses since each item is assumed to convey specific, differentiated information about the individual's HRQOL level.

In this regard, item response theory offers several potential advantages. IRT permits not only item responses to inform the scale score assigned to a person, but also person responses to inform the estimation of a scale score for each item; thus, fundamentally more information is brought to the table than with CTT. The latter paradigm is simply not geared to garner and deploy empirical information about the performance of items in a way that allows one prospectively to tailor the choice of items to persons. Nor does CTT facilitate analysis of the functional relationship between items on the same (unidimensional) scale or between different items on different scales. The IRT measurement framework, on the other hand, allows one to model the item-person relationship, in such a way that (1) item parameters are independent of the particular respondent sample, while (2) person parameters – central to inferring the individual's position, or score, on the latent construct – are independent of the particular item set selected.

This leads proponents to claim that IRT can:[19,24]

• Generate measurement models that are more reliable because, with joint knowledge of person fit *and* item fit, it becomes possible to ensure that scales have an adequate number of good performing items across the entire construct continuum (including, by implication, scale regions where the population of interest might be concentrated). In CTT, there is one overall estimated level of reliability (typically, Cronbach's alpha), which can be increased merely by adding additional survey items, irrespective of whether they contribute substantially to increasing measurement precision in under-populated regions of the scale, e.g., towards the upper and lower extremes. In IRT, each item has an associated reliability (precision, or information conveyed) estimate, so it is possible to select items in concert to ensure adequate precision across the continuum.

- Generate measurement models that are potentially more valid – or, more precisely, whose construct and criterion validity can be assayed with greater confidence – because again one can ensure that scales are appropriately populated with items that perform well so that the underlying construct is well delineated and illuminated. But of course this does not then guarantee that the resulting HRQOL scale will demonstrate construct or criterion validity. What is arguably enhanced is the statistical confidence one has in those validity calculations, whatever the verdict.

- Facilitate the cross-walking of instrument scores between two instruments measuring the same construct by providing both the theory and analytical machinery to equate scores for selected items from the instruments, thereby creating the linkage needed for mapping one total score to another.

- Provide the appropriate theoretical and empirical framework for item banking and computer-adaptive testing (CAT). As Hambleton[19] and Reise[24] point out, item banking with CAT can significantly reduce respondent burden compared with traditional fixed-item survey instruments – the only format possible under CTT. With an item banking-CAT approach, items are selected sequentially and strategically, with each choice driven by the respondent's pattern of answers to that point in the interview. This reduces the number of items required to achieve any targeted level of measurement precision. By implication, the sometime difficult issue of choosing among competing fixed-item instruments in a given application (e.g., measuring HRQOL in lung cancer initial therapy) is resolved, in principle, if one is confident the item content of the bank adequately encompasses the construct (e.g., the regions of the HRQOL continuum most relevant to those lung cancer patients).

- Permit a statistically rigorous examination of whether a given instrument performs the same or differently (i.e., measurement equivalence) across cultures, geographic borders, or population subgroups through analysis of "differential item functioning" (DIF), as Aaronson also emphasizes.[18]

These and related points (e.g., the intellectual property issues that may arise with item banking) are explored by McHorney and Cook.[41]

Constructs like HRQOL that are generally thought to comprise several sub-constructs, or dimensions, can pose particular challenges whether the measurement model is IRT or CTT. Suppose the objective is to obtain separate scores for each of the posited dimensions (that is, a summary score for the HRQOL construct is not needed). Both CTT and the most common IRT models assume that each subscale is unidimensional. If multiple dimensions are being measured separately, the total number of survey items needed to capture all sub-domains (assuming a traditional pencil-and-paper administration) may be large enough to create concerns about respondent burden or excessive administrative costs. In response, Wilson[40] proposes an IRT-based (in fact, Rasch model-based) multidimensional item response model that economizes on the number of items for each subscale, with no loss in estimation precision, by extracting information strategically from responses to items on the instrument's other correlated subscales. Likewise, for any given number of items on the instrument as a whole, such a model leads to more precise estimation for each subscale.

The advantages of IRT notwithstanding, Hambleton[19] cautions that it, ". . . is not a magic wand to wave over poorly defined constructs and items to produce valid and reliable instrumentation." The full benefits are realized only when the underlying assumptions hold. (This is clearly true also for CTT, but because these models arguably ask less of the data, they impose less demanding assumptions.) Moreover, IRT does not readily address all potential issues related to a latent construct of interest, e.g., how to generate a completely defensible summary score for a multidimensional construct like HRQOL. IRT is conceptually challenging and relatively difficult to communicate, which can pose barriers to its adoption and appropriate use in multidisciplinary team research. Similarly, estimating these models requires sophisticated, relatively complex software (though more user-friendly programming packages are becoming increasingly available) and also comparatively large sample sizes (e.g., several hundred) to estimate model parameters reliably.[19,24,40]

All the while, we await hard evidence from the field that IRT's impressive potential for outcomes research can be fulfilled. As Reise[24] observes, additional analyses are required to determine whether IRT models (including the one-parameter Rasch variant and the multiparameter specifications) when applied to patient-reported outcomes lead to substantially different, and more valid, findings than CTT approaches. Given the technical demands of IRT, Reise predicts that outcomes researchers will not migrate away from traditional measurement approaches without compelling evidence that the benefits exceed the costs. At present, many psychometricians would recommend that both CTT and IRT be applied, when possible, in order to provide complementary perspectives on the estimation of scale scores for a difficult construct like HRQOL. However, there is virtual consensus that IRT provides the most (if not only) sound theoretical basis for item banking, computer-adaptive testing, cross-walking scale scores via item linking, and investigating differential item functioning.

There is another area where new approaches to IRT may be particularly useful. While HRQOL is generally regarded as multidimensional, on many occasions a single, summary score is needed. The most prominent case in point arises in cost-effectiveness analyses (CEA), where the CEA calculus demands a single-dimensional effectiveness measure, such as life-years saved or (for cost-utility analysis) quality-adjusted life years. A summary measure of HRQOL may prove useful in other contexts as well, whether for population surveillance or providing an overall picture of patient outcome in a trial. Standard CTT and IRT approaches, both geared to producing unidimensional scales, do not readily offer a conceptually clean resolution to this issue, in our view. True, it is possible to put all items from all subscales onto one grand summary scale labeled "HRQOL" and derive an aggregate score. Indeed, by establishing a sufficiently liberal item-fit inclusion criterion, one can effectively create "support" for the critically important assumption of unidimensionality. But what is one then to make of the prior assumption, ideally supported by the appropriate conceptual model, that HRQOL is multidimensional? Is it really possible to have it both ways, especially when the component scale and summary scale analyses are carried out with the very same pool of items?

The "multidimensional" IRT models introduced by Wilson[40] are designed to enhance insight and informational efficiency in the estimation of individual scale scores, not to derive a summary score across scales. But as Feeny[42] implies, this is precisely the role that patient utility weights play in the derivation of preference-based summary measures of HRQOL, when the latter is regarded as multidimensional. Future research should investigate alternative approaches to deriving summary scores for multidimensional HRQOL, including the possibility of using preferences or other external criteria to weight the separate unidimensional domain scores emerging from either IRT- or CTT-based analyses.

An important new direction in the analysis of cancer outcome measures is proposed by O'Brien,[43] who urges that greater consideration be given to Bayesian statistical modeling. He argues that Bayes provides a unifying framework (consistent with modern statistical decision theory) for conducting cost-effectiveness and cost-utility analyses in a way that facilitates: (1) assessing the impact of uncertainty on the choice of cancer interventions, (2) conducting meta analyses to integrate findings from multiple trials and also observational studies, and (3) calculating the expected payoff from acquiring additional information to inform intervention choice – thus providing a rational basis for setting priorities among competing new studies. O'Brien also discusses recent methodological advances for transforming any cost-utility analysis-based assessment of interventions into a corresponding determination of which of these interventions (if any) would pass a cost-benefit analysis test for adoption. The linchpin requirement here is a controversial one, as he notes: the decision maker must explicitly consider what monetary value to attach to gaining (or losing) a quality-adjusted life year (QALY).

Does the purpose of a study affect the choice of assessment tools, and is there a standard core assessment module to be used in all studies?

One of the most frequent comments heard at COMWG meetings and one that is found in many chapters of this book as well, is that the purpose of a study influences the choice of questionnaires, and that no single questionnaire is best for all purposes. In other words, the objective of a study should determine the best instrument to measure HRQOL and other patient variables, and we need outcome measures that are appropriately sensitive (for cross-sectional group comparisons) or responsive (for longitudinal comparisons). HRQOL measures have been used, or considered for use, across various groups, going from individuals to the entire population and for a variety of purposes. These include patient-physician communication,[44] assessing the outcomes of clinical trials and modifying them in response to HRQOL concerns,[45,46] monitoring the HRQOL of specified population groups,[47] and policy decision making, including deliberations by the US Food and Drug Administration concerning the approval and marketing of pharmaceutical

agents.[48–50] It seems clear that different audiences and different study purposes are likely to require different approaches to outcomes assessment.

At the same time, it seems equally clear that having a common measure across various applications would greatly facilitate comparability across studies and would enable HRQOL and other patient outcomes to be used more readily in policy decisions, which are rarely as specific as a given clinical trial. This is a complex issue, and it is only as HRQOL measures are used more frequently in the various arenas of application that the appropriate rules of thumb will become apparent.

For the moment, the following observations seem warranted:

• In studies, or applications, that seek to use HRQOL data at the bedside – whether for the benefit of patients or their family members – the ability of the instrument to provide clear and interpretable data is paramount. While issues of patient burden are important, these may be less significant than the instrument's capacity to provide clinically meaningful and understandable data, which may be possible by using multiple instruments. As discussed earlier in this chapter, there have been positive developments with respect to identifying minimally important differences but these are still somewhat embryonic with respect to translating these differences into appropriate interventions.

• When the study objective is to compare interventions in clinical trials or observational studies, very specific and highly targeted measures may be most likely to detect differences across groups. However, investigators need to ask themselves candidly if finding small, targeted differences – even when they are statistically significant – is always sufficient to gauge the merit of an intervention. For example, a labor-intensive psychological intervention might indeed lead to a gain of a few points on a depression index; but this finding should immediately trigger the question: Is this difference large enough to be important for decision making? Clearly, patient values and perceptions of costs and benefits are critical to this query.

- Research questions that investigate patient or provider decision making may best be addressed through preference-based measures. Feeny[42] discusses how preference-based measures, which account for patients' values of outcomes, are commonly used in other disease areas and applications but were not frequently found in the cancer literature. This may result from the nature of the literature reviewed, primarily clinical trials and observational studies comparing treatment interventions. However, measures of patient utility are required for other applications, such as decision-analytic modeling, cost-utility analysis, and population health surveys. These measures allow calculation of quality-adjusted life years, capturing the trade-off between quantity and quality of life so important in cancer. Current efforts to develop cancer-specific utility measures may increase their use in cancer.[42]
- When the study objective is to compare HRQOL of a study population to the population at large (as, for example, in a study of cancer prevention or cancer survivors), a generic HRQOL measure with normative data available on healthy populations seems appropriate.
- Finally, when the objective is to use data for policy purposes (such as monitoring the cancer burden at the national level to inform budgetary discussions), having a metric that is comparable with those used in other diseases and perhaps in the population more generally may be optimal.

The authors of this chapter have given considerable thought to the question of whether there is a set of core measures that should be used across applications. In fact, one of the NCI's initial expectations of the COMWG effort was that the group would evaluate the merit of identifying a core set of outcome measures that could be used across cancer outcomes research. Such core instruments would have a number of advantages: they would enable pooling data across studies and meta-analysis, allowing examination of effects in subgroups of individuals across studies; they would provide a common metric that

would guide assessment and interpretation across the spectrum of applications, from prevention to end of life; and they would focus efforts of outcomes researchers in the same direction, to increase communication and attention to common methodological and analytic issues.

While such aims have merit, there was not a consensus among COMWG members that establishing core outcome measures was desirable. Our distillation of the working group's commentary suggests that those reluctant to support the pursuit of core measures would likely embrace one or more of the following observations: (1) Each study needs to include measures that are appropriate to its distinct hypotheses and patient population. (2) The field of patient reported outcomes research is sufficiently new that determining core measures and expecting most researchers to use them is premature. (3) While a number of current measures, both generic (e.g. SF-36) and cancer-specific (e.g., QLQ-C30, FACT) meet many of the criteria that a "gold standard" would be expected to demonstrate, none of these measures stands out above the rest. (4) There are currently analytic methods being developed, such as IRT, that could make this issue moot, since in the future, IRT-based item banks may facilitate computer-adaptive assessments that would draw from the constellation of available items that mix and sequence items most appropriate for each respondent. Under this scenario, there is no need for a "core" (traditional, fixed-item) instrument – though there would obviously need to be some judgment about the items appropriate for the bank.

As discussed elsewhere in the book and indicated above, the application of IRT to outcomes such as HRQOL has considerable appeal and promise. However, such approaches rely on defining one or more dimensions on which relevant items can be classified and ranked. The identification of these dimensions requires a notion of "core constructs" or domains, as they are often referred to in the HRQOL literature. As discussed previously, such core constructs need to be identified and defined and receive consensus endorsement. However, it may be that researchers need to return to some of the central conceptual issues previously discussed before definitive progress in this area can be made.

We believe there are currently two things that might be done to strike a useful, acceptable balance or else to develop instrumentation that promotes both sensitivity to detect differences in focused studies as well as to promote comparability across different studies: (1) Further development of modular instruments, with core items that would be invariant across applications (ideally across the full arena of applications, as defined here) and supplementary items that would be specific to cancer disease site, phase of care, or other distinguishing features.[9] (2) Development of item banks and computer-adaptive testing, which would optimize the amount of useful information obtainable at acceptable levels of respondent burden. This may be especially important, given that the survey must yield sufficient data to locate the respondent on both the (possibly multidimensional) core HRQOL construct and also on the module(s) selected for inclusion.

The next phase

For cancer outcomes research to contribute optimally to the goal of reducing the death and suffering due to cancer, at least three instrumental objectives must be successfully pursued. Specifically, we need:[51] outcome measures that are valid, reliable, and feasible (and, indeed, that satisfactorily meet the MOT criteria); sound evidence about the impact of interventions on such outcome measures; and both the capacity and commitment to translate this evidence (about efficacy, effectiveness, and cost-effectiveness) into findings useful to the full spectrum of decision makers. From this vantage point, we can say that outcomes assessment in cancer is concerned with identifying, developing, and applying scientifically sound and appropriate outcome measures in support of studies to identify effective interventions and other information that can usefully inform choices about cancer care.

Consistent with this perspective, the chapters comprising this volume, taken together, provide an appraisal of the state of the science in cancer outcomes measurement of unprecedented depth and comprehensiveness. By design, members of NCI's Cancer Outcomes Measurement Working Group and additional invited authors were charged with examining the extant published literature. The resulting wealth of findings and recommendations has been assayed selectively in this chapter, reported in detail throughout the book, and provide the ingredients for a robust research agenda. That said, it became ever clearer as the COMWG's work progressed that virtually all of the literature on cancer outcomes measures to date focuses either on empirical research applications (e.g., in clinical trials) or methodological matters. By contrast, surprisingly little has been published, and even anecdotal information is hard to uncover, about the day-to-day use of outcome measures for actual decision making.

The stage is set now to embark upon the "next phase" of activities to improve the scientific quality and usefulness of cancer outcome measures, not only in the USA but internationally. This work should build naturally on findings from the COMWG and also other significant outcomes research assessment efforts, public and private, as noted in earlier chapters. While not attempting to chart, at this juncture, the step-by-step journey through that next phase, we can identify three broad areas requiring continuing attention in any comprehensive agenda to enhance cancer outcomes assessment:

- *Sustaining scientific advancement* to accelerate progress towards improving both the scientific soundness of cancer outcomes measures and their application to evaluate the effectiveness of cancer care. Indeed, virtually every chapter of this volume has made specific recommendations to strengthen the quality and research relevance of the outcome measures of particular interest here – HRQOL, patient perceptions and evaluations of care, and economic burden. Following the COMWG's final meeting, in December 2002, NCI polled each member about the required next steps. A number of members recommended conducting a follow-up state-of-the-science meeting to take stock of

COMWG findings; lay the groundwork for formal consensus development, if natural pockets of agreement were evident; and formulate a research agenda for the outcomes measurement field. That agenda would clearly include a systematic examination of HRQOL and other patient-reported outcomes in cancer disease sites beyond the four examined here. Perhaps the most ambitious recommendation submitted called for the creation of Cancer Outcomes Research Teams (CORTs) to conduct multi- and interdisciplinary studies on a range of topics, while also training the next generation of cancer outcomes researchers.

All the while, outcomes measurement continues to be a major research component within NCI's Quality of Cancer Care Initiative.[52] Most recently, the National Institutes of Health (within which NCI resides) announced a $20 million, 5-year extramural research project to support innovative applications of item response theory, including item banks and computer adaptive testing for chronic diseases like cancer.[53] These are encouraging developments, to be sure. However, both the vision to guide and the resources to support research in cancer outcomes assessment can and should come from many quarters – not only US public agencies but their international counterparts, as well as from private cancer organizations and professional associations both in the USA and abroad.

- *Improving the empirical base* for cancer outcomes research by enhancing the accuracy, timeliness, and "linkability" of the major data sources: cancer registries; medical records; administrative files including claims information; and surveys of patients, at-risk individuals, and providers of care.[54] Advances in information technology are expected to accelerate the adoption of electronic health systems, including but extending beyond the medical record proper. While patient protection issues must continue to be addressed, there has never been a more opportune time to encourage the creation, testing, and expansion of linked data systems to support cancer outcomes monitoring, evaluation, and improvement.

- *Investigating the actual, and potential, role of outcome measures in cancer care decision making*, focusing on the patient and family, providers, payers, regulators, and other policy makers. We still await (in mid 2004) explicit guidelines or guidance documents from the US Food and Drug Administration and the European Medicine Evaluation Agency on the use of HRQOL information in submissions for product approval and advertising. In a 2003 article,[50] FDA officials concluded that among the 57 regular (non-accelerated) approvals for cancer drugs over the 1990–2002 period, tumor response was the approval basis for 26, with relief of tumor-specific symptoms bringing added support in 9 of these 26. Overall, symptom relief "provided critical support" for approval of 13 of the 57, while "no approvals were based on instruments measuring health-related quality of life." The authors cited poor study design and execution as key reasons for HRQOL's lack of influence. They concluded by urging the "development of additional endpoints to describe symptom-based clinical benefit in cancer patients."

It remains to be seen in what ways these conclusions adumbrate the scope, tone, and specific provisions of the agency's forthcoming guidelines on the use of patient-reported outcomes for drug approval and marketing decisions. Such guidelines will undoubtedly influence, over time, the types of patient-reported outcomes included in many clinical trials and other intervention studies; payer decisions about coverage (if not reimbursement); and provider recommendations about treatments. (We note that the definition of HRQOL employed by the COMWG, both in the selection of published research for analysis and conclusions about the value of patient-reported outcomes, encompasses patient-provided symptom reports and evaluations.)

What is clear at this point is that we have scant systematic knowledge about how real decision makers go about sorting out and synthesizing information on biomedical outcomes, patient-reported outcomes, cost considerations, and other factors to arrive at judgments related to cancer care. To remedy this, we must acquire a better understanding of how cancer-related decisions, at all levels, are made. A multi-faceted research strategy may be required: field surveys, analyses of previous decisions including case studies, focus groups, and in-depth interviews of decision participants. The appropriate definition and measurement of such subjective concepts as HRQOL will likely vary by study purpose and design, and need to be tailored accordingly.

Reducing the death and suffering due to cancer is a compelling and daunting challenge – one being pursued not only by the US National Cancer Institute, but a worldwide community of cancer researchers, providers, patients, survivors, families, caregivers, and volunteers. With basic and clinical scientific discoveries now accelerating the development of promising new interventions, and with a heightened public and private focus on delivering quality cancer care to all who need it, there are good reasons to expect substantial and sustained progress in reducing the cancer burden. Through cancer outcomes assessment, we can monitor the progress being achieved at any point in time, while conducting the research needed to inform decisions that will have a direct impact on reducing the burden over time.

REFERENCES

1 Lipscomb, *et al.*, this volume, Chapter 1.
2 Lohr, K. N. (for the Scientific Advisory Committee of the Medical Outcomes Trust) (2002). Assessing health status and quality-of-life instruments: attributes and review criteria. *Quality of Life Research* 11:193–205.
3 Ganz, Goodwin, this volume, Chapter 5.
4 Moinpour, Provenzale, this volume, Chapter 8.
5 Earle, Weeks, this volume, Chapter 7.
6 Litwin, Talcott, this volume, Chapter 6.
7 Ferrell, this volume, Chapter 12.
8 Snyder, this volume, Chapter 16.
9 Erickson, this volume, Chapter 3.
10 Darby, this volume, Chapter 14.
11 Gustafson, this volume, Chapter 15.
12 Zebrack, Cella, this volume, Chapter 11.
13 Potosky, A. L., Harlan, L. C., Stanford, J. L. *et al.* (1999). Prostate cancer practice patterns and quality of life: the Prostate Cancer Outcomes Study. *Journal of the National Cancer Institute* 91(20):1719–24.
14 Gotay, C. (2004). Assessing cancer-related quality of life across a spectrum of applications. *Journal of the National Cancer Institute Monograph* 33:126–33.
15 Spilker, this volume, Invited Paper A.
16 Fairclough, this volume, Chapter 17.
17 Sloan, this volume, Chapter 18.
18 Aaronson, this volume, Chapter 20.
19 Hambleton, this volume, Chapter 22.
20 Mandelblatt, Selby, this volume, Chapter 10.
21 Holland, J. C. (2003). Psychological care of patients: psycho-oncology's contribution (American Cancer Society Award lecture). *Journal of Clinical Oncology* 21 (23 Suppl.): 253s–65s.
22 Ferrans, this volume, Chapter 2.
23 Fayers, P. M., Machin, D. (2002). *Quality of Life: Assessment, Analysis and Interpretation*. Chichester: John Wiley & Sons.
24 Reise, S., this volume, Chapter 21.
25 Hornbrook, this volume, Chapter 24.
26 Williams, this volume, Chapter 13.
27 Willis *et al.*, this volume Invited Paper C.
28 Barry, Dancey, this volume, Chapter 9.
29 Schwartz, C. E., Sprangers, M. A. G. (2000). *Adaptation to Changing Health: Response Shift in Quality-of-Life Research*. Washington, DC: American Psychological Association.
30 Sprangers, M. A. G., Schwartz, C. E. (1999). Integrating response shift into health-related quality of life research: a theoretical model. *Social Science and Medicine* 48:1507–15.
31 Patrick, D. L., Kinne, S., Engleberg, R. A. *et al.* (2000). Functional status and perceived quality of life in adults with and without chronic conditions. *Journal of Clinical Epidemiology* 53:779–85.
32 Osoba, this volume, Chapter 19.
33 Sloan, J. A., Cella, D., Frost, M. H. *et al.* (2002). Assessing clinical significance in measuring oncology patient quality of life: introduction to the symposium, content overview, and definition of terms. *Mayo Clinic Proceedings* 77:367–70.
34 Dowie, J. (2002). Decision validity should determine whether a generic or condition-specific HRQOL measure is used in health care decisions. *Health Economics* 11:1–8.
35 Wasson, J. H. (2003). Office practice today: as good as it gets? tomorrow: as good as it can be? International Society for Quality of Life Research, 10th Annual Conference, Prague, Czech Republic.

36 Gotay, C. C., Wilson, M. E. (1998). Use of quality of life out-come assessments in current cancer clinical trials. *Evaluation and the Health Professions* **21**:157–78.

37 Gotay, C. C. (2003). Quality of life assessment in cancer clinical research: current status and a look to the future. *Expert Review of Pharmacoeconomics and Outcomes Research* **3**:479–86.

38 Lindley, C., Vasa, S., Sawyer, W. T. *et al.* (1998). Quality of life and preferences for treatment following systemic adjuvant therapy for early-stage breast cancer. *Journal of Clinical Oncology* **16**:1380–7.

39 Slevin, M. L., Stubbs, L., Plant, H. J. *et al.* (1990). Attitudes to chemotherapy: comparing views of patients with cancer with those of doctors, nurses, and general public. *British Medical Journal* **300**:1458–60.

40 Wilson, this volume, Chapter 23.

41 McHorney, Cook, this volume, Invited Paper B.

42 Feeny, this volume, Chapter 4.

43 O'Brien, this volume, Chapter 25.

44 Donaldson, M. S. (2004). Taking stock of health-related quality-of-life measurement in oncology practice in the United States. *Journal of the National Cancer Institute Monograph* **33**:155–67.

45 Barofsky, I., Sugarbaker, P. H. (1990). Cancer. In *Quality of Life Assessments in Clinical Trials*, ed. B. Spilker, pp. 419–39. New York: Raven Press.

46 Sugarbaker, P. H., Barofsky, I., Rosenberg, S. A. (1982). Quality of life assessment in patients with extremity sarcoma clinical trials. *Surgery* **91**:17–23.

47 Clauser, S. B. (2004). Use of cancer performance measures in population health: a macro-level perspective. *Journal of the National Cancer Institute Monograph* **33**:142–54.

48 Revicki, this volume, Chapter 27.

49 Copley-Merriman *et al.* this volume, Invited Paper D.

50 Johnson, J. R., Williams, G., Pazdur, R. (2003). End points and United States Food and Drug Administration approval of oncology drugs. *Journal of Clinical Oncology* **21**:1404–11.

51 Lipscomb J., Snyder C. F. (2002). The outcomes of cancer outcomes research: focusing on the National Cancer Institute's quality-of-care initiative. *Medical Care* **40** [supplement]:III:3–10.

52 National Cancer Institute. "Improving the quality of cancer care" in *The Nation's Investment in Cancer Research: a Plan and Budget Document for Fiscal Year 2005*. Available at http://plan.cancer.gov. Last accessed on September 18, 2004.

53 National Institutes of Health. "Dynamic Assessment of Patient-Reported Chronic Disease Outcomes." NIH Roadmap Initiative RFA-AR-04–007, released November 18, 2003. Available at http://grants.nih.gov/grants/guide/rfa-files/RFA-RM-04-011.html. Last accessed on September 18, 2004.

54 Gotay, Lipscomb, this volume, Chapter 26.

Invited Paper A
The world of outcomes research:
yesterday, today, and tomorrow*

Bert Spilker, Ph.D., M.D.

Bert Spilker and Associates, Bethesda, MD

This paper presents an informal look at some of the peaks and valleys of the past, present, and future of outcomes research. It is not intended to be a comprehensive history or summary of the subject, but it describes some highlights of this important area. Additional details can be found in the book *Quality of Life and Pharmacoeconomics in Clinical Trials*.[1]

One of the overall themes over the last 25 years is the progress from considering patient satisfaction to a more careful evaluation of functional states, which in turn led to the use of scales and instruments for evaluating quality of life. Because of the various types of quality of life, this term evolved, in turn, to become health-related quality of life. In recent years, the umbrella term "patient-reported outcomes" (PROs) has become accepted and is becoming widely used to describe this field. PROs cover a continuum from patient satisfaction through measures of functional states through health-related quality-of-life assessments. The terminology has been standardized by a PRO harmonization group, composed of academic, government, and industry members of various trade associations, professional societies, and government agencies (European Regulatory Issues on Quality of Life Assessment [ERIQA], International Society for Pharmacoeconomics and Outcomes Research [ISPOR], International Society for Quality of Life Research [ISOQOL], and the Pharmaceutical Research and Manufacturers of America [PhRMA] Health Outcomes Committee, plus Food and Drug Administration [FDA] observers). Their report is available on-line at www.mapi-research-inst.com.

Below, this paper provides a brief history of PRO research and a discussion of the challenges ahead.

Yesterday (1960s, 1970s, 1980s)

The initial years of PRO research were a "lawless time" when few rules existed to place constraints on those who conducted research or made claims. It was the "Wild West" where an astute practitioner of this craft would often try to prove any product (regardless of price) was the most cost-effective one. The trick was choosing the comparator drug and/or parameter to study very carefully and seeking an aspect to emphasize that would make one's case.

This approach involved starting with the conclusion one sought and then working backwards to find the parameter or comparator that would produce that response. Then, the researcher would write and design a study or test with knowledge of the result, conduct the study, and, unsurprisingly, achieve perfect results every time. By the decade of the 1990s, this practice had mostly disappeared and is seldom encountered at present.

There were skeptics during this period who claimed that patient-reported outcomes and

---

*For the initial meeting of the Cancer Outcomes Measurement Working Group in February 2001, the NCI invited Bert Spilker, M.D., Ph.D. – analyst, editor, and pharmaceutical industry executive – to offer a broad, impressionistic perspective on the continuing evolution of health outcomes research. This chapter expands upon that presentation.

pharmacoeconomics were a passing fad: "They won't last, my friend!" However, those who understood the relevance and importance of this area realized that patient well-being represents the ultimate clinical endpoint for chronic disease. Improving quality of life is the goal of many treatments.

Over time, a series of new questions were frequently asked, and increasing importance was gradually assigned to the answers. Questions asked included, "Is the treatment (e.g., drug, transplant, new modality) really worth it?" These questions were asked in terms of actual costs, comparative costs, medical value, and patient benefits.

Clinicians began to recognize the obvious fact that the real goal of therapy is not to improve a laboratory value or test number but to improve a patient's well-being. It also was apparent that patient well-being is a general concept that cannot be objectively measured with a single clear parameter. It was recognized, however, that one could measure different domains (categories) of quality of life to make comparisons of different treatments (e.g., two drugs, drug and placebo, non-drug treatment and no-treatment) between two or more groups of patients. One could also study a single group of patients who receive different drugs during a clinical trial. This conceptual breakthrough was substantial. Leading drug development decision makers began to consider adding outcomes research studies and tests in their development plans.

The past was also a time when a group of people might get together and decide to create a quality-of-life instrument in a very short period. It was not uncommon for analysts (with little or no outcomes research experience) to say, in effect, "Let's create a quality-of-life instrument this weekend." Such was the naiveté about types of validation required and even the need for validation. A related problem during this period was the focus on a single overall score for PROs rather than examining the individual domain scores. The latter scores provide greater information and ability to interpret the influence of various interventions.

Common sense (and possibly large egos) led many physicians and scientists to say that a patient's physician could rate that patient's well-being, and certainly one's spouse would be able to score 100% on any such test. Yet, studies confirmed that there were significant differences between patient- and physician-reported outcomes. Neither physicians nor spouses can reliably rate their patients' or partners' quality of life. Unfortunately, many physicians were not convinced of these findings and only in recent years have they come to realize this basic truth.

During much of this period it was not clear whether well-being was a safety or efficacy parameter and whether it was a secondary or primary endpoint. This question was settled when well-being was defined as part of efficacy. There was a period in the 1970s when virtually anything that affected a patient was said to be indicative of "quality of life." For example, the number of blood transfusions was said, by one group, to be an indication of quality of life. The assumption was made that the fewer the number of transfusions the better off one would be.

The sensation of pain was realized to be intimately related to patient well-being. Persons in moderate or severe pain focus on little else and find that their quality of life is directly related to their pain. There is undoubtedly no other single characteristic that is as closely and directly related to quality of life as is pain.

In measuring quality of life, there are many apparently obvious parameters to use as surrogates, but almost all can be misleading in some cases. For example, a new drug for treating asthma was evaluated for its effect on well-being a few years ago. A parameter chosen as a major clinical endpoint was the number of visits to a hospital emergency room (ER). The children taking the drug appeared to both parents and physicians to be doing much better clinically, but their number of ER visits did not decrease and, in fact, increased. This puzzle was solved when the children were interviewed. A significant number of them were so greatly improved that they could play outdoors with their friends, sometimes for the first time in a long period. The children knew that this type of play was likely to lead to an asthma attack and an ER visit, but they did not mind this visit because being able to play outside and act more "normal" with their friends made the ER visit a worthwhile trade-off.

Today (1990s and the first years of the new millennium)

Currently, there is increasing application of pharmacoeconomic models – using cost-benefit, cost-effectiveness, cost-utility, cost-of-illness, and cost-consequence methods – to evaluate new interventions. The theoretical underpinnings of these approaches are now well understood, and accepted, by most outcomes researchers.[2]

A few years ago, there was little agreement on the appropriate guidelines for applying these evaluation methodologies to real-world decision problems. But, in the last 5 to 10 years, organizations and experts in numerous countries have put forward various sets of guidelines (see Mullins and Ogilvie[3] for descriptions and references, and Pritchard[4] for comparisons among guidelines) for designing, conducting, and reporting the application of these principles to clinical trials and other types of studies. The acceptance of these guidelines is growing, and it is widely acknowledged that they serve to increase the standards of the field.

At the present time, there is a widespread acceptance of PRO evaluations as true efficacy measures. In addition, many older PRO instruments that have been adequately, or even well, validated in one or more populations are currently being tested and validated in new patient populations. It is important, if not essential, for researchers to understand when and where the instrument may or may not be used. Occasionally, it is found that one or more subscales of an existing (validated) instrument may be used to evaluate one or more specific outcome domains; for example, all eight subscales of the SF-36 have been individually validated, although the subscales

cannot be modified and the entire instrument is usually given. In most cases, however, such multidimensional instruments have been validated "as a whole," and it is not appropriate to pull out and use selected domain scales simply to improve the measured responsiveness of the study subject to the intervention being examined. As research continues, the best outcomes instruments for each disease or condition will eventually be determined.

In some outcomes evaluations, there may not exist a well-validated instrument appropriate for the problem at hand. In those situations, another approach to evaluating patient outcomes is needed. It is best to begin by first determining the key research questions that are not answered by a standard instrument. A few (say, two to six) such questions can be posed in a clinical trial. The data obtained in response to these questions may be analyzed statistically and the results compared between groups. If those questions are important (or will be important), the data collected can be used exactly as any other clinical data, whether in a regulatory submission or in a publication. It is important not to refer to these questions collectively as an "outcomes instrument" or to combine the results of multiple, disparate questions into a single score. To do so is to invite serious criticism, and rightfully so.

Currently, many key decision makers in government and managed care organizations are seriously questioning what these PROs contribute to their decisions. This critical question must be satisfactorily answered if PROs are to assume their place as a factor in influencing major health care policies.

Challenges for tomorrow (after 2005)

The most important goals for outcomes research are presented below using two categories. First, methodological and definitional considerations are presented. Then, the influences of outcomes research on (1) the practice of medicine, (2) national health care policy, and (3) media reporting are described. Within these categories, the specific challenges mentioned are not listed in any order.

Some of these goals may be achieved within the next few years, but all are expected to be achieved eventually.

Methodological and definitional challenges

(1) Standard guidelines for designing, conducting, and reporting pharmacoeconomic studies will achieve widespread acceptance. Achieving this goal will prevent people from designing trials that are guaranteed to yield desired results or that are substandard in one or more aspects. Using scientific standards assures a fair approach to the design, conduct, analysis, and interpretation of results. Achievement of this goal will result from pressure by journal editors, formulary committees, and peers to adhere to current standards.

(2) Terms that are often misused will consistently be used correctly (e.g., "pharmacoeconomics," which refers to the entire field and "cost-effectiveness," which refers to a single specific methodology). The latter term is often mistakenly applied to the entire field. This issue is a relatively minor point that can be readily addressed through common usage making the correct terminology a matter of habit.

(3) A set of well-established and well-validated disease-specific and generic patient-reported outcomes instruments will be established. It is widely agreed by professionals in this field that better validated instruments of both types are needed. Achieving this goal will take significantly more time for some diseases than for others. Progress towards this goal will result from methodologists developing and validating measures for those diseases where specific instruments are lacking.

(4) More research will be conducted on how other aspects of life outside health (e.g., life events such as birth, marriage, or death) affect patient's reported outcomes. It is likely that major unanticipated life events (e.g., severe illness, winning the lottery) and other aspects of life outside health (e.g., career) strongly affect some aspects of a patient's reported outcomes. Studying this influence may be of significant value in learning how to control or factor-in these variables and in determining what this relationship means in terms of appropriate therapy. Greater attention to this issue by professional societies and publishers will be key in achieving this goal.

(5) The role of the spiritual/ethical domain in outcomes measurement will attain its appropriate place in patient-reported outcomes instruments. In some situations, the spiritual domain is relevant to consider, but it is missing from most instruments. Progress towards this goal will result from professional pressure and encouragement at meetings, in journals, and from instances where its use added important interpretations and contributions to the field.

(6) Professionals who design clinical trials focused on outcomes research will not be permitted by an institutional review board to work backwards from a desired conclusion to determine which specific protocol elements and design will yield the desired result. This goal will be achieved through the critical review of protocols and results submitted for publication.

(7) All domains of patient-reported outcomes will be studied in a clinical trial and will be reported, even if most data are negative. When trials are reported and only a few domains are mentioned, it is not always known if others were measured (possibly with another unreported scale) and yielded negative or contrary results. This goal will be achieved as professional societies, funding bodies, and professional journals insist on full reporting.

Influence of outcomes research on the practice of medicine, on national health care policy, and on the media

(1) Patient-reported outcomes data will have an appropriate influence on national health planners and legislators who, collectively, guide the allocation of a nation's health care resources.

This goal represents one of outcomes scientists' major hopes. Health planners include people in numerous areas of the US government (e.g., the Department of Health and Human Services (DHHS), including its Centers for Medicare and Medicaid Services (CMS); the Office of Management and Budget; and Congress). Progress towards achieving this goal will be made as the field of outcomes research becomes more widely respected as a key influence in health care.

(2) Regulatory authorities and national organizations like the National Institute for Clinical Excellence (NICE) in the UK will only conditionally (and not permanently) pass judgment on a drug's therapeutic value at the time it is initially marketed. Understanding unanticipated benefits and assessing incompletely known or unknown risks is not possible at the time of first marketing because all costs, cost estimates, and outcomes are not truly known and cannot be identified. Thus, it is necessary to wait at least about five years before attempting definitive interpretation of a drug's value. Authorities will not (as they sometimes do now) keep a promising therapy out of the market because, and only because, the available outcomes data are not regarded as sufficiently complete or comprehensive. Rather, they will work creatively to use the market to garner the outcomes data needed for making sound long-term decisions about the intervention's effectiveness, cost, and cost effectiveness. This goal will be achieved through pressure on NICE, and other such agencies, by patients who are unable to receive the drugs they need and possibly also from government pressures.

(3) Evidence-based data from outcomes research from observational studies as well as from traditional clinical trials will be used by physicians as the basis for a far greater proportion of their clinical decisions. The importance of using evidence as the basis for clinical decision making is widely endorsed, but in most areas of medicine, lags far behind the potential application. Use of outcomes data will be facilitated by widespread dissemination of validated decision trees, professional guidelines, and other tools. Achieving this goal will result from pressure from peers, professional societies, managed care organizations, journals, and other groups.

(4) Private insurance companies and public payers (e.g., Medicare and Medicaid) will be more willing to pay for new treatments with demonstrated or expected patient-reported outcomes benefits. As more interventions to improve lifestyle are developed, there will be increased pressure on payers to cover such drugs. Prices of drugs, together with costs and savings in other health care areas (e.g., physician visits, monitoring, hospital visits), are essential factors to be included in a cost-effectiveness analysis. Otherwise, one is only observing increases in drug prices without measuring if savings are being realized elsewhere in the health care system. This goal will be achieved through the growing importance of outcomes research and its eventually attaining the influence it deserves.

(5) The media, politicians, and the public will use the terms "prices" and "costs" correctly when referring to drugs, devices, and other interventions generally. With media headlines blaring about "double digit cost increases" without an explanation of how costs differ from prices, many people blame the pharmaceutical industry for "high prices." The annual cost for a nation's (or other group's) health budget rises because of many reasons, only one of which is the price increase for a specific drug. Other factors include hospital costs, physician and other health care professional costs, new drugs introduced on the market, and greater use of older drugs, to mention only a few of the most important factors. In 2001, for instance, the most significant source of increase in US health care spending was the hospital sector, not the pharmaceutical. It is essential for the public to understand that drug costs (for hospitals or the nation) generally increase for several reasons independent of the price of

a drug. The two most important reasons for this increase are greater use of existing drugs and the introduction of new drugs.

All of this points to the important role that outcomes research can play in providing an accurate perspective on the true net economic costs of innovative therapies, as well as a fair consideration of the health benefits being purchased with these dollars. In particular, if a new drug leads to an increase in a payer's outpatient pharmacy bill but also a decrease in hospital costs, it is the net cost impact that obviously should matter.

This brief "tour" of patient outcomes issues of the past and present highlights many of the future challenges that must be addressed and that require a great deal of effort on the part of scientists, health care professionals, and policy makers. Progress in this field requires novel, independent thinking to better obtain, interpret, and use outcomes data. No

timeline can be established to achieve these results, but if most (if not all) of these goals are used as beacons, they will guide us as we progress on a meaningful journey.

REFERENCES

1 Spilker, B. (ed.) (1996). *Quality of Life and Pharmacoeconomics in Clinical Trials* (2nd Edition). Philadelphia, PA: Lippincott-Raven.

2 Weinstein, M. C., Toy, E. L., Sandberg, E. A. *et al.* (2001). Modeling for public policy decisions: uses, roles and validity. *Value in Health* 4:348–61.

3 Mullins, C. D., Ogilvie, S. D. (1998). Emerging standardization in pharmacoeconomics. *Clinical Therapeutics* 20:1194–202.

4 Pritchard, C. (2001). Pharmacoeconomic guidelines around the world. In *Spectrum Reimbursement, Pharmacoeconomics, and Disease Management Issue 5*, pp. 5–1 to 5–12. Waltham, MA: Decision Resources Inc.

Invited Paper B
The ten Ds of health outcomes measurement for the twenty-first century*

Colleen A. McHorney, Ph.D.[1] and Karon F. Cook, Ph.D.[2]

[1]Indiana University School of Medicine and Roudebush Veterans Affairs Medical Center, Indianapolis, IN
[2]Baylor College of Medicine and Houston Veterans Affairs Medical Center, Houston, TX

Introduction

The origins of health status assessment can be traced to the 1960s and the need at that time for a new armamentaria of health statistics to measure outcomes above and beyond mortality and morbidity. The state of health outcomes assessment in the 1960s has been characterized by the five Ds: death, disease, disability, discomfort, and dissatisfaction.[1] In the USA, death registration was standardized in most states by 1930[2] and disease surveys had been underway since the late 1880s.[3-6] Measurement of disability began in the 1930s[7-9] but earnestly gained momentum in the late 1950s.[10-12] The National Health Interview Survey, which is a major source of information on disease and disability, was instituted in 1957[13] and continues today. Measurement of discomfort (subjective and objective sickness impacts) began in the 1940s[14,15] and continues to constitute a significant component of health-related quality of life (HRQOL) surveys. Measurement of patient satisfaction commenced in the 1950s for mental health care[16,17] and the 1960s for general medical care.[18]

We have made great progress in measuring patient health outcomes since the five Ds were first propounded. There are over 85 tools that measure basic and instrumental activities of daily living.[19] Myriad measures of depression exist.[20] Close to two dozen generic HRQOL instruments have been developed.[21] Hundreds of disease-specific instruments abound.[22,23] In cancer, over 75 different HRQOL measures exist.[24] The vast majority of these measures have been created under the umbrella of classical test theory (CTT). CTT is a set of assumptions and procedures that has been used to develop tests for much of the twentieth century.[25,26]

There are a number of problems that arise in developing tests and in using test scores that CTT cannot overcome. First, the statistics used to describe item performance are dependent on the particular sample of respondents on which they are calculated.[26,27] Thus, items and scales will have different statistics if the measured samples do not have similar distributions of ability. Second, CTT is *test*-driven rather than *item*-driven. Different sets of items will differ in difficulty and will provide different estimates of ability. Unless the tests have been equated, the scores of respondents taking one test cannot be compared to those of respondents taking another. To date, the bolus of health status measures have rarely been equated,[19,28] and thus have not been placed on a common metric of ability.

*As the COMWG chapters on psychometric topics strongly suggest, modern measurement theory has the potential to revolutionize the way that patient-reported outcomes are conceptualized, analyzed, and interpreted. To examine further the promises, and possible pitfalls, in rapidly incorporating such developments as item response theory into cancer outcomes measurement, NCI invited two leading experts in the field – Colleen A. McHorney, Ph.D., and Karon F. Cook, Ph.D. – to reflect on the issues that lie ahead. Preparation of this chapter was supported in part by the Department of Veterans Affairs (RR&D C-2488-R).

In recent years, item response theory (IRT) has been increasingly used in health outcomes assessment.[21,29–31] IRT is a theoretical framework and a collection of quantitative techniques for test construction, scaling, and equating, as well as for identifying item bias and supporting computerized adaptive testing. If its assumptions are met, IRT can overcome some of the limitations of CTT by providing item parameters that are theoretically invariant with respect to the sample of examinees and ability parameters that are theoretically invariant with respect to the set of items used.[27,32,33]

Given the simultaneous growth of patient-centered measures and the increasing use of IRT in health outcomes assessment, it is timely to take stock of our measurement progress. The purpose of this chapter is to suggest advances for the *process* of outcomes measurement in distinctive and informative manners. As a way of doing so, we propose and discuss the ten Ds of health outcomes measurement for the twenty-first century.

The ten Ds

Definitions of quality of life

Two seminal pieces of work have lamented the state of conceptual affairs in health outcomes assessment. Gill and Feinstein[34] argued that no unified approach has characterized HRQOL assessment and that there is little conceptual agreement on exactly what HRQOL means. They found researchers to be deficient in defining HRQOL and in justifying the selection of HRQOL instruments. The same criticism applies to instrument developers. Leplege and Hunt[35] have elegantly argued that:

. . . a clear conceptual basis for quality-of-life measures is lacking, and the few attempts to develop models or operational definitions of quality of life have been woefully inadequate . . . It is difficult to progress in any field if there is no shared definition of the concept or phenomenon under study . . . assessment of quality of life measures too often has been based on arguments of authority rather than on rational debate. (p. 47)

Disease-specific measures often have biomedically driven measurement models based upon

known or hypothesized manifestations of the underlying pathology. Conceptual frameworks for generic measures can generally be characterized as insubstantial, usually attributing conceptual models to the World Health Organization (WHO)[36] trinity of physical, social, and mental health. Yet, the WHO definition is just that – only a definition (not a conceptual framework), and one that is at the same time both vague and idealistic.[37] Unfortunately, adherence to the WHO definition has led researchers to implicitly ignore what they seek to measure – the patient point of view. Both Gill and Feinstein and Leplege and Hunt take issue with the fact that many HRQOL measures do not ask patients what is important to them. As Gill and Feinstein[34] argue:

. . . quality of life can be suitably measured only by determining the preferences of patients and supplementing (or replacing) the authoritative opinions contained in statistically "approved" instruments. (p. 624)

Leplege and Hunt[35] resonate with this assessment by contending that:

. . . there has been some confusion between questionnaires that are completed by patients and those that reflect the concerns of patients. . . . most of the currently used questionnaires do no more than force patients to address themselves to the concerns of physicians and/or social scientists and statisticians. (p. 49)

We are in a transition phase from fixed-length, one-size-fits-all assessment to more tailored assessment. This transition will involve the construction and calibration of item banks and the use of IRT and computerized adaptive testing to assess HRQOL.[19,21,28] As we make this transition, we should not repeat the mistakes we have made over the past 30 years by having unbridled promulgation of myriad item banks, myriad redundant banks, and myriad redundant banks that, as Gill and Feinstein assert, possess psychometric elegance but are far removed from the subjects they purport to assess – the individual patient.

Discovery methods

The thin conceptual cornerstone that has characterized many health status measures may have impelled instrument developers to use existing items rather than develop them de novo. Only two generic measures (the Sickness Impact Profile and the Nottingham Health Profile) obtained their items from consumers themselves.[21] Otherwise, items for generic measures have been recycled from the literature, often gleaned from clinically oriented tools.[38] Disease-specific tools derive their items from three sources: (1) existing generic tools;[39-41] (2) clinical expertise;[42] and (3) patient testimony about the impact of disease and treatment on health status.[43-45]

Use of existing items to construct HRQOL surveys has benefits and drawbacks. As to the former, one can theoretically select items with desirable psychometric properties. In reality, however, item characteristics are a combination of the item itself and the group in which it is tested.[21,46,47] As to the latter, many older items violate contemporary standards for item writing, insofar as they often contain multiple attributions (e.g., do you have difficulty *bending, kneeling, or stooping*, or how much of the time have you been in firm control of your *behavior, thoughts, emotions, feelings*?). Cognitive interviewing has revealed the sources of invalidity that these practices can yield.[48,49] Older, recycled items often have antiquated language. For example, in the Sickness Impact Profile, there is an item "I get sudden frights," a phrase which is not common today.

We should be true to our intent – to measure patient-centered outcomes – which means using patients and their caregivers as active participants in the item generation, selection, and pretesting phases of instrument development. Patients should be used to generate items, whether it be through semi-structured interviews,[50-53] ethnography,[54,55] phenomenology,[56-58] existentialist methods,[59] or the more efficient focus group approach.[43-45,60-62] Importance ratings provided by patients[63-67] should be used in item selection and reduction to complement psychometric criteria. Pretesting needs to be more patient-centered, with greater use of cognitive testing methods[68-72] in addition to standard psychometric analysis. There are two measurement applications for which discovery methods should prove critical in the years ahead.

First, the field has given scant attention to differential item functioning (DIF) (see below). The purpose of DIF analyses is to identify items that exhibit dissimilar response patterns for persons having equal ability but different group membership (such as age, gender, race, and ethnicity). Once DIF is identified, one needs to discover the potential causes of the DIF. Psychometric methods do not easily lend themselves to such discovery research. Qualitative researchers, however, have a repertoire of methods that is better suited to understand the reasons *why* persons of equal ability answer questions differently. Thus, discovery methods should prove useful in understanding the myriad reasons for DIF. Once identified, DIF can be corrected at the item writing stage.

Second, item banking and computerized adaptive testing (CAT) is on the measurement horizon.[21] CAT requires the calibration of a large bank of items. Items can be assembled through expert opinion or by cutting and pasting from the literature. However, many published items themselves were constructed by cutting and pasting from even earlier measures, thus perpetuating a long lineage of items that may have lost their relevance, salience, or discriminability over time. It would be appropriate, indeed essential, to inform the development of item banks by using discovery methods that enlist patients and consumers in identifying new items to fill in known or hypothesized gaps in the functioning and well-being continuum, as well as using the patient point of view in helping to eliminate or cull out redundant items.

Dimensionality

Unidimensionality is an important, but underdiscussed, aspect of health status assessment. Unidimensionality concerns the extent to which the ability being measured is a single unitary trait or dimension. Unidimensionality is important for score interpretation. If a score is composed of more than one dimension, it is impossible to determine what is contributing to the score.

The development of superordinate summary scales, like those for the Sickness Impact Profile,[73] the SF-36,[74] and other measures,[75-80] directly challenges the property of unidimensionality by factor scoring diverse profiles into a limited number of composite scores, often deriving orthogonal structures along the way. In this scoring scheme, a good "physical health" summary score is achieved by having high scores on physical scales (e.g., good physical and role functioning and no pain) and low scores on mental scales (e.g., anxious and depressed). The same applies to the summary mental scale, whereby a high score is achieved by having good mental health status but poor physical health status. This orthogonalized scoring practice has been criticized on methodological and conceptual grounds.[81,82]

Summary scales have been derived, in part, to address problems related to multiple comparisons in hypothesis testing.[29,83] Despite the desire for parsimony in hypothesis testing, the use of superordinate summary scales can often complicate inferential testing more than it simplifies it. Numerous studies have reported summary scores that yield quite different substantive findings than their more unidimensional profile scales.[81,82,84-98] These discrepancies occur because different scoring weights (often derived from factor analytic procedures) are given to individual profile scores. When combined into a superordinate score, the effects of individual, substantively meaningful profiles can be blurred, obscured, under-estimated, or over-estimated because of the sign and direction of the scoring coefficients. As an example, Figure B.1 shows the eight SF-36 health profiles for three persons with the normative mean score of 48.3 for the physical component summary (PCS) and 50.2 for the mental component summary (MCS). As the figure shows, persons with the same exact score at the sample mean level have dramatically different individual health profiles. HRQOL measures should inform, rather than complicate or obfuscate, studies of treatment effectiveness. If we cannot attribute an observed treatment effect (i.e., whether it is due to deterioration in pain or improvement in anxiety), then we cannot confidently use HRQOL findings to support labeling and promotional claims for medical procedures or devices or pharmaceutical products. If we cannot attribute HRQOL effects in clinical trials, then those data will not be of measurable use to physicians when advising their patients on alternative therapies. If we cannot attribute HRQOL effects in treatment studies, then policy makers and payers will not consider such data in policy development.

The final issue about unidimensionality is its use as an underlying assumption for IRT analysis. Investigators utilizing IRT need to assess unidimensionality, preferably using more than one method. Unidimensionality is also a strong requisite for item banks and, thus, computerized adaptive testing.[99] Unidimensionality also plays a significant role in studies of DIF because items could be statistically flagged as being DIF if they are multidimensional. Thus, for both old and new applications of measures, unidimensionality assessment needs to become a more standardized aspect of instrument development and validation.

Disparities and determinants

One of the national health goals in Healthy People 2010 is to eliminate health disparities.[100] The National Institutes of Health (NIH) defines health disparities as "differences in the incidence, prevalence, mortality, and burden of diseases and other adverse health conditions that exist among specific population groups in the United States."[101] Health status and HRQOL fall squarely under the burden of disease umbrella.

Research over the past 40 years has consistently underscored the role of non-medical factors in determining individual and population health.[102,103] It is now well established that social, lifestyle, and psychological factors account for 50% of preventable morbidity and mortality, environmental factors and human biology account for another 20% each, and medical care only 10%.[104] The unique signature of the outcomes movement is that it broadened the scope of our dependent variables to include functioning, well-being, and patient satisfaction, in addition to more traditional indicators of mortality, morbidity, and costs. A shortcoming of the outcomes movement is that it has implicitly adopted the medical model's reductionistic view of health because it has focused on what works in *medicine* – thus, the independent variables are the same ones we

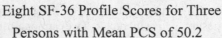

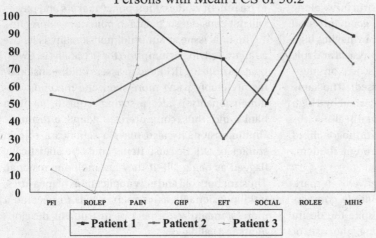

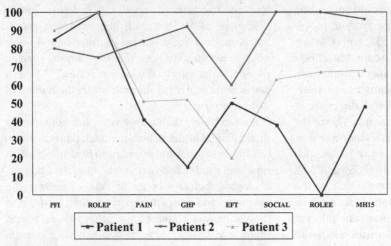

Figure B.1.   Individual health profiles of three patients with the same mean physical component summary (PCS) and mental component summary (MCS).

have been studying for years. As a result, our knowledge base is rich in terms of the impact of disease, severity, comorbidity, symptoms, and treatment on health status and HRQOL, but less so in terms of the non-medical determinants. Further, clinically-

driven outcomes research has tended to view health status in an episodic manner, with most studies being cross-sectional or having limited longitudinal designs. However, health status and HRQOL are dynamic phenomena that change in response to aging, illness adaptation, treatment, and natural history. Thus, future research needs to address the life-course character of health status above and beyond disease and treatment episodes.

Individuals and populations vary greatly in health status when they are free of pathological disease,[105] as well as when they are matched on pathophysiologic disturbance. This occurs because social factors (e.g., socioeconomic status, stress, environment) exert an important influence on health status.[103] As Leplege and Hunt[35] argue:

> . . . the concept of health-related quality of life implies that people can analyze quality of life into its health and non-health related components. This view fails to acknowledge the interconnectedness of health status with other aspects of existence. (p. 48)

Since HRQOL is the illness-impact iceberg underlying disease, morbidity, and disability, future research needs to expand its explanatory potential by studying health determinants vis-à-vis HRQOL outcome measures. In part, this could be accomplished in the context of validity assessment. Generic measures are intended for use across population segments. Thus, one important validity test should be whether they exhibit the same patterns of social differentials (by age, gender, race, and socioeconomic status[106–113]) as has been observed with mortality and morbidity. Put differently, generic measures should reflect predominant social patterns of inequality in health, especially if they are to be used at the population level for planning and evaluation purposes. The same case can be made for disease-specific measures. The co-modeling and co-presentation of social with clinical variables will help to situate the relative importance of both determinants. More profound analysis of social variables will contribute to a deeper and more meaningful understanding of health determinants.

Disadvantaged populations, disenfranchisement, and the digital divide

Relatively few health outcomes assessment tools have been assessed in disadvantaged or vulnerable populations.[114] That is, most reliability and valid-ity studies have been conducted in white, middle-class populations. Few investigations have even superficially assessed the myriad conditions under which measures may become degraded in disadvantaged populations. Such psychometric ethnocentrism is regrettable because the USA is becoming a more diverse society. Its population is aging and is becoming more ethnically diverse.[115] Because of the growing cultural pluralism, there is, more so than ever before, a need for evidence that health outcome tools exhibit measurement equivalence across diverse population groups.[114]

For group comparisons to be meaningful, one must establish that the variable(s) measured in different groups is parallel enough to be considered the same behavior, attitude, symptom, or feeling.[116] Tests of *psychometric equivalence* (determination of whether the derived scale provides equivalent measurement across groups) are often undertaken. However, they vary in their breadth and depth of analysis, ranging from simple group comparisons of means or Cronbach's alpha coefficients to structural equation modeling of factor structures to IRT-based analyses of DIF. Most investigators assess psychometric equivalence and then assert conceptual equivalence if no psychometric differences are found. This "absolutist approach"[117] begs the question as to whether the construct under investigation is meaningful and relevant across different groups.

Conceptual equivalence involves assessing whether the construct under consideration has identical meaning, relevance, and significance across groups. It could be that the feelings or behaviors assessed are differentially salient across groups, that the selected items only partially represent the construct as defined by a group, or that some experiential aspects of the construct are omitted altogether.[114,118] Studies of conceptual equivalence should assess the extent to which the operationalization of the construct, and the specific items used to represent the construct, are portable across groups.[119,120] Assessing conceptual equivalence ideally involves qualitative discovery research to gain knowledge of people's vocabularies and terminology and to understand the attributions or qualities they assign to feelings and behaviors.[121]

Disenfranchisement can occur through several mechanisms, such as failing to ensure conceptual equivalence and cultural appropriateness of an instrument, failing to adequately sample disadvantaged and vulnerable respondents, and failing to provide respondents with a user-friendly mode of administration. The reading level of instruments must be appropriate for poor readers. The field has been moving toward computerized assessment. For example, computerized surveys have been used for preoperative testing[122] and mental health assessment,[123–128] and computerized HRQOL assessment is increasingly used.[129–138] However, the nature and extent of the digital divide by age, race, and socioeconomic status is well documented.[139,140] Accordingly, we need to ensure that disadvantaged and vulnerable patient groups are not disenfranchised from computerized outcomes assessment, including the anticipated use of computerized adaptive testing for health outcomes assessment.

Differential item functioning (DIF)

Identification and correction of DIF items has a long history in achievement and educational testing. If items in an achievement test (or qualification, promotion, or certification tests) are answered differently by women versus men, or minorities versus majorities, when their underlying ability is the same, then the test scores would not be comparable and educational placement decisions would unfairly hurt one group and unfairly favor another. If items in such tests are biased, then inequitable treatment may likely result, thus materially affecting lives of the test takers.[141] In educational and achievement testing and professional credentialing, item writers and instrument developers purify their items a priori.[142] Unfortunately, in health outcomes assessment, instrument developers have tended to ignore DIF or have identified it long after the measure has been in use.

DIF has been identified in a large number of health assessment tools, including measures of functional status[19,143–150] cognitive status,[151–154] HRQOL,[155] satisfaction,[156,157] and many mental health and personality measures.[118,158–178] Across all of these studies, DIF has been identified by age, gender, race, ethnicity, socioeconomic status, language, and nationality. DIF has been large enough to cause meaningful shifts in group means or case rates when DIF items are removed from the scale.[143,144,159,161,165,172,173,175,177,179,180]

Identifying, understanding, and correcting DIF is fundamental to developing assessment instruments, to testing hypotheses, to theory building, to screening and diagnosing individuals, and to implementing and evaluating health service delivery programs. Culturally fair health outcomes assessment (with "culture" defined broadly as gender, age, racial, ethnic, socioeconomic, geographic, and language variations[181]) are crucial when individual decisions are in balance, such as with mental or physical health screening, diagnostic, placement, and referral decisions. If items in a health assessment instrument are biased, detection rates will be biased (over-estimated or under-estimated), leading to over- and under-detection and over- and under-treatment. Item bias in health outcomes assessment tools can have implications at the policy level (e.g., under- and over-utilization of health services, erroneous prevalence rates) and at the individual patient level.

Research on DIF will not "throw the baby out with the bath water." DIF items have been identified in many health assessment tools and will surely be identified in others. Such identification in and of itself will not call for the mass abandonment of current assessment tools. Rather, advances in DIF identification and amelioration will help to polish current instruments and iron out measurement kinks,[182] so that current and future assessment tools become more culturally applicable and fair across the board.

Item difficulty

Item difficulty gets its name from the educational context in which IRT was developed. In this context, it is common to think of some items as "harder" or "easier" than other items. In scaling medical outcomes, however, the parameter name often does not communicate well. An alternative is to think of the difficulty of an item as the item's *intensity*. On a headache pain scale, for example, the item, "my headaches kept me from being productive at work: yes/no" is more intense (harder to endorse) than, "my headaches caused me little interruption in my daily activities: yes/no." All IRT models estimate an item difficulty parameter.

As described elsewhere,[21] the field has been entrenched in a paradigm of psychometric efficiency over the past decade, with an emphasis on constructing measures with as few items as possible. Acceptable standards of reliability with few items can best be achieved by selecting items that are fairly homogeneous. Thus, selected items are often in the middle range of item difficulty and are near alternate forms of one another. There is one major consequence of this measurement standard: the endpoints of the health continuum tend to be poorly defined, yielding substantial ceiling effects.[21] Score imprecision has two principal consequences. First, it is impossible to distinguish among individuals at the ceiling, even though they likely vary in the underlying construct. Thus, ceiling effects paint a more favorable image of population health than is true. For researchers, ceiling effects produce Type II errors in hypothesis testing. For clinicians, ceiling effects yield false-negative outcomes. Second, it is impossible to measure improvement in health over time for those at the ceiling. Thus, score distributions that are skewed at baseline will underestimate (or miss) the effects of effective treatment or natural history on health status.

The most common source of imprecision is the selection of items whose difficulty is incongruent with the *ability* of the population of interest.[21] Simply put, floor and ceiling effects derive from a poor marriage between the difficulty of an item and the ability of the targeted population. Ceiling effects occur when easy items are administered to high-ability populations, and floor effects happen when difficult items are administered to low-ability populations. Few positive well-being scales exhibit ceiling effects,[183–185] which is the result of two factors. First, they are often comprised of items having multiple categorical rating points (five to seven response cat-

egories). Compared to dichotomous items, polytomous items provide information across a broader range of the measurement continuum and more precisely differentiate individuals on the underlying construct. Second, positive well-being measures often have balanced items (those tapping negative and positive health states). Items that tap positive health states tend to have very low ceiling effects (i.e., few individuals report that they are a "happy person" all of the time).

Thus, problems with precision pertain largely to measures of physical, role, and social function. How can we "raise the bar" for the measurement of function? Recent work on calibrating basic and instrumental activities of daily living[19,28,147,186,187] has indicated obvious redundancies in measuring lower-level functioning and conspicuous gaps in measuring higher-order functioning. This is a clear beacon for future measurement development. Even for elderly populations, it is not necessary to oversample lower-level functioning because many items are redundant in terms of item difficulty and item discrimination.[19,28,147,149,186–192] The challenge is to more effectively sample and distribute the lower-level items while concurrently adding items to fill in known gaps at the difficult end of the continuum (e.g., higher-order functioning, productive activities, executive functioning, leisure exercise, and physical fitness). These are activities that will raise the ceiling while also being consistent with national health objectives and public health recommendations.[100]

The challenges for future advances in functional status assessment are both conceptual and methodological. Conceptually, qualitative methods should be used to glean from consumers themselves facets of contemporary functioning. For example, Porter[57] discovered numerous nuances about ADL performance in the context of qualitative research. The same applies to role and social functioning. The content of these concepts has been fairly narrow to date. A combination of focus group, diary, and time-use methods might yield valuable insights into what types of basic, intermediate, and advanced activities are performed on a regular basis, as well as what types of activities are abandoned and in what sequence.

Further, qualitative methods would be useful to understand how people adapt to occult or incipient disability. A crucial area for future research is to more profoundly understand the physical, economic, and social compensatory strategies used by the elderly in maintaining independence. Future advances in functional assessment might benefit from developing rating scales that tap compensation rather than difficulty per se.

Methodologically, a better way of matching item difficulty with the ability of the targeted population is needed. If we want to know how well persons are with respect to function, the most efficient procedure is to ask them about activities that are close to their level of ability. What is required is some means of functionally relating performance on each test item to a person's ability. IRT is well designed for this purpose in the context of item banking and computerized adaptive testing. Thus, a logical extension for health status assessment is to move from pen-and-paper tools to computerized adaptive assessment of health status.[21] Computerized health status assessment could: (1) reduce the human capital involved in administering and scoring questionnaires; (2) challenge patients at their targeted level of ability instead of boring or discouraging them; (3) provide researchers with the exact amount of precision required for each patient sample and each specific application; and (4) provide "real-time" scores to clinicians for use at the individual patient level in clinical practice.

Development of an adaptive framework would require four phases of methodological work.[21] The first task would be to assemble item banks on different health concepts (concept-specific banks). The second task would involve conducting cognitive interviews with a variety of patient groups to obtain in-depth information about respondent understanding and acceptance of the banked items. The cognitive interviews could also obtain input from patients/consumers on gaps in content coverage in each underlying continuum. The third task would be to employ IRT to calibrate items and to select a subset of items that comprehensively, and evenly, tap the underlying construct of interest. The

final phase would be to develop and implement algorithms for adaptive testing (e.g., starting and stopping rules).

Item discrimination

Item discrimination refers to an item's ability to distinguish among individuals who have different levels of the trait being measured. In the headache example above, we would expect the items to discriminate between those with severe headaches and those with mild headaches. A group of respondents with severe headache should be more likely than those with mild headaches to endorse the item, "my headaches kept me from being productive at work: yes/no." If this is not the case, the item is a poorly (low) discriminating item. In polytomous IRT models, the discrimination parameter is related to the item characteristic curves (ICC) for an item. The ICCs are the functions obtained by plotting the probability of scoring in a particular response category against the latent trait being measured. For very discriminating items, the probability function rises sharply; for low discriminating items, the function remains relatively flat across the measured continuum.

The discrimination parameter is related to another important construct in IRT, *information*. Information is defined as the reciprocal of the square root of the standard error of measurement. More highly discriminating items yield greater information and have smaller standard errors than lesser discriminating items. In the development of a scale, low discriminating items tend to be deleted from the pool of potential items since such items do not "cooperate" well in the measurement of the trait of interest. This is roughly analogous to deleting items that do not correlate with their hypothesized construct of interest (item convergent validity).

In Rasch models, items are assumed to have equal discriminations. If the data do not fit this assumption, estimates of the information functions and standard errors of measurement can be artificially inflated or deflated depending upon whether the value of the assumed discrimination is an over- or under-estimate of the actual discrimination of the item. Items with unequal discriminations tend to be identified as "misfitting" items in a Rasch model and, therefore, would be dropped from the developmental item pool. Items with common item discrimination values would exhibit better model fit and, therefore, be more likely to be retained in the final Rasch-based scale.

The heterogeneity of the construct being measured affects the value of the discrimination parameter. Items in a scale are a sample of the hypothetical universe of all items that could be chosen to measure the construct. The selected items should adequately represent the domain being measured. The more narrow the domain, the more homogenous will be item discriminations and vice versa. It is often difficult to distinguish between item heterogeneity due to the breadth of the domain sampled from item heterogeneity due to multidimensionality. However, the distinction is important because the most widely used IRT models assume the measurement of a unidimensional construct. Researchers who favor the use of Rasch models argue that high discrimination values result from multidimensionality and, therefore, indicate items inappropriate for scaling using unidimensional IRT models. It also is conceivable that the Rasch requirement that items equally discriminate could inadvertently restrict the content coverage of the set of items that comprise a scale.

As discussed earlier, to be useful, an item bank must contain items that differ in difficulty. However, items with good discrimination are also desired to differentiate between persons close together on the ability distribution (i.e., to yield more information about persons of seemingly contiguous ability). Thus, a challenge for compilers of item banks is to write discriminating items. Ambiguity can degrade an item's potential discrimination.[28] In one of our studies,[28] highly discriminating functional status items (e.g., put underclothes on, move between rooms, take pants off, get into bed) were almost behavioral measures – they targeted daily activities that were specific, explicit, and unequivocal. In short, they were questions that respondents could understand (because they were simple and concrete) and evaluate with respect to their range of

function (because they were in the realm of daily experience). Improvements in item writing efforts may be facilitated by scrutiny of low and high discrimination items.[163,193-195] Also, adherence to conventional item writing standards[196,197] (such as write items that can only be interpreted in one way; use clear, simple, direct language; and avoid multiple attributions) may go far towards improving item discrimination.

Dispute and divisiveness

A researcher who chooses to use IRT instead of CTT in the measurement of health outcomes has many IRT models from which to choose. For the outcomes researcher new to the use of IRT models, the heat of the debates regarding model selection can come as a surprise. At the extremes, there exist two "camps": one comprised of those who favor the one parameter (1-pl) Rasch model and the other comprised of those who favor the two parameter (2-pl) models.

The debates in IRT model selection center largely on whether an item discrimination parameter is estimated or not. Those who favor Rasch models argue that theoretical considerations as well as empirical ones should govern the choice of IRT models.[198] They claim that the Rasch model obeys "the rules of measurement."[199] An example of this "obedience" is the fact that, with Rasch models, persons who have higher raw scores also have higher calibrated scores. This is not necessarily the case with the 2-pl models. On a 5-item scale with 3 response categories for each item, a person may obtain a given raw score in many different ways. Response strings of "3,2,2,1,1" and of "3,1,2,1,2" both yield a raw score of "9." If the scale were calibrated using a 1-pl model, both response patterns would yield the same calibrated score. If the scale were calibrated using a 2-pl model, however, this would not necessarily be the case because the discrimination of the items would be factored into the computation of the calibrated score.

In scale construction using the Rasch model, emphasis is placed upon finding data (items) that fit the model. For proponents of the 2-pl camp, emphasis is placed on finding a model to fit the data (items). Proponents of the 2-pl models note that, within medical outcomes, item discrimination can vary substantially.[28,151,158,163,166,172,174,194,195,200–207] They argue that the Rasch approach is too simplistic to model the kinds of measures frequently encountered in outcomes research. From this perspective, the Rasch criteria for items is too selective and, therefore, too much of the data (items) are "thrown away" because they do not fit the model.

It is in scale construction where fundamental differences between the 2-pl and 1-pl camps become particularly evident. In response to the question, "how should a latent trait be measured?" the 2-pl camp's answer is statistical in its approach – *model the data; don't force the data to fit the model*. For the Rasch camp, the answer more closely follows the approach used in tool development and quality assurance – *build an instrument with the properties most desirable for measurement*.

Despite the heat of the arguments from both camps, the arguments of neither side are conceptually pure. Two illustrations suffice. With the partial-credit model,[208] reversals in calibrated step difficulties occur; that is, a person higher on the trait level being measured can be more likely than a person lower on the trait to endorse an easy item category. Such a reversal would appear to be counter to "the rules of measurement." Among those in the 2-pl camp, indignation is sometimes offered regarding the Rasch approach of "throwing away data." No similar objection is made to discarding items that fail to load on the desired factor in a factor analysis.

For medical outcomes researchers trying to root through the arguments between measurement camps, it may be helpful to recall that all models, by definition, are wrong. The questions of practical importance to the medical outcomes researcher are "how wrong are our models?" and "what is the impact of specific kinds of "wrongness?". In other words, how robust are IRT models in health outcomes applications? These questions have yet to be addressed adequately.

The selection of an IRT model should be supported by careful consideration of the measurement application. We suggest two applications, one in which a 2-pl model would be the more appropriate and another in which a 1-pl model would be more appropriate. A way in which IRT models have been applied in outcomes research is in the development of new measures. In the psychometric tradition, a large pool of items is developed and administered to a sample of respondents. The pool is refined based on factor analysis, measures of inter-item consistency, and estimates of item-to-total correlations. The scale developer could also choose to select only items that are homogenous with respect to discrimination, i.e., items that fit a Rasch model. Fitting to the Rasch model may provide advantages. As discussed above, the Rasch model has some desirable measurement properties that are particular to it. Also, because there are fewer item parameters, stable parameter estimation can be achieved with smaller sample sizes. Before settling on a Rasch model for a scale's calibration, however, the scale developer should verify that the selection of homogenously discriminating items has not had a deleterious impact on the content coverage of the items. Content coverage affects the construct validity of the measure being developed and should be privileged over parsimony in the selection of an IRT model.

Another way in which IRT has been applied is in the evaluation and/or equating of well known and often used measures.[19,28,209,210] For such applications, the pool of items has already been selected, and the onus is on the IRT model to adequately estimate the items properties. Within health outcomes assessment, items can vary substantially in discrimination.[28,151,158,163,166,172,174,194,195,200–207] Therefore, except in the improbable case in which the set of pre-existing items happens to have equal discrimination, a 2-pl model would be the better choice. A 2-pl model might also be preferred in computerized adaptive testing (CAT) applications. The promise of CAT is to achieve maximum information with as few items as possible, conditional on the desired precision of the obtained ability estimates. The efficiency of CAT increases as item informativeness increases,[211] and item information is directly related to item discrimination.[205,212,213]

Debate

The intellectual and technical infrastructure for item banking, computerized adaptive testing, and test equating under IRT is at hand. What is not clear is whether it is desirable for health outcomes assessment to move toward item banking. Health status and HRQOL assessment can both be praised and faulted for the number of tools that have been generated in the last 35 years. There have been both innovations and repetitions. The same, of course, could apply in the future to item banks, where investigators argue about the extent to which "my bank is better than yours." Applications of IRT in education have been led by world-renowned scholars in measurement at the Educational Testing Service (ETS), a not-for-profit enterprise. Because it is not-for-profit, conflict of interest due to profit motive is less salient. As movements begin in health outcomes assessment toward the development of item banks, linking studies, and computerized adaptive testing,[21,30,214–216] earnest thought will need to be given to whether profit motive will corrupt or enhance the measurement developments that are on the cusp.

A bank is a composite of the work of hundreds of individuals over time. For the most fair and productive use, it would be desirable to have health banks reside in the public domain, since their constituent parts were developed with public monies in one form or another. Health banks could reside within the National Center for Health Statistics, or the Agency for Healthcare Research and Quality, or they could be operated by a non-profit organization, similar to the ETS. Regardless, item banks require regular attention in terms of retiring items that become outdated or obsolete or whose item parameters change over time. New items need to be added to the bank in response to natural history and would need to be linked into the bank and calibrated. The population invariance property of IRT makes it possible to update item parameters using different samples of examinees.[217]

In health status assessment, where there exist over two dozen generic measures[21] and hundreds of disease-specific measures,[22,23] dialogue among measurement specialists has sometimes resembled a childhood fistacuffs with claims of "my tool is better than yours." However, at least these dialogues have taken place within the context of peer-reviewed science. If measurement developments move from the halls of academia to the private sector, we may continue to hear the polemic of "my item bank is better than yours," but without the safeguard of peer review. As Shapiro[218] argues, privatization can be problematic in that it results in a loss of openness among scholars, a failure to completely disclose the methods and results of research, and a tendency to not publish at all or to only publish results that make the "product" look good.

Conclusion

Much has been accomplished in health assessment and HRQOL assessment in the last 40 years. Measurement specialists are at the cusp of a paradigm shift[21] away from sizable reliance on classical test methods to broader use of IRT methods. There is much to be both excited and cautious about as IRT methods are used for test construction, scaling, and score equating, as well as for identifying item bias and supporting functions such as computerized adaptive testing. It may be desirable to reach consensus among stakeholders – methodologists, users, policy makers, and funders – about the relative merits of any alternative course which outcomes measurement could assume in the years ahead before any one road is definitively taken. We offer the ten Ds herein as a platform for informing and stimulating discussion about how and where measurement advances might proceed.

REFERENCES

1 White, K. L. (1967). Improved medical care statistics and the health services system. *Public Health Reports* **82**(10):847–54.

2 Trask, J. (1935). Vital Statistics. In *Preventive Medicine and Hygiene*, ed. M. Rosenau, pp. 1175–220. New York, NY: D. Appleton-Century Company.

3 Cumming, H. (1936). Chronic disease as a public health problem. *The Milbank Memorial Fund Quarterly* **14**:125–31.

4 Hailman, D. (1941). Health status of adults in the productive ages. *Public Health Reports* **56**:2071–87.

5 Collins, S. (1949). Sickness Surveys. In *Administrative Medicine*, ed. H. Emerson, pp. 511–35. New York: Thomas Nelson & Sons.

6 Logan, W., Brooke, E. (1953). The Survey of Sickness 1943 to 1952. *Studies on Medical and Population Subject*s **12**:1–43.

7 Sheldon, M. (1935). A physical achievement record. *Journal of Health and Physical Education* **30**:1.

8 Deaver, G., Brown, M. (1945). *Physical Demands of Daily Life: An Objective Scale for Rating the Orthopedically Exceptional*. New York, NY: Institute for the Crippled and Disabled.

9 Bennett, R., Stephens, H. (1949). Functional testing and training. *The Physical Therapy Review* **29**(3):99–107.

10 Moskowitz, E., McCann, C. B. (1957). Classification of disability in the chronically ill and aging. *Journal of Chronic Diseases* **5**(3):342–6.

11 Mahoney, F., Wood, O., Barthel, D. (1958). Rehabilitation of chronically ill patients. *Southern Medical Journal* **51**:605–9.

12 Staff of the Benjamin Rose Hospital (1959). Multidisciplinary studies of illness in aged persons: II. A new classification of functional status in activities of daily living. *Journal of Chronic Diseases* **19**(1):55–62.

13 US Department of Health, Education, and Welfare (1964). Health survey procedure: Concepts, questionnaire development, and definitions in the health interview survey. *Vital and Health Statistics: Programs and Collection Procedures* **1**(2):1–66.

14 Hoffer, C. R., Schuler, E. A. (1948). Measurement of health needs and health care. *American Sociological Review* **13**:719–24.

15 Brodman, K., Erdmann, A., Wolff, H. (1949). The Cornell Medical Index. *Journal of the American Medical Association* **140**(6):530–4.

16 Souelem, O. (1955). Mental patients' attitudes toward mental hospitals. *Journal of Clinical Psychology* **11**:181–5.

17 Klopfer, W. G., Wylie, A. A., Hillson, J. S. (1956). Attitudes toward mental hospitals. *Journal of Clinical Psychology* **12**:361–5.

18 Hecker, J., Lewis, C. E. (1965). Factors determining attitudes towards medical care – study of a metropolitan area. *Journal of the Kansas Medical Society* **66**:123–8.

19 McHorney, C. (2002). Use of item response theory to link three modules of functional status items from the Asset and Health Dynamics among the Oldest Old Study. *Archives of Physical Medicine and Rehabilitation* **83**(3):383–94.

20 Task Force for the Handbook of Psychiatric Measures (2000). *Handbook of Psychiatric Measures*. Washington, DC: American Psychiatric Association.

21 McHorney, C. (1997). Generic health measurement: past accomplishments and a measurement paradigm for the 21st century. *Annals of Internal Medicine* **127**:743–50.

22 McHorney, C. (1999). Health status assessment methods for adults: past accomplishments and future challenges. *Annual Review of Public Health* **20**:309–35.

23 Bowling, A. (2001). *Measuring Disease: A Review of Disease-Specific Quality of Life Measurement Scales* (2nd Edition). Buckingham: Open University Press.

24 McHorney, C. A. (2001). Prospects and Problems Associated with Item Banking and Computerized Adaptive Testing in Cancer Clinical Trials. National Cancer Institute, Cancer Outcomes Working Group Symposium, February 2001, Bethesda, MD.

25 Gulliksen, H. (1950). *Theory of Mental Tests*. New York: John Wiley & Sons.

26 Lord, F. M., Novick, M. R. (1968). *Statistical Theories of Mental Test Scores*. Reading, MA: Addison-Wesley Publishing Company.

27 Hambleton, R., Swaminathan, H. (1985). *Item Response Theory: Principles and Applications*. Boston, MA: Kluwer Nijoff Publishing.

28 McHorney, C., Cohen, A. (2000). Equating health status measures with item response theory: illustrations with functional status items. *Medical Care* **38**(9, Suppl. II):II43–59.

29 Cleary, P. D. (1996). Future directions of quality of life research. In *Quality of Life and Pharmacoeconomics in Clinical Trials* (2nd Edition), ed. B. Spilker, pp. 73–8. Philadelphia, PA: Lippincott-Raven.

30 Hambleton, R. (2000). Emergence of item response modeling in instrument development and data analysis. *Medical Care* **38**(9):II60–5.

31 Teresi, J. (2001). Statistical methods for examination of differential item functioning (DIF) with applications to cross-cultural measurement of functional, physical and mental health. *Journal of Mental Health and Aging* **7**(1):31–40.

32 Lord, F. M. (1980). *Applications of Item Response Theory to Practical Testing Problems*. Hillsdale, NJ: Lawrence Erlbaum Associates.

33 Baker, F. (1992). *Item Response Theory: Parameter Estimation*. New York: Springer-Verlag.

34 Gill, T. M., Feinstein, A. R. (1994). A critical appraisal of the quality of quality-of-life measurements. *Journal of the American Medical Association* **272**(8):619–26.

35 Leplege, A., Hunt, S. (1997). The problem of quality of life in medicine. *Journal of the American Medical Association* **278**(1):47–50.

36 World Health Organization (1947). *Chronicle of the World Health Organization* **1**(1–2):13.

37 Ahmed, P., Kolker, A. (1973). The role of indigenous medicine in WHO's definition of health. In *Toward A New Definition of Health: Psychosocial Dimensions*, ed. P. Ahmed, G. Coelgo, pp. 113–28. New York: Plenum Press.

38 Stewart, A. L., Ware, J. E. (1992). *Measuring Functioning and Well-Being: The Medical Outcomes Study Approach.* Durham, NC: Duke University Press.

39 Meenan, R. F., Gertman, P. M., Mason, J. H. (1980). Measuring health status in arthritis. *Arthritis and Rheumatism* **23**(2):146–52.

40 Roland, M., Morris, R. (1983). A study of the natural history of back pain part I: development of a reliable and sensitive measure of disability in low-back pain. *Spine* **8**(2):141–4.

41 Wu, A. W., Rubin, H. R., Mathews, W. C. *et al.* (1991). A health status questionnaire using 30 items from the Medical Outcomes Study: preliminary validation in persons with early HIV infection. *Medical Care* **29**(8):786–98.

42 Ingersoll, G., Marrero, D. (1991). A modified quality-of-life measure for youths: psychometric properties. *The Diabetes Educator* **17**(2):114–18.

43 Marks, G. B., Dunn, S. M., Woolcock, A. J. (1992). A scale for the measurement of quality of life in adults with asthma. *Journal of Clinical Epidemiology* **45**(5):461–72.

44 Hyland, M., Bott, J., Singh, S. *et al.* (1994). Domains, constructs and the development of the breathing problems questionnaire. *Quality of Life Research* **3**:245–56.

45 McHorney, C., Bricker, D., Kramer, A. *et al.* (2000). The SWAL-QOL outcomes tool for oropharyngeal dysphagia in adults: I. Conceptual foundation and item development. *Dysphagia* **15**:115–21.

46 McHorney, C. Methodological and psychometric issues in health status assessment across populations and applications. In *Advances in Medical Sociology,* Vol. 5, ed. G. L. Albrecht, R. Fitzpatrick, pp. 281–304. Stamford, CT: JAI Press.

47 McHorney, C. A., Ware, J. E., Lu, J. F. R. *et al.* (1994). The MOS 36-item short-form health survey (SF-36): III. Tests of data quality, scaling assumptions and reliability across diverse patient groups. *Medical Care* **32**(1):40–66.

48 Jobe, J. B., Mingay, D. J. (1990). Cognitive laboratory approach to designing questionnaires for surveys of the elderly. *Public Health Reports* **105**(5):518–24.

49 Lessler, J. (1995). Choosing questions that people can understand and answer. *Medical Care* **33** (4 Suppl.):AS203–8.

50 Weitzner, M., Meyers, C., Steinbruecker, S. *et al.* (1997). Developing a care giver quality-of-life instrument. *Cancer Practice* **5**(1):25–31.

51 Moore, K. N., Estey, A. (1999). The early post-operative concerns of men after radical prostatectomy. *Journal of Advanced Nursing* **29**(5):1121–9.

52 Hobart, J., Lamping, D., Fitzpatrick, R. *et al.* (2001). The Multiple Sclerosis Impact Scale (MSIS-29): a new patient-based outcome measure. *Brain* **124**:962–73.

53 Kadam, U. T., Croft, P., McLeod, M. *et al.* (2001). A qualitative study on patients' views on anxiety and depression. *British Journal of General Practice* **51**(466):375–80.

54 Ware, N., Tugenberg, T., Dickey, B. *et al.* (1999). An ethnographic study of the meaning of continuity of care in mental health services. *Psychiatric Services* **50**(3):395–400.

55 Angel, R., Frisco, M. (2001). Self-assessments of health and functional capacity among older adults. *Journal of Mental Health and Aging* **7**(1):119–35.

56 De Geest, S., Abraham, I., Gemoets, H. *et al.* (1994). Development of the long-term medication behaviour self-efficacy scale: qualitative study for item development. *Journal of Advanced Nursing* **19**:233–8.

57 Porter, E. (1995). A phenomenological alternative to the "ADL Research Tradition". *Journal of Aging and Health* **7**(1):24–45.

58 Krasner, D. (1998). Painful venous ulcers: themes and stories about their impact on quality of life. *Ostomy/Wound Management* **44**(9):38–49.

59 Koch, T., Webb, C., Williams, A. (1995). Listening to the voices of older patients: an existential-phenomenological approach to quality assurance. *Journal of Clinical Nursing* **4**:185–93.

60 Spies, J., Coyne, K., Guaou, N. *et al.* (2002). The UFS-QOL, a new disease-specific symptom and health-related quality of life questionnaire for leiomyomata. *Obstetrics and Gynecology* **99**(2):290–300.

61 Lerner, D., Amick, B., Rogers, W. *et al.* (2001). The Work Limitations Questionnaire. *Medical Care* **39**(1):72–85.

62 Wu, A., Fink, N., Cagney, K. *et al.* (2001). Developing a health-related quality-of-life measure for end-stage renal disease: The CHOICE Health Experiences Questionnaire. *American Journal of Kidney Diseases* **37**(1):11–21.

63 Juniper, E. F., Guyatt, G. H., Epstein, R. S. *et al.* (1992). Evaluation of impairment of health related quality of life in asthma: development of a questionnaire for use in clinical trials. *Thorax* **47**:76–83.

64 Wilde, B., Larsson, G., Larsson, M. *et al.* (1994). Quality of care: development of a patient-centred questionnaire based on a grounded theory model. *Scandinavian Journal of the Caring Sciences* **8**:39–48.

65 Launois, R., Reboul-Marty, J., Henry, E. (1996). Construction and validation of a quality of life questionnaire in chronic lower limb venous insufficiency (CIVIQ). *Quality of Life Research* **5**:539–54.

66 Rubin, H., Jenckes, M., Fink, N. *et al.* (1997). Patient's view of dialysis care: development of a taxonomy and rating of importance of different aspects of care. *American Journal of Kidney Diseases* **30**(6):793–801.

67 Cronin, L., Guyatt, G., Griffith, L. *et al.* (1998). Development of a health-related quality-of-life questionnaire (PCOSQ) for women with polycystic ovary syndrome (PCOS). *Journal of Clinical Endocrinology and Metabolism* **83**(6): 1976–87.

68 Jabine, T., Straf, M., Tanue, J. *et al.* (1984). *Cognitive Aspects of Survey Methodology.* Washington, DC: National Academy Press.

69 Fienberg, S., Loftus, E., Tanur, J. (1985). Cognitive aspects of health survey methodology: an overview. *Milbank Memorial Fund Quarterly* **63**(3):547–64.

70 Lessler, J. T., Sirken, M. G. (1985). Laboratory-based research on the cognitive aspects of survey methodology: the goals and methods of the National Center for Health Statistics study. *Milbank Memorial Fund Quarterly. Health and Society* **63**(3):565–81.

71 Loftus, E., Fienberg, S., Tanur, J. (1985). Cognitive psychology meets the national survey. *American Psychologist* **40**(2):175–80.

72 Jobe, J. B., Mingay, D. J. (1989). Cognitive research improves questionnaires. *American Journal of Public Health* **79**(8):1053–5.

73 Bergner, M., Bobbitt, R. A., Pollard, W. E. *et al.* (1976). The Sickness Impact Profile: validation of a health status measure. *Medical Care* **14**(1):57–67.

74 Ware, J., Kosinski, M., Bayliss, M. *et al.* (1995). Comparison of methods for the scoring and statistical analysis of SF-36 health profile and summary measures: Summary of results from the MOS. *Medical Care* **33** (4 Suppl.):AS264–79.

75 Bozzette, S., Hays, R., Berry, S. *et al.* (1994). A perceived health index for use in persons with advanced HIV disease: derivation, reliability, and validity. *Medical Care* **32**(7):716–31.

76 Bozzette, S. A., Hays, R. D., Berry, S. H. *et al.* (1995). Derivation and properties of a brief health status assessment instrument for use in HIV disease. *Journal of Acquired Immune Deficiency Syndromes and Human Retrovirology* **8**(3):253–65.

77 Devinsky, O., Vickrey, B., Cramer, J. *et al.* (1995). Development of the quality of life in epilepsy inventory. *Epilepsia* **36**(11):1089–104.

78 Vickery, B., Hays, R., Garooni, R. *et al.* (1995). A health-related quality of life measure for multiple sclerosis. *Quality of Life Research* **4**:187–206.

79 Revicki, D., Sorensen, S., Wu, A. (1998). Reliability and validity of physical and mental health summary scores from the Medical Outcomes Study HIV health survey. *Medical Care* **36**(2):126–37.

80 Varni, J., Seid, M., Kurtin, P. (2001). PedsQL 4.0: Reliability and validity of the pediatric quality of life inventory version 4.0 generic core scales in healthy and patient populations. *Medical Care* **39**(8):800–12.

81 Simon, G., Revicki, D., Grothaus, L. *et al.* (1998). SF-36 summary scores. Are physical and mental health truly distinct? *Medical Care* **36**(4):567–72.

82 Rubenach, S., Shadbolt, B., McCallum, J. *et al.* (2002). Assessing health-related quality of life following myocardial infarction: is the SF-12 useful? *Journal of Clinical Epidemiology* **55**:306–9.

83 Fairclough, D. (1997). Summary measures and statistics for comparisons of quality of life in a clinical trial of cancer therapy. *Statistics in Medicine* **16**:1197–209.

84 Beusterien, K., Nissenson, A., Port, F. K. *et al.* (1996). The effects of recombinant human erythropoietin on functional health and well-being in chronic dialysis patients. *Journal of the American Society of Nephrology* **7**(5):763–73.

85 Jenkinson, C., Gray, A., Doll, H. *et al.* (1997). Evaluation of index and profile measures of health status in a randomized controlled trial. *Medical Care* **35**(11):1109–18.

86 Ruhland, J., Shields, R. (1997). The effects of a home exercise program on impairment and health-related quality of life in persons with chronic peripheral neuropathies. *Physical Therapy* **77**(10):1026–39.

87 Gartsman, G., Brinker, M., Khan, M. *et al.* (1998). Self assessment of general health status in patients with five common shoulder conditions. *Journal of Shoulder and Elbow Surgery* **7**(3):228–37.

88 Gartsman, G., Khan, M., Hammerman, S. (1998). Arthroscopic repair of full-thickness tears of the rotator cuff. *Journal of Bone and Joint Surgery* **80-A**(6):832–40.

89 Wiklund, I., Junghard, O., Grace, E. *et al.* (1998). Quality of life in reflux and dyspepsia patients. Psychometric

documentation of a new specific questionarie (QOLRAD). *European Journal of Surgery* **583**(Suppl.):41–9.

90 Reuben, D. B., Frank, J. C., Hirsch, S. H. *et al.* (1999). A randomized clinical trial of outpatient comprehensive geriatric assessment coupled with an intervention to increase adherence to recommendations. *Journal of the American Geriatrics Society* **47**:269–76.

91 Revicki, D., Crawley, J., Zodet, M. *et al.* (1999). Complete resolution of heartburn symptoms and health-related quality of life in patients with gastro-oesophageal reflux disease. *Alimentary Pharmacology and Therapeutics* **13**:1621–30.

92 Stavem, K., Erikssen, J., Boe, J. (1999). Performance of a short lung-specific health status measure in outpatients with chronic obstructive pulmonary disease. *Respiratory Medicine* **93**:467–75.

93 Taylor, S., Taylor, A., Foy, M. *et al.* (1999). Responsiveness of common outcome measures for patients with low back pain. *Spine* **24**:1805–12.

94 Adler, D., Bungay, K., Cynn, D. *et al.* (2000). Patient-based health status assessments in an outpatient psychiatry setting. *Psychiatric Services* **51**(3):341–8.

95 Hughes, S., Weaver, F., Giobbie-Harder, A. *et al.* (2000). Effectiveness of team-managed home-based primary care: a randomized multicenter trial. *Journal of the American Medical Association* **284**(22):2877–85.

96 Mayo, N., Wood-Dauphinee, S., Cote, R. *et al.* (2000). There's no place like home: an evaluation of early supported discharge for stroke. *Stroke* **31**:1016–23.

97 Nortvedt, M. W., Riise, T., Myhr, K.-M. *et al.* (2000). Performance of the SF-36, SF-12 and RAND-36 summary scales in a multiple sclerosis population. *Medical Care* **38**(10):1022–8.

98 Hobart, J., Freeman, J., Lamping, D. *et al.* (2001). The SF-36 in multiple sclerosis: why basic assumptions must be tested. *Journal of Neurology, Neurosurgery, and Psychiatry* **71**(3):363–70.

99 Roznowski, M., Tucker, L., Humphreys, L. (1991). Three approaches to determining the dimensionality of binary items. *Applied Psychological Measurement* **15**(2):109–27.

100 US Department of Health and Human Services. *Healthy People 2010 [Web Page]*. Available at http://www.healthypeople.gov/document/. Accessed September 18, 2004.

101 National Institutes of Health. *Addressing Health Disparities: The NIH Program of Action*. Available at http://healthdisparities.nih.gov/whatare.html. Accessed September 18, 2004.

102 McKinlay, J. B., McKinlay, S. M., Beaglehole, R. (1989). A review of the evidence concerning the impact of medical measures on recent mortality and morbidity in the United States. *International Journal of Health Services* **19**(2):181–208.

103 Evans, R., Stoddart, G. (1992). Producing health, consuming health care. *Social Science and Medicine* **35**:1347–63.

104 U.S. Department of Health and Human Services. (1979). *Risks to good health. Healthy People – the Surgeon General's Report on Health Promotion and Disease Prevention*. Hyattsville, MD: U.S. Department of Health and Human Services, Public Health Service, Office of the Assistant Secretary for Health and Surgeon General, (PHS) 79-55071.

105 McHorney, C. (1999). Concepts and Measurement of Health Status and Health-Related Quality of Life. In *The Handbook of Social Studies in Health & Medicine*, ed. G. L. Albrecht, R. Fitzpatrick, S. Scrimshaw, pp. 339–58. London: Sage.

106 Blaxter, M. (1987). Evidence on inequality in health from a national survey. *Lancet* **2**(8549):30–3.

107 House, J. S., Kessler, R. C., Regula, A. (1990). Age, socioeconomic status, and health. *Milbank Memorial Fund Quarterly* **68**(3):383–412.

108 Arber, S., Ginn, J. (1993). Gender and inequalities in health in later life. *Social Science and Medicine* **36**(1):33–46.

109 Guralnik, J. M., Land, K. C., Blazer, D. *et al.* (1993). Educational status and active life expectancy among older blacks and whites. *New England Journal of Medicine* **329**(2):110–16.

110 Sorlie, P., Backlund, E., Keller, J. (1995). US mortality by economic, demographic, and social characteristics: the national longitudinal mortality study. *American Journal of Public Health* **85**(7):949–56.

111 Schoenbaum, M., Waidmann, T. (1997). Race, socioeconomic status, and health: accounting for race differences in health. *Journal of Gerontology* **52B**(Special Issue): 61–73.

112 Kind, P., Dolan, P., Gudex, C. *et al.* (1998). Variations in population health status: results from a United Kingdom national questionnaire survey. *British Medical Journal* **316**:736–41.

113 Adams, P., Hendershot, G. E., Marano, M. (1999). *Current Estimates from the National Health Interview Survey, 1996. Data from the National Health Survey; Vol. 10*. Hyattsville, MD: U.S. Department of Health and Human Services; (PHS) 99–1528.

114 Stewart, A., Napoles-Springer, A. (2000). Health-related quality-of-life assessments in diverse population groups in the United States. *Medical Care* **38**(9, Suppl.):II-102–24.

115 Day, J. (1996). *Population Projections of the United States by Age, Sex, Race, and Hispanic Origin: 1995 to 2050*. Washington, DC: US Government Printing Office.

116 Liang, J. (2001). Assessing cross-cultural comparability in mental health among older adults. *Journal of Mental Health and Aging* **7**(1):21–30.

117 Herdman, M., Fox-Rushby, J., Badia, X. (1997). 'Equivalence' and the translation and adaptation of health-related quality of life questionnaires. *Quality of Life Research* **6**:237–47.

118 Byrne, B., Campbell, T. (1999). Cross-cultural comparisons and the presumption of equivalent measurement and theoretical structure. A look beneath the surface. *Journal of Cross-Cultural Psychology* **30**(5):555–74.

119 Kleinman, A. (1977). Depression, somatization and the new cross-cultural psychiatry. *Social Science and Medicine* **11**:3–10.

120 Flaherty, J., Gaviria, F., Pathak, D. *et al.* (1988). Developing instruments for cross-cultural psychiatric research. *Journal of Nervous and Mental Disease* **176**(5):257–63.

121 Pelto, P., Pelto, G. (1997). Studying knowledge, culture, and behavior in applied medical anthropology. *Medical Anthropology Quarterly* **11**(2):147–63.

122 Lutner, R., Foizen, M., Stocking, C. (1991). The automated interview versus the personal interview. *Anesthesiology* **75**:394–400.

123 Rozensky, R., Honor, L., Rasinski, K. *et al.* (1986). Paper-and-pencil versus computer-administered MMPIs: a comparison of patients' attitudes. *Computers in Human Behavior* **2**:111–16.

124 Greist, J., Klein, M., Erdman, H. *et al.* (1987). Comparison of computer- and interviewer-administered versions of the Diagnostic Interview Schedule. *Hospital and Community Psychiatry* **38**(12):1304–11.

125 Kobak, K., Reynolds, W., Rosenfeld, R. *et al.* (1990). Development and validation of a computer-administered version of the Hamilton Depression Rating Scale. *Psychological Assessment* **2**(1):56–63.

126 Baer, L., Brown-Beasley, M., Sorce, J. *et al.* (1993). Computer-assisted telephone administration of a structured interview for obsessive-compulsive disorders. *American Journal of Psychiatry* **150**:1737–8.

127 Kobak, K., Reynolds, W., Greist, J. (1993). Development and validation of a computer-administered version of the Hamilton Anxiety Scale. *Psychological Assessment* **5**(4):487–92.

128 Baer, L., Jacobs, D. G., Cukor, P. *et al.* (1995). Automated telephone screening survey for depression. *Journal of the American Medical Association* **273**(24):1943–4.

129 Roizen, M. F., Coalson, D., Hayward, R. S. A. *et al.* (1992). Can patients use an automated questionnaire to define their current health status? *Medical Care* **30**(5 Suppl.):MS74–84.

130 Newell, S., Girgis, A., Sanson-Fisher, R. *et al.* (1997). Are touch-screen computer surveys acceptable to medical oncology patients? *Journal of Psychosocial Oncology* **15**(2):37–46.

131 Taenzer, P., Speca, M., Atkinson, M. *et al.* (1997). Computerized quality-of-life screening in an oncology clinic. *Cancer Practice* **5**(3):168–75.

132 Buxton, J., White, M., Osoba, D. (1998). Patients' experiences using a computerized program with a touch-sensitive video monitor for the assessment of health-related quality of life. *Quality of Life Research* **7**:513–17.

133 McBride, J., Anderson, R., Bahnson, J. (1999). Using a hand-held computer to collect data in an orthopedic outpatient clinic. *Medical Care* **37**(7):647–51.

134 Velikova, G., Wright, E. P., Smith, A. B. *et al.* (1999). Automated collection of quality-of-life data: a comparison of paper and computer touch-screen questionnaires. *Journal of Clinical Oncology* **17**(3):998–1007.

135 Lofland, J., Schaffer, M., Goldfarb, N. (2000). Evaluating health-related quality of life: cost comparison of computerized touch-screen technology and traditional paper systems. *Pharmacotherapy* **20**(11):1390–5.

136 Taenzer, P., Bultz, B., Carlson, L. *et al.* (2000). Impact of computerized quality of life screening on physician behavior and patient satisfaction in lung cancer outpatients. *Psycho-Oncology* **9**:203–13.

137 Carlson, L., Speca, M., Hagen, N. *et al.* (2001). Computerized quality of life screening in a cancer pain clinic. *Journal of Palliative Care* **17**(1):46–52.

138 Ernst, M., Doucette, W., Dedhiya, S. *et al.* (2001). Use of point-of-service health status assessments by community pharmacists to identify and resolve drug-related problems in patients with musculoskeletal disorders. *Pharmacotherapy* **21**(8):988–97.

139 Brodie, M., Fournoy, R., Altman, D. *et al.* (2000). Health information, the internet, and the digital divide. *Health Affairs* **19**(6):255–65.

140 Burstin, H. (2000). Traversing the digital divided. *Health Affairs* **19**(6):245–9.

141 Ree, M. (1993). Foreword: Differential Item Functioning (DIF): A perspective from the Air Force Human Resources Laboratory. In *Differential Item Functioning*, ed. P. Holland, H. Wainer, pp. xi–xii. Hillsdale, NJ: Lawrence Erlbaum Associates.

142 Hambleton, R. (2001). The next generation of the ITC test translation and adaptation guidelines. *European Journal of Psychological Assessment* **17**(3):164–72.

143 Teresi, J., Cross, P., Golden, R. (1989). Some applications of latent trait analysis to the measurement of ADL. *Journal of Gerontology* **44**(5):S196–204.

144 Groenvold, M., Bjorner, J. B., Klee, M. C. *et al.* (1995). Test for item bias in a quality of life questionnaire. *Journal of Clinical Epidemiology* **48**(6):805–16.

145 Avlund, K., Era, P., Davidsen, M. *et al.* (1996). Item bias in self-reported functional ability among 75-year-old men and women in three Nordic localities. *Scandinavian Journal of Social Medicine* **24**(3):206–17.

146 Kempen, G., Miedema, I., Ormel, J. *et al.* (1996). The assessment of disability with the Groningen Activity Restriction Scale. Conceptual framework and psychometric properties. *Social Science and Medicine* **43**(11):1601–10.

147 Spector, W., Fleishman, J. (1998). Combining activities of daily living with instrumental activities of daily living to measure functional disability. *Journal of Gerontology* **53**(1):S46–57.

148 Custers, J., Hiujtink, H., van der Net, J. *et al.* (2000). Cultural differences in functional status measurement: analyses of person fit according to the Rasch model. *Quality of Life Research* **9**:571–8.

149 Wolfe, F., Hawley, D., Goldenberg, D. *et al.* (2000). The assessment of functional impairment in fibromyalgia (FM): Rasch analyses of 5 functional scales and the development of the FM Health Assessment Questionnaire. *Journal of Rheumatology* **27**(8):1989–99.

150 Jagger, C., Arthur, A., Spiers, N. *et al.* (2001). Patterns of onset of disability in activities of daily living. *Journal of the American Geriatric Society* **49**(4):404–9.

151 Teresi, J. A., Golden, R. R., Cross, P. *et al.* (1995). Item bias in cognitive screening measures: Comparisons of elderly White, Afro-American, Hispanic and high and low education subgroups. *Journal of Clinical Epidemiology* **48**(4):473–83.

152 Teresi, J., Kleinman, M., Ocepek, K. (2000). Modern psychometric methods for detection of differential item functioning: application to cognitive assessment measures. *Statistics in Medicine* **19**:1651–83.

153 Teresi, J., Kleinman, M., Ocepek-Welikson, K. *et al.* (2000). Applications of item response theory to the examination of the psychometric properties and differential item functioning of the comprehensive assessment and referral evaluation dementia diagnostic scale among samples of Latino, African American, and white non-latino elderly. *Research on Aging* **22**(6):738–73.

154 Teresi, J., Holmes, D., Ramirez, M. *et al.* (2001). Performance of cognitive tests among different racial/ethnic and education groups: findings of differential item functioning and possible item bias. *Journal of Mental Health and Aging* **7**(1):79–89.

155 Bjorner, J. B., Kreiner, S., Ware, J. E. (1998). Differential item functioning in the Danish translation of the SF-36. *Journal of Clinical Epidemiology* **51**(11):1189–202.

156 Collins, W., Raju, N., Edwards, J. (2000). Assessing differential functioning in a satisfaction scale. *Journal of Applied Psychology* **85**(3):451–61.

157 Morales, L., Reise, S., Hays, R. (2000). Evaluating the equivalence of health care ratings by whites and Hispanics. *Medical Care* **38**(5):517–27.

158 Schaeffer, N. (1988). An application of item response theory to the measurement of depression. In *Sociological Methodology*, ed. C. Clogg, pp. 271–307. San Francisco, CA: Jossey-Bass.

159 Ellis, B. B., Minsel, B., Becker, P. (1989). Evaluation of attitude survey translations: an investigation using item response theory. *International Journal of Psychology* **24**:665–84.

160 Ellis, B. E., Kimmell, H. (1992). Identification of unique cultural response patterns by means of item response theory. *Journal of Applied Psychology* **77**(2):177–84.

161 Stommel, M., Given, B., Given, C. *et al.* (1993). Gender bias in the measurement properties of the Center for Epidemiologic Studies Depression Scale (CES-D). *Psychiatry Research* **49**:239–50.

162 Dancer, L., Anderson, A., Derlin, R. (1994). Use of log-linear models for assessing differential item functioning in a measure of psychological functioning. *Journal of Consulting and Clinical Psychology* **62**(4):710–17.

163 Flannery, W., Reise, S., Widaman, K. (1995). An item response theory analysis of the general and academic scales of the Self-Description Questionnaire II. *Journal of Research in Personality* **29**:168–88.

164 Hammond, S. (1995). An IRT investigation of the validity of non-patient analogue research using the Beck Depression Inventory. *European Journal of Psychologic Assessment* **11**(1):14–20.

165 Huang, C., Church, A., Katigbak, M. (1997). Identifying cultural differences in items and traits. *Journal of Cross-Cultural Psychology* **28**(2):192–218.

166 Panter, A., Swygert, K., Dahlstrom, W. *et al.* (1997). Factor analytic approaches to personality item-level data. *Journal of Personality Assessment* **68**(3):561–89.

167 Suh, T., Gallo, J. (1997). Symptom profiles of depression among general medical service users compared with specialty mental health service users. *Psychological Medicine* **27**:1051–63.

168 Coelho, V., Strauss, M., Jenkins, J. (1998). Expression of symptomatic distress by Puerto Rican and Euro-American patients with depression and schizophrenia. *Journal of Nervous and Mental Disease* **186**(8):477–83.

169 DeRoos, Y., Allen-Meares, P. (1998). Application of Rasch analysis: exploring differences in depression between African-American and white children. *Journal of Social Science Research* **23**(3/4):93–107.

170 Gallo, J., Cooper-Patrick, L., Lesikar, S. (1998). Depressive symptoms of whites and African Americans aged 60 years and older. *Journal of Gerontology* **53B**(5):P277–86.

171 Santor, D., Ramsay, J. (1998). Progress in the technology of measurement: applications of item response models. *Psychological Assessment* **10**(1):345–59.

172 Smith, L., Reise, S. (1998). Gender differences on negative affectivity: an IRT study of differential item functioning on the multidimensional personality questionnaire stress reaction scale. *Journal of Personality and Social Psychology* **75**(5):1350–62.

173 Christensen, H., Jorm, A., MacKinnon, A. *et al.* (1999). Age differences in depression and anxiety symptoms: A structural equation modeling analysis of data from a general population sample. *Psychological Medicine* **29**(2): 325–39.

174 Cooke, D., Michie, C. (1999). Psychopathy across cultures: North America and Scotland compared. *Journal of Abnormal Psychology* **108**(1):58–68.

175 Grayson, D., Mackinnon, A., Jorm, A. (2000). Item bias in the Center for Epidemiologic Studies Depression scale: effects of physical disorders and disability in an elderly community sample. *Journal of Gerontology* **55B**(5):P273–82.

176 Waller, N., Thompson, J., Wenk, E. (2000). Using IRT to separate measurement bias from true group differences on homogeneous and heterogeneous scales: An illustration with the MMPI. *Psychological Methods* **5**(1):125–46.

177 Azocar, F., Arean, P., Miranda, J. *et al.* (2001). Differential item functioning in a Spanish translation of the Beck Depression Inventory. *Journal of Clinical Psychology* **57**:355–65.

178 Santor, D., Coyne, J. (2001). Evaluating the continuity of symptomology between depressed and nondepressed individuals. *Journal of Abnormal Psychology* **110**(2):216–25.

179 Drasgow, F., Hulin, C. (1987). Cross-cultural measurement. *Interamerican Journal of Psychology* **21**(1–2):1–24.

180 Walstad, W. B., Robson, D. (1997). Differential item functioning and male-female differences on multiple-choice tests in economics. *Journal of Economic Education* **28**(2):155–71.

181 Guarnaccia, P. (1996). Anthropological perspectives: the importance of culture in the assessment of quality of life. In *Quality of Life and Pharmacoeconomics in Clinical Trials*, (2nd Edition), ed. B. Spilker, pp. 523–7. Philadelphia, PA: Lippincott-Raven.

182 Rogler, L. (1989). The meaning of culturally sensitive research in mental health. *American Journal of Psychiatry* **146**(3):296–303.

183 McHorney, C. A., Ware, J. E., Rogers, W. *et al.* (1992). The validity and relative precision of MOS short- and long-form health status scales and Dartmouth COOP Charts: Results from the Medical Outcomes Study. *Medical Care* **30**(Suppl.):MS253–65.

184 McHorney, C., Tarlov, A. (1995). The use of health status measures for individual patient level applications: problems and prospects. *Quality of Life Research* **3**(1):43–4.

185 McHorney, C. (1996). Measuring and monitoring general health status in elderly persons: practical and methodological issues in using the SF-36 health survey. *The Gerontologist* **38**(5):571–83.

186 Haley, S. M., McHorney, C. A., Ware, J. E. (1994). Evaluation of the MOS SF-36 physical functioning scale (PF-10): I. Unidimensionality and reproducibility of the Rasch item scale. *Journal of Clinical Epidemiology* **47**(6):671–84.

187 Prieto, L., Alonso, J., Lamarca, R. *et al.* (1998). Rasch measurement for reducing the items of the Nottingham Health Profile. *Journal of Outcome Measurement* **2**(4):285–301.

188 Finch, M., Kane, R., Philp, I. (1995). Developing a new metric for ADLs. *Journal of the American Geriatrics Society* **43**:877–84.

189 Grimby, G., Andrén, E., Holmgren, E. *et al.* (1996). Structure of a combination of functional independence measure and instrumental activity measure items in community-living persons: a study of individuals with cerebral palsy and spina bifida. *Archives of Physical Medicine and Rehabilitation* **77**:1109–14.

190 Nordenskiold, U. (1996). *Daily Activities in Women with Rheumatoid Arthritis*. Goteborg, Sweden: Goteborg University.

191 Doble, S. E., Fisher, A. G. (1998). The dimensionality and validity of the older Americans resource services (OARS) activities of daily living (ADL) scale. *Journal of Outcome Measurement* **2**(1):4–24.

192 Grimby, G., Andren, E., Daving, Y. *et al.* (1998). Dependence and perceived difficulty in daily activities in community-living stroke survivors 2 years after stroke. *Stroke* **29**:1843–9.

193 Carter, J., Wilkinson, L. (1984). A latent trait analysis of the MMPI. *Multivariate Behavioral Research* **19**:385–407.

194 Steinberg, L., Thissen, D. (1995). Item response theory in personality research. In *Personality, Research, Methods, and Theory: a Festschrift Honoring Donald W. Fisk*, ed. P. E.

Shrout, S. T. Fisk, pp. 161–81. Hillsdale, NJ: Lawrence Erlbaum Associates.

195 Gray-Little, B., Williams, V., Hancock, T. (1997). An item response theory analysis of the Rosenberg Self-Esteem Scale. *Personality and Social Psychology Bulletin* **23**(5):443–51.

196 Payne, S. (1951). *The Art of Asking Questions.* Princeton, NJ: Princeton University Press.

197 Wesman, A. (1971). Writing the test item. In *Educational Measurement*, ed. R. Thorndike, pp. 81–129. Washington, DC: American Council on Education.

198 Andrich, D. (1995). Distinctive and incompatible properties of the common classes of IRT models for graded responses. *Applied Psychological Measurement* **19**(1):101–19.

199 Wright, B., Masters, G. (1982). *Rating Scale Analysis.* Chicago, IL: MESA Press.

200 Gibbons, R., Clark, D., Cavanaugh, S. *et al.* (1985). Application of modern psychometric theory in psychiatric research. *Journal of Psychiatric Research* **19**(1):43–55.

201 Steinberg, L. (1994). Context and serial-order effects in personality measurement: limits on the generality of measuring changes the measure. *Journal of Personality and Social Psychology* **66**(2):341–9.

202 Kirisci, L., Clark, D., Moss, H. (1996). Reliability and validity of the State-Trait Anxiety Inventory for Children in adolescent substance abusers: Confirmatory factor analysis and item response theory. *Journal of Child and Adolescent Substance Abuse* **5**(3):57–69.

203 Kirisci, L., Moss, H., Tarter, R. (1996). Psychometric evaluation of the situational confidence questionnaire in adolescents: fitting a graded item response model. *Addictive Behaviors* **21**(3):303–17.

204 Cooke, D. J., Michie, C. (1997). An item response theory analysis of the Hare psychopathy checklist-revised. *Psychological Assessment* **9**(1):3–14.

205 Kim, Y., Pilkonis, P. A. (1999). Selecting the most informative items in the IIP scales for personality disorders: an application of item response theory. *Journal of Personality Disorders* **13**(2):157–74.

206 Waller, N. (1999). Searching for structure in the MMPI. In *The New Rules of Measurement*, ed. S. Embretson, S. Hershberger, pp. 185–217. Mahwah, NJ: Lawrence Erlbaum Associates.

207 Marshall, G., Orlando, M., Jaycox, L. *et al.* (2002). Development and validation of a modified version of the Peritraumatic Dissociative Experiences Questionnaire. *Psychological Assessment* **14**(2):123–34.

208 Masters, G. (1982). A Rasch model for partial credit scoring. *Psychometrika* **47**(2):149–74.

209 Kolen, M., Brennan, R. (1995). *Test Equating: Methods and Practices.* New York: Springer-Verlag.

210 Feuer, M., Holland, P., Green, B. *et al.* (1999). *Uncommon Measures: Equivalence and Linkage among Educational Tests.* Washington, DC: National Academy Press.

211 Reise, S., Henson, J. (2000). Computerization and adaptive administration of the NEO PI-R. *Psychological Assessment* **7**(4):347–67.

212 Green, B. F. (1983). The promise of tailored tests. In *Principles of Modern Psychological Measurement*, ed. H. Wainer, S. Messick, pp. 69–80. Hillsdale, NJ: Lawrence Erlbaum Associates.

213 Hambleton, R. K., Jones, R. W. (1993). Comparison of classical test theory and item response theory and their applications to test development. *Education Measurement: Issues and Practice* Fall:38–47.

214 Waller, N., Reise, S. (1989). Computerized adaptive personality assessment: an illustration with the Absorption Scale. *Journal of Personality and Social Psychology* **57**(6):1051–8.

215 Koch, W. R., Dodd, B. G., Fitzpatrick, S. J. (1990). Computerized adaptive measurements of attitudes. *Measurement and Evaluation in Counseling and Development* **23**:20–30.

216 Dodd, B., De Ayala, R., Koch, W. R. (1995). Computerized adaptive testing with polytomous items. *Applied Psychological Measurement* **19**(1):5–22.

217 Hambleton, R., Slater, S. (1997). Item response theory models and testing practices: current international status and future directions. *European Journal of Psychological Assessment* **13**(1):21–8.

218 Shapiro, M. (1994). Is the spirit of capitalism undermining the ethics of health services research? *Health Services Research* **28**(6):661–72.

Invited Paper C
The use of cognitive interviewing techniques in quality-of-life and patient-reported outcomes assessment*

Gordon Willis, Ph.D.,[1] Bryce B. Reeve, Ph.D.,[1] and Ivan Barofsky, Ph.D.[2]

[1]National Cancer Institute, Bethesda, MD
[2]The QOL Institute, East Sandwich, MA

As pointed out by multiple researchers, including several contributors to this volume, the designers of any health-related quality-of-life (HRQOL) questionnaire must consider the viewpoint of the individual who is asked to complete that instrument.[1-4] In particular, it is imperative that we understand the *cognitive aspects of the response process* – what the respondent understands the questions to be asking, his or her recall of relevant information (or failure to recall it), and other judgment and decision processes that influence the nature of the given answers that constitute our raw data. HRQOL instrument developers appear to vary widely in the extent to which they explicitly take into account respondent cognition, and several questionnaires have been either developed or evaluated through means that emphasize the respondent point of view or that empirically investigate key cognitive processes.[3,5]

However, the application of cognitive principles and techniques is inconsistent, often unsystematic, or not well documented. Ganz and Goodwin have suggested that instrument development is generally not a high priority in the peer-review process.[6] The purpose of the current chapter is to suggest means for enhancing both practice and communication between researchers in this regard by: (a) advocating the explicit use of the cognitive interviewing method as a systematic means for studying cognition, and (b) describing the ways this technique can be used to inform several key design decisions that confront HRQOL questionnaire developers. This chapter is not intended to review extant quality-of-life instruments (see Chapter 3 by Erickson in this volume).[7] Rather, we focus on the further development, evaluation, and pretesting of questionnaires having an HRQOL or patient-reported outcomes emphasis. Although we have chosen to focus on relatively general HRQOL measures that may not specifically encompass cancer outcomes, we note that such measures are frequently used within cancer-oriented studies.[7,8] Further, the interviewing methods to be described are fully applicable to cancer-specific HRQOL measures and may be applicable more broadly.

Background: cognitive interviewing and questionnaire design

Starting in the early 1980s, a series of conferences were convened to examine the cognitive aspects of survey methodology, or CASM.[9] Subsequently, cognitive psychologists and survey researchers developed an interdiscipline which asserts that standardization, field testing, and even psychometric

---

*The validity and interpretability of any patient-reported outcome measure hinges in part on whether the respondent understands what is being asked and can successfully recall and synthesize the appropriate information. For an examination of important cognitive aspects of outcomes assessment, the NCI turned to three noted measurement experts: Gordon Willis, Ph.D., cognitive psychologist; Bryce B. Reeve, Ph.D., psychometrician; and Ivan Barofsky, Ph.D., a psychologist who has written widely on health-related quality of life measurement in cancer.

testing of questionnaires are insufficient to ensure that respondents understand the questions asked and that the investigator appropriately interprets the answers given. A major approach to bridging the gap between the respondent and investigator was to encourage the development of the *cognitive interview* as a means for reducing measurement error. Briefly, cognitive interviewing consists of survey questionnaire pretesting or evaluation through the use of interviews in which a specially trained interviewer administers draft survey questions to the subject. However, in addition to eliciting answers, the interviewer delves into the subject's cognitive processing of the questions to obtain information relevant to potential sources of response error. A basic assumption underlying this approach is that in order to answer a survey question meaningfully the respondent must enact a sequence of cognitive processes including: (a) question comprehension, (b) information retrieval (recall), (c) decision and judgment processes (e.g., decisions about whether to give a truthful answer), and (d) response processes (such as mapping an internal representation of the answer to the list of response categories printed on the questionnaire).[10]

Verbal probing versus think-aloud

In practice, cognitive interviewing consists of the use of both *verbal probing* by the interviewer ("*What does the term mental health mean to you*"), and *think-aloud*, in which the respondent is induced to not simply report an answer but to verbalize whatever comes to mind as he/she goes through the mental process of answering the question.[11] The following example illustrates an idealized think-aloud response to a single tested survey question:

INTERVIEWER How many times have you talked to a doctor in the last 12 months?
SUBJECT I guess that depends on what you mean when you say "talked." I talk to my neighbor, who is a doctor, but you probably don't mean that. I go to my doctor about once a year, for a general

check-up, so I would count that one. I've been to a specialist a couple of more times in the past year – once to get a bad knee diagnosed, and I also saw an ENT about a chronic coughing thing, which I'm pretty sure was in the past year, although I wouldn't swear to it. I've also talked to doctors when I brought my kids to the pediatrician – I assume that you don't want that? Also, I saw a chiropractor, but don't know if you consider that to be a doctor. So, I don't know what number to give you, because I'm not sure what you want.

Note that pure forms of think-aloud require a significant capacity to externalize one's thoughts. In part because many individuals lack this ability, the current practice of cognitive interviewing largely consists of verbal probing by the interviewer,[11] although it has also been suggested that think-aloud may be particularly useful for quality-of-life questions.[12]

Detecting and fixing problems with questions

A cognitive interviewing team typically conducts one or more *rounds* of interviews with 8–12 subjects who are specifically recruited for their suitability (e.g., a questionnaire intended for the elderly might target individuals 65 and over). Interviewers normally audio- or video-record interviews and use these recordings, as well as written notes, to identify questions that appeared to produce significant problems across interviews. For example, questions may consistently pose interpretation challenges (as the think-aloud example above), require retrieval of information that subjects simply do not have at their disposal, contain subtle forms of bias likely to provide misleading responses, or include response categories that do not match the answers that subjects tend to provide.

On the basis of these results, the investigators make recommendations concerning question modification, deletion, re-ordering, or other alterations, and ideally submit the revised questions to a further round of cognitive testing,[a] in iterative fashion. Cognitive testing is most effective when combined with other forms of pretesting: prior to cognitive interviewing, focus groups can be conducted to guide content development, and expert review used to evaluate the draft questionnaire. Subsequent to cognitive testing, the instrument is normally tested within a field environment. However, note that cognitive interviewing is not limited to pretesting, and can be carried out as an ongoing feature of quality assessment, at multiple points.

Cognitive interviewing has been used widely to fashion specific changes to questions, even beyond the domain of questionnaire development. As an illustration of one such change, the first author has used this technique to study the problem-solving behavior of young children engaged in solving math word problems, such as:

The poodle has 9 puppies.
The collie has 5 puppies.
How many more puppies does the poodle have?

Cognitive testing was accomplished by administering simple probe questions such as "*How did you get that answer?*" This approach was useful in solving the riddle of why several children had initially answered "None;" upon probing, the justification given was, to paraphrase, that the poodle already had 9 puppies; because she had no more, the answer was obviously zero. The investigators concluded that some children had interpreted the term "more" only in terms of an increase in quantity, as opposed to comparison (i.e., "more than . . ."), and, as a result, the information related to the collie was viewed as irrelevant. The indicated solution was to rephrase the question to better direct item comprehension: "*How many more puppies does the poodle have than the collie?*" This example illustrates the general model of questionnaire design as informed by cognitive interviewing – a question is empirically tested, a source

of error detected, and a potential modification then proposed.

General versus specific application of cognitive interviewing

Cognitive testing has been advocated for a wide range of self-report questionnaires, and its general uses are well documented.[13,14] Further, researchers have begun to investigate the utility of cognitive interviewing for predicting problems observed in the field environment.[13,15] However, virtually all of the existing literature is generic in nature; even detailed texts on how to conduct such testing fail to pay explicit attention to the way in which cognitive techniques might vary with the nature of questionnaire content.[11] Clearly, HRQOL instruments may pose different cognitive problems than do, for example, surveys of income or childhood immunization (and, in fact, a few recent studies have examined methods relevant to HRQOL instrument formatting or provider-related health outcomes).[16,17] Just as importantly, although a variety of cognitive probing techniques exists, published descriptions of cognitive interviewing rarely indicate exactly *how* to conduct this activity to best examine each relevant design issue. We turn next to these topics.

Applying cognitive interviewing to HRQOL outcomes

To organize our discussion, we examine four design issues to be considered when developing or evaluating HRQOL questionnaires and, in each case, suggest how cognitive interviewing can best be used to inform decisions related to these issues:

(1) Item selection – definition and specification of key terms and response categories within HRQOL questions
(2) Reference period selection
(3) Sensitive and socially desirable behaviors
(4) Frame-of-reference effects.

---

[a] The terms "cognitive interviewing," "cognitive testing," "laboratory interviewing," and "intensive interviewing" are used interchangeably in the survey methods field.

Where possible, we also cite the results of both cognitive interviewing investigations and field evaluations of HRQOL items, in order to tie cognitive testing results to those from the environment in which the question will ultimately be administered.[b]

Issue 1: Item selection in the context of respondent interpretation of HRQOL questions

Investigator and respondent characterization of concepts

First, the study of respondent interpretation of survey questions presumes that the investigators have a firm grasp of the key concepts, especially with respect to basic issues such as whether the questions implicitly involve behavioral, attitudinal, or knowledge measures. Such distinctions are often relatively straightforward within self-response surveys. For example, researchers (and respondents) would likely agree that questions on levels of participation in physical activities over the past month are purely behavioral/autobiographical in nature, and they can be contrasted with attitudinal and knowledge questions that relate to the respondent's opinions about physical activity. However, the process of defining HRQOL, and then selecting items and determining issues to examine through cognitive testing of respondent interpretations, presents a complex and sometimes contentious issue. In Chapter 2 in this volume, Ferrans[5] reviews issues of defining HRQOL and suggests that there is little consensus on key definition within the health outcomes research field; HRQOL scales differ markedly in terms of whether they emphasize patient self-assessment of overall health, physical functioning, clinical symptoms, or other variables.

Such diversity of definition may reflect the wide variation in application of HRQOL assessments. To the extent that quality of life is considered to be an underlying, latent construct as opposed to a directly observable manifestation of health, there is a tendency by some researchers to define HRQOL as a (subjective) attitudinal variable; in effect, "*How is your health?*"[18,19] Alternatively, HRQOL and outcome measures might be viewed as more objective, observable, and factual in nature, especially where summary measurement is based on statistical aggregation over a number of discrete items[5] (e.g., in terms of behaviors such as ". . . have you vomited" in the European Organization for Research and Treatment of Cancer Core Quality of Life Questionnaire, or EORTC QLQ-C30).[20] Finally, van der Veer, Hak, and Jansen consider HRQOL to be neither a behavior nor attitude, but rather a form of self-evaluation.[12]

The distinction between factual and attitudinal emphasis is important for cognitive evaluation, largely because the testing of attitudinal questions presumes that there is no "right" answer, that is, there is no gold standard or objective source of information that can (even in theory) be used to validate a response.

As an explicit example of cognitive testing of attitudinal HRQOL questions, consider what is sometimes labeled *the general health question*[c]: *In general, would you say your health is excellent, very good, good, fair, or poor?* In evaluating this question, a key issue is not factual accuracy, as for strictly behavioral variables, but rather the determination of the subjective basis for the person's response. A vital area to investigate is therefore the respondent's conception of key terms, as the (latent) construct of health is somewhat abstract and does not naturally involve a well-defined observable behavior (such as vomiting) that can be assumed to be mutually agreed upon by the investigator and respondents. Further, note that the response categories (excellent . . . poor) may also be subject to variability in interpretation, as these

---

[b] Although other researchers have conducted similar forms of testing, these results are generally not documented in the literature in a way that makes them easy to review. The evidence presented in this chapter therefore relies heavily on work previously done by one of the authors (Willis); we present these examples partly as an effort to place specific cognitive testing results into the research literature.

[c] We note that this general health status item has sometimes been viewed as measuring a domain that is distinct from quality of life, per se.[5] Rather than sorting through this debate, we choose instead to present this item only for illustrative purposes, in order to demonstrate how cognitive interviewing techniques are applied.

consist of vague (ill-defined) quantifiers. Hence, to investigate comprehension of these item features, two types of probe questions are appropriate: (a) those investigating conceptions of the key issue of health, and (b) those involving response category selection. Though these overlap, we discuss potential means for assessing them in turn.

How do respondents conceive of health?

Regarding the first issue, it would be appropriate to cognitively test the general health question through the use of simple probe questions that target a latent, subjective concept: *"This question asks about your health – can you tell me in your own words what that makes you think of?"* By being unbiased and fairly general, the interviewer can determine whether the respondent is able to think of health in a coherent fashion that matches the investigator's intent.[d] In conducting cognitive testing in this way, researchers have often found that respondents have a tendency to mention only facets of their physical health without making reference to mental health,[21] let alone the additional social or existential domains sometimes viewed as fundamental components of HRQOL.[2,5] If the investigator is mainly concerned with physical health (e.g., where cancer treatment is intended for purposes of improving physical aspects of functioning), this focus may be acceptable. However, it is sometimes important to consider multiple aspects of health, particularly the mental and emotional. Hence, one alternative would be to address the cognitive testing results by providing an introduction that induces respondents to consider both categories of health, explicitly (e.g., *"The next question is about health, which includes your physical health as well as how you are feeling mentally or emotionally"*).

A second resolution would be to take one further step: Dividing the initial question into a series of two (or more) items, similar to the approach used in the Centers for Disease Control and Prevention Behavioral Risk Factor Surveillance System Survey[8] (CDC BRFSS):

(a) The first question is about your PHYSICAL health, which includes physical illness and injury. In general would you say that your physical health is excellent . . . poor?

(b) Now, how about your MENTAL OR EMOTIONAL health. In general would you say that your mental or emotional health is excellent . . . poor?

There is empirical evidence that decomposing general health in this way is meaningful. In testing of a related question on days in the past 30 that the respondent had either not-good physical or not-good mental health, it has been repeatedly found that ratings of physical health decline with age, whereas self-reports related to quality of mental health tend to increase.[8,22] Further, data from the CDC BRFSS indicate that the majority of individuals report substantially different numbers of physically versus mentally unhealthy days (for example, in 1998, about 68% reported only one of the two types of unhealthy days, and only about 5% reported equal numbers).[8] That is, there is a basis for believing that, within the general population, these two facets of health are meaningfully differentiable, and that cognitive testing results are indirectly validated by field outcomes.

However, it would be interesting to extend this research to the cancer-related HRQOL domain, especially by applying cognitive interviewing to examine the relationship between physical and mental health for cancer survivors. It may be that specific physical effects (e.g., urinary incontinence) directly influence social life and, therefore, emotional health within this population.[2] Hence, independence of physical and mental health might not be exhibited within this population, due to differential experiences and conceptions related to health that in turn influence question comprehension.

Cognitive probing can assist in studying HRQOL item comprehension in several other fundamental ways. First, by probing the degree to which

---

[d] Comparison of respondent interpretation to investigator intent depends on the clear specification of the latter, and highlights the importance of well-specified measurement objectives. On the other hand, one function of cognitive testing may be to identify concepts that have been insufficiently specified and require further development.

respondents view particular experiences, such as diarrhea or depression, as constituting core components of their health as opposed to factors that influence their health, we may be able to contribute to theoretically oriented efforts to disentangle *causal* and *indicator* variables[2,5,23] and to avoid mixing these in our analyses. More generally, cognitive testing results may assist in making decisions about whether to use global HRQOL measures (e.g., your health in general) versus a longer series of questions targeting specific domains. Barofsky[24] has argued that researchers sometimes develop summary indices that are limited by either failing to include the dimensions that are important to respondents or including dimensions that are unimportant. By asking subjects about how they perceive of their health, we can fashion instruments that are positioned at the appropriate level of aggregation or specificity.

Overall, our experience suggests that questions that are very general and that give rise to multiple interpretations (such as the general health item featured in this paper) may be useful mainly for global health assessment, as in the BRFSS. On the other hand, if the major research objective is to track specific changes in HRQOL due to treatment intervention, such general items may suffer from excessive comprehension variance and associated measurement noise.[6,25] Again, decisions concerning whether a question functions appropriately must be made with respect not only to whether it appears to pass the cognitive tests to which it is submitted, but also whether it meets the measurement objectives of the investigation.

How does the respondent select a response category?

Darby[3] discusses issues related to item response category selection. Cognitive testing of the general health question above also provides a useful example related to selection of response categories, in particular, whether these should consist of imprecise verbal labels (excellent . . . poor), or quantifiably precise labels (". . . for how many days during the past 30 days was your physical health not good"). Effective cognitive interviewing practice to this end depends on asking unbiased probe questions such as:

You said there were 10 days in the past 30 that your physical health wasn't good – how did you arrive at that answer?

Why do you say that your health is good?

Under what conditions would you say that your health was only fair, as opposed to good?

To you, what does it mean to have poor health?

In this way, the interviewer can examine subjective definitions concerning the terms used to divide health into ordinal levels, and this reveals whether subjects use a measurement system that involves a single dimension reliably. It may be found, for example, that a particular sub-population has a strong tendency to equate poor health with one focal subdimension, such as needing frequent inpatient hospital visits over a long time period, but to consider good, very good, and excellent health to be synonymous concepts that simply confer a generalized absence of medical problems. One would conclude that for this group the general health question does not serve as a unidimensional construct corresponding to overall HRQOL status.

As an example of the use of cognitive probing to examine response category interpretation, Schechter *et al.* carried out an extensive set of cognitive interviews to determine how well these different response categories appeared to function.[22] In particular, does the nominal increase in specificity obtained through use of a "number-of-not-good-days" approach result in better data than would the use of descriptive verbal labels? The authors found that older respondents in particular had difficulty in providing precise estimates that matched the open-ended responses they either provided spontaneously or gave when answering probes such as "*Why do you say X days?*" In contrast, they had little trouble choosing a response of "excellent" . . . "poor" for the general health item. Further, data from a follow-up field study revealed that the proportion of "Don't Know" responses for the 30-day questions was higher for the elderly than for non-elderly (approximately 7% versus 0.7%), yet non-response for the general health item was almost nonexistent in both groups.

Though not definitive, the combined results suggested that a move toward precise response categories was not particularly effective for elderly respondents. Although the more specific 30-day measures might be perfectly appropriate for a study involving young adults, one might conclude that a study protocol involving the elderly would be best served by using a more general response task. For purposes of developing or evaluating HRQOL scales, the most relevant point is that cognitive testing was useful in identifying relevant measurement issues and providing a basis for decision-making concerning the nature of response category selection.

Finally, an interesting example of the use of cognitive techniques to examine respondent interpretation of response categories within the cancer HRQOL domain, to determine whether these match investigator intent, is provided by a fairly extensive study by Groenvold et al.[26] The investigators evaluated the EORTC QLQ-C30 through a process that made heavy use of cognitive interviewing techniques (although the authors did not label their techniques as such). Using techniques designed to induce respondents to provide answers to the questions in their own words rather than relying on the response categories provided in the instrument, interviews were conducted with 95 cancer patients who had previously completed the instrument through self-administration. An independent rater then completed a blank questionnaire while listening to an audio-tape of the open-ended version of the interview, attempting to code the elaborated answers into the instrument's response categories. Finally, a comparison was made of the respondent's unaided responses and those as interpreted by the rater to assess degree of agreement for each questionnaire item. Overall, obtained values of kappa were very high (median 0.85), indicating that similar information was obtained from either source. By implication, the authors concluded that the instrument as designed (self-administered, closed-ended response categories) was able to represent respondents' thought

processes, and that there was little misinterpretation of the closed-ended response categories. Such an approach points a way for other cancer-related HRQOL researchers to evaluate their instruments.

Issue 2: Reference periods and asking about the present versus the past

Probing the present

A second cognitive issue that may be particularly germane to HRQOL measurement is the potential effectiveness of various reference periods. Some HRQOL measures mainly concern current health, as opposed to long-term retrospective assessment. As such, for questions on health status – that is, current functioning or self-perception – cognitive probing need not focus excessively on the basis for respondent recall and whether retrieval failure contributes heavily to response error. Further, to the degree that health status is considered to be an attitude rather than a behavior, one might not be particularly concerned with whether the respondent is able to accurately enumerate particular events, as for a question such as "In the past 12 months, how many times have you visited a doctor?" and the cognitive interviewer therefore would not probe intensively to determine whether the person had actually visited the doctor three versus four times during that period.

On the other hand, cognitive testing could be used to target the more general timeframe the respondent spontaneously selects when formulating a response to a general health question. For example, if the individual believes her overall physical health to be "good" because she has rarely visited the doctor in the past year, it might be concluded that she has adopted a roughly 12-month retrospective period when thinking about current health. Similarly, if the individual answered "Excellent – I've hardly been sick a day in my life," this would constitute evidence that she conceives of health status as a static, long-term trait as opposed to a dynamic attribute. Such findings have led some question designers to conclude that, whenever possible, questions should specify a reference period (e.g., "In the past 30 days, would you *say that your health in general has been excellent . . . poor?*").[27] Further, where the topic of interest is found to vary significantly over time, it is sometimes best to use short reference periods. For example, through cognitive testing of a Chronic Prostatitis Symptom Index, Litwin *et al.*[28] determined that a 1-week reference period was better suited to the ability to recall changes in pain and urinary symptoms than was the more typical 4-week period.

Probing the past

Rather than considering only current status, some HRQOL measures incorporate a more distant reference period. Investigators interested in infrequent events (like falling in the elderly) may therefore choose a longer period, such as 12 months. Further, HRQOL assessment sometimes involves *relative* status with respect to a time prior to a disease, treatment, or other significant process or event, as opposed to current status. For example, the investigator may ask about relative changes in urinary functioning over time (better, worse, or the same) due to a treatment such as prostate surgery. Such judgments may be cognitively complex, because, in addition to recall of a previous state or behavior, they require an assessment of the current state and finally a comparison between the two.

Cognitive probing can be especially useful in determining the relative difficulty of making such assessments. For example, it may be that the judgment is easy to make because subjects provide clear and immediate replies such as "It's much worse now." Appropriate probing at that point would seek elaboration by asking *"What is it exactly that is worse now than before?"* On this basis, the individual might recount prior experiences of sleeping through the night without needing to urinate and how this has changed drastically. An astute interviewer would further inquire about time course by asking when the person noticed the biggest changes in order to determine whether a hidden assumption (that the change was due to a treatment intervention) is satisfied. It might be determined, especially over multiple interviews, that this assumption is perfectly appropriate,

and the question as written poses no particular difficulties.

The above example is presented not to make the case that comparative pre-post judgments of function are easy (as the entire point of cognitive interviewing is to empirically test such notions). Rather, the aim is to illustrate where cognitive testing might be used to examine a potential cognitive issue, so the designer can determine whether the target question presents clear problems. Note that the overall purpose of cognitive testing is not, as is sometimes believed, to find flaws with every question, but to differentiate between those questions that cause major problems from those that appear not to.

Based on past cognitive interviewing experience, we recommend that HRQOL investigators pay particular attention to issues of reference period specification, and empirically assess respondent interpretation of time periods such as "the past year" or "the past month." Often, the past year is variably interpreted as "the past 12 months," "last year" (e.g., 2002), or "since January 1." Overall, it seems advisable to rely on well-specified periods such as "the past 12 months," "the past 30 days," or "the last 7 days."

Issue 3: Investigating responses to sensitive and socially desirable behaviors

In the HRQOL domain, some topics may be either overtly sensitive (e.g., sexual function and behavior), or else present subtle issues related to social desirability (e.g., ability to walk upstairs without resting). Further, within HRQOL domains, item sensitivity often appears to center around the issue of what respondents are able to *do* (e.g., sexual functioning, activities of daily living) as opposed to what they *have done* (e.g., had sex with a prostitute, taken heroin, or evaded income taxes); this is sometimes referred to as the distinction between *capacity* and *performance*. For example, the EORTC QLQ-C30 includes items asking whether the individual has any trouble taking a long walk; needs help with eating, dressing, washing; and is completely unable to work or do household jobs.[20] Potential response error associated with answering these questions may be exacerbated because they do not concern single behavioral events, but require the respondent to compose a summary judgment of his or her own abilities (again, *can* you do something, as opposed to *do you* do them).

A clear requirement of cognitive testing is to determine whether the use of questions concerning capacity (self-evaluation) presents cognitive tendencies that differ from those associated with performance or function (behavioral) questions. Related to our earlier discussion, one obvious difference is that function questions tend to have unspecified reference periods, which leads to a range of subjective definitions. A second issue relates to the complexities imposed by variability in function over time; capacity questions often (incorrectly) assume a static situation. Finally, the questions often combine a list of functions (e.g., eating, dressing, and so forth), and are therefore classically double-barreled. Cognitive interviewing therefore provides a mechanism for determining whether division of the question into constituent parts relieves the respondent of the burden of determining which inherent question to decide to answer. Note that the recommendation to decompose items in order to reduce potential for error is a common outcome of cognitive testing. To illustrate, testing of the question *"During the past year, have you had any serious personal or emotional problems?"* has revealed a double-barreled confounding effect; cognitive laboratory subjects tended to consider personal and emotional problems as separate issues that differ in level of sensitivity.[29] In any event, such testing frequently makes evident the complex and varied nature of thinking that goes into influencing the seemingly simple process of choosing a "Yes" versus a "No" answer to an HRQOL question.

Issue 4: Investigating frame of reference effects in HRQOL measures

The frame-of-reference phenomenon involves questions that do not have absolute answers, but rather can be defined only relative to an implicit comparison standard. Put simply, the item as posed begs the further question: "Compared to what . . .?" (or to whom?). HRQOL instruments often pose questions of this nature, so this issue is particularly worthy of cognitive testing. The general health question again serves as an illustration: When asked during the cognitive interview whether one's health is excellent . . . poor, elderly respondents, or others in apparently poor health, may respond "Excellent" or "Very Good" much more frequently than the interviewer expects. For example, when the lead author probed an octogenarian cognitive interview subject who had multiple health problems why he thought his health was excellent, his response was *"I got up this morning, didn't I?"* Further discussion clarified that, given his age (as the frame of reference), he felt that any health state other than death was worthy of the label "Excellent." The same interviewer has also experienced instances in which, for example, a much younger subject reported that his health was only "Good" because he had strained a hamstring muscle and was unable to engage in marathon training that week. One cannot draw the conclusion that either subject's answer is "wrong," but simply that they use different subjective measurement systems to describe the absolute level of health to be associated with a particular verbal label.

A closely related argument within the quality-of-life literature involves the notion of "Response Shift" involving a change in one's internal standard of measurement over time.[30] In response to evidence that this phenomenon is pervasive, one proposed solution has been to use a modification of the general health question:[31] *Compared to other people your age, would you say that your health in general is excellent, very good, good, fair, or poor?* Upon further testing, this version may appear to remove the tendency towards age-based frame-of-reference effects. However, choosing between this version and the more general formulation must be based on several factors: the range of ages to be included in the study (for an age-homogenous group, the standard question may be sufficient); the need for comparability to an external standard (again, the general form of the question is much more frequently administered); and whether the objective is to grade individuals along a continuum or to select a certain sub-group based on a cut-point (it might be that individuals selecting "poor" constitute a unique group of interest, no matter how the question is asked). Note that *cognitive testing cannot necessarily be used to prove which version of a question is "better." Rather, it serves to externalize the trade-offs that are implicit in the use of each of several question versions, for the purposes of fulfilling measurement objectives.*[32]

Zebrack has argued that the concept of cognitive frame-of-reference is particularly relevant to the HRQOL assessment of cancer survivors. He found that the meaning (frame) that long-term survivors of leukemia and lymphoma apply to their experience involves a number of positive outcomes that may not apply to the general population;[33] hence, questions about general health might not function in the same manner for this group. Below we note the implications of such findings as they suggest the need to test questions on the appropriate respondent populations.

Strengths, weaknesses, and extensions of the cognitive interviewing approach to HRQOL and outcomes measurement

We have discussed features of HRQOL measures that are especially important when making questionnaire design decisions, and have described how cognitive interviewing techniques can be used to influence these decisions. In closing, we review limitations of these techniques, and potential future directions.

Logistics: what investment is required to do cognitive interviewing?

Cognitive laboratories have been established by Federal agencies that routinely pretest questionnaires, such as the National Center for Health Statistics, the US Census Bureau, and the Bureau of Labor Statistics, and by private contract research organizations. Given that it is generally not feasible for HRQOL researchers to establish or make use of such laboratories, can they practically apply cognitive testing techniques? We believe that if cognitive interviewing

is seen as a flexible process, as opposed to a formal laboratory-based capability, then this is certainly feasible. Training in cognitive techniques has frequently been accomplished through self study,[11,34] and cognitive techniques can be conducted in any private setting, without specialized equipment. Further, we have found that as few as five cognitive interviews can be extremely effective in revealing covert problems with survey questions that are simply not apparent in the absence of empirical investigation involving live subjects.

Potential for bias: is a small sample representative of the population?

First, note that statistical representativeness cannot be a feature of cognitive interviewing due to sample size constraints. Rather, the investigator endeavors to carefully select subjects who are representative of the target population in a qualitative sense. In particular, one should recruit as wide a range of eligible individuals as possible to maximize the chances of detecting potential problems. It is advisable to include subjects who are likely to represent several levels of HRQOL, as conceptualized by the investigator, in order to determine whether the questionnaire functions effectively across this range. Finally, because cognitive test subjects tend to be better educated than the general population, it is useful to include individuals from across the educational spectrum by recruiting some individuals having, at most, a high school education.

The possibility of misleading results due to small or biased samples always exists, of course; a single subject's responses, if taken literally, might markedly skew the interpretation. For this reason, an important mediating step between the review of cognitive interviewing results and modification of the instrument is the judicious application of the investigative team's "clinical" judgment. That is, the investigators should temper the obtained results according to how typical the tested individuals appear to have been, and on the basis of expert knowledge concerning questionnaire item functioning in the intended field environment. Cognitive interviewing does not serve as the singular driving force; rather, it provides one source of information.

Does cognitive interviewing replace other forms of evaluation?

As discussed initially, although resources for pretesting and evaluation are generally limited, the process of item development appears to work best when cognitive interviewing is integrated into a development system that involves several steps.[35] In addition to other forms of qualitative pretesting, investigators are advised to use procedures such as psychometric analysis in order to further evaluate item function (see Chapter 21 in this volume by Reise[36]). Extensions to Item Response Theory (IRT) may represent a particularly useful means for enhancing the degree of interplay between questionnaire evaluation techniques and to serve as an effective construct validation mechanism. For example, consider a hypothetical result from cognitive testing indicating that a scale containing the categories Always, Most of the time, Usually, A good bit of the time, and Never appears to be flawed due to respondent difficulty in matching their subjective responses to the given categories, and that a revised scale (e.g., All or most of the time, Some of the time, A little of the time, Never) functions better. Based on field data, IRT analysis could then be invoked to evaluate both responses scales. To the degree that cognitive testing and IRT analysis produce consistent results, it should be found that item functioning, as described by IRT category and information curves, is superior for the latter scale.

Conversely, findings from (quantitative) IRT analysis that are not easily interpretable on their own could be submitted to (qualitative) cognitive laboratory assessment. For example, IRT provides an excellent analytical tool for detecting Differential Item Functioning (DIF), in which two groups respond differently to a question even after controlling for the population differences on the measured construct.[36] As an illustration, an IRT-based study of adolescent attitudes toward smoking by Panter and Reeve revealed that non-smokers endorsed the item "Smoking helps people feel more comfortable at parties and other social events" as one of the main benefits of smoking, whereas smokers believed this social feature to be a much less important issue.[37] Further, this difference of beliefs between smokers and non-smokers persisted when controlling for overall differences in attitudes towards smoking. IRT can be used to evaluate DIF across age group, race, and administration modes (e.g., paper vs. computer-based), and between different language translations of an instrument. Once DIF is detected, cognitive testing can help researchers understand the cognitive processes involved in guiding this behavior. *We propose that advances in HRQOL measurement will largely depend on this type of flexible integration of qualitative (cognitive) and quantitative (psychometric) techniques.*

Can cognitive interviewing be used for self-administered instruments?

The examples within this chapter mainly involve interviewer-based question administration: the interviewer reads the survey question, the respondent answers it, and the interviewer then asks further probe questions to obtain additional information. However, HRQOL instruments are frequently designed as self-administered (paper or computer-based) questionnaires, and the issue arises of how cognitive testing can be done for such instruments. First, cognitive interviewing of self-administered questionnaires is sometimes conducted as if the questionnaire were interviewer administered (as in the Groenvold et al. study[26] discussed earlier), and it appears that useful information is obtained in this way to the extent that cognitively-oriented problems are not strictly associated with mode of administration.[11] Further, specific methods for cognitive testing of self-administered forms have been developed. Investigators sometimes allow the respondent to complete the questionnaire unaided, and then conduct a retrospective cognitive interview in which the questions are immediately revisited; the same types of probe questions as referenced throughout this paper are administered. Again, flexibility in use of procedure is a key feature of the cognitive approach.

Can cognitive interviewing be used in cross-cultural HRQOL assessment?

Increasingly, researchers are addressing the complex issue of assessing quality of life from a cross-cultural perspective, an endeavor that is complicated not only by language but also by potential differences in conceptions of health.[38,39] Hence, it is very difficult to make the argument that HRQOL items exhibit measurement equivalence, such that results from different groups can be directly compared. Although this is a relatively new area of questionnaire development, pretesting, and evaluation, the use of cognitive interviewing to establish such equivalence is becoming increasingly prevalent (for example, to evaluate HRQOL and symptom-related questions for a French-language cystic fibrosis instrument[40]). Further, as mentioned above, cognitive testing and IRT can be used together to ascertain cross-cultural equivalence.

Conclusions

This chapter has emphasized several key points:

(1) HRQOL instrument assessment must be done in the context of an understanding, and an active investigation, of respondent cognitive processes.

(2) Cognitive interviewing procedures provide a useful and efficient means for investigating key cognitive processes associated with item comprehension, recall, decision, and response processes.

(3) We again sound one note of caution: Cognitive testing can establish that the questions we pose are meaningful to respondents, ask for information that they can provide, are minimally biasing, and overall, are likely to minimize response error. What this technique cannot do, however, is to determine whether we are asking the right questions in the first place. As Gotay has pointed

out,[25] asking about inappropriate or irrelevant variables, experiences, and facets of health status may render an instrument useless for the purpose of detecting differences due to variation in cancer treatment. Similarly, Ganz and Goodwin make the case that questions querying relatively static attributes that are unlikely to change are not useful for purposes of measuring temporal changes in health status.[6] Ultimately it is the researcher's responsibility to ensure that the instrument is both appropriately targeted and is designed to be well-received by the targeted population.

REFERENCES

1 McHorney, Cook, this volume, Invited Paper B.

2 Zebrack, Cella, this volume, Chapter 11.

3 Darby, this volume, Chapter 14.

4 Cohen, S. R., Leis, A. (2002). What determines the quality of life of terminally ill cancer patients from their own perspective? *Journal of Palliative Care* 18(1):48–58.

5 Ferrans, this volume, Chapter 2.

6 Ganz, Goodwin, this volume, Chapter 5.

7 Erickson, this volume, Chapter 3.

8 Centers for Disease Control and Prevention (2000). *Measuring Healthy Days.* Atlanta, GA: CDC.

9 Jobe, J. B., Mingay, D. J. (1991). Cognition and survey measurement: history and overview. *Applied Cognitive Psychology* 5:175–92.

10 Tourangeau, R., Rips L. J., Rasinski, K. (2000). *The Psychology of Survey Response.* Cambridge: Cambridge University Press.

11 Willis, G. B. (1994). *Cognitive Interviewing and Questionnaire Design: A Training Manual.* Hyattsville, MD: National Center for Health Statistics: Cognitive Methods Staff, Working Paper No. 7.

12 van der Veer, K., Hak, T., Jansen, H. (2002). The Three-Step Test-Interview (TSTI): An observational instrument for pretesting self-completion questionnaires. Paper presented at the International Conference on Questionnaire Development, Evaluation, and Testing Methods (QDET), Charleston, SC.

13 Jobe, J. (2003). Cognitive psychology and self reports: models and methods. *Quality of Life Research*, 12(3):219–27.

14 Lessler, J. T. (1995). Choosing questions that people can understand and answer. *Medical Care* 33(4, Suppl.):AS203–8.

15 Willis, G. B., Schechter, S. (1997). Evaluation of cognitive interviewing techniques: do the results generalize to the field? *Bulletin de Methodologie Sociologique* **55**:40–66.

16 Mullin, P. A., Lohr, K. N., Bresnahan, B. W. *et al.* (2000). Applying cognitive design principles to formatting HRQOL instruments. *Quality of Life Research* **9**(1):13–27.

17 Harris-Kojetin, L. D., Fowler, F. J., Brown, J. A. *et al.* (1999). The use of cognitive testing to develop and evaluate CAHPS(R) 1.0 core survey items. *Medical Care* **37**(3, Suppl.): MS10–MS21.

18 Sehulster, J. R. (1994). Health and self: paths for exploring cognitive aspects underlying self-report of health status. In *Proceedings of the 1993 NCHS Conference on the Cognitive Aspects of Self-Reported Health Status*, ed. S. Schechter, pp. 89–105. Hyattsville, MD: National Center for Health Statistics, Cognitive Methods Staff Working Paper Series, No. 10.

19 Fowler, F. J. (1995). *Improving Survey Questions: Design and Evaluation*. Thousand Oaks, CA: Sage.

20 Aaronson, N. K., Ahmedzai, S., Bergman, B. *et al.* (1993). The European Organization for Research and Treatment of Cancer QLQ-C30: a quality of life instrument for use in international clinical trials in oncology. *Journal of the National Cancer Institute* **85**(5):365–76.

21 Beatty, P., Schechter, S. (1998). *Questionnaire Evaluation and Testing in Support of the Behavioral Risk Factor Surveillance System (BRFSS), 1992–1998*. Hyattsville, MD: National Center for Health Statistics, Cognitive Methods Staff Working Paper No. 26.

22 Schechter, S., Beatty, P., Willis, G. B. (1999). Asking survey respondents about health status: judgment and response issues. In *Cognition, Aging, and Self-reports*, ed. N. Schwarz, D. Park, B. Knauper, S. Sudman, pp. 265–83. Washington, DC: Psychology Press.

23 Fayers, P. M., Machin, D. (2000). *Quality of Life: Assessment, Analysis and Interpretation*. Chichester: John Wiley & Sons.

24 Barofsky, I. (1996). Cognitive aspects of quality of life assessment. In *Quality of Life and Pharmacoeconomics in Clinical Trials* (2nd Edition), ed. B. Spilker, pp. 107–15. New York: Lippincott-Raven Press.

25 Gotay, C. C. (1996). Trial-related quality of life: using quality-of-life assessment to distinguish among cancer therapies. *Journal of the National Cancer Institute Monographs* **20**:1–6.

26 Groenvold, M., Klee, M. C., Sprangers, M. A. G. *et al.* (1997). Validation of the EORTC QLQ-C30 Quality of Life Questionnaire through combined qualitative and quantitative assessment of patient-observer agreement. *Journal of Clinical Epidemiology* **50**(4):441–50.

27 Willis, G. B., Lessler, J. (1999). *The BRFSS-QAS: A Guide for Systematically Evaluating Survey Question Wording*. Research Triangle Park, NC: Research Triangle Institute.

28 Litwin, M. S., McNaughton-Collins, M., Fowler, F. J. *et al.* (1999). The National Institutes of Health Chronic Prostatitis Symptom Index: development and validation of a new outcome measure. *Journal of Urology* **162**:369–75.

29 Willis, G. B. (1994). *Results of NCHS Cognitive Testing: 1995 Year 2000 Objectives Questionnaire*. Hyattsville, MD: National Center for Health Statistics.

30 Lepore, S. J., Eton, D. T. (2000). Response shifts in prostate cancer patients: an evaluation of suppressor and buffer models. In *Adaptation to Changing Health: Response Shifts in Quality-of-Life Research*, ed. C. E. Schwartz, M. A. G. Sprangers, pp. 37–51. Washington, DC: American Psychological Association.

31 Abeles, N. (1998). *What Practitioners Should Know About Working with Older Adults*. Washington, DC: American Psychological Association.

32 Beatty, P. (2002). The dynamics of cognitive interviewing. Paper presented at the International Conference on Questionnaire Development, Evaluation, and Testing Methods (QDET), Charleston, SC.

33 Zebrack, B. (2000). Quality of life of long-term survivors of leukemia and lymphoma. *Journal of Psychosocial Oncology* **18**(4):39–59.

34 US Bureau of the Census (1993). *Protocol for Pretesting Demographic Surveys at the Census Bureau*. Suitland, MD: U.S. Bureau of the Census.

35 Esposito, J. L., Rothgeb, J. M. (1997). Evaluating survey data: making the transition from pretesting to quality assessment. In *Survey Measurement and Process Quality*, ed. L. Lyberg *et al.*, pp. 541–71. New York, NY: John Wiley & Sons.

36 Reise, this volume, Chapter 21.

37 Panter, A. T., Reeve, B. B. (2002). Assessing tobacco beliefs among youth using item response theory models. *Drug and Alcohol Dependence* **68**:521–39.

38 Lankenau, B. H., Hennessy, C. H., Moriarty, D. G. *et al.* (1995). Health-related Quality of Life: A New Approach to Measuring the Health Status of a Population. Paper presented at Ninth World Productivity Congress, Istanbul, Turkey.

39 Aaronson, this volume, Chapter 20.

40 Quittner, A. L., Sweeny, S., Watrous, M. *et al.* (2000). Translation and linguistic validation of a disease-specific quality of life measure for cystic fibrosis. *Journal of Pediatric Psychology* **25**(6):403–14.

Invited Paper D
Industry perspective regarding outcomes research in oncology*

Kati Copley-Merriman, M.S., M.B.A.,[1] Joseph Jackson, Ph.D.,[2]
J. Gregory Boyer, Ph.D.,[3] Joseph C. Cappelleri, Ph.D., M.P.H.,[1]
Robert DeMarinis, Ph.D.,[4] Joseph DiCesare, M.P.H., R.Ph.,[5]
M. Haim Erder, Ph.D.,[6] Jean Paul Gagnon, Ph.D.,[7] Lou Garrison, Ph.D.,[8]
Kathleen Gondek, Ph.D.,[9] Kim A. Heithoff, Sc.D.,[10] Tom Hughes, Ph.D.,[11]
David Miller, Ph.D.,[12] Margaret Rothman, Ph.D.,[13]
Nancy Santanello, M.D., M.S.,[14] Richard Willke, Ph.D.,[3] Bruce Wong, M.D.[2]

[1]Pfizer Inc., [2]Bristol-Myers Squibb, [3]Pharmacia Corp, [4]Wyeth-Ayerst Research, [5]Novartis Pharmaceuticals Corp., [6]Amgen Inc., [7]Aventis Pharmaceuticals Inc., [8]F. Hoffman-La Roche AG, [9]Bayer Corp., [10]Schering-Plough Pharmaceuticals, [11]Eli Lilly and Company, [12]GlaxoSmithKline, [13]Johnson & Johnson Pharmaceutical Services, LLC, [14]Merck Research Laboratories

Introduction

The goal of treatment for many persons with cancer is not cure but improvement or maintenance of functioning and well-being during their remaining period of life. This is particularly true for patients with advanced or metastatic cancers. Trials to produce evidence of effectiveness or for regulatory approval may include patient assessments of benefit as well as classical clinical endpoints used in oncology settings. These patient assessments of treatment benefit may or may not be related to the traditional measures of treatment success such as survival, tumor shrinkage, or time to tumor progression. For this reason, additional outcome measures to estimate benefit or risk/benefit trade-offs have been developed. Outcomes measures in this category of health assessment are referred to as patient-reported outcomes (PROs) because they are used to collect data directly from the patient.

It is increasingly recognized that the patient's perspective is unique and represents a valuable contribution to drug evaluation and treatment processes. This is particularly important when studying the effects of treatments on cancer symptoms such as pain and fatigue, outcomes not accurately measured by observers. Recent changes in the health care system have greatly empowered patients who are now considered partners rather than passive consumers. To maximize their contribution, they need to be informed about the outcomes associated with treatment. Patients are not always concerned with the same questions as treating physicians or clinical researchers. While the clinical researcher may focus on evaluating change in tumor size, patients may be more concerned with questions such as: What is my

*The drug industry clearly has an important stake in the development and application of valid, reliable, and responsive outcomes measures that can inform public and private decision making about the effectiveness, and cost-effectiveness, of new products. In this regard, NCI invited the Health Outcomes Committee of the Pharmaceutical Research and Manufacturers of America to provide an industry perspective on the role, actual and potential, of outcomes research in cancer.

life likely to be like if I take these drugs? What will I be able to do? How will I feel? It is important that the patient's concerns be addressed in any comprehensive attempt to understand the impact of treatment. Lindley *et al.*[1] have reported that patients' health-related quality of life (HRQOL) can even influence their willingness to continue cancer therapy. Eighty-four percent of patients who had little or no disruption in HRQOL during chemotherapy were willing to receive additional chemotherapy, while only 58% of those patients experiencing severe negative impacts on their HRQOL during chemotherapy were willing to receive additional chemotherapy.[1]

In a recent survey of oncologists, 51% indicated that PRO study findings had an impact on their recommendations for treatment.[2] Currently, much of the available PRO information related to treatments is developed within the context of clinical trials. The pharmaceutical industry is associated with many of these efforts. The industry works with regulatory authorities, academics, and professional organizations to plan, conduct, and report PRO evaluations. This collaboration normally begins early in the drug development process with the initial small trials in which experimental drugs are first tested for tolerability in human beings and continues throughout the product life cycle. It is in later phases of drug development, often after the initial approval, when confirmatory effectiveness studies are completed, often in additional indications or optimized treatment regimens.

New drug development usually involves studies in advanced-stage patients first, followed by studies in early-stage patients. The reason for this development approach is related, in part, to the ethics of giving an early-stage patient an unproven therapy. Thus, the initial proof of effectiveness dictates a conservative approach. It is also quicker to document survival advantages in advanced-stage patients, who exhibit greater risk of mortality. This approach is still the gold standard for efficacy of a new therapy. However, advanced-stage patients often score fairly low on the PRO measures at baseline, and they also tend to progress rapidly to worse HRQOL scores over time. Therefore, the objective of treatment is often to maintain HRQOL rather than improve it.

In any drug development program, it is important to provide the conceptual framework for the clinical assessments that is relevant to the clinical setting targeted by the therapy. Regulators are interested in the relationships among and between endpoint measures, including PRO, HRQOL, and clinical endpoints. Thus, the usefulness and relatedness of clinical assessments, including PRO assessment, will be considered during the drug approval process in the context of standards of care for a given clinical setting.

To maximize the health care benefit to everyone, policy makers and payers must consider the value of each intervention as well as the health care benefit. Industry is committed to showing the value of pharmaceutical products as well as the health care benefit. However, the ultimate value of oncology agents is demonstrated better post-launch (i.e, when a drug is first marketed following regulatory approval), after doses, schedules, and tumor types have been optimized.

Patient-reported outcomes

The successful generation of PRO findings requires careful attention to the research design and implementation to ensure reliability, validity, and responsiveness as an indicator of treatment impact. Pharmaceutical companies have invested heavily in this area as indicated by their use of generic and oncology-specific measures to assess PROs in clinical trials. The use of validated instruments builds on previous research experience across programs and may enable access to normative data to facilitate historical benchmarking. New approaches are focused on the development of measures, usually targeted at the impact of symptoms, function, adverse events, patient satisfaction, and treatment preference, in a specific disease setting.

Definitional considerations

A PRO measure comprises one or more self-reported items that reflect an underlying concept. While PROs may encompass a wide variety of patient-perceived assessments of health status, they should include items that are relevant and important to the patient. HRQOL instruments, symptom scales, work productivity measures, and other assessments that evaluate self-perception of the impact of illness are all examples of PROs. PROs may be symptom specific, such as the Rotterdam Symptom Checklist[3] or the Memorial Symptom Assessment Scale,[4] or they may combine several domains or concepts in a multidimensional measure such as the EORTC[5] and FACT[6] measures which include items related to symptoms, functional status, and well-being.

The term "quality of life" is widely used in oncology, but its connotation varies depending on the nature of the measure and the research perspective. Regulators have often related "QOL assessment" to improvement in cancer-related symptoms. Conversely, they also contend that the use of the QOL term as a claim to represent findings limited to the symptom impact is tantamount to 'semantic inflation.' In other words, symptom improvement alone does not demonstrate that patients' health-related quality of life has been improved. Many physicians and patients believe quality of life represents the trade-off between efficacy and side effects. The term "HRQOL" has a specific, somewhat different meaning to outcomes researchers, generally indicating a composite assessment of impact on symptoms, function, and well-being in a multidimensional context. The non-specific use of the term, however, has led to confusion and some concern by regulators. In response to this situation, the term "Patient-Reported Outcomes" has been adopted by many outcomes researchers to represent a more diverse set of outcomes representing the patient's perspective. PRO is an umbrella concept that includes symptoms, bother, functional status, well-being, HRQOL, satisfaction with treatment, treatment adherence, and other patient–relevant dimensions of disease and/or treatment. Data are collected from patients via structured questionnaires. Conceptualization and definition of the "PRO" term was established by the PRO Harmonization Group, which brought together members of four groups: European Regulatory Issues on Quality of Life Assessment (ERIQA), International

Society of Pharmacoeconomics and Outcomes Research (ISPOR), International Society for Quality of Life Research (ISOQOL), and the Pharmaceutical Research and Manufacturers of America (PhRMA) Health Outcomes Committee.[7] The term "Patient-Reported Outcomes" has been adopted by both industry and the US Food and Drug Administration (FDA), but its use has not diffused widely into the academic and clinical communities yet.

PROs and product labeling

The 2002 Physician Desk Reference (electronic version)[8] was used to assess PRO measures, including HRQOL claims that are currently included in cancer product labeling and selected products within supportive care (Table D.1). For example, we did not review all products that are used in the treatment of cancer pain. There has been a movement in cancer trials to address clinical benefit that includes supportive care such as reduced disease- or treatment-related symptoms. Because the benefits of supportive care require substantial evidence for claims, these are also included in Table D.1.

Both cancer and chemotherapy may cause a variety of cancer-related symptoms and chemotherapy-related toxicities, including pain, fatigue, cachexia, bone marrow suppression, cardiac and gastrointestinal abnormalities, which potentially affect an individual's quality of life.[9] Cancer pain can largely be controlled with available therapies. Weight loss is a concern since it can reduce the patient's ability to tolerate chemotherapy and increase morbidity, thus having secondary impacts on the success of treatment strategies and aspects of HRQOL. Nausea and vomiting, mucositis, pulmonary and cardiotoxicity, reproductive complications, bone marrow suppression, and fatigue similarly play an important role in patient well-being and affect successful outcomes for the patient.

Fatigue occurs frequently in cancer patients and has demonstrable impact on the activities of daily life. Fatigue is one manifestation of anemia. Epoetin alfa has been shown to be an effective therapy for anemia and various PROs (Table D.1). Three community-based studies in 5000 patients have

Table D.1. Patient reported outcomes in oncology product labeling and selective review of supportive care labeling

Drug Brand Name	Generic Name	Manufacturer	Label
ONCOLOGY PRODUCTS			
Aredia® for Injection	pamidronate disodium	Ciba Geigy Corp Pharm	**Osteolytic Bone Metastases of Breast Cancer and Osteolytic Lesions of Multiple Myeloma** In addition, decreases in pain scores from baseline occurred at the last measurement for those Aredia patients with pain at baseline (p = .026) but not in the placebo group. At the last measurement, a worsening from baseline was observed in the placebo group for the Spitzer quality-of-life variable (p < .001) and ECOG performance status (p < .011) while there was no significant deterioration from baseline in these parameters observed in Aredia-treated patients. Pain and analgesic scores, ECOG performance status and Spitzer quality of life index were measured at baseline and periodically during the trials. The changes from baseline to the last measurement carried forward are shown in the table.
Taxol®	paclitaxel	Bristol-Myers Squibb	**Non-Small-Cell Lung Cancer** In the ECOG study, the Functional Assessment of Cancer Therapy-Lung (FACT-L) questionnaire had seven subscales that measured subjective assessment of treatment. Of the seven, the Lung Cancer Specific Symptoms subscale favored the TAXOL 135 mg/m²/24 hour plus cisplatin arm compared to the cisplatin/etoposide arm. For all other factors, there was no difference in the treatment groups.
Gemzar®	gemcitabine HCI	Eli Lilly & Co	**Non-Small-Cell Lung Cancer** Quality of Life (QOL) was a secondary endpoint in both randomized studies. In the Gemzar plus cisplatin versus cisplatin study, QOL was measured using the FACT-L, which assessed physical, social, emotional, and functional well-being, and lung cancer symptoms. In the study of Gemzar plus cisplatin versus etoposide plus cisplatin, QOL was measured using the EORTC QLQ-C30 and LC13, which assessed physical and psychological functioning and symptoms related to both lung cancer and its treatment. In both studies no significant differences were observed in QOL between the Gemzar plus cisplatin arm and the comparator arm. Eleven patients on the Gemzar arm and two patients on the 5-FU arm showed improvement in analgesic consumption and/or pain intensity with stable performance status. Two patients on the Gemzar arm showed improvement in analgesic consumption or pain intensity with improvement in performance status. One patient on the 5-FU arm was stable with regard to pain intensity and analgesic consumption with improvement in performance status. No patient on either arm achieved a clinical benefit response based on weight gain.
Hycamtin®	topotecan hydrochloride	SmithKline Beecham Pharm	**Small-Cell Lung Cancer** Changes on a disease-related symptom scale in patients who received Hycamtin or who received CAV are presented in Table 3 of the package insert. It should be noted that not all patients had all symptoms nor did all patients respond to all questions. Each symptom was rated on a four category scale with an improvement defined as a change in one category from baseline sustained over two courses. Limitations in interpretation of the rating scale and responses preclude formal statistical analysis.

Table D.1. (*cont.*)

Drug Brand Name	Generic Name	Manufacturer	Label
Camptosar®	irinotecan HC	Pharmacia & Upjohn	**Metastatic Carcinoma of Colon or Rectum** In the two randomized studies, the European Organization of Research and Treatment of Cancer Quality of Life Questionnaire (EORTC QLQ-C30) instrument was utilized. At each visit, patients completed a questionnaire consisting of 30 questions, such as "Did pain interfere with daily activities?" (1 = Not at All, to 4 = Very Much) and "Do you have any trouble taking a long walk?" (Yes or No). The answers from the 30 questions were converted into 15 subscales that were scored from 0 to 100. The global health status subscale was derived from two questions about the patient's sense of general well being in the past week. The results as summarized in Table 4 are based on patients' worse post-baseline scores. In Study 1, a multivariate and univariate analyses of the individual subscales were performed and corrected for multivariate testing. Patients receiving irinotecan reported significantly better results for the global health status, on two of five functional subscales, and on four of nine symptom subscales. As expected, patients receiving irinotecan noted significantly more diarrhea than those receiving best supportive care. In Study 2, the multivariate analysis on all 15 subscales did not indicate a statistically significant difference between irinotecan and infusional 5-FU. (Functional Subscales: Cognitive, Emotional, Social, Physical, Role) (Symptom Subscales: Fatigue, Appetite Loss, Pain Assessment, Insomnia, Constipation, Dyspnea, Nausea/Vomiting, Financial Impact, Diarrhea).
Nolvadex®	tamoxifen	Zeneca	**Metastatic Breast Cancer, Adjuvant Treatment of Breast Cancer** The table in the package insert, entitled "NSABP P-1 Trial: All Adverse Events" has a reference to number with Quality of Life Questionnaires under self-reported symptoms. No reference to what the QoL questionnaire is.
Navelbine®	vinorelbine	Glaxo Wellcome	**Non-Small-Cell Lung Cancer** Quality of life (QoL) was also an endpoint in this study. Patients completed a modified Southwest Oncology Group QoL questionnaire which assessed the domains of role functioning, physical functioning, symptom distress, and global QoL. Quality of life was not adversely affected by NAVELBINE when compared to control.
Zoladex®	gosereline acetate	AstraZeneca	**Breast Cancer** Subjective responses based on measures of pain control and performance status were observed with both treatments; 48% of the women in the Zoladex treatment group and 50% in the oophorectomy group had subjective responses.
Casodex®	bicalutamide	Zeneca	**Metastatic Carcinoma of Prostate** Quality of life was assessed with self-administered patient questionnaires on pain, social functioning, emotional well-being, vitality, activity limitation, bed disability, overall health, physical capacity, general symptoms, and treatment related symptoms. Assessment of the quality-of-life questionnaires did not indicate consistent significant differences between the two treatment groups.

(*cont.*)

Table D.1. (*cont.*)

Drug Brand Name	Generic Name	Manufacturer	Label
Photofrin®	porfimer sodium	QLT Phototherapeutics Inc	**Non-Small-Cell Lung Cancer** Patient symptoms were evaluated using a 5- or 6-grade pulmonary symptom severity rating scale for dyspnea, cough, and hemoptysis. Patients with moderate to severe symptoms are those most in need of palliation. Improvements of 2 or more grades are considered to be clinically significant. Table 3 of the package insert, shows the percentages of patients with moderate to severe symptoms at baseline who demonstrated a 2-grade improvement at any time during the interval evaluated. Dyspnea was graded on a 6-point severity rating scale; cough and hemoptysis on 5-point scales. Clinically significant improvement was defined as a change of at least two grades from baseline.
			In a separate retrospective analysis, patients were individually evaluated to identify those patients whose benefit to risk ratio was most favorable, ie., those who obtained clinically important benefit with minimal adverse reactions. Clinically important benefit was defined as one of the following:
			1. a substantial improvement in pulmonary symptoms at Month 1 or later (dyspnea $>/=2$ grades, hemoptysis $>/=3$ grades, cough $>/=3$ grades or increase in $FEV_1 >/=40\%$);
			2. a moderate improvement in symptoms at Month 2 or later (dyspnea 1 grade, cough 2 grades, hemoptysis 2 grades or increase in FEV $1>/=20\%$); or
			3. a durable objective tumor response (CR or PR maintained to Month 2 or longer).
			Thirty-six (36) of the 99 PDT-treated patients (36%) and 23 of the 99 Nd: YAG-treated patients (23%) received clinically important benefit with only minimal or moderate toxicities of short duration. 34 of 99 PDT-treated patients demonstrated improvements in 2 or more efficacy endpoints (dyspnea, cough, hemoptysis, sputum, atelectasis, pulmonary function tests of FEV1 or FVC, Karnofsky Performance Score or tumor response) and 29 patients had improvements in 3 or more.
SUPPORTIVE THERAPY			
Neupogen®	Filgrastim	Amgen	Treatment with Neupogen® significantly reduced the median time to absolute neutrophil count (ANC) recovery and the median duration of fever, antibiotic use, and hospitalization following induction chemotherapy. In the Neupogen® treated group, the median time from initiation of chemotherapy to ANC recovery was 20 days vs 25 days in the control group, p = 0.0001, the median duration of fever was reduced by 1.5 days (p = 0.009) and there were statistically significant reductions in the durations of IV antibiotic use and hospitalization.
Marinol®	dronabinol	Unimed Pharmaceuticals	The appetite stimulant effect of Marinol (dronabinol) in treatment of AIDS-related anorexia associated with weight loss was studied in a randomized, double-blind, placebo-controlled study involving 139 patients. The effect of Marinol on appetite, weight, mood, and nausea was measured at scheduled intervals during the six-week treatment period.

Table D.1. (*cont.*)

Drug Brand Name	Generic Name	Manufacturer	Label
			As compared to placebo, Marinol treatment resulted in a statistically significant improvement in appetite as measured by visual analog scale. Trends toward improved body weight and mood, and decreases in nausea were also seen.
			Marinol treatment of chemotherapy-induced emesis was evaluated in 454 patients with cancer, who received a total of 750 courses of treatment of various malignancies. The antiemetic efficacy of Marinol was greatest in patients receiving cytotoxic therapy with MOPP for Hodgkin's and non-Hodgkin's lymphomas.
Epogen®/Procrit®	epoetin alfa	Amgen /Ortho Bio	Changes in the quality of life of adult patients treated with Procrit were assessed as part of a phase 3 clinical trial. Once the target hematocrit (32% to 38%) was achieved, statistically significant improvements were demonstrated for most quality of life parameters measured, including energy and activity level, functional ability, sleep and eating behavior, health status, satisfaction with health, sex life, well-being, psychological effect, life satisfaction, and happiness. Patients also reported improvement in their disease symptoms. They showed a statistically significant increase in exercise capacity Vox max, energy and strength with a significant reduction in aching, dizziness, anxiety, shortness of breath, muscle weakness, and leg cramps.
Actiq®	fentanyl citrate	Anesta Corp	Actiq produced statistically significantly more pain relief compared with placebo at 15, 30, 45 and 60 minutes following administration. In this same study patients also rated the performance of medication to treat their breakthrough cancer pain using a different scale ranging from "poor" to "excellent." On average, placebo was rated "fair" and Actiq was rated "good."
Sandostatin LAR® Depot	octreotide acetate for injection suspension	Novartis Pharm	Overall, mean daily stool frequency was as well-controlled on Sandostatin LAR® Depot as on Sandostatin® Injection (approximately 2 to 2.5 stools/day). Mean daily flushing episodes were similar at all doses of Sandostatin LAR® Depot and on Sandostatin® Injection (approximately 0.5 to 1 episode/day).
Thyrogen®	thyrotropin alfa for injection	Genzyme Corporation	Quality of Life: Following Thyrogen, no change was observed in any of the 8 domains of the SF-36 Health Survey, a patient-administered quality-of-life measurement instrument. Following thyroid hormone withdrawal, statistically significant negative changes in quality of life parameters were observed in 4 of the 8 SF-36 domains. These 4 domains were: physical functioning, physical role, bodily pain and emotional role. No change was observed in the following scales: general health, vitality, social functioning and mental health. Thyrogen administration was not associated with the signs and symptoms of hypothyroidism that accompanied thyroid hormone withdrawal as measured by the Billewicz scale. Statistically significant worsening in all signs and symptoms were observed during the hypothyroid phase ($p<0.01$).
			Thyrogen is indicated for use as an adjunctive diagnostic tool for serum thyroglobulin (Tg) testing with or without radioiodine imaging in the follow-up of patients with well-differentiated thyroid cancer.

Source: PDR@ Electronic Library ™ Copyright © 2002 Medical Economics Company, Inc.[8]

found that epoetin alfa can significantly increase hemoglobin levels, reduce transfusion requirements, and improve patient quality of life. These benefits appear to be independent of tumor response.[10]

The FDA approved gemcitabine for patients with pancreatic carcinoma refractory to fluorouracil and mitoxantrone for hormone-refractory prostate carcinoma. In these two examples, clinical benefit addressed the positive effects of a treatment in improving disease-related symptoms beyond the classic cancer outcomes of partial or complete response.[11] In two gemcitabine studies, clinical benefit was defined as a composite assessment of the treatment's effect on pain (measured by intensity and analgesic consumption), Karnofsky Performance Status, and changes in body weight. Gemcitabine was shown to induce a clinical benefit in over 20% of patients, a rate statistically significantly superior to the clinical benefit obtained with fluorouracil (Table D.1).

In the mitoxantrone study, the clinical benefit was defined as a two-point reduction in pain on a six-point scale. This level of pain reduction was achieved by 29% of patients receiving mitoxantrone plus prednisone, compared to 12% of patients receiving prednisone alone. In this example, patient-reported pain was the primary endpoint of the study.

PRO labeling has been achieved for several other prescription medicines. Table D.1 provides specific information from the product labels for 16 drugs. In summary, Hycamtin®, Aredia®, Actiq®, and Zoladex® all demonstrated improvement in pain control; Procrit®, Epogen®, and Taxol® demonstrated improved quality of life as well as symptom control; Sandostatin® LAR reported reduced flushing and stool frequency; and Photofrin® demonstrated an improvement in symptom control. Marinol® has been shown to decrease wasting and control nausea. Thyrogen®, used as a diagnostic tool for patients with thyroid cancer, demonstrated a significant decrease in quality of life in patients who were hypothyroid. One product contains information regarding economic outcomes in the label:

Neupogen® is associated with reduced intravenous antibiotic use and decreased hospitalizations.

There has been a growing body of research on the cognitive impact of standard versus high-dose chemotherapy.[12] Adults with cancer experience cognitive deficits associated with a variety of treatments. A study by van Dam et al.[13] evaluated breast cancer patients an average of two years post-treatment who were randomized to high-dose chemotherapy plus tamoxifen or standard-dose (5-fluorouracil, epidoxorubicin, and cyclophosophamide) plus tamoxifen. A control group included stage I patients who had local therapy only. Cognitive impairment appeared dose related with 37% in the high-dose arm, 17% in the standard-dose arm, and 7% of those receiving local therapy only demonstrating cognitive impairment. Other studies support this finding.[14–16] Many cytotoxic drugs commonly used in standard-dose chemotherapy regimens have documented neurotoxicity affecting both the central nervous system and peripheral nerves. Data and reports from cancer survivors suggest that cognitive difficulties, although subtle, may have significant impacts on quality of life.

While the list in Table D.1 does not represent all PRO labeling for oncology drugs, it is clear from recent trends in labeling that more specificity is apparent concerning PRO claims. That is, PRO research is increasingly more focussed. There is recognition that HRQOL instruments aimed at a broad overall view may miss subtle changes that are relevant to cancer patients. Much progress has been made in determining the impact of chemotherapy and supportive care on the patient's quality of life. More attention is being paid to the clinical benefit and symptom assessment components of PRO measures. Questions remain regarding cognitive impairment and other disease- and treatment-specific approaches.

Drug advertising and promotion

When a new drug is approved in the US, the promotion of the drug must conform to standards set forth in the Federal Food Drug and Cosmetic Act. The promotional standards are guided by the content in the approved labeling. If a specific promotion is supported by substantial evidence and is associated with a labeled claim or the specific mention of the findings in the package insert, then the dissemination of this information and of the evidence supporting the claim is straightforward. Under the Federal Food Drug and Cosmetic Act Sec. 505(d), substantial evidence means evidence consisting of adequate and well-controlled investigations, usually deemed to mean two or more. A single adequate and well-controlled investigation with confirmatory evidence can be sufficient to establish substantial evidence in special circumstances; these are usually large and convincing studies. Companies are permitted to promote PRO findings if they are adequately supported and not inconsistent with the product label. When the FDA grants a labeled claim, they warrant that there is sufficient evidence to support promotion. If the information is supported by substantial evidence and consistent with the product label, but is not noted in the package insert, promotion is acceptable. However, the sponsor may be required to provide supporting evidence at the request of the FDA. If the promotion is not related to a labeled indication or claim, it is considered to be off limits for general promotion, in journal ads and by pharmaceutical sales representatives, for example.

Statistical considerations

For the labeling and advertising of pharmaceutical products, the analysis of PROs generally should meet the same standards as other clinical outcomes considered for claims and be integrated into the drug development process.[17,18] The analysis of PRO data should be pre-specified as part of the overall statistical analysis plan and be in accordance with sound statistical principles. The analysis plan should pre-specify the objectives and hypotheses, sample size calculations, methods of analysis including the handling of missing data and multiple testing, and expectation of a clinically meaningful difference. Simplicity of analyses should be the rule when appropriate.

Missing data

In oncology clinical trials, especially in advanced disease, it is evident that not all patients will complete the same number of assessments because of illness, death, study constraints, and other reasons. Given the multidimensional, prospective, and longitudinal nature of PRO data, missing data and multiple testing are key considerations in the analysis of such data. A distinction should be made between situations where all responses are missing and where responses to specific items are missing. When all responses are missing, there are several ways to proceed: prospectively document reasons for missing data, collect covariates to help analyze the missing data pattern, conduct sensitivity analyses with different models or strategies, and pre-specify in the data analysis plan the use of selected methods.[19,20] When items are missing, the data analysis plan should address how missing items will be handled.

Multiple testing

Because assessments on measures of PRO data often involve several variables (domains or items), multiple testing is required, and it is therefore important to first identify and rank the domains or items in order of importance. For example, if a new therapy is intended to alleviate problems with cognitive functioning, then cognitive functioning could be regarded as the most important PRO domain and, hence, would be used for sample size determination in a clinical trial. Pre-specification of the analytic approach consistent with the objectives for the PRO research targets aids interpretation of the results at the end of the study. If more than a few variables have equal and prime importance, one of several multiple comparison procedures ought to be considered.[20,21]

Clinically important effects

Another important topic for PROs is the concept of the clinically meaningful difference. No industry consensus exists regarding a single research approach for determining the minimal magnitude of effect needed for clinical relevance.[17] Anchor-based methods and distribution-based methods are steps in the right direction, and may prove useful, but are not perfect.[22] Statistical thresholds for effect sizes are also used to evaluate differences.

Evaluation for clinical significance of a given PRO measure should be based on solid evidence that can withstand peer review and regulatory scrutiny and is generally done case-by-case. Instruments with published results on clinical meaningfulness, like the EORTC QLQ-C30[23] and FACT-L,[24] are likely to increase the chance of being chosen for not only powering studies but also establishing promotional claims. After a range of clinical significance is established from pre-marketing studies, phase IV studies can serve to test the generalization of clinical significance in special populations and specific clinical situations not examined fully in earlier studies.

Bayesian approaches

Several other major statistical issues currently confront industry, regulators, and purchasers of health care, and they will receive increasing attention in the years ahead. Among the most prominent are Bayesian approaches and the role of decision modeling. Their methodologies apply to PROs and especially to economic evaluations.

Three basic components in the Bayesian framework are the prior distribution, likelihood function, and posterior distribution.[25-27] The prior distribution describes a parameter or quantity of interest (e.g., a treatment effect) based on evidence not derived from the study under analysis. The likelihood function captures summary information concerning the same quantity available from the data collected in the study. The posterior distribution synthesizes both prior and likelihood information, providing an update to the quantity of interest.

Differences exist between classical (frequentist) and Bayesian approaches.[27] Unlike frequentist methods, Bayesian methods formally specify a prior probability distribution. With Bayesian methods, interpretation of the parameter (quantity) of interest is taken as an unknown quantity with a probability distribution; with frequentist methods, on the other hand, interpretation of a parameter is considered a fixed state of nature. The basic objective in Bayesian methods concerns how likely is a particular value of the parameter given the data, whereas the fundamental objective in frequentist methods concerns how likely is the data given a particular value of the parameter. These differences help to explain why Bayesian analysis is said to provide results and interpretations that are naturally amenable to decision-making in ways that classical analysis is not intended.

A key benefit of the Bayesian approach is that it can make use of prior information in addition to the sample data for the purpose of drawing inferences in the context of economic evaluation. The Bayesian approach can incorporate all available sources of evidence (e.g., randomized controlled trials, databases, expert judgments) into a single model that can be used to evaluate the cost-effectiveness of alternative treatments. Information from Bayesian analysis offers the potential for pharmaceutical companies to justify, and policy makers to decide, whether the analysis provides a sufficient basis for preferring or recommending a treatment, or whether there remains a need for more information.

Before the potential can be fully realized, however, Bayesian approaches need to be made more transparent and accessible. Moreover, philosophical differences and especially practical issues need to be understood and overcome.[28,29] The essence of Bayesian logic is that concerning estimates of effectiveness – close is good enough. While this logic is clear in some settings such as thrombolytic therapy where the mechanism of action is well characterized, the clinical effects are highly predictable, and the ancillary concerns are known; in settings where the clinical and biological course is not so well characterized, hormone replacement therapy or inflammatory bowel disease, for example, the use of Bayesian methods may be more tenuous. Analysts should consider the relative certainty of key effectiveness parameters in applications of Bayesian techniques.

The application of frequentist approaches to estimation and inference for PROs has gradually gained mainstream acceptance. The adoption of Bayesian methods has been slowed somewhat by a reluctance to use prior information, unfamiliarity, mathematical complexity, conservativism, and lack of software. Current international guidelines for statistical submissions to drug regulatory authorities state, "the use of Bayesian and other approaches may be considered when the reasons for their use are clear and when the resulting conclusions are sufficiently robust."[30]

Receptivity to Bayesian methodology has increased over the last few years with the advent of publicly available software,[31] as well as with educational efforts that have minimized mathematical details. Educational efforts have included the following: (1) sensitivity analyses with different types of prior information (including a non-informative prior) to strengthen conclusions or examine their robustness; (2) case studies with practical import; (3) comparisons between Bayesian analyses and existing frequentist analyses; and (4) enhanced interpretation of results in clinical trials and other studies on outcomes research.[27,32-37] Bayesian analyses of phase IV studies can benefit considerably from the prior information, as well as the amenability of modeling assumptions, garnered from phase II and phase III studies.

Decision modeling

The pharmaceutical industry uses decision modeling in pharmacoeconomic evaluations for purposes of marketing and advertising.[38] Here, the industry is faced with dual challenges. One challenge is how best to report and disseminate information for health economic decision makers. The twin challenge is how to encourage the use and acceptance of the information by principal stakeholders such as journal editors, regulatory agencies, and payers and providers of health care.

Some degree of modeling is generally necessary to assess clinical and economic consequences beyond the restrictions of a randomized controlled trial. For example, extrapolation models are usually necessary to assess clinical and economic consequences beyond the period observed in a clinical trial. Any decision model that relies on assumptions about a drug's efficacy that are not based on data from randomized controlled trials must be prominently disclosed in any promotion. Large and simple trials to measure resource utilization in early phase IV studies is one way to improve randomized controlled studies as tools for health economic decision-making. Whenever possible, models should be validated against other data sets.

Economic studies for new oncology products

As with all decisions where economics plays a role, appropriate utilization of medicines depends on whether their benefits exceed their costs. At an aggregate level, there is an extensive body of evidence showing that medicines have provided substantial societal benefits, at costs below those acceptable for other types of interventions (safety, environmental), and that new medicines provide incremental benefits over older medicines.[39-41] There are also many studies documenting the cost-effectiveness of individual medications, including oncology medicines. Most of this evidence is based on research into the actual benefits and costs of medicines once used in common practice.

However, there is an ever-growing demand for evidence on the economic value of newly marketed medicines, including oncology products. National health services as well as hospital and managed care formularies often require economic assessments and estimates of value of new oncology products. As a result, pharmaceutical companies commonly conduct economic assessments of oncology products during their development to have evidence ready at the time of launch. These assessments present many challenges, some of which are discussed below. Due to these challenges, it is often difficult to make a definitive statement about the cost-effectiveness, and thus the true value, of the product before it is used in a real-world setting in the general population of oncology patients. Thus, it is important to consider the appropriateness of economic analyses in the initial, early decisions about pricing, reimbursement, and use of oncology products. Definitive value estimates for oncology agents are best performed when the optimal tumor types, dosing, patient populations, and combination therapy agents are all known, which is usually several years post-launch.

Challenges and timing of economic evaluations

The challenges present in early economic evaluation for oncology products are due to both the nature of clinical trials needed to gain approval to market a new drug and the particular characteristics of oncological medicine. They can occur in other areas as well, but generally not in the same degree or combination. These challenges include but are not limited to the following:

- evolution of the role of an agent in therapy (2nd line, 1st line, adjuvant . . .)
- use of combination and sequential therapy
- relatively small clinical trials
- relevance of the quality of life vs. survival trade-off
- prevalence of off-label use
- need for long-term modeling due to short trial duration and use of surrogate endpoints.

As previously mentioned, oncology is somewhat unique in that few newly diagnosed cancer patients are willing to be treated with anything but proven therapy. Thus, most experimental oncology products are first tested on patients who have failed the more standard treatments for their type of cancer. A product that proves to be efficacious in 2nd or 3rd line therapy immediately becomes a valuable part of the oncologist's armamentarium and generally first gets marketing approval as a backup agent. However, it then also becomes a proven therapy and, depending on the efficacy of existing first-line agents and comparative side-effect profiles, may become an option for first-line therapy as well. New clinical trials may or may not be conducted to obtain an indication as a first-line agent officially. The product may also be considered for adjuvant therapy. If a drug progresses from last-resort to front-line use in this way, many aspects of the economic evaluation will change as well (e.g., survival estimates). As a result, the best economic evaluation that can be done at the time of launch may be largely irrelevant within a few years.

It is also fairly uncommon for cancer patients to be treated with just one therapy during the course of their disease. Drug therapies are often given in combination with each other or with other treatments such as radiation or surgery. Even if a drug is initially successful, cancer patients often relapse and may be given a different treatment subsequently. Even though randomized trials can test the efficacy of a therapy in a particular treatment situation, an economic assessment should analyze the therapy's incremental cost and effectiveness at least over the disease episode, and probably over the patient's remaining lifetime, either of which, in cancer, may be many years.[42,43] Measuring the incremental effects of a single treatment under these conditions can be very difficult; rarely is there efficacy data available to model all the possible treatment alternatives, much less actual cost data – and certainly not before the drug is introduced to the market.

It is well recognized that, to a greater degree than in most other drug classes, a significant proportion of the use of oncology drugs may be off-label, in unregistered indications or doses. This is partly due to the desire of oncologists to try agents that have demonstrated efficacy in one tumor type or combination in other settings to explore rapidly the full efficacy of the new agent beyond what the drug company may examine for registration (i.e., regulatory approval for initial marketing) purposes. Because of this tendency, estimating the full cost impact of an oncology drug once it is available for use can be very problematic. Related to this point is the fact that, as with many other therapies, clinical knowledge about how best to use a cancer drug is limited at the time of introduction. It may take several years of collective experience with a product for practicing physicians to be experienced and skillful in selecting patients most likely to respond favorably to the drug and its dosing, or in recognizing or mitigating side effects before they become significant problems. In the hands of a physician who can adapt this collective learning to the individual patient, a drug may become significantly more cost-effective than initial estimates, based on limited data, would indicate.

Pre-launch economic analysis is further hindered by the fact that many oncology drugs are approved on the basis of relatively small clinical trials, at least in comparison to other therapeutic areas. Patients in these trials are often relatively homogenous and may have characteristics not representative of the more general population in which the product may be used. Also, as discussed above, once a drug has shown efficacy in a population that has failed other therapies, it is often eligible for registration. Only a few hundred patients may be needed to demonstrate such efficacy, and having a large patient basis for safety evaluation is less necessary when patients are already in life-or-death medical situations. Such patients are also often hospitalized or require other costly care, resulting in costs not only with a high mean but also high variance. Obviously, the combination of small samples and high variance data poses major problems for deriving precise estimates of costs or cost-effectiveness.

Modeling in economic evaluations

A final challenge for economic evaluation in oncology, which is also present for most chronic diseases, is the need to use mathematical models to project the long-term outcomes over the patient's remaining lifetime.[44–46] Trials are necessarily of limited duration, but the disease's effects may be lifelong, usually affecting the survival chances of oncology patients. The outcomes observed in trials are generally censored at some point or are based on surrogate measures, such as time to another stage of disease progression. Economic assessments will usually need to be based on assumptions about how these observed measures relate to long-term clinical outcomes, including patient survival.

The challenges above are mainly related to the availability of appropriate data. Methodological concerns are also present but are less unique to oncology. In general, methods for economic assessment as applied to oncology have been described in detail,[47] with some further points, in Chapter 24 by Hornbrook[48] and Chapter 25 by O'Brien[49] in this volume.

This discussion of these issues in the economic assessment of oncology products is not meant to argue that these assessments should not be done. Medical resource allocation decisions must be made at all stages of the product life-cycle, but it is important to recognize and consider the uncertainties at all stages. Early assessments are still important; they can be helpful in identifying the nature of the cost impacts to be expected during the initial marketing period for the product, as well as in guiding future economic assessments. The future assessments, done post-marketing, will be better able to consider many of the issues discussed above and will support more mature judgments about the cost-effectiveness of the product and how that may affect its place in the order of therapy.

Ongoing medical and economic assessments of a therapy are a joint responsibility of the demand and supply side of the information equation, since both the producers and users of the products have a vested interest in the proper valuation of the therapy.[50] Pharmaceutical companies commonly run phase IV trials and may include economic assessments as part of them; they may also sponsor database and other studies to investigate real-world experiences. Government organizations, such as the (US) National Cancer Institute, are important representatives of the public's health in further investigations of the health economic aspects of therapy. Their sponsorship and/or involvement in both pre-marketing and post-marketing studies have played a key role in cancer medical research and an increasing role in economic assessment. More recently, the (UK) National Institute for Clinical Excellence (NICE) has issued several guidances regarding cancer therapies to stimulate more rational and uniform utilization of therapies across the UK.[51–53] Private sector organizations, including both academic centers and the cooperative oncology groups in the US, can and do contribute significantly to this effort. Managed care organizations have tended to be only a secondary partner in most post-marketing oncology studies, but have the patient population and data to play a much larger role.

Conclusions

Although the desired goal of any new oncology drug regimen is to eliminate cancer completely, most tumor types remain resistant to total elimination. Therefore, from the patient's perspective, assessments of clinical benefit of new therapy regimens are more complex in oncology than in diseases where cure or effective management is achievable. The new umbrella term for this type of assessment is "Patient-Reported Outcomes." Clinical trials aimed at the registration of new oncology drugs generally include structured assessments designed to measure PROs, symptoms, function, or HRQOL improvements, for example. If the trials are well designed and demonstrate a result important to prescribing physicians, the PRO findings may be included in the patient drug label and/or drug advertisements. The analysis of PROs should meet the same standards as other clinical outcomes. This is true whether the focus is approval standards, labeling, or promotion.

In today's cost-conscious environments, the value proposition for new drugs must be demonstrated to payers. The value proposition for oncology drugs is complex. The therapy must be positioned relative to the current standard of care and relative to the clinically relevant gains in health status that can be demonstrated in well-controlled studies.

The NCI is in a unique position to further the development of outcomes research in oncology. There are many questions that deserve further research, such as:

- What do patients think is important to measure and improve regarding new oncology drugs?

- How are various cancers managed over a lifetime?
- What evidence is needed to prove the value of a new oncology drug?

It is clear that the oncology field has led the way in quality of life/outcomes research concerned with the patient's perspective. It is only with the combined resources of all the stakeholders that high-quality health technology assessments of existing therapy can be accomplished and then can be incorporated into evolving standards of care.

REFERENCES

1 Lindley, C., Vasa, S., Sawyer, W. T. *et al.* (1998). Quality of life and preferences for treatment following systemic adjuvant therapy for early-stage breast cancer. *Journal of Clinical Oncology* **16**(4):1380–7.

2 Bezjak, A., Ng, P., Skeel, R. *et al.* (2001). Oncologists' use of quality of life information: results of a survey of Eastern Cooperative Oncology Group physicians. *Quality of Life Research* **10**(1):1–13.

3 de Haes, J. C. J. M., van Knippenberg, F. C. E., Neijt, J. P. (1990). Measuring psychological and physical distress in cancer patients: structure and application of the Rotterdam Symptom Checklist. *British Journal of Cancer* **62**: 1034–8.

4 Chang, V. T., Hwang, S. S., Feuerman, M. *et al.* (2000). The Memorial Symptom Assessment Scale Short Form. *Cancer* **89**:1162–71.

5 Aaronson, N. K., Ahmedzai, S., Bergman, B. *et al.* (1993). The European Organization for Research and Treatment of Cancer QLQ-C30: a quality of life instrument for use in international clinical trials in oncology. *Journal of the National Cancer Institute* **85**(5):365–76.

6 Cella, D. F., Tulsky, D. S., Gray, G. *et al.* (1993). The Functional Assessment of Cancer Therapy Scale: development and validation of the general measure. *Journal of Clinical Oncology* **11**(3):570–9.

7 Acquandro, C. (2001). Important issues in patient reported outcomes (PROs) research. *Quality of Life Newsletter*, MAPI Research Institute, No. 27.

8 PDR@ Electronic Library™ Copyright (©) 2002 Medical Economics Company, Inc.

9 Khayat, D. (2000). The main causes of quality of life in cancer patients. *International Journal of Pharmaceutical Medicine* **14**:70–3.

10 Sabbatini, P. (2000). Treating cancer symptoms improves quality of life: Part I: treatment of anemia and fatigue. *International Journal of Pharmaceutical Medicine* **14**: 88–91.

11 Roila, F., Cortesi, E. (2001). Quality of life as a primary end point in oncology. *Annals of Oncology* **12** (Suppl. 3):S3–6.

12 Ahles, T. A., Saykin, A. (2001). Cognitive effects of standard-dose chemotherapy in patients with cancer. *Cancer Investigation* **19**(8):812–20.

13 Van Dam, F. S. A. M., Schagen, S. B., Muller, J. M. *et al.* (1998). Impairment of cognitive function in women receiving adjuvant treatment for high risk breast cancer: high dose versus standard dose chemotherapy. *Journal of the National Cancer Institute* **90**(3):210–18.

14 Wienie, M. H., Diets, E. R. (1995). Neuropsychological assessment of cognitive functioning following chemotherapy for breast cancer. *Psycho-Oncology* **4**:61–6.

15 Schagen, S. B., van Dam, F. S. A. M., Muller, M. J. *et al.* (1999). Cognitive deficits after postoperative adjuvant chemotherapy for breast carcinoma. *Cancer* **85**(3):640–50.

16 Ahles, T. A., Saykin, A., Furstenber, C. *et al.* (2002). Cognitive impact of standard-dose chemotherapy in long-term survivors of breast cancer and lymphoma. *Journal of Clinical Oncology* **20**(2):485–93.

17 Santanello, N. C., Baker, D., Cappelleri, J. C. *et al.* (2002). Regulatory issues for health-related quality of life – PhRMA Health Outcomes Committee Workshop, 1999. *Value in Health* **5**:14–25.

18 Chassany, O., Sagnier, P., Marquis, P. *et al* for the European Regulatory Issues on Quality of Life Assessment Group (2002). Patient-reported outcomes: The example of health-related quality of life – A European guidance document for the improved integration of health-related quality of life assessment in the drug regulatory process. *Drug Information Journal* **36**:209–18.

19 Curran, D., Fayers, P. M., Molenberghs, G. *et al.* (1998). Analysis of incomplete quality of life data in clinical trials. In *Quality of Life Assessment in Clinical Trials: Methods and Practice*, ed. M. J. Staquet, R. D. Hays, P. M. Fayers, pp. 249–80. New York, NY: Oxford University Press.

20 Fairclough, D. L. (2002). *Design and Analysis of Quality of Life Studies in Clinical Trials*. New York: Chapman & Hall/CRC.

21 Zhang, J., Quan, H., Ng, J. *et al.* (1997). Some statistical methods for multiple endpoints in clinical trials. *Controlled Clinical Trials* **18**:204.

22 Guyatt, G. H., Osoba, D., Wu, A. W. *et al.* (2002). Methods to explain the clinical significance of health status measures. *Mayo Clinic Proceedings* **77**:371–83.

23 Osoba, D., Rodrigues, G., Myles, J. *et al.* (1998). Interpreting the significance of changes in health-related quality-of-life scores. *Journal of Clinical Oncology* **16**:139–44.

24 Cella, D., Eton, D. T., Fairclough, D. L. *et al.* (2002). What is a clinically meaningful change on the Functional Assessment of Cancer Therapy-Lung (FACT-L) Questionnaire? Results from Eastern Cooperative Oncology Group (ECOG) Study 5592. *Journal of Clinical Epidemiology* **55**:285–95.

25 Harrell, F. E., Jr., Shih, Y. C. (2001). Using full probability models to compute probabilities of actual interest to decision makers. *International Journal of Technology Assessment in Health Care* **17**:17–26.

26 Hornberger, J. (2001). Introduction to Bayesian reasoning. *International Journal of Technology Assessment in Health Care* **17**:9–16.

27 Spiegelhalter, D. J., Myles, J. P., Jones, D. R. *et al.* (1999). An introduction to Bayesian methods in health technology assessment. *British Medical Journal* **319**:508–12.

28 Sheingold, S. H. (2001). Can Bayesian methods make data and analyses more relevant to decision makers? A perspective from Medicare. 2001. *International Journal of Technology Assessment in Health Care* **17**:114–22.

29 Winkler, R. L. (2001). Why Bayesian analysis hasn't caught on in healthcare decision making. *International Journal of Technology Assessment in Health Care* **17**:56–66.

30 International Conference on Harmonization. *Statistical Principles for Clinical Trials*, 1998. Available at: www.ich.org/pdfifpma/e9.pdf. Accessed October 31, 2002.

31 Fryback, D. G., Stout, N. K., Rosenberg, M. A. (2001). An elementary introduction to Bayesian computing using WinBUGS. *International Journal of Technology Assessment in Health Care* **17**:98–113.

32 Fryback, D. G., Chinnis, J. O. Jr., Ulvila, J. W. (2001). Bayesian cost-effectiveness analysis: An example using the GUSTO trial. *International Journal of Technology Assessment in Health Care* **17**:83–97.

33 Briggs, A. H. (2001). A Bayesian approach to stochastic cost-effectiveness analysis: an illustration and application to blood pressure control in type 2 diabetes. *International Journal of Technology Assessment in Health Care* **17**:69–82.

34 Claxton, K., Neumann, P. J., Araki, S. *et al.* (2001). Bayesian value-of-information analysis: an application to a policy model of Alzheimer's disease. *International Journal of Technology Assessment in Health Care* **17**:38–55.

35 Spiegelhalter, D. J., Myles, J. P., Jones, D. R. *et al.* (2000). *Health Technology Assessment* **4**:1–130.

36 O'Hagan, A. O., Stevens, J. W., Montmartin, J. (2000). Inference for the cost-effectiveness acceptability curve and cost-effectiveness ratio. *Pharmacoeconomics* **17**:339–49.

37 O'Hagan, A. O., Stevens, J. W., Montmartin, J. (2001). Bayesian cost-effectiveness analysis from clinical trial data. *Statistics in Medicine* **20**:733–53.

38 Hay, J., Jackson, J., Luce, B. *et al.* (1999). Panel 2: Methodological issues in conducting pharmacoeconomic evaluations – modeling studies. *Value in Health* **2**(2):78–81.

39 Meyer, J. A. (2002). *Assessing the Impact of Pharmaceutical Innovation: A Comprehensive Framework*. Washington, DC: New Directions for Policy.

40 Tengs, T. O., Adams, M. E., Pliskin, J. S. *et al.* (1995). Five-hundred life-saving interventions and their cost-effectiveness. *Risk Analysis* **15**:360–90.

41 Lichtenberg, F. R. (2001). Are the benefits of newer drugs worth their cost? Evidence from the 1996 MEPS. *Health Affairs* **20**:241–51.

42 Weinstein, M. C., Siegel, J. E., Gold, M. R. *et al.* (1996). Recommendations of the Panel on Cost-Effectiveness in Health and Medicine. *Journal of the American Medical Association* **276**:1253–8.

43 Meltzer, D. (1997). Accounting for future costs in medical cost-effectiveness analysis. *Journal of Health Economics* **16**:33–64.

44 Hutton, J., Brown, R., Borowitz, M. *et al.* (1996). A new decision model for cost-utility comparisons of chemotherapy in recurrent metastatic breast cancer. *Pharmacoeconomics* **9**: 8–22.

45 Nuitjen, M., McCormick, J., Waibel, F. *et al.* (2000). Economic evaluation of letrozole in the treatment of advanced breast cancer in postmenopausal women in Canada. *Value in Health* **3**:31–9.

46 Weinstein, M. C., Toy, E. L., Sandberg, E. A. *et al.* (2001). Modeling for health care and other policy decisions. *Value in Health* **4**:348–61.

47 Brown, M., Glick, H. A., Harrell, F. *et al.* (1998). Integrating economic analysis into cancer clinical trials: the National Cancer Institute – American Society of Clinical Oncology economics workbook. *National Cancer Institute Monographs* **24**:1–28.

48 Hornbrook, this volume, Chapter 24.

49 O'Brien, this volume, Chapter 25.

50 Bennett, C. L., Smith, T. J., George, S. L. *et al.* (1995). Free-riding and the prisoner's dilemma: problems in funding economic analyses of phase III cancer clinical trials. *Journal of Clinical Oncology* **9**:2457–63.

51 National Institute for Clinical Excellence (2000). *Guidance on the Use of Taxanes for Breast Cancer, Technology Appraisal Guidance No. 6, June 2000*. London: National Institute for Clinical Excellence.

52 National Institute for Clinical Excellence (2001). *Guidance on the Use of Docetaxel, Paclitaxel, Gemcitabine and Vinorelbine for the Treatment of Non-Small Cell Lung Cancer, Technology Appraisal Guidance No. 26, June 2001*. London: National Institute for Clinical Excellence.

53 National Institute for Clinical Excellence (2001). *Guidance on the Use of Topotecan for the Treatment of Advanced Ovarian Cancer, Technology Appraisal Guidance No. 28, August 2001*. London: National Institute for Clinical Excellence.

Index

ability to work 396
Activities of Daily Living (ADL), survivorship studies 249
Acute Radiation Morbidity Scoring Criteria 206
adjuvant therapy, breast cancer 93, 95
   cost-effectiveness study 507–8
   HRQOL studies 106–7, 109
   long-term late effects 115
administrative data 526–8
   enhancements to support outcomes research 529
   strengths and limitations 528–9
Affect Balance Scale (ABS) 249
Agency for Healthcare Research and Quality (AHRQ)
   Healthcare Cost and Utilization Project (HCUP) 534, 537
   Integrated Delivery System Research Network (IDSRN) 543
   Medical Expenditure Panel Survey (MEPS) 534, 537
   Primary Care Practice-Based Research Networks (PBRNs) 543
aggregated scores 392, 465
   derivation for multidimensional instruments 476–7, 577
     item aggregation 476
     subscale aggregation 476–7
   see also summary scales and scores
allowed amounts 488–9
ambulatory care costing algorithms 490
American Cancer Society, Study of Cancer Survivors-II
      (SDS-II) 532, 536
American Society of Clinical Oncology (ASCO), National
      Initiative on Cancer Care Quality (NICCQ) 540–1
analytical techniques 10
   see also statistical analyses in outcomes research
androgen deprivation 127–8, 203
   see also hormonal therapy
anemia 625–30
Appraisal of Caregiving Scale (ACS) 338, 339
Area Resource File (ARF) 537
area under curve (AUC) statistic 374

Assessment of Patients' Experience of Cancer Care (APECC) Study 533, 536
Asset and Health Dynamics (AHEAD) Study 493, 535, 538
audio-CASI (computer-assisted self-interview) 352

balance billing 489
balance of error 474
Bayesian methodology 379–80, 515, 561, 577–8, 632–3
  in cost-effectiveness analysis 515–16
  in patient-reported outcome analysis 632–3
Behavioral Risk Factor Surveillance System 530, 531
billed charges 488
bisphosphonates, symptom control in breast cancer 110
blood pressure measurement 2
bowel symptoms
  with prostate cancer treatment 131, 150
    survivorship studies 245
  see also colorectal cancer
BRCA1/BRCA2 genes 222–4
breast cancer 5
  chemoprevention 220–1
    short-term outcome measurement 219
  economic burden 485
  epidemiology 93
  genetic testing 222–4
    short-term outcome measurement 223
  HRQOL studies 9, 94, 107–8, 570
    added benefits of 111–13
    adjuvant drug therapy 106–7, 109, 115
    advanced disease treatment 107–8, 109–10
    follow-up studies 108, 110
    future research needs 113–16
    history of 94–5
    in clinical trials 95, 105–11, 114–15, 116
    instrument selection 104–5
    instruments used 96–7, 101, 105–6
    literature review 96
    primary breast tumor treatment 106, 107
    psychosocial interventions 108, 110–11, 115
    recommendations 113–16
    studies using more than one instrument 101–5
    symptom control 108, 110
  prognosis 93–4
    outcome prediction 112

psychological impacts 94–5, 115
screening 228–9
  false positive screening results 228–9
  negative screening results 228
  short-term outcomes measurement 225–7
survivorship studies 243–4
  instruments used 245–53
treatments 93, 202–3
  adjuvant drug therapy 93, 95, 106–9, 115
  advanced disease 109–10
  cost-effectiveness analysis 507–8
  cost-utility analysis 505
  impact on patients 204–5, 210
  primary breast tumor 106
  treatment decisions 93, 106–10, 112, 115–16
  see also cancer treatments
Breast Cancer Chemotherapy Questionnaire (BCQ) 95, 101, 105
Breast Cancer Prevention Trial (BCPT) 219, 220
Breast Cancer Surveillance Consortium 541
Brief Hospice Inventory (BHI) 267–9, 274, 277
Brief Male Sexual Function Inventory (BSFI) 126, 146–7
Brief Symptom Inventory-53 (BSI-53) 247, 252
burden, concept of 480
  see also economic burden of cancer
Burden Scale 339

California Health Interview Survey (CHIS) 530, 531
cancer
  disease focus 5
  epidemiology 1
  impact on individual 1, 24
  outcomes see outcomes research
  see also breast cancer; colorectal cancer; economic burden of cancer; lung cancer; prostate cancer
cancer care
  continuum of care 5
    HRQOL assessment across 9–10
    patient perspective across 297
    prostate cancer 346
  defining cancer care episodes 486–8
    concurrent episode coding 486–7
    retrospective computerized episode algorithms 488
    retrospective episode coding 487–8
  long-term care costs 491–2
  medical care costs 1, 482–91
  quality of care 3
    categories of 291
    patient perspectives 290–2

see also cancer treatments; caregivers; patient perspectives on cancer care

Cancer Inventory of Problem Situations (CIPS) 96–8

see also Cancer Rehabilitation Evaluation System (CARES)

Cancer Outcomes Measurement Working Group (COMWG) 3–4, 568–9

common approach establishment 7–8

approach to tables 8

categorization of HRQOL measures 7–8

defining HRQOL 7

evaluation of outcome measurement instruments 7

data sources 6–7

development of 4

focus groups 6–7

future directions 580–2

sustaining scientific advancement 580–1

membership 4

operations of 6

outcomes assessment framework 4–6

arenas of application 5

continuum of care 5

disease focus 5

outcome measures of prime interest 4–5

Cancer Outcomes Research and Surveillance Consortium (CanCORS) 538, 540

Cancer Outcomes Research Teams (CORTs) 581

Cancer Patient Need Questionnaire (CPNQ) 310

Cancer Patient Need Survey (CPNS) 309, 310

cancer patients 10

needs of 310, 320–2

see also needs; needs assessment

terminally ill patients *see* end-of-life (EOL) care

treatment impact on 201–2, 210–13, 550

domains of HRQOL affected 204–5

late effects 115, 244

patient-reported instruments 207

treatment preferences 115–16, 288

direct studies 77–8

proxy assessment of patient preferences 349

see also patient perspectives on cancer care; patient-reported outcomes (PROs)

cancer prevention 216, 217

decision making 217

HRQOL studies 9

prophylactic surgery 224

short-term outcomes 217, 231–2

literature review 218

measurement of 229–31

measures 218

see also chemoprevention

cancer registries 523–6

enhancements to support outcomes research 525–6

strengths and limitations 525

Cancer Rehabilitation Evaluation System (CARES) 15, 45–54, 95

breast cancer studies 97, 98, 105

features 45–54

needs assessment 310, 316

performance across the cancer continuum 54

prostate cancer studies 126

psychometric data and validation 46–53

quality-of-life dimensions 16

Short Form (CARES-SF) 54, 95, 310, 316, 320–2

measuring importance of needs 322

translation and cultural adaptation 408–9

survivorship studies 246, 251

translation and cultural adaptation 408–9, 419, 420

psychometric performance 409

usage 54

Cancer Research Network (CRN) 541

cancer treatments 1

economic cost of 1

goal of 623

impact on cancer patients 201–2, 210–13, 550

domains of HRQOL affected 204–5

late effects 115, 244

measurement 206–13

patient-reported instruments 207

outcomes *see* outcomes research

survivor's perspective 287

treatment decisions 201, 389–90

breast cancer 93, 106–10, 112, 115–16

colorectal cancer 193, 194–5

lung cancer 160

prostate cancer 147, 148–50, 558

see also clinical decision making

treatment preferences 115–16, 288

direct studies 77–8

proxy assessment of patient preferences 349

see also cancer care; chemotherapy; drug development; radiation therapy; *specific types of cancer*; surgical treatment

Cancer Worry Scale 249

Caregiver Appraisal Scale 339

Caregiver Quality of Life Index (CQLI) 339–40

Caregiver Quality of Life Index-Cancer (CQOLC) 334, 335–6, 338, 340–1, 342–3
  comparison with Caregiver Reaction Assessment (CRA) 340–1
  construct validity 338, 341
  reliability 338, 341
  responsiveness 338, 339, 341

Caregiver Reaction Assessment (CRA) 334–6, 338, 340–1, 342–3
  comparison with Caregiver Quality of Life Index-Cancer (CQOLC) 340–1
  construct validity 337, 341
  reliability 337, 341
  responsiveness 337, 341
  subscales 337

caregivers 10, 331
  at-risk caregivers 342
  impacts on 10, 329–30, 331, 332, 340
    analysis 330–1
    conceptual model 331–4
    data abstraction 330
    economic burden 493–4
    emotional domain 331–3
    end-of-life care 264–5
    future research 341–2
    literature search 330
    objective impacts 329
    physical domain 333
    positive impacts 333, 341
    social/role domain 333
    spiritual domain 333–4, 341–2
    subjective impacts 329–30, 331, 332
    uses of caregiver impact information 342
  measures of caregiver impact 334–6, 340, 342–3
    overall description 334
  needs of 310, 320–2
  proxy measures of patient-oriented outcomes 348–9
  see also family members and friends

CARES see Cancer Rehabilitation Evaluation System (CARES)

cascading 231

category response curves (CRCs) 431, 448–51

ceiling effects 597

Center for Epidemiologic Studies-Depression (CES-D)
  survivorship studies 247, 252

cervical cancer
  chemoprevention 221–2
    short-term outcome measurement 219
  screening 228–9
    false positive screening results 228–9
    negative screening results 228
    short-term outcomes measurement 225–7

chaining 231

Charlson Index 151

chemoprevention 217, 218–22
  breast cancer 219, 220–1
  cervical cancer 219, 221–2
  colorectal cancer 219, 221
  impact on HRQOL 219–22, 230
  prostate cancer 126, 219, 221
  short-term outcomes 217, 231–2
    literature review 218
    measurement of 219, 229–31
    measures 218
  see also cancer prevention

chemotherapy
  breast cancer 202–3
    cost-effectiveness analysis 507–8
    HRQOL studies 95, 109
    symptom control 110
  colorectal cancer 178, 203
    HRQOL studies 185, 193, 194–5
  impact on cancer patients 201–2, 550, 625–30
    cognitive impact 630
    domains of HRQOL affected 205
    HRQOL endpoint data 559
    measurement 208–10
    patient-reported instruments 207
    toxicity criteria 206–7
    see also specific types of cancer
  lung cancer 203
    cost-effectiveness analysis 504
    HRQOL studies 166
  prostate cancer 128, 203
  see also adjuvant therapy; cancer treatments; drug development; hormonal therapy

Chemotherapy Symptom Assessment Scale (C-SAS) 208–9

childhood cancers 346–7

City of Hope (COH)
  model 17
  Quality of Life Scale (QOLS) 271–3, 275, 277

Clarke and Talcott prostate cancer specific questionnaire 126, 135, 136
  psychometric properties 135

classical test theory (CTT) 425, 590–1
  comparison to item response theory (IRT) modeling 433–8,
      575–8, 591
    computerized adaptive testing 439
    differential item functioning 439–40, 576
    information 436–8
    invariance 435–6
    optimal scaling/scale score interpretation 440–1
    scale development and analysis 438–9
  limitations 445, 469, 590
clinical decision making 389–90
  cost-effectiveness plane 506–7
  in cancer prevention 217
  in screening 217
  levels of 391
    macro level 391
    meso level 391
    micro level 391
  use of HRQOL information 10, 389–90, 554, 558–9,
      581
    from observational studies and clinical trials 588
    instrument selection 578–9
    interpretation of HRQOL data 397
  see also cancer treatments
clinical response benefit 368, 379
clinical significance 370, 631–2
  assessment 379, 560–1
clinical trials 11
  breast cancer 95, 105–11, 114–15, 116
  design of 587
  economic analyses 347
    see also cost-effectiveness analysis (CEA)
  economic studies for new products 633–6
    challenges and timing 634–5
    modeling in economic evaluations 635–6
  HRQOL instrument selection 578
  incorporation of patient-reported outcomes 346–7, 552–3,
      624
    data collection modes 348–53
    decision modeling 633
    measurement across phases of drug development 348
    measurement across stages of disease 346–8
    missing data 353–5, 631
    multiple testing 631
    recommendations 358–9
    regulatory perspective 552–3
    timing and administration 355–6
  lung cancer 169
  prostate cancer 148–50

cognitive aspects of survey methodology (CASM) 610
cognitive interviewing technique 610, 611, 621
  detecting and fixing problems with questions 611–12
  general versus specific application 612
  investigating frame-of-reference effects 618–19
  item selection related to respondent interpretation 613–16
    how respondents conceive of health 614–15
    investigator and respondent characterization of
        concepts 613–14
    selection of response category 615–16
  reference periods 616–17
    probing the past 617
    probing the present 616
  responses to sensitive topics 617–18
  responses to socially desirable behaviors 617–18
  strengths and weaknesses 619–21
    logistics 619
    potential for bias 619–20
    replacement of other evaluation methods 620
    use in cross-cultural assessment 621
  use in self-administered instruments 620–1
  verbal probing versus think-aloud 611
cognitive testing 301
colon cancer 178
  treatment 178
  see also colorectal cancer
colonoscopy 224
  cost-effectiveness analysis 512
colorectal cancer (CRC) 5
  chemoprevention 221
    short-term outcome measurement 219
  economic burden of 485
  epidemiology 178
  HRQOL studies 9, 571
    clinical implications 193–5
    future research needs 195
    instruments used 179–84
    literature search 179
    measurement issues 184–5
    performance of HRQOL measures 192–3
    qualitative findings 190–1
    recommendations 195
    treatment impact 185–90
    value added 191–2
  screening 178, 224–8, 536
    cost-effectiveness analysis 512
    short-term outcomes measurement 225–7
  survivorship studies 245
    instruments used 245–53

colorectal cancer (CRC) (*cont.*)
   treatments 9, 178, 187, 203
      impact on patients 185–90, 205
      metastatic disease 186–7, 188–90
      mixed treatments 185–8
      treatment decisions 193, 194–5
      see also cancer treatments
Common Toxicity Criteria 206
communication issues
   facilitation of communication 390–1
   in end-of-life care 280
   interaction analysis 291–2
   survivor's perspective 287–8
   see also interpersonal care
comparator therapy 511–12
Comprehensive Assessment of Satisfaction with Care
      Questionnaire (CASC) 293–4
computer use for patient-reported data collection 351–2
   digital divide significance 596
   hand-held computers 352
computer-assisted preference elicitation 86–7
computer-assisted self-interview (CASI) 352
computerized adaptive testing (CAT) 439, 445–6, 459–61, 576,
      592
   health status assessment 598
   model selection 600
conceptual equivalence 595
concurrent episode coding 486–7
conjoint analysis 322–4
   hybrid conjoint model 324, 325
ConQuest program 477
construct map 466–8
Consumer Assessment of Health Plans (CAHPS) survey 292,
      295, 299, 300, 530, 532
   response options 296
continuum of care 5
   HRQOL assessment across 9–10, 570
   patient perspective across 297
   prostate cancer 126–8
   see also cancer prevention; end-of-life (EOL) care; screening
core constructs 579–80
cost management information systems (CMISs) 489
Cost of Cancer Treatment Study 495
cost-benefit analysis (CBA) 505–6
cost-effectiveness analysis (CEA) 70–1, 347–8, 398, 494, 503, 504
   Bayesian methods 515–16
   decision analytic models 507–11
      data incorporation 508
      data modeling 508–10

      model structure 507–8
      model validation 510–11
   expected value of information 516
   integration of trials and models 516–18
   net benefit analysis 514–15
   randomized cost-effectiveness trials 511–13
      efficacy versus effectiveness endpoints 512
      integration of evidence 513
      protocol effects 512
      truncated follow-up time 512–13
      wrong comparator therapy 511–12
   sensitivity analysis 513–14
   summary score 577
   see also economic evaluation
cost-effectiveness plane 506–7
cost-minimization analysis (CMA) 504
cost-utility analysis (CUA) 70, 504–5
costing algorithms 490
costs
   assigning costs to specific procedures and services
      488–90
      allowed amounts 488–9
      balance billing 489
      costing algorithms 490
      list prices/billed charges 488
      paid amounts 489
      production costs 489–90
      revenues 489
   drug costs 490
      versus prices 588–9
   hospitalization costs 485
   household costs induced 492–4
   long-term care costs induced 491–2
   lost productivity costs induced 492–4
   measurement of attributable costs 485–8
      comparison sample strategy 486
      defining cancer care episodes 486–8
      microcosting strategy 486
      top-down strategy 485–6
   medical care costs induced 1, 482–91
   societal costs 495–6
counseling *see* genetic counseling; psychosocial interventions
Cronbach's alpha 316–17
cross-cultural use of HRQOL assessments 406–7
   Cancer Rehabilitation Evaluation System (CARES) 408–9, 420
      psychometric performance 409
      Short Form (CARES-SF) 408–9
   EORTC QLQ-C30 411–12, 419, 420–1
      psychometric performance 412–13, 416

Functional Assessment of Cancer Therapy-General
    (FACT-G) 416, 419, 420–1
    psychometric performance 416–18
Functional Living Index Cancer (FLIC) 407–8
    psychometric performance 407–8
    recommendations 418–21
Rotterdam Symptom Checklist (RSCL) 409–10
    psychometric performance 410–11
cultural issues 296, 596
    cognitive interviewing 621
    disenfranchisement 595–6
    see also cross-cultural use of HRQOL assessments

Dale *et al.* prostate cancer specific questionnaire 126, 135,
    136
    psychometric properties 135, 136
data collection from patients *see* patient-reported outcomes
    (PROs)
data sources 6–7, 11, 522
    administrative data 526–8
        enhancements to support outcomes research 529
        strengths and limitations 528–9
    cancer registries 523–6
        enhancements to support outcomes research 525–6
        strengths and limitations 525
    enhancement 581
    focus group 523
    literature search 522–3
    mechanisms 523–6, 539–44
        consortia and networks 540–4
        industry-supported mechanisms 544
        single organizations 539–40
    medical records 526, 528
        enhancements to support outcomes research 529
        strengths and limitations 529
    surveys 530–3, 539
        enhancements to support outcomes research 539
        health knowledge, practices, and outcomes 530–6
        resource use and cost 534–5, 536–8
        strengths and limitations 538
        towards a national cancer data system 544–6
decision analytic models 507–11
    data incorporation 508
    data modeling 508–10
    model structure 507–8
    model validation 510–11
decision making *see* clinical decision making
decision modeling 633
decision significance 573

decision trees 507, 508, 509
Department of Defense (DoD), Military Cancer Institute 539
Department of Veterans Affairs (VA) 539
    Colorectal Cancer Quality Enhancement Research Initiative
        (CRC QUERI) project 539–40
depression
    genetic counseling and 222
    Hospital Anxiety and Depression Scale (HAD) 32–3
Derdiarian Informational Needs Assessment (DINA) 312
diagnosis, survivor's perspective 286–7
Diagnosis Related Groups (DRGs) 490
differential item functioning (DIF) 439–40, 576, 592, 596,
    620
    alternative language instrument evaluation 412, 419
digital divide 596
dimensionality 592–3
    multidimensional approach 11, 456, 465, 576–7
    unidimensionality 432–3, 446–8, 465, 592, 593
disability measurement 590
disability-adjusted life years (DALYs) 485, 496–7
disadvantaged populations 595
    disenfranchisement 595–6
disaggregated scores 392
discomfort measurement 590
discovery methods 591–2
disenfranchisement 595–6
    digital divide 596
distance 469–70
drug costs 490
    versus drug prices 588–9
drug development 624, 636
    development phases 551
        phase I studies 551
        phase II studies 551
        phase III studies 551
        phase IV studies 551
    economic studies for new products 633–6
        challenges and timing 634–5
        modeling in economic evaluations 635–6
    promotional claims 553–4, 555, 556–7, 559–60
        patient-reported outcomes and 630–1
    regulatory issues 552–4
        drug evaluation 588
    use of HRQOL data 11–12, 550, 551–4, 555
        industry perspective 554–5, 624
        patient-reported outcome measures 348
    see also clinical trials
drug labeling 552, 553–4, 555, 559–60
    patient-reported outcomes and 625–9, 630

drug therapy *see* chemotherapy
Dyadic Adjustment Scale (DAS) 249

Eastern Cooperative Oncology Group (ECOG) measure 369–70, 386
economic analysis *see* economic evaluation
economic burden of cancer 1, 11, 480–1, 572
  applications 482
  challenges 496–9
    equity issues 496, 498–9
    total societal value-loss 496–8
  economic evaluations 482, 490–1, 494
  formal long-term care costs induced 491–2
  formal medical care costs induced 1, 482–91
  household costs induced 492–4
  lost productivity costs induced 492–4
  methodological approaches 481–2
    macrocosting 481, 485–90, 492
    microcosting 481, 485, 486, 487, 492
    modeling 481–2
  patient-level burden 482, 485–90, 493–4
    assigning costs to procedures and services 488–90
    measuring attributable costs 485–8
  population-level burden 482, 492–3
  prostate cancer 485
  see also cost-effectiveness analysis; costs
economic evaluation 480, 482, 503–7
  clinical trials 347
  cost-benefit analysis (CBA) 505–6
  cost-effectiveness plane 506–7
    see also cost-effectiveness analysis
  cost-minimization analysis (CMA) 504
  cost-utility analysis (CUA) 70, 504–5
  household costs 494
  lost productivity costs 494
  medical care costs 490–1
  new oncology products 633–6
    challenges and timing 634–5
    modeling in economic evaluations 635–6
  rationale 503–4
Edmonton Symptom Assessment System (ESAS) 269–71, 275, 277
Educational Testing Service (ETS) 601
effectiveness studies 398, 512
efficacy studies 398, 512
emotional impacts *see* psychological impacts
end results 1–2
  see also endpoints

end-of-life (EOL) care 23, 264
  domains of HRQOL affected 265–6
    physical well-being 266
    psychological well-being 266
    social well-being 266
    spiritual well-being 266
  HRQOL studies 10, 264, 276
    barriers to EOL research 279
    in health services research 279
    instruments used 17, 266–73, 276
    longitudinal designs 278–9
    moving away from narrow symptom focus 276–7
    posthumous approach 278
    qualitative versus quantitative methods 279
    role in palliative care research 279–80
    subject burden 277–8
  impact on caregivers 265
  importance of HRQOL 264–5
  prostate cancer 128
  see also palliative care
end-of-scale aversion 72
endpoints 1–2, 386
  clinical response benefit 368, 379
  construction and validation of 379
  efficacy versus effectiveness endpoints 512
  end-of-life care 276–7
  identification and measurement of 367–8
  multiple endpoints 356–7, 370–1
  see also health-related quality of life (HRQOL)
EORTC QLQ-C30 15, 54–5, 95
  breast cancer module (BR-23) 97, 98, 99–100
  breast cancer studies 97, 98, 105
    representative scores 102
  changes in scores 394–5
  colorectal cancer module (CR-38) 179–80, 182, 194
  colorectal cancer studies 179, 180, 188–9
    performance of instrument 192
    treatment impact 185
  end-of-life studies 275–6, 277
  features 54
  lung cancer module (LC-13) 161, 162–4, 171
    construct validity 164
    content validity 162–4
  lung cancer studies 161–2
  performance across the cancer continuum 54–5
  profiles 31
  prostate cancer module 135, 136–45
    psychometric properties 135

prostate cancer studies 126, 145, 148, 151
　representative scores 141
psychometric data and validation 46–53, 99–100, 412–13,
　　414, 415, 416
quality-of-life dimensions 16
Subjective Significance Questionnaire (SSQ) 394–5
survivorship studies 246, 251, 255
translation and cultural adaptation 411–12, 419, 420–1
　psychometric performance 412–13, 416
type of information elicited 21
usage 54–5
epoetin alfa 625–30
equity issues
　conceptual equivalence 595
　digital divide 596
　disadvantaged populations 595
　in economic burden measurement 496, 498–9
　psychometric equivalence 595
European Organization for Research and Treatment of Cancer
　　(EORTC)
　Core Quality of Life Questionnaire see EORTC QLQ-C30
　toxicity criteria 206
European Randomized Study of Screening for Prostate
　　Cancer 127
EuroQol EQ-5D 78–80, 179
　colorectal cancer studies 190
　components 78–9
　measurement properties 79–80
　　construct validity 79
　　content validity 79
　　practical aspects 80
　　reliability 79–80
　　responsiveness 80
　strengths and limitations 85
evaluations, in subjective assessment 19–23, 27
　changes over time 23
　in definitions of quality of life 20–2
　influencing factors 22–3
　measurement of 22
Expanded Prostate Cancer Index Composite (EPIC) 126, 135–7,
　　146, 152
　psychometric properties 135–7
　representative scores 144
expectations 297–8
　influence on patient evaluations 297–8, 299
expected utility theory 73
expected value of perfect information (EVPI) 516,
　　517
expected value of sample information (EVSI) 516

face-to-face interviews 350
FACT see Function Assessment of Cancer Therapy (FACT)
FAMCARE Scale 293, 314
Family Inventory of Needs (FIN) 314
　Husbands (FIN-H) 314
family members and friends
　HRQOL assessment 288
　needs assessment 306
　proxy measures of patient-oriented outcomes 348–9
　see also caregivers
fatigue 625–30
Feeling Thermometer (FT) 71–3
Ferrans and Powers Quality of Life Index (QLI) 16–17, 21,
　　23
　psychometric data and validation 34–42
　quality-of-life dimensions 16
　survivorship studies 246, 251
　type of information elicited 21
　see also Quality of Life Index (QLI)
Ferrans model 17
field testing 301
Fieller's Theorem 514
final endpoints see endpoints
finasteride 221
FLIC see Functional Living Index – Cancer (FLIC)
focus groups 6–7
Food and Drug Administration (FDA) 550, 552–4
　regulatory perspective on HRQOL endpoints 552–4
　　guidance and standards 555, 556–7, 581
foreign language questionnaires see translation
forms, design of 354
Forrest plot 375, 377
Fowler Prostate Cancer Outcomes Assessment 250
frame-of-reference effects 618–19
friends see family members and friends
Function Assessment of Cancer Therapy (FACT) 21, 23,
　　95
　breast cancer module (FACT-B) 97, 98, 99–100, 105
　　representative scores 102
　colorectal cancer module (FACT-C) 179–84, 194
　　construct validity 81
　end-of-life studies 276, 277
　endocrine subscale 210
　FACIT 251, 276
　General (FACT-G) 55, 98
　　breast cancer studies 97, 98, 99–100
　　changes in scores 395
　　colorectal cancer studies 180–4
　　features 55

Function Assessment of Cancer Therapy (FACT) (*cont.*)
  performance across the cancer continuum 55
  prostate cancer studies 126, 135, 145, 148, 151
  psychometric data and validation 46–53, 99–100, 135,
    418
  translation and cultural adaptation 416, 417, 419, 420–1
  usage 55
  lung cancer module (FACT-L) 162, 163–5, 171
    construct validity 165
    content validity 165
    criterion-related validity 165
    Trial Outcome Index 164–5
  profiles 31
  prostate cancer module (FACT-P) 126, 135, 146, 148
    psychometric properties 135
    representative scores 142
  quality-of-life dimensions 16
  survivorship studies 246, 251, 255
  type of information elicited 21
functional assessment 386, 597–8
Functional Living Index – Cancer (FLIC) 55–6, 95
  breast cancer studies 96, 97, 105
    representative scores 103
  colorectal cancer studies 179, 189
  features 55–6
  performance across the cancer continuum 56
  prostate cancer studies 126, 150–1
  psychometric data and validation 46–53
  quality-of-life dimensions 16
  survivorship studies 247, 251
  translation and cultural adaptation 407–8, 419
    psychometric performance 407–8
  usage 56
functional status 26
  assessment 386, 597–8
  measures 7
  see also health status

GBU (Good-Bad-Uncertain) Index 369–70
gemcitabine 630
genetic counseling 222–4
  short-term outcome measurement 223
genetic testing 217, 222–4
  breast cancer 222–3, 224
  negative test result 222
  ovarian cancer susceptibility 223
  positive test result 222–4
    prophylactic surgery and 224
    subsequent surveillance and 222–4

short-term outcomes 217
  literature review 218
  measurement of 223, 229–31
  see also screening
Gibbs Sampling 515
Giesler *et al.* prostate cancer specific questionnaire 126, 135,
  136
  psychometric properties 135–7
global rating measures 7, 394–6
  relationship to magnitude of HRQOL change
    394–6
goserelin *see* hormonal therapy
graded response model (GRM) 430–2, 448–51
graphical presentation of data 375, 376, 377
grief 280
Group Health Cooperative of Puget Sound 539

health
  conception of 614–15
  determinants of 593–5
  physical versus mental health 614
  see also health status
health care policy, influence of patient-reported
    outcomes 587–8
health care utilization 396
Health, Eating, Activity, and Lifestyle (HEAL) Study 532,
  536
Health Insurance Portability and Accountability Act
    (HIPAA) 545
health state preference measurement 8–9, 496–7
  hypothetical health states 77
    see also disability-adjusted life years (DALYs);
      preference-based outcome measures; quality-adjusted
      life years (QALYs)
health status 593–5
  marker states 72
  model 24
  quality of life relationship 25, 26, 558
    functional status 26
  see also functional status; health state preference
      measurement
Health Utilities Index (HUI) 80–3
  Mark 1 (HUI1) 80
  Mark 2 (HUI2) 79, 80
  Mark 3 (HUI3) 79, 80–1, 82
  measurement properties 81–3
    construct validity 81
    content validity 81
    practical aspects 83

reliability 82
responsiveness 82–3
strengths and limitations 85
health-related quality of life (HRQOL) 14–15, 27, 584,
    625
  added value of HRQOL data 555–9, 574–5
    prognostic value 559
    relationship with clinical status 558
    treatment differences 558–9
  breast cancer studies 105–6, 107–8, 570
    added benefits of HRQOL measurement 111–13
    adjuvant drug therapy 106–7, 109, 115
    advanced disease treatment 107–8, 109–10
    follow-up studies 108, 110
    primary breast tumor treatment 106, 107
    psychosocial interventions 108, 110–11, 115
    survivorship studies 243–4
    symptom control 108, 110
    see also health-related quality of life (HRQOL)
      assessment
  causal models 23–7
    Patrick and Chiang model 25–6
    Ware health status model 24
    Wilson and Cleary model 24–5, 26
  chemoprevention impact 219–22
  colorectal cancer studies 571
    qualitative findings 190–1
    treatment impact 185–90
    value added 191–2
    see also health-related quality of life (HRQOL)
      assessment
  cultural variation 421
  definitions 7, 8, 18–19, 568, 571
    as attitudinal versus objective variable 613
    categories of 18–19
    diversity of 613
    issues 591
    selection of 19
  domains of 15–18, 571–2
    impact of cancer therapy 204–5
    in instruments for cancer care 16
  end-of-life studies 264
    domains of HRQOL affected 265–6
    importance of HRQOL at end of life 264–5
    role in palliative care research 279–80
  HRQOL outcomes 389–90
    classification based on level of decision making 391
    health determinants and 595
    primary outcomes 389

    relationship among different outcomes 573–5
    role in palliative care 279–80
    secondary outcomes 389–90
    see also patient-reported outcomes (PROs)
  HRQOL profile 388–9
  impact of cancer therapy 204–5, 210–13, 550
    chemotherapy 208–10
    radiation therapy 207–8
    surgery 207
    see also patient perspectives on cancer care
  interpretation of HRQOL data 391–8, 399–400, 573
    aggregated versus disaggregated scores 392
    anchor-based interpretations 393–6
    by clinicians 397
    by regulatory agencies 397–8
    decision significance 573
    distribution-based interpretations 392–3
    in efficacy, effectiveness or cost-effectiveness studies
      398
    recommendations 398–9
  lung cancer studies 166, 571
    survivorship studies 244
    value added 166–9
  measurement of see health-related quality of life (HRQOL)
      assessment
  mortality relationship 396
  needs relationships 308
  prostate cancer studies 128–9, 571
    survivor's perspective 286–9
    see also health-related quality of life (HRQOL) assessment
  regulatory perspective 552–4
  survivors see survivorship studies
  use of HRQOL information
    by patients and caregivers 10, 554
    by regulatory agencies 11–12, 397–8, 550, 552–4
    current situation 586
    future directions 559–61
    guidance and standards 555, 556–7, 559–60, 581
    in clinical decision making 10, 389–90, 554, 581, 588
    in drug development 11–12, 550, 551–5, 624
    in drug labeling 552, 553–4, 555, 559–60
    patient monitoring 390
  versus quality of life 14–15
  see also quality of life
health-related quality of life (HRQOL) assessment 2–3, 306–8,
    387, 399–400
  across the cancer continuum 9–10, 570
    see also cancer prevention; cancer treatment; end-of-life
      (EOL) care; screening; survivorship studies

health-related quality of life (HRQOL) assessment (*cont.*)

breast cancer 9, 94

added benefits of HRQOL measurement 111–13

future research needs 113–16

history of 94–5

in randomized clinical trials 95, 105–11, 114–15, 116

instrument selection 104–5

instruments used 96–7, 101, 105–6

literature review 96

recommendations 113–16

studies using more than one instrument 101–5

see also health-related quality of life (HRQOL)

classification according to purpose of assessment 387–91

clinical decision making 389–90

communication facilitation 390–1

preference (utility) assessment 390

profile description 388–9

screening 388

cognitive interviewing application 612–19

colorectal cancer 9

clinical implications 193–5

future research needs 195

instruments 179–84

measurement issues 184–5

performance of HRQOL measures 192–3

recommendations 195

targeted assessments 195

see also health-related quality of life (HRQOL)

distinction from symptom assessment 387, 552

during treatment 9

colorectal cancer 9

domains of HRQOL affected by cancer therapy 204–5

lung cancer 9

prostate cancer 9

end-of-life studies 10, 264, 276

instruments used 17, 266–73, 276

methodological considerations 277–9

moving away from narrow symptom focus 276–7

role in palliative care research 279–80

families and friends of patients 288

feasibility 569

frame-of-reference effects 618–19

funding issues 113–14

future needs 399

in clinical trials 346, 551–3

assessment after discontinuation of therapy 355–6

data collection modes 348–53

duration of HRQOL assessment 355

frequency of evaluations 355

instrument selection 578

measurement across phases of drug development 348

measurement across stages of disease 346–8

regulatory perspective 552–3

timing of follow-up assessments 356

timing of initial assessment 356

timing when therapy is cyclic 356

instruments 15–16, 17, 27, 31, 32, 406, 570

adaptation of 10–11

balance of error 474

challenges 571–3, 587, 591–2

construct validity 573

content validity 572

core set of measures 579

crosswalking scores between instruments 458–9, 576

evaluation of 453–5, 560–1

future research issues 57–8, 114, 580

general cancer instruments 45–53, 57

generic instruments 32–42, 45

in survivorship studies 245–53

incorporation of patients' concerns 16–17

item bias 461–2, 463

nonstandard use of 379

positive accomplishments of 367–8

profiles 31

psychometric data and validation 34–42, 46–53, 99–100, 587

quality of 569

redesign of 453–5, 572–3

reliability 573

responsiveness 560–1

selection of 17, 578–9

types of information elicited 21

validity assessment 595

see also instrument construction; item banks; patient-reported outcomes (PROs); *specific instruments*

lung cancer 9, 170–2

analytic concerns 169–70

curative treatment 166–9

instruments 161–4, 166, 167–8

non-randomized studies 169

randomized studies 169

see also health-related quality of life (HRQOL)

measurement approaches 11

item response theory modeling 11

multidimensional approach 11, 456, 465, 576–7

see also item response theory (IRT)

measures 8–9, 25
  cancer-specific measures 8
  functional status measures 7
  general cancer measures 7–8, 45–53, 57
  generic measures 7, 32–42, 45
  global rating measures 7
  symptom measures 7
  see also patient-reported outcomes (PROs)
methodological issues 114
new directions 575–8
objective assessment 19
prostate cancer 9, 130–1
  added value of HRQOL assessments 147–8, 288
  future research needs 152–3
  instruments used 126, 131–47, 148, 150–2, 288
  ongoing assessment 288
  performance of HRQOL measures 148–52
  see also health-related quality of life (HRQOL)
proxy measures of patient-oriented outcomes 349
qualitative approaches 254–5
recommendations 398–9
statistical issues 368–9
subjective assessment 19–23
  evaluations 19–22, 23, 27
  perceived status 19–21, 22, 27
unanticipated findings 17–18
see also cognitive interviewing technique; health-related
    quality of life (HRQOL); patient-reported outcomes
    (PROs); quality of life
Healthcare Cost and Utilization Project (HCUP) 534,
  537
HMO Cancer Research Network (CRN) 541
Hodgkin's disease 17–18
Home Care Study
  Caretaker Form (HCS-CF) 315
  Patient Form (HCS-PF) 311
Home Caregiver Need Survey (HCNS) 314
hormonal therapy
  breast cancer 202–3, 210
    HRQOL studies 109
  impact on patients 205
    measurement 210
  prostate cancer 127–8, 203
  survivorship studies 245
Hospital Anxiety and Depression Scale (HADS) 32–3
  breast cancer studies 97, 98, 105
  colorectal cancer studies 179, 189
  features 32–3
  lung cancer studies 161

performance across the cancer continuum 33
prostate cancer studies 126, 134–45
psychometric data and validation 34–42
survivorship studies 249
usage 33, 45
hospitalization costs 485
household costs induced by cancer 492–4
  economic evaluations 494
  patient-level burden 493–4
  population-level burden 492–3
human papilloma virus (HPV) 221–2
hybrid conjoint model 324, 325

Impact of Event Scale (IES) 248, 252
Index of Coexistent Disease (ICED) 151
Indian Health Service, Resource and Patient Management
    System 539
informal caregivers see caregivers
information 598
Information and Support Needs Questionnaire (ISNQ) 315
instrument construction 453–5, 477, 575–6
  discovery methods 591–2
  Four Building Blocks 466–72, 477
    construct map 466–8
    items design 468
    measurement model 469–72
    outcome space 468–9
  see also specific instruments
Instrumental Activities of Daily Living (IADL)
  survivorship studies 249
insurance claims data 526–8
  see also administrative data
Integrated Delivery System Research Network (IDSRN) 543
intent-to-treat (ITT) analysis 372–4
interaction analysis 291–2
International Breast Cancer Study Group (IBCSG) 101
International Index of Erectile Function (IIEF) 126, 146–7
International Prostate Symptom Score (IPSS) 126, 147
  survivorship studies 250
international studies 406
  see also cross-cultural use of HRQOL assessments
interpersonal care 291
  patient perspectives 291–2
    evaluations 291–2
    reports 291–2
  see also communication issues
interviews
  face-to-face 350
  telephone 350

Inventory of Complicated Grief (ICG) 315
item aggregation 476
item banks 439, 445, 455, 592
  adding items 456–8
  debate 601
  development of 455–6, 576, 580, 601
item bias 461–2, 463, 596
item difficulty 596–8
item discrimination 598–9
item information function (IIF) 436–7, 453
item response theory (IRT) modeling 11, 425–7, 445, 561, 575; 591
  applicability 379
  applications 425, 445, 446, 462–3, 561
    computerized adaptive testing (CAT) 439, 459–61, 576, 579–80
    crosswalking scores between instruments 458–9, 576
    detecting potentially biased test items 461–2, 463
    instrument construction and evaluation 453–5, 572–3, 575–6
    item bank development 455–8, 576
    model selection and 600
    optimal scaling/scale score interpretation 440–1
    reducing patient burden 369
    scale development and analysis 438–9
    summary scores 577
    see also differential item functioning (DIF)
  assumptions 432–3, 446–53
    assessment of 446–53
    local independence 433
    model fit 448–53
    monotonicity 432
    unidimensionality 432–3, 446–8, 465
  basics 427–32
    dichotomous response data 428–30
    polytomous response data 430–2
  category response curves (CRCs) 431, 448–51
  comparison with classic test theory (CTT) approach 434–8, 575–8, 591
  estimation of item and person parameters 433–4
    item-fit 434
    person-fit 434
  evaluation of fit 434
  extensions to 620
  future role in outcomes assessment 441–2
  information concept 436–8
    applications 438–41
    item information function (IIF) 436–7, 453
    scale information function (SIF) 437–8, 453–5

    target information function 453
    trait score estimation 454–5
  invariance property 435–6
    applications 438–41
  item characteristic curve (ICC) 598
  item response curve (IRC) 427–8, 434
  model selection 599–600
  multidimensional approach 11, 456, 465, 576–7
    see also multidimensional item response modeling (MIRM)
  obstacles to greater use 426
  standardized residuals (SRs) 451–3
  terminology 427
items design 468

Japanese Quality of Life Research Group 209

Kaiser Permanente 539
Karnofsky Performance Status Scale (KPS) 386

labeling *see* drug labeling
Late Effects of Normal Tissues/Subjective-Objective Management Analytic (LENT/SOMA) scales 206
Late Morbidity Scoring Criteria 206
levels of evidence 386
linear analogue self-assessment (LASA) scales
  breast cancer 101
Lipscomb, Joseph 4
list prices 488
local independence 433
long-term care costs 491–2
Long-Term Quality of Life (LTQL) 254
  survivorship studies 247, 251–2
longitudinal analysis 301, 374–5
lost productivity costs 492–4
  economic evaluations 494
  patient-level burden of cancer 493–4
  population-level burden of cancer 492–3
lung cancer 5
  HRQOL studies 170–2, 571
    analytic concerns 169–70
    curative treatment 166–9
    findings 166
    instruments used 161–4, 166, 167–8
    literature search 160–1
    non-randomized studies 169
    randomized studies 169
    value added 166–9

mortality 160
non-small-cell (NSCLC) 160, 203
small-cell (SCLC) 160, 203
survivorship studies 244
    instruments used 245–53
treatments 160, 203
    cost-effectiveness analysis 504
    curative treatment 166–9
    decision-making 160
    HRQOL studies 9, 166–9
    impact on patients 205
    see also cancer treatments
Lung Cancer Symptom Scale (LCSS) 162, 163–4, 165–6,
    171
    construct validity 165
    content validity 165
    criterion-related validity 165–6
    reliability 165

M-Plus program 477
McGill Quality of Life Questionnaire (MQOL) 15–16, 274–5
    end-of-life studies 269–71, 274–5, 277
    quality of life dimensions 16
macrocosting 481, 485–90
    long-term care costs 492
mammography see breast cancer
Mammography Questionnaire 294
marker states 72
Markov State-Transition models 507–8, 510
Massachusetts Male Aging Study 146–7
mastectomy 202–3
    HRQOL studies 106
    impact on patients 204, 205
    treatment decisions 93
Medicaid 588
    claims files 527
    see also administrative data
Medical Care Attitude Scale (MCAS) 294
medical care costs 482–91
    economic evaluations 490–1
    patient-level burden of cancer 485–90
    population-level burden of cancer 483–5
Medical Expenditure Panel Survey (MEPS) 534, 537, 539
Medical Outcomes Studies Short Form Health Survey see Short
    Form 36 (SF-36)
Medical Outcomes Trust (MOT) 7, 569
medical records 526, 528
    computer-based systems 529
    enhancements to support outcomes research 529

incorporation of patient-reported outcomes 529
    strengths and limitations 529
Medicare 588
    claims data 526–7
        see also administrative data
    Cost Reports (MCRs) 489
    Current Beneficiary Survey (MCBS) 535, 537–8, 539
    Health Outcomes Survey (HOS) 530, 532
Memorial Symptom Assessment Scale (MSAS) 271–3, 275,
    277
    Global Distress Index (GDI) 275
Mental Adjustment to Cancer (MAC) Scale 248, 252
microcosting 481, 485
    assigning costs to specific procedures and services 488
    attributable cost measurement 486, 487
    long-term care costs 492
minimum important difference (MID) 394
mirror image stream plot 375, 376
missing data 353–5, 372, 373, 561, 631
    analysis approaches 356–8, 371–2, 561, 631
    avoidance of 353–4, 569
        education and training 354
        form design 354
        primary prevention 353–4
        secondary prevention 354
    colorectal cancer studies 191–2
    data collection and management 353
    follow-up procedures 354–5
    lung cancer studies 169–70, 171
Missoula-VITAS Quality of Life Index (MVQOLI) 268–9, 274,
    277
mitoxantrone 630
Montreal Prostate Cancer Model 511
multi-attribute preference-based measures see
    preference-based outcome measures
Multiattribute Health Status (MAHS) 190
multidimensional approach 11, 456, 465, 576–7
multidimensional item response modeling (MIRM) 465, 474–6,
    477
    aggregate score derivation 476–7, 577
        item aggregation 476
        subscale aggregation 476–7
    comparison with unidimensional approaches 466
    future research and applications 477–8
    software options 477
multidimensional random coefficients multinomial logit
    (MRCML) model 475
multinational studies 406
    see also cross-cultural use of HRQOL assessments

multiple endpoints 356–7, 370–1
Multiple Outcomes of Raloxifene Evaluation (MORE) Trial
    220

National Cancer Data Base (NCDB) 524, 525
    strengths and limitations 525
national cancer data system 544–6
National Cancer Institute (NCI) 3
    Assessment of Patients' Experience of Cancer Care (APECC)
        Study 533, 536
    Breast Cancer Surveillance Consortium 536
    Clinical Trials Cooperative Group 541–2
    Community Clinical Oncology Programs (CCOPs) 541–2
    Comprehensive Cancer Centers (CCC) 543
    Health, Eating, Activity, and Lifestyle (HEAL) Study 532, 536
    Physician Survey of Cancer Susceptibility Testing 533, 536
    Survey of Colorectal Cancer Screening Practices 533, 536
    toxicity criteria 206
    see also Cancer Outcomes Measurement Working Group
        (COMWG)
National Cancer Institute of Canada Clinical Trials Group
        (NCIC-CTG) 206
National Center for Health Statistics (NCHS)
    National Ambulatory Medical Care Survey (NAMCS) 534,
        537
    National Hospital Discharge Survey (NHDS) 534, 537
National Comprehensive Cancer Network (NCCN) 541
National Health and Nutrition Examination Survey 530,
        531
national health care policy see health care policy
National Health Interview Survey (NHIS) 530, 531, 590
National Hospital Discharge Survey (NHDS) 534, 537
National Initiative on Cancer Care Quality (NICCQ) 540–1
National Institute for Clinical Excellence (NICE), UK 588
National Long-Term Care Survey 536
National Program of Cancer Registries (NPCR) 524
    strengths and limitations 525
National Survey of Colorectal Cancer Screening Practices 533,
        536
National Survey of Mammography Facilities 536
nausea assessment 19
Need Evaluation Questionnaire (NEQ) 311
needs 305, 310, 320–2
    hierarchy of 305
    identification of 318–19, 324–5
        critical incident technique 318
        person-focused techniques 318–19
    importance of
        influencing factors 319–22

measurement 322–4
    trade-offs 322
of caregivers 310, 320–2
relationships among needs 308, 325
relationships with satisfaction and HRQOL 308, 325
needs assessment 10, 306–8, 573–4
    developing and conducting a needs assessment 317–24
        factors influencing the importance of needs 319–22
        measuring importance of needs 322–4
        needs identification 318–19, 324–5
    distinction from satisfaction and HRQOL assessment 306–8
    family members 306
    importance of 305–6
    instruments review 308–15, 317
        domains 309–17
        instrument characteristics 309
        literature search 308–9
    recommendations 324–5
Needs Near the End-of-Life Care Screening Tool (NEST) 313
net benefit analysis 514–15
net monetary benefit (NMB) 514–15
    Bayesian methods 515–16
non-steroidal anti-inflammatory agents (NSAIDs) 221
Nottingham Health Profile (NHP) 34–42
    colorectal cancer studies 179, 185
    survivorship studies 248
nursing home care costs 490

objective assessment 19
On-Line Guide to Quality-of-Life Assessment (OLGA) 32
Oncology Treatment Toxicity Assessment Tool (OTTAT) 207
1-parameter logistic model (1PLM) 429–30
optical scanning 351
outcome space 468–9
outcomes measurement 2–4, 590–1
    desirable characteristics of outcome measures 3
        identification of 7
    Five D's 590
    new directions 575–8, 580–2
        sustaining scientific advancement 580–1
    outcomes assessment framework 4–6
        arenas of application 5
        continuum of care 5, 570
        disease focus 5
        outcome measures of prime interest 4–5
    proxy measures of patient-oriented outcomes 348–9
    see also health-related quality of life (HRQOL) assessment;
        patient-reported outcomes (PROs); preference-based
        outcome measures

outcomes research 1–2, 522
  common clinical outcomes 386
  current situation 586
  endpoints 1–2, 386
    construction and validation of 379
    end-of-life care 276–7
    identification and measurement of 367–8
    multiple endpoints 356–7, 370–1
  future research needs 445, 580–2, 586–9
    data source enhancement 581
    role of outcome measures in decision making 581
    sustaining scientific advancement 580–1
  HRQOL outcomes 389–90
    primary outcomes 389
    secondary outcomes 389–90
    see also health-related quality of life (HRQOL) assessment
  influence on health care policy 587–8
  literature review 3, 6–7, 364
  methodological challenges 10–11, 587
    analytical techniques 10
    study guidelines 587
  psychometric theory in 11
  statistical issues see statistical analyses in outcomes
      research
  see also data sources; outcomes measurement
ovarian cancer susceptibility testing 223

paid amounts 489
pain
  assessment in prostate cancer palliative treatments 147
  management of 265
  quality-of-life relationship 585
palliative care 264
  lung cancer 170–1
  prostate cancer 147
  role for HRQOL outcomes 279–80
  see also end-of-life (EOL) care
Palliative Care Assessment (PACA) 313
pancreatic cancer economic burden 485
Pap smear test see cervical cancer
Paradox of Cancer Survivorship 255
patient education 288–9
patient expectations 297–8
  influence on patient evaluations 297–8, 299
Patient Information Need Questionnaire (PINQ) 312
Patient Needs Assessment Tool (PNAT) 312, 316
patient perspectives on cancer care 10, 290–1, 623–4
  challenges with patient evaluation measures 297–9
    influence of expectations 297–8, 299

    influence of patient characteristics 298–9
    predispositions 298
  evaluations versus reports 291–2, 299
  instrument review 292–5, 297
    cancer specific versus general measures 296–7
    continuum of care and cancer site 297
    cultural and language differences 296
    domains 295
    reference period 296
    reliability and validity 296
    respondents 296
    response options 296
    sensitivity of measures 296
    weighting the importance of domains 295–6
  interpersonal care 291–2
  literature search 292
  measurement of 292
  questionnaire development 300–1
    cognitive testing 301
    domain development and refinement 300–1
    field testing 301
    longitudinal research 301
    new item construction 301
  ratings 291
  recommended strategy 300–1
    questionnaire content 300
  reports 291–2
    potential usefulness of 299–300
  satisfaction 291
    needs relationships 308
  technical care 291
  value of 623–4
  see also patient-reported outcomes (PROs)
patient satisfaction see patient perspectives on cancer care;
      satisfaction surveys
patient satisfaction with medical care (PSMC) item bank 456
  development of 456–8
Patient Satisfaction with Medical Care Questionnaire
      (PSQ-III) 446, 447, 449, 456–7, 460
  principal components analysis 448
  scale information function 453–5
patient well-being see well-being
patient-oriented prostate utility scale (PORPUS) 84–5
patient-reported outcomes (PROs) 530–6, 584, 623, 624–31
  clinically important effects 631–2
  current usage of 586
  data collection modes 348–53
    cost considerations 351
    face-to-face interview 350

patient-reported outcomes (PROs) (*cont.*)
    mailed self-assessment 351
    proxy measures from caregivers/family 348–9
    self-administration versus interviewer
      administration 349–50
    telephone interview 350
  definitional considerations 624–5
  drug advertising and promotion and 630–1
  history of research 584–6
  in clinical trials 346–7, 551–3, 587, 624
    assessment after discontinuation of therapy 355–6
    duration of HRQOL assessment 355
    frequency of evaluations 355
    measurement across phases of drug development 348
    measurement across stages of disease 346–8
    multiple testing 631
    recommendations 358–9
    regulatory perspective 552–3
    timing of assessments when therapy is cyclic 356
    timing of follow-up assessments 356
    timing of initial assessment 356
  in medical records 529
  influences on 587
  media for data collection 351–2
    computer-assisted self-interview (CASI) 352
    computers 351–2
    cost considerations 352
    hand-held computers (PDAs) 352
    optical scanning 351
    pencil and paper 351
  missing data 353–5, 631
    analysis approaches 356–8, 371–2, 631
    avoidance of 353–4
    data collection and management 353
    follow-up procedures 354–5
  of HRQOL 7, 16–17, 21, 69
    prostate cancer 149–50
  of treatment-related toxicity 169, 207
  product labeling and 625–9, 630
  significance for health care policy 587–8
  statistical considerations 631–3
    Bayesian approaches 632–3
  study quality 352–3
  value added 107–8
  see also health-related quality of life (HRQOL); patient
    perspectives on cancer care; subjective
    assessment
patients *see* cancer patients
PCOS Prostate Index 250

perceived status 19–21, 27
  in definitions of quality of life 20–2
  measurement of 22
Person Trade-Off (PTO) technique 498
personal data assistants (PDAs), for patient-reported data
    collection 352
pharmaceutical industry *see* drug development
Physician Estimate of Survival 33
Physician Survey of Cancer Susceptibility Testing 533, 536
Picker Survey 295, 300
Policy Analysis Institute Questionnaire 249
policy issues *see* health care policy
POLYFIT program 451–2
Post-Traumatic Stress Disorder (PTSD) Checklist 249
preference-based outcome measures 69–71, 87
  direct 69, 71–8, 86
    hypothetical health states 77
    standard gamble (SG) 73, 74, 75–7
    strengths and limitations 85
    surrogate informants 77
    time trade-off (TTO) 74, 75–7
    visual analogue scale (VAS) 71–3
  employment of in cancer intervention studies 70–1
  implications for research agenda 85–7
    computer-assisted preference elicitation 86–7
    direct versus multi-attribute measures 86
    future directions 87
    importance of choice-based preference elicitation 86
    preference-based measures as complement to other
      approaches 86
  indirect (multi-attribute approach) 69–70, 78–85, 86
    disease-specific multi-attribute systems 84–5
    EuroQol EQ-5D 78–80
    Health Utilities Index (HUI) 80–3
    Quality of Well-Being Scale (QWB) 83–4
    selection of multi-attribute system 84
    strengths and limitations 85
  see also outcomes measurement; patient-reported outcomes
    (PROs)
prevention *see* cancer prevention
prices, versus costs 588–9
Primary Care Practice-Based Research Networks (PBRNs)
  543
Princess Margaret Hospital Patients Satisfaction with Doctor
  Questionnaire 293
principal components analysis (PCA) 446, 448
privacy regulations 545
probabilistic sensitivity analysis 513–14
probability (P) value 393

problem-oriented medical record (POMR) 486–7
production costs 489–90
Profile of Mood States (POMS) 43
  alternative language studies 417
  breast cancer studies 97, 98–101, 105
  colorectal cancer studies 179
  features 43
  performance across the cancer continuum 43
  prostate cancer studies 126, 134–45, 150–1
  psychometric data and validation 34–42
  survivorship studies 248, 252–3
  usage 43
prophylactic surgery 224
prostate cancer 5
  chemoprevention 126, 221
    short-term outcome measurement 219
  continuum of care 126–8
  economic burden of 485
  end-of-life care 128
  HRQOL studies 128–9, 571
    added value of HRQOL assessments 147–8
    during treatment 9
    future research needs 152–3
    instruments used 126, 131–47, 148, 150–2, 288
    literature search 129
    measurement of HRQOL 130–1
    multi-attribute preference systems 84–5
    ongoing assessment 288
    performance of HRQOL measures 148–52
  need for 287–8
  screening 126–7, 228
    short-term outcomes measurement 225–7
  support groups 289
  survivor's perspective 286–8
    diagnosis 286–7
    long-term survivorship 287–8
    potential contributions of HRQOL assessment 288
    recommendations 288–9
    treatment 287
  survivorship studies 128, 244–5
    instruments used 245–53
  treatments 127–8, 203
    HRQOL endpoints 147–8
    impact on patients 9, 131, 150, 205
    quality of life issues 129
    treatment decisions 147, 148–50, 558
    treatment preferences 288
    see also cancer treatments
Prostate Cancer Index 23

Prostate Cancer Intervention Versus Observation (PIVOT)
    trial 148
Prostate Cancer Needs Assessment (PCNA) 312
Prostate Cancer Prevention Trial (PCPT) 126, 149, 219,
    221
Prostate Cancer Specific Quality of Life Instrument
    (PROSQOLI) 126, 135
  psychometric properties 135
Prostate Cancer Treatment Outcome Questionnaire 250
Prostate, Lung, Colon and Ovary Trial (PLCO) 127
prostate-specific antigen (PSA) screening 126
Psychological Adjustment to Illness Scale (PAIS)
  survivorship studies 248, 253
psychological impacts
  breast cancer 94–5
  end-of-life studies 266
  on caregivers 331–3
  prostate cancer 134–45
    survivor's perspective 287–8
  survivorship studies 243, 254
    late effects of cancer treatment 244
  see also Profile of Mood States (POMS)
psychometric equivalence 595
psychosocial interventions, breast cancer 108, 110–11,
    115

qualitative approaches 254–5
  colorectal cancer studies 190–1
  end-of-life studies 279
  survivorship studies 253, 254–5
quality of care 3
  categories of 291
  patient perspectives 290–2
    evaluations 291–2
  instrument review 292–7
  reports 291–2
quality of life 14, 15, 625
  definitions 19–21, 22, 591
  health status relationship 25, 26, 550
    functional status 26
  versus health-related quality of life 14–15
  see also health-related quality of life (HRQOL); well-being
Quality of Life and Well-being Questionnaire 179
Quality of Life-Cancer Survivors (QOL-CS) 247, 252, 254
Quality of Life Index (QLI) 43–4
  features 43–4
  performance across the cancer continuum 44
  prostate cancer studies 126
  psychometric data and validation 34–42

Quality of Life Index (QLI) (*cont.*)
  quality-of-life dimensions 16
  usage 44
  see also Ferrans and Powers Quality of Life Index
Quality of Life Inventory 23
Quality of Life Questionnaire for Cancer Patients Treated with
    Anticancer Drugs (QOL-ACD) 209–10
Quality of Life Questionnaire-C30 *see* EORTC
    QLQ-C30
Quality of Life-Radiation Therapy Instrument
    (QOL-RTI) 207–8, 209
Quality of Life Scale for Cancer (QOL-CA) 16–17
  quality-of-life dimensions 16
  type of information elicited 21
Quality of Well-Being Scale (QWB) 79, 83–4
  measurement properties 83–4
    construct validity 83
    content validity 83
    practical aspects 84
    reliability 83–4
    responsiveness 81
quality-adjusted life years (QALYs) 70, 398, 504–5
  cancer burden measurement 485, 496–7
  equity issues 498
quality-adjusted time without symptoms or toxicity
    (Q-TWIST) 78

radiation therapy
  breast cancer 93, 202–3
    cost-utility analysis 505
    HRQOL studies 106
    treatment decisions 93
  colorectal cancer 178, 203
  impact on cancer patients 201–2
    domains of HRQOL affected 204–5
    measurement 207–8
    patient-reported instruments 207
    toxicity criteria 206–7
  lung cancer 203
  prostate cancer 203
    survivorship studies 245
  see also cancer treatments
Radiation Therapy Oncology Group (RTOG) toxicity criteria
    206
raloxifene 220–1
RAND Mental Health Index 150–1
randomized clinical trials *see* clinical trials
randomized cost-effectiveness trials *see* cost-effectiveness
    analysis (CEA)

Rasch model 17, 266–76, 430, 470, 598–9
  model selection 599–600
recall bias 395
rectal cancer treatment 178
  see also colorectal cancer
reference periods 296, 616–17
  probing the past 617
  probing the present 616
reframing 188
regulatory agencies
  interpretation of HRQOL data 397–8
  use of HRQOL data 11–12, 550
    guidance and standards 555, 556–7, 559–60, 581
    regulatory perspective on HRQOL endpoints 552–4
Research Association of Practicing Physicians (RAPP)
    543
Resource-Based Relative Value Scale (RBRVS) 490
response shift 378–9, 395, 573, 618–19
retrospective computerized episode algorithms 488
retrospective episode coding 487–8
revenues 489
Revised Grief Experience Inventory (RGEI) 315
Rotterdam Symptom Checklist (RSCL) 56–7
  breast cancer studies 96, 97, 105
  colorectal cancer studies 179, 189
  features 56
  lung cancer studies 161
  performance across the cancer continuum 56–7
  prostate cancer studies 126
  psychometric data and validation 46–53
  survivorship studies 249
  translation and cultural adaptation 409–10, 419
    psychometric performance 410–11
  usage 56–7
RSCL *see* Rotterdam Symptom Checklist (RSCL)

sample attrition 371–2
satisfaction surveys 291, 306–8, 590
  use in needs assessment 322
  see also patient perspectives on cancer care
scale information function (SIF) 437–8, 453–5
scales
  development and analysis 438–9
  optimal scaling/scale score interpretation
    440–1
screening 216, 217, 224–9
  breast cancer 225–7, 228–9
    false positive screening results 228–9
    negative screening results 228

cervical cancer 225–7, 228–9
  false positive screening results 228–9
  negative screening results 228
colorectal cancer 178, 224–7, 228, 536
  cost-effectiveness analysis 512
decision making 217
HRQOL status 388
HRQOL studies 9
negative test result 217–18, 228
  false negative 217–18
positive test result 217, 218
  false positive 217, 228–9
prostate cancer 126, 225–7, 228
short-term outcomes 217, 218, 231–2
  literature review 218
  measurement of 225–7, 229–31
  measures 218
see also genetic testing
selection bias 375
selective estrogen receptor modulators (SERMs) 220
  see also raloxifene; tamoxifen
Selenium and Vitamin E Cancer Prevention Trial (SELECT)
  221
self-explicated utility model 324
  hybrid conjoint model 324, 325
sensitivity analysis 513–14
sexual dysfunction
  measurement 146–7
  prostate cancer treatment and 131, 150
  survivorship studies 245
Short Form 6D (SF-6D) 87
Short Form 36 (SF-36) 21, 31, 33–43, 465–6, 472–6
  breast cancer studies 97, 98, 105
    representative scores 103
  features 33
  item response theory (IRT) modeling 426–7, 430–2
  Mental Health (MH) subscale 426–7, 428, 430–2
    dimensionality 432–3
    scale information function 437
    standard error of measurement function 438
  multidimensional item response modeling (MIRM)
    approach 474–6, 477
  Omnibus Summary Scale 476
  performance across the cancer continuum 33–43
  Physical Functioning (PF-10) subscale
    construct map 467–8
    construct validity 470–2
    items design 469
    outcome space 469

prostate cancer studies 126, 134, 150–1
  representative scores 143
psychometric data and validation 34–42
quality of life dimensions 16
reliability coefficients 473
subscales perspective 473–4, 477
summary scale perspective 473–4, 477
survivorship studies 245–50, 255
type of information elicited 21
usage 33–43, 45
short-term outcomes 217
  measurement of 219, 223, 225–7, 229–31
  see also cancer prevention; genetic testing; screening
Sickness Impact Profile (SIP) 31, 44–5, 179
  colorectal cancer studies 189–90
  features 44
  performance across the cancer continuum 44–5
  psychometric data and validation 34–42
  Short Form (SF-SIP) 44
  usage 44–5
skilled nursing facilities (SNF) costs 490
slope parameter 470
Snyder, Claire 4
social impacts
  end-of-life care 266
  on caregivers 333
social well-being 266
societal costs 495–6
societal value 481
  total societal value-loss 496–8
soft-tissue sarcoma 346–8
Southwest Oncology Group Quality of Life Questionnaire 190
Specific Disease and Continence-Related Symptoms
  questionnaire 179
specific objectivity 430
spiritual domain 266, 587
  caregivers 333–4
  end-of-life care and 266
Spitzer Quality of Life (QL-Index)
  colorectal cancer studies 179, 189
  quality-of-life dimensions 16
  survivorship studies 249
standard deviation (SD) 393
standard error of measurement (SEM) 393, 436, 438
standard gamble (SG) 73, 74, 75–7
  measurement properties 75–7
    construct validity 72, 75–6
    content validity 75
    practical aspects 73, 77

standard gamble (SG) (*cont.*)
    reliability 76
    responsiveness 76
standardized residuals (SRs) 451–3
statistical analyses in outcomes research 10, 362–4, 365, 380–1,
      569–70
  aggregated versus disaggregated scores 392
  anchor-based interpretations 393–6
    ability to work 396
    global ratings 394–6
    health care utilization 396
    mortality 396
    relationship to disease status and treatment 396
  challenges 363–5, 366
  distribution-based interpretations 392–3
  future research needs 378–80
    Bayes methodology role 379–80, 561, 577–8
    clinical significance assessment 379, 560–1
    endpoint construction and validation 379
    item response theory applicability 379
    nonstandard use of instruments 379
    response shift 378–9
    training needs 379
  gold standard 365–6, 367
  issues 367–78
    clinical response benefit 368, 379
    clinical significance 370, 631–2
    graphical presentation of results 375, 376, 377
    HRQOL assessment 368–9
    identifying and measuring endpoints 367–8
    intent-to-treat (ITT) analysis 372–4
    longitudinal analysis 374–5
    missing data and sample attrition 371–2, 373
    multiple endpoints 370–1
    role of complex statistical methods 375–8
    selection bias 375
    stratification 369–70
  patient-reported outcomes 631–3
  see also item response theory (IRT)
stratification 369–70
structural equation modeling (SEM) 572
Study of Cancer Survivors-II (SDS-II) 532, 536
subjective assessment 19–23
  evaluations 19–23, 27
    changes over time 23
    in definitions of quality of life 20–2
    influencing factors 22–3
    measurement of 22

perceived status 19–21, 27
  in definitions of quality of life 20–2
  measurement of 22
subjective significance 394–5
Subjective Significance Questionnaire (SSQ) 394–5
subscales 465, 466
  aggregation 476–7
  Four Building Blocks 466–72, 477
    construct map 466–8
    items design 468
    measurement model 469–72
    outcome space 468–9
  multidimensional item response model approach 474–6
  reliability 473, 475, 477
  validity 466, 475
  see also specific instruments
summary scales and scores 465, 466, 577, 592–3
  see also aggregated scores
support groups, prostate cancer 289
  need for 287–8
Support Team Assessment Schedule (STAS) 313
Supportive Care Needs Survey (SCNS) 311, 316
  measuring importance of needs 322
surgical treatment
  breast cancer 93, 202–3
    HRQOL studies 106
    treatment decisions 93, 115–16
  colorectal cancer 178, 203
    clinical implications of HRQOL studies 193, 194
    impact on HRQOL 185–8, 192
  impact on cancer patients 201–2
    domains of HRQOL affected 204–5
    measurement 207
    toxicity criteria 206–7
  lung cancer 203
  prophylactic surgery 224
  prostate cancer 150, 203
    survivorship studies 245
  see also cancer treatments
Surveillance, Epidemiology, and End Results (SEER)
    program 485, 523–4
  combined SEER/administrative data 526–8, 529
  strengths and limitations 525
surveys 530–3, 539
  enhancements to support outcomes research 539
  health knowledge, practices, and outcomes 530–6
  resource use and cost 534–5, 536–8
  strengths and limitations 538

survival curves 33
survivorship studies 241–2, 243
  breast cancer 243–4
  colorectal cancer 245
  data abstraction techniques 242
  HRQOL assessment 9–10, 241–2, 243–5
    adding value 253
    future research needs 255–6
    instruments used HRQOL 245–53
    performance of instruments 253–5
    positive outcomes 242
    qualitative approaches 253, 254–5
  late effects of cancer treatment 244
  literature search 242
  lung cancer 244
  Paradox of Cancer Survivorship 255
  prostate cancer 128, 244–5
    survivor's perspective 286–9
SWOG Prostate Outcomes Questionnaire 250
Symptom Checklist 179
symptoms 264–5
  control of 265
    breast cancer 110
    end-of-life care 279–80
  impact on HRQOL 265
  measures of 7
    distinction from HRQOL assessment 387, 552

T scores 101
tamoxifen
  breast cancer chemoprevention 220
  HRQOL impact 220–1
  see also hormonal therapy
target information function 453
taxanes, cost-effectiveness 503
technical care 291
  patient perspectives 291
telephone interviews 350
terminally ill patients see end-of-life (EOL) care
test characteristic function (TCF) 458, 459
Therapy-Related Symptom Checklist (TRSC) 207, 208
think-aloud responses 611
  see also cognitive interviewing technique
TIME (Toolkit of Instruments to Measure End of life care) 266
time trade-off (TTO) 74, 75–7
  measurement properties 75–7
    construct validity 72, 75–6

content validity 75
  practical aspects 73, 77
  reliability 76
  responsiveness 76
Tobacco Use Supplement, Current Population Survey, US Census Bureau 530
Toronto Informational Needs Questionnaire-Breast Cancer (TINQ-BC) 313
Total Mood Disturbance (TMD) score 98
toxicity data 386
  patient-reported measures 169, 207
  toxicity criteria 206–7, 212
training
  missing data avoidance 354
  statisticians 379
trait scores
  computerized adaptive assessment 459–61
  estimation of 454–5
  statistically equating scores 458–9
translation
  Cancer Rehabilitation Evaluation System (CARES) 408–9, 419, 420
    psychometric performance 409
    Short Form (CARES-SF) 408–9
  EORTC QLQ-C30 411–12, 419, 420–1
    psychometric performance 412–13, 416
  Functional Assessment of Cancer Therapy-General (FACT-G) 416, 419, 420–1
    psychometric performance 416–18
  Functional Living Index Cancer (FLIC) 407–8, 419
    psychometric performance 407–8
  recommendations 418–21
  Rotterdam Symptom Checklist (RSCL) 409–10, 419
    psychometric performance 410–11
treatment decisions see cancer treatments; clinical decision making
2-parameter logistic model (2PLM) 428–9

UCLA Prostate Cancer Index (UCLA PCI) 126, 135–7, 146, 151, 152
  psychometric properties 135–7
  representative scores 144
  survivorship studies 250
unidimensionality 432–3, 446–8, 465, 592, 593
urinary function
  measurement 147
  prostate cancer treatment and 131, 150
    survivorship studies 245

utilities 231
    cost-utility analysis 70
    expected utility theory 73
    measurement of 231, 390
    utility scores 71, 390
    see also Health Utilities Index (HUI)

value scores 71
verbal probing 611
    see also cognitive interviewing technique
Veterans Affairs Information Resource Center (VIReC) 539
video-CASI (computer-assisted self-interview) 352
visual analogue scale (VAS) 71–3
    measurement properties 72–3
        construct validity 72
        content validity 72
        practical aspects 73
        reliability 72–3
        responsiveness 73
vomiting assessment 19
von Neumann–Morgenstern expected utility theory 73

well-being 585
    physical 266
    psychological 266
    social 266
    spiritual 266
    see also quality of life
willingness-to-accept (WTA) approach 498
willingness-to-pay (WTP) approach 497–8,
        505–6
    equity issues 498–9
withholds 488
working group 4
    see also Cancer Outcomes Measurement Working Group
        (COMWG)
World Health Organization Quality of Life Questionnaire
        (WHOQOL-BREF) 417
Worthington Chemotherapy Satisfaction Questionnaire
        (WCSQ) 210, 293–4
Wright map 470–2, 477

Zarit Burden Interview/Inventory 340